The Complementary Therapist's Guide to Conventional Medicine

For Elsevier:
Commissioning Editor: Claire Wilson
Development Editor: Carole McMurray
Project Manager: Nayagi Athmanathan
Designer: Kirsteen Wright
Illustration Manager: Bruce Hogarth
Illustrator: Graeme Chambers

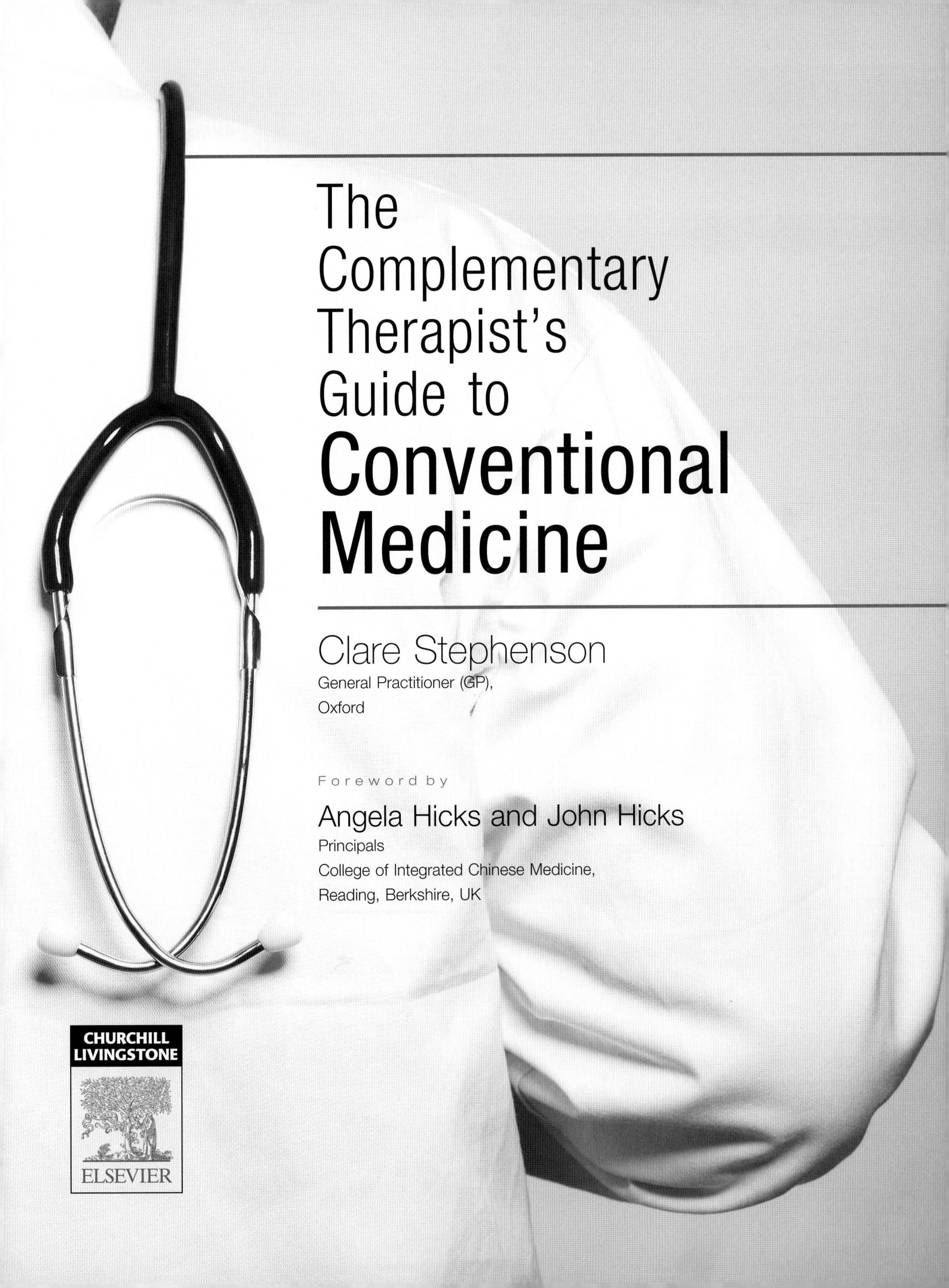

The Complementary Therapist's Guide to Conventional Medicine

Clare Stephenson
General Practitioner (GP),
Oxford

Foreword by

Angela Hicks and John Hicks
Principals
College of Integrated Chinese Medicine,
Reading, Berkshire, UK

CHURCHILL LIVINGSTONE
ELSEVIER

CHURCHILL
LIVINGSTONE
ELSEVIER

ISBN 978-0-7020-3428-2

British Library Cataloguing in Publication Data
A catalogue record for this book is available from the British Library

Library of Congress Cataloging in Publication Data
A catalog record for this book is available from the Library of Congress

Notices

Knowledge and best practice in this field are constantly changing. As new research and experience broaden our understanding, changes in research methods, professional practices, or medical treatment may become necessary.

Practitioners and researchers must always rely on their own experience and knowledge in evaluating and using any information, methods, compounds, or experiments described herein. In using such information or methods they should be mindful of their own safety and the safety of others, including parties for whom they have a professional responsibility.

With respect to any drug or pharmaceutical products identified, readers are advised to check the most current information provided (i) on procedures featured or (ii) by the manufacturer of each product to be administered, to verify the recommended dose or formula, the method and duration of administration, and contraindications. It is the responsibility of practitioners, relying on their own experience and knowledge of their patients, to make diagnoses, to determine dosages and the best treatment for each individual patient, and to take all appropriate safety precautions.

To the fullest extent of the law, neither the Publisher nor the authors, contributors, or editors, assume any liability for any injury and/or damage to persons or property as a matter of products liability, negligence or otherwise, or from any use or operation of any methods, products, instructions, or ideas contained in the material herein.

The Publisher's policy is to use **paper manufactured from sustainable forests**

Printed in China

Dedication

This book is dedicated to my son Adam, without whom this book would have been completed far earlier than it has been, and to my infinitely patient partner John, without whom it would not have been finished at all.

Many thanks also go to Di Eckersley and Pam Batten for their meticulous attention to the text in its early stages, and for the feedback and enthusiasm of successive classes of students at the College of Integrated Chinese Medicine, Reading.

Contents

Foreword

The College of Integrated Chinese medicine brings together two styles of Chinese Medicine. We had not thought, however, of bringing together Chinese and Western medicine. Until, that is, Clare Stephenson joined the staff. She saw the potential for something different.

As both a Western doctor and a practitioner of Chinese medicine, Clare immediately recognised the huge areas of similarity, as well as differences, between these two systems of medicine. She graduated from the College, and subsequently became the programme leader for conventional medicine. This started her on the path of writing what was later to become this textbook.

From the moment we saw the first texts for the study course, it became clear that she was writing something very special, unique even. The students agreed. Their evaluations sang the praises of the course. Staff who had not done the course clamoured for the text. They had recognised its potential for deepening their learning and as a reference tool.

It soon became obvious to us that this should and would become a textbook at some stage. It took over five years for Clare to fully complete what was then an in-depth study course for our students. We are now delighted that from its first conception as a course in 1998, through its extensive development, it has finally been born as a book.

Before this book the only in-depth texts available were those written for Western medicine practitioners such as doctors, nurses and physiotherapists. Clare's innovative vision for complementary therapists was to enable them to learn Western medicine but from their own perspective.

Chinese medicine and Western medicine are two substantial yet very different medical models. Complementary medicine practitioners can often search for connections and relationships between the two models but find more differences than similarities. This book bridges that gap and brings the two closer. This enables practitioners of both medical models to understand how the other thinks.

In this textbook Clare takes complementary practitioners through the basics of Western physiology and pathology and compares and contrasts it with the underlying theory of Chinese medicine. It helps complementary medicine practitioners to understand the workings of the mind of a conventional doctor: how they question patients, what tests they might carry out, how the results might be interpreted, as well as possible Western treatments and their effects.

Throughout the text each subject is discussed not only from the Western but also from the Chinese medical perspective. For instance, she examines holistic versus reductionist theories, are examined, the underlying philosophy of both medical models are summarised medications are explained both in Western terms and in terms of their Chinese energetic effects. On top of this, and perhaps most striking, is how she thoughtfully compares each Western disease is compared to a possible Chinese medicine diagnosis.

For a holistic practitioner, comparing diseases from these two perspectives might be seen as slightly risky. We might worry that it could encourage practitioners to treat only what in Chinese medicine terms is called the *biao*, or outward manifestation, rather than the *ben*, or root cause of the problem. Clare's rich understanding prevents this from happening. Whilst remembering that this is primarily a conventional medicine textbook, she comments on Chinese Medicine differentiations of disease, without being too prescriptive. This gives practitioners useful insights but doesn't narrow their holistic point of view.

Each part of this clear text is complemented by learning-points, self-tests and case histories as well as numerous additional comments and comparisons between Western and complementary medicine.

This book will be of use to students of complementary therapies as an in-depth step-by-step study course with timed and specified sections of study. Equally it is extremely useful to qualified practitioners as a reference book. Although this book was not written for Western practitioners, those who read it with an open mind might also find it arouses their interest. The discussion about the Chinese medicine approach might resonate with their experience of patients.

This book is immensely dense and at the same time exceedingly readable. It will be hard for another textbook to match in breadth and depth. We have no doubt that it will soon be a standard text for Chinese and other complementary medicine students as well as a standard reference for practitioners. It has so much embedded in the text that the reader might find, as we did, valuable gems popping out at every visit. It has left us more interested in, as well as much more informed about, Western medicine, whilst remaining proud of our own Chinese medicine.

Angela Hicks and John Hicks
Principals, College of Integrated Chinese Medicine,
Reading, Berkshire, UK, September 2010

Introduction

This text has been written primarily to meet the needs of people who are studying or practising a complementary health discipline. The author is a medical doctor who also trained in and practised Chinese medicine for a number of years before then returning to conventional medical practice. Over this time she learned that the process of embracing more than one philosophical medical framework in clinical practice could ultimately enrich the medical consultation. Patients seemed to benefit from the insights and wisdom inherent in the best aspects of each of the medical disciplines to which they were exposed.

The overarching aim of the book is that complementary therapists might develop an understanding of conventional medicine that will enable them to make links between conventional and complementary medical concepts. Further aims are to encourage a clear understanding of why doctors behave they way they do, and to instil greater confidence in the management of 'red flag' conditions – those situations when a patient is likely to benefit from, or even urgently need, referral for conventional medical treatment.

Many institutions involved in training complementary healthcare practitioners in the conventional medical sciences currently rely on source texts designed for doctors and nurses in training. These texts are generally excellent in informing about the knowledge base of conventional medical practice, but were never intended to answer questions about how medical facts and approaches may relate to a complementary health discipline. For this reason, many students find the conventional medical aspects of their training dry and irrelevant, and the material difficult to retain.

What this text offers in addition to the material found in standard medical texts is that it presents medical information in a systematic way, whilst continually referring to how this information might relate to complementary medical practice. The comparisons and discussions about complementary medical practice are largely confined to Chinese medicine concepts, but these illustrate a process that it is very possible to undertake in any of the complementary medical disciplines.

To achieve this aim there are frequent references to aspects of the practice of a 'conventional medical practitioner' which are then compared to the practice of a 'complementary medical practitioner' (and specifically a practitioner of Chinese medicine). In doing this the conventional practitioner is ascribed a reductionist world view – one in which the body is seen as a series of systems that can be objectively measured and objectively treated. To the complementary medical practitioner is ascribed a more holistic world view – one in which the body is seen as a dynamically integrated organism and in which body, mind and soul are intimately related and underpinned by an understanding of a vital force such as the Chinese idea of Qi. It must be stressed that this polarisation is for the purposes of illustration only. In real-life practice many medical doctors adopt a more holistic world view, and some complementary health practitioners work from a more structural or reductionist view of the body.

The attempted translation from one medical language to another in this text is based on the premise that there is one reliable constant irrespective of the world view of the health practitioner. This reliable constant is the patient's experience of disease (the symptoms), and how the patient demonstrates a response to the disease process in their body (the signs). All medical approaches respond to these fixed points, which can be recognised by practitioners from all disciplines. Moreover, although conventional and complementary medical approaches may seem to have different languages, they all respond to a patient's symptoms and signs in predictable ways. For this reason, in theory, it can become possible to 'translate' from one medical language to another, even when the underlying theoretical framework of the two medical approaches appears to be startlingly different. The patient's symptoms and signs become the point at which a medical description from one discipline, 'inflammation', for example, can be mapped onto a medical description from another such as 'Wind-Heat'.

This text is for the main part, however, a conventional medical textbook. It presents information about clinical medicine that is both up to date and relevant to clinical practice in the UK, and to the structure and practice of conventional medicine in any developed country. The most significant area in which the text may differ from texts from other developed countries is in that of drug nomenclature, with many countries having their own unique systems for naming drugs. The names used in this text are based on the International Non Proprietary Name (rINN) system recommended by the World Health Organization and used in the British National Formulary of medications.

The text has been designed for two modes of use. First, it will stand alone as a medical textbook, which can be referred to in the course of clinical practice. The language in which it is written has been chosen to act as a bridge for a practitioner with little or no scientific background to help to make a conceptual link between the patient's medical diagnosis with what might be written in medical language about that diagnosis in standard medical texts. Initially designed as a study course for students of Chinese medicine in the UK, the text has been studied in detail by hundreds of students, who have provided valuable feedback and confirmed the accessibility of the information it presents.

Second, the text has been written in such a way that it can be followed systematically as part of a study course in clinical medicine. To this end, study aids such as in-text questions and end of chapter assessment tests have been designed to relate to the material in each chapter. These feature as prompts in the body of the chapter, which link to study material on the CD which accompanies the text. The CD also contains additional images that are not necessary for the understanding of the text, but will enrich the appreciation of the detail of each topic to which they relate.

The text is structured in six stages, each of which is subdivided into chapters. Each chapter begins with a list of learning intentions and ends with a self-assessment test to help the student ensure that the learning intentions have been met. Each chapter also offers an estimated time for study so that a study schedule can be planned. If teaching institutions choose to adopt this text as a study course then a pace of one stage per semester provides continual challenge without becoming too overwhelming. Ideally, if the course is taught in this way, home study can be supported by 2–4 teaching sessions per stage of the course, and setting the students an end-of-stage written assignment as a form of summative assessment of their learning. More information about suggested lesson plans and assessment tools to support the use of this text as a study course can be obtained from the author (clarestephenson@doctors.org.uk).

This book is packed with information intended to enrich the clinical encounter with a patient in need of healing. It is always good, however, to retain a degree of perspective when dealing with such information; there is often a danger that the weight of the information distracts the practitioner to the detriment of the potential of the healing encounter. For this reason, this introduction concludes with the words of a wise healer:

> *I say to any beginner – learn your theories as well as you can, but put them aside when you touch the miracle of the living soul. Not theories but your own creative individuality must decide.*
>
> C. G. Jung

These words encourage the practitioner developing a mastery of information to allow those theories to work quietly from only the background of their consciousness during the profound time when the patient has entered the clinic room.

Clare Stephenson
Didcot Health Centre, Oxfordshire

Note to the reader

The rationale and method used for the mapping of western medical diagnoses to chinese medicine theory

The meeting of two independent systems of medicine is a great opportunity for enriching and developing each. As explained in the Introduction, the primary focus of this book has been to introduce to practitioners of complementary medicine the basic principles, pathological interpretations and clinical approaches of western medicine. It also offers throughout the text 'translations' of some of the signs and symptoms of western medicine into the descriptive language of Chinese medicine. In places these translations suggest possible Chinese medicine interpretations of physiological and pathological process about which the ancient Chinese could not have known. Modern patients, however, will present more than just a complex of symptoms and signs to their practitioners, often arriving with a portfolio of test results and western medical diagnoses. It is intended that the interpretations offered in the Chinese medicine sections may deepen the understanding of the patient from at least one complementary medicine perspective, and encourage this additional medical information to be embraced as something that may enrich a complementary medical diagnosis.

All physicians observe and describe symptoms and signs in their patients, whatever their philosophical background. They will place different degrees of emphasis on different symptoms and signs. The pulse qualities that are described and considered significant in Chinese medicine, for example, are very different from those considered clinically significant in western medicine. Nevertheless, physicians are unlikely to disagree that an individual patient has nausea, fever, a rash and swollen joints, if indeed these are the symptoms and signs present in that particular case.

The links suggested between western and Chinese medicine in this text are forged on the basis that western and Chinese practitioners share this common ground – they both recognise the consistency and value of symptoms and signs as indicators of disease. In this text, when a translation is attempted from western to Chinese medicine language, the symptoms and signs form the bridge that enable this leap between western and Chinese medicine language.

Western medical diagnoses are, in keeping with their reductionist roots, based on very subtle and detailed analyses of symptoms and signs, as well as pathological changes and test results. For example, an early diagnosis of rheumatoid arthritis is hinted at by hot symmetrically swollen joints and fever, but is confirmed by blood tests that demonstrate the measurable presence of characteristic autoantibodies and inflammatory markers. These distinguish this inflammatory polyarthritis from a number of similar conditions.

Chinese medicine diagnoses, however, are often based on taking in quite broad sweeps of information, which are qualitatively rather than quantitatively assessed. The diagnosis is based on the answers to questions such as 'Is the patient hot?' 'Is there dryness?' 'Is there swelling?' and 'Is the pain fixed and boring, or dull and improved by movement?' The answers to these questions are supported by characteristic changes in the pulse and tongue. The fine distinctions made within western diagnoses may not be so apparent in Chinese diagnoses. A case of early rheumatoid arthritis is likely to be described on the basis of hot swollen painful joints and fever as manifesting Heat and Blood and Qi Stagnation (in this case in the form of a manifestation of Bi syndrome). These descriptions may also be applied to any number of forms of polyarthritis that involve hot symmetrically swollen and painful joints.

In Chinese medicine the very subtle distinctions in diagnosis will emerge as a consequence of the uniqueness of the patient who is displaying the symptoms. While all patients with a symmetrical hot polyarthritis may safely be described as manifesting Heat and Blood and Qi Stagnation, this tells us nothing about the aetiology of the development of the Heat and the Stagnation, or indeed if these need to be treated directly. It may be more important in such a case to assess the degree of underlying deficiency (e.g. of Heart Qi or Kidney Yin), which could be the most appropriate focus of treatment.

In this text, attempts to make linguistic links between western and Chinese medicine have been made using the consistent constellation of symptoms and signs as an enabling between the two. There is nothing remarkable or controversial about this. Once symptoms and signs are clearly described by western medicine (e.g. fever, constipation, depression, rash, etc.), then Chinese theory very readily allows for a range of possible diagnoses to be suggested. It is important to emphasise, however, that these 'translations' are intended to enrich understanding of how western and Chinese medicine diagnoses may be linked. They are not intended as guides to treatment.

While all forms of symmetrical polyarthritis might be described in terms of Heat and Stagnation of Blood and Qi, this does not mean that a Chinese medicine practitioner will focus only on Clearing Heat and Moving Stagnation in the treatment of such patients. The Chinese medicine practitioner will need to base treatment on the outcome of a traditional diagnosis, involving questioning, observation, and the pulse and tongue characteristics. However, there is no doubt that the knowledge that certain Chinese medicine syndromes are consistently linked with certain medical diagnoses may enrich the understanding of the pathology and aetiology of disease.

A perhaps more controversial aspect of the text is the attempt to make statements about Chinese energetic interpretations on the basis of internal or microscopic changes in the body, which would not have been directly observed in the patient by the ancient practitioners of Chinese medicine. For example, a pathological process that involves blood clotting might be equated to Qi and Blood Stagnation, or inflammation to Heat and Stagnation, even if the process is going on deep within the body rather than on the surface. A process involving withering and loss of vitality of tissues, such as the degenerative changes seen in the lung in emphysema, might be equated to Yin Deficiency and a process in which the dynamic function of a body structure is compromised, such as inefficient pumping of the failing heart to Qi or Yang Deficiency.

The compelling factor about assumptions that western pathology can be equated to Chinese descriptions is that, very often, what can be assumed about what is happening at a microscopic level in a disease from a Chinese medicine perspective is made manifest in the symptoms and signs commonly associated with that disease. For example, a coronary thrombosis might suggest Heart Blood Stagnation on the basis of there being a blood clot in a coronary artery. This conjecture is then corroborated by the fact that the common symptoms and signs of coronary thrombosis of intense fixed central chest pain and irregular pulse rate are consistent with those described in the Chinese medicine syndrome of Heart Blood Stagnation.

Again it must be emphasised that statements linking western pathology with Chinese descriptions of disease process (a blood clot suggests Blood Stagnation; an accumulation of fluid suggests Damp) are not intended to be guides for treatment or exact equivalences. Treatment always needs be planned in the light of the unique constellation of symptoms and signs with which an individual patient presents and which inform the complementary medical discipline in which the practitioner works.

A similar process has been undertaken in the Chinese medicine interpretation of the actions of medical treatments (explained in more detail in Section 1.3b, Drugs from an Alternative Viewpoint). Again, the Chinese medicine descriptions of drug actions are drawn from what is known in conventional medicine about how those drugs relieve symptoms and signs and their side effects. It must also be taken into consideration that drugs tend not to directly nourish or replenish the body (nutritional supplements and replacement hormones being possible exceptions), but instead often subdue or boost bodily processes, be they physiological or pathological. For example, the oral contraceptive pill subdues the natural bodily process of ovulation, and the ovulatory drug clomiphene stimulates or boosts ovulation, which would not have happened without medical assistance. Beta blockers (such as propranolol) subdue the action of the heart and result in slowed heart rate and reduced blood pressure. Beta agonists (such as adrenaline and salbutamol) boost the action of the heart and lead to increased heart rate and blood pressure.

What the text postulates is that such interruption of bodily processes, even if they are pathological processes, carries an energetic cost. Subduing bodily functions might manifest in an imbalance, such as the Stagnation of Qi or Heat at another level in the body. This has some resonance with the classical homeopathic concept of suppression of symptoms where, as a result of the suppression, the imbalance becomes manifest at a deeper level in the body. This assumption is based on the Chinese medicine theory that the pathological bodily process, such as overforceful pumping of the heart leading to hypertension, may be the result of a deeper imbalance (e.g. sustained high levels of stress-related emotions such as anger or anxiety), and simply stopping this outer expression of the imbalance will not allow the deeper imbalance to dissipate.

Moreover, it is suggested that the boosting of bodily functions by a medical treatment might be beneficial in the short term, but ultimately draining for the body. For example, the stimulation of heart rate and blood pressure by beta agonists may in the short term profoundly benefit a body system in which these functions might be failing to rally round, and can be literally life saving. From an energetic perspective, a system that was deficient in Yang has been boosted. But this is not the same as nourishing Yang, as might be the consequence of careful attention to diet, sleep and exercise. This instantaneous boosting may well be at the cost of drawing on deep bodily reserves, and so ultimately draining. At a deep level this boosting of Yang is possibly actually quite the opposite, as the deep reserves of Yang are depleted. It makes sense that in this situation that patient will also benefit from some additional treatment approaches to nourish the depleted reserves in the long term. This theory fits with the common experience of the use of any of the stimulatory substances in the diet, such as sugar, caffeine or chocolate. After a temporary high, overuse of these substances may leave a person feeling even more drained and out of balance than before.

These ideas have been drawn into the interpretation of drug energetics. What is happening on the surface may be accompanied by a paradoxical effect at a deeper level. A drug that clearly seems to be Cooling in nature (e.g. an anti-inflammatory medication) may demonstrate a range of side-effects that are Hot in nature (e.g. rash, fever, inflammation of the stomach). While some of these side-effects may be a consequence of the toxic nature of the drug to body tissues, evidenced by the fact that the effects will be experienced by people who take these medications irrespective of the nature of the underlying disease, it is noteworthy that many drugs do seem to generate side-effects that have an energetic interpretation which is the opposite of that of their therapeutic action.

Again the point needs to be made that these interpretations of drug energetics are intended to enlighten the understanding about complex symptoms and enrich the diagnostic process. They are not intended as guides to Chinese medicine treatment, which always needs to be based on the outcome of the traditional Chinese medicine diagnostic process. Drugs may cause dramatic symptoms and signs in a patient, but often it is careful attention to the individual's root imbalance, and the one that probably preceded any drug treatment, which can lead to the most profound shifts in that patient's health.

In summary, the meeting of two independent systems of medicine is a great opportunity to enrich and develop each of them. It is hoped that the interpretations offered in the Chinese medicine sections may deepen the complementary medical practitioner's understanding of the patient from a Chinese medicine perspective. Moreover, a Western medical doctor who has begun to embrace the Chinese medicine understanding of the grouping and interrelationship of signs and symptoms may well add to their medical diagnoses the sophisticated understanding of the environmental, emotional and spiritual correlates of physiological and pathological processes which are at the heart of Chinese medicine as a system, and in so doing enrich their conventional medical practice.

The structure of the text

This book is structured in six stages, each of which consists of 15–20 chapters ordered into topic sections. The checklists in Appendix V summarise the main topic areas covered in the chapters. These checklists together form the syllabus of any study course that is structured around this book as the core text.

The first two stages relate to topics at the foundation of the understanding of clinical medicine, including basic principles of physiology, pathology and pharmacology. These stages also introduce the theoretical basis used throughout the text for the 'translation' of conventional medical language into Chinese medicine language, as described above. The next four stages focus on the description of all the important medical conditions and their treatment as they relate to conventionally recognised body systems or patient groups. The conclusion focuses on the practical details of the complementary medical clinical practitioner dealing with patients who have received medical diagnoses. This part of the text attends to subjects such as the referral of patients with 'red flag' conditions, managing withdrawal from conventional medication, and the ethico-legal aspects of treating a patient who is also under the care of a medical practitioner.

Introduction to medical sciences

1.1

Chapter 1.1a Introduction to physiology: the systems of the body

LEARNING POINTS

At the end of this chapter you will be able to:

- define the term 'physiology'
- understand the physiological levels of organisation of the body
- list the systems and the associated organs that constitute the human body
- outline the functions of each system.

Estimated time for chapter: 60 minutes.

Introduction to physiology

The term 'physiology' is derived from the Greek words meaning 'study of nature', and is used to describe how all living organisms work or function. The study of physiology has to underpin the study of clinical medicine, as it is only through knowledge of how biological processes function in health that the mechanisms and outcomes of disease may be understood. Throughout this text, physiological descriptions of the body systems precede the descriptions of how disease manifests in those systems. The introduction and explanation of the key concepts necessary to understand these descriptions is the purpose of this first chapter.

The study of physiology offers more to the complementary medical practitioner than simply the building blocks for the foundation of the further study of medical sciences. Central to all healing modalities is the development of an understanding and respect for the human body in health and disease. This respect enriches the way in which the practitioner communicates with patients and handles their bodies. It may well, indeed, add to the healing potential of the encounter, as through this respect the patient will feel recognised and understood. Respect comes with knowledge, and although the perspective of many complementary medical modalities is of the human body as more than a mere collection of physical parts, it is very helpful for their practitioners to acquire a sound understanding of the structure and normal functions of these physical parts. Only then can they appreciate in greater detail the importance of the functions of each part, and exactly how all the parts need to work together in a harmonious way in the healthy body viewed as a whole.

An additional benefit of a physiological understanding of the body is that it may also enhance the understanding of the energetic nature of the body parts, as understood by a number of complementary medical systems. Bodily functions are recognised and described in diverse ways, but some elements remain constant. All medical systems recognise major functional details – the lungs take in air, the heart pumps blood, the blood clots and the skin produces sweat. Although the processes of these various functions may be described very differently, an awareness that all disciplines recognise the same summary descriptions can help when translating from the language of one medical discipline to another.

As an illustration of this, in this text physiological concepts are, from time to time, translated into the language of the complementary medical discipline of Chinese medicine. In Chinese medicine the body is understood in terms of constantly interchanging and interdependent forms of Qi, the underlying energetic principle on which that system of medicine is founded. The comparisons with Chinese medicine's concepts of physiology described in this text clearly illustrate not only the internal consistency of thought in Chinese medicine but also the possibility of translation. This process of translation has the potential to promote increased understanding and respect between conventionally trained practitioners and those complementary medical practitioners who use the language of energetics to describe the philosophical basis of their practice.

The systems of the body

Physiologists consider the human body to be a collection of functionally integrated systems. Although these systems

Table 1.1a-I The 12 physiological functional systems of the body

- Integumentary (skin)
- Muscular
- Skeletal (bone)
- Neurological (nervous)
- Endocrine (hormone secreting)
- Cardiovascular/circulatory (heart and blood vessels)
- Respiratory (breathing)
- Gastrointestinal (digestive)
- Lymphatic (immune)
- Haematological (blood)
- Urological/renal/urinary (kidneys and bladder)
- Reproductive

cannot work in isolation, each can be defined in terms of its structure (anatomy) and function (physiology).

The physiological systems of the body are listed in Table 1.1a-I. Some of the terms may appear unfamiliar (the more commonly used descriptions follow in brackets). However, as they are fundamental to the organisation of most conventional medical textbooks, it is important that their names and functions are clearly recognised and understood.

Most conventional general medical textbooks are written with chapter headings that refer to these systems. This is because conventional practitioners have learned to classify diseases as they affect each system. The in-depth study of diseases according to a physiological system is known as a 'medical speciality' (often spelled speciality). Usually, the term for the speciality is the name of the system together with the suffix '-ology'. For example, the medical speciality devoted to diseases of the endocrine system is known as endocrinology (see Q1.1a-1).

Sometimes two or more systems are considered together because their functions are related. For example, the urinary and reproductive systems may be considered together as the urogenital system, and the blood and the cardiovascular system can be considered together as the circulatory system.

Conversely, a system can be broken down into component 'subsystems' for study in depth. This leads to terms such as ophthalmology (the study of the eye), otorhinolaryngology (the study of the ear, nose and throat), hepatology (the study of the liver) and cardiology (the study of the heart).

The organs

Each system in the body comprises organs that work together to enable the system to perform its role in the physiology of the whole body (see Q1.1a-2).

Information box 1.1 a-1

The organs: comments from a Chinese medicine perspective

Chinese medicine describes twelve Organs, all but one of which are given the same name as the solid organs which are described in physiology. However, these Organs, such as the Heart, Lung and Kidneys, do not correspond directly to the physiological structures, after which all but the Sanjiao (Triple Heater) are named. The organs in physiology are defined primarily in terms of their structure and location, and also by their function. In contrast, the Organs in Chinese medicine are not recognised to have a physical structure. They are defined in terms of the functions that they have in the body, some of which have emotional or spiritual aspects as well as physical ones. They are recognised to have a dominant, but not exclusive, influence over the physical organ after which they are named.

The physiologist is talking about a physically tangible reality when discussing organs, but a Chinese medicine practitioner is describing energetics when using the same term. The term 'energetics' is used here to refer to any description of a manifestation of the Chinese concept of the energetic body, and also the action of a drug on this body. In Chinese medicine, this energetic body may be defined in terms of Yin and Yang, the five Elements and the vital substances of Qi, Blood, Essence (Jing) and also the Pathogenic Factors (such as Cold and Damp), which may impact upon it.

In this text, to minimise possible confusion between terms used differently in Chinese and Western medicine, all Chinese medicine terms that have a meaning which is particular to Chinese medicine theory are ascribed an upper-case initial letter.

The differences may be briefly summarised as follows:

Physiological organs	Chinese medicine Organs
Solid physical structures	Terms to describe a collection of functions
The structure and function of the organs can be assessed by scientific means: dissection, physical examination, blood tests, ultrasound, x-ray imaging, etc.	The functions of the Chinese medicine Organs are assessed subjectively by checking the state of the Qi–using techniques such as pulse and tongue diagnosis
The function of the organ can be related to the structure of the organ. (e.g. the pumping action of the heart organ can be related to its muscular shape, electrical activity and valves)	The function of the Chinese medicine Organs is not related to any structure, although the Chinese medicine Organ may dominate the function of a physiological organ (e.g. the Qi of the Heart Organ, as interpreted in Chinese medicine, supports the heart organ)
For any one organ there is not necessarily a counterpart Chinese medicine Organ (e.g. pituitary)	For any one Chinese medicine Organ there is not necessarily a counterpart physiological organ (e.g. Triple Burner)

It is probably best never to consider that the physiological and Chinese medicine use of a term might correspond. Although there are some similarities (e.g. the function of the stomach is to store food both in physiological and in Chinese medicine), there are many more differences (e.g. the physiological spleen has nothing to do with the digestion of food, whereas this is a significant function of the Spleen in Chinese medicine).

Appendix I demonstrates in much more detail the nature of the differences between the functions of the physiological and Chinese medicine organs. The appendix gives a set of 'Correspondence Tables', each relating to a particular organ, and shows how the various functions of the physiological and Chinese medicine organs map onto one another (see Q1.1a-3).

The physiological levels

The distinct systems of the body described earlier can in turn be broken down (in some cases) into subsystems, each of which represents a collection of interrelated organs. From a physiological perspective, the body as a collection of functionally integrated physiological systems is considered the most complex level of organisation of the body. The various organs around which the systems function represent the next level of organisation of the body.

To descend further to even less complex levels, organs can be considered in terms of the different tissues of which they are made. Tissues, of which there are four main types, comprise the range of basic living materials with which organs can be built. Finally, the most simple level of organisation is the organisation of the cell. This is viewed as the single building block out of which all tissues, and therefore all organs, systems, and the body itself are made.

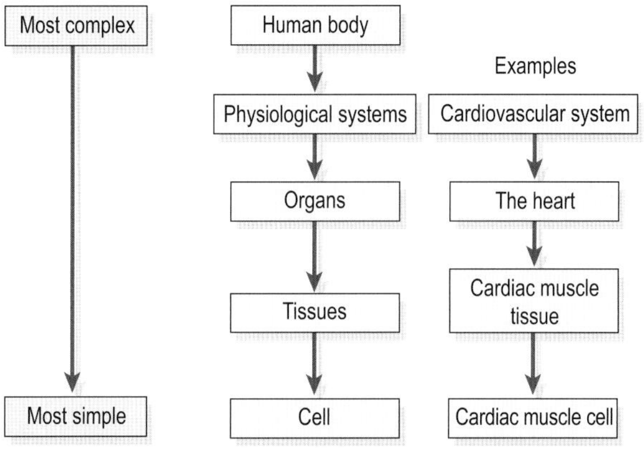

Figure 1.1a-I • The levels of organisation of the body.

The physiological levels are summarised in Figure 1.1a-I.

Self-test 1.1a

Introduction to physiology: the systems of the body

1. What is the definition of the term physiology?
2. Name two organs that form part of the following physiological (functional) systems:
   (i) gastrointestinal system
   (ii) cardiovascular system
   (iii) endocrine system
   (iv) skin.
3. List the physiological levels of organisation from least complex to most complex.
4. Describe one function of each of the following systems:
   (i) urinary system
   (ii) reproductive system
   (iii) the blood
   (iv) nervous system.

Answers

1. Physiology refers to the study of the function of all living organisms.
2. (i) Gastrointestinal system – any two of: mouth, oesophagus, stomach, duodenum, small intestine, large intestine, liver, gallbladder, pancreas.
   (ii) Cardiovascular system – blood vessels, heart.
   (iii) Endocrine system – any two of: pancreas, thyroid, pituitary, pineal, adrenal, ovaries, testes.
   (iv) Skin – any two of: skin, hair, nails, glands which open into the skin.
3. Physiological levels of organisation from least complex to most complex: the cell tissues, the organs, the systems, the body.
4. (i) Urinary system – any one of: excretion of waste products into the urine, control of the fluids in the body, and maintenance of balance of chemicals and acidity in the blood.
   (ii) Reproductive system – propagation of the species.
   (iii) The blood – any one of: transport of oxygen and nutrients, removal of wastes, and carriage of immune cells, proteins and clotting factors for healing.
   (iv) Nervous system – any one of: communication between distant parts of the body, regulation of bodily activity, perception of the outside world and response to the outside world.

Chapter 1.1b The cell: composition, respiration and division

LEARNING POINTS

At the end of this chapter you will be able to:

- recognise the structure of a typical cell and name the main parts
- describe in simple terms how the cell uses nutrients to produce energy
- understand how the energy from nutrition is used by the cell
- describe how the cell replicates, and differentiate between the processes of mitosis and meiosis.

Estimated time for chapter: 60 minutes.

The cell

The cell is the building block that lies at the most simple of the levels of organisation of all plants and animals. It is important to understand how the cell functions in order to make sense of the physiology of those more complex organisational levels of the body, the tissues, the organs and the physiological systems.

Most cells are too small to be seen with the naked eye, but a simple microscope can reveal certain details of their structure. If some tissue from the body is examined under a microscope, the boundaries between cells, the plasma membranes, and also the largest structure within the cell, the nucleus, may be distinguished.

Figures 1.1b-I to 1.1b-IV are diagrammatic representations of how cells in different tissues can appear under the light microscope. These diagrams indicate the wide variety of shapes of cells found in different tissues and how each cell within these tissues contains a large central structure, the nucleus. The nucleus also has a characteristic shape in cells of different tissues.

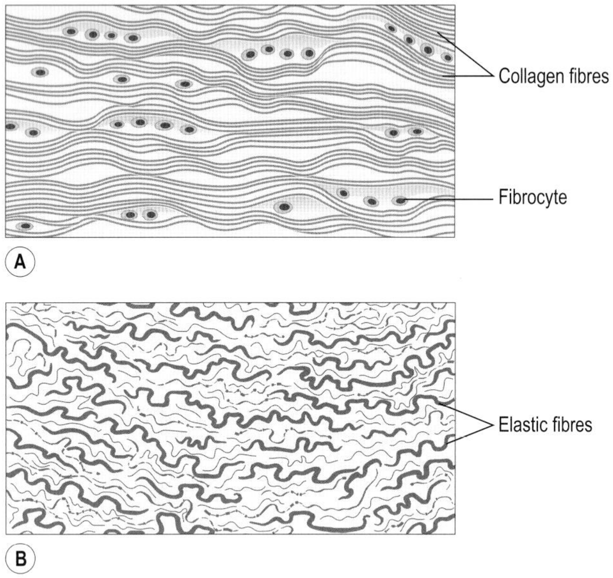

Figure 1.1b-I • Fibrous tissue, illustrating fibre-generating cells (fibrocytes) and collagen fibres.

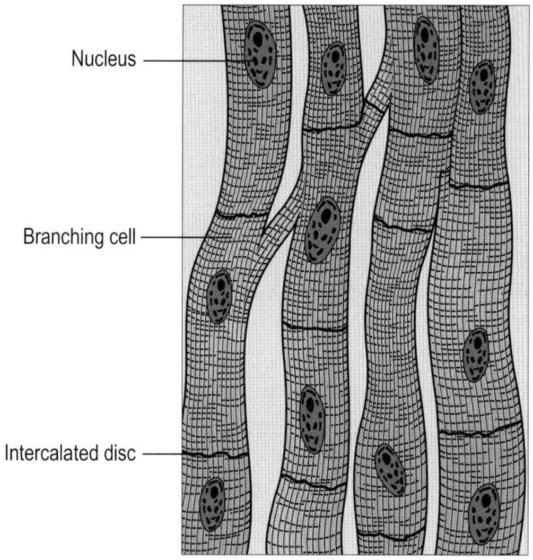

Figure 1.1b-IV • Cardiac muscle tissue, illustrating the fibre-like cardiac muscle cells linked by connecting 'intercalating discs'.

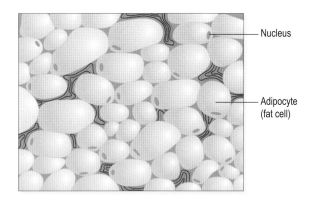

Figure 1.1b-II • Adipose (fat) tissue, illustrating fat-filled adipose cells and minimal connective fibres.

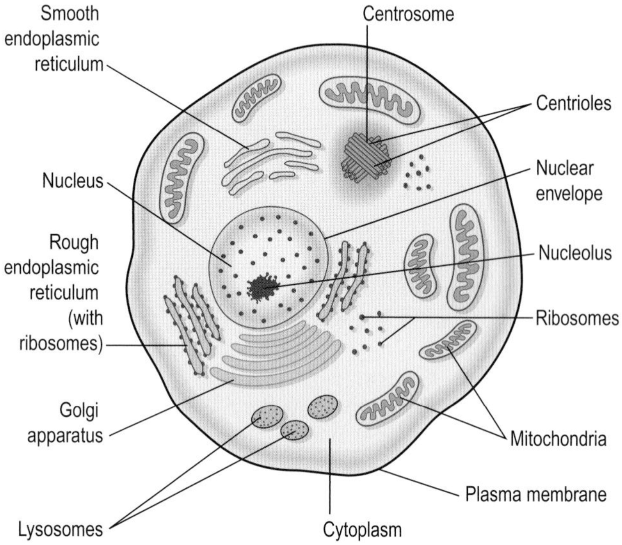

Figure 1.1b-V • The structure of a generalised animal cell.

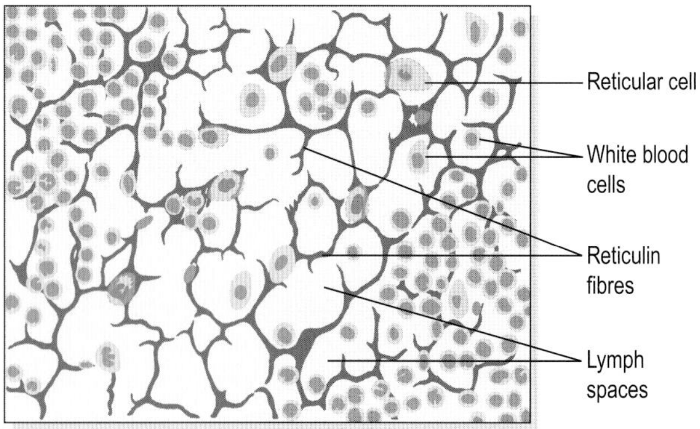

Figure 1.1b-III • Tissue from a lymph node, illustrating immune cells (white blood cells and reticular cells) and supportive reticulin fibres.

The electron microscope is a more powerful microscope that has enabled much more detail to be discovered about the structure of the cell. It has revealed that all animal cells have some basic features in common. Although the precise structure of each cell is different, depending upon the tissue in which it is found and the role it has to play, all cells in the human body have these basic features in some form. This makes sense when considering that every cell in the body has originated from the first unique cell formed at the moment of conception.

It can be helpful to use the idea of a generalised cell to study how all cells are made up and function. No single cell will be *exactly* like this generalised cell, but most cells will have the features portrayed in the generalised cell depicted in Figure 1.1b-V.

The structure of the cell

Each cell contains a plasma membrane and a number of different internal structures known as the organelles ('little organs'). This terminology reflects the fact that a single cell can be seen as a living unit in isolation, with the organelles corresponding to the organs of the body. The organelles are fluid in nature, being bound by oily fluid membranes and suspended within a fluid matrix known as the cytosol.

Each cell is bounded by an oily fluid plasma membrane, otherwise known as the cytoplasm. Cytoplasm is a term used to describe all the fluid contents of the cell, with the exception of the nucleus.

The plasma membrane acts as the link between the cell and the outside world. Large molecules, called proteins, in the membrane make the cell unique (they give the cell its 'immunological identity'), and respond to various chemicals in the cell's environment to bring about changes within the cytoplasm. In addition, the membrane allows the passage of nutrients into the cell and waste out of the cell (transport across the membrane) but is able to retain essential fluids and substances within the cell. This important feature of cell membranes, known as 'semipermeability' is described in Chapter 1.1c.

The nucleus is the largest structure found within the cell. It contains genetic material in the form of chromosomes, which consist of strands of a very complex molecule called DNA (deoxyribonucleic acid). DNA is the template for making (synthesising) essential building materials (proteins) in the cell, which are necessary for its functions. Another complex molecule with a similar structure, RNA, takes the role of the 'messenger', which transfers the information coded on DNA out to the cytosol and to the ribosomes, where the proteins are actually made.

The other large rounded structures in the cytosol are the numerous cigar-shaped mitochondria, which utilise oxygen to break down the basic nutrients obtained from carbohydrates and fats (and sometimes proteins) to form an energised compound called ATP (adenosine triphosphate). ATP can be likened to a battery as it holds a readily available store of energy to 'power' all processes of the cell. This process of using oxygen and nutrients to form energy is called cellular respiration. The waste product of respiration is carbon dioxide.

A large part of the remaining cytosol consists of many layers of oily membrane called the endoplasmic reticulum, on which the dense ribosomes are situated. Where the ribosomes are numerous the endoplasmic reticulum is described as rough (rough ER), and where they are less numerous it is described as smooth (smooth ER). Ribosomes are the site at which the long molecule of RNA is used as a template to guide the production of proteins from simple chemicals called amino acids, out of which all proteins are made. Proteins made on the rough ER pass into the space between its membranes in preparation for transport out of the cell.

The Golgi apparatus is an extension of the ER. It takes the proteins made on the ribosomes and covers them with a membrane coating to make 'vesicles' (also known as secretory granules). These vesicles can travel to the plasma membrane, so that proteins can be released into the outside environment when necessary.

Microfilaments and microtubules are fibres that can contract and cause the movement of substances from one part of the cell to another. These fibres, also known as the cytoskeleton, maintain the structure of the cell and link the various organelles (see Q1.1b-1-Q1.1b-3).

The essential information about the 'generalised' cell is listed in Table 1.1b-I.

Table 1.1b-I The important characteristics of the cell

- The cell is a self-contained living unit
- It is bounded by a membrane, which is studded with characteristic proteins
- The membrane allows communication with the outside world
- The cell takes in nutrients and oxygen to produce energy to 'power' its activities
- It contains genetic material in its nucleus, which allows the manufacture of specific cellular building materials, the proteins
- These proteins can be 'exported' out of the cell to the outside environment

Information Box 1.1b-I

The production of cellular energy: comments from a Chinese medicine perspective

It is an interesting exercise to consider the cell as a small body and the organelles as small organs, and then to reflect how this small body may be described in terms of the 12 Organ systems of Chinese medicine in the same way in which the human body is described. One interesting parallel between the Chinese description and the physiological insight is that of the production of cellular energy. According to Chinese medicine, the formation of True (Zhen) Qi is derived from Gathering (Zong) Qi, which in turn is a product of Food Qi and Air. According to Chinese medicine theory, vitality from the food, Food Qi, is transported by the Spleen to the Lungs, where it is combined with vitality from the air to form Zong Qi. It is under the catalytic action of original Qi that the Zong Qi is transformed into Zhen Qi, which then circulates in the channels and nourishes the organs in the form of Nutritive (Ying) Qi and Protective (Wei) Qi.

Physiologists recognise that cellular energy is similarly derived from a catalytic process involving food (which is broken down into the essential components of simple sugars and amino acids) and oxygen drawn into the body from the air breathed into the lungs. When explained in this way, there is a clearly an interesting parallel with the production of cellular energy, stored in the form of energised ATP as the source of energy for all tissues, and the Chinese description of the production of True (Zhen) Qi.

Cell replication

The replication of cells is a fundamental process within the body that begins with the first division of the fertilised egg (zygote). It is essential both for growth and for the repair of ageing and damaged tissues. There are two ways in which cells can divide, known as mitosis and meiosis. Mitosis is the process whereby a single cell divides into two identical cells following the replication and separation of the chromosomes in the nucleus. Meiosis is the process whereby a single cell divides into daughter cells, each of which carries exactly half of the genetic material of the parent cell.

Mitosis and meiosis are illustrated in Figure 1.1b-VI. In this diagram, for the sake of clarity, only a single pair of the human cell's complement of 23 chromosomal pairs is illustrated. The diagram shows how mitosis results in two identical daughter cells, whereas meiosis results in the production of four genetically unique daughter 'half-cells' or gametes.

Mitosis reproduces the parent cell for the purposes of the growth of the tissue or the repair of damaged tissue, while meiosis produces the reproductive cells (spermatozoa and ova), also known as gametes. When the gamete is fertilised, the resulting zygote (the very first cell, which will later divide to form the embryo) will have a unique combination of genetic material, half from the mother and half from the father. It is the process of meiosis that leads to the uniqueness of every human being (see Q1.1b-4 and Q1.1b-5).

Both meiosis and mitosis are involved in the development of the fertilised egg (zygote) into an adult human being. Meiosis in the sex organs of the parents leads to the production of the gametes. When a male gamete (spermatozoan) and female gamete (egg or ovum) meet, they fuse through the process of fertilisation. The resulting zygote divides and grows by the process of mitosis.

Mutation

When the genetic material of the daughter cells from mitosis and meiosis has become damaged during the process of cell division, this is referred to as a mutation. There are three possible consequences of this. First, the mutation is so minor that the resulting cell is very similar in function to its parent. Second, the mutation disturbs the function of the daughter cells so much that they die. Third, and most significantly the mutation may lead to disturbed function in the daughter cells, although these cells continue to live and replicate. This disturbed function may or may not have a significant effect on the tissue of which the parent cell is a part.

If the parent cell is one of the cells in an embryo, a single mutation can have devastating effects, as the daughter cells may have been destined to develop into major body parts. The thalidomide tragedy resulted from the use of a drug developed in the early 1960s as an anti-nausea medication in early pregnancy. It was later found that this drug causes mutations in the embryo. The mutation caused by thalidomide taken in the first trimester of pregnancy affected embryonic cells that were destined to develop into limbs. A mutation in mitosis can also lead to cancerous change in the daughter cells and can occur at any stage of life. This means that the mutated cells have abnormal and uncontrolled growth patterns, and can take over and destroy neighbouring tissues.

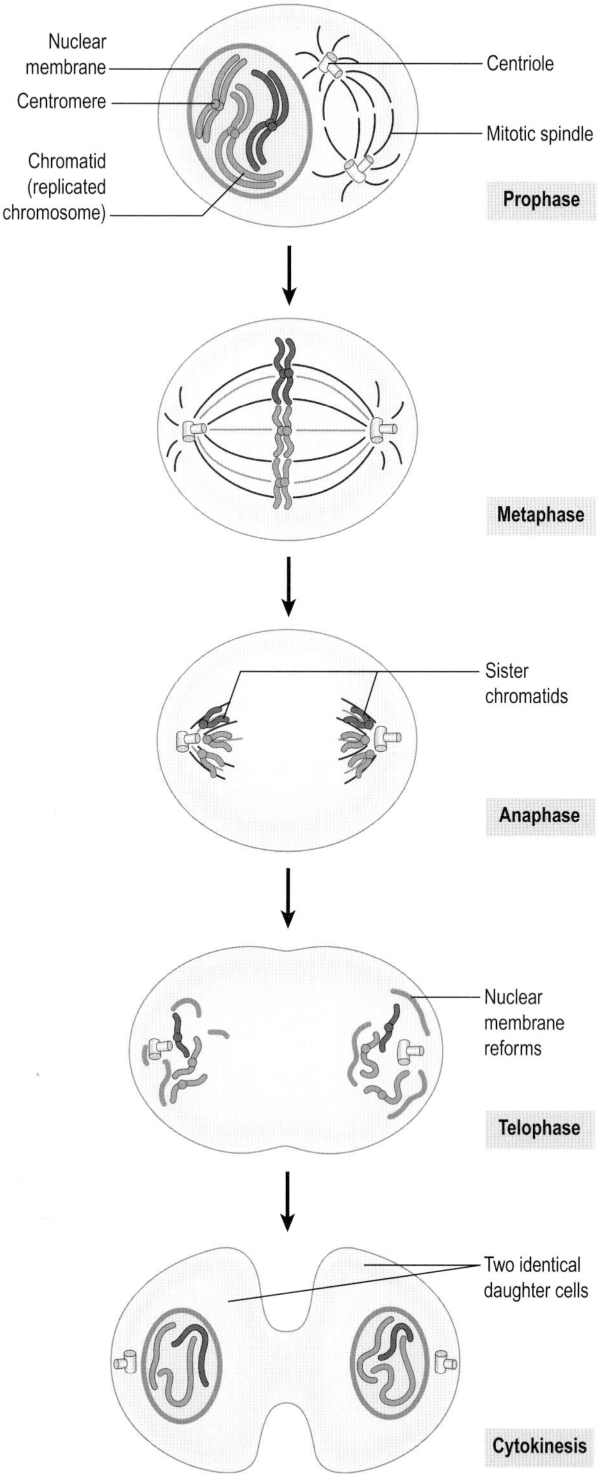

Figure 1.1b-VI • The stages of mitosis.

Mutation in meiosis may result in gametes that carry a defect in the genetic code formed by the DNA. Sometimes this means that the gametes cannot be fertilised. In some cases of mutation of the gamete, fertilisation is possible and the DNA of the resulting zygote will also carry the defect. This will mean that every cell of the developing embryo will also carry the mutation. This may lead to an insignificant or minor change in the function of the adult, such as colour blindness, but can also result in very severe disease, such as sickle cell anaemia or haemophilia (see Q1.1b-6).

Mutation is an important process to understand in the study of pathology. Mutation in mitosis can cause cancer, and mutation of the gametes and the embryo is the cause of congenital disease.

Self-Test 1.1b

The cell

1. What is the name of the cell part (organelle) that is responsible for producing energy?
2. Name two main internal cell parts that are composed almost entirely of membrane. How are their functions linked?
3. (i) What ingredients does the cell require to produce energy?
   (ii) How is this energy stored?
   (iii) What is the waste product?
   (iv) What is the whole process called?
4. In what way does the cell use this energy (in very general terms)?
5. What is the role of the nucleus in cell replication?
6. List two major differences between the processes of meiosis and mitosis.

Answers

1. The mitochondrion is the organelle responsible for producing energy.
2. The ER (endoplasmic reticulum), the Golgi apparatus and the secretory vesicles are made almost entirely of membrane. Their roles are linked because all three use membrane to enclose proteins (manufactured by ribosomes) that are in the process of being exported to the outside of the cell.
3. (i) The cell requires nutrients from food (especially carbohydrates and fats) and oxygen to produce energy.
   (ii) The energy is stored within a substance called ATP.
   (iii) The waste product is carbon dioxide.
   (iv) The process is called cellular respiration.
4. The cell uses energy to power all the activities of the cell. Without this energy the cell would die.
5. The nucleus contains the chromosomes, which are the first parts of the cell to divide in replication. The chromosomes replicate before moving, with the aid of microtubules, to opposite ends of the cell. These separated chromosomes are destined to become the nuclei of the daughter cells
6. Mitosis: leads to two cells identical to the parent cell.
   Mitosis: requires a single division of the chromosomes.
   Meiosis: leads to four gametes, each containing half the genetic material of the parent cell.
   Meiosis: requires two divisions of the chromosomes.

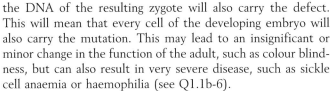

Chapter 1.1c Cell transport and homeostasis

LEARNING POINTS

At the end of this chapter you will be able to:

- list the different mechanisms by which substances can pass through the cell membrane
- differentiate between diffusion, osmosis and active transport
- define the principle of homeostasis and explain how this is central to the health of the human body.

Estimated time for chapter: 80 minutes

Cellular transport processes

Chapter 1.1b introduced the cell membrane and its particular property of allowing the passage of some substances but not of others. This characteristic is called 'semipermeability'. The cell takes in nutrients and expels wastes via the cell membrane. It can also respond to changes in the outside world. An example of this is the nerve cell, which picks up information from one part of the body (e.g. an image in the eye) and relays this to another part of the body (e.g. to the brain, for recognition of the image). This property of 'response to stimuli' is also dependent on the passage of substances across the cell membrane.

The cell membrane is both fluid and oily in nature, and may be pictured as a mobile, slippery and very thin layer surrounding the cell, rather like the wall of a soap bubble. The oily nature means that substances that are soluble in fat, such as gases (oxygen and carbon dioxide) and steroids, can pass through the membrane by first dissolving in it. This oily (phospholipid) layer also contains pathways made through the membrane by large protein molecules embedded within it. These pathways are of a sufficient size to allow the slow, but free, passage of small molecules such as water and salt (Figure 1.1c-I).

Simple diffusion

Movement of substances within the body, whether inside cells, outside cells or across cell membranes, always involves movement through body fluids. When substances are dissolved or suspended in water they tend to move from an area of high concentration to one of low concentration, and the movement continues until the differences in concentration are evened out as much as is physically possible. This form of movement of substances dissolved or suspended within water is called 'diffusion'. When orange squash concentrate is poured into a glass of water, the eventual even mix of orange and water occurs as a result of diffusion.

When a semipermeable membrane such as the cell membrane separates two regions of fluid of different concentrations, the process of diffusion for small molecules is slowed down but not prevented. For example, if there is a strong salt

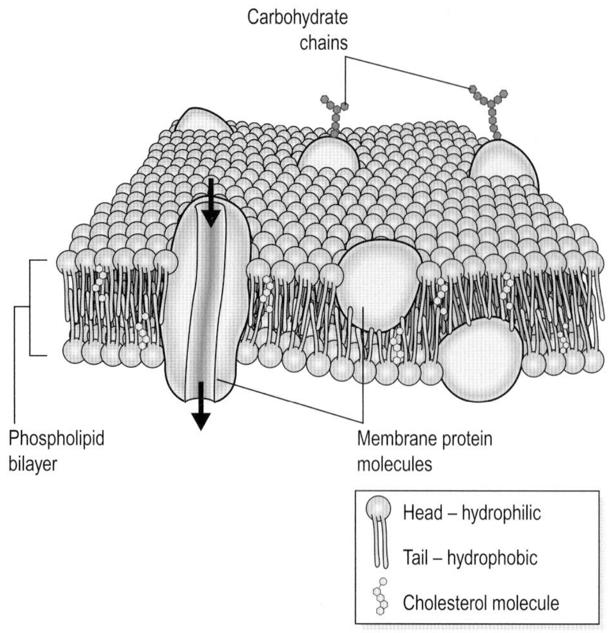

Figure 1.1c-I • A section of the fluid plasma membrane.

solution on one side of a membrane and water on the other, water molecules will cross the membrane via the protein channels to mix with the salt solution. Eventually, the solutions on each side will be of equal concentration. The process may take some time but, as with the orange squash, the result is a solution of an even concentration on either side of the membrane.

Diffusion of certain fat-soluble substances can actually occur through the membrane itself rather than through the protein membrane channels. This is because the membrane is made of an oily substance and permits the free passage of molecules that can dissolve in it. Therefore, because of diffusion, a difference in concentration of oxygen on either side of a semipermeable membrane will eventually become evened out. This will be as a result of the movement of the oxygen between the oily molecules, which make up the membrane, from the more concentrated side to the less concentrated side.

The slow movements of small molecules, such as water and oxygen molecules across the cell membrane are examples of simple diffusion across membranes.

Facilitated diffusion

In addition to the protein channels (holes), there are also 'gates' (also made of protein) that allow the passage of slightly larger substances such as glucose and amino acids. Movement of larger molecules via these gates is known as 'facilitated diffusion'. The gates restrict the free passage of these substances, so that this form of diffusion is extremely slow. This means that, if one of these substances is contained by a membrane, such as the glucose dissolved within the cytoplasm of a cell, only a small amount will be able to pass through.

Some molecules, such as proteins, are so large that they cannot pass across the membrane by the process of diffusion. This means that any large molecules contained within a membrane, such as proteins forming the microfilaments in the cytoplasm, will be unable to leave.

In summary, the membrane is permeable to water and fat-soluble molecules, slightly permeable to glucose, and impermeable to large molecules. This illustrates the meaning of 'semipermeable'. Understanding the concept of semipermeability is a prerequisite for making sense of the process of osmosis.

Osmosis

The process of osmosis in action is evident when limp flowers are placed in some water and the floppy stems become, after a length of time, much more sturdy. What is happening in this example is that the water in the vase is moving across the plasma membranes of the plant cells into the cells themselves. This causes the cells to swell, and then the whole stem to regain its firmness. The water is moving into the cells by diffusion, because the cytoplasm contains a concentrated solution of glucose and large molecules. These larger molecules have a tendency to move in the opposite direction out of the cells, but they are unable to do this because of the semipermeable membrane. Therefore, most of the movement is of water passing one-way across the membrane, and of course this benefits the plant.

In physiology, the term 'osmosis' refers to the process of the transfer of water from a dilute solution across a membrane to a more concentrated solution.

Osmotic pressure

In osmosis, the tendency of the water is to continue moving until the solutions on each side of the are of equal strength (isotonic solutions). However, the movement of water into a concentrated solution of large molecules does not always occur indefinitely. Otherwise, in the example of limp flowers placed in water, the cells in the stems of the flowers would eventually burst. What happens is that, eventually, the process slows down to reach a stable state; the plant cells are firm, but not overfull.

This example illustrates the idea of osmotic pressure. The tendency of the water to dilute the solution on the other side of the membrane can be likened to it being moved under a pressure. However, there are opposing pressures to this movement. In the case of the plant cell, the opposing pressure is the tautness of the fibrous skin of the stem. Eventually, the osmotic pressure is matched by the opposing pressures, and the one-way movement stops at a 'steady state'. This explains how plant cells in a stem can contain a concentrated solution of large molecules, but do not burst when placed in water.

However, the force of osmotic pressure can, in some situations, be strong enough to rupture cells. Red blood cells are not supported by fibrous tissue. If a drop of blood is placed in pure

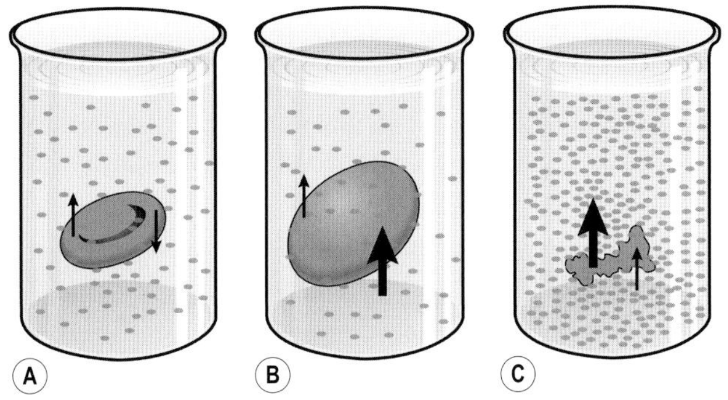

Figure 1.1c-II • The process of osmosis.

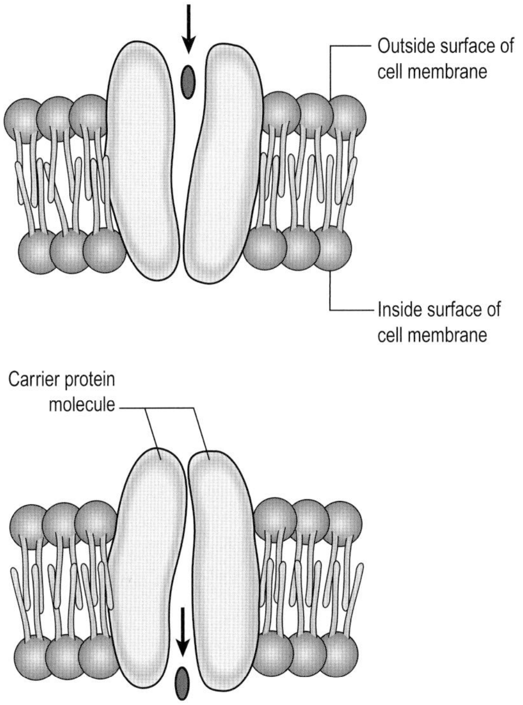

Figure 1.1c III • The role of the carrier protein in active transport and facilitated diffusion across membranes.

water (which is much more dilute than the plasma in which these cells normally circulate), the red blood cells will swell as water molecules move by osmosis into their cytoplasm. Eventually, these cells will burst under the force of the osmotic pressure.

Figure 1.1c-II illustrates what could happen to a red blood cell if it is placed into (a) a solution of the same strength (isotonic) as the fluid in its cytosol, (b) a much more dilute (hypotonic) solution, and (c) a more concentrated (hypertonic) solution. In (a) the movement of water across the cell membrane is balanced inwards and outwards, and the cell remains the same size. In (b) there is a tendency of the more dilute solution to move into the red blood cell and cause it to swell; if the solution is very dilute, the red cell might even burst. In (c), the tendency is for the fluid to move out of the cytosol, across the cell membrane and into the surrounding solution; the red blood cell will tend to shrivel as a result.

This powerful effect of osmosis explains why hospital patients are given intravenous 'saline' in a drip. Saline is a salt solution made to be precisely the concentration of the cytoplasm of all cells, and thus the cells will neither burst nor shrivel when mixed with it.

Osmosis also explains why the bouncy and firm quality of the skin is lost in cases of dehydration. Lack of water means the blood becomes more concentrated. The cells are bathed in the fluid derived from blood. Therefore, when the body is in a state of dehydration, the fluid within the cells will be less concentrated than the surrounding fluid. Water will then move out of the cells by osmosis. This leaves the whole tissue limp, as each cell has slightly shrivelled due to the cellular dehydration caused by the osmosis.

Active transport

Larger molecules, such as complex proteins and glucose, cannot pass readily through the holes and gates formed by membrane proteins. Instead, for rapid movement, these large molecules rely on a 'pump', in the form of a specialised membrane protein powered by the energy stored by the chemical ATP, to permit them to pass. The energy released by the ATP powers a change in the shape of the pump proteins, and this change allows the carriage of the large molecule from one side of the membrane to the other, rather akin to a turnstile that can take a person from one side of a gateway to the other once the entry fee has been inserted (Figure 1.1c-III). Osmosis and diffusion are known as 'passive transport' because they require no added input of energy to take place. In these processes, the movement of molecules occurs simply as a result of the natural tendency of these molecules to be in movement. When added power in the form of ATP is required to move substances from one side of a membrane to another, this is known as 'active transport'.

Bulk transport

The term 'phagocytosis' (literally 'cell-eating') describes the process whereby the cell membrane forms 'arms' that can reach out and engulf external substances so that they can be drawn into the cell. Exocytosis is the process whereby an intracellular vesicle containing complex substances can fuse with the external membrane of the cell so that those substances can be released. Both are forms of active transport, because the movements of the vesicles in both are enabled by the contraction of ATP-powered microfilaments and tubules.

These four simple processes are at the foundation of all that enables a cell to work as part of a living organism. Transport across membranes is what allows a cell to take in nutrients and excrete wastes. It also permits a response to changes in the environment, and therefore communication between cells and the ability of one cell to alter the behaviour of another (see Q1.1c-1-Q1.1c-3).

Homeostasis

Homeostasis refers to the body's ability to maintain a state of balance despite changing external circumstances. The term 'homeostasis' comes from the Greek meaning 'staying the same'.

Two important concepts in physiology that relate to homeostasis are those of the 'internal environment' and the 'external environment'. The internal environment describes all parts of the body that are contained by an epithelial layer, the outside surface of which has a direct connection with the external environment. The external environment includes those parts of the body connected to the outside by orifices. Therefore, parts of the body such as the air passages leading to the lungs, the long space enclosed by the tube of the gut, and the inside of the bladder are all part of the external environment. The external environment, of course, is unpredictable and prone to change in temperature, composition of the air and other substances such as food and liquids.

The principle of homeostasis is that, despite changes in the external environment, the internal environment is always maintained at a steady state. For example, it is a consequence of homeostatic mechanisms that our body temperature remains the same whatever the outside weather (except in the case of illness). Homeostatic processes ensure that diverse variables, including the concentration of the blood (tonicity), the levels of hormones, oxygen, carbon dioxide, blood sugar and mineral salts, the density of the bone and the muscle tone remain controlled within very narrow limits that maximise function and health (see Q1.1c-4).

The process of homeostasis is underpinned by a system of negative feedback loops, which respond to changes in the internal balance by effecting change to re-establish balance. This requires a detector to recognise a move away from balance, a control centre that recognises when the move has been so great that something has to be done about it, and an effector that brings about a change in the body to reverse the imbalance. A thermostat is a mechanical example of a negative feedback loop in action. The detector in this case is a thermometer. The control centre is the mechanism that is set to recognise when the temperature falls outside a desired range. The negative feedback loop is based on the maximum desired temperature. When the temperature becomes higher than this maximum, the effector, in this case the heating element, is switched off until the time when the temperature drops within the desired range once again.

It is clear that in chronic (long-term) illness, and also in ageing, these feedback systems no longer work as effectively. In chronic illness the body never quite achieves the ideal internal environment for optimal function. For example, the blood glucose concentration of a person with untreated diabetes is at a level that is too high for the cells to remain undamaged, and in chronic rheumatoid arthritis the inflammatory processes of the body are always too overactive to be wholly beneficial. With this perspective, it is easy to understand how being in a state of ill health can lead to progressively worsening ill health. The way to stop this would be to reset in some way the 'thermostat' of the feedback loop. Unfortunately, most scientifically derived treatments for chronic illness cannot do this; they tend to work much more on the consequences of the imbalance in homeostasis, and not its underlying cause (see Q1.1c-5).

This chapter has explored how the physiological view of the workings of the healthy body is dependent on the idea that the body has a natural tendency to remain in balance. Illness is the result of a failure in this delicate system.

Self-test 1.1c

Cellular transport and homeostasis

1. Name:
   (i) three processes of passive transport
   (ii) three processes of active transport across cell membranes.
2. What is the fundamental difference between active and passive transport?
3. Match the following processes with one of the six underlying methods of transport across the cell membrane (i.e. diffusion, osmosis, facilitated diffusion via protein channels, active transport via protein gates, phagocytosis and exocytosis):
   (i) removal of bacteria in a wound
   (ii) absorption of water from the stomach
   (iii) absorption of sugar (glucose) from the stomach
   (iv) absorption of oxygen from the air passages of the lungs.
4. Write a definition of the term 'homeostasis'.
5. Can you think of one bodily response, triggered by each of the following states, which will lead to the return of homeostatic function?
   For example, shivering is one bodily response triggered by low body temperature that will lead the temperature to rise towards normal.
   (i) fever
   (ii) dehydration
   (iii) low blood sugar
   (iv) too little oxygen.

Answers

1. (i) Simple diffusion, facilitated diffusion, osmosis.
   (ii) Protein pumps in the cell membrane, pinocytosis and phagocytosis.
2. Active transport requires an external input of energy from ATP, whereas passive transport relies on the internal energy contained in the movement of molecules in fluids.
3. (i) Phagocytosis
   (ii) osmosis
   (iii) facilitated diffusion, and active transport
   (iv) diffusion (across the lungs membrane itself)
4. Homeostasis is the process by which the healthy body maintains a stable internal environment.
5. (i) The responses to fever include sweating, dilatation of blood vessels in the skin and increased blood flow at the surface of the body.
   (ii) The responses to dehydration include production of more concentrated urine, reduced sweating and a strong desire to drink.
   (iii) The responses to low blood sugar include a desire to eat sweet things, and release of hormones that cause glucose stored in the body to enter the bloodstream (these include glucagon and adrenaline).
   (iv) The responses to too little oxygen include increased rate of breathing and increased heart rate.

Chapter 1.1d The tissue types

LEARNING POINTS

At the end of this chapter you will be able to:
- list the four main types of tissue
- explain how the tissue types are specially adapted to perform their individual roles
- name some of the tissue types that can be found in the major body organs.

Estimated time for chapter: 60 minutes.

Specialisation

This chapter explores in more detail about how individual cells are specialised to perform different roles, and how specialised cells are grouped together to form the different tissue types.

Single-celled organisms, such as the amoeba, can survive without specialisation because all parts of the cell membrane are in contact with the external environment. It is therefore possible for a single-celled organism to obtain the food and oxygen it needs, to excrete wastes and to respond to other changes in the environment simply as a result of the fact that all of its boundaries are in touch with the outside world. Specialisation is necessary in larger organisms because most cells are not in contact with the external environment. Cells buried deep within a large organism are unable on their own to be in contact with nutrients and oxygen, and to excrete their wastes into the external environment. They will also be unable to detect changes in the external environment and to respond to maintain homeostasis.

Specialisation is necessary in larger organisms to overcome this problem of the internally situated cells being unable to 'fend for themselves'. In larger organisms, specialised organs take over the role of functions such as nutrition, respiration, excretion and sensing the environment. In this way they support all the other cells in the body.

For example:
- the digestive tract is specialised to obtain food for all cells in the body
- the lungs are specialised to obtain oxygen and excrete carbon dioxide for all cells in the body
- the liver and kidney are specialised to excrete other wastes for all cells in the body
- the nervous system is specialised to sense changes in the environment for all cells in the body (see Q1.1d-1).

Tissue types

There are four recognised categories of specialised tissues:
- epithelial tissue
- connective tissue
- muscle tissue
- nervous tissue.

All these can be subdivided into different tissue subtypes within each category, but this chapter will focus only on the main characteristics of the four types.

Epithelial tissue

All parts of the body that are in direct contact with the external environment are epithelial in nature, whether they are on the outside surface of the body or form the linings of the cavities and passageways of internal organs, such as the lung. Epithelial cells are specialised to protect, secrete and absorb. These are the functions that would be required of an external lining to the body, which has to perform the role of protection, taking in nutrients from the environment and the excretion of wastes.

Epithelial cells are also found lining the heart, blood and lymph vessels. Here they are known as 'endothelium', reflecting the fact that these epithelial cells are deep within the body rather than on the surface.

Epithelial cells develop from a connective-tissue basement membrane that overlies connective tissue underneath. They usually form a single layer of cells, akin to paving stones, but in some regions and organs, including the skin, they develop in layers. These cells tend to multiply rapidly, as they are easily damaged through wear and tear. Figure 1.1d-I illustrates five different forms of epithelium that are found throughout the body (see Q1.1d-2 and Q1.1d-3).

Connective tissue

Connective tissue is specialised to have a structural role in the body. In its various forms it supports and protects the organs both from within and without. The six types of structural connective tissue are areolar (loosely structured) tissue, adipose (fat) tissue, fibrous tissue, elastic tissue, cartilage and bone.

The remaining two types of connective tissue are less to do with structure, and instead comprise the organs of the blood and the lymphatic systems. These have been classed as connective tissue, because the cells found in the blood and lymphoid tissues have similarities with the macrophages, plasma cells and mast cells found in structural connective tissue. All these cells, which include the red and white blood cells, have originated from one common type of immature cell found in the bone marrow.

Connective tissue usually underlies all epithelial tissue. In general, it consists of living cells embedded in a 'matrix' consisting of structural strand-like proteins and a semisolid or solid ground material (which together confer both strength and flexibility akin to reinforced concrete). This complex range of tissues forms the padding and support that separates the internal organs from the epithelial linings. Therefore, it is the next line in defence if the epithelium fails to prevent the occurrence of either a wound or the entry of infection. The presence of the immune cells, such as the macrophages, plasma cells and mast cells, whose functions are to work in the processes both of wound healing and fighting of infection, makes structural connective tissue a very important aspect of the body's defence mechanisms. Figure 1.1d-II illustrates the diversity of the structure of connective tissues (see Q1.1d-4 and Q1.1d-5).

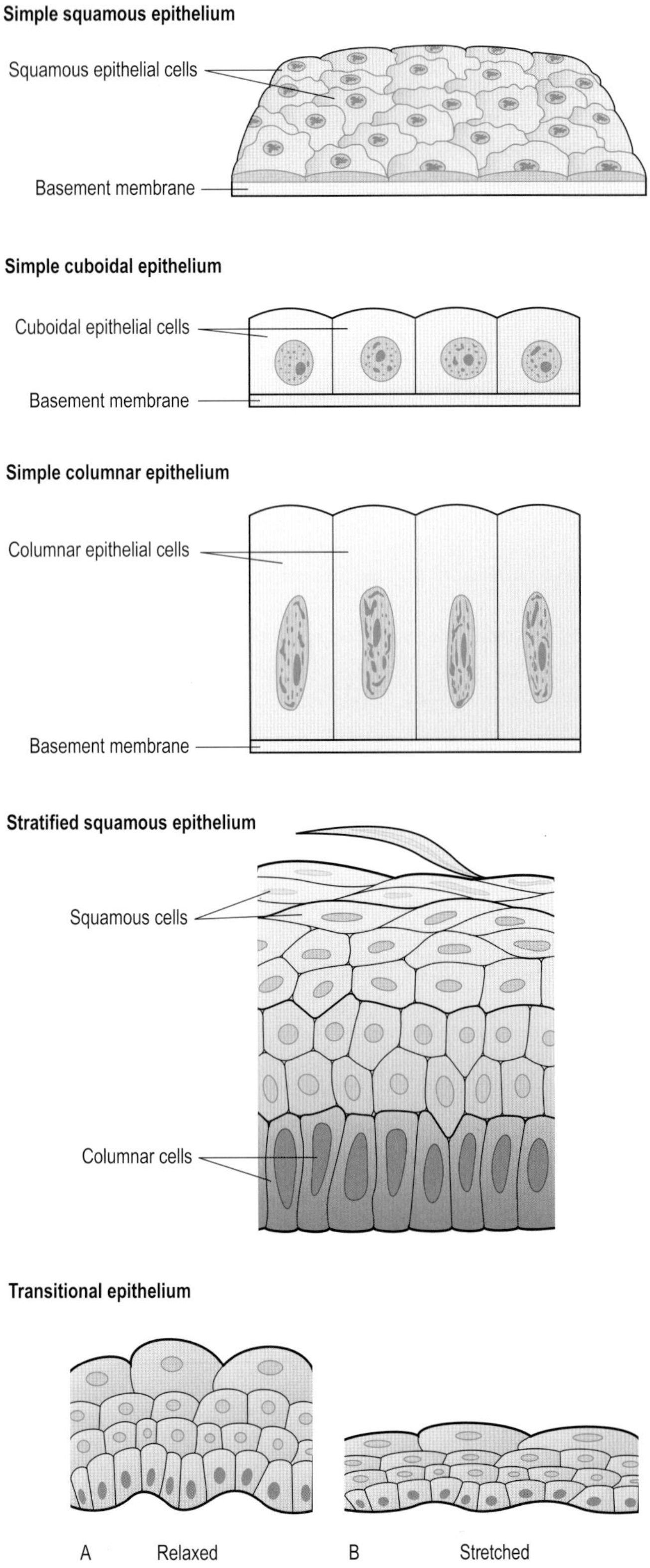

Figure 1.1d-I • The five important categories of epithelium found in the body.

Muscle tissue

Muscle cells are characterised by the fact they all contain protein fibres that can contract. The energy for contraction comes from ATP. Muscle cells also contain another sort of protein, called 'myoglobin', which is specialised to store the large amount of oxygen required to produce sufficient ATP in the muscle cell. There are three types of muscle tissue: striated, smooth and cardiac. Each is specialised for different roles.

Striated muscle tissue (Figure 1.1d-III) is primarily found in skeletal muscle. It has cells in the form of long fibres and responds only to impulses from motor nerves. The cells are bound together in parallel, and can contract together as a unit to increase the available power.

Smooth muscle tissue (Figure 1.1d-IV) is mainly found in the hollow organs and consists of sheets of spindle-like cells, which have a natural tendency to contract. Although not dependent on motor impulses, smooth muscle can contract in response to the autonomic nerves, which run to the hollow organs. Their contraction of smooth muscle is slow and sustained.

Cardiac muscle tissue (Figure 1.1d-V) is specially adapted for the heart wall, with fibres arranged in sheets and the cells arranged with 'joints' that allow for a wave-like contraction across the sheet rather than a single contraction as a unit. Heart muscle tissue also has a natural tendency to contract and is not dependent on motor impulses (see Q1.1d-6).

Nervous tissue

Unlike the other physiological systems which, with the exception of blood, are composed of more than one of the first three tissue types, the nervous system is composed entirely of nervous tissue.

The tissue of the nervous system is composed of two types of cells:

- 'excitable cells' (ordinarily called nerve cells, or neurons)
- 'non-excitable cells' (supportive cells), which can be likened to a specialised form of structural connective tissue.

The structure of this tissue is described in detail in Chapter 4.1.

Membranes and glands

The membranes and glands are specialised forms of epthelial tissue.

There are three main types of membrane – mucous, serous and synovial – each of which has an important structural role in the body, in that they line and protect the organs.

Mucous membranes are characterised by the presence of mucus-secreting cells, which provide the lining of the gut, respiratory tract and genitourinary tracts with a protective coating. They are, therefore, in contact with the external environment.

In contrast, serous membranes are deep within the internal environment. They both surround the body of organs and line the cavities in which they sit. They provide a fluid-filled space to separate the organ from the wall of its cavity.

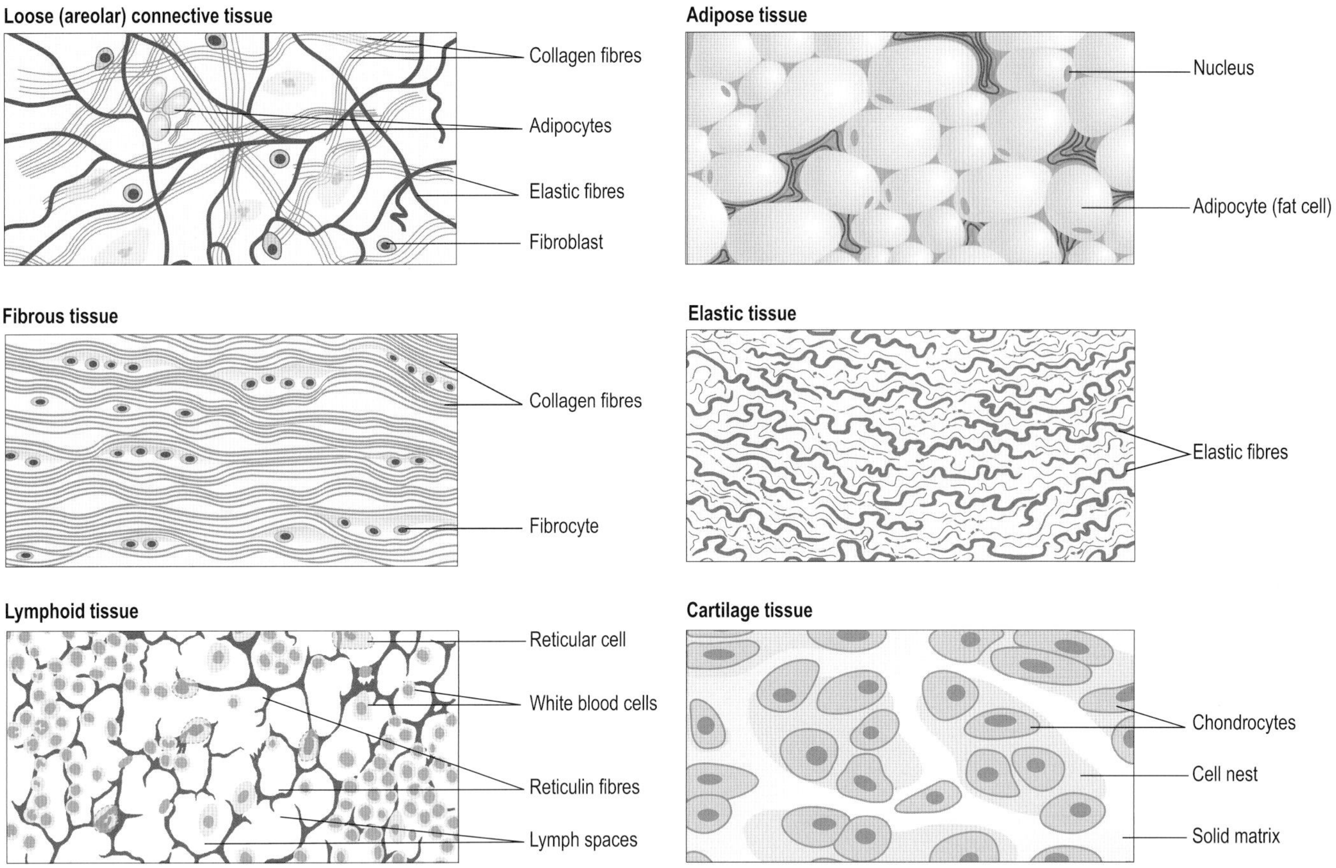

Figure 1.1d-II • Six examples of connective tissue found in the body.

Synovial membrane is the layer that separates the cartilage-covered ends of bone from the space in the joint. It secretes the fluid that nourishes the cartilage and lubricates the joint.

Glands fall into two broad categories: endocrine and exocrine. Endocrine glands are collections of epithelial cells that secrete hormones. Endocrine glands have no ducts; instead, their secretions are released directly into the fluid surrounding the cells (lymph), and from there to the bloodstream. Exocrine glands secrete specialised substances that are discharged towards the epithelium of the organs via a duct. The secretion therefore ends up in the external environment (e.g. on the skin, or in the gut, respiratory passages or genitourinary tract) (see Q1.1d-7-Q1.1d-9).

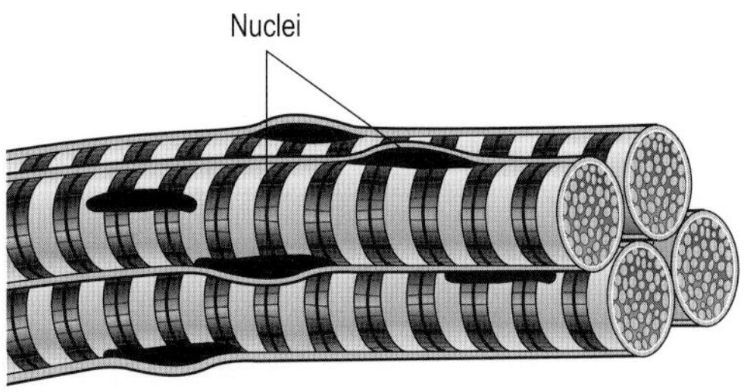

Figure 1.1d-III • Skeletal (striated) muscle fibres.

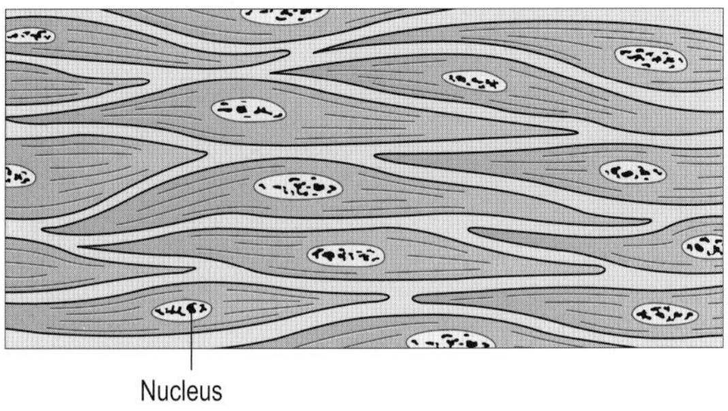

Figure 1.1d-IV • Smooth muscle fibres.

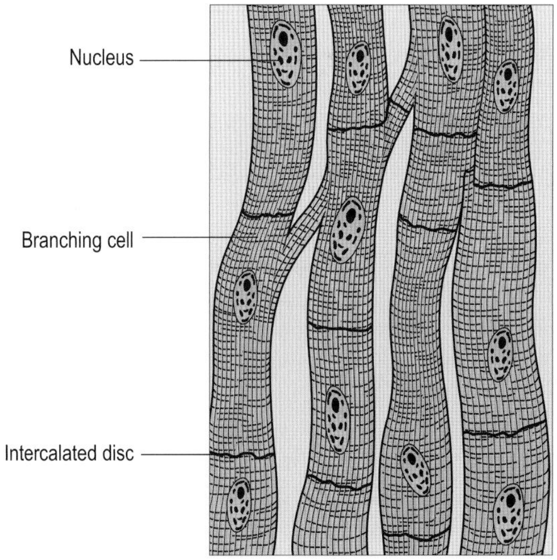

Figure 1.1d-V • Cardiac muscle fibres.

Self-test 1.1d

Tissue types

1. List two characteristic features of each of the four main tissue types.
2. Out of which main tissue types are the following body parts made:
   (i) the linings that surround the lung (the pleura)
   (ii) the conjunctiva of the eye
   (iii) the external muscles of the eye (i.e. those muscles that allow movement of the eyeball)
   (iv) the pancreas
   (v) the olecranon process
   (vi) the platelets.
3. How is the large amount of genetic material in a zygote different from that within a specialised cell?

Answers

1. Epithelial tissue:
   - covers the body and lines cavities, tubes and glands
   - it is the tissue in contact with the external environment
   - cells are specialised to protect, secrete and absorb.

   Connective tissue:
   - forms the structural support of the body
   - is important in immune response.

   Muscle tissue:
   - contains cells that can contract
   - energy for contraction comes from ATP
   - contains myoglobin to store oxygen.

   Nervous tissue:
   - consists of nerves and supportive cells only
   - the nervous system is composed entirely of nervous tissue.
2. (i) The pleura are serosal membranes: epithelial tissue.
   (ii) The conjunctiva of the eye is in contact with the external environment: epithelial tissue.
   (iii) The external muscles of the eye are voluntary muscle: muscle tissue.
   (iv) The pancreas is largely both endocrine and exocrine glands: epithelial tissue.
   (v) The olecranon process is the elbow bone: connective tissue.
   (vi) The platelets are part of the blood: connective tissue.
3. Through the process known as 'differentiation', parts of the genetic material in the daughter cells in the zygote become inactivated while other parts are activated.

The process of differentiation

The various manifestations of the tissue types illustrate the diversity of ways in which the few identical cells of the very early embryo become differentiated into cells with unique and enduring characteristics. Once a cell of an embryo starts to develop into a squamous epithelial cell or a striated muscle fibre, this is the form in which its daughter cells will continue to appear as long as health is maintained.

Although each cell that is produced by mitosis in the embryo contains the same genetic code, through the process of differentiation parts of the genetic code are 'switched off' and other parts are activated. A cell destined to develop into nerve tissue will have the genetic code relevant to the structure of nerve tissue 'switched on' and all of that part of the code relevant to other types of tissue 'switched off'. The way in which this intricate process, known as 'differentiation', is controlled is by no means clearly understood.

It is worth bearing in mind that although the nucleus-containing cells in every tissue in a single human being may look very different, they all contain the same genetic material as the zygote, even though some of it may have been inactivated in some way. Each cell in all the diverse types of tissue is recognised to contain the blueprint for the whole human being.

Chapter 1.1e Introduction to pathology and pharmacology

LEARNING POINTS

At the end of this chapter you will be able to:
- define 'pathology'
- define 'pharmacology'
- explain the different approaches used in conventional medicine to manage disease.

Estimated time for chapter: 60 minutes.

A significant proportion of this text is concerned with how the body responds to disease. This is known as 'pathology'. The chapters in this book associated with each physiological system in turn also explore how conventional medicine has developed approaches to manage disease. The study of drug-based treatments is known as 'pharmacology'.

Pathology

The word 'pathology' is derived from the Greek terms for 'disease' and 'study' (the word 'pathogenic' has the same root – meaning 'disease causing'). During their training, conventional practitioners study the way in which diseases affect the body in great depth. The science of pathology involves understanding the various ways in which the homeostasis of the perfectly functioning body can be moved out of balance (see Q1.1e-1 and Q1.1e-2).

Conventional pathologists understand that disease arises in the body for a range of reasons, some of which are the result of endogenous factors and some a result of the interaction of a body with the external environment.

From a medical perspective, the internal causes of disease include:

- constitutional weakness (inherited disease)
- autoimmune disease
- cancerous change (although some cancers are understood to be triggered by external causes)
- degeneration of age
- negative emotions (the relation of chronic anger, depression and 'stress' to ill health have all been studied in detail)

and the external causes of disease include:

- infections
- inadequate diet
- overeating/obesity
- underexercise
- physical trauma
- excessive heat or cold and dampness
- chemical damage/poisoning (including dietary and recreational factors such as caffeine, tobacco and alcohol) and radiation
- stressful living and working conditions (see Q1.1e-3-Q1.1e-5).

Medical approaches to management of disease

The full breadth of the role of a medical professional is not easily appreciated by a layperson, as certain very technical aspects of medical care, such as drug treatment and surgery, tend to stand out as the most prominent and memorable defining features. However, it may well be that other more simple or mundane aspects of medical care have the most profound effects in terms of improving the health of individuals or populations. To help with the understanding of the breadth of medical approaches, these are now considered within three categories: prevention of disease, cure of disease and treatment of symptoms.

Prevention of disease

Preventive medicine is an essential aspect of any medical care provided by a doctor, irrespective of the medical speciality in which the doctor has trained. At the foundation of any medical approach to preventive medicine is an ever-expanding evidence-based wealth of knowledge on the diverse determinants of disease listed above. In preventive medicine, the physician is concerned with developing this knowledge base and developing effective methods of influencing medical practice and, at a wider level, national and international health and economic policy, so that the important causes of disease are readily recognised and managed appropriately.

Methods of prevention include:

- social change (e.g. banning tobacco advertising, improved sanitation)
- counselling and advice to the public (e.g. healthy eating)
- use of medications (e.g. vaccination, antibiotics during surgery)
- surgery (e.g. removal of a breast in someone considered to be at high risk of cancer)
- routine screening for treatable risk factors for disease (e.g. tests performed in antenatal care).

Prevention can be focused at the level of stopping a disease event from developing (e.g. encouraging cardiac health by focusing on exercise and smoking cessation, with the aim of preventing heart attacks), in which case it may be termed 'primary prevention'. Alternatively, efforts to prevent disease may be concentrated on a patient who has suffered from a disease so that progression of the disease is minimised (e.g. the prescription of aspirin to someone who has suffered from a heart attack), in which case it may be known as 'secondary prevention'.

Confusingly, the terms 'primary', 'secondary' and 'tertiary prevention' are used by the medical profession in a slightly different way also, and it is important to be clear about this, as both forms of nomenclature appear in current respected texts. Some medical authors use the term 'primary prevention' to mean the practice of preventing any aspect of a disease from developing. An example of 'primary prevention' used in this sense is the recent UK policy of administering the human papilloma virus vaccine to young teenage girls. This practice has the aim of preventing wart virus infection, now strongly associated with cervical cancer, from taking hold with the onset of sexual activity in later teenage years. 'Secondary prevention' is the practice of detecting early treatable markers of disease so that early curative treatment can be instigated. The national cervical screening programme in the UK is an example of this, in which all women aged between 25 and 60 years are offered regular cervical smear tests to look for early precancerous changes, which can then be treated to prevent the development of cervical cancer. In this form of naming of prevention of disease, 'tertiary prevention' refers to the approaches used to deal with established disease. Following on from the earlier examples, tertiary prevention would include the surgical and medical treatment of established cervical cancer

According to this nomenclature, many of the approaches used by doctors to screen for disease, such as mammography for breast cancer, blood tests for markers of prostate and ovarian cancer, and examination of the testicles for testicular cancer, are all examples of secondary prevention of disease.

It is currently generally accepted that the greatest impact that modern medicine may have on health is in the realm of the promotion of the general health of a population and the prevention of disease.

Cure of disease

Although prevention of disease may have the most significant impact on health, it is the doctor's ability to cure diseases that often attracts the greatest respect. Moreover, while medical and surgical approaches often have the most dramatic results in terms of cure, it is important to remember that healing modalities requiring less technical expertise, such as the giving of simple advice or the administration of basic nursing care, may be all that is needed to effect a full return to health.

Methods of cure include:

- medication that reverses the process of disease
- physical therapies (e.g. physiotherapy)
- lifestyle advice
- talking therapies (i.e. psychotherapy)
- surgery
- basic needs supplied through hospital care
- treatment of distressing symptoms or disability resulting from disease.

Treatment of disease

Most diseases that impact on the health of western populations are chronic conditions such as coronary heart disease, diabetes, depression, cancer and dementia. These sorts of conditions are not necessarily amenable to cure. In a developed country, the bulk of medical care is devoted to the management of these chronic conditions and preventing their progression as far as is possible.

Methods of treatment of the symptoms of chronic disease include:

- medication that alleviates symptoms or hinders progression of disease
- surgery
- physical therapies (e.g. physiotherapy)
- advice
- talking therapies (e.g. psychotherapy)
- occupational therapy and rehabilitation
- nursing home/hospital care
- referral to other agencies (e.g. social services) (see Q1.1e-6).

Pharmacology

The term 'pharmacology' is derived from the Greek meaning 'medicine' and 'study '. It is another science that is studied in depth by doctors during their training. Pharmacology embraces the study of all drugs that are prescribed for each disease. In addition, it involves the understanding of the complex way in which each drug interacts with the chemical and cellular processes of the body. Pharmacologists are interested in predicting possible side-effects and 'contraindications' (the situations when a drug should not be prescribed) (see Q1.1e-7).

Accessing information in medical textbooks

This text is written with the aim of making medical information more accessible to health practitioners with a non-medical background or focus. An important skill to acquire is a facility for using medical texts and for interpreting the language used within such texts. Very often the information presented by medical textbooks and on websites is organised in a way that follows a predictable pattern. A familiarity with this pattern can greatly assist in the process of extracting important information.

Texts on physiology and pathology

Medical textbooks are generally structured around the 12 physiological systems, and this will also apply to texts on physiology and the pathology of disease. When reading any textbook it is important to question the reliability of the information presented. Physiology and pathology are descriptive subjects, and the information found in pathology texts can generally be trusted as established fact derived from scientific observation. For example, a phrase from a pathology textbook such as '...bone is a connective tissue with cells (osteocytes) surrounded by a matrix of collagen fibres...' has its origins in the scientific observation of the microscopic structure of bone. Most readers probably would not dispute such facts, even though they might hold an alternative view of the body based on an energetic foundation of bone. This technical description is simply a way to describe the material nature of healthy bone.

In a similar fashion, most statements about pathology are also facts based on the observation of diseased tissue. For example, the sentence, 'In Paget's disease osteocytes resorb excess bone, softening the tissue, and then overactive osteoblasts deposit abnormal new bone that is thickened or enlarged or structurally weak', reflects a process that has been observed using scientific methods, including microscopy.

Information box 1.1e-1

Western descriptions of pathology: comments from a Chinese medicine perspective

Facts concerning pathological processes can be surprisingly relevant and helpful to the practice of a complementary health practitioner. Not only can they assist in providing the language for communicating the conventional view of disease to patients, but they can also provide valuable information about a possible energetic interpretation of a particular condition.

For example, consider the sentence about Paget's disease quoted earlier in the body of the text: 'osteocytes resorb excess bone, softening the tissue, and then overactive osteoblasts deposit abnormal new bone that is thickened or enlarged or structurally weak'. It is feasible that a Chinese medicine energetic interpretation be drawn from such a description. Overactive cells and rapid growth of bone might suggest the presence of Heat, possibly springing from Yin Deficiency. It also suggests Phlegm (if the bone growth is irregular). Paget's disease is, in fact, a condition of ageing bones. It presents with deformed hot areas of bone, and these areas carry a risk of undergoing cancerous change. This suggests that it is presumably a condition of Phlegm/Heat, with underlying Kidney Yin deficiency of old age as the possible origin of the Heat. Here it can be seen that the detail of the pathology may be reflected in the energetic understanding of the symptoms and signs of this condition.

This process of learning the descriptions of pathological processes as aids to the energetic interpretation of disease (according to Chinese medicine theory in particular) is explored further in Stage 2.

Texts on clinical medicine

'Clinical medicine' is the term used to describe the practice of medicine in the setting of the clinic or hospital. Texts on clinical medicine are also generally structured around the 12 physiological systems, and may include some introductory physiology and pathology to introduce the description of clinical medical approaches system by system.

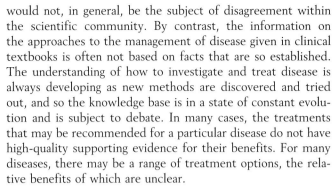

Doctors use the term 'medicine' to describe the discipline that aims to treat diseases by means of non-surgical techniques. Drug treatments are a principal therapy in the practice of medicine. For mainly historical reasons, the practice of surgery is considered by doctors to be a separate, albeit complementary, discipline to medicine. For this reason, most specialists in clinical medicine are not trained to perform even the most basic of surgical operations, and many surgeons will have only a relatively basic knowledge of clinical medicine.

Textbooks of general clinical medicine do not, therefore, describe in detail those conditions that are primarily managed by surgeons. In particular, the specialties of orthopaedics (surgical conditions of the bones and joints), otorhinolaryngology (ear, nose and throat diseases), obstetrics and gynaecology (diseases of pregnancy and women's health), urology (diseases of the urinary tract) and plastic surgery are not embraced within many conventional texts. Specialist aspects of clinical medicine, such as paediatrics (children's diseases), ophthalmology (diseases of the eye), and gerontology or geriatrics (medicine of old age), are also not necessarily found in general clinical textbooks.

The information relating to each disease in medical texts, be they medical or surgical in bias, is ordered according to a structure that is familiar to conventional health practitioners. This method relies on classifying information about the disease under the following sorts of subheading:

- Disease name.
- Definition.
- Epidemiology: the study of the causes and manifestations of disease within populations (as distinct from individuals). (For example, 'rheumatoid arthritis affects 2% of the UK population' is a statement about the epidemiology of the disease.)
- Aetiology: the causation of disease.
- Screening: the approaches used for the prevention of disease. (For example, the cervical smear and mammography are used in two national screening programmes to detect early treatable cervical and breast cancer respectively.)
- Pathogenesis: the processes that have instigated the development of disease.
- Pathology/pathophysiology: the processes that maintain the disease.
- Clinical features: the experience of the patient (the symptoms), and features that can be found on medical examination (the signs).
- Investigations: the tests that might reveal abnormal results for this disease.

  Differential diagnoses: the range of conditions that might present with similar symptoms, signs and test results. (For example, central crushing chest pain suggests a heart attack, but the differential diagnoses include angina, severe indigestion, bronchial infection, broken rib, etc.).
- Treatment/management (see Q1.1e-8).

In terms of reliability of information, it has already been explained how descriptions of physiology and pathology found in medical texts are generally based on established facts that would not, in general, be the subject of disagreement within the scientific community. By contrast, the information on the approaches to the management of disease given in clinical textbooks is often not based on facts that are so established. The understanding of how to investigate and treat disease is always developing as new methods are discovered and tried out, and so the knowledge base is in a state of constant evolution and is subject to debate. In many cases, the treatments that may be recommended for a particular disease do not have high-quality supporting evidence for their benefits. For many diseases, there may be a range of treatment options, the relative benefits of which are unclear.

For the sake of simplicity, many clinical texts, particularly those aimed at medical students or the general public, frequently present the information on diagnosis and treatment as if they are undisputed fact. They may occasionally open a discussion on how beneficial a particular treatment is likely to be. In reality, there is a wide variation in clinical practice, and not all doctors will manage their patients in the way described in respected texts. Increasingly, however, clinical texts will present the considered opinion of a body of specialists on what would be the most evidence-based and cost-effective approaches to the clinical management of a

Self-test 1.1e

Introduction to pathology and pharmacology

1. Define the terms 'pathology' and 'pharmacology'.
2. What are three important differences between the way conventional practitioners and practitioners of Chinese medicine view the causes of disease?
3. What are the three categories of ways in which a conventional practitioner might manage disease?

Answers

1. Pathology is the study of disease processes. Pharmacology is the study of the use and action of therapeutic drugs.
2. In Chinese medicine, emotions are seen as primary in the causation of disease, whereas the emotions are only considered as a secondary factor, if at all, by conventional practitioners.

   Climatic factors are considered important sources of pathogens in Chinese medicine, but only extremes of cold, heat and dampness are considered harmful by conventional practitioners.

   The following can be seen as potentially beneficial in conventional terms, but not necessarily conducive to health in Chinese medicine:
   - plenty of fresh fruit and salad
   - a low calorie diet
   - aerobic exercise
   - outdoor exercise, whatever the weather
   - frequent sexual intercourse
   - vaccinations.
3. - preventive approaches
   - treatments aimed at cure
   - approaches to relieve symptoms/disability.

condition. The UK National Institute for Health and Clinical Excellence (NICE) is one such body. NICE has published a wide range of statements on evidence-based treatment guidelines for various diseases.

It is also important to be aware that information in texts on clinical medicine, including this one, is likely to become out of date very rapidly. For this reason, new editions of popular clinical medical texts are produced every 3–4 years.

Conventional clinical practice

1.2

Chapter 1.2a The conventional medicine approach

LEARNING POINTS

At the end of this chapter you will be able to:
- describe the three conventional steps in diagnosing a disease
- classify a disease according to a conventionally recognised method
- explain how treatments are chosen for a patient with a recognised disease.

Estimated time for chapter: 60 minutes.

This chapter explores more closely how a patient with a disease is diagnosed and treated by a conventional medicine practitioner. It is important to be familiar with the steps involved in the management of disease before going on to study specific diseases and their treatment.

Conventional medical training

Conventional training in medicine (and also the paramedical professions such as nursing, physiotherapy and occupational therapy) is based largely on scientific method and how this applies to health. From the outset of the training, medical 'knowledge' is taught as fact, with relatively little emphasis on the history of medicine or on the philosophy that underlies current medical thought.

The early years of medical school training are focused on the sciences of anatomy, biochemistry, physiology, pathology, pharmacology and psychology. As the training progresses, medical students are given increasing contact with patients in a hospital setting. It is in this clinical setting that the skills of case history taking, clinical examination, diagnosis and treatment are taught. Much of the learning in this clinical part of training is by example, as students accompany doctors in their practice in the clinic or on the ward.

One highly valued setting for learning in the UK is the 'ward round', in which the teaching doctor takes students to the bedside. The patient is the stimulus for the teaching, which is often in the form of encouraging rapid recall of relevant facts about the case in question. For example, on a ward round, the teaching doctor might ask: 'This patient has renal failure. What are the causes of renal failure?' The student is expected to reply with a systematic and complete list of causes of the condition in question. In this way, the diagnostic process becomes ingrained as a reflex in which, with the stimulus of characteristic symptoms and signs in a patient, appropriate diagnoses can be made and treatment selected.

The emphasis in medical training is that the skills of a fine clinician should include the ability to elicit the symptoms and signs of disease by careful questioning and sensitive clinical examination, and to have mental access to a complex series of lists of possible diagnoses and treatment options. To be successful, hospital clinicians require an analytical mind and an ability to structure facts in a rigorous way.

Interpersonal skills are also considered important to enable the rapport necessary to elicit symptoms from a patient, and the foundations of skills in communication are laid down in the early years of training of a medical student. More in-depth training in communication skills plays an important role in later aspects of medical training, particularly in the more person-centred specialities of general practice and psychiatry.

How disease is defined in conventional medicine

Most medical textbooks will describe a disease according to a system that lists the defining characteristics of the disease within a series of categories. For example, the characteristics of chickenpox could be presented as shown in Box 1.2a-I.

By having information structured in this way, each disease can be assessed in terms of its cause, symptoms and signs,

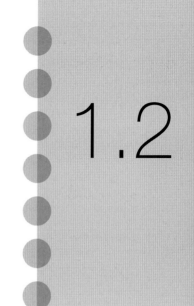

Box 1.2a-I

Chickenpox: defining characteristics

Name:	Primary herpes zoster (chickenpox)
Epidemiology:	Universal; 95% of people in metropolitan communities have had infection by adulthood
Aetiology/cause:	Herpes zoster virus infection. Droplet spread of vesicle fluid
Symptoms and signs:	13–17 day incubation period followed by sudden onset of fever, mild constitutional malaise and, after 2 days, a widespread vesicular rash with lesions appearing in crops mainly on the trunk. Lesions leave a scab after rupturing in 3–4 days. Symptoms can be more severe in adults. Complications include bacterial infection of lesions, pneumonia and encephalitis. Can manifest later in life as secondary herpes zoster (shingles)
Investigations:	Can be diagnosed by clinical features alone. Rising antibodies can be assayed after 3–4 days (blood test)
Treatment:	For symptoms only. Treat infected lesions with oral flucloxacillin
Prognosis:	Usually mild and self-limiting. Case fatality: 2/100,000 in children; 30/100,000 in adults
Prevention:	Live attenuated vaccine available for susceptible children. Varicella zoster immune globulin can be given within 4 days of exposure to reduce risk of contracting severe disease in the immunocompromised (e.g. patients with leukaemia or AIDS)
Differential diagnosis:	No other illnesses present in this way, but other infectious diseases such as measles, rubella and scarlet fever may be considered in the differential diagnosis

investigations, etc. The differential diagnosis alerts the diagnosing doctor to other diseases that might have similar characteristics.

In forming a definition such as this one for chickenpox, the focus is on the characteristic pattern of the disease as it might affect any person, and not on the individual characteristics of the patient.

This model is often termed 'reductionist', because of the way in which the body is seen as a collection of smaller parts, and the characteristics of disease reduced down to tangible facts. The reductionist aspects of modern medicine are explored in more detail in Section 1.3.

How disease is diagnosed

Disease is diagnosed in three stages. These enable the doctor to match the individual patient with the descriptions of diseases that become so familiar through the course of medical training. The three stages of diagnostic information gathering are questioning for the presence of symptoms, examining the body for signs and checking the results of tests. Although a great deal of emphasis can be placed on the results of tests, medical students are taught that over 70% of diagnoses can be made with skilful history taking (questioning of the patient) alone. Adding in the results of physical examination will bring this diagnosis rate up to about 90%.

Thus, together, symptoms and signs will offer the necessary information for narrowing down the diagnosis. Medical students are trained to respond to characteristic symptoms and signs (e.g. central chest pain or a painless red rash) by generating a list of possible causes. To ensure the list of possible diagnoses is complete, students are taught to consider methodically the systems of the body and then important aetiological factors in turn. A full list will consider causes that might affect the circulatory, respiratory, digestive, urinary, nervous, endocrine, musculoskeletal and reproductive systems. Additional categories of causes that might be considered include infective, inflammatory, degenerative, malignant, social and psychological causes. This technique relies on memorisation of facts (see Q1.2a-1 and Q1.2a-2).

With a list of possible diagnoses to hand, the doctor is then ready to ask more questions to narrow down the diagnosis and also to consider whether any investigations might provide further diagnostic information. However, it is noteworthy that test results are only essential in less than 10% of diagnoses, as the majority of diagnoses can be confidently made on the basic of skilful history taking and examination alone.

Tests should, ideally, be used to confirm a diagnosis and to help with the monitoring of treatment. An example would be the use of blood levels of thyroid-stimulating hormone (TSH) to confirm hypothyroidism in somebody with tiredness, weight gain and a slow pulse. An initial measurement that is well above the normal range would confirm the diagnosis. TSH levels would be expected to drop as the patient is given thyroid replacement therapy, thus showing a good treatment response (see Q1.2a-3).

To summarise, the three steps to reaching a diagnosis are:

- questioning to elicit symptoms
- physical examination to elicit signs
- performing tests ('investigations') and obtaining the results.

These stages will be familiar to anyone who has trained in complementary medicine. However, in most forms of complementary medicine, the emphasis is very much on the symptoms (which are the patient's own subjective experience), and there is far less emphasis on performing tests. Nevertheless, many practitioners of complementary medicine will make use of objective tests, such as blood pressure assessment, peak-flow assessment, x-ray imaging and analysis of the urine, to give more information about the patient's condition.

Questioning for symptoms

The approach to the questioning of the patient in conventional medicine is very similar to the approach taught to many practitioners of complementary medicine. For example, conventional doctors use a very similar checklist to the one that many Chinese medicine practitioners often use to guide them through the questioning of patients about their symptoms. The major difference in conventional medicine is that there are often serious time limitations that constrain this aspect of diagnosis.

Medical students are trained to ask nine questions that can be used to clarify the details about any one symptom. In using these questions, the doctor is undertaking detective work, looking for the clues that will help to narrow down the diagnosis. The nine questions relate to:

- site
- radiation (i.e. to what body parts does the experience of the symptom extend?)
- character
- severity
- onset
- frequency
- duration
- accompanying symptoms
- what makes the symptom better or worse?

Examination for signs

A doctor is trained to take a systematic approach to the physical examination of the body. This examination is intended to reveal any bodily changes that might indicate the presence of physical disease. This approach to physical examination is, therefore, quite different to the examination performed by many complementary therapists, which may focus more on the subjective interpretation of energetic imbalance.

The case scenario presented in Box 1.2a-II illustrates these first two stages of the diagnostic process (see Q1.2a-4).

Performing tests

Medical investigations or tests are performed to narrow down a diagnosis and also to monitor the progress of treatment.

The diagnostic aspect of tests can be best illustrated by continuing with the case scenario given in Box 1.2a-II, as described in Box 1.2a-III. This case history illustrates the process of diagnosis and choice of treatment. Many doctors find this process a pleasing one to follow. The diagnosis is made by a logical process of elimination, and the treatment for a clear diagnosis is usually obvious from the current textbooks or guidelines.

However, in practice, diagnosis is rarely that straightforward. Some of the problems that beset doctors in the diagnostic process relate to the reliability of diagnostic signs as indicators of disease. Medicine is a discipline that is dogged

Box 1.2a-II

Case scenario

Ian, a 63-year-old man, has noticed that he has started to get up at night to urinate and goes to see his doctor.

The doctor remembers the checklist for the possible causes of this symptom, known as nocturia, which includes:

- endocrine causes such as diabetes
- urinary causes such as chronic renal failure
- degenerative disease such as benign enlargement of the prostate gland
- malignant causes such as prostate cancer
- social causes such as drinking too much alcohol or caffeine late at night
- psychological causes such as anxiety with insomnia

Ian's doctor uses questioning and examination to find out more about the nocturia. In response to her questions, Ian tells her that he has had the problem for some months, when it started with having to get up just once in the night. Now he gets up three or more times, but more often than not just passes a few dribbles of water, even though he has to wait at the toilet for some time. Otherwise he is well, so there are no accompanying symptoms. He finds that to cut down on all fluids in the evening improves the chances of a less disturbed night.

The doctor performs a physical examination, which involves examination of the prostate gland. This can be felt just inside the anus. Ian's prostate gland feels smoothly enlarged and has a rubbery texture. There are no other physical abnormalities.

The task of Ian's doctor is to start to match the symptoms and signs of Ian's condition with the conditions that she knows can cause nocturia. The physical findings, together with a characteristic history, alert her to the possibility that constriction of the urethra by an enlarged prostate gland might be the cause of the problem.
She reaches this conclusion because she knows that a common cause of nocturia in men of Ian's age group is benign enlargement of the prostate gland, also known as prostatic hypertrophy (BPH).

BPH results in gradual obstruction of the urethra, which is the tube that leads from the bladder to the penis. This means that efficient emptying of the bladder is no longer possible, and this leads to a frequent urge to pass small amounts of urine.

The main similarities of BPH with prostate cancer lie in the symptoms, which are those of 'lower urinary tract obstruction'. Both tend to occur in older men, although BPH is more likely to first present at an earlier stage in life than cancer. Another similarity is that a sign of prostate cancer is an enlarged prostate gland, but in cancer the prostate is often irregular and hard. In contrast, in BPH it is smooth and rubbery.

A medical textbook might systematically define BPH as follows:

Name:	Benign prostatic hypertrophy (BPH)
Aetiology/ cause:	Degenerative (ageing) disease of unknown cause
Incidence:	In most men over 60 years of age
Symptoms:	Nocturia, difficulty in urination, dribbling, poor stream
Signs:	Smooth enlarged prostate gland felt on rectal examination
Investigations:	Test urine for infection (culture), blood test for kidney problems and assessment of prostate-specific antigen to exclude cancer. Detailed imaging of the kidneys and bladder (x-ray and ultrasound) to exclude the kidney problems that can result from prolonged BPH
Treatment:	Drug treatment if mild, surgical resection of the prostate gland if severe
Differential diagnosis:	Prostatic cancer

It is clear that Ian's doctor needs first to eliminate the diagnosis of prostate cancer before treating Ian for BPH.

Box 1.2a-III

Continuation of case scenario in Box 1.2a-II

It is clear that Ian's doctor needs first to eliminate the diagnosis of prostate cancer before treating Ian for BPH, and so she arranges for some tests to be performed, including blood tests for prostate-specific antigen (PSA) and markers of renal function, and an ultrasound scan of the bladder and kidneys.

On completion of the investigations, Ian's bladder and kidneys do not appear to be damaged, and the PSA test is negative.

The doctor can then explain to Ian the purpose and the outcome of the tests, that it appears that it is most likely he has a mild form of BPH, which is part of the normal ageing process for some people. She might then explain the current treatments for BPH, according to current professional guidelines, which include drug treatments or surgery. She might discuss the pros and cons of these options. This is intended to leave Ian with sufficient information to make a decision about which treatment options he might follow.

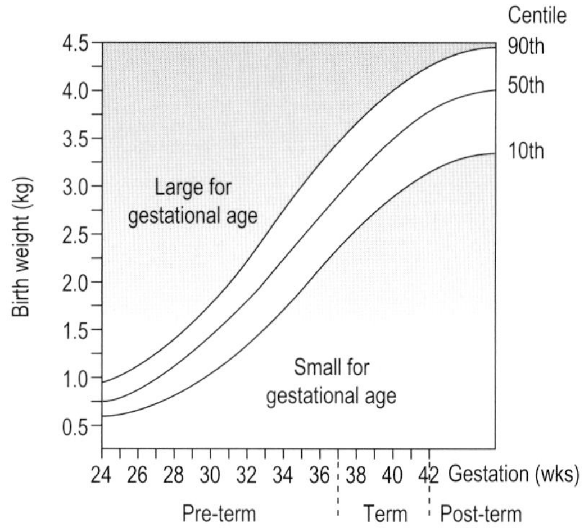

Figure 1.2a-I • Graph illustrating mean birthweight according to stage of pregnancy at delivery • The mean birthweight is indicated by the 50th centile line. (From Lissauer and Clayden 1997, p. 78, with permission).

with uncertainty. Not all symptoms, signs and positive test results indicate disease, as they can occur in healthy people (these are known as 'false-positive' findings). Similarly, not all normal measurements are indicative of health; in some people with disease, tests results are within the normal range (this would be described as a 'false-negative' result). Some of the uncertainty in diagnosis stems from limitations in the measurability of bodily functions.

Measurability in medicine

From a conventional medicine perspective, all functions of the parts of the body should be measurable, because they are believed to stem from something that is physical in nature. Although conventional doctors appreciate that the physical basis of some aspects of function, such as the emotions, are still unclear, there is still an underlying fundamental belief that, in the course of time, and with the results of high-quality research, all aspects of the body are potentially quantifiable.

The use of symptoms and signs is a form of measurement. For some symptoms and signs, the measurement is crude and rather subjective, as for example in the visual assessment of the redness of a sore throat. For other signs, however, such as pulse rate or temperature, the measurement can be more precisely recorded and then expressed in comparison to a 'normal range'. Normal ranges are derived by taking measurements of a variable, height for example, from a large population. For many variables, the measurements are found to cluster around the most common, or mean, value.

An example of this is shown in Figure 1.2a-I, which illustrates how the birthweight of babies varies according to the week of pregnancy in which they were born. The graph shows three almost parallel curves. The central curve (labelled 50th centile) indicates the average or mean birthweight at any length of gestation. For example, an average baby born at the normal time (the 40th week of gestation) will have a birthweight of about 3.5 kg. The two outer curves (labelled 90th and 10th centiles) are an indication of the range of birthweights of most babies (80% to be precise) born at a particular time. For example, at 40 weeks of gestation, 90% of babies will have a birthweight less than 4.0 kg, and only 10% will have a birthweight less than 2.75 kg.

According to the graph, the normal range for birthweight at 40 weeks of pregnancy is 2.75–4.0 kg. In other words, 80% of babies will have a birthweight between 2.75 and 4.0 kg. Conversely, the 20% of babies who have birthweights either greater or less than this range are 'outside the normal range'. This implies that 20% of babies born at the normal time are, according to their birthweight, abnormal in some way. Logically speaking, this statement has to be true if a normal birthweight has been defined as 2.75–4.0 kg. Of course, it does not follow that one-fifth of all babies born at 40 weeks of gestation are unhealthy in any way. Some might be, but others might be small or large because of a familial tendency to be of a small or large build. The important point to draw from this example is that 'abnormal' as defined by a measurement that falls outside the normal range does not necessarily mean unhealthy.

The value of such an approach is that a baby whose weight falls outside the normal range will be examined more carefully to check that there are no underlying problems that might account for the abnormality. Conversely, the disadvantage of such an approach is that some healthy babies will be labelled as 'abnormal', and this can be a cause of unnecessary anxiety.

Most commonly, normal ranges express the range of values into which 95% of a population might fall for any one variable. This means that, for every possible variable, only 5% of the population will be considered to be outside this normal range. However, whatever the percentage of the population that has been selected to express the normal range, it would be very unlikely for anyone to be normal in every respect.

To summarise, this approach to defining normality has consequences that are not always appreciated by either the patient or the doctor. These are:

- some healthy people will, as a consequence of chance, fall outside the normal range
- unhealthy people can fall within the normal range
- if the population from which the normal range is derived is unhealthy, what can be said about normality and how it equates to health?

The issue of the definition of 'normality' is relevant when a seemingly well patient undergoes a health check. In a typical health check the patient undergoes a physical examination and some routine tests of bodily functions. Health checks involving a large number of tests are promoted particularly within the private health sector. Such tests raise problems. Does a 'pass' on all the tests included in the check really confirm 'health'? It is well recognised that a person who feels very unwell, for example someone with recurrent migraine, may fall within the normal range for all the tested variables. The doctor might give such a person a clean bill of health on the basis of a health check. The problem here is that what is being measured is not necessarily related to any disease that the person may be experiencing.

Another problem that arises from health checks is the question of what should be done if a previously healthy person has an abnormal test result. This is complex territory, not only for patients but also for most practitioners. An abnormal test is always a worrying finding, despite the fact that in a large proportion of cases there may be no actual abnormality in terms of disease. Conversely, a negative test may give false reassurance as, despite a value in the normal range, the disease may still be present.

An additional problem with many tests is that they cannot be wholly reliable because of inevitable errors in the processing of the test. This is another reason for an abnormal test result in someone with no actual disease. Conversely, an unreliable test can fail to reveal actual disease. Both these types of error are well recognised to affect any screening procedure, and doctors have to account for them when they interpret test results.

The prostate-specific antigen (PSA) test for prostate cancer is a good example of these points. If the PSA test is positive, this suggests a cancer is present, but it can be positive in some cases of benign prostatic hypertrophy (BPH) (i.e. a false-positive result). The PSA test can also be negative in some cases of cancer (i.e. a false-negative result), so giving a false sense of reassurance. The same applies to the sign of a smooth prostate. A smooth prostate suggests a benign cause, but is not a reliable indicator that a cancer is not present (i.e. it could be a false-negative).

To return to the scenario of Ian, the 63-year-old man with nocturia (see Box 1.2a-II), although he may feel that he has been given the 'all clear' from cancer, Ian's doctor cannot totally be sure that the smooth prostate is not hiding a small cancer, and that the PSA result is not a false-negative. Given Ian's age, together with the signs and test result, cancer would seem unlikely, but remains possible. The doctor has a dilemma whether or not to discuss this small possibility with Ian. It would actually be a very difficult discussion, because most textbooks do not offer information on the certainty of symptoms, signs and test results as predictors of disease. Without undertaking some in-depth research of the literature, the doctor would not be able to put any figure on the probability of an undiagnosed cancer in Ian's case. Therefore, most doctors choose not to worry the patient about a serious, but unlikely, outcome.

This aspect of the diagnostic process is not completely satisfactory. In Ian's case it is very likely he has a benign problem, but in other cases the diagnosis may be far less certain (see Q1.2a-5 and Q1.2a-6).

The problem of functional disease

The scenario of 'normal tests in an unwell patient' is an all too familiar one in practice. Many people have had the experience of being reassured by a doctor that, despite their symptoms, all tests are normal. All general practitioners have to deal with unusual symptoms for which there are few or no physical abnormalities to be found on examination and all test results are normal. There are a large number of recognised syndromes of uncertain physical basis described in medical textbooks. Because the underlying disease process in many of these syndromes is poorly understood treatments for such conditions can only be targeted at relieving symptoms.

The term given to these syndromes of uncertain cause in which physical examination and test results are generally normal is 'functional diseases'. The functional diseases include irritable bowel syndrome, migraine, low back strain, fibromyalgia, and chronic fatigue syndrome (CFS). Although such conditions are never seen as 'serious', in that they are not a threat to life, they are extremely important in terms of the degree to which they impair well-being.

Functional diseases are a problem for the medical profession because they are poorly understood, difficult to categorise and often do not respond well to treatment. Doctors often find them less satisfying to treat, and patients learn they cannot expect to achieve a cure for their condition from their doctor. Often, functional diseases result in the patient being referred from one specialist to another to exclude any possible more serious disease. Many patients in the west who turn away from conventional medicine to seek benefit from complementary medical therapies would be classified as suffering from functional disease.

Self-test 1.2a

The conventional medicine approach

1. What are the three stages in the diagnosis of disease?
2. Access a medical textbook or website to determine the characteristic features of the following diseases, and list the (i) symptoms (ii) signs and (iii) one test result:
   - meningococcal meningitis
   - rheumatoid arthritis
   - kidney (urinary tract) stones (calculi).
3. If a patient has a negative 'rheumatoid factor' does this rule out the possibility of rheumatoid arthritis?
4. A doctor diagnoses the following diseases by determining, symptoms, signs and test results. Access a medical textbook or website to determine what treatments the doctor could prescribe to treat:
   - gonorrhoea
   - hay fever
   - eczema (atopic/endogenous in type).

Continued

Self-test 1.2a—Cont'd

Answers

1. • Questioning for symptoms.
   • Examining for signs.
   • Performing tests/investigations.
2. Meningococcal meningitis:
   (i) nausea, vomiting, headache
   (ii) fever, petechial (bruising) rash, altered consciousness, neck rigidity
   (iii) tests on blood and cerebrospinal fluid (CSF) for meningococci (bacteria).

   Rheumatoid arthritis:
   (i) joint pain, morning stiffness, fatigue, malaise
   (ii) swelling, warmth, tenderness, limitation of movement, deformities, nodules
   (iii) X-ray changes including erosions, rheumatoid factor in the blood, blood count shows anaemia.

   Kidney stone:
   (i) maybe none (asymptomatic), sharp or dull, colicky or constant pain, can be very severe with sweating, vomiting
   (ii) occasionally haematuria (blood in the urine), pallor, restlessness
   (iii) culture of urine may show blood, x-ray may reveal a stone, excretion urography will show abnormal damming of urine behind a blockage in the ureter.
3. No. Rheumatoid factor is positive in 80% of people with rheumatoid arthritis, so in 20% (one fifth) the result will be a false-negative.
4. • Gonorrhoea: antibiotics.
   • Hay fever: avoidance of allergens (pollen), antihistamines, decongestants, anti-inflammatory drugs and steroids.
   • Atopic (endogenous) eczema: emollients (moisturisers), exposure to ultraviolet (UV) light, corticosteroid creams, coal tar creams.

Chapter 1.2b Conventional medical prescribing

LEARNING POINTS

At the end of this chapter you will be able to:

- list the different factors that can influence a conventional practitioner when prescribing medication
- appreciate which of these are likely to be the most important factors for patients taking prescribed medication.

Estimated time for chapter: 60 minutes.

This chapter explores the conventional medical approach to prescribing medication. It is a common situation for a complementary practitioner to be working with patients who are concurrently taking prescribed conventional drug therapy. For this reason, it is helpful to understand not only the medical reasons behind a prescription choice, but also what other factors might have prompted a doctor to consider giving a prescription.

The reasons why conventional practitioners prescribe medication

From a complementary medicine perspective, the situation of a patient taking a number of medically prescribed drugs may be a difficult one to manage. A practitioner trained in the philosophy of a complementary therapy may be considering the energetic nature of a prescribed drug, and how this might interfere with the delicate energetic state of a patient who is already likely to be out of balance in some way. However, it is important to remember that, in practice, most prescriptions are given by doctors with the intention that the drug will benefit the patient according to conventional medical thought. It is helpful, therefore, for the complementary therapist to be very clear about the reasons why the drug may have been prescribed.

Some patients who seek complementary medical treatment may not be happy about their medications and may wish to stop them. Others, however, may believe, like their doctor, that they are following the best course of action for their health. These patients may have a good understanding of the medical reasoning that underlies their treatment and trust in their doctor's good intentions. In these cases, if the complementary practitioner starts to discuss the potentially adverse energetic consequences of medication without a clear understanding of what has led the doctor to prescribe them, there is a risk of losing rapport.

An understanding of the factors that lead doctors to prescribe can help the complementary therapist to explore with patients the pros and cons of their medication, from both the conventional and complementary viewpoints. In some cases, a clear understanding of why the drug has been prescribed may lead to the conclusion that, for that patient, the possible negative energetic side-effects are far outweighed by the benefits of the medication. Conversely, a clear understanding might bring the confidence that to withdraw the drug is the best thing to do.

There are many different factors that influence a medical doctor to prescribe. In most cases the overriding influential factor is that the practitioner wishes either to follow what is believed to be good medical practice, or to do something positive for the patient in a situation when it is unclear what treatment is necessary.

On rare occasions, in a situation in which it is unclear which of a range of treatments is the best option for a patient, a treatment may be prescribed as part of clinical research. On a less positive note, a decision to prescribe may, at least in part, have arisen as a response to the powerful advertising techniques used by pharmaceutical companies. Financial gain cannot influence most prescribing in the UK, although there are a few exceptions to this. Conversely, cost saving may influence the decision to prescribe one treatment, or no treatment, instead of another more costly one.

Prescribing as good practice

Every medical diagnosis will be associated with one or more 'textbook' methods of treatment. Increasingly, many of these methods will have been rigorously assessed in clinical trials, and there will be a strong evidence base supporting the fact that they are likely to offer benefit in a significant proportion of patients. For other methods, although the evidence is less strong, there is at least a clear consensus from an expert panel on the 'correct' approach to treatment (e.g. the British Thoracic Society guidelines on the management of asthma). A practitioner who chooses a treatment on the basis of either high-quality research evidence or expert guidelines would be considered to be working according to good practice.

However, there are many other treatments for which there is only poor evidence of effectiveness, and often less agreement on the best approach to management (e.g. a sore throat may lead to a prescription of linctus, soluble aspirin, antibiotics or nothing at all). In a situation in which the value of a particular treatment choice is uncertain, the prescribing doctor may have developed a personal preference for one approach, for a variety of reasons. As long as the treatment is one of the range recognised in textbooks for use in that clinical situation, this too would be considered to be good practice, even though the treatment may be of uncertain benefit to the patient (see Q1.2b-1).

The case scenario presented in Chapter 1.2a illustrates well some problems that can arise from prescribing as part of good practice. Ian is the 63-year-old man who has been diagnosed with benign prostatic hypertrophy after telling his doctor that he was having to get up at night to pass urine. The doctor is thinking about starting Ian on treatment with a drug called finasteride. This counteracts the effect of the male hormone testosterone, and can lead to a reduction in prostate size. Current textbooks are not able to be conclusive on whether this treatment has any advantages over the surgical option of transurethral resection. The medical formulary gives information about the potential side-effects of the drug, which include impotence and breast swelling in men.

With this information to hand, the doctor decides to prescribe the drug. In doing this, she is behaving entirely correctly according to her professional norms. Ian experiences a slight improvement in his symptoms, but unfortunately suffers from the side-effect of impotence. He does not initially link this to his treatment, and is distressed about its effect on his current relationship.

Medical treatments are chosen because they are known to benefit the majority of people. However, there may be a significant minority who do not do so well with the treatment. Distressing side-effects are seen as an unavoidable consequence of the risk that has to be accepted when taking a recommended treatment. The treatment has been recommended because it is believed professionally that the benefits to most patients outweigh the risk of side-effects in the few.

Good practice includes counselling a patient about a prescription. Doctors should prepare a patient for the possibility of common side-effects. The dilemma for the doctor is which side-effects, if any, should be discussed. Some are very rare, and there is limited time in the consultation. In this case scenario, Ian's doctor could be criticised if it was shown that she had failed to warn Ian about the possibility of impotence. As this side-effect is at the top of the list in the medical formulary, this suggests it is a well-documented occurrence.

To summarise, it is clear that, while it is intended to help the patient, prescribing as good practice may not necessarily benefit the patient. However, good practice always means that the majority of patients have been shown to benefit from the treatment and/or the practice is consistent with professional norms.

Prescribing in response to pressure to do something positive

Conventional medicine deals best with clear diagnoses with explainable pathology. However, many conditions are 'functional'. As described in Chapter 1.2a, functional conditions have no clearly understood physical cause. They give rise to symptoms, rarely have objective signs, and test results come back showing no abnormalities. In these conditions a specific therapy cannot be directed towards the causative process as the cause is unclear.

Examples of 'functional' conditions commonly encountered in general practice are chronic fatigue syndrome ('tired all the time'), recurrent sore throats/colds, irritable bowel syndrome, and many cases of low back pain. In these cases it is difficult for a doctor to say to a patient, 'There is nothing I know of that I can do for you'. The patient wants treatment in recognition of the symptoms, and the doctor wants to be of some help.

Often the doctor is constrained by time, or may know that the patient is expecting a tangible treatment. A prescription may follow, even when it seems not to be the ideal thing to do. This would be an example of doctors prescribing because of a perceived pressure to do something positive for the patient (see Q1.2b-2).

Prescribing as part of clinical research

Very occasionally, a doctor will be involved in clinical research requiring the prescription of a treatment of as yet unproven benefit to patients. However, there are strict ethical guidelines in the UK that protect patients' rights, so that in the performance of high-quality research informed consent will always be ensured. There should be no situation in which a patient is, without their knowledge, prescribed a treatment that is still undergoing clinical trials of effectiveness. In addition, the guidelines state that patients involved in a research project should never be denied any treatment that is known to be more beneficial than the experimental therapy.

The more serious a disease, the more likely it is that new therapies will be part of current treatment for that disease. All new therapies are initially introduced within controlled research programmes. This means that many patients with conditions such as HIV or cancer will receive therapy that is the subject of research. This does not mean that they are experimental 'guinea-pigs'. It usually means that a therapy has been developed that looks as though it may have more benefits or fewer side-effects than other treatments. However, this will not be known for sure unless the first prescriptions are monitored very carefully and results compared against patients on the old treatment within a research setting.

Prescribing in response to advertising

This fourth factor has an insidious and unmeasurable influence on prescribing. The pharmaceutical industry clearly recognises that it is worth the enormous financial investment required to advertise drug products to the medical profession. There is strict legislation in the UK that controls how drug companies are allowed to influence practitioners. This is intended to inhibit overt bribery. Nevertheless, it is very common for free samples and equipment to be supplied by companies. Ostensibly these gifts come with 'no strings attached', but can range from customised ballpoint pens to state-of-the-art operating equipment.

The promotion of brand names may well encourage doctors to prescribe the advertised product in a situation in which there are a number of possible treatment options, and in which there is little evidence to suggest that one option is superior to all the others.

Perhaps more importantly, most research on new drug therapies is funded by the pharmaceutical companies. Often the research is of a high standard, and cannot be accused of bias in methodology. However, there commonly is bias in the choice of research topic. A pharmaceutical company is more likely to have been stimulated by potential financial gain rather than clinical need. This means that the range of drugs available for prescription is very much influenced by the pharmaceutical companies, and naturally this will influence prescribing decisions.

Self-test 1.2b

Conventional prescribing

1. Give three examples of reasons for prescribing medication which would be seen by a conventional doctor as aspects of good practice.
2. Consider the following two scenarios:
   - Joe, aged seven, has been diagnosed with mild eczema on his arms and legs which is not improving with moisturising cream. His doctor prescribes 1.0% hydrocortisone cream (a low-dose steroid preparation) to be applied regularly until the rash improves.
   - Jim, aged 24, has developed an itchy rash on the inside of one arm which the doctor does not recognise. Jim thinks that it is because he keeps scratching it that it is not getting better. The doctor prescribes 1.0% hydrocortisone cream to try to settle the rash down.

What do you think might be the differences in motivation behind these two prescriptions?

Answers

1. All the following would be considered good practice:
   - prescribing the recommended treatment for a known diagnosis
   - prescribing within a research programme to test the benefits of a new therapy
   - prescribing in the NHS in any of the situations according to a Quality Outcome Framework, as this programme is intended to benefit the health of the population
   - prescribing of non-proprietary medications in place of proprietary medications
   - rationing of prescribing to ensure cost-effectiveness.
2. Although it may sound extreme to prescribe such medications for a mild condition, corticosteroid creams are one recommended treatment for childhood eczema.
   - Joe's doctor was therefore following good practice.
   - Jim's doctor is unsure of the diagnosis, and therefore cannot know what the recommended treatment for Jim's rash would be. By prescribing a steroid cream, the chances are the rash will become less itchy, although there is a possibility Jim's rash could get worse if, for example, it is due to a fungal infection. Jim's doctor is trying to do something positive for Jim in an uncertain situation.

Prescribing in response to financial incentives and disincentives

Financial incentives are far less prominent as an influence on prescribing in the UK than is popularly believed. Many people suspect, incorrectly, that their doctor has written a prescription because there is some sort of financial incentive. In the UK National Health Service, this cannot be the case. Hospital doctors are on a fixed wage according to their professional grade, and according to the 2003 General Medical Services contract general practitioners are funded in a complex way, largely dependent on the number of patients and their assessed needs and also on the demonstration of good practice according to a Quality Outcomes Framework. Most prescriptions bring no financial reward to practitioners.

There are some exceptions to this rule in general practice in the UK. In the UK, remuneration follows the achievement of good-practice targets, such as immunising a certain percentage of the infant population, or prescribing anticoagulants to people who have been diagnosed with an irregular heartbeat. However, these incentives are explicitly offered so that they can be used to benefit further the population served by the practice, and evidence demonstrates that they really do improve medical care according to expert guidelines on best practice.

Conversely, many current expert guidelines, such as those produced by the UK National Institute for Health and Clinical Excellence (NICE), focus on cost-effectiveness, and will tend to recommend the least expensive of the effective therapies for a particular condition. Some hospitals and general practices have developed local formularies that ensure only the cheapest of the effective drugs can be prescribed by their practitioners. Cost-effectiveness does not necessarily mean poor practice, although this can be interpreted by the media and public as a form of short-changing patients. Often, cheap therapies are perfectly adequate and comparable to more expensive recently developed drugs. The cost-effectiveness approach is intended to redirect limited resources to those therapies that can achieve the most overall benefit for the whole population.

Some very expensive therapies may be overtly 'rationed' in the UK. This means that they are either unavailable for prescription, or available only in special clinical circumstances. Rationing is intended to direct limited resources to those treatments that are most likely to bring the most benefit to the most people. Rationed treatments are often of uncertain benefit. The principle of rationing is fraught with ethical dilemmas, as it is often someone who is disadvantaged because of serious illness who misses out on the opportunity of the treatment.

Financial or material incentives are likely to carry much more weight in prescribing decisions in countries in which the doctor receives some remuneration for each treatment given or in which the rewards offered by pharmaceutical companies are less tightly regulated.

Chapter 1.2c Introduction to conventional drugs

LEARNING POINTS

At the end of this chapter you will be able to:
- understand how drugs are categorised and described in medical formularies
- categorise drugs in the way they are conventionally seen to work in order to begin to develop an energetic interpretation of their action.

Estimated time for chapter: 90 minutes.

Introduction

A formulary (or pharmacopoeia) is a book or document that categorises and summarises the characteristics of all drugs used in a certain setting. This chapter focuses on the way drugs are categorised in conventional medicine, and specifically on how they are listed and described in the formulary most widely used by medical practitioners in the UK, the *British National Formulary* (BNF). However, the principles of categorisation and description of prescribed medication explored in this chapter will be applicable to the structure of any formulary. The BNF can be accessed online (http://www.bnf.org).

Description of drugs

When the characteristics of a particular drug or class of drug are described in a formulary, they are often structured under the following headings: indications, cautions, contraindications, side-effects, dosages, nomenclature and prices.

Indications

The term 'indications' describes the conditions for which a drug preparation may be prescribed. For example, the BNF lists the indications for the antibiotic penicillin as chronic bronchitis, middle-ear infections, urinary infections, gonorrhoea and endocarditis prophylaxis.

Cautions

'Cautions' describes those situations in which the drug needs to be prescribed with caution as there is an increased risk of adverse reaction.

Contraindications

'Contraindications' describes those situations in which it is advisable not to prescribe the drug because of a very high risk of adverse reaction.

Side-effects

Side-effects are unwanted additional effects of the drug on the body that will affect some, but not necessarily all, people. For example, the BNF lists one side-effect of penicillin as a maculopapular rash (i.e. a rash consisting of flat round spots akin to the rash of measles or rubella), which is most likely in people with glandular fever.

Dose

The dose is the recommended amount and frequency of taking the drug. This is usually expressed in terms of metric weight and daily regimen; for example, 500 milligrams every 8 hours (three times a day).

Nomenclature

Drugs are named in three ways. First, the drug may be described by means of its chemical name, and this would be an internationally recognised term that indicates the structure of the compound that is the active part of the drug. For example, salicylic acid, sodium bicarbonate and lithium carbonate are all chemical names for commonly prescribed drugs.

Second, drugs may be known by a generic name, which is an often less complicated term than the chemical name and is assigned to the drug for ease of reference. For example, aspirin is the generic name recognised in the UK for salicylic acid. In the past, generic names have varied according to country of use, which means that a doctor from one country may not recognise the names of drugs commonly prescribed in another country. For this reason, the World Health Organization (WHO), because of its constitutional mandate to 'develop, establish and promote international standards with respect to biological, pharmaceutical and similar products', advocates an international naming system for drugs known as rINN (Recommended International Non-proprietary Names). There are now over 7000 rINNs, which have been chosen to be easily recognisable terms and which in many cases link drugs of the same class by the same suffix. For example, the SSRI (selective serotonin re-uptake inhibitor) group of antidepressants are assigned names that end with the syllable '-ine' (e.g. fluoxetine, sertraline, paroxetine and fluvoxamine).

As a result of ongoing collaboration of countries with the WHO, and also of international legislation (e.g. European law), national naming systems such as British Approved Names (BAN), Dénominations Communes Françaises (DCF), Japanese Adopted Names (JAN) and United States Adopted Names (USAN) are increasingly adapting to match the rINN system.

The third way in which a drug may be named is by a proprietary name. This is a name chosen by the pharmaceutical manufacturer for the purposes of branding and marketing the drug. The proprietary name is chosen to appeal to the ears of the culture to which it is intended to be sold, and so may be unique to a single country. For example, Disprin, Amoxil, Remegel, Zantac, Prozac and Ibuleve are proprietary names used in the UK for the commonly used medications soluble aspirin, amoxicillin, calcium carbonate, ranitidine, fluoxetine and ibuprofen gel, respectively. Drugs are marketed under their proprietary name and often cost a lot more than the same drug sold under the generic name.

For example, the proprietary name for amoxicillin is Amoxil. According to the 57th edition of the BNF (March 2009), 21 capsules of 500 mg Amoxil cost £7.19, whereas the same quantity of the same drug sold under the generic name of amoxicillin costs £1.56. The proprietary drug Amoxil therefore costs over six times the price of the non-proprietary (generic) version of the same antibiotic. The prescribing of marketed drugs can obviously be a major source of expense to the prescriber, but offers no added benefit to the patient.

The origins of conventional drugs

Some drugs have their origins in antiquity, and are derived directly from herbal preparations or other natural sources. Contrasting examples of prescribed drugs originally derived from natural substances are oil of evening primrose (gamma linoleic acid), derived from the seeds of the evening primrose plant, penicillin, derived from mould, and insulin, extracted from the dog pancreas. However, almost all drugs can be manufactured synthetically, so that the natural source is no longer necessary to produce the same chemical. For example, human insulin is now available by a process involving genetic engineering.

Some drugs are modifications of the original naturally derived substance. The modifications are an attempt to make the drug more suited to its role. It may be found that a natural substance, although effective, has very severe side-effects. Modification, which is the work of research chemists, may give rise to a substance that is as effective, but has fewer side-effects. Nowadays, many drugs are modifications of natural substances. Amoxicillin, for example, is chemically derived from the naturally occurring substance penicillin. Natural penicillin can only be taken by injection, and is effective against fewer types of bacteria. Amoxicillin has activity against a broad spectrum of bacteria and can be taken by mouth. This is obviously preferable for both the patient and the prescribing doctor.

Increasingly, new drugs are being developed for which there are no natural predecessors. As more is known about the chemistry of the body, drugs can be tailor-made to suit a particular requirement. Sometimes these drugs are termed 'designer drugs'. For example, the development of the SSRI antidepressant fluoxetine (Prozac) was based on the knowledge that a certain natural chemical in the brain, called serotonin (5HT), is important in depression. Fluoxetine is a chemical that causes 5HT to be reabsorbed by brain cells more slowly than usual, and this leads to a lifting effect on mood.

Whatever their origins, all drugs have to go through a very rigorous testing process before being released for public use. This invariably requires multiple testing on animals, many of which die in the process. If no problems are revealed by animal testing, the drug is then tested on humans within 'clinical trials'. These trials have to conform to a rigorous ethical framework, so that the participants are extremely unlikely to suffer any measurable harm from being involved. However, sometimes serious side-effects are not revealed by this testing process, as was the case in the development of Vioxx (refecoxib), for example. Vioxx was an anti-inflammatory drug for arthritis developed by the company Merck. It was withdrawn from public use in 2004 as an ongoing clinical trial revealed an increased incidence of cardiovascular side-effects, including heart attacks and strokes, in people taking this drug for more than 18 months. This outcome was not revealed by the results of earlier trials conducted over a shorter timescale by the company, which had all suggested that the drug would be safe for public use.

A system for classification of conventional drugs

The vast range of drug types presented in formularies such as the BNF may be daunting for complementary therapists. However, it is possible to simplify the way in which drugs are categorised by grouping them into nine categories according to the way in which they are conventionally seen to act in the body. These categories have been chosen for this text because all the drugs within each category have ways in common of affecting the body, and such a categorisation is particularly useful for comparing the way in which drugs act in an energetic sense. Ordering drugs into these categories can provide a means by which drug action can be interpreted according to a complementary medical system, such as Chinese medicine.

The information provided by a formulary such as the BNF about any one drug will be all that is required to decide the category in which that drug can be placed.

The categorisation of drugs according to mode of action in the body is shown in Table 1.2c-I. Each of the categories listed will now be explored in more detail.

Table 1.2c-I The categorisation of drugs according to mode of action in the body

	Mode of action of drug	Examples of drugs
1	Replaces a deficient substance that is normally obtained from the diet	Iron (ferrous sulphate) in iron-deficiency anaemia
2	Replaces a deficient substance that is normally produced by the body	Insulin in diabetes mellitus
3	Kills or suppresses the growth of infectious agents (microbes and other life forms that cause infection)	Penicillin in meningitis
4	Counteracts the damage caused by toxins	Acetyl cysteine in paracetamol overdose
5	Toxic to rapidly dividing human cells, in particular cancer cells	Vincristine in cancer chemotherapy
6	Specifically stimulates the immune response by the introduction of an antigen	Polio vaccine
7	Other drugs that artificially stimulate natural bodily functions	Clomifene to stimulate ovulation
8	Suppresses natural bodily functions	Corticosteroids to suppress the immune response
9	Other drugs that directly counteract the symptoms (manifestation) of a disease process rather than its root cause	Digoxin in heart failure; paracetamol in headache

1 Drugs that replace a deficient substance that is normally obtained from the diet

These drugs are synthetic forms of the nutrients, vitamins and minerals that the body requires for full health, and which for dietary and other reasons (e.g. impaired digestion) are not available to the patient in sufficient quantities to meet his or her needs.

Examples include iron, vitamin C and fluid replacement (see Q1.2c-1).

2 Drugs that replace a deficient substance that is normally produced by the body

These drugs are used to treat disorders in which the body fails to manufacture the basic chemicals (including hormones) that are essential for healthy homeostasis.

One example is thyroxine replacement in thyroid deficiency. The thyroid gland in this condition is diseased and no longer able to produce thyroxine, which is essential for life. The drug is chemically synthesised to be exactly the same as, or very similar to, the natural hormone (see Q1.2c-2).

3 Drugs that kill or suppress the growth of infectious agents (microbes and other life forms that cause infection)

This category includes all drugs that work against microbes and life forms that are 'foreign' to a normally healthy body. They are listed together in Section 5 of the BNF, 'Infections'.

Examples include antibiotics such as amoxicillin. Some antibiotics are known only to suppress the growth of some infectious agents rather than kill them outright. This is true for the antiviral drugs such as oseltamivir (Tamiflu).

4 Drugs that counteract the damage caused by toxins

This is a category of drugs that generally are used in the emergency treatment of poisoning or overdose. They are not, therefore, likely to be encountered in usual complementary medical practice. The category is included here for completeness.

In general, these drugs prevent the absorption of drugs and poisons from the digestive tract (e.g. charcoal given by mouth), or enable the transformation of the drug within the body to a less toxic form (e.g. acetyl cysteine given by intravenous injection in paracetamol overdose).

5 Drugs that are toxic to rapidly dividing human cells, in particular cancer cells

This category includes the cytotoxic anticancer drugs. When human cells are recognised to have become diseased, particularly in the case of cancer, the conventional response is to remove them. This can either involve the surgical removal of a lump, or the use of radiation or drugs that are chemically designed to attack cells with the particular properties of cancer cells. One important characteristic of the cytotoxic drugs used to kill cancer cells is that they are also toxic to some extent to all other human cells in the body.

For example vincristine is a cytotoxic drug that is commonly used in chemotherapy. It works by blocking the physiological process of cell division, and so rapidly dividing cancer cells will be most affected. However, hair loss and diarrhoea are signs that rapidly dividing hair and gut cells have also been damaged by the drug. The development of numbness and weakness in a patient on vincristine is a sign that vital nerve cells are being damaged. In this case the drug should be stopped.

6 Drugs that specifically stimulate the immune response by introduction of an antigen

This category of drugs includes all the vaccines. Vaccines are designed to mimic natural infections, and so stimulate a natural bodily process. In this way the action of the vaccine can be compared to that of an infectious agent.

7 Other drugs that artificially stimulate natural bodily functions

Drugs in this category are used to bring about a bodily process that is not occurring naturally, usually because of underlying disease. This category actually also embraces drugs in categories 2 and 6. However, the drugs in these categories have been separated from category 7 because they have additional unique energetic characteristics.

Examples of drugs that artificially stimulate natural bodily functions include drugs, such as clomifene, which are used in infertility to stimulate ovulation. Other examples include oxytocin, which is used to stimulate labour, and hormone replacement therapy, which is given to delay a natural menopause (this 'stimulates' the continued maintenance of the female secondary sexual characteristics, including pubic hair growth, vaginal moistness and fleshiness of breast tissue).

8 Drugs that suppress natural bodily functions

This category includes a wide range of drugs that suppress natural bodily functions. In some cases the bodily function (e.g. ovulation or menstruation) is simply not wanted because it interferes with the person's perceived needs. In other cases the bodily function is a natural response to disease (e.g. the pain of a fractured leg) and leads to unpleasant symptoms.

Examples include the contraceptive pill, which suppresses ovulation, corticosteroids, which suppress the immune response, anaesthetics in surgery, which suppress consciousness, painkillers, which suppress the pain of injury, and anti-sickness medication given with chemotherapy.

9 Other drugs that directly counteract the symptoms of a disease process rather than deal with its root cause

Strictly speaking, drugs in categories 2, 5, 7 and 8 also fall into this very broad category, as do some of the drugs from all the other categories. The important energetic interpretation of any drug that deals with the symptoms (manifestation) rather than the root of a disease is that it is likely to lead to energetic suppression of the root imbalance. The concept of energetic suppression is discussed in more detail in Chapter 1.3b.

Many of these drugs in this category have been developed as a result of the detailed understanding that has evolved of the nature of non-infectious disease. For example, in coronary heart disease, it is recognised that the heart muscle may be failing to pump efficiently. This may be the result of a lifetime's damage to the blood supply of that muscle from hardening of the arteries (atherosclerosis). However, drugs can used to boost the contracting energy of the heart muscle cells (e.g. the cardiac glycosides, such as digoxin) or reduce the pressure of the blood against which the heart has to pump (e.g. the ACE inhibitors, such as ramipril). Neither of these types of drug remedy the original disease, but they will remedy, at least in the short term, the symptoms that are distressing for the patient. In some cases, drugs in this category have been shown in clinical trials to prolong life, for example the ACE inhibitors.

Other examples of drugs in this broad category include fluoxetine for depression, omeprazole for duodenal ulcer, salbutamol for asthma and lamotrigine for epilepsy (see Q1.2c-3 and Q1.2c-4).

Chapter 1.3b explores in more depth how this categorisation of how drugs are conventionally seen to act can be used to develop an energetic perspective of their action.

Self-test 1.2c

Introduction to conventional drugs

1. Use the BNF to find out the names of:
   (i) two combined oral contraceptives ('the pill')
   (ii) two progesterone-only contraceptives (the 'minipill').
2. List two major side-effects for:
   (i) combined oral contraceptives
   (ii) progesterone-only contraceptives.
3. Name four of the subsections into which the antidepressants are classed.
4. What is the Committee of Safety of Medicines' (CSM) advice about treating with minor tranquillisers (benzodiazepines)?
5. In consideration of the nine categories of how drugs are seen to work, which three categories of drugs, if prescribed appropriately, are least likely to have negative energetic consequences on the body?
6. Which category includes the drugs which, in general, are most likely to cause extreme energetic disturbance?

Answers

1. Possibilities include:
   (i) Loestrin, Mercilon, Microgynon 30, Logynon, and many more
   (ii) Femulen, Micronor, Cerazette, Noriday, and more.
2. Possibilities include:
   (i) nausea, vomiting, breast tenderness, weight changes, thrombosis, change in sex drive, and more
   (ii) irregular periods, nausea and vomiting, headache, depression, skin problems, weight gain, and more.
3. The BNF lists three distinct classes of antidepressants and then adds a class that embraces those which do not fit into these three categories.
   4.3.1 Tricyclic antidepressants (e.g. amitriptyline (Tryptizol))
   4.3.2 Monoamine oxidase inhibitors (e.g. phenelzine (Nardil))
   4.3.3 SSRIs (e.g. fluoxetine (Prozac)).
   4.3.4 Other antidepressants
4. CSM advice is given throughout the BNF to encourage safe prescribing by doctors. The advice given for tranquillisers is intended to reduce the risk of addiction: i.e. only give for short-term relief of severe anxiety, and only for insomnia if it is leading to extreme distress in the patient.
5. Drug categories 1 and 2, which represent *nutrients and replacement therapy*, include drugs that are similar to substances that the body requires for natural healthy functioning, and so if prescribed appropriately are not likely to cause great energetic disturbance.
   Drugs in category 4, which *counteract the effect of toxins*, are likely to leave the body in a more energetically balanced state than had they not been prescribed. Therefore, these drugs can also be seen as having a positive energetic effect.
   Nevertheless, all three categories include preparations with powerful energetic properties that, if the drug is taken inappropriately, would cause extreme imbalance (e.g. use of male sex steroids by athletes).
6. Category 5, drugs that *kill certain types of human cells*, includes drugs that invariably have a wide range of severe side-effects, which is always an indication of profound energetic disturbance.

Comparisons with alternative medical viewpoints

1.3

Chapter 1.3a Contrasting philosophies of health

LEARNING POINTS

At the end of this chapter you will be able to:

- discuss the differences between a reductionist and a holistic philosophy of health
- explain how a philosophy of health might affect a practitioner's interactions with their patients.

Estimated time for chapter: 90 minutes.

This chapter is intended to promote the recognition that different health systems are built upon unique philosophical perspectives of the physiology of the body and pathology of disease. The approaches can be broadly categorised as 'reductionist' and 'holistic'. There are crucial differences between these two approaches, and without asserting that either has greater or lesser value, these differences need to be clarified before the work of trying to compare one discipline with another can begin.

The term 'reductionist' refers to the principle of analysing complex things by considering them in terms of a collection of parts. Simply speaking, a reductionist view of the body will tend to examine and describe the workings of individual parts, without necessarily having to draw upon an understanding of the working of the body as an integrated whole. From a mechanistic perspective, this is similar to the approach of the engineer who, by identifying and replacing a faulty part, such as a distributor or fuel pump, can transform a faltering vehicle into an adequately working model. The process involves testing clearly defined systems within the malfunctioning vehicle and then identifying and making good the faulty part.

From a reductionist perspective, the body may be viewed as akin to a wonderfully intricate machine. In this model, illness or disease in one part of the body will not necessarily be manifest in or experienced by other parts. The faulty part will, however, like the vehicle, trigger warnings in the form of signs and symptoms, and the diagnosis of disease is then made by a thorough examination of all body parts and systems. The whole assembly is just a collection of individual parts, no more and no less.

By contrast, the term 'holistic' is used to refer to a view that sees each part of a complex system as being inextricably linked with all the other parts of the system, and the whole system being more than just the sum of the parts. A problem in one part will resonate widely throughout the system. Furthermore, this immediately brings the non-material aspects of life into the equation, the thoughts and emotions that form a part of the 'whole person'. Some medical systems that might be described as holistic according to this definition are underpinned by the idea that the individual parts are linked and vivified by an underlying non-measurable energetic state. This energetic state is made manifest in the material body, but is more than just the physical body. This understanding of an underlying state has been described as the 'vitalistic principle'. Terms such as 'life force', 'Qi', 'Ki' and 'Prana' are used to describe this energetic state in different health disciplines (see Q1.3a-1).

With a holistic model of health, the body, the emotions, the mind and the spirit are seen as interdependent and intercommunicating. An illness of the body will impact on the function of the emotions, the mind and the spirit, and, conversely, a sickness of the spirit or mind will have repercussions that become manifest in the physical body.

This belief is the basis for diagnostic systems that focus on just one body part such as the pulse, tongue, iris, sole of the foot or abdomen (hara). The interconnections within the body, mind and spirit will mean that every illness is reflected throughout all parts of the system. By following diagnostic systems such as these, the focus of a skilled practitioner on a single body part is understood to reveal information not just about the health of the body but also about the state of the mind and spirit (see Q1.3a-2).

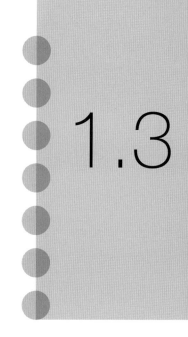

One important corollary of this 'holistic' view of health is that symptoms of a disease may become manifest in a different body part, or indeed at a different level, from that in which a disease first developed. For example, the grief following a bereavement, which might be expected to be experienced at an emotional or spiritual level, may instead manifest in the body in the form of an asthma attack or skin rash. These emotional or spiritual correlates of physical disease are of great interest to many holistic practitioners. Some go as far as to suggest that all physical diseases have emotional or spiritual roots, and that some diseases consistently reflect specific emotional or spiritual 'blocks'. A pain in the shoulders, for example, may be considered to represent a difficulty in shouldering the burdens imposed by a busy and complicated lifestyle.

The idea that symptoms are expressions of imbalances throughout all levels of the body, emotions, mind and spirit has implications when symptoms are treated medically. From a holistic perspective, if symptoms are not treated at their root origin then any other treatment of them may be described as suppressive. If the root imbalance persists, then it makes sense to a holistic practitioner that it will find an outlet at another body site or within another level of the body. This idea, that symptoms suppressed in this way might re-emerge in a different form at a different body site or level, is a concept that is not tenable within a purely reductionist health system.

Conventional medicine as a reductionist system

It might be easy to comment that conventional medicine is a purely reductionist health system, and this is often suggested in pejorative tones by proponents of complementary health disciplines. It is true that many of the ideas of modern medicine have sprung from the reductionist view of the world that dominated scientific thought in the 18th to 20th centuries. The 'Linnaean' approach to classification of illness, which modern doctors use to define disease according to body system, is one good example. The tendency of doctors to specialise so that their focus is directed at single body systems or subsystems is also evidence of this approach. Medical training largely focuses on the diseases of body parts and diseases of the mind, and categorises them as distinct entities that merit defined and agreed treatment approaches.

However, an ever-deepening scientific understanding of the workings of the body and the mind over the latter part of the 20th century has begun to erode the more simplistic reductionist approach to disease. Increasingly, conventional practitioners recognise that the different body parts and the workings of the brain are inextricably interrelated and interdependent. Moreover, factors such as social class and standing, education, ability to deal with stress, and general happiness are now recognised to have very powerful effects on health and well-being. The healthy human being is no longer seen as a well-oiled machine that responds to a regular service of all parts. Instead it is seen as a complex entity, the health of which depends on delicate physiological internal relationships and on relationships that exist within the context of the community in which the individual is placed.

This more holistic perspective of health is expressed clearly in the 1948 constitution of the World Health Organization, where health is defined as 'a state of physical, mental and social well-being and not merely the absence of disease or infirmity'. The medical model can now more accurately be described as a biopsychosocial model in which biological, psychological and social determinants are readily accepted as contributing to the development of disease. It is also now accepted that treatment focused on a body symptom in isolation may not deal fully with the real root of the problem.

However, there remain important differences, and these can lead to misunderstandings between practitioners of conventional medicine and practitioners of those complementary health disciplines that hold to a more holistic perspective. One author and alternative medicine practitioner has summarised the differences between 'alternative medicine' and conventional medicine as shown in Table 1.3a-I.

This rather stark comparison perhaps unfairly places conventional medicine firmly in the reductionist camp. However, the comparison does illustrate some key differences between the conventional medical view of health and healing and those of medical disciplines such as Chinese medicine, Ayurvedic medicine, homeopathy and craniosacral therapy. All these disciplines adhere to concepts of a vitalistic principle and the interrelationship of the physical with spiritual as well as emotional and mental levels of health.

The major difference here is that modern medicine does not hold to the idea of a unifying vitalistic principle and a spiritual level of health. While modern medicine understands that the mind can affect the body, and vice versa, it attempts to explain this in terms of neural and endocrine connections rather than by means of a non-measurable energetic principle. In conventional medicine the two domains of mind and body are in practice not seen as totally enmeshed and interdependent, as the levels of health are understood to be from the more holistic medicine viewpoint.

A discipline such as Chinese medicine, for example, recognises that when the Heart is imbalanced, then symptoms will always manifest in the physical, emotional, mental and spiritual realms. A conventional practitioner will be less ready to

Table 1.3a-I A comparison between alternative and conventional medicine according to Gascoigne (2000)

Alternative medicine	Conventional medicine
Energetic	Physical
Holistic	Separatist/reductionist
Transforms	Eliminates
Cures	Suppresses
Patient centred	Disease centred
Symptoms are useful pointers	Symptoms are to be removed
Disease is a group of symptoms (a syndrome)	Disease is a fixed entity
Cure is a move towards balance	Cure is removal of symptoms

make this claim. A conventional doctor may be very ready to accept that heart disease can lead to low mood and troubled thoughts, but the conceptual link made between the two will be less immediate. For the conventional medical doctor, the low mood of a patient with heart disease will be more a result of having to deal with the pain and disability that accompany heart disease and of carrying the weight of a poor prognosis. This contrasts with the holistic practitioner's expectations that a disease of the heart will manifest naturally in the realms of emotions, mind and spirit because these are part of what defines the function of the Heart.

However, while the stereotypical conventional and alternative practitioner may practise within very different conceptual frameworks, this does not necessarily mean that either has a more accurate grasp of an absolute truth. This book has been written from the perspective that conventional and complementary practitioners are working with different aspects of the same essential truth.

A helpful analogy is that of a concert violinist and a sound engineer who are both listening to a performance of a violin concerto. The concert violinist may be attentive to the sensitivity of the interpretation of the music, and may be deeply moved as he listens. The sound engineer may recognise the physical characteristics of the harmonics she hears and can comment on the acoustics of the concert hall. No one can deny that they have both been listening to the same piece of music, but their 'philosophies' for interpreting the music mean that their individual perceptions, what they actually 'hear', will differ markedly.

This is the case when a complementary and a conventional practitioner consider health and disease in an individual. Both can offer valid insights about what is happening for that individual, although it is not always the case that either comprehends or can appreciate the view of the other (see Q1.3a-3).

It is important to recognise, however, that no practitioner, nor indeed medical practice, is wholly reductionist or holistic in focus, although the conventional/reductionist, complementary/holistic labels are frequently misused in this way. Many conventional practitioners adhere strongly to the holistic management of their patients, and many complementary medicine practitioners practise in a way that relies on a reductionist conceptual framework as its foundation (see Q1.3a-4).

For the patient seeking appropriate healthcare, it is important to recognise that the philosophical framework of any medical practitioner will have both strengths and weaknesses. Just as the violinist and the sound engineer both have a great deal to contribute to the production of a beautiful musical performance, so practitioners with different medical and philosophical frameworks can have truly complementary insights and skills to offer in promoting healing. Clarity about where these strengths and weaknesses lie will enable a patient to make an informed choice of medical treatment appropriate to their specific needs at any particular time.

Tables 1.3a-II and 1.3a-III summarise some of the potential advantages and disadvantages of seeking treatment from complementary and conventional medical practices. These lists have been drawn up from a patient's perspective. Not all

Table 1.3a-II Complementary medical treatment: advantages and disadvantages

Advantages	Disadvantages
• In-depth consultation	• Seems expensive
• Recognises and will treat a wide range of contributory factors in the disease process – holistic approach	• May not recognise features of serious disease
• Will be open to the patient's point of view	• Difficult to find out whether therapy is appropriate or if therapist is adequately qualified
• Will clarify to patient how lifestyle may have contributed to problem	• Makes the patient responsible in part for the cause of the problem
• Empowers patient to be involved in own healing	• Requires the patient to be active in changing lifestyle to enable healing
• Unlikely to harm	• May not be powerful enough to cure advanced disease
• Should result in a change at a deep personal level	

Table 1.3a-III Conventional medical treatment: advantages and disadvantages

Advantages	Disadvantages
• Usually available as part of nationally or insurance funded health service	• May not be time or willingness to allow patient to be listened to or valued • Minor 'functional' symptoms may be ignored
• Directed towards excluding serious disease	• The practitioner may be inflexible if the patient requires an approach that is contrary to the medically accepted view
• The practitioner is likely to be following the recognised approach as accepted by the medical profession	• May not be tailored to the complex needs of the individual patient
• Will often be consistent with the patient's expectations	• Lifestyle factors are not addressed adequately, and so root of problem is perpetuated
• Will often focus on the disease rather than causation, and so the patient need not change lifestyle	• Patient may feel out of control within the healing process
• Practitioner takes responsibility for the healing process	• The risk of iatrogenic disease (disease resulting from side-effects of treatment) is high
• Powerful treatments available	
• Is not expected to challenge the patient at a deep level	• May ignore the need for deep personal change, which could be ultimately the most health giving

patients want to be actively involved in their treatment, nor wish to have their world view challenged, and both these things may occur in some complementary therapies. This explains why a statement such as 'Requires the patient to be active in changing lifestyle to enable healing' is listed as a possible disadvantage of complementary therapy, and 'Treatment is not expected to challenge the patient at a deep level' as a possible advantage of conventional medical treatment.

Being clear about the distinctions between the philosophical foundations of conventional and complementary thought is essential when practitioners of different medical disciplines seek to develop a meaningful dialogue. It is important to be both clear and respectful about essential differences, and avoid the tendency to overgeneralise. This clarity becomes perhaps most useful in building up relationships with patients who have complex health needs, many of whom are likely to benefit by receiving the best aspects of treatment from contrasting medical perspectives.

Self-test 1.3a

Contrasting philosophies of health

1. Write down your own definitions of the words 'reductionist' and 'holistic' as used to describe philosophies of health.
2. Alice is a gardener and has a lot of work to do. She is finding that hay fever is really reducing the effectiveness of her work. The antihistamine tablets prescribed by her doctor do not seem to touch the problem. She turns to acupuncture as she has heard it has good results in hay fever.

How do you feel Alice's philosophy of health may affect her first experience of acupuncture?

Answers

1. Your definitions could be similar to the following:
   Reductionist: considers the human organism as separable into distinct parts. A disease or a treatment need not affect all these parts
   Holistic: the human organism is considered as a range of interrelated functions that cannot be separated. Disease or a treatment may be focused at one of these functions but will necessarily affect the whole organism.
2. It is likely that Alice has a conventional view of health, as her first choice for treatment was the conventional drug, an antihistamine. She may well be hoping that acupuncture can likewise suppress her uncomfortable symptoms and let her get on with her life. This could have the following consequences:
   - Alice may not expect to be questioned about all aspects of her lifestyle or to receive a full physical examination
   - she may be confused to hear her condition being diagnosed in terms such as weakness of the Lung and Kidney 'energy' and Wind invasion
   - she may have understood that a single treatment or course of treatments was all that would be required
   - she may be disturbed about the cost of a series of treatments
   - she may not expect to feel a bit worse before she improves (an 'aggravation')
   - she may not expect to experience change in other aspects of her life.

All these could lead to Alice feeling dissatisfied with her experience unless these issues are explained to her sensitively and in familiar language.

Chapter 1.3b Drugs from a complementary medical viewpoint

LEARNING POINTS

At the end of this chapter you will be able to:
- begin to think in broad terms about the energetic effects of modern drugs
- discuss the concepts of suppression and cure
- arrive at an energetic interpretation of an individual drug.

Estimated time for chapter: 120 minutes.

Chapter 1.2c introduced a method of categorising drugs by mode of therapeutic action and the concept of iatrogenic disease (illness as a result of medical treatment). This chapter presents some complementary perspectives on the beneficial and adverse effects of drugs in the body. It also describes some principles of mapping Chinese medicine concepts to western medical theory. These are explored in some detail under the heading 'The Rationale and Method Used for the Mapping of Western Medical Diagnoses to Chinese Medicine Theory' in the Note to the Reader contained in the preliminary pages of this book.

Suppression of symptoms

The concept of suppression of symptoms in homeopathic theory refers to the idea that the disappearance of symptoms or signs of a disease may not necessarily mean 'cure', but instead may be a consequence of the disease moving to a deeper, less immediately manifest level. This concept has a parallel with the Chinese medicine idea of disease having a manifestation (Biao) and a root (Ben). According to Chinese medicine theory, treatment that is targeted at the level of the manifestation, and which does not simultaneously attend to the root causes, may actually lead to a worsening of the root imbalance.

The Chinese medicine description of treating the manifestation is analogous to the homeopathic idea of suppression. In both there is a suggestion that, although treatment may cause an alleviation of symptoms, there may be a worsening of disease at a deeper level. In Chinese medicine, however, this is most often seen as not attending to the factors that cause the root imbalance, as a consequence of which it will become more pronounced and may generate further symptoms. Homeopaths take this a stage further, and argue that the symptom may actually serve a useful purpose by providing some sort of release for the deeper root imbalance. When it is prevented from serving this purpose, it may directly cause the root imbalance to deepen and be expressed in a different and potentially more damaging form. In both cases the unattended root imbalance is believed to create more serious problems.

Figure 1.3b-I illustrates the complementary medicine concept of suppression. The bathtub with a running tap has a problem; it is leading to a dripping overflow pipe, and thus causing damp to the exterior wall. This ideally would be treated by turning off the taps, the root of the problem. However, someone outside the house might be tempted to deal

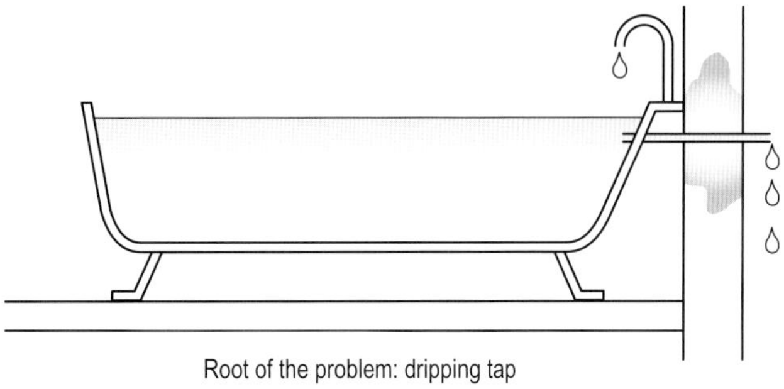

Root of the problem: dripping tap
Treating the root (turning off the tap) cures the problem
Manifestation of problem: overflowing pipe and damp wall
Treating the manifestation (stopping the pipe) suppresses the problem and may cause a worse problem at a deep level

Figure 1.3b-I • An illustration of the concept of suppression.

with the manifestation of the problem. They could stop the dripping overflow and allow the wall to dry out by blocking the overflow pipe with a cork. This treatment would indeed solve the problem of the dripping pipe, but of course would result in a more catastrophic problem inside the house as the bath then proceeds to overflow onto the bathroom floor.

The case of an overworked businesswoman self-medicating every day with paracetamol for recurrent tension headaches provides an example of suppression of symptoms by medication. When questioned, the woman readily admits that she feels dependent on her painkillers, because if she cannot take one for any reason she really suffers with a couple of days of severe headaches.

This patient's underlying condition might have been diagnosed in Chinese medicine as Liver Yang Rising resulting from Kidney Yin deficiency. Tonification of the Kidneys would be considered to be beneficial, but alongside this an appropriate treatment of the root of the problem might also include a re-evaluation of working habits, the taking of appropriate rest and ensuring a diet containing appropriately nourishing foods. All these treatments target the root problem and not the symptom.

However, the painkiller does not work in this way. Although it removes the symptoms (i.e. it subdues the symptoms of Liver Yang rising), it does not deal with the root problem of depleted Kidney Yin. Its recurrent use may lead the businesswoman to ignore the reasons why her headache might have developed. In her case, one reason is very probably her stress-inducing lifestyle, which is likely to be depleting of Kidney Yin.

The concept of suppression suggests that the underlying imbalance that has led to the headache may now become more pronounced. One obvious reason for this is that the root cause, the pressured lifestyle, is left untreated. A further reason, in line with the homeopaths' beliefs, is that the Heat which was being released in the symptom of a headache now has nowhere to go and actively forces the root to express itself as, for example, anxious depression, a feature of Kidney and Heart Yin deficiency. As this symptom is seen in Chinese medicine to be at the level of the spirit rather than the body, this could suggest progression of the imbalance to a deeper energetic level.

The recognition that suppressive treatment may have deleterious effects pervades complementary medical practice. Many complementary medicine practitioners advocate the ideal of patients withdrawing from suppressive medical treatment so that deep imbalance can be exposed and treated appropriately. The healing of suppressed disease might also be associated with the emergence of suppressed symptoms, as a consequence of which the patient might be expected to get worse before he or she gets better. Suppressed disease, although pervasive in nature, is often thought to be subtle, and therefore very difficult to assess or quantify. It could simply manifest in a general sense of malaise or lack of vitality rather than in symptoms and signs that can be studied objectively using the scientific method.

The use of treatment that suppresses symptoms and signs is very commonplace in conventional medical pharmacology. Conventional medicine practitioners do not, in general, recognise that symptoms may be a necessary expression of an underlying imbalance, the suppression of which would be harmful. This view is reinforced by the fact that there is no obvious physiological or pathological theory to explain why preventing the expression of a symptom such as headache or a sign such as high blood pressure would be harmful.

No conventional doctor would deny that treatments such as paracetamol for chronic pain or atenolol for high blood pressure are actually suppressing these symptoms and signs. These treatments do indeed suppress symptoms, as is evidenced by the fact that when they are withdrawn the original condition tends to recur. However, the fact that drugs are available that can suppress unpleasant symptoms of chronic disease is seen only to be positive from a conventional viewpoint. Moreover, without any physiological or pharmacological proof that suppression of symptoms might be harmful, the homeopathic understanding of the effects of suppressive medication is incomprehensible to a conventional physician, whose beliefs rest on scientifically proven certainties.

Conventional practitioners do, of course, recognise that drug treatment is not without risks, but they see these risks in entirely physical terms – as the harm that a drug may do because it is in some way toxic to the body. The likely benefits and risks of harm caused by a drug can be studied by means of observations of how the drug affects the physiology of the body and also by observing populations of patients who have been given the drug. In these ways the effects of drugs can be evaluated quantitatively. The risks and benefits associated with a particular drug treatment can thus be predicted.

The complementary medicine idea of suppression can be expanded further to help explore the different effects that a drug might have on the body in energetic terms. The term 'energetics' is used in this text to describe the interpretation within certain complementary medicine disciplines of the action of a drug on the energetic body. In Chinese medicine, for example, the energetic body may be defined in terms of Yin and Yang, the Five Elements and the vital substances of Qi, Blood, Essence (Jing), and also the Pathogenic Factors (such as Cold or Damp) which may impact upon it.

The energetic effects that may result from any form of treatment may be one or more of the following:

- cure
- suppression
- drug-induced disease
- placebo.

Cure

Within holistic complementary medical thought, when a treatment leads to 'cure', it is the appropriate remedy for the condition. The curative treatment deals with the root of the problem, and so leads to a move towards energetic balance, and an overall improvement in health.

In conventional medical treatment, replacement of iron in certain cases of anaemia (i.e. those cases that are due to lack of iron in the diet) is an example of cure. Other examples of medical treatments that are aimed at restoring the body to balance by reversing the effects of an external cause of disease include the setting of a fractured bone, the surgical repair of a road-traffic injury, the treatment of burns, administration of fluids in dehydration and the treatment of poisoning. All these are treating the root problem and are examples of curative approaches.

In some cases, the appropriate treatment of an acute infection with antibiotics will restore the body to balance and might also be interpreted as curative.

Suppression

In suppression (illustrated earlier with the analogy of the overflowing bath), the drug causes the disappearance of symptoms, but the underlying imbalance, the root of the symptoms, has not been rectified. Within many holistic medicine systems, symptoms may even be seen as a natural expression of a particular energetic imbalance, and one through which the imbalance may be healed, or at least stabilised. A suppressive treatment targeted at the symptoms alone is believed, particularly in homeopathic thought, to prevent this natural mode of expression, and to force the imbalance to express itself in another way, often at a deeper level. A similar concept is found within Chinese medicine, with the differentiation between the manifestation (Biao) and the root (Ben) of a syndrome. According to Chinese medicine, the ideal approach, except in emergencies, is always to focus treatment at the root of the problem.

Suppression can be illustrated in a diagrammatic way in the form of a negative cycle of events, in which suppression of symptoms leads to worsening of the root imbalance (Figure 1.3b-II).

To the holistically minded complementary therapist, a marker of suppression would be that, if a drug is withdrawn, the original symptoms can reappear and may be even worse than before treatment because the underlying imbalance has worsened. This may lead the patient to have to rely on the drug to feel well; in other words, to become dependent on the drug.

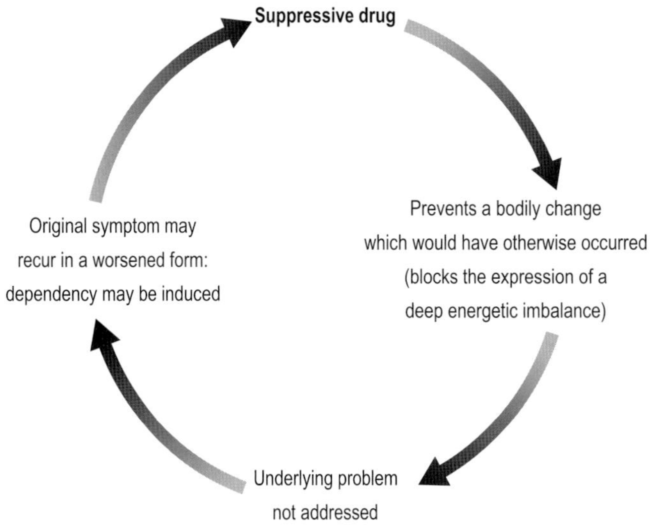
Suppressive drug
Prevents a bodily change which would have otherwise occurred (blocks the expression of a deep energetic imbalance)
Underlying problem not addressed
Original symptom may recur in a worsened form: dependency may be induced

Figure 1.3b II • The negative cycle of suppression.

Introduction of drug-induced disease

When considering the energetic effects of medication, not all harmful effects of a drug need be attributed to suppression. Few drugs target a particular symptom alone. They will often have other effects on the body. Aspirin, for example, recognised in conventional medicine to alleviate headaches because of its anti-inflammatory properties, also has an adverse effect on the lining of the stomach. In most people aspirin will cause inflammation and some degree of bleeding of the stomach lining. This effect is a direct result of the action of aspirin on the function of inflammatory chemicals (the prostaglandins) in the stomach lining. The term 'drug-induced disease' will be used in this text to describe the generation of a side-effect as a direct consequence of a physiological property of the drug.

The latter two categories of suppression and drug-induced disease may be difficult to distinguish in practice. In both situations the symptoms of the original condition have been improved, but at the cost of the appearance of other, newer symptoms. These other symptoms may either be a consequence of suppression (an old imbalance expressed at a deeper energetic level) or a drug-induced disease.

One important distinguishing characteristic of drug-induced disease is that it will affect even a person who has no disease to suppress. If a 'well' person were to take a high-dose aspirin on a regular basis, they would be very likely to experience symptoms of irritation of the stomach lining after some time. In contrast, a condition that results from suppression, as in the example of worsened Yin deficiency in the case of the business woman taking paracetamol, would not necessarily develop in a well person taking the same drug. Taking paracetamol does not in itself lead to anxiety and depression.

Placebo

The 'placebo effect' is well recognised in conventional medicine. It is seen to occur when symptoms improve even when a prescription contains no active ingredient. In the case of the placebo effect, symptoms recover measurably more often than if no prescription had been given at all. As a placebo tablet is better than no tablet at all, it seems that the simple act of receiving and taking a prescription has a benefit in terms of health. Before the advent of antibiotics, brightly coloured placebo tablets (made of a pharmacologically inactive substance such as sugar) were an important part of the doctor's armamentarium.

The placebo effect is a manifestation of the induction of healing within a therapeutic relationship. In all treatments, be they complementary or conventional, the placebo effect will play a part.

Is suppression always bad?

Sometimes suppressive treatment is the only option available to enable a person to cope with intolerable circumstances. Conventional medicine has adopted many suppressive treatments where there appears to be no available alternative to improve an intolerable or rapidly deteriorating situation.

Examples of this sort of 'necessary' suppression include:

- chemotherapy in childhood leukaemia (now known to save lives in a high proportion of cases)
- strong pain relief and other palliative measures in terminal cancer
- antidepressants or tranquillisers in an acutely suicidal person
- 'clot-busting' medication to reverse the blockage in an artery that is causing an acute heart attack (also known to be life-saving).

Less extreme, and therefore more controversial, examples include:

- antidepressants prescribed to an overburdened single mother, who lives in a district in which social care is underfunded and waiting lists for supportive counselling are full – the prescription has undoubtedly helped her to cope when no other care was available.
- a contraceptive injection for someone who would be physically or emotionally traumatised by pregnancy.
- antibiotics to reduce the disfigurement of acne in an underconfident and bullied teenager.

Many conventional medical treatments can be classed as suppressive in nature. It is important to remember that often the conventional practitioner will also recognise these treatments as suppressive, and therefore not choose them as the ideal option. Nevertheless, suppressive treatments may be a necessary aspect of coping with the human condition. Before making negative judgements about the choice of suppressive treatments, it is often advisable to consider what other choices were available for the patient at that time. In many cases it may be found that suppressive treatment was the only feasible option to relieve the patient's distress.

The energetic effects of the nine categories of drugs

The categorisation of conventional drugs introduced in Section 1.2 can help with interpreting whether or not a medical treatment is likely to be curative or suppressive in action. Table 1.3b-I demonstrates how an energetic interpretation can be matched to each of the nine categories of mode of drug action as described in Section 1.2.

It is noteworthy that stimulant drugs are also categorised as suppressive according to this interpretation of drug energetics. Although the term 'suppression' evokes pictures of damping something down rather than stimulating it, the stimulant drugs do in fact also suppress a more natural state of events. For example, the stimulant drug caffeine suppresses tiredness, the stimulant drug salbutamol suppresses constricted breathing when inhaled, and the ovulatory stimulants suppress the state of infertility.

The difference with stimulants is that these drugs force, or 'boost', a bodily state that otherwise would not have occurred.

Table 1.3b-I Energetic interpretation of each of the nine categories of mode of drug action

	Mode of action of drug	Energetic interpretation
1	Replaces a deficient substance that is normally obtained from the diet	Usually returns the body to a state of more balance: **energetic cure** However, if given without attention to a deeper underlying cause of deficiency, for example iron replacement given to treat anaemia due to blood loss: **suppression**
2	Replaces a deficient substance that is normally produced by the body	In cases in which the body will never be able to produce the essential substance ever again, the replacement treatment moves the body towards a state of more balance: (e.g. insulin replacement in type 1 diabetes mellitus due to total failure of the insulin cells of the pancreas): **energetic cure** In cases when the body is underproducing an essential substance as a result of an ongoing deeper disease process, the replacement of that substance is suppressive (e.g. thyroxine replacement in mild hypothyroidism): **suppression**
3	Kills or suppresses the growth of infectious agents (microbes and other life forms that cause infection)	In infections due to a strong Pathogen (in Chinese medicine terms) in a relatively balanced individual, the drug may enable full clearance of the Pathogen, and will enable the restoration of balance: **energetic cure** In infections that have occurred due to an underlying imbalance in the individual, the treatment does not target the root cause, and so tends to be suppressive, even with full clearance of the Pathogen: **suppression** In some cases the Pathogen is not fully cleared but persists to lead to symptoms at a deeper energetic level: **suppression**
4	Counteracts the damage caused by toxins	These treatments reverse the damage that would have been caused by an external toxic substance: **energetic cure**
5	Toxic to rapidly dividing human cells	These treatments always target the manifestation (a tumour) of a deep underlying imbalance: **suppression**
6	Specifically stimulates the immune response by introduction of an antigen	Vaccines are given to well people. They involve the administration of a foreign substance, which primarily stimulates a natural immune response. This has to be classed as drug-induced disease. In some cases this disease leads to serious symptoms, but in other cases, the individual regains a healthy state of balance as the artificial 'infection' is overcome: **drug-induced disease**
7	Other drugs that artificially stimulate natural bodily functions	These drugs firstly may stimulate a bodily function that perhaps should be occurring (e.g. a lack of ovulation in female infertility) but is not, due to an underlying imbalance. By ignoring the underlying imbalance and treating the symptom, these treatments will be depleting. Also, any drug that causes an increase in a natural bodily response (e.g. alertness induced by caffeine, or relaxation of the airways by inhaled salbutamol in asthma) could also be described as a stimulant. If stimulants mask the symptoms of an imbalance then this is **suppression** Stimulants can be used when there is no disease (e.g. in the case of occasional recreational drug use), in which case they induce **drug-induced disease**
8	Suppresses natural bodily functions	The suppression of a natural bodily function, either in a well or an unwell person, will of course move the individual away from a healthy state of balance: **suppression**
9	Other drugs that directly counteract the symptoms (manifestation) of a disease process rather than its root cause	All these drugs are suppressive by definition: **suppression**

As drugs carry no nutritive value, they do not actually introduce energy into the body. Because of this, any boosting of a bodily state is very likely to be at the expense of reserves of the energy that would be descried as Qi in Chinese medicine. Figure 1.3b-III illustrates the effect of stimulant drugs in the form of a cycle.

Figure 1.3b-III illustrates how, from a Chinese medicine perspective, a stimulant drug may actually cause an impression of improving the energetic state of the body by the 'boosting' of substances such as Qi, Jing, or Yang. A good example might be the action of salbutamol, which reduces the wheeze of asthma. This action might be described as the 'boosting' of Lung and Kidney Qi. However, this drug is not curative of asthma, except in the short term. The theory of suppression would suggest that repeated use might actually tend to deplete reserves of Lung and Kidney Qi, and in this way cause the patient to become dependent on the medication.

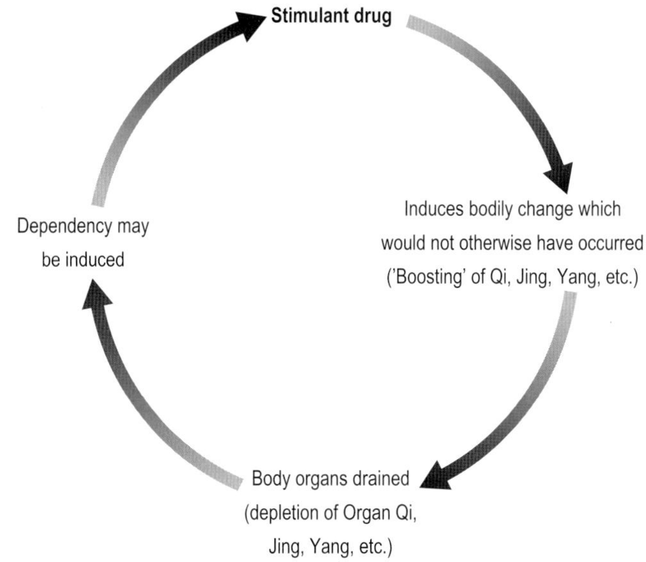

Figure 1.3b III • The negative cycle of stimulant drugs.

It is important to clarify at this point that describing salbutamol as suppressive does not suggest that this drug is potentially harmful. There is no doubt that, in severe asthma, drugs such as salbutamol are potentially life saving, and are a good example of how suppressive treatment may be the best option for some patients. However, in mild asthma, alternative treatment for the root of the problem may well reduce or negate the need for a patient to rely on medication.

In a similar way, other stimulant drugs can be described as boosting. Caffeine could be described as boosting of Heart Qi, and ovulatory stimulants could be thought of as boosting of Blood and Essence.

The energetic action of drugs: from theory to practice

Some fictional case histories from conventional medicine will help this theory of the energetics of drug action come to life. These case histories present different examples of drugs leading to cure, drug-induced disease and suppression. Each case history is followed by a brief discussion of the energetic interpretations of the action of the drugs described (see Q1.3b-1).

Case history 1

Case History 1

Joe, a previously fit teenager, rapidly becomes very unwell and is rushed to hospital nearly unconscious with bacterial meningitis. However, he makes a dramatic recovery after 5 days of treatment with intravenous antibiotics. He is tired for a few days following his illness, but returns to playing football for the school within 3 weeks. Six months later, he continues to appear lively and healthy.

This is a case describing the use of antibiotics. Antibiotics are believed to be Cold in nature according to Chinese Medicine. Evidence for this is that they can 'Cool' the Heat of bacterial infections and may lead to loose stools or vaginal discharge (thrush) as unwanted side-effects. Meningitis is a condition of strong Wind and Heat, and so requires a strong treatment for the Pathogens to be cleared. Joe was basically healthy and so has good Upright Qi. With antibiotic treatment the Pathogen was cleared and, possibly as a result of resilient Upright Qi, he was able to tolerate the negative aspects of the drugs and experienced no side-effects.

As the Pathogen is cleared and there is no feature to suggest suppression, this does seem to be an example of cure (see Q1.3b-2).

Case history 2

Case History 2

Alf, the elderly grandfather of the teenager in Case History 1, also contracts the infection. He is increasingly confused for 5 days before the condition is recognised. With the same treatment, the older man makes a much slower recovery. He develops a prolonged case of diarrhoea following the antibiotics, and even when this is better after 3 weeks, he is never quite as sprightly again.

Alf is an elderly man and his Upright Qi will not be as strong as that of his grandson. For this reason, Alf's body does not respond as dramatically to the infection as his grandson's body, and so the diagnosis is delayed. The diarrhoea is a common side-effect of antibiotics, and in Alf's case may be a consequence of having relatively weak Spleen Qi. For these reasons he takes much longer to recover.

Moreover, Alf is never quite the same again after the infection has cleared. He has been left in a less healthy state than he was previously. However, without the treatment he is likely to have died. This is, therefore, an example of cure, but with 'drug-induced disease' complicating the old man's recovery.

The depletion following the illness (possibly a result of Full Heat consuming Yin) is more likely mostly due to the effect of the meningitis than the antibiotics. However, in view of the prolonged diarrhoea, the antibiotics possibly may have contributed to Alf's reduction in overall health. A possible Chinese description for this is that antibiotics have led to the accumulation of Damp (see Q1.3b-3).

Case history 3

Sue has also been prescribed antibiotics. Unfortunately, this anxious teenager has developed a well-recognised side-effect of antibiotics, vaginal thrush. From a conventional perspective, this is believed to occur because the antibiotic destroys natural 'protective' bacteria (lactobacilli) in the vagina as well as those causing the sore throat. From a Chinese medicine perspective, the antibiotics were too cooling for someone with (exam-related) depleted Spleen Qi, and led to the formation of a

Case History 3

Joe's sister Sue is worrying about GCSE exams, and has a distracting sore throat. She receives a prescription for the broad-spectrum antibiotic (amoxicillin) from her GP. Her sore throat gets better, but she develops vaginal thrush, and is extremely uncomfortable. She buys some medication for this from the chemist. Although her vaginal infection gets better in 2 days, it recurs just before the exams, and continues to do so for the next few months. Each time it responds less well to the chemist's treatment. A year into the sixth form she goes to her GP feeling depressed and exhausted. She doesn't like to mention the thrush. All her blood tests come back as normal, but she is worried that she is developing ME (chronic fatigue syndrome).

Case History 4

Meanwhile, Sue's best friend Ann had been experiencing similar symptoms of exhaustion, and also sweats at night. She had also been putting these symptoms down to stress in the sixth form, but one evening she felt a firm swelling on one side of her neck. Her doctor was concerned to discover that Ann had markedly swollen lymph nodes on that side. Urgent investigations revealed that Ann had developed a rare form of tumour of the lymph glands called Hodgkin's disease. She was started on chemotherapy, which made her feel nauseous and caused her hair to fall out. Also she had radiotherapy to certain groups of lymph nodes in her body. Ann felt awful on this regimen and had to drop behind a year at school.

After the course of treatments the doctor said that she was 'in remission'. This meant there was no evidence of any tumour in any of her glands, but 'cure' could not be proven. Ann would have to return for yearly check-ups. Nevertheless, she was determined to fight against a possible recurrence, and paid careful attention to eating a diet free of any processed food or addictive substances. Within 2 years she had raised money for Cancer Research by cycling from John O'Groats to Land's End.

Now, 5 years later, she is completing her training at medical school, feeling well, still clear of disease, and keen to be an oncologist (cancer doctor). Ann now says that her current problems are that her teeth need frequent dental attention, and that she is worried that she may be infertile.

discharge with characteristics of Cold and Damp. This can be interpreted as drug-induced disease resulting from the energetic effect of the antibiotic.

However, the fact that the symptoms persisted, and only temporarily responded to antifungal treatment suggests that suppression is also part of the picture. As time goes on Sue develops more symptoms, but this time at a deeper physical and also emotional level, and this is further evidence of suppressed symptoms becoming expressed at different levels to the original imbalance.

Looking back, it may have been the stress of Sue's exams that led to an energetic imbalance such Yin deficiency, which was then followed by Wind Heat invasion. The medication just 'treated' the manifestation of the imbalance, so possibly allowing the root cause to worsen, and may also have led to incomplete clearance of the Pathognomic Factor and the emergence of the syndrome of Residual Pathogenic Factor (both of these are examples of suppression). The treatment also induced additional imbalance from Cold and Damp (drug-induced disease) (see Q1.3b-4).

Case history 4

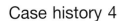

Ann has received chemotherapy and radiotherapy for her lymphoma. Radiotherapy and chemotherapy are toxic to dividing cells and so fit into Category 5 of drug action as summarised in Table 1.3b-I. Therefore, it can be assumed that the action of the treatment is suppressive. The fact that the treatment caused severe side-effects at the time is an indication of additional significant drug-induced disease.

However, there is no doubt, from the historical understanding of the prognosis of lymphoma before treatment, that Ann would have died without therapy. Therefore, this case is an example of how a powerfully suppressive treatment, and one that also causes marked drug-induced disease, has prevented death and given a person the opportunity to continue to live life to the full.

A lymphoma is an initially painless mass, which might be considered as Phlegm (or possibly Blood Stagnation) in Chinese medicine. In Chinese medicine the aetiology of cancer would be that there must have also been a pre-existing deficiency in terms of Yin and/or Yang to allow such a substantial mass to develop.

Chemotherapy has a range of side-effects, which suggests that it is energetically Heating: it causes angry inflamed tissue if it leaks out of the infusion needle, it leads to a painful sore tongue and mucous membranes, and also increases the risk of bleeding. From a Chinese medicine perspective, it is possibly the heating effect that, almost literally, burns the tumour away (there are Chinese herbs, known as escharotics, used in cancer that work in this way). This aspect of the treatment attends only to the manifestation of Ann's underlying imbalance, but does not treat the root deficiency. This is the nature of suppressive treatment.

Chemotherapy also appears to damage Spleen Qi, in that vomiting and diarrhoea are very common side-effects. There is a known risk of infertility and also of impairment of the immune system, which implies damage to Kidney Qi or Jing. So here is some evidence for additional drug-induced disease. This drug-induced disease is likely to compound further the pre-existing deficiency.

However, in Ann's case, although drug-induced disease and suppression are not in themselves desirable, it is clear they were a price worth paying in the face of a rapidly progressive disease process. This could be described as an example of 'necessary suppression'.

It is helpful to remember the strong tendency of the human body/spirit to be healed despite the presence of suppressed symptoms. Perhaps Ann's determination to fight and her subsequent attention to her health enabled her body to resolve the original deficiency (which in her case is possibly congenital) that had led to the cancer.

The systematic interpretation of the energetics of individual drugs

The case histories have provided examples of the energetic effects of the nine broad categories of drugs, and have illustrated how their effects can fall into one or more of five categories (i.e. no effect, cure, placebo effect, suppression or drug-induced disease). It is possible to work through cases such as these in a systematic way in order to arrive confidently at a simple interpretation of the energetics of the drugs being used.

This method will now be introduced, drawing upon the Chinese medicine language of energetics. By way of illustration, the energetic properties of two common drugs are explored. This method involves gathering information about the action of a drug in a particular scenario in six steps. Each step involves a question, the answer to which will contribute towards a final energetic interpretation. As Case Histories 1–3 illustrate, the energetic interpretation of the same drug might be different according to the clinical setting of its use (e.g. antibiotics may either be curative or suppressive in action), so it is important when using this method to first be clear about the clinical setting.

Although Chinese medicine language has been drawn upon as an illustration, this method can be readily adapted to the theoretical structures of most complementary therapies.

The six steps relate to the following aspects of treatment:

1. *Relief of symptoms*. Ask: 'In what way does the drug relieve symptoms physiologically?'
2. *Chinese medicine interpretation of disease*. 'What is a simple Chinese medicine interpretation of the disease being treated?'
3. *How does the drug alleviate disease in Chinese medicine terms*. Explain the alleviation of this disease in Chinese medicine terms.
4. *Common side-effects*. Ask: 'What are the common side-effects listed in the BNF?'
5. *Simple Chinese medicine interpretation of side-effects*. Explain these in Chinese medicine terms.
6. *Category of mode of action*. Ask: 'Is there any likelihood of the drugs leading to suppressed symptoms in addition to drug-induced disease?'

To help make sense of this, the process will be followed for a commonly taken painkiller, ibuprofen, which is classed as a non-steroidal anti-inflammatory drug (NSAID). The name NSAID describes the fact that, even though it is not a corticosteroid preparation, ibuprofen will act to calm down the natural process of inflammation in the body. It gives relief for swollen painful joints, but is also very effective in headache and period pain (see Q1.3b-5).

Each of the six questions will now be answered for ibuprofen in the clinical setting of it being used to relieve pain and inflammation

1. *How does ibuprofen give relief of symptoms?* The answer to this question need only be given in the most simple descriptive terms, and will be obvious as long as it is understood why the drug has been prescribed. Ibuprofen in this clinical setting relieves pain, stiffness and dysmenorrhoea.
2. *What is a possible Chinese medicine interpretation of pain and inflammation?* The answer to this question requires some understanding of how symptoms relate to Chinese medicine syndromes. In Chinese medicine, the pain and inflammation for which ibuprofen may be prescribed is generally described in terms of Stagnant Qi and Blood together with Heat.
3. *How does ibuprofen alleviate pain and inflammation in Chinese medicine terms?* The answer to this question relates to the alleviation of the syndromes, given as the answer to question 2. A simple answer in this clinical setting would be that ibuprofen moves Qi and Blood and clears Heat.
4. *What are the common side-effects of ibuprofen?* To answer this question requires access to a formulary such as the BNF. The most common side-effect for ibuprofen listed in the BNF is inflammation of the stomach lining, which in turn can lead to indigestion, slight oozing of blood, and occasionally a stomach ulcer. Rare side-effects that can affect susceptible people include headache, tinnitus (ringing in the ears), dizziness, liver and kidney damage, and asthma.
5. *What is a possible simple Chinese medicine interpretation of the side-effects?* Like the answer to question 3, to answer this question requires some basic knowledge of how Chinese medicine syndromes relate to symptoms. However, this is a more difficult question to answer because the information given in the BNF is not presented in the detail with which a complementary medical practitioner might describe symptoms. Because of the paucity of details of symptoms, often only a guess at the most likely possible syndrome can be made on the basis of a few key symptoms such as headache, depression and abdominal disturbance.

Sometimes, knowledge of the pathological process at play can offer helpful additional information; for example, local inflammation and bleeding suggests Heat, painless overgrowth of tissues suggests Phlegm, degeneration of the substance of tissues suggests Yin Deficiency, and impairment of function might suggest Qi or Yang deficiency. The rationale for these assumptions is explained in more detail under the heading 'The Rationale and Method Used for the Mapping of Western Medical Diagnoses to Chinese Medicine Theory' in the Note to the Reader contained in the preliminary pages of this book

The common gastric side-effects of ibuprofen imply depletion of Stomach Yin, a key symptom of which is epigastric discomfort. If a painful stomach ulcer develops, the more intense fixed pain characteristic of this condition implies the development of Blood Stagnation. Bleeding from the stomach suggests Heat.

Headaches and dizziness and tinnitus may imply Stagnation of Liver Qi and Liver Yang Rising. Deep organ damage to the kidneys and liver tell us that the drug in some way has the potential to damage Liver and Kidney Qi and Yin.

6. *Into what category of mode of action does ibuprofen fall?* This question relates to the nine categories of modes of action listed in Table 1.3b-I. As the pain is always the symptom of some other underlying condition, such as arthritis or injury, ibuprofen fits into category 8 or 9, depending on the situation of its use. Its action is therefore suppressive. As the condition being treated is one of Heat and Stagnation, then the two common side-effects (depletion of Stomach Yin and Headaches) may also be exacerbated as a result of suppression of these Pathogenic factors.

   Summary. We can say that ibuprofen is a drug with properties of moving Qi and Blood and is Heating, but may damage Stomach Yin, and also the Liver and Kidney Qi in susceptible people. Its side-effects indicate it has the potential to cause severe drug-induced disease, as well as suppression of symptoms.

Because it is possible to make only very general energetic interpretations from the limited information given in the BNF, one key to keeping this approach a manageable tool is to aim for the Chinese energetic interpretations to be as simple as possible.

A similar process is now followed for caffeine, a drug that is commonly included in cold and pain remedies, but is much more familiar as a prominent component of the western diet.

Caffeine is considered as a mild stimulant – it slightly speeds up the pulse and metabolic rate. It is recognised to help move the bowels and promote urination. It is claimed to have slight painkilling properties, although this is disputed in the BNF. It appears to lift the mood (the poet William Cowper described tea as 'the cup that cheers but not inebriates'). For some people caffeine can cause indigestion, a migraine-type headache or palpitations. Regular caffeine intake is recognised as a cause of tiredness. Caffeine has a known withdrawal syndrome of severe headaches and reduced mood for days after suddenly stopping intake. In Chinese medicine, coffee is recognised to be Warming, but in excess to harm Spleen and Kidney Yang and Stagnate Liver Qi (see Q1.3b-6).

Each of the six questions is now answered for caffeine in the clinical setting of it being used as a 'pick me up' at a time of lethargy and lack of enthusiasm.

1. *How does caffeine give relief of symptoms?* In this setting caffeine lifts the mood and induces wakefulness.
2. *What is a possible Chinese medicine interpretation of lethargy and lack of enthusiasm?* Caffeine may be taken in times of lethargy, and also may lift the spirits. Lethargy could have a range of causes, but at its simplest could be accounted for by Qi Deficiency or Stagnation. Likewise, low spirits could be attributed to Heart Qi Deficiency or Qi Stagnation.
3. *How does caffeine alleviate lethargy and lack of enthusiasm in Chinese medicine terms?* Caffeine acts possibly by Boosting and Moving of Qi, and in particular of the Heart. Tea and Coffee are Warming in nature according to Chinese Medicine, and Warming substances have the tendency to move Qi.
4. *What are the common side-effects of caffeine?* In susceptible people caffeine can cause indigestion, headaches, palpitations and tiredness.
5. *What is a possible simple Chinese medicine interpretation of the side-effects?* In some modern interpretations of Chinese medicine, coffee is recognised to harm Spleen and Kidney Yang and Stagnate Liver Qi. This fits with the observed side-effects of caffeine. Caffeine also can 'boost' Heart Qi, and this could explain the palpitations experienced by some when caffeine is taken in excess. In addition to impaired Spleen Yang, indigestion might relate to the Heating properties of caffeine.

   The headaches that might result from caffeine may imply Stagnation of Liver Qi and Liver Yang Rising. The occurrence of these side-effects might suggest that suppression of the original symptom might be leading to the emergence of these Liver-related symptoms, as the 'condition' being treated by caffeine is often one of Stagnation of Liver Qi.
6. *Into what category of mode of action does caffeine fall?* Caffeine primarily masks the natural bodily response of tiredness. This fits into category 8. In those who are dependent on caffeine, it relieves a craving for caffeine, headaches and low mood, which all are symptoms of a deeper imbalance. This fits into category 9. The energetic action is suppressive.

   Summary. Caffeine is a substance that has both Moving and Warming properties, which seem to result in Boosting of Qi, in particular Heart Qi. In the case of coffee, it has also been described to deplete Spleen and Kidney Yang, and Stagnate Liver Qi. These are signs of drug-induced disease. The presence of a marked withdrawal syndrome tells us it has a suppressive action. In this case, caffeine suppresses an underlying condition of depleted Heart Qi and Stagnant Liver Qi.

These two summaries of the six-step approach to summarising the energetic action of drugs illustrate that this simple process can be applied to two very different treatments. To further illustrate the simplicity and flexibility of this approach, some more worked examples of energetic interpretations of drug actions are given in Appendix II.

Self-test 1.3b

Drugs from an alternative viewpoint

Consider the nine categories in which modern drugs are conventionally seen to work, and also the five ways in which we can understand them to exert energetic effects (i.e. no effect, cure, placebo, suppression and introduction of drug-induced disease).

Now think about:

(i) how the treatment described is seen to work conventionally (including which of the nine categories best fits the treatment), and

(ii) in which of the five ways that treatment may be working energetically and apply this to the following scenarios.

1. Ben develops a crop of inflamed boils on his back and is feverish. He has been feeling generally run down for some time now. The GP does some tests to check for serious diseases such as diabetes, and gives Ben the all clear. Ben takes a prescription of flucloxacillin, and within 2 days is feeling a bit better. Weeks later, however, he is still feeling out of sorts, although the boils have disappeared.
2. Marjorie is proud that she doesn't need to go to the doctor when she is feeling a little off colour. All she has to do is go to the chemist for some of her vitamin tonic. After a glass of that, within hours she feels better.
3. Jim was prescribed amitriptyline for 6 months at a time in his life when he was feeling really down and couldn't see a way out. He has to admit it really helped him see some solutions to his problems, although he wasn't so happy about some of the side-effects, particularly drowsiness and dry mouth. He has been off the drug for 3 months now, and is still so much better, but is feeling that since the winter has come his mood is getting lower again.

Answer

1. (i) Flucloxacillin is a drug that kills or suppresses bacteria; category 3.

   (ii) In this case the drug is suppressive, and may have introduced drug-induced disease in terms of Damp.

   Explanation. Boils in Chinese medicine are Fire Poison/Damp Heat, and are a manifestation of Internal Heat. Conventional medicine recognises that boils tend to occur in people who are run down (i.e. the cause is not purely external). Ben in given antibiotics to treat the overgrowth of usually harmless bacteria which is known to occur in boils. The treatment is not therefore treating the root cause, which is possibly dietary and emotional. The symptoms have been suppressed, and could manifest again in Ben. He may feel run down as the root cause has not been dealt with, and also the antibiotic may have led to increased Damp Accumulation.

2. (i) A vitamin tonic is a nutritional drug; category 1.

   (ii) The tonic may have no effect, and Marjorie would have felt better anyway. It may also have acted as a placebo, or may have been the appropriate energetic remedy and led to cure. It is unlikely to have caused suppression.

   Explanation. Marjorie has faith in the fact that her tonic will sort her out. She is also proud that she doesn't have to depend on the doctor. Here are two reasons why, at a deep level, her ability to heal herself could become active as she takes her tonic. It may also be that the tonic contains an ingredient that is the correct energetic remedy for her condition. We cannot say what this might be without more information. This would be understood conventionally in terms of a vitamin or mineral deficiency.

3. (i) Amitriptyline, like fluoxetine, treats a chemical imbalance recognised to contribute to in depression, and so is a drug that treats symptoms but does not deal with the root imbalance; category 9.

   (ii) Although there may be an initial placebo effect, 6 months of lifted mood is unlikely to be placebo induced. The primary effect is suppression of symptoms (possibly by Boosting and Moving of Qi), and side-effects are due to drug-induced disease.

   Explanation. Jim suffered from a deep depression, and was treated with an antidepressant. The theory behind prescribing a 6-month course of antidepressants is that it allows the mood to be lifted for a sufficient time for the individual to start sorting out the issues that brought about the depression. This would be commendable if the person is able to do that sort of personal healing work. Too often, however, symptoms recur after treatment is withdrawn, and although antidepressants are not considered to be addictive, they do induce a dependency syndrome in some cases. Often, treatment is not withdrawn at all; the 'crutch' becomes a permanent fixture. We can presume from the way amitriptyline is seen to work that it is suppressive; by removing the manifestation, the root is less likely to be healed.

   The side-effects of amitriptyline suggest that it has Heating and, ultimately, Yin-depleting properties: rapid pulse, sweating, dry mouth and difficulty with urination. It appears to have a particular effect on the heart, and can induce palpitations. In some people, it can cause manic states that suggest Phlegm Obstructing the Heart. The paradoxical side-effect of sedation may be a reflection of Phlegm-forming properties. Multiple other side-effects imply additional Liver Stagnating and Wind-inducing properties. The side-effects should give us no doubt that amitriptyline causes drug-induced disease.

Barriers to disease and susceptibility

2.1

Chapter 2.1a Health and susceptibility: what makes us vulnerable to disease?

LEARNING POINTS

At the end of this chapter you will be able to:
- define susceptibility from a conventional viewpoint
- understand the conventional view of barriers to disease
- list the factors that increase susceptibility to disease
- appreciate the role of preventive medicine
- compare and contrast the conventional and alternative views of susceptibility.

Estimated time for chapter: 60 minutes.

Introduction

In this first half of Stage 2 of the course there is a progression from the introductory topics of Stage 1 to an exploration of the foundations of pathology, the study of how the body responds to disease.

Susceptibility as vulnerability to disease

Chapter 1.1e introduced the basic causes of disease from the perspective of both conventional and more holistic approaches to medicine, and looked at their similarities and differences.

This chapter explores in more detail the topic of causation of disease, and what factors influence susceptibility to disease. 'Susceptibility' is a term used commonly in conventional medicine to refer to vulnerability to disease. From a holistic perspective, susceptibility might more accurately be defined as vulnerability to imbalance, as within a holistic paradigm reduced health tends to be considered in terms of imbalance rather than as disease (see Q2.1a-1).

The conventional view of barriers to disease

Conventional medicine considers susceptibility in terms of weakness of one or more of a series of levels of defences, or barriers to disease. The body is conventionally understood to have several methods of protection against disease. Some of these are located in the superficial layers of the body, within the skin and mucous membranes. Some protect from the more deep levels of the tissues beneath the skin and from within the organs (see Q2.1a-2).

Conventional medicine recognises mechanical and immune barriers to disease. Mechanical barriers are those that confer protection as a result of the physical structure of the barrier (e.g. the keratinised squamous epithelium of the skin). Immune barriers are those that protect by a complex interaction of the immune cells and proteins (including antibodies) that circulate in the body fluids and can move into tissues when required. Examples of these are summarised in Table 2.1a-I.

Table 2.1a-I summarises those parts or functions of the body that have a protective role. Most of the mechanical barriers serve as a protective method for the body literally by providing physical protection against damage. Healing of wounds and the blood-clotting mechanism may be more difficult to picture as a mechanical barrier, as a chain of physiological responses has to be set in action for them to exert their protective effect. The role of the immune system in protection is even more complex. For this reason, wound healing, blood clotting and the immune system are each discussed in more detail in the following chapters in this section.

Health and susceptibility

Table 2.1a-I lists those body parts or functions that have a specific role in protection against disease. However, overarching the protection that these specific barriers provide is the

Table 2.1a-I Examples of the barriers to disease

Depth	Name of barrier	Type
Superficial	Skin, and body hair	Mechanical
	Oily secretion of skin (sebum)	Mechanical
	Antibodies in sweat	Immune
	The structures which protect the orifices (e.g. eyelids, nostrils, urethra)	Mechanical
	Mucous membranes	Mechanical
	Mucus secreted from mucous membranes	Mechanical
	Antibodies in mucus and tears	Immune
	The cushioning of subcutaneous tissues (fat)	Mechanical
	The bony skeleton	Mechanical
	The supportive and protective nature of other types of connective tissue in all parts of the body	Mechanical
	The ability of wounds to heal	Mechanical
	The ability of blood to clot	Mechanical
Deep	Immune cells and antibodies in the blood and lymph	Immune

general health of the body. In fact, health in any organ or body part will in itself provide a barrier against disease. For example, a perfectly structured heart organ will be less susceptible to heart disease than one with damaged heart valves or a weakness in the heart muscle (see Q2.1a-3).

Periods of naturally increased susceptibility

There are times within a healthy lifespan when these barriers to disease are less effective. These can be seen as periods of naturally increased susceptibility to disease (see Q2.1a-4).

The three periods when a healthy person is more than usually susceptible to disease are during infancy, pregnancy and old age. In infancy, the barriers to disease, such as the immune system or the ability to maintain a steady body temperature, are not fully mature. In pregnancy, the vitality required to maintain the healthy barriers to disease is diverted to the growing fetus (e.g. calcium is diverted to the fetus and the mother's teeth become more vulnerable to decay). In old age, all barriers to disease are in a state of degeneration (e.g. the skin and bones become less strong and are more vulnerable to damage by trauma).

Moreover, in ill-health susceptibility is increased because one or more of these barriers will not be functioning as they should be. The susceptibility that results from ill-health can be categorised as either congenital (dating from the time of birth) or acquired (developing at a later stage in life as a result of deficiency, disease or injury).

Congenital susceptibility

Congenital susceptibility means that one or more of the barriers to disease are not functioning well from birth (see Q2.1a-5). Examples of congenital disease conferring susceptibility include albinism, haemophilia and congenital heart disease. In albinism an inability to produce the skin pigment melanin leads to vulnerability to sunburn and skin cancer. In haemophilia an inability to produce sufficient blood-clotting proteins leads to vulnerability to bleeding into joints and muscles. In congenital heart disease poorly formed heart valves and gaps in the internal muscle wall of the heart lead to a vulnerability to poor heart pumping action, breathlessness and, over time, lung damage. The important congenital diseases are described in detail in Chapter 5.4c.

Some forms of congenital susceptibility are more subtle. Although a named inherited condition, such as cystic fibrosis, may not be present, it is clear that some people fall ill more often than others, and for some, this has been the case since infancy. The term 'weak constitution' might be applied in such a situation. This is because the inherited barriers to disease are not as strong as they could be, but are not so damaged as to constitute a named disease.

Acquired susceptibility

Acquired susceptibility is the consequence of a weakening of the barriers to disease after birth. Any one of the conventionally accepted causes of disease (Chapter 1.1e), such as poor diet, lack of exercise, obesity and smoking, is understood to contribute to increased susceptibility before disease is seen to occur.

For example, a long-term smoker may appear to be very fit but in fact is very likely to have sustained damage to a number of the barriers to disease, thus meaning that he or she has a higher risk of succumbing to disease. Reasons for this include the fact that smoking damages the protective lining of the lungs, so lung infections are more likely to take hold, and also that it impairs the free circulation of blood and increases the tendency of the blood to clot, which mean that diseases of the cardiovascular system such as heart attack are more likely to occur. However, the fact that some smokers do not develop smoking smoking-related diseases tells us that susceptibility is not the same as disease (see Q2.1a-6).

A smoker will always increase his or her risk of developing smoking-related disease by smoking because cigarette smoke invariably damages the lungs and circulation to some degree. If the smoker's constitution is strong, the damage from smoking may not be so severe as to lead to a very high risk of disease, although his or her personal risk of disease has undoubtedly increased. A smoker with a poor constitution manifesting in weakness in the lungs or circulation (e.g. someone with asthma or diabetes) already has an increased risk of developing lung and heart disease. The risk of these diseases therefore becomes even higher if such a person smokes.

Nevertheless, both types of smoker may avoid disease, because other factors may be present that reduce susceptibility. For example, in the case of smokers, living in a warm, dry climate may reduce the risk of bronchitis, and eating a healthy, low-fat diet may reduce the risk of circulatory problems. Such factors are known as 'protective factors'. Some protective factors may be far less easy to assess clinically than others. For example, personality traits such as a generally positive attitude or a calm approach to the vicissitudes of life may well be protective against illness.

Risk factors

The term 'risk factor' is used medically to describe anything that increases the risk of disease. For example, high blood pressure is a risk factor for stroke, and unprotected sex is a risk factor for developing human immunodeficiency virus (HIV) infection.

Therefore, the presence of a risk factor means that the susceptibility to disease is increased. In fact, any of the conventional external causes of disease (e.g. inadequate diet, insufficient exercise, exposure to radiation and smoking) can also be seen as a risk factor for disease.

Preventive medicine

Conventional doctors aim to reduce risk factors in order to prevent disease. Preventive medicine therefore aims to decrease susceptibility to disease.

Disease prevention may be directed at an individual patient, in the form of personalised health education advice to a patient, screening for early signs of preventable disease, or by prescribing medication to reduce the impact of risk factors such as high blood pressure. Alternatively, changes can be instituted at a national, or even international level to prevent disease. Such changes may require political reform. The advances in sanitation in the UK made in the 19th century are an example of this sort of wide-scale 'public health' measure. Other examples include legislation concerning the advertising of tobacco products, and supplementation of foods with nutrients, such as folic acid in breakfast cereals (see Q2.1a-7). Table 2.1a-II lists some more examples of approaches to the prevention of disease.

Table 2.1a-II Examples of preventive measures against known risk factors for disease

Risk factor	Preventive measure
Meningitis outbreak	Information to the public about warning signs Antibiotics prescribed to close contacts of person with disease
Unprotected sex	Education campaign about safe sex Free condoms at family-planning clinics
High-fat diet	Education about healthy eating Provision of healthy foods in schools Government subsidies of healthy foods
Sedentary lifestyle	Encouragement to exercise by providing cheap access to leisure centres, cycle tracks, etc.
Tendency to accidents in childhood	Education of parents about risks House alterations: smoke alarms, stairgates, etc.
Smoking tobacco	Stop-smoking campaigns Prescription of nicotine patches
Alcohol	Restriction on the sale of alcohol to children

Self-test 2.1a

Health and susceptibility: what makes us vulnerable to disease?

1. Define susceptibility from the perspectives of conventional and holistic medicine.
2. What is the more popular term for what is understood as an inherited susceptibility to disease?
3. Name three types of mechanical barrier to disease, and for each one:
   (i) describe how this barrier may be weakened by a risk factor
   (ii) name one disease/condition for which there is increased susceptibility as a result of the weakened barrier.

(For example, subcutaneous fat is a barrier to disease. (i) This barrier is weakened by weight loss and this (ii) leads to susceptibility to injury from falls.)

4. Name two risk factors that predispose to skin cancer.
5. Name two factors that are protective in road safety.
6. List four possible conventional medical approaches to the prevention of heart disease. Include in your list at least one approach that is aimed at the individual patient and at least one public health approach.

Answers

1. Conventional medicine: vulnerability to disease.
   Holistic medicine: vulnerability to imbalance.
2. Poor constitution (constitutional vulnerability) is the more popular term for an inherited susceptibility to disease.
3. Possible examples include (there are many):

Barrier	Risk factor	Disease
Bony skeleton	Low calcium in diet Inactivity Menopause	Tendency to fracture (osteoporosis)
Skin	Long-term sun exposure	Early ageing Skin cancer
Wound healing	Diet low in vitamin C	Scurvy (poor wound healing)
Immune system	Unprotected sex	HIV infection

4. Possibilities include:
   (i) prolonged sun exposure/repeated sunburn
   (ii) use of sun beds
   (iii) fair skin.
5. Possibilities include:
   (i) seat belt legislation
   (ii) speed cameras
   (iii) prohibition of drink-driving.
6. Conventionally accepted risk factors for heart disease include smoking, a high-fat diet and physical inactivity. Preventive medicine would therefore attempt to reduce susceptibility to heart disease by focusing on smoking reduction, reducing fatty foods in the diet and increasing levels of activity.
   There are many possible preventative approaches. These include:
   (i) Aimed at the individual: counselling to stop smoking, prescription of nicotine patches, dietary advice, exercise instruction.
   (ii) Public health measures: banning cigarette advertising, health warnings on cigarette packets, food labelling to show fat content, provision of low-cost access to leisure centres.

Chapter 2.1b Barriers to disease: wound healing

LEARNING POINTS

At the end of this chapter you will:
- be able to describe the stages in the healing of a wound
- be familiar with the pathology of poor wound healing, chronic skin ulcers and keloid scars.

Estimated time for chapter: 60 minutes.

Introduction

From now on the content of the text is focused much more on the diseases that affect the human body. The contents of this and many of the future chapters will have the following structure:

- the physiology of a particular topic or physiological system is described
- based on this understanding of how the healthy body should function, the pathology relevant to the topic or system (i.e. what happens when disease causes imbalance) is explored
- the conventional medicine approach to treatment of the diseases that have been described is discussed
- comparisons with the language of one holistic medical perspective, that of Chinese medicine, are brought in wherever possible. These 'translations' relate to physiology, pathology and the effects of medical treatments. To distinguish these from the main part of the text, this text is be presented in characteristic boxes. The rationale for these comparisons is explained in detail in the Note to the Reader in the preliminary pages of this book.

The role of wound healing and clotting

The processes of wound healing and clotting were introduced in Chapter 2.1a as two of the mechanical barriers to disease. It was pointed out that these are different from the purely structural barriers of skin, mucous membranes and bone. Instead, they are both dynamic processes that are set in motion after injury has occurred. They prevent the damage from worsening, and enable repair to take place. In this way, their role is similar to that of the immune system.

This chapter focuses on wound healing. The principles of blood clotting are studied in Chapter 2.1c.

The physiology of wound healing

A description of the mechanism of wound healing is fundamental to a full understanding of how the body responds to disease. There are many situations in disease when the healthy structure of the body tissues is damaged and has to be repaired by means of this delicate process. The formation of a blood clot is the first stage of wound healing, and this is described in more detail in Chapter 2.1c.

Wound healing is least complicated when the injury is clean and there has been a simple cut or puncture to the tissues rather than a loss of tissue. With a clean cut or a puncture the edges of the wound can stay in alignment with each other, and this provides the conditions for the process known as 'primary wound healing' (or healing by first intention). If there has been loss of skin and underlying tissue, then the wound healing has to fill and repair a gaping hole. The reparative process is more complex, takes longer and is prone to complications resulting from trauma and infection. This is known as 'secondary wound healing' (or healing by second intention).

Primary wound healing

Primary wound healing can take place when the edges of a cut or puncture are in close opposition. Figure 2.1b-I illustrates the three stages of primary wound healing. The edges of the wound ooze blood from the broken capillaries, and the blood rapidly forms into a clot in the confined space. The blood clot releases chemicals that stimulate the process of 'chemotaxis', i.e. the attraction of the cells of the immune system (the leukocytes) and the fibroblasts (the connective tissue repair cells) into the region of the clot. The phagocytic ('engulfing') leukocytes move into the clot and absorb and remove cell debris, dirt and bacteria. Fibroblasts lay down a delicate network of fibrous strands that begin to bridge the gap formed by the wound. Into this meshwork the broken ends of the capillaries start to re-grow a new network of tiny vessels so that this developing scar tissue has a rich blood supply. At the same time, the deepest layer of the epithelium of the broken skin grows through the upper regions of the blood clot to close the breach formed by the injury. This stage is one of proliferation, and when the fibrous and capillary network is sufficiently strong it causes the scab, the dried blood clot overlying the wound, to drop away, leaving the pink and delicate scar tissue protected by a layer of new epithelium beneath. The proliferative stage takes 5–30 days. Over the next few days to weeks the maturation phase involves the delicate scar tissue becoming strengthened and more organised due to increasing amounts of fibrous tissue. The initially complex network of tiny capillaries is simplified in this phase. At the end of this phase what remains is a stronger, more densely structured and paler tissue than the newly formed scar.

Secondary wound healing

Secondary wound healing is the process that takes place when the wound leaves a gap in both the skin and the underlying connective tissue. Figure 2.1b-II illustrates the three stages of secondary wound healing. As is the case with primary wound healing, the first stage is the lining of this breach with a blood clot originating from blood that has oozed from the

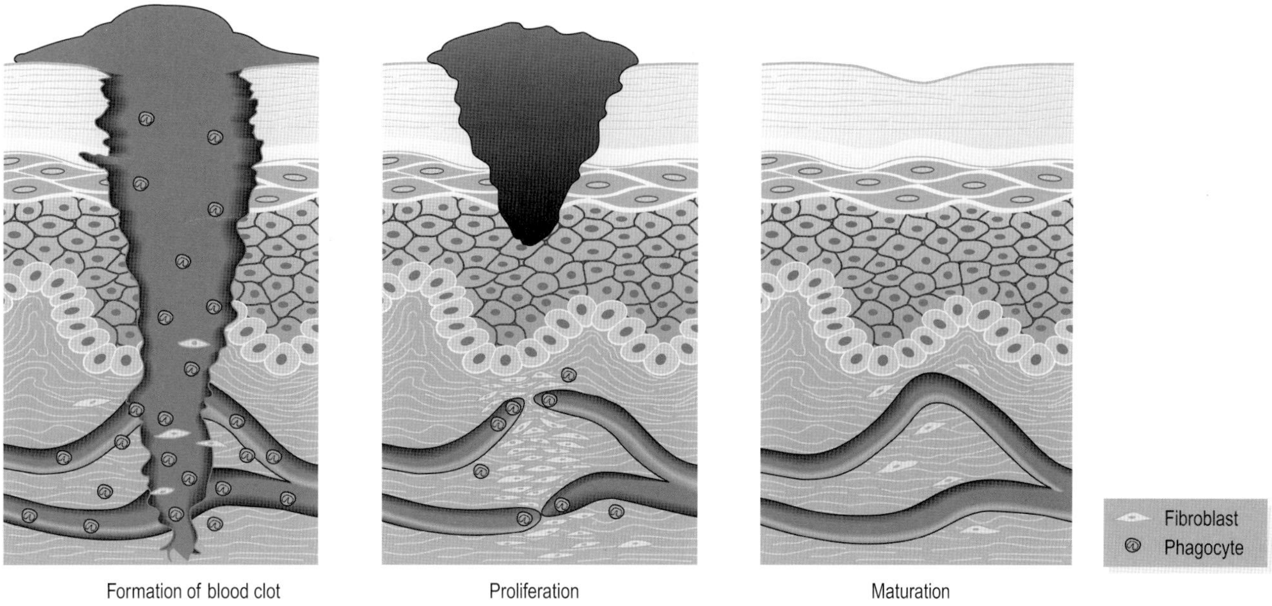

Figure 2.1b-I • The stages of primary wound healing (healing by first intention).

remaining damaged tissue. The clot encourages the ingrowth of new fibrous tissue and capillaries and the appearance of phagocytic cells to remove debris and bacteria. This delicate new tissue is known as 'granulation tissue'. This proliferative stage takes longer than the corresponding stage in primary wound healing, the time to healing being dependent on the size of the breach in the tissue, and the health and quality of blood supply to the underlying tissue. If foreign bodies (dirt) and bacteria are present they can be the focus for ongoing damage, and will further slow this stage of the healing process. The initially shallow layer of proliferating new tissue cannot yet be lined by epithelium and, once the scab drops away, it is instead covered by a moist yellowing layer of dead cells called 'slough'. Like the old blood clot, slough continues to be a stimulus for the chemotaxis of fibroblasts, leukocytes and new capillaries. Once the new scar tissue reaches the level of the edges of the broken skin epithelium, the new epithelium can grow inwards, closing the breach by degrees. Any breach in an epithelium is called an 'ulcer', which means that secondary wound healing always involves the formation of an ulcer. Ideally, the ulcer is gradually reduced in size until it is has been closed over entirely by new epithelium. Following the closure of the ulcer the maturation phase continues to strengthen and organise the new fibrous tissue until the healed wound eventually appears as a pale, shiny patch of tough new scar (see Q2.1b-1 and Q2.1b-2).

The pathology of wound healing

In general, secondary wound healing is more likely to become problematic than is primary wound healing. This is because, in the former, the area of exposed wound is larger, and the new delicate granulation tissue is more likely to become damaged or infected.

There are a number of factors that can negatively affect the healthy course of wound healing. These include the state of nutrition of the body, the richness of the blood supply to the damaged tissue, and the age of the person. In malnutrition, the response of the immune system, and also the connective tissue healing, is less efficient. Scurvy, the disease resulting from vitamin C deficiency, is particularly associated with poor wound healing.

In old age, the connective tissue supporting the skin is less vital and is more easily damaged, and the healing response is less rapid. A compromised blood supply, such as occurs in arteriosclerosis (see Chapter 3.2c), will also reduce the speed and effectiveness of healing, as it is the blood that is the source of nutrients and immune cells to the tissues.

Diabetes mellitus (see Chapter 5.1d) is a condition in which the blood supply to the tissues may be compromised. In addition, there are two other factors in diabetes that have an impact on wound healing. First, the nerve supply to the tissues may be deficient, meaning that injuries are more easily sustained; and, secondly, there is an increased risk of minor infections taking hold. For these three reasons, wound healing can be very problematic for a person with diabetes.

Finally, a wound may not heal if it becomes infected or if it becomes repeatedly damaged. This is why such careful attention is given to the application of sterile, strong and breathable dressings in the surgical management of wounds (see Q2.1b-3).

Chronic skin ulcer

If a patient has a condition that leads to impaired wound healing, a wound may reach a state of becoming resistant to becoming fully healed. This is particularly likely if it is secondary rather than primary wound healing that is taking place. In such patients, the granulation tissue can easily become

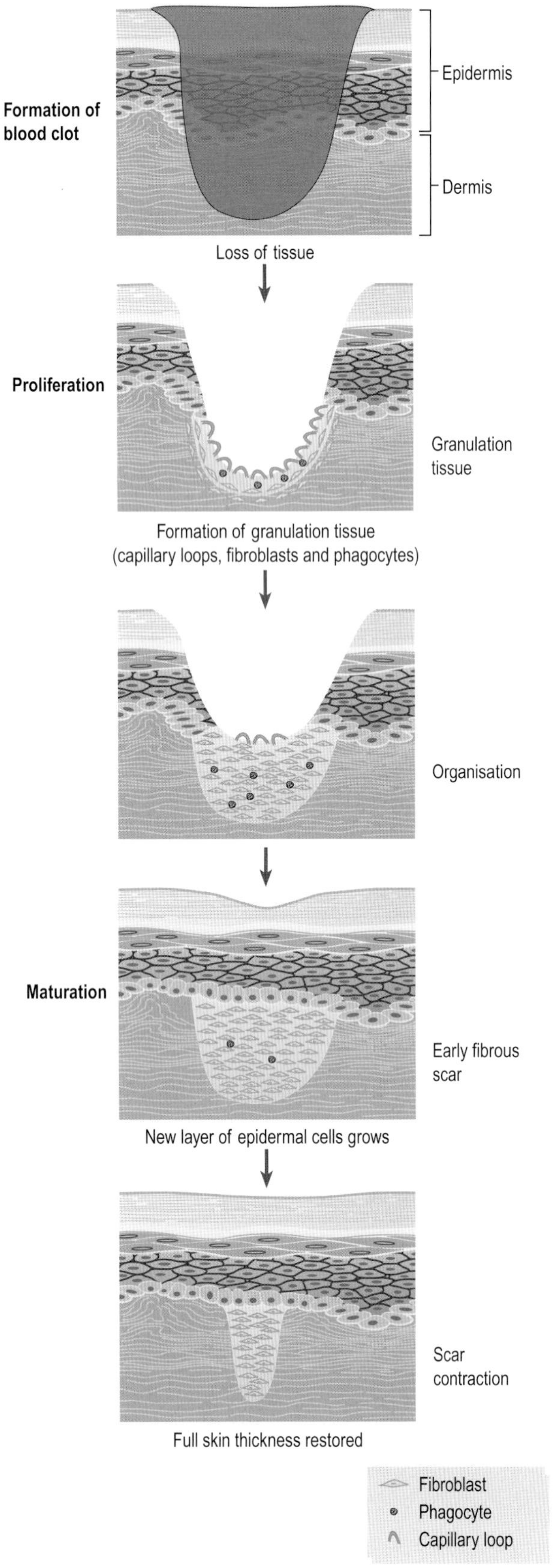

Figure 2.1b-II • The stages of secondary wound healing (healing by second intention).

infected or damaged, and the wound repeatedly oozes or bleeds. This prevents new skin from growing to close the gap. Such a condition is known as a 'chronic skin ulcer'.

The term 'chronic' refers to the fact that a condition is of long standing. The opposite of the term chronic is 'acute', meaning 'short lived'. Contrary to popular understanding, the medical use of these terms does not tell us anything about severity of a condition.

A chronic skin ulcer is a condition that is a cause of great disability, because a continually discharging wound is both exhausting and painful. Ulcers also carry a long-term risk as a source of infectious organisms, and may result in the need for amputation. Patients with diabetes, poor circulation, immobility and/or malnutrition are particularly at risk of developing a chronic ulcer. The lower legs and areas in which there is repeated damage (e.g. the feet) or pressure (e.g. the buttocks) are the most common sites for ulcers to develop.

Keloid scars

In some people, scars can heal in an abnormal way, with an excessive production of fibrous tissue. This poorly understood condition leads to raised lumps of scar tissue at the site of even minor wounds. These overgrown areas of scarring are known as 'keloid' scars. These can be a cause of distress for the patient, because they can be cosmetically unsightly. Keloid formation appears to be more common in black skin.

Keloid scars are considered very difficult to treat, as simple surgical removal may lead to a scar that produces another keloid. Injection of a corticosteroid preparation into the scar may reduce the swelling in some people.

Conventional and treatment of wounds

There are some basic principles that are conventionally followed to enable wounds to heal. These include:

- prevent infection by removing any foreign matter or dead or dying tissue
- encourage primary wound healing if possible by opposing and stitching the sides of clean wound
- protect the healing area with a sterile, breathable, dry dressing
- treat any infection rapidly by cleaning and the use of antibiotics, which are either applied to the wound or taken by mouth.

Prevention and treatment of poor wound healing and ulcers

In general, there are four broad approaches to someone who is at risk of poor wound healing:

- Prevention of injury: e.g. attentiveness to skin care in diabetes, and prevention of falls in the elderly.
- Treatment of the underlying cause: e.g. vitamin supplements and increased carbohydrate and protein in the

diet in malnutrition, and improvement of blood supply by means of vascular surgery or drugs that affect the circulation.

- Attentive care to any wound that occurs: the basic principles of enabling wound healing are essential to support healing in vulnerable groups such as the elderly or diabetics.
- A chronic ulcer requires regular sterile dressing and cleansing of the open wound area: there can be increasing problems with recurrent infection as the bacteria become resistant to the repeated use of antibiotics. Methicillin-resistant *Staphylococcus aureus* (MRSA) has become a particular problem in chronic wounds in recent years, as this form of the normally harmless skin bacterium is now resistant to all the common antibiotics and can become a life-threatening condition in the immunocompromised. Ideally, the patient should be under the care of a specialist nursing team, as there is now great expertise in approaches to the healing of ulcers (see Q2.1b-4).

Chapter 2.1c Barriers to disease: blood clotting

LEARNING POINTS

At the end of this chapter you will:
- understand the principles of how the blood clots
- be familiar with the pathology of insufficient platelets
- be familiar with the pathology of haemophilia.

Estimated time for chapter: 60 minutes.

The physiology of blood clotting

It is a common experience to observe blood clotting rapidly if the skin or mucous membranes become damaged. Gradually, and particularly if the wound is held closed or is padded, the flow of blood from the wound slows down and is replaced by a dark, initially rubbery, mass of congealed blood.

If a syringe of fresh blood is left untouched at room temperature, within a few minutes the blood within it will have separated into a solid clot and a clear fluid known as 'serum'. The serum is the original fluid component of the blood, whereas the clot contains all the blood cells within its solid mass.

For the purposes of this chapter, it is helpful to understand that the blood consists of a clear fluid (plasma) that contains a vast range of nutrients, salt and proteins, and three broad groups of cells: the red blood cells (erythrocytes), the white blood cells (leukocytes) and much smaller cells called 'platelets' (thrombocytes). This composition of the blood is described in some detail in Chapter 3.4a.

The role of the platelets in clotting

Platelets are tiny cells without nuclei that are continually produced within the bone marrow. Their function is to work together with the clotting-factor proteins in the plasma to enable an efficient and controlled clotting reaction. Platelets circulate for only a few days in the blood before they start ageing and are removed and broken down in the spleen. If the platelet level falls too low, the kidneys release a hormone

Information box 2.1b-1

Wound healing: comments from a Chinese medicine perspective

The Chinese medicine view is that a wound, by disruption of Qi and Blood flow in local Channels, causes impaired flow of Qi and Blood, and thus local Qi and Blood Stagnation. The pain and formation of the blood clot are physical reflections of this. However, here is an example of when Qi and Blood Stagnation perhaps may not necessarily signify a wholly negative energetic state, because in this case from a conventional perspective the pain and blood clot are both essential to help the healing process.

The intricate processes of healthy wound healing may be seen as manifestations of strong Upright Qi and Blood, and these permit a return to normal flow of the vital substances.

An area of scarring will always be left with a degree of Qi and Blood Deficiency (indicated by the lack of elasticity and patches of numbness associated with scars), but this will be minimal if healing by first intention is possible. This should make sense from the perspective of Chinese medicine, because if the edges of the wound can be brought together it will mean that the natural flow of the Qi and Blood in the area is less likely to be disrupted.

If the damage to the area is large and the original shape of the tissues cannot be restored, Qi and Blood Stagnation is likely to be prolonged, and long-term Qi and Blood Deficiency in the area more marked. In the case of scars that remain painful, this suggests persisting Qi and Blood Stagnation.

Wound healing is dependent on healthy tissues with a rich blood supply and an ability to fight infection. This would suggest that any conditions that involve poor wound healing might point to either a local or a general Blood and Qi Deficiency. In addition, an inherited tendency to poor healing or the poor wound healing seen in old age could indicate an underlying factor such as Jing (Kidney Essence) Deficiency.

Healing wounds sometimes ooze blood and fluid. This could suggest the presence of local Heat and/or Damp. However, in western medicine people with local problems such as this often manifest a number of other symptoms such as poor circulation and cold extremities. This might suggest that the poor wound healing is connected with wider systemic problems such as Deficiency of Spleen Qi and Spleen not Holding Blood. This is particularly the case in a chronic ulcer, in which poor healing of the underlying flesh might well point to the involvement of the Spleen, which is responsible for the tone and quality of flesh in general.

By contrast, the lumpiness of keloid scars might be interpreted as a manifestation of Phlegm. Preventing a keloid from forming with steroid injections could be interpreted as reducing local Stagnation and Phlegm, but may be a suppressive treatment, as described in Chapter 1.3b. Steroid injections are recognised to cause thinning and weakening of tissues, and so the benefits of local improvements may come at the price of subsequent local deficiencies of Qi and Yin.

called 'thrombopoietin', which stimulates the bone marrow to generate more platelets to redress the balance. The spleen serves as a store for platelets and can release these in time of stress, such as during a haemorrhage.

Platelets are very sensitive to changes in the blood vessel walls. If a blood vessel wall becomes damaged in any way, the platelets that move past the damaged area respond by adhering to it and then forming a clump around the damaged area. This change is also accompanied by a release of a hormone called serotonin (5HT), which stimulates the damaged vessel to constrict. The sticky platelets also release a chemical called adenosine diphosphate (ADP), which attracts more platelets to the site of damage so that the platelet clump enlarges.

Both these changes, the platelet clumping and the narrowing of the passage through the blood vessel, serve to block the blood flow and reduce any bleeding that might be occurring at the site of the damage. If the wound is small, the platelet plug may be sufficient to stem the bleeding totally in the short term.

The role of the clotting factors in clotting

The platelet plug is not sufficiently strong to stem the bleeding from larger wounds or to be maintained for any length of time. Under these circumstances the clotting proteins, a family of 12 different proteins produced by the liver and dissolved in the plasma of the blood, come into play. These proteins undergo a dramatic series of changes at the site of injury that enable the platelet plug to be strengthened.

There are two stimuli that encourage the clotting factors to undergo change. The first is tissue damage and the release of certain chemicals that result from this. These chemicals react rapidly with some of the clotting factors to result in the change of factor II (prothrombin) into an activated form called 'thrombin'. Thrombin then stimulates the change of factor I (a soluble protein called 'fibrinogen') into the fibrous and insoluble fibrin.

The second stimulus that affects other clotting factors, but less rapidly, is triggered by the formation of the platelet plug. The end result of this change in this other group of clotting factors is the same as that triggered by tissue damage (i.e. the formation of activated thrombin and then insoluble fibrin).

The change of fibrinogen to fibrin can be compared to the change that occurs when heat is applied to the soluble albumin contained in egg white, which then becomes the white solid of cooked egg – a small change in the external environment generates an irreversible change in the molecular structure and physical nature of the protein. So it is with fibrinogen; a small change induced by thrombin causes the production of insoluble fibres that are deposited as a network at the site of tissue damage. This fibrin network traps blood cells and thereby forms the familiar rubbery mass of a blood clot.

This process would carry on unchecked without an opposing process known as 'fibrinolysis'. In fibrinolysis, chemicals released through the activation of clotting factors and from the lining of blood vessels lead to the activation of a plasma protein called 'plasmin'. Plasmin acts to break down fibrin fibres, and so its production helps to ensure that the clotting process is never excessive.

The balance of clotting is so delicate that its precise control is not clearly understood in conventional medicine. It seems that, with these closely opposed mechanisms of clotting and fibrinolysis, it is almost as if the body can sense when a clot is of sufficient size for the positive feedback process of its formation to stop, and the opposing process of fibrinolysis to begin.

The miraculous nature of this degree of sensitivity and balance in the control of clotting becomes apparent when the balance is lost in certain disease states. In some conditions the blood does not clot sufficiently, and this results in excessive bleeding and bruising. In other conditions, excessive blood clot formation is the problem, as it impairs the free circulation of blood in the vessels (see Q2.1c-1-Q2.1c-3).

The pathology of insufficient clotting

Clotting will be impaired if either the number of platelets or the amount of blood clotting factors is insufficient.

Insufficient platelets (thrombocytopenia)

The condition wherein there are insufficient platelets is known as 'thrombocytopenia' (literally meaning 'too few thrombocytes'). This can be the result of a poorly understood immune reaction, when it is called 'autoimmune thrombocytopenic purpura' (AITP), or can be a rare side-effect of some drug treatments. As platelets are formed in the bone marrow, any condition that damages the bone marrow will also reduce the platelet numbers, as well as the numbers of all the other types of blood cells. Thrombocytopenia, therefore, also occurs in bone marrow failure. The causes of bone marrow failure include cancer spreading in the bone marrow, and toxic reactions to drugs and radiation (see Chapter 3.4c). An enlarged spleen can also cause thrombocytopenia. This is because one of the roles of the spleen in health is to store excess platelets, and when the size of the spleen is excessive, too many platelets become hidden from the circulation within the spleen.

The main symptoms and signs of thrombocytopenia are those that result from insufficient stemming of bleeding from broken blood vessels. These include easy bruising, nosebleeds and heavy periods in women. Purpura are clusters of tiny pinpoint bruises that are a characteristic of thrombocytopenia, and can appear in 'showers' on areas of skin that are exposed to minor trauma.

The treatment of thrombocytopenia is dependent in part on the underlying cause. In AITP and drug-related thrombocytopenia, mild cases may settle on their own or may respond to oral corticosteroid medication (prednisolone tablets). In severe, chronic (long-standing) cases, a surgical option is the removal of the spleen (splenectomy) so that the reduced numbers of platelets are not reduced further by this organ (this operation is described in Chapter 3.4d). In cases when the numbers of platelets are so low as to lead to a risk of life-threatening bleeding, platelets can be extracted from donated blood and given by transfusion (see Q2.1c-4).

Clotting (coagulation) disorders

Diseases involving insufficiency of one or more of the 12 clotting factors are known as the 'coagulation (clotting) disorders'. 'Haemophilia' is a term used to describe the range of disorders of blood coagulation that result from defective production of clotting factors. The three most common forms of haemophilia are haemophilia A, haemophilia B (Christmas disease) and von Willebrand's disease.

Haemophilia A is an X-linked recessive condition, affecting 1 in 5,000 of the male population. X-linked recessive inheritance means that the gene defect is carried on the X chromosome, and so is rarely expressed in girls because a defective gene from both parents is required for this to happen. As boys only have one X chromosome, they need inherit the defect from only one parent or to have a single spontaneous mutation to develop the condition. The disorder results from defective production of clotting factor VIII. The gene that codes for the production of this factor is found on the X chromosome. Some gene defects lead to more severe forms of the disease than others.

Bleeding in factor VIII deficiency tends to manifest in the joints and within muscles much more than is the case in thrombocytopenia. This means that a person with haemophilia might suddenly experience an acutely hot swollen joint (haemarthrosis) or a painful swelling in a muscle (haematoma). As free blood stimulates a powerful reaction from the immune system, it can cause damage and scarring when confined in a joint capsule or in the body of the muscle. Serious long-term complications include joint deformity and contracted muscles. Some patients become wheelchair bound.

The bleeding in haemophilia A is usually treated by means of replacement of factor VIII. This has to be given intravenously (by means of injection into a vein). Factor VIII can also be obtained from the plasma of pooled donated blood. This is now recognised to carry the risk of transmission of as yet uncharacterised infectious disease that may originate from donated blood. The risk is all the greater because clotting factors have to be derived from pooled blood donated by many people.

In the 1980s and 1990s it became clear that thousands of people with haemophilia had contracted HIV and hepatitis C infections through receiving contaminated factor VIII. Many people died, or are continuing to suffer from the consequences of these infections. The treatment was given before these diseases were recognised or their mode of transmission was clearly understood. Although blood products are now screened and treated for these viruses, there is still a possibility that they contain as yet uncharacterised transmissible agents. A genetically engineered form of factor VIII (recombinant) has been developed that does not carry this risk, although this is not yet universally available.

Haemophilia B (Christmas disease) is clinically very similar to haemophilia A. It too is an X-linked recessive condition, but results from the absence of clotting factor IX. It affects 1 in 30,000 males.

Von Willebrand's disease results from a deficiency of a factor that aids in both platelet adherence and the action of factor VIII. This rare form of haemophilia is a recessive condition because the defective gene is found on chromosome pair 12 rather than on an X chromosome.

In all three of the above described conditions, the severity of the condition depends on the precise nature of the genetic defect (see Q2.1c-5).

Information box 2.1c-1

Insufficient clotting: comments from a Chinese medicine perspective

In Chinese medicine, abnormal bleeding may be described in terms of four syndromes. These are Spleen Qi Deficiency with Spleen not holding Blood (bleeding tends to be in lower parts of the body), Full Heat, (causing profuse bleeds), Yin Deficiency with Empty Heat (less profuse blood; can be a cause of purpura) and Blood Stagnation (dark blood with pain).

Thus the characteristics of these syndromes may be observed in varying degrees in different patients with problems in blood clotting. It would make sense that Yin Deficiency underlies the bleeding in both thrombocytopenia and haemophilia, as the cause of both is a deficiency in the components of the blood. Blood as a body substance carries many of the properties that the Chinese equated with Yin (being for example fluid in nature and nourishing in action).

The purpura in thrombocytopenia might be described in terms of Empty Heat causing blood to leave the blood vessels, whereas profuse bleeds are more in keeping with a diagnosis of Full Heat. It is interesting to note that the site of the destruction of the platelets is the Spleen. It would make sense from this observation that Spleen not holding Blood may also be an aspect of the diagnostic picture in clotting disorders.

The clotting factors are manufactured in the liver, so this would support a suggestion that Liver Qi Stagnation could be part of the diagnostic picture in the bleeding in haemophilia. Haemophilia can lead to painful joint bleeds and fixed deformities and contractures of the muscles, which in Chinese medicine are likely to be attributed to Stagnation of Liver Qi and Blood.

Treatment of both involves replacing the missing blood components with a transfusion of concentrates from donated blood. This could be described as a form of Nourishing Yin. Transfusion, however, has a wide range of possible side-effects, including allergic reactions, suggesting that there is a risk that Pathogenic Factors may be introduced at the same time.

Disorders of excessive clotting

The disorders of excessive or inappropriate clotting are thrombosis, embolism and infarction. These together are classed as one of the seven basic processes of disease, and are introduced in Chapter 2.2a and discussed in detail in Chapter 2.2d.

Chapter 2.1d Barriers to disease: the immune system

LEARNING POINTS

At the end of this chapter you will be able to:

- recognise the lymphatic system as the structural basis of the immune system
- understand the role of white blood cells and antibodies in the immune response
- understand the principles of immunity and immunisation.

Estimated time for chapter: 100 minutes.

Self-test 2.1c

Barriers to disease: blood clotting

1. What components of the blood are essential in the clotting process?
2. What might your treatment principles be for a 15-year-old patient with haemophilia?
3. What precautionary measures do you think should be taken before using acupuncture to treat someone with haemophilia or thrombocytopenia?

Answers

1. The platelets and the 12 clotting factors are the essential components involved in the building up of a blood clot. The process of fibrinolysis (involving tissue plasminogen activator and plasminogen) keeps the size of clot under control.
2. A 15-year-old patient with haemophilia may have suffered joint damage and muscle contractures as a result of joint bleeds in childhood. A fundamental treatment principle will be to Nourish Blood and Yin. There may be need to move Liver Qi and Blood, both local to the painful joints, and generally to Nourish Tendons.
3. In both patients, you should be aware that there is an increased risk of bleeding from points. It is impossible for you to assess the full risk of bleeding in your patient, and so you should always discuss your plans for treatment with the patient's doctor before you consider needling.

It may be worth considering the non-puncture treatment alternatives in Chinese medicine such as the use of moxa, external stimulation of points and herbs.
Cupping should be avoided as this promotes bleeding under the skin.

Introduction

A healthy immune system protects against diverse infectious diseases and the development of cancer. It also plays a vital role in the removal of dead or damaged tissues. If it is out of balance, intractable infections, allergies, autoimmune disease and cancer can result.

This chapter explores the physiology of the immune system and immunity in health. The consequences of deficiency in the immune system, including infections, cancer, allergies and autoimmune disease, are described in Section 2.2.

The physiology of the immune system

A crucial difference between the immune system and the other physical barriers to disease is that it is able specifically to distinguish foreign material (e.g. a microbe) within the body and initiate a series of events to neutralise and remove that foreign material.

The structure and function of the immune system can be summarised very broadly as follows:

- the immune system is made up of six different types of white blood cells (leukocytes) that work together to perform the role of protection
- the immune system is able to recognise foreign material
- recognition of foreign material enables the immune cells to make the foreign material harmless to the body through a series of events known as the 'immune response'
- the lymphatic system can be considered to be the home of the immune system.

The lymphatic system

All tissues are bathed in fluid that originates from blood capillaries. This tissue fluid is drained away via vessels called 'lymphatic vessels'. The lymphatic vessels are a complex network of streams that eventually converge to return 3 litres of fluid a day back to the blood circulation at a meeting with the major veins deep in the thorax. As they start to converge, the lymphatic vessels pass through lumps of tissue called 'lymph nodes'. The lymph nodes act as filters for this fluid, and their role is to cleanse the lymph of any foreign matter such as microbes, cancer cells and cell debris.

The network of lymphatics approximately follows the course of the arteries and veins in the body. Like the arteries and veins, the lymphatic system consists of larger vessels deep within the body, which branch repeatedly outwards to form tiny networks of vessels lined only with a single layer of flattened epithelial cells at the periphery of each of the organs and other body parts. Figure 2.1d-I illustrates the distribution of the lymphatic vessels and the lymph nodes in the body and the way in which the lymphatic system drains into the subclavian veins within the upper thorax.

Apart from the lymphatic vessels, the bulk of lymphatic tissue is in the form of lymph nodes, which can be found in deep and superficial groups throughout the body. The large superficial nodes cluster in groups that, when enlarged, can be felt through the skin in the neck (cervical nodes), the elbow and the armpit (trochlear and axillary nodes), at the back of the knee (popliteal nodes) and in the groin (inguinal nodes). There are other important lymph node groups deep within the chest (thoracic cavity), abdomen and pelvis. The structure of a typical lymph node is illustrated in Figure 2.1d-II. This figure demonstrates the fact that the lymphatic vessels contain valves that enable a one-way circulation of fluid throughout the lymphatic system and the nodes. It also shows that a lymph node consists of islands of dense 'lymphoid tissue' supported by looser ('reticular') connective tissue. This lymphoid tissue is the site of maturation of some of the white blood cells (leukocytes).

In addition to these nodes, lymphatic tissue is found in the form of the tonsils, appendix, spleen and thymus gland, as well as in clusters of cells, called 'follicles', distributed under the mucous lining of the respiratory and gastrointestinal tracts (mucosa-associated lymphoid tissue, or MALT). Each of these regions of the lymphatic system contains islands of lymphoid tissue similar to that found in the lymph nodes. The lymphatic system is structured in such a way that all fluid from the tissues drains through a series of nodes containing lymphoid and reticular tissue before being returned to the blood stream (see Q2.1d-1).

Figure 2.1d-I • The lymphatic system.

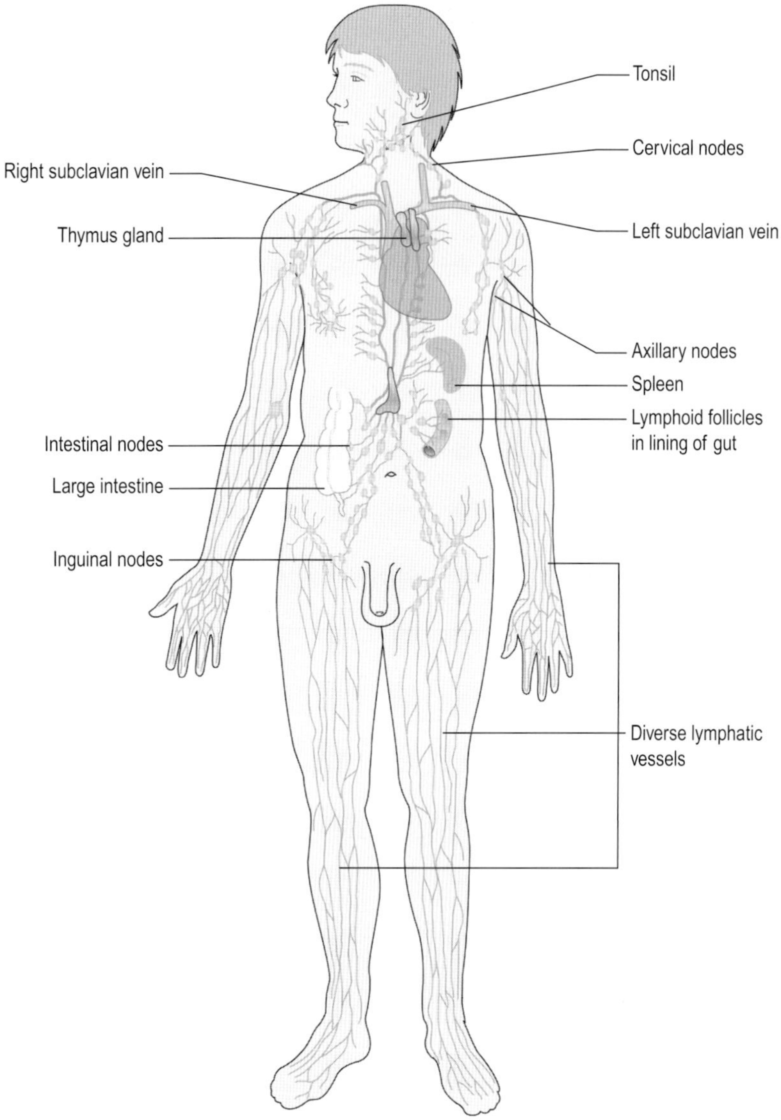

The leukocytes (white blood cells)

The three types of blood cells – red cells, white cells and platelets – are derived from a parent blood cell line that is continually dividing and maturing in the bone marrow. Various subtypes of immature white blood cells emerge from the bone marrow to enter the blood stream. Some of these subtypes that are important in the immune response are the T-lymphocytes, B-lymphocytes and phagocytes (e.g. the macrophages and neutrophils). Phagocytes are cells that have the amoeba-like ability to engulf and digest debris and other cells.

T-lymphocytes

The T-lymphocytes are so called because they undergo further maturation in the thymus gland, situated deep in the thorax (see Figure 2.1d-I). While still in the bone marrow, each T-lymphocyte acquires an ability to recognise a very specific molecular shape (known as an 'antigen'). Myriad variations of the T-lymphocyte are formed at this stage in development, each with the ability to recognise a different antigen. It is understood that any T-lymphocytes that develop an ability to recognise a molecular shape that is found in healthy body tissue (i.e. a 'self' antigen) are rapidly inactivated, so that only those that recognise non-self antigens (e.g. proteins on viruses, bacteria, cancer cells and foreign cells) remain to emerge from the thymus gland and to re-enter the circulation.

B-lymphocytes

The B-lymphocytes develop in a similar fashion the bone marrow, so that myriad subtypes develop. The B-lymphocytes are not just able to recognise foreign antigens, but can also produce and export a protein with a precise structure that enables it to adhere to particular non-self antigens, and so is specifically targeted, rather like a guided missile. The protein manufactured by B-lymphocytes is called 'immunoglobulin'. The individual, specifically shaped immunoglobulin structures that the B-lymphocytes produce are known as 'antibodies'. The molecular shape of the antibody is such that it fits the shape of the antigen rather like a lock fits around a key.

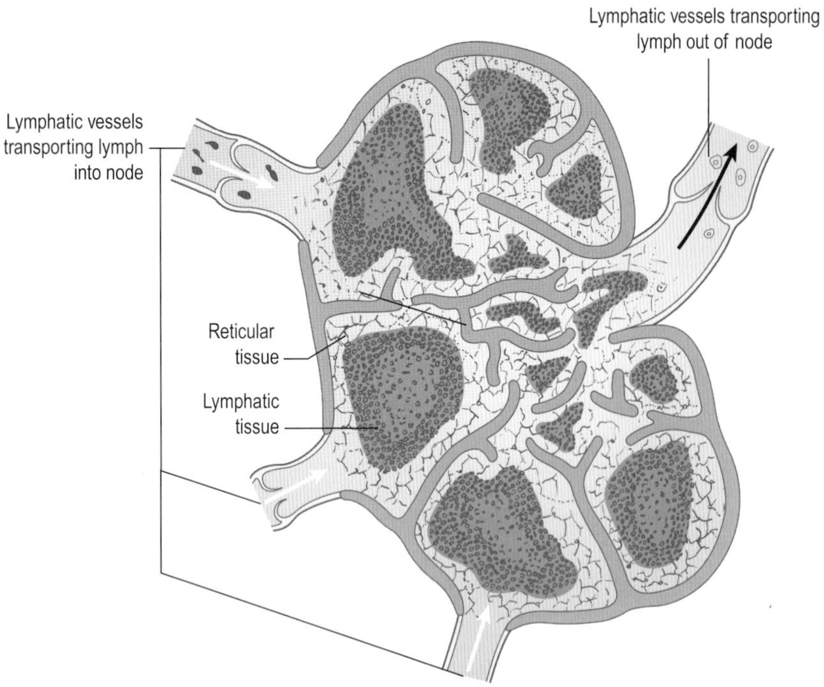

Figure 2.1d-II • Section through a lymph node.

The response of lymphocytes to antigens

When both B- and T-lymphocytes first meet up with a foreign antigen that they have a specific ability to recognise, they become 'sensitised' to it and are stimulated to multiply so that, in time, large numbers of antibodies and T-lymphocytes specific to that foreign antigen are produced. The immune system has a 'memory' for foreign antigens, which is reflected in the fact that if an antigen should be encountered a second time, this response of the sensitised immune cells to multiply and produce antibodies is much more rapid. For T-lymphocytes sensitisation occurs in the thymus gland, and for B-lymphocytes it occurs in the lymphoid tissue of the lymph nodes.

When the antigen 'key' fits the 'lock' of the T-lymphocyte surface or the circulating antibody produced by B-lymphocytes, a chain of events, known as the 'immune response', is triggered.

In the case of a T-lymphocyte, the connection with an antigen may first require the antigen to be 'presented' to the T-lymphocyte by means of one other immune cell, the macrophage. This intermediary role of the macrophage is not necessary for antigens on the surface of large cells, such as cancer cells. The recognition and connection with the non-self antigen triggers a change within the T-lymphocyte so that it will then act in diverse ways to enable the removal of the foreign matter. Subtypes of T-lymphocytes act in different ways to do this. Cytotoxic T-lymphocytes recognise and respond to foreign, cancerous and infected cells, and inject toxins to destroy them. Helper T-lymphocytes multiply to produce chemicals to support the other immune cells. These 'cytokines', which include interleukins and interferons, stimulate the action of cytotoxic T-lymphocytes and macrophages. Helper T-lymphocytes also appear to be important in enabling the role of the B-lymphocytes in the production of antibody in the lymph nodes. Again, the cytokines are important in this role. A third category, the suppressor T-lymphocyte, is important in modulating the immune response so that it is not too excessive and is not directed towards self antigens. Finally, the memory T-lymphocyte persists to stimulate the production of specific cytotoxic, helper and suppressor T-lymphocytes when the need arises. The different roles of the T-lymphocytes are illustrated in Figure 2.1d-III.

The B-lymphocytes that leave the bone marrow migrate and lodge in lymphoid tissue, and here they stay. In the presence of foreign antigens, sensitised helper T-lymphocytes drawn from the circulation encourage the expansion of specific B-lymphocytes into specific antibody-producing 'plasma cells'. The plasma cell has a very short life of less than a day, but in this time produces antibody that can circulate in the blood stream and target the foreign antigens. The short life of the plasma cell means that, once the antigen has been removed, the antibody response ceases. Memory B-lymphocytes persist to stimulate the production of more plasma cells should the need for more antibody continue. The production of the two forms of B-lymphocytes is illustrated in Figure 2.1d-IV.

The immune complex and activation of complement

When antigen-specific antibody is circulating in the blood stream the connection of antibody with the antigen on the surface of the foreign matter forms a structure called an 'immune complex'. The characteristic shapes of immune complexes are recognised by phagocytic (cell-engulfing) leukocytes such as neutrophils and macrophages, which are then stimulated to surround and digest the foreign matter. The antibody–antigen immune complex is also a trigger for the activation of a group of proteins in the blood stream called 'complement'. Activated complement is toxic to cells that are bound by antibodies, and it stimulates the healing response of inflammation (see Chapter 2.2b).

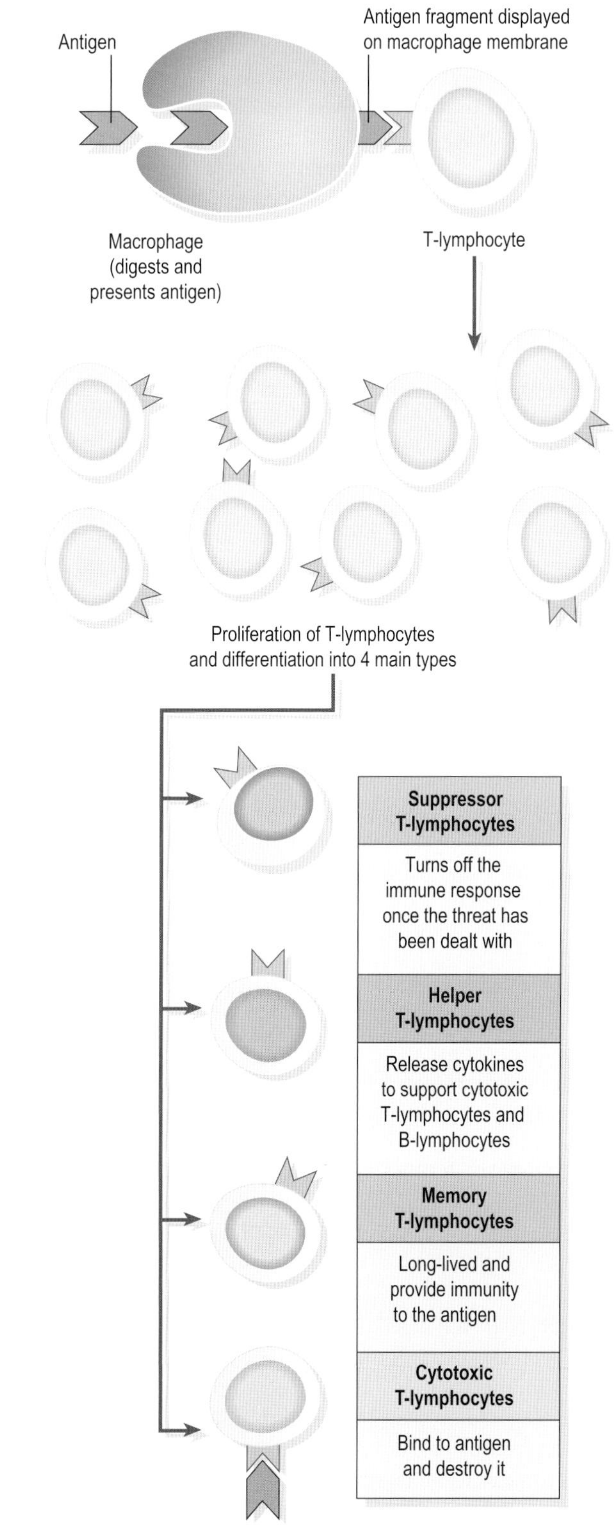

Figure 2.1d-III • The four types of T-lymphocyte.

Different forms of antibodies

Different forms of antibody are recognised, although each has a similar immunoglobulin (Ig) structure. Immunoglobulin M (IgM) is the antibody produced when a foreign antigen is first encountered by B-lymphocytes. A raised level of specific

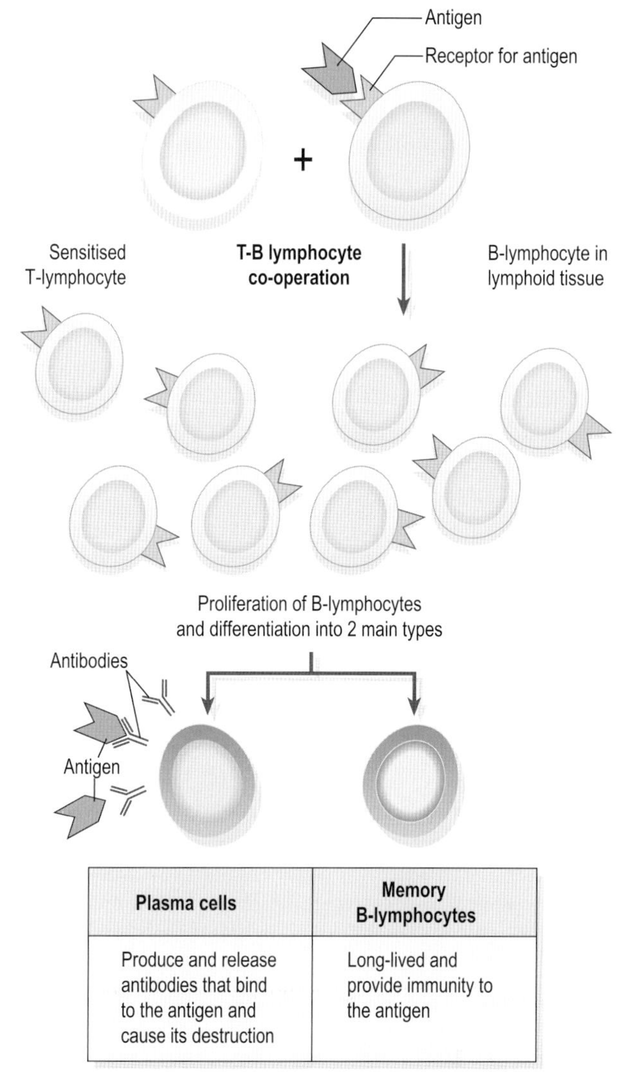

Figure 2.1d-IV • The two types of B lymphocytes.

IgM detected by a blood test tells the doctor that the patient is showing a first response to an infection. IgM is a particular trigger for the activation of the complement proteins that enable destruction of foreign organisms and stimulate inflammation, another very important aspect of the healing response to foreign material (see Chapter 2.2b).

IgG is the antibody that is produced once B-lymphocytes have been sensitised, and this will persist after an infection has settled down. If specific IgG levels are raised, this tells a doctor that a person has immunity to a condition.

IgA is a particular form of antibody produced in body fluids such as tears, saliva and breast milk. IgE is present on the surface of other leukocytes called 'basophils', 'eosinophils' and 'mast cells', which when they encounter antigens release chemicals that also stimulate inflammation.

The effect of the immune response

The immune response is a chain of reactions that culminates in the removal of the foreign material. To summarise, the aspects of the immune response that enable the foreign material to be removed include:

- the release of chemicals to attract more immune cells around the foreign material (complement and 'cytokines' from helper T-lymphocytes)
- the release of chemicals in response to immune complexes, which can break down and digest foreign material that has been bound by antibodies (complement)
- direct killing of foreign or damaged human cells (cytotoxic T-lymphocytes)
- phagocytosis of microbes and particles of other foreign material that have been bound by antibodies (neutrophils and macrophages)
- stimulation of the production of more antibodies (helper T-lymphocytes and plasma cells)
- the release of chemicals (complement, basophils, eosinophils and mast cells) to stimulate inflammation (a process that provides the best possible environment for the immune response to take place).

These reactions have the effects that are experienced by a patient suffering a microbial infection. The attraction of more immune cells and inflammation at the lymph nodes leads to swollen and tender lymph nodes (glands). In a generalised infection, all nodes can be affected. If the infection is in only one part of the body, for example in the thigh, only the local lymph glands, in this case the inguinal nodes, will be affected.

Release of various chemicals by the leukocytes into the blood stream can lead to the symptoms of fever and malaise. These may have a protective function in that they cause the patient to rest while the infection is being dealt with.

Immunity

'Immunity' describes the ability of the immune system to recognise foreign material, such as a microbe, and to produce an effective immune response. Immunity is the consequence of the B- and T-lymphocytes being able to become sensitised to foreign antigens and thereafter develop a memory to a specific infectious agent. Immunity enables a rapid immune response to an infection. In an immune person large quantities of IgG antibody can be produced so quickly that the infection may not be allowed to take hold. This ability of the immune system to respond tends to wear off with time, but the memory can be reinforced if the body has repeated encounters with a microbe in a short period of time.

The development of immunity explains why there are certain illnesses, such as chickenpox, which are usually experienced only once in a lifetime. During the initial infection, the immune system learns to develop very effective antibodies to the chickenpox virus. When the body next encounters chickenpox, these antibodies are reproduced so rapidly that the virus is destroyed and removed from the body before the infection can take hold (see Q2.1d-2).

Active immunisation

Active immunisation (vaccination) is a process through which the tendency of the body to develop a memory to foreign antigens is encouraged. The aim of active immunisation is to induce immunity to a certain disease, but without the risks inherent in first developing that disease.

Active immunisation involves the exposing the patient to a foreign material (a vaccine) that is very like a particular infectious agent or a toxic product of that agent. However, the ideal vaccine contains an infectious agent that has been altered so that it no longer has the properties that cause the original disease, and thus carries no risk of disease. The ideal vaccine still retains the antigens of the original infectious agent, so that the immune response is stimulated. In most cases the vaccine is administered by injection into a muscle or just under the skin. The exception to this rule is the live poliovirus vaccine (Sabin vaccine), which is administered by mouth. Vaccines usually need to be given more than once, as they are unlikely to stimulate as strong an immune response as the infectious disease itself. For example, in the UK the combination vaccine containing diphtheria, pertussis, tetanus, inactivated polio, and *Haemophilus influenzae* B vaccines (DTaP-IPV-Hib vaccine) is given to infants in a course of three successive injections separated by 4 weeks. All but the Hib component are then repeated at the preschool entry, and the DTa components may also be boosted at 10-yearly intervals thereafter.

Vaccines may come in the form of live, but attenuated, strains of the original infectious agent. The measles, mumps and rubella (MMR) vaccine contains three live attenuated viruses. These all induce an immune response, and can cause fever and even a rash in the recipient, but have been modified in a way that means a dangerous contagious infectious disease will not develop. Nevertheless, each of the three strains is sufficiently similar to measles, mumps and rubella that immunity to the diseases will result in 95% of those who receive the vaccination (this involves giving two doses separated by a minimum of 3 months).

Alternatively, some vaccines consist of agents that have been treated so that they no longer have infectious potential. For example, the tetanus immunisation carries no risk of causing infectious disease. This is because it contains formaldehyde-modified tetanus toxin ('toxoid'), which is sufficiently like the tetanus toxin to stimulate immunity, but modified as to no longer be toxic.

Passive immunisation

'Passive immunisation' is a term used to describe the administration of antibodies that confer immunity but do not stimulate an immune response or an immunological memory. Passive immunisation is achieved by preparing concentrates of immunoglobulin from the plasma of donated blood. Passive immunisation is useful when the risk of infection is high and there is no time to stimulate immunity by means of a course of vaccination, for example to prevent rabies after a bite from an infected dog.

Babies are born in a state of passive immunisation, as their mother's IgG antibodies remain circulating in their blood stream for a few weeks after birth. The protection these offer is reinforced by IgA antibodies present in breast milk (see Q2.1d-3-Q2.1d-5).

Information box 2.1d-1

The immune system: comments from a Chinese medicine perspective

A healthy immune system protects against diverse infectious diseases and the development of cancer. If it is out of balance it can lead to infections, cancer, allergy and autoimmune disease. According to Chinese medicine theory, healthy Wei (Defensive) Qi and its foundation, Kidney Yang, are required to protect against invasions of external Pathogenic Factors, so it might be an easy assertion to make that a healthy immune system suggests flourishing Wei Qi and Kidney Yang. The basis of Wei Qi and Kidney Yang is healthy Kidney Essence (Jing), which according to Chinese theory is the basis of constitutional strength.

However, from a broader perspective the health of the Qi of all the Organs, and in particular Zheng (Upright) Qi, is necessary for good health. In this way it is reasonable to suggest that there is no one Substance or Organ in Chinese medicine that directly corresponds to the immune system. A healthy immune system corresponds to a body with good Upright Qi and healthy Organs.

Wei Qi is the superficial defence against invasion of Pathogenic Factors. If strong, then invasions of Pathogenic Factors, and in particular Exterior Wind, cannot penetrate, and the person is protected from coughs, colds, chills and fevers. As defences from coughs and colds are considered to reside in the immune cells of the circulation and lymph nodes, as well as the integrity of the defences of the respiratory system, a physiological counterpart to the defensive Wei Qi might be the leukocytes of the immune system and the health of the tissues of the nose, throat and the respiratory tree.

The Chinese medicine view of the aspect of the immune function that protects against autoimmune disease and cancer is less easy to describe. The conventional view of these conditions is discussed in more detail in later chapters. Briefly, from a Chinese medicine viewpoint, both conditions occur on a background of long-standing deficiency of Blood, Kidney Yang and/or Yin. These two complex diseases are manifestations of the additional presence of Pathogenic Factors, including Heat, Damp, Blood Stagnation or Phlegm, which have accumulated as a consequence of the long-standing background deficiency.

With this understanding we can also see that the healthy immune system depends not only on healthy Wei Qi and Jing, but also healthy Vital Substances, Yin and Yang. This would fit with the general observation that any form of slight imbalance (e.g. feeling stressed or run down) can increase susceptibility to infections, irrespective of the nature of the imbalance.

The concept of acquired immunity following an infectious disease is also difficult to describe in Chinese medicine terms. On that basis it would have to be asserted that, following an infection, Wei (Defensive) Qi is actually strengthened. As a febrile disease is perceived as an invasion of an External Pathogenic Factor like Wind Heat, it appears that, when immunity is strengthened as a result of an infectious disease, this infection has, in the long term, had a beneficial outcome. It has been suggested, for example by Gascoigne (2000), that in some infectious diseases the appearance of a Pathogenic Factor on the Exterior is potentially beneficial because it represents the release of deeply rooted Heat Toxins. In this way minor infectious disease is seen as a potentially beneficial experience, through which deeper Pathogenic Factors can be expelled and Upright Qi strengthened.

Self-test 2.1d

Barriers to disease: the immune system

1. A patient of yours has noticed tender swollen lymph nodes in her left armpit for the past few days. She is worried that this might mean cancer of the breast. What is the common cause that might explain this finding?
2. Define the terms 'antigen' and 'antibody'.
3. How, in simple terms, does the invasion of a microbe lead to an immune response, clearance of the infection and acquired immunity?
4. Why, in conventional terms, do you think a vaccine has not been developed for the common cold?
5. What vital substances in Chinese medicine could play a role in immunity to:
   (i) the common cold
   (ii) measles infection
   (iii) onset of cancer.

Answers

1. Swollen lymph nodes in one part of the body suggest that there is activity of the immune system in the region of the body drained by those nodes. A short history and tender swelling is most likely the result of infection rather than a response to cancer cells. You could question and examine for any signs of infection in the left arm and hand and left breast (e.g. an inflamed insect bite).
2. An antigen is a protein on the surface of a foreign cell or other material that can trigger an immune response by being recognised as foreign by immune cells.
   An antibody is (an immunoglobulin) protein that is produced by B-lymphocytes in response to an antigen. The shape of the antibody matches that of the antigen like a lock fits around a key.
3. The invasion of a microbe introduces foreign proteins into the body.
   The microbe is drained from the tissue fluid of the body through lymphatics to lymph nodes, where the foreign protein is recognised (as antigen) by the lymphocytes.
   Antigen presented by macrophages is recognised by T- and B-lymphocytes, and this triggers the chain of reaction in the immune response.
   Part of this response involves the production of more antibody by B-lymphocytes. The immune response increases and the microbes are eventually destroyed and removed from the body. The immune system is left with a memory of the microbe antigens that will enable a much more rapid and effective response next time.
4. There are many different types of cold virus, each with different antigens. A vaccine would have to include all these antigens. This is not possible because of the great variety of cold viruses.
5. (i) Wei (Defensive) Qi and Jing.
   (ii) Wei (Defensive) Qi and Jing. Also, according to one theory, active acquired immunity against measles may be a consequence of elimination of toxic heat.
   (iii) Cancer is avoided by maintaining a healthy balance of the vital substances and Yin and Yang. It is considered to be preceded by depletion of one or more of these substances such as Blood or Kidney Yin.

2.2

Processes of disease

Chapter 2.2a Processes of disease

LEARNING POINTS

At the end of this chapter you will be able to:

- list the seven processes of disease
- describe which of the seven processes underlie the pathology of a given disease.

Estimated time for chapter: 30 minutes.

Introduction

This chapter introduces some ideas that lie at the foundation of how conventional medicine starts to classify disease. Within conventional medical thought, diseases can be classified according to different criteria. All systems of classification share the potential benefit of clarifying those features that disparate diseases may have in common, and thus aiding communication about these diseases.

Diseases may be classified according to cause, and this is known as 'classification by aetiology'. Understanding the language of aetiology is an essential prerequisite if the prevention of disease is to be considered. A classification system that focuses on the disease mechanisms (pathogenesis of disease) is a prerequisite for beginning to understand which treatments may be most effective for different diseases and also for predicting outcome (prognosis).

All systems of medicine, be they holistic or conventional, have their own systems of classification of aetiology and pathogenesis.

Aetiology of disease

'Aetiology', literally meaning 'the study of causes', is the term used to describe the cause of disease. From a conventional medical viewpoint, the cause of disease can be simplified into a few distinct categories, including:

- congenital defects (acquired between the time of conception and birth)
- infectious agents
- physical trauma (including extremes of temperature and radiation)
- effects of drugs, chemicals and toxins
- degeneration (resulting from overuse and ageing)
- psychological stressors
- unknown cause (idiopathic or essential)
- iatrogenic (caused by medical treatment) – this category will of course overlap with any one of the others.

The terms 'idiopathic' and 'essential' may be ascribed to diseases of unknown cause (e.g. idiopathic thrombocytopenic purpura and essential thrombocythaemia) (see Q 2.2a-1).

Processes of disease

'Pathogenesis' (literally 'the birth of disease') is the term used to describe the pathology of how disease develops. The diverse forms of the disease process can be grouped into seven broad categories:

- inflammation (redness, swelling, heat, pain and loss of function of tissues)
- tumours (excessive and inappropriate growth of cells)
- abnormal immune mechanisms (either under- or overactive immune responses)
- thrombosis, embolism and infarction (excessive and inappropriate clotting)
- degeneration (wearing out of tissues through ageing or trauma)
- metabolic abnormalities (homeostatic biochemical functions of the cells become imbalanced)
- genetic abnormalities (the cells carry defective genetic material that means they function in a less than healthy way)

From the perspective of the study of clinical medicine, classification of the processes of disease is important because it generates principles of causation of disease that can then be applied to all diseases. For example, if the process of inflammation is understood, then this will aid in the study of any one of the diseases that involves inflammation, such as arthritis, dermatitis, meningitis and pneumonia. Because the understanding of these basic processes of disease is fundamental to the study of the pathology of all diseases, they are explored in some depth in this text. The topics of inflammation, abnormal immune mechanisms, thrombosis, embolism and infarction, and tumours (cancer) are the subjects of the next four chapters.

Degeneration is the result of ageing. In general, ageing involves cell loss and atrophy of tissues. Rapidly regenerating active tissue may become replaced with tough, fibrous, less-active tissue, and organs may cease to function as effectively. Deformities (e.g. of skin, joints or bones) become commonplace. Degenerative diseases will be discussed in later chapters according to the physiological system which they affect.

The category of metabolic abnormality embraces all diseases that develop when the homeostatic function for metabolism (the chemical processes that go on continuously in living cells) becomes imbalanced. Again, the metabolic disorders are discussed throughout the text according to the physiological system which they affect.

The principles of genetic (congenital) abnormalities are presented in Chapter 1.1b, under the heading 'Mutation'.

An understanding of the processes of disease can also aid thinking about disease from the perspective of another medical system. If it is possible to consider each process of disease in terms of corresponding pathological descriptions described in another medical system, then it is possible to take these correspondences and use them to help describe pathological processes in all manner of diseases. For example, inflammation always involves the generation of redness and heat in tissues. According to Chinese medicine, redness and local heat always corresponds to the Pathogenic Factor of Heat. Therefore, it would be reasonable to conclude that all inflammatory diseases will be described, amongst other things, in terms of Heat in Chinese medicine. In this chapter, all the processes of disease are also interpreted in terms of Chinese medicine, and this will provide the foundation for the Chinese medicine interpretations of all the individual diseases described later in the text (see Q2.2a-2).

In summary, it cannot be overstated how much the understanding of the basic processes of disease can enrich the understanding of conventional pathology and how it might relate to another medical system such as Chinese medicine.

Information Box 2.2a-I

Processes of disease: comments from a Chinese medicine perspective

As a general introduction, it is important to explain the rationale for comparing the conventional view of the processes of diseases with a Chinese medicine understanding of pathology. As stated in the text, in the study of clinical medicine classification of the processes of disease is important because it generates principles of causation of disease, which can then be applied to all diseases. For example, an understanding of the process of inflammation will aid in the study of any disease that involves inflammation, such as arthritis, dermatitis, meningitis and pneumonia.

The important aspect of this system of classification is that, although the understanding of conventional processes would have involved knowledge that would not have been known to the ancient Chinese, the manifestations of the processes in signs and symptoms are consistent within each process. It is these that are the bridge between the two systems of medicine.

Inflammation will always have characteristics of heat and swelling, and degeneration will always involve a drying and withering of tissue. As observable phenomena, these would form the basis for making a diagnosis in Chinese medicine. However, the way in which the heat and swelling is generated in each individual case does not share the same consistent internal process as understood in the conventional view, and looking for parallels of process is a trap for the unwary.

When a patient presents with a condition that results from one or more of the seven processes of disease, it can reasonably be expected that the symptoms and signs normally associated with those processes are evident. The meaning and importance of the signs and symptoms can then be assessed within the entirely different understanding of the manifestation of symptoms and signs described in Chinese medicine. What this means is that the symptoms and signs of the conventionally described processes of disease will help point to the Chinese medicine syndromes that might be expected to be discerned in any medical condition, first assuming the underlying process of disease is recognised.

A Chinese energetic interpretation of inflammation

Inflammation is a basic response to tissue damage that results in increased blood flow to the tissues, swelling from increased tissue fluid, pain as a result of release of irritant cell contents and loss of function of the body part as a result of pain and swelling. Together these factors result in the five characteristics of inflamed tissue described in medicine as redness, swelling, heat and pain (or in Latin as rubor, tumour, dolor, calor), and loss of function.

In Chinese medicine the characteristics of redness and heat would automatically point to Heat. The excess tissue fluid would often be associated with an underlying Pathogenic Factor such as Damp, especially if there was any oozing of liquids or the swelling was considerable. The swelling in a clearly defined area would itself point to local stagnation, usually of Qi or Blood, and the character of the pain would indicate which. If inflammation is confined to one peripheral body part, the term 'Bi Syndrome' may be applied in Chinese medicine, as this describes localised manifestations of Pathogenic Factors, particularly in the region of the joints.

In conclusion, inflammation in the body might be described as evidence of Heat with Qi or Blood Stagnation, often with underlying Damp.

Continued

Information Box 2.2a-I—Cont'd

A Chinese energetic interpretation of tumours

Tumours result from excessive and inappropriate overgrowth of tissue cells. The underlying problem from a conventional medicine perspective is that the genetic control of cell multiplication has become disordered and the immune system has failed to recognise and control the growth of these disordered cells.

In Chinese medicine, substantial masses that do not move easily are usually regarded as manifestations of either Phlegm or Blood Stagnation (or sometimes a combination of both). Blood Stagnation is characterised by hardness and intense boring pain with violaceous colour changes. Phlegm is more often associated with numbness, and will usually develop against a backdrop of Heat and Damp, which will manifest in other signs and symptoms. For long-standing masses to develop there is often a pre-existing state of deficiency of Qi, as it is only healthy Qi moving freely that prevents the development of Stagnation and Phlegm. However, some masses can manifest against a background of good Upright Qi, the strength of which is often used to determine priorities in treatment.

In conclusion, tumours in the body might be described as evidence of Phlegm and/or Blood Stagnation on an underlying background of marked deficiency of Qi.

Chinese energetic interpretation of abnormal immune mechanisms

Abnormal immune mechanisms fall into two broad categories: those involving an insufficient response to infection, and those involving inappropriate responses, where there is hypersensitivity to specific stimuli or the misrecognition of the body's own cells as a threat.

In Chinese medicine, the functions of a healthy immune system are reflected in the concept of Healthy Upright Qi. The foundation of Healthy Upright Qi lies in Kidney Essence, and both are essential in maintaining Wei Qi. Some of the patterns of abnormal immune responses, for example, type I allergic hypersensitivity, are reflected in recognised patterns of disruption of Wei Qi, and suggest deficiencies either in Wei Qi or in the underlying Kidney Essence itself. Others, for example in multisystem autoimmune disease, present much more of a pattern of Full Pathogenic Factors against a background of long-term deficiency of Upright Qi or Kidney Essence.

In conclusion, inappropriate immune responses might be described as evidence of Deficiency of Upright Qi, Deficiency of Wei Qi and/or Kidney Essence.

Chinese energetic interpretation of thrombosis, embolism and infarction

Excessive blood clotting in the body is characterised by intense pain, coldness, violaceous coloration and loss of function. All these symptoms are associated with what is described in Chinese medicine as Stasis of the flow of Blood, with associated Stagnation of Qi in the affected tissues.

In conclusion, thrombosis, embolism and infarction might be described as evidence of Blood Stasis and Qi Stagnation.

Chinese energetic interpretation of degeneration

In conventional medicine, degeneration of tissues involves excessive cell death, poor healing responses and the formation of less vital tissues, with excessive fibrous tissue and deposits of substances such as calcium salts that impede healthy function. The resulting tissues tend to be less springy and soft and resilient, and also may manifest with deformities ('lumps and bumps').

In Chinese medicine language, all these changes, if seen across large areas of the body, would be primarily described in terms of broad deficiencies of Yin and Yang. More particularly, they are linked with a deficiency rooted in the Kidneys, and are characteristic of the ageing process as Kidney Essence depletes. The deposits and deformities are evidence of a widespread lack of flow of Qi, leading to an accumulation of Pathogenic Factors such as Phlegm and Damp and Blood Stagnation. If these are localised, there may be evidence of local Qi or Blood Stagnation impairing the flow of Qi to a part of the body.

In conclusion, degeneration of a body part might be described as evidence of Deficiency or Yin and/or Yang, in particular of Kidney Qi/Essence, leading to an accumulation of Phlegm/Damp and other Pathogenic Factors.

Chinese energetic interpretation of metabolic abnormalities

The metabolic diseases are complex and have diverse symptoms depending on the fundamental abnormality. Most metabolic diseases will be manifest in the function of all the body tissues and so reflect a fundamental and profound state of imbalance.

Chinese interpretations of metabolic disease will be equally complex, and are likely to describe deep deficiency. However, in Chinese medicine a profound and prolonged deficiency can often result in full Pathogenic Factors, which create complex patterns of signs and symptoms. As in conventional medicine, however, the effects are likely to be widespread in the system.

Chinese energetic interpretation of genetic abnormalities

A genetic abnormality may affect every cell in the body (if present from the time of conception), or may be the result of a developmental problem in the womb and thus affect some body parts and not others. From a conventional medicine perspective, there is no doubt that a congenital abnormality will compromise the health of the child and, unless carefully managed, is likely to affect the growth and development of the affected child.

The ancient Chinese interpreted congenital disease (i.e. a condition present from the time of birth) as a deficiency of Kidney Essence (Jing). To the Chinese, Kidney Essence was what determined a person's constitutional strength and is fundamental to healthy growth and development. Kidney Essence underlies the health of all the organs, and so more specific imbalances will often be present as the visible sequelae of the congenital disorder (e.g. of Spleen and Lung Qi in cystic fibrosis).

In conclusion, a congenital problem might be described as evidence of Primarily Jing deficiency, but may be described as a specific organ deficiency, depending on where the underlying genetic defect manifests.

Self-test 2.2a

Processes of disease

1. In your own words, describe each of the seven processes of disease.
2. Give one example of a disease with pathology resulting from each of the seven processes of disease.
3. Name one Chinese medicine diagnosis that might be associated with each disease process.

Answers

1. *Inflammation*: a response of tissues to damage.
   Tumours: excessive cell production leading to the development of a mass.
   Abnormal immune mechanisms: due to the normally protective immune system producing undesirable effects.
   Thrombosis, embolism and infarction: due to increased clotting of blood or abnormal changes in the blood vessel walls.
   Degeneration: due to deterioration of the body structures.
   Metabolic abnormalities: a loss of balance of the usual chemical processes that comprise metabolism.
   Genetic abnormalities: disease that is present in the fetus before birth, either due to a mutation of one of the gametes or to a mutation occurring during the development of the fetus.
2. Examples of diseases are too various to list. Refer to the table in the answer to the last question to check your answers.
3. Simple energetic interpretations of the seven process of disease are:
   Inflammation: Heat, Qi and Blood Stagnation with Damp.
   Tumours: Phlegm and/or Blood Stagnation on an underlying background of marked deficiency of basic substances (e.g. Yin and Yang).
   Abnormal immune mechanisms: deficiency of Kidney Qi and/or Wei Qi, and often underlying deficiency of basic substances (e.g. Yin and Yang, Blood, Jing, etc).
   Thrombosis, embolism and infarction: Blood and Qi Stagnation.
   Degeneration: deficiency, particularly of Kidney Qi.
   Metabolic abnormalities: complex.
   Genetic abnormalities: primarily Jing deficiency, but can manifest as a specific organ deficiency, depending on the underlying genetic defect.

Chapter 2.2b Inflammation

LEARNING POINTS

At the end of this chapter you will be able to:
- list the five characteristics of inflammation
- describe the essential role of inflammation in healing
- describe how inflammation can lead to symptoms of disease
- describe the pathology of boils and abscesses
- describe the pathology of fibrosis.

Estimated time for chapter: 90 minutes.

Physiology of acute inflammation

'Inflammation' is the term used to describe a complex bodily response to damage. The word is derived from the Latin words meaning 'to set on fire', because two manifestations of inflammation are heat and redness. Two other important features are swelling and pain. These characteristics of inflammation have been familiar to doctors over many centuries. They were noted by the 1st century Roman medical encyclopaedist Celsus as calor (heat), tumour (swelling), rubor (redness), dolor (pain).

Inflammation has one other major characteristic in that it leads to 'loss of function' of the affected body part. Swelling and pain largely contribute to this loss of function. In mild disease, loss of function can be beneficial, as it encourages the patient to rest the inflamed area, and this should promote healing. For example, inflammation of the voice box (laryngitis) may give rise to discomfort and malaise. This means that the patient avoids talking, and may wish to rest in bed. Both these responses will promote healing.

In severe disease, the loss of function can jeopardise the health of the whole body, and is not necessarily so beneficial. For example, inflammation of the lining of the brain resulting from bacterial infection (meningitis) leads to swelling of the brain and carries the risk of coma and death.

The five characteristics of inflammation are listed in the Table 2.2b-I.

When a body part is inflamed, it is often medically described by the suffix '-itis'. This suffix may be added on to the common name for the affected organ or, more usually, to the Latin term for the organ. Hence in tonsillitis, dermatitis, laryngitis, osteomyelitis and tendonitis we would expect to find inflammation of the tonsils, skin, larynx, bone marrow and tendons, respectively (see Q2.2b-1).

The trigger for inflammation is always tissue damage. When tissues are damaged, cells are ruptured and release their contents. The presence of cell contents in the extracellular space has a powerful effect on the immune system and the capillary cells. The released chemical contents of cells signal to the immune system and capillary cells that there is cell debris that needs removing, that repairs may need to be performed, and that there might be foreign bodies and infectious organisms to be eradicated. Their presence induces responses in immune and epithelial cells that bring about the inflammatory

Table 2.2b-I The characteristics of inflammation

- Redness
- Heat
- Swelling
- Pain or tenderness
- Loss of function

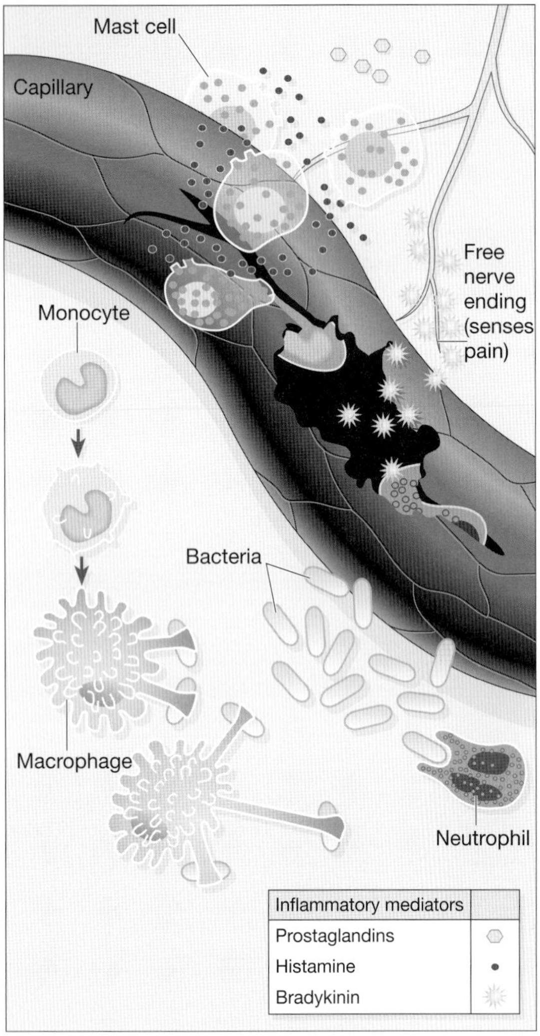

Figure 2.2b-I • The inflammatory response.

response, and thus begins the process of healing. The chemicals released include the prostaglandins, histamine, serotonin (5HT) and bradykinin.

The purpose of inflammation in the body is protective. It enables isolation and inactivation of foreign material and damaged tissue, and leads to its removal from the body.

Some of the changes that occur in inflammation are summarised in Figure 2.2b-I.

Hyperaemia

A cardinal response in inflammation is that blood flow to the damaged area increases, a result of widening of the small blood vessels (vasodilatation). This response is termed 'hyperaemia' (literally meaning 'more blood'). Hyperaemia leads to the increased warmth and redness that are characteristic of inflammation. Hyperaemia also contributes to tissue swelling.

Exudation

Another response of the blood vessels to inflammatory chemicals is that gaps form between the epithelial cells of the vessels so that molecules and fluids move out of capillaries into the fluid surrounding the tissue cells. In this way important proteins such as antibodies and fibrinogen enter the site of the damage. This reaction, known as 'exudation', leads to the swelling that is characteristic of inflammation. Fibrinogen, one of the 12 clotting factors in the blood, is converted to fibrin once it enters tissue fluid, and in this way it forms a meshwork that contains the inflamed area and thus prevents the spread of any infection that may be present. Antibodies bind to foreign antigens at the site of the inflammation and so form immune complexes that are then engulfed by phagocytic cells such as neutrophils.

Migration of leukocytes

Various forms of leukocytes, which are the basis of the immune system, are attracted from the blood and the tissue fluid to the site of the damage by the chemicals (chemotaxins) that have been released as a consequence of the damage. Neutrophils are amoeba-like white cells that appear rapidly at the site of inflammation. These have the capacity to engulf and digest any material that presents foreign antigens in the form of an immune complex. In this process, the phagocytic cells may die, releasing their greenish cell contents. It is these discharged cell contents that contribute to the green colour of pus, which is usually only formed as a consequence of a heavily infected wound. Macrophages are slower moving, larger phagocytic cells, which after a few hours also enter the site of inflammation to engulf and digest cell debris, microbes and dead neutrophils.

Increased body temperature

If the bodily response of inflammation is sufficiently large, then interleukin-1, a chemical released by macrophages, can lead to an increase in the core temperature of the body. The fever that results leads to more efficient activity of phagocytes and also encourages the patient to rest. Fever is thus understood to be beneficial to the healing process in inflammation.

Pain

The chemicals released by damaged and inflammatory cells tend to irritate the local nerve endings, so leading to the acute pain and intense tenderness associated with inflammation (see Q2.2b-2 and Q2.2b-3).

Resolution of acute inflammation

In uncomplicated situations, the inflammatory process leads to removal of damaged cells, dirt and infectious organisms, and provides a clean environment for the process of wound healing. The redness, swelling, pain and heat resolve, function of the area is restored and healing is complete, with or without scar formation.

Chronic Inflammation

The resolution of inflammation may be hindered by a poor blood supply, the presence of a foreign body or as a response to certain organisms. In the case of chronic inflammation, after a time increasing numbers of lymphocytes get attracted to the area and the scar-tissue forming cells, the fibroblasts, are continually activated meaning excess scar tissue may be formed. The chronic skin ulcer described in Chapter 2.1b is an example of chronic inflammation. Tuberculosis (TB) is an example of an infection in which the slow-growing infectious organism *Mycobacterium tuberculosis* encourages a chronic inflammatory response and the formation of clusters of immune cells around foci of infection known as granulomas (see Q2.2b-4). These tiny clusters of immune cells are characteristic of this disease and are evidence to the pathologist of its ability to induce damaging chronic inflammation.

Information Box 2.2b-I

Inflammation: comments from a Chinese medicine perspective

Redness and heat signify the presence of Heat in Chinese medicine. The characteristics of pain, with aversion to pressure, and a purplish discoloration suggest a degree of Blood Stagnation. In Chinese medicine, Blood Stagnation can lead to Heat, and Heat can be a cause of Blood Stagnation. Therefore, these Pathogenic Factors are inextricably interrelated in inflammation.

Excess tissue fluid and the swelling and oozing which result could be equated with the Pathogenic Factor of Damp. This may be localised or may be systemic, in which case there may well be underlying patterns of Spleen Deficiency.

Pathology of inflammation

Boils and abscesses

Boils and abscesses occur when excess pus is formed and collects within the tissues at a site of inflammation. Abscesses are simply big boils; there is no clear-cut difference between the two. Pus is more likely to collect if a foreign body is present at the site of inflammation and also if certain 'pyogenic' organisms are present. The most common pyogenic organism to cause medical problems is *Staphylococcus aureus*, one of the many normal and healthy (commensal) skin bacteria.

Pus is a problem because it is a reservoir of microbes, and thus a source of chemicals that act as pyrogens (i.e. lead to fever and malaise), and it inhibits full resolution of the inflammation.

A boil or abscess ideally heals by means of discharge of pus to the surface. For example, a stye (a boil of the edge of the eyelid) usually comes to a point after a few days and this then breaks open to release the pus and allow healing.

This ideal outcome is not always achieved. In some cases the pus does not discharge fully, and the channel leading from the pus to the skin does not heal fully, remains as a sinus that discharges pus long term. This can lead to long-term ill-health, as the body is always in a state of fighting infection. An infection in bone (osteomyelitis) can easily lead to sinus formation, because the bone is relatively protected from the immune system and thus chronic inflammation can easily develop in bone. This is a particular problem with shrapnel wounds in wartime, which may lead to a continual discharge of pus from the bone through a sinus to the skin.

When a sinus is formed, the discharge of pus can go two ways: into closely apposed organs (e.g. stomach and bowel, or bladder and bowel) so that a permanent channel is formed between them (fistula). This can have severe consequences. One common cause of a fistula is the inflammatory bowel disease Crohn's disease. Diverticulitis of the bowel is another cause.

If the pus is not discharged at all it is eventually phagocytosed. This is a common occurrence with small boils (pustules) such as occur in severe acne. Instead of discharging fully, these form tender lumps that gradually become less painful. This form of healing is more likely to lead to scarring resulting from chronic inflammation, as fibrous tissue is formed to fill the cavity formed by the pus, and this can have severe cosmetic consequences (see Q2.2b-5).

The most appropriate medical treatment of boils and abscesses promotes natural resolution. Astringent medication in the form of hot packs (poultices) can be applied to the site of a superficial abscess to encourage the pus to discharge outwards.

Resolution can be assisted surgically by lancing, where a clean wound is made in the skin to allow natural drainage of the pus. A larger abscess may be drained by inserting a sterile

Information Box 2.2b-II

Boils and abscesses: comments from a Chinese medicine perspective

In Chinese medicine, boils and abscesses are manifestations of Damp and Heat, and in severe cases of Fire-Poison. Full resolution represents clearance of these Pathogens; therefore, poultices, lancing and drainage are energetically appropriate treatments that can facilitate full cure.

Antibiotics may actually suppress full cure in the conventional sense of the term, as the causative microorganisms may remain relatively protected from the drug deep within the walled-off centre of the abscess. From an alternative medicine perspective this outcome may be interpreted as suppression, as the root cause has not been treated directly (e.g. Spleen Qi Deficiency leading to poor health of the tissues). Nevertheless, there are situations in which antibiotic treatment is necessary to allow healing of an abscess while preventing the dangerous spread of infection (e.g. in a brain abscess).

A discharging sinus or fistula suggests Chronic Damp Heat, usually on a background of marked deficiency such as Qi or Yin Deficiency.

An abscess that does not discharge, but instead resolves to form a hard painless lump under the surface of the skin, might be described in Chinese medicine in terms of accumulation of Phlegm, which is usually the consequence of the action of Heat on Damp.

tube to connect with the outside for a few days. When the pus has drained, the tube is removed and, ideally, the cavity will then heal by the process of primary wound healing.

Often antibiotics are given to prevent spread of infection whilst the abscess is healing, although in some cases this treatment may be inappropriate. With adequate drainage, most abscesses will resolve without the need for antibiotics. Paradoxically, antibiotics can prevent full drainage of an abscess, as they may inhibit the process of pointing of the abscess to the surface, thus leading to a more chronic situation.

Fibrosis (scar tissue formation)

Chronic inflammation may be characterised by excessive scar-tissue formation (fibrosis). This can be damaging, as scar tissue can cause shrinkage of tissues and damage to the integrity of organs. Cirrhosis is an example of the result of chronic inflammation of the liver. In cirrhosis, scar tissue takes over the space of the healthy liver cells and may result eventually in liver failure. Scar tissue in the abdominal or pelvic cavity can cause adhesions between organs, and may promote obstruction of organs and infertility (see Q2.2b-6).

The main treatment for fibrosis is surgical removal of scar tissue, in as much as this is possible. Physiotherapy and massage may be used to encourage the stretching of contracted areas of skin and muscle.

Information Box 2.2b-III

Fibrosis: comments from a Chinese medicine perspective

Scar tissue is unyielding and relatively dry in contrast to the springy, moist nature of healthy tissue. For this reason, scars are often described in terms of local Qi and Yin deficiency. If the scar tissue is more bulky than the healthy tissue would have been, this could be interpreted as an accumulation of Phlegm.

A more detailed Chinese medicine interpretation would depend also on the site and on the consequences of the fibrosis. For example, intra-abdominal adhesions may lead to intermittent griping abdominal pain, suggesting Stagnation of Qi in Middle and Lower Jiao, while fibrosis of the heart muscle may lead to inefficient pumping of the heart and accumulation of fluid in the lower body (oedema), suggesting Heart and Kidney Yang Deficiency.

Self-test 2.2b

Inflammation

1. A patient has a reddened, hot, painful, and swollen thumb after a splinter of wood punctured the skin. Although he managed to remove the splinter, he is now unable to use the thumb because of the discomfort. Describe what processes might be going on at the puncture site to cause these five characteristics of inflammation.
2. What might your treatment principles be if this patient comes to you for acupuncture treatment?
3. How might the inflammation be beneficial to your patient?
4. Another patient has developed a large boil on the buttock (a relatively common site for a boil). She is generally run down, and you have previously diagnosed long-standing Damp and Yin Deficiency. She says that the doctor wants to perform a minor operation to lance the boil, and is asking your advice about whether or not to go ahead with this treatment.
   (i) What might you advise?
   (ii) Would you treat this patient with Chinese medicine?

Answers

1. Redness, heat and swelling result from the increased blood flow to the inflamed area (hyperaemia).
   Exudation of fluid from the capillaries also contributes to the swelling.
   Swelling and release of chemicals causes pain by stimulation of sensory nerves.
   Swelling and pain mean that your patient cannot use his thumb (loss of function).
2. If the patient is unable to use his thumb it would be prudent to ensure he first seeks medical advice and ensure that there is no deep infection or damage to delicate structures such as joints or tendons. Acupuncture can be offered to complement medical treatment. In this case, the patient has a form of Hot Bi (painful obstruction syndrome). The treatment principles could include those to:
   - clear Heat
   - move local Stagnant Blood and Qi.
3. The patient may have damaged his thumb tissues and also allowed the entry of some dirt and bacteria through the injury. Inflammation is beneficial because it aids healing in the following ways:
   - fluid and antibodies enter the damaged area so that toxins can be diluted and washed away, and antibodies can bind to bacteria and foreign material to form immune complexes.
   - leukocytes are attracted to the area to engulf and digest unwanted material and immune complexes
   - fibrin is formed to wall off the area and to prevent the spread of infection
   - pain and swelling encourage the patient to rest his thumb.
4. (i) Lancing of a boil is an energetically appropriate treatment because it will allow the release of the pus and thus permit clearing of the Pathogen of Damp Heat. You could tell the patient that the minor operation may well help the abscess to resolve naturally.
   You could also advise her that she could avoid taking antibiotics, as often full resolution will occur with adequate drainage of pus alone (unless the inflammation around the abscess appeared to be spreading after the operation).
   (ii) There is no reason why you should not also treat this patient, both for her long-term problems of Damp and Yin Deficiency, but also to clear Damp Heat.

Chapter 2.2c Disorders of the immune system

LEARNING POINTS

At the end of this chapter you will be able to:
- discuss the pathology of immunodeficiency
- discuss the pathology of allergy
- describe the action of antihistamines and decongestants
- discuss the pathology of autoimmune disease
- describe the action of corticosteroids and other drugs that can suppress the usual immune response.

Estimated time for chapter: 120 minutes.

Introduction

Immune-related disease can be grouped into two broad categories:
- Disease resulting from an insufficient immune response
  - immunodeficiency (also termed 'immune deficiency') syndromes
- Disease resulting from an inappropriate immune response
  - allergy
  - autoimmune disease.

In this chapter, these broad categories of immune related disease are discussed in turn.

Pathology of immunodeficiency syndromes

An insufficient immune response occurs when the complex interaction of the six types of lymphocyte fails to function in a balanced way. A person with immunodeficiency will therefore be less able to fight off infection.

Immunodeficiency may be a congenital condition, and if so results from specific problems in the function of the leukocytes, the production of antibodies or deficiencies in the complement proteins. The severity of inherited immunodeficiency can vary. In severe forms, a patient may be susceptible to life-threatening infections. In milder forms, the patient may just experience a few more colds and other minor infections than the average person.

Immunodeficiency can also be the result of illness acquired in later life. Illness affecting the ability of the bone marrow to produce white blood cells (bone marrow failure) can manifest in devastating immunodeficiency. This state can become apparent in conditions such as leukaemia and secondary bone cancer. Acquired immunodeficiency syndrome (AIDS) is a particular form of immunodeficiency that is the result of infection with the human immunodeficiency virus (HIV). HIV targets T-lymphocytes and impairs their action in the immune response, and the result is a characteristic pattern of opportunistic infections and vulnerability to tumours (see below), including pneumocystis pneumonia, candidal fungal infections and Kaposi's sarcoma.

A patient with immunodeficiency can develop unusual infections that most healthy people would be able to resist. Often these 'opportunistic' infections do not manifest in a dramatic way. Instead, there may be a gradual development of symptoms that are not very specific, such as mild fever or slight sweats. Also characteristic of immunodeficiency are low-grade fungal infections of the skin and the mouth lining, and long-standing but slight diarrhoea. The vagueness of the symptoms and signs of opportunistic infections means that there can be a delay in their diagnosis. However, even though symptoms of opportunistic infections may not be marked, the infection can take hold and rapidly become life-threatening. The infectious agents that cause opportunistic infections are often resistant to common antibiotics. and this can further complicate their treatment.

The other major health risk that faces a person with an immunodeficiency syndrome is cancerous change, as new cancerous cells are usually destroyed by a healthy immune system (see Q2.2c-1).

Information Box 2.2c-I

Immunodeficiency: comments from a Chinese medicine perspective

A patient with an immunodeficiency syndrome does not have a strong response to pathogens. From the perspective of Chinese medicine, this suggests that the Upright Qi is weak. More specifically, as many of these infections manifest on the exterior, with skin rashes and sweats, it points in these cases to the Wei Qi, and its foundation, Kidney Essence, being deficient.

The symptoms of immunodeficiency can also include low-grade fever, night sweats, enlarged lymph nodes, and a tendency to diarrhoea and fungal skin problems such as athlete's foot and thrush. There is a tendency to develop cancer. Taken together, the wide range of potential symptoms usually reflects an underlying Kidney Qi Deficiency, with a consequent effect on many of the other organs. Spleen Qi Deficiency, Damp and Phlegm are all possible outcomes, as are specific symptoms arising from Kidney Yin and Yang Deficiency.

Although it is likely that each of these components is present to some degree in a case of immunodeficiency, the symptom picture in each patient will be unique, and it is the skill of the practitioner in tracing the complex aetiology of the patterns that will point to a more precise Chinese diagnosis.

Pathology of allergy

Allergy (also termed 'hypersensitivity') is seen to occur when there is an excessive immune response to a substance that does not normally provoke such a reaction in healthy people. The substance that provokes the allergic response is called the 'allergen'. The allergic response may be localised to the part of the body that has been exposed to the allergen (e.g. in contact allergic eczema or hay fever), or it may be a generalised response to an allergic trigger (e.g. an anaphylactic response to a bee sting or a penicillin-induced rash).

Many people commonly use the term 'allergy' to mean that they do not react well to certain substances, and will complain of symptoms such as fluctuating digestive or respiratory disturbances or headaches. However, conventional medicine tends to recognise only those situations in which a definite abnormality of the immune system can be detected. This is why doctors may deny that there is an allergic component to conditions such as chronic tiredness and irritable bowel syndrome. Nevertheless, many patients with these conditions will notice a consistent adverse relationship between their symptoms and coming into contact with substances to which they feel they are allergic.

Examples of diseases that doctors would agree are the result of allergic reactions are listed in Table 2.2c-I. It is clear from the information presented in the table that allergic reactions can have very different presentations. This is because for each type of allergic reaction different aspects of the immune system may be over-reacting. The two broad ways in which the immune response can result in allergic disease are termed type I and type IV hypersensitivity.

Type I hypersensitivity

In some people the white blood cells that release histamine in the inflammatory response, the mast cells and basophils, react excessively to the antigens on certain trigger substances such as house dust, pollen, animal dander, bee stings and specific dietary components (commonly eggs, peanuts, fish). Histamine in excess causes itching, exudation of fluid into tissues and constriction of the airways of the lungs. If extreme, the result is anaphylactic shock, in which the dramatic exudation of fluid causes a drop in blood pressure and life-threatening asthma can develop within a matter of minutes of exposure to the allergen. In less severe reactions the person might just experience temporary itching, sneezing or breathlessness. This histamine-mediated allergy is known as type I hypersensitivity. Hay fever, rhinitis, urticaria (nettle rash) from eating shellfish and bee sting allergy are all examples of type I hypersensitivity.

Type IV hypersensitivity

Another form of allergy involves the T-lymphocytes reacting excessively to externally originating antigens. The antigens cause a delayed reaction, as lymphocytes are slow to accumulate at the site of injury. Over time, this sort of allergic reaction will cause a local area of inflammation, with itching. The skin can react in this way to contact with substances such as latex, nickel, leather and certain plants. The result is a localised area of skin irritation, with itch and thickening of the skin (contact allergic eczema). This is also the allergic reaction that can cause some forms of transplant operation to fail (e.g. skin graft). This form of T-lymphocyte-mediated allergy is known as type IV, delayed-type hypersensitivity.

Type III (immune-complex-mediated) hypersensitivity

Type III hypersensitivity is a less common mechanism for an allergic reaction. It describes the excessive formation of immune complexes (antibody–antigen complexes), which can circulate in the blood stream before becoming deposited in the kidneys, skin and joints. They then trigger inflammatory damage in these tissues, leading to symptoms and signs such as blood in the urine, a bruising rash and joint aches. The allergic response to penicillin is understood to be a type III response.

Treatment of allergy

It is helpful before treating allergies to diagnose the cause. In some cases this is obvious, but certain hospital tests can clarify a range of potential allergens that might cause reactions in an individual. Skin-prick tests involve the injection of tiny amounts of allergen under the surface of the skin, and monitoring for a 'wheal' response. These tests are used to diagnose

Table 2.2c–I Allergic conditions recognised by conventional medicine

Condition	Symptoms	Allergen
Anaphylactic shock	Extreme bodily reaction, including severe asthma, and swelling and rash of skin	Can be various; common ones include bee stings, peanuts, egg, antibiotics
Worsening of childhood eczema and asthma	Symmetrical itchy rash distributed all over the body	Various, including dairy products, egg, wheat and oranges. Sometimes no allergen is found
Hay fever	Streaming eyes and nose, sneezing, itchy throat	Grass and tree pollen
Contact eczema	Rash on the skin at the site of contact with the allergen	Metals, including nickel, detergents, garden plants, sticking plaster
Perennial rhinitis and chronic sinusitis	Blocked and runny nose, sneezing, facial pain	House dust and moulds
Urticaria (nettle rash)	Blotchy, raised rash widely distributed over the skin	Dietary allergens such as shellfish and eggs are common triggers
Migraine	Unilateral headache, nausea and neurological symptoms and signs	Cheese, chocolate and red wine are common dietary triggers

type I hypersensitivity. A blood test, known as the RAST test, can also be used to test for antigen-specific immunoglobulin E (IgE) antibody in type I allergic conditions.

Skin-patch tests involve holding an allergen against the skin by means of an adhesive plaster, and assessing the reaction over the next few days. These test for type IV hypersensitivity. Skin-prick and skin-patch tests are usually designed to test for sensitivity to a battery of potential antigens at the same time.

The first principle in treatment is to avoid the offending allergen, or to protect the skin if avoidance is not possible. This is often very difficult to do, as many allergens, such as pollen and house dust mite, are impossible to remove totally from the environment.

Antihistamines, anti-inflammatories and corticosteroids are all drugs that reduce the effect of the overactive immune and inflammatory responses.

Antihistamines (e.g. cetirizine and loratidine) counteract the effect of the excessive release of histamine that occurs in type I allergic reactions. Side-effects include dry mouth, rashes and palpitations in some people. The more sedating, older antihistamines (e.g. promethazine) can also reduce nausea, and may be prescribed to prevent travel sickness and for sedation in children.

There is a wide range of anti-inflammatory drugs, many of which are used to reduce pain. Those that are used in allergy and asthma (e.g. sodium cromoglicate) appear to reduce the release of histamine from the mast cells.

Corticosteroids (commonly known as 'steroids') can be taken by mouth, applied to the skin or inhaled into the nose according to the type of allergy. These are known to suppress the function of immune cells (in particular the T-lymphocytes) and also the inflammatory response by reducing the production of proinflammatory chemical mediators such as interleukin-2. They are, therefore, both anti-inflammatory and immunosuppressant.

Decongestants (such as oxymetazoline, the active constituent of Vicks Sinex nasal spray) are available in the UK in various forms "over-the-counter" from pharmacists. Because of the ease of their availability they are commonly used preparations. They act by causing constriction of blood vessels in the nose which, in the case of runny nose, reduces the amount of fluid that can ooze out. The main problem with these drugs is that, when they wear off, the nasal drip can be worse than before, so that people can become dependent on using them. Constriction of blood vessels in the head can cause headache, and may increase the blood pressure in some people.

Information Box 2.2c-II

Allergy: comments from a Chinese medicine perspective

Most 'true' allergic reactions have characteristics of what the Chinese describe as Wind invasion. The runny nose, itchy eyes, itchy skin and rashes characteristic of many allergies often come on suddenly, and change rapidly. The rash of urticaria can move across the body from site to site dramatically. This suggests that the allergic person has a specific Deficiency of Wei Qi, which in some way is exacerbated by the contact with the particular allergen.

The allergen can be seen as a form of Xie (Pathogenic) Qi. An allergic person does not necessarily succumb to more colds, which indicates that the Wei Qi deficiency is specific to particular forms of Xie Qi.

Allergic reactions that affect the skin often manifest as pallor and dryness, symptoms usually ascribed to Blood Deficiency. This, in turn, may also predispose the sufferer to Wind invasions.

Antihistamines reduce the response to the allergen, although this returns when the drug is stopped. There are usually no obvious long-term side-effects or worsening of the condition if these drugs are taken for a long time. As the allergy is usually in the form of acute invasion of Wind Heat/Cold, this suggests that the drugs in some way prevent the invasion (i.e. expression) of the Pathogen. Subduing the Pathogenic Factor in the Interior is a possible energetic mechanism. If this is the case, then in theory the root imbalance will have worsened as a result of the suppression of symptoms, but this might not become immediately apparent in symptoms that are significant medically. Subdued Heat, for example, may just become apparent in the form of mental agitation or restlessness, which may not be attributed directly to the drug treatment.

Drug-induced disease could occur with the older forms of antihistamine. These often caused drowsiness and were chemically related to the stronger first-generation major tranquillisers, such as chlorpromazine used to sedate and suppress thought in severe mental illness. This effect suggests a tendency to Obstruct the Shen, and generate Non-Substantial Phlegm.

Although newer forms of antihistamine do not have this property, both types can cause dryness of the mouth and difficulty urinating. These both suggest depression of Kidney Yin. The palpitations that can be caused by the newer antihistamines also suggest depression of Heart Blood/Yin.

Decongestants are chemically related to the ephedrine in the Chinese medicine herb *Ephedra*. These do seem to have a suppressive action, as the runny nose that they help to resolve returns in a more pronounced form on withdrawal. The headache and hypertension that they can cause suggests that they might stimulate Yang and lead to the expression of the syndrome of Liver Yang Rising in susceptible people.

Food intolerances are not considered to be true allergies according to conventional medicine. However, many patients report that certain foods will worsen conditions such as bloating and irritable bowel syndrome (IBS). From a Chinese medicine perspective, conditions that manifest in bloating, abdominal discomfort and unstable bowel habit often have Spleen Qi Deficiency as their foundation. In these conditions it would appear that the symptoms brought about by offending dietary substance (e.g. wheat, citrus or dairy products) are characteristic of weakened Spleen Qi and Stagnated Liver Qi. These syndromes also allow the generation of a Pathogen such as Heat or Damp, and describe the process by which the patient manifests symptoms such as flushing or vaginal discharge.

In contrast to most patients with 'true' allergies, patients with food intolerances may notice that their sensitivity to certain foods fluctuates significantly over time. This is possibly a reflection of the quality and harmony of their Spleen and Liver Qi at a given point in time.

Pathology of autoimmune disease

Autoimmune disease occurs when antibodies are produced that bind to antigens which are part of the body itself. These antibodies are called 'autoantibodies'. This means that the immune response, which leads to inflammation, is directed toward normal body tissue, and leads to damage that includes swelling, pain, heat and loss of function. Fibrosis (scarring) of the affected tissue can also occur.

Type II (cytotoxic) hypersensitivity

Strictly speaking, autoimmunity is also viewed from a conventional perspective as a manifestation of hypersensitivity. Much autoimmune disease is the consequence of type II (cytotoxic) hypersensitivity, in which there is a deleterious immune response to the self antigens present on tissue cells. This results in the death of the cells that carry the antigens. The T-lymphocytes are the cytotoxic cells in this disease process, but their action in cell damage is supported by the helper B-lymphocytes (see Chapter 2.1e).

In some autoimmune diseases there is further tissue damage resulting from circulating antibody–antigen immune complexes (for example, this type III hypersensitivity is the cause of the kidney damage in systemic lupus erythematosus).

Organ-specific autoimmune diseases

In organ-specific autoimmune diseases, the autoantibodies are targeted usually at only one type of tissue cell, and so the damage is located within a single organ. Table 2.2c-II illustrates the diversity of some of the common organ-specific autoimmune diseases.

People with one organ-specific autoimmune disease are slightly more likely than an average person to develop another one. It is not uncommon that a person with diabetes, for example, may also develop hypothyroidism. In general, the damage in organ-specific autoimmune disease is mediated by type II (cytotoxic) hypersensitivity.

Table 2.2c-II Some of the organ-specific autoimmune diseases

Autoimmune disease	Tissue affected
Diabetes mellitus	Insulin-producing cells of the pancreas gland (endocrine tissue)
Thyrotoxicosis (Graves' disease) and hypothyroidism (some antibodies stimulate the gland, and some cause destruction of the gland)	Thyroxine-producing cells of the thyroid gland (endocrine tissue)
Pernicious anaemia (anaemia due to vitamin B_{12} deficiency)	Cells in the stomach that secrete a chemical called 'intrinsic factor', which is essential for the absorption of vitamin B_{12}
Vitiligo	The cells in the skin that produce melanin. Vitiligo leaves symmetrical pale patches of unpigmented skin
Addison's disease (a deficiency of cortisol, a natural corticosteroid)	Cells in the adrenal gland that secrete a steroid hormone called cortisol

Multisystem autoimmune diseases

In the multisystem autoimmune diseases, a wider range of tissues are damaged as a result of excessive immune reactions, which means that the symptoms are much more diverse. Multisystem autoimmune disease is also termed 'rheumatic autoimmune disease', because in many of these conditions the joints are affected, leading to joint pain and swelling (arthritis). Another commonly applied term for a subclass of these conditions is 'connective-tissue diseases'.

Other tissues commonly affected in the multisystem autoimmune diseases include the arteries, the kidney and the skin. This can lead to the development of thrombosis, kidney failure and rashes, respectively.

These conditions are often progressive and debilitating, and can lead to death from kidney failure. Rheumatoid arthritis is the most common multisystem autoimmune disease. Systemic lupus erythematosus ('lupus' or SLE) is another important multisystem disorder. The immune damage in the multisystem disorders is mediated by a combination of type II (cytotoxic) and type III (immune complex mediated) hypersensitivity.

Treatment of autoimmune disease

In the organ-specific autoimmune diseases the damage done to an organ may be irreversible. The treatment in these conditions tends not to be targeted at the autoimmune process. Instead, the important aspect of treatment is to deal with the imbalance resulting from the loss of organ function. For example, in type 1 diabetes mellitus an autoimmune process has caused irreversible damage to the insulin-producing beta cells of the pancreas. The treatment is insulin, given to replace the deficiency resulting from damage to the insulin-producing cells of the pancreas.

In the multisystem autoimmune diseases, significant damage to widespread tissues is ongoing and progressive, and so treatment is targeted towards the overactive immune system. Drugs are used that inhibit the immune response. These are known as 'immunosuppressants'. Immunosuppressant drugs are also used commonly as part of cancer chemotherapy as they seem to inhibit the multiplication of cancer cells. They are also essential in preventing the 'rejection' of an organ that has been transplanted. This rejection is the result of a normal immune response to the foreign tissue, but has to be suppressed to ensure the viability of the transplanted tissue.

Corticosteroids

Corticosteroids are a commonly prescribed class of immunosuppressant drugs that also have the property of inhibiting inflammation. They are, therefore, doubly effective in autoimmune disease. They act by reducing the production of the chemical mediators that promote the immune response, and this has a particular impact on the phagocytic immune cells the neutrophils. In this way they can slow down the damage caused by autoantibodies throughout the tissues of the body, and can prevent the development of life-threatening conditions such as kidney failure and thrombosis.

Corticosteroids can be given by mouth or by intravenous injection. The two most commonly prescribed oral preparations are dexamethasone and prednisolone.

Corticosteroids are closely related to a natural hormone called cortisol, which is produced by the cells of the cortex (outer layer) of the adrenal gland. Cortisol is essential for life, and people with the organ-specific immune condition Addison's disease will die if their deficient cortisol is not replaced by synthetic corticosteroids. It is known that under conditions of stress cortisol is released in increased amounts by the adrenal gland. Its role includes ensuring that the body cells can have ready access to the sugar that is present in the diet and stored in the liver, and also that extra sugar is manufactured (by breaking down proteins) if necessary. Cortisol also acts at the kidney to ensure that sufficient salts and water are maintained in the circulation to keep the blood pressure adequately high. These responses are essential in the short term, but may contribute to the development of diseases such as diabetes and hypertension in people who are continually under stress.

Cortisol also influences the inflammatory mediator chemicals and thus the leukocytes, which bring about a normal immune response and assist in wound healing. However, when in excess, cortisol leads to a suppressed immune response and poor wound healing. This effect could offer one reason why stressed people tend to succumb to illness more often, and also may not recover from injury so rapidly.

Patients on corticosteroids prescribed to suppress immune responses will experience problems consistent with the physiological effects of cortisol in excess. These include:

- high blood sugar (can lead to diabetes mellitus)
- high blood pressure and fluid retention due to the effects on the kidney
- excessive loss of muscle because muscle protein is broken down to make sugar
- impaired generalised immune response leading to increased risk of infection and poor wound healing.

Other important side-effects of corticosteroids include:

- alteration of mood (they can cause depression and manic states)
- impaired growth in children
- thinning of tissue under the skin leading to easy bruising, stretch marks and damage to skin
- thinning of the bones (osteoporosis) in adults
- weight gain, particularly around the face, on the shoulders and over the abdomen.

One important side-effect of synthetic corticosteroids is that they suppress the body's natural production of cortisol. For this reason corticosteroids should never be withdrawn suddenly, because their sudden removal can lead to a condition similar to Addison's disease, and there is a risk that the patient may develop a coma and die.

The constellation of serious side-effects of corticosteroids was first described by a doctor called Cushing, and so is called Cushing's syndrome (Figure 2.2c-I). Cushing's syndrome will

Figure 2.2c-I • The features of Cushing's syndrome.

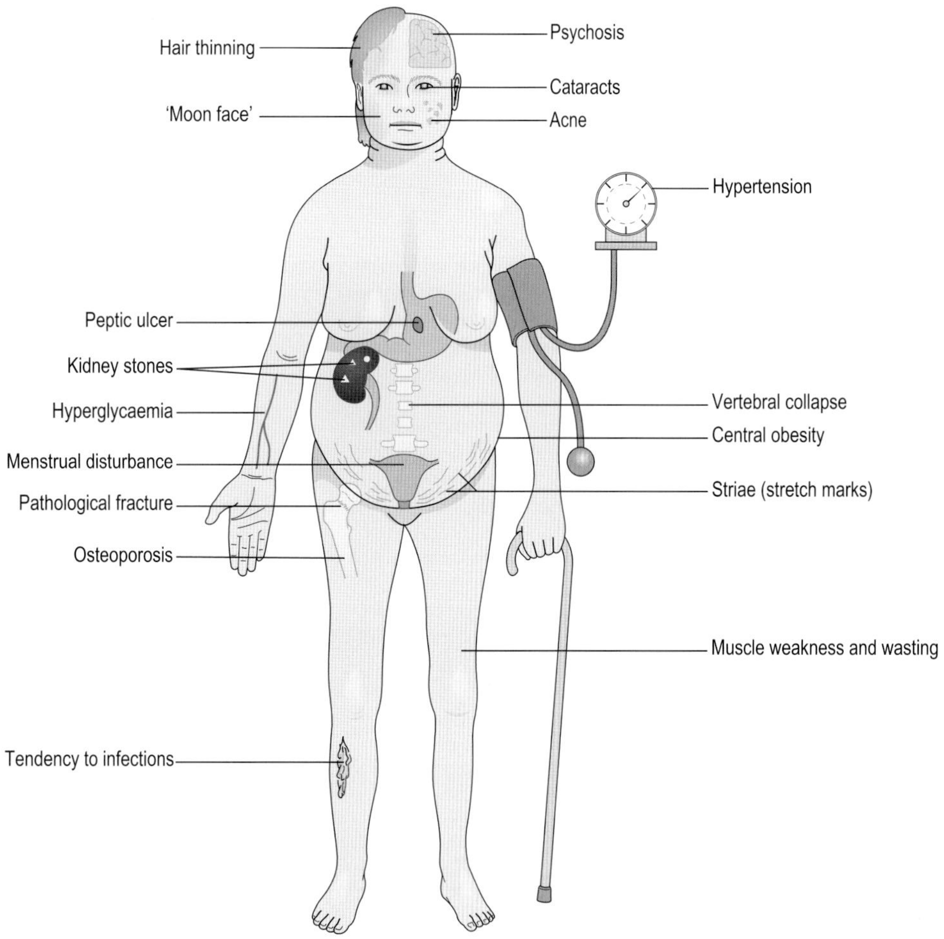

only become apparent after weeks of treatment with high-dose corticosteroids.

When corticosteroids are being considered for treatment of an allergic or autoimmune disease, the potential benefits will always be weighed against the risks of Cushing's syndrome. Patients on corticosteroid therapy should be clearly warned about the side-effect of an impaired response to infection, as a minor infection can lead to a life-threatening situation in a person on this form of steroid treatment. They should also be warned never to stop their medication suddenly.

Other immunosuppressant drugs

The immunosuppressant drugs are a diverse group of drugs that act by inhibiting various aspects of the immune response. They may be prescribed to reduce the need for high doses of corticosteroid (so-called 'steroid-sparing' effects). In severe autoimmune disease they are often used in combination with corticosteroids. Some of the more commonly used immunosuppressant drugs include methotrexate, cyclophosphamide and azathioprine. These act by inhibiting the production and action of the lymphocytes. They are also used for their cytotoxic effects in cancer chemotherapy. Because they cause a degree of damage to healthy cells they have a wide range of toxic side-effects.

Ciclosporin and tacrolimus are immunosuppressants that have a more powerful effect on lymphocyte function and are commonly used to prevent transplant reactions. Both are associated with an impressively long list of potentially serious side-effects.

More recently introduced immunosuppressants include immunologically derived products such as immunoglobulin (antibodies) targeted against white blood cells and inflammatory mediators such as tumour necrosis factor (TNF) (see Q2.2c-2).

Information Box 2.2c-III

Autoimmune disease and its treatment: comments from a Chinese medicine perspective

In the organ-specific autoimmune diseases, the main symptoms come from the reduced function of the affected organ. The syndromes that result are diverse. The Chinese medicine view of the main organ-specific autoimmune conditions such as diabetes and thyroid disease is discussed in later chapters.

The multisystem autoimmune diseases (such as rheumatoid arthritis and SLE) have some common energetic features. In these diseases, the common cause of damage to the body tissues is inflammation, which suggests Heat as an important common Pathogenic Factor. In many of these conditions there is also a degree of joint swelling and deformity, and also thickening of the tissues or formation of nodules. The Damp and Phlegm with which these are associated are, therefore, usually also prominent in multisystem autoimmune disease.

Such profound energetic disturbance would not occur without there being a background history of marked depletion. Autoimmune disease does run in families, and this suggests that an inherited Jing deficiency plays a part in the susceptibility to autoimmune disease. If this is the case, imbalances such as Kidney Yin Deficiency and Spleen Qi deficiency are also likely to be present, and these in turn may create a susceptibility to Pathogenic Factors such as Heat, Damp and Phlegm.

The energetic interpretation of the action of corticosteroids (steroids) is very complex. When the treatment of keloid scars was described in Chapter 2.1b, the local action of injected steroids was interpreted as clearing of Heat, Phlegm and Stagnation. This would also be a reasonable interpretation of the effect when steroids are injected into inflamed and swollen joints.

The action of steroids taken into the whole body by tablet or intravenous injection might also, at one level, be described in terms of clearance of these Pathogenic Factors, as inflammation, swellings and pain are ameliorated. However, the side-effects embraced by Cushing's syndrome suggest there is a range of less beneficial energetic effects. Possible energetic interpretations of these side-effects are summarised in the following table:

Side-effect of corticosteroid drugs	Possible Chinese medicine energetic interpretation
High blood sugar/diabetes (which leads to excessive thirst and urination, and damage to blood vessels)	Internal Heat leading to Kidney Yin Deficiency
High blood pressure	Kidney Yang and Yin Deficiency leading to water retention and Accumulation of Damp and Phlegm
Retention of fluids	Kidney Yang Deficiency
Muscle wastage and thinning of flesh beneath the skin	Spleen Qi Deficiency
Poor growth in children	Jing Deficiency
Thinning of the bones	Kidney Deficiency
Acne	Damp Heat
Elevated mood, mania, depression	Phlegm/Heat obstructing Heart Orifices
Weight gain	Damp
Poor wound healing	Blood and Qi Deficiency
Poor response to infection	Wei Qi and Jing Deficiency

In summary, the symptomatic benefit of corticosteroids may come at a cost of serious side-effects. Many of these may be described in terms of depression of the function of the Kidney Qi and Kidney Essence from a Chinese medicine perspective. The corticosteroids also have side-effects that would suggest accumulation of Heat, Damp and Phlegm. It is noteworthy that these are the Pathogenic Factors that are cleared when corticosteroids have a therapeutic effect. According to the theory of suppression introduced in Chapter 1.3b, this might point to the possibility that the apparent clearance of Pathogenic Factors is actually suppression of imbalance to deeper levels in the body.

Self-test 2.2c

Disorders of the immune system

1. Pat is receiving chemotherapy, which includes corticosteroids and immunosuppressant drugs, for a cancer called 'lymphoma'. She wakes one morning with a slight cough and breathlessness. Her temperature is 38°C. What should you advise her to do about her symptoms?
2. (i) How might a patient with hay fever be treated by their doctor?
   (ii) How would you treat the same patient (list treatment principles only)?
3. Maria has experienced an early menopause at the age of 35. Her doctor tells her that she has a condition called 'ovarian failure'. Her mother Alice has a condition called 'polymyositis', which manifests as a slight fever, weak muscles, and a red skin rash. Both have types of autoimmune disease.
   (i) What is the broad distinction between the two conditions?
   (ii) What sort of conventional treatments might be chosen for the two women?

Answers

1. You should be concerned that Pat may have developed an opportunistic infection, because she is taking medication and has a condition that will lead to a state of immunodeficiency. Mild symptoms and slight fever are consistent with this. She should be recommended to contact her specialist, who will arrange to see her for investigations as soon as possible.
2. (i) The patient could be advised to avoid going out on days when the pollen count is high (avoidance of allergen). They might be prescribed an antihistamine preparation such as cetirizine, which they could either take by mouth twice a day or when required if their symptoms are not too bad.
   A preparation of corticosteroid, such as beclometasone, or an anti-inflammatory called sodium cromoglicate may be prescribed as an inhaler to be taken through the nose. Some doctors may prescribe a single injection of long-acting dose of corticosteroid, although this is currently considered bad practice because of the risk of side-effects.
   (ii) The primary treatment principles might be to Clear Wind–Heat or Wind–Cold in a current attack (manifestation), and Strengthen Wei Qi (by nourishing lungs and kidneys) to benefit the root of the problem.
3. (i) Maria has an organ-specific autoimmune disease in which antibodies have caused permanent damage to her ovaries. Alice has a multisystem autoimmune disease in which a wider range of tissues is affected.
   (ii) Maria will be treated with hormone replacement therapy, to attempt to replace the oestrogen that should have been produced by the ovary. Alice's condition reflects ongoing inflammation due to antibodies, and will be treated with corticosteroids and other immunosuppressant drugs.

Chapter 2.2d Thrombosis, embolism and infarction

LEARNING POINTS

At the end of this chapter you will:
- be familiar with the pathology of thrombosis, embolism and infarction
- understand the pharmacology of aspirin and warfarin.

Estimated time for chapter: 60 minutes.

Introduction

Chapter 2.1c described clotting as a barrier to disease. This chapter focuses on what happens when clotting is excessive to bodily requirements. When this happens, the conditions of thrombosis, embolism and infarction may be the result. In conventional pathology, these together are considered as one of the basic processes of disease.

The causation of thrombosis, embolism and infarction

The term 'thrombosis' describes a blood clot (thrombus) that forms within a blood vessel, and which then stops the usual flow of blood within that vessel.

'Embolism' is a term used to describe the situation when any substance (known as an 'embolus'; plural 'emboli') is transported within the bloodstream until it wedges in a narrow artery from where it can then stop the flow of blood. The most usual cause of an embolus is a piece of clot that has broken away from the site of a thrombosis.

'Infarction' describes what happens to tissue that is damaged as a result of the blockage caused by a thrombosis or the lodging of an embolus in an artery. The tissue normally nourished by the blocked blood vessel becomes suddenly deprived of nutrients, most importantly oxygen. Sensitive tissues such as the brain or the heart muscle can only survive for a short amount of time without these essential nutrients. If the blockage is prolonged, the tissue cells die, release their contents and the process of inflammation is triggered.

Infarcted tissues become acutely painful and swollen. However, if infarction occurs in an external part of the body, in the first instance the body part (e.g. a limb) becomes cold and purplish rather than hot and red, because its blood supply has been cut off.

Together, these disease processes account for more than half of all adult deaths, as they are the cause of conditions such as heart attacks (myocardial infarction), strokes (cerebral infarction) and blood clots in the lung (pulmonary embolism). These conditions are explored in more detail in later chapters, while this chapter focuses on the general features of these disorders of excessive clotting.

Thrombosis and embolism occur for four main reasons:

- damage to a vessel wall
- damage to the heart and atrial fibrillation
- increased platelet adherence
- thrombophilia – an inherited tendency to increased blood clotting.

Thrombosis resulting from damage to a vessel wall

As is described in Chapter 2.1c, damage to a vessel wall stimulates the formation of a blood clot. Usually this is a useful bodily response, as the blood clot will stem bleeding from a damaged vessel. However, the lining of the vessel can be damaged not just by traumatic injury but also by deposits of fatty atheroma (one of the causes of 'hardening' of the arteries) or by external compression, such as might occur in an injury. In these cases, a blood clot forms in the region of the damaged vessel, even though there is no bleeding.

Embolism resulting from damage to the heart or atrial fibrillation

Like the blood vessels, the heart is lined with smooth epithelial tissue. Compromise of this tissue by disease, which most commonly occurs as a result of a heart attack (coronary thrombosis), may stimulate the formation of a blood clot within one of the chambers of the heart. The pumping action can then cause particles of blood clot to dislodge and form emboli, which are ejected into the circulation. Similarly, irregular or artificial heart valves cause abnormal turbulence in the jets of blood that are pumped through the heart, and this also can, through damage to the platelets, stimulate the clotting cascade and lead to embolism. Finally, atrial fibrillation, a condition in which the wall of the heart muscle of the atria pumps irregularly, can also stimulate the formation of small clots within the chambers of the heart.

Thrombosis resulting from increased platelet adherence

In certain bodily states, the platelets tend to adhere to each other and the vessel wall more readily than they should. Platelets become more sticky in many conditions of serious ill-health, such as cancer and systemic infection, as a result of increased levels of inflammatory chemicals in the circulation. This is also the cause of increased platelet adherence after major surgery and trauma.

Pregnancy is another condition in which this can occur. The use of hormone-containing drugs such as the contraceptive pill also carries a risk of thrombosis because it causes increased platelet adherence.

Smoking also increases platelet adherence and is often contributory in a case of thrombosis.

Platelets are more likely to adhere in cases of dehydration, when the proteins and cells in the plasma become more concentrated.

All these factors may become more significant in a situation in which there is physical immobility, which of course is more likely in serious illness, after surgery or trauma, and during pregnancy. If there is physical immobility, the circulation in the peripheries of the body is sluggish and there is an increased risk of thrombosis.

Thrombophilia

'Thrombophilia' is a term used to describe any condition in which there is an increased susceptibility to thrombosis and embolism. There are several inherited forms of thrombophilia, in which gene defects lead to abnormalities in the function of the clotting factors. The most common form, which may affect up to 5% of the population to some degree, affects factor V (Leiden) and causes it to persist in the circulation longer than it normally should. Protein C and S mutations hinder the clearance of factors V and VIII from the circulation, and a prothrombin (factor II) mutation leads to abnormally high levels of this clotting factor. Antithrombin deficiency is a rare but serious genetic abnormality of a protein that aids in the breakdown of thrombin (activated factor II).

A thrombophilia can result from the development of autoantibodies. Antiphospholipid syndrome is a condition characterised by thrombosis and recurrent miscarriage, which is sometimes associated with the multisystem autoimmune disease systemic lupus erythematosus (SLE). In this condition autoantibodies are directed towards anticoagulant proteins present both in the general circulation and the placenta.

The consequences of thrombosis and embolism

The consequences of thrombosis and embolism depend very much on the site of the blood clot. Thrombosis may occur either in arteries, which bring blood to tissues, or veins, which drain blood away from the tissues. Because of the way in which they are transported in the blood stream, emboli always lodge within a vessel in the narrowing network of the arterial tree.

Arterial thrombosis or embolism has serious and immediate consequences because it suddenly cuts off the blood supply to tissues. It is blockage of an artery which causes infarction. The bigger the artery that is blocked, the greater is the amount of tissue that is deprived of its blood supply. 'Ischaemia' is the term given to a poor blood supply. Ischaemic tissue is at risk of infarction unless the blood supply is regained rapidly. Infarction is more likely to occur in areas of tissue that are dependent on a single blood vessel for their supply of oxygen and nutrients.

Arterial thrombosis can occur anywhere in the body. The most common sites for severe arterial thrombosis are the vessels supplying the heart muscle (coronary arteries) and the vessels supplying parts of the brain (cerebral arteries). The consequences of these are heart attack (myocardial infarction) and stroke (cerebral infarction), respectively. These are particularly serious occurrences, because both the brain and the myocardial tissues have high demands for oxygen and nutrients and so suffer very rapidly when deprived of these. Significant arterial thrombosis can also occur in the main vessel supplying a limb or in a vessel supplying a segment of bowel. If the blood supply to a limb is suddenly compromised, the limb becomes cold and acutely painful. Thrombosis of the bowel will lead to acute abdominal pain and collapse (the syndrome of 'acute abdomen').

'Deep venous thrombosis' (DVT) is a term given to a thrombosis of a deep vein, which usually occurs in the deep veins of the calf, thigh or pelvis. DVT prevents the free drainage of blood from the tissues, and leads to swelling and discomfort behind the thrombosis. The discomfort is not as severe as the intense pain that results from an arterial thrombosis. It is particularly likely to occur in veins where the blood flow is sluggish. DVT most commonly occurs in the calf muscle vein after long periods of inactivity.

The serious problem that results from DVT is that the obstructing thrombus can enlarge and clot particles can break off to become emboli. These are then carried through the large veins in the blood supply towards the heart. Because the chambers in the heart are relatively large, the emboli are pumped through the heart and end up lodging in the blood vessels of the lungs. This is called pulmonary embolism (a term derived from the Latin 'pulmo', meaning lung) (see Q2.2d-1).

The treatment of thrombosis and embolism

The treatment of thrombosis and embolism depends on whether the event has just happened (acute thrombosis or embolism) or whether the treatment is required to prevent the formation of a blood clot in someone at high risk.

Treatment of acute thrombosis or embolism

Acute (sudden) thrombosis or embolism in a major artery is a serious threat to the life of the tissue supplied by that artery. If the artery is accessible, the first choice of treatment is surgery, in which the artery is opened, the thrombosis or embolus removed, and the cut in the artery repaired.

Another less invasive surgical approach is angioplasty. In this case a tube is passed into the blocked artery via the large artery in the groin or the neck (a bit like rodding a blocked drain), and with the help of x-ray imaging, guided into the clot. The end of the tube is then expanded, which compresses the clot against the wall of the vessel, ideally leaving a passage through which the blood circulation can continue. This procedure is used most commonly in heart disease, to open up narrowed coronary vessels that have become blocked with thrombus, but also may be employed if there has been thrombosis of a major limb artery.

If the clot is large and has occurred within 24 hours of access to treatment, patients may be given a 'clot-busting' (thrombolytic) drug by intravenous injection. The most commonly used of these are streptokinase and tissue plasminogen activator (tPA). These drugs act in the same way as the body's natural process of fibrinolysis, by activating plasminogen to form plasmin, and so can cause fresh clots to dissolve. The thrombolytic drugs carry the risk of causing embolism as the clot breaks up, and sometimes lead to life-threatening bleeding at other sites in the body.

In the case of DVT and pulmonary embolism, rapid anticoagulation is achieved by means of a drug called 'low-molecular-weight heparin', which has to be given by injection. This drug may also be used to prevent thrombosis in patients who are in high-risk situations.

In the long term, almost all patients who have experienced thrombosis or embolism will receive treatment with either aspirin or warfarin. These drugs are commonly believed to 'thin' the blood. This is not exactly the case, as it is not the blood cells, but rather the clotting mechanism, that is affected.

Aspirin acts by reducing the adherence of platelets, and is known to be effective at a daily dose of 75 mg (one-quarter of a proprietary aspirin tablet). Aspirin has a moderate effect on reducing clotting, without a markedly increased risk of bleeding. It is generally given in a dose of 300 mg in acute cases such as heart attack and stroke, both to treat the acute event by prevention of the spread of the clot, and to prevent future events. At the low dose, aspirin has few side-effects. The most common side-effect of aspirin is inflammation/bleeding of the stomach lining.

Warfarin (a drug infamous as being related to the active component of rat poison) acts by inhibiting the manufacture of four of the clotting factors in the liver. This reduces the effectiveness of the clotting cascade, and therefore reduces the formation of clots. Patients with thrombosis or embolism may be started on this drug in hospital. As warfarin takes a few days to reach therapeutic levels in the blood, the patient is treated with injections of low-molecular-weight heparin until this time. The dose of warfarin is adjusted in accordance with the results of regular blood tests (the international normalised ratio (INR) test is used) to check that the clotting time of the blood has been increased, but not by too much.

Patients remain on warfarin for 6 weeks to 6 months in the case of a single episode of thrombosis/embolism, but may have to be on lifelong treatment if the problem recurs, or if there is a long-term risk such as from a damaged heart valve. The main problem with warfarin is difficulty achieving ideal levels of the drug in the blood, and an increased risk of severe bleeding. Patients are advised to avoid alcohol and drugs that can affect the liver and alter the effect of warfarin. Other rare side-effects of warfarin include rashes, nausea and jaundice.

Prevention of thrombosis/embolism

Lifestyle factors that may be discussed with a patient with regard to prevention of thrombosis and embolism include:

- weight loss
- avoidance of long periods of immobility
- smoking cessation

- stopping the combined oral contraceptive pill
- strict attention to control of blood lipids and diabetes.

Aspirin and warfarin are both used for the long-term prevention of thrombosis in patients who are more susceptible to thrombosis and embolism.

Low-dose aspirin is advised for patients with angina, some patients with atrial fibrillation, and patients who have had a heart attack or stroke.

Warfarin is advised for patients who have had recurrent DVT/embolism, patients with damaged or replacement heart valves, and some patients with atrial fibrillation.

Low-molecular-weight heparin is given by injection to some patients who are undergoing surgery. This acts in a similar way to warfarin, but is rapid acting and the effects wear off very quickly. Heparin cannot by given by mouth, so is generally confined to hospital use.

Information Box 2.2d-I

Thrombosis, embolism and infarction: comments from a Chinese medicine perspective

In Chinese medicine inappropriate clotting could be described in terms of Blood Stagnation. The characteristics of this Pathogenic Factor described by Chinese medicine include severe stabbing pain, fixed masses and purple discoloration, all of which may commonly accompany thrombosis/embolism.

The recognised causes of Blood Stagnation in Chinese medicine include Liver Qi Stagnation, Blood and Qi Deficiency, Interior Cold and Heat in the Blood. It is likely, therefore, that one or more of these syndromes will be apparent in the case of an individual patient who is at risk of thrombosis/embolism.

Aspirin relieves symptoms by reducing platelet stickiness, and common side-effects include bleeding from the stomach lining and asthma and allergic reactions. By preventing the blood from clotting, the action of aspirin might be described as movement Blood and Qi. The movement of Blood and Qi has been interpreted as resulting from the Warming action of aspirin. Aspirin is also recognised to play a role in releasing the Exterior in the treatment of febrile disease.

The side-effect of gastrointestinal bleeding, however, suggests that aspirin causes Stomach Heat. The other recognised side-effect of aspirin, asthma, has associations with an allergic response. As noted above, this suggests that aspirin might also have a depressive effect on Wei Qi in susceptible people, and so permit the invasion of Wind.

In summary, broad statements about aspirin in terms of Chinese energetics are that it is Warming in nature and that it also seems to cause Heat in the Stomach. In susceptible people it may result in depression of Wei Qi (leading to allergic asthma).

Warfarin relieves symptoms by increasing the clotting time of blood. This is through the action it has on the liver in which it inhibits the formation of clotting factors. Side-effects listed in the British National Formulary (BNF) include bleeding, rash, hair loss, low red blood cell count (haematocrit), diarrhoea, purple toes and death (necrosis) of skin, liver and pancreatic disorders.

In Chinese medicine, the syndromes related to an increased tendency to bleed include Full Heat, Yin Deficiency with Empty Heat, Spleen not holding Blood and Blood Stagnation.

Bleeding resulting from warfarin anticoagulation can be profuse. Profuse bleeding would be in keeping with the Chinese medicine description of Heating the Blood. The purple toes and skin necrosis suggest that warfarin can also cause Blood Stagnation. This may be a consequence of Liver Qi Stagnation, and thus it is of interest that this drug acts directly on the liver, and can cause liver disorders. The remaining side-effects imply that the function of the Spleen is also affected, explaining, for example, the diarrhoea.

In summary, broad statements about warfarin in terms of Chinese energetics are that it is Heating in nature and that it also seems to cause disharmony of the Liver and Spleen.

Self-test 2.2d

Thrombosis, embolism and infarction

1. List five risk factors for thrombosis and embolism (thromboembolic disease).
2. A patient is keen to come off her anticlotting medication. How would you advise her in each of the following scenarios:
   (i) she has been prescribed low-dose aspirin following a heart attack to prevent recurrence
   (ii) she has been prescribed daily warfarin medication to prevent embolism after heart-valve replacement.

Answers

1. Risk factors include:
   - immobility
   - factors that increase platelet stickiness (severe illness, surgery, pregnancy, the contraceptive pill, smoking, dehydration)
   - factors that lead to distortion of the vessel wall (atheroma, trauma, damaged or prosthetic heart valves, atrial fibrillation)
   - inherited tendency to clotting (thrombophilia).
2. The problem in withdrawing from a preventive medication and treating instead with a form of complementary medicine is that there is no definite way of knowing whether or not your treatment has reduced the previous risk of thrombosis/embolism.

   As both aspirin and warfarin have been scientifically shown to reduce the risk of clotting, it is important to be circumspect in all cases before making a decision to withdraw the drug. Such a decision would almost universally be opposed by the patient's doctor.

   In both cases (i) and (ii) it would be wise to suggest your patient remains on the medication: (i) because the adverse energetic effect of low-dose aspirin is not great and the potential benefit is significant; and (ii) the risk of embolism in valvular heart disease is very high, and most people tolerate warfarin fairly well.

Cancer

2.3

Chapter 2.3a Cancer

LEARNING POINTS

At the end of this chapter you will be:

- familiar with the principles of how cancer develops
- able to recognise the difference between benign and malignant tumours
- able to recognise the role of surgery, chemotherapy and radiotherapy in the treatment of cancer
- able to understand the pharmacology of chemotherapy
- able to understand the principles of palliative care
- able to recognise the red flags of cancer.

Estimated time for chapter: 90 minutes.

Introduction

In developed countries, the impact of cancer on health is enormous. Cancer accounts for approximately one-third of all deaths in the western world, second only to cardiovascular disease.

Many people who have been offered conventional therapy for cancer will also seek complementary medical treatment. Increasingly, and perhaps more so for cancer than for other chronic diseases, the conventional medical approach is embracing complementary treatments, such as acupuncture, reflexology and visualisation, as part of the normal provision of care for a patient with cancer. This is very common in the context of cancer care centres or hospices. It is particularly important that those practitioners of complementary medicine who may be working in a conventional medical setting have a clear understanding of the conventional understanding of the causation of cancer and how it can be treated.

This chapter focuses on the broad principles of pathology and treatment that apply to all forms of cancer. Each type of cancer has its own particular features. More detail about the most important types of cancer can be found in later chapters, when the diseases of the physiological systems in which they arise are discussed.

The pathology of cancer

The initiation of cancer

As explained under the heading Mutation in Chapter 1.1b, cancer is the result of mutation in mitosis. A cancer cell develops when damage to the chromosomes during mitosis leads to defective control of cell growth in the daughter cells.

A healthy cell responds to the cells around it such that it only self-replicates in a controlled way. There are many proteins produced within the cell that control its replication. These are coded for by genes called 'proto-oncogenes' located within the chromosomes of the cell's nucleus. The delicate function of these proteins within the cell is disordered if the proto-oncogene becomes mutated or moved during mitosis, or if it loses its relationship to another controlling gene on a chromosome as a result of insertion of the genetic material from a virus. When the function of a proto-oncogene is altered so that cell replication is no longer so well controlled, it is then known as an 'oncogene'.

There are other genes that are important in the development of cancer. These provide the information that codes for the manufacture of the cell tumour-suppressor proteins. Tumour-suppressor proteins have diverse roles, including the recognition and repair of damaged DNA in the nucleus. Some activate the process of apoptosis ('programmed cell death') in cells that have sustained too much damage. Apoptosis is a controlled form of cellular suicide that does not involve an inflammation-inducing release of cell contents. If tumour-suppressor genes lose their function through mutation, then cancerous multiplication of cells is more likely. One tumour-suppressor mutation in the gene coding for the protein known as p53 has been identified in all forms of human tumour. It is now known that, in health, p53 is activated by damaged DNA, and when activated it halts the normal process of mitosis and in doing so initiates apoptosis. It is also recognised that some viruses can inactivate tumour-suppressor proteins, another mechanism for promoting cancerous growth.

In summary, cancer cells have lost the ability for ordered growth because of the presence of oncogenes and ineffective tumour-suppressor proteins. As cancer cells continue to multiply, more mutations may arise and the growth can become inexorably chaotic and the cancer may eventually invade neighbouring tissues. The result is an irregular mass of cells called a 'tumour' (meaning 'swelling') or 'neoplasm' (meaning 'new growth').

In order to sustain continued growth, tumours require a blood supply. Invasive tumours do this by secreting proteins that promote the ingrowth of new blood vessels, a process known as 'angiogenesis'. These proteins are also the by-product of cancerous mutations.

Most mutated cells are recognised by the immune system as abnormal because they present unfamiliar patterns of proteins in their cell membranes. As a result they are removed by cytotoxic T-lymphocytes as part of the immune response. It is only those cells that slip through this protective net which develop into tumours. Some tumours effectively paralyse this protective action of the immune system by secreting immunosuppressive proteins. These contribute to the general immunodeficiency seen in some patients with cancer.

The generation of an established cancer is called 'carcinogenesis' (literally meaning 'the creation of cancer'). For carcinogenesis to occur, a complex series of mutations must have occurred in proto-oncogenes and the genes that provide the information which codes for the manufacture of tumour-suppressor proteins and angiogenesis-promoting factors. These mutations may have developed over many cycles of cell division, sometimes taking years, until they eventually give rise to a cancerous growth. Moreover, the newly mutated cancer cells need to bypass the safety net provided by the immune system. Cancer is, therefore, more likely in those people who have impaired immune systems, or in those in whom the rate of spontaneous mutation of the genetic material in certain cells is higher than normal.

Table 2.3a-I Some common carcinogens and the cancers they cause

Carcinogen	Cancer caused
Tobacco smoke	Mouth, oesophagus, larynx, lung, bladder
Alcohol	Mouth, oesophagus, larynx, colon, rectum
Dietary factors:	
High-fat diet	Colon, rectum
Naturally occurring environmental factors:	
ultraviolet light	Skin
radon gas	Lung
Industrial exposure:	
asbestos	Lung
vinyl chloride	Liver
radiation	Leukaemia, thyroid
Infectious agents:	
hepatitis B and C infection	Liver
Helicobacter pylori	Stomach
human papilloma virus	Cervix
human immunodeficiency virus	Kaposi's sarcoma. lymphoma
Medications:	
oestrogens	Endometrial
androgens	Prostate
cytotoxic drugs	Bladder, bone marrow

The cause of increased mutation: carcinogens

It is known that mutation can occur simply by chance. Cells are dividing all the time and some of these divisions are not perfect, resulting in a mutation in the genetic material of the daughter cells. As described earlier, in most cases all these defective cells are removed either by the action of tumour-suppressor proteins or by the cytotoxic cells of the immune system.

However, under certain conditions the number of mutations arising in a tissue will increase, and the risk of the formation of cancerous cells will also increase. Such conditions are described by the term 'carcinogenic' (literally meaning 'cancer causing'). When this happens there is an increased susceptibility to the development of established cancer, as the sheer numbers of cancer cells being produced increases the risk of failure of the tumour-suppressor and immune mechanisms to eliminate every single abnormal cell.

Diverse environmental factors, including tobacco smoke, alcohol, dietary factors, ultraviolet light, chemicals in the environment, infectious microbes and drugs, have all been shown to be carcinogenic. Most of these are carcinogenic because they tend to promote mutations, either of proto-oncogenes or of tumour-suppressor-protein genes. There are other mechanisms of carcinogenesis. Certain viruses can insert cancer-promoting sections of DNA into the chromosome or, as described earlier, can inhibit the action of tumour-suppressor proteins. Other carcinogens, such as X-radiation and cancer chemotherapeutic agents, impair the protective action of the immune system (see Q.2.3a-1). Table 2.3a-I summarises some of the common carcinogens and the diverse forms of cancer that can result from exposure to them.

Congenital susceptibility to cancer

It is recognised that a tendency to develop cancers may be inherited. In some cases the tendency to suffer from particular cancers can run very strongly in families. For example, there is one rare form of breast cancer that will develop in over 80% of the daughters of women who have been diagnosed with that cancer. This cancer develops as a result of the transmission of the *BRCA1* and *BRCA2* gene defects. These defects result in inefficient DNA repair mechanisms in breast and ovarian tissues.

In such inherited cases, there is increased susceptibility to cancer, either because of an inherited relative deficiency of the immune system, or because the cells of certain tissues are genetically more prone to mutation.

Acquired susceptibility to cancer

The susceptibility to the effect of carcinogens also depends on the health of the immune system. This is impaired in conditions that cause immunodeficiency, as described in Chapter 2.2c. In addition, factors such as stress and ageing will also contribute to impaired immune responses, and may permit a cancer cell to divide and form a malignant tumour.

The development and spread of cancer

Tumours may be considered as benign or malignant. Benign growths are areas of overgrowth of normal tissue in which the replication of the individual cells remains orderly. Common benign growths include the fatty subcutaneous lump, the lipoma, and the leiomyoma (the muscular fibroid commonly found in the womb). Benign growths tend to be very slow growing and, because they are non-invasive, have a smooth distinct boundary that separates them from neighbouring tissue. They do not spread to distant sites.

In general, the term 'cancer' is used to describe malignant tumours only. Malignant tumours demonstrate much more chaotic growth and may contain a number of different cell forms (a state described as 'pleomorphic') as a result of repeated mutations. The spread of the primary malignant tumour tends to be invasive and irregular as it finds its way through the normal tissues from which it has arisen. The name cancer is derived from the Latin word for crab. This term embodied for early pathologists the claw-like growth of the cancer tissue into neighbouring tissues (see Q2.3a-2).

The term 'primary cancer' describes a malignant growth that demonstrates local spread at the site of the original cancer cell. 'Secondary', or 'metastatic', cancer describes new cancerous growths that have spread to other sites from the original location of the primary cancer. Secondary spread can occur by seeding of malignant cells via the lymphatic system, the circulation or within the body cavities such as the intra-abdominal space. For example, a primary lung cancer is situated within the lung, but secondary lung cancer might develop in the thoracic lymph nodes, the brain and the adrenal glands. Lung cancer tends to metastasise by means of lymphatic spread to lymph nodes, and via the circulation to the brain and adrenal glands.

The effects of malignant tumours

As malignant tumours continue to grow they can exert a diverse range of symptoms. Pain is a much feared symptom of cancer, although is not a significant cause of distress in some cases. Pain can result from the pressure of a tumour in an enclosed space, blockage of a hollow organ causing the organ to distend, and invasion of or pressure on nerves.

'Cachexia' is the term used to describe the loss of appetite, weight loss and generally feeling of malaise which affects many patients with advanced cancer. Nausea and constipation can also be very distressing symptoms of advanced cancer.

The immune system is often depressed in advanced cancer, partly because of the malnutrition that accompanies cachexia, and partly because of the tumour's ability to produce immunosuppressant proteins. Moreover, if the cancer invades the bone marrow (leading to bone-marrow failure), then the production of leukocytes will be impaired. Immune deficiency leaves to body open to infectious diseases which may give rise to symptoms such as cough, fever and cloudy urine. These symptoms may have characterisitic of opportunistic infections.

Organ failure (e.g. failure of parts of the brain, kidney, or liver) can lead to severe life-threatening symptoms. Additional consequences of bone-marrow failure are anaemia and bleeding from thrombocytopenia.

Information Box 2.3a-I

Cancer: comments from a Chinese medicine perspective

From a conventional medicine perspective, tumours result from excessive and inappropriate overgrowth of tissue cells. The underlying problem is that the genetic control of cell multiplication has become disordered and the immune system has failed to recognise and control the growth of these disordered cells.

It is important to note that the category of cancer was not one recognised in ancient Chinese medicine. Instead, the various manifestations were described according to the individual constellation of symptoms and signs presented. The terms used in the Nei Jing, for example, of 'Intestinal mushroom', 'dysphagia and weight loss', and 'breast boil and abscess' probably described rectal, oesophageal and breast cancer, respectively.

Modern Chinese medicine oncology dates only from the 20th century and recognises four aetiological factors: disordered emotions, poor diet, external attack by Pathogens and weakened Zang-Fu organs. The most important syndromes predisposing to cancer that these aetiological factors can lead to are considered to be Stagnation of Qi and weak Spleen and Kidney Qi. These contribute to accumulation and stasis of Blood and Fluids and the formation of tumours.

In Chinese medicine any substantial masses that do not easily move are usually regarded as manifestations of either Phlegm or Blood Stagnation (or sometimes a combination of both). Blood Stagnation is characterised by hardness and intense boring pain, with violaceous colour changes. Phlegm is more often associated with numbness, and will usually develop against a backdrop of Heat and Damp, which will manifest in other signs and symptoms. For long-standing masses to develop there is often a pre-existing state of Deficiency of Qi, as it is only healthy Qi moving freely that prevents the development of Stagnation and Phlegm.

However, some masses can manifest against a background of good Upright Qi, the strength of which is often used to determine priorities in treatment.

In contrast to the western medical approach, which is to remove the tumours, generally the focus of treatment in Chinese medicine oncology is at the root of strengthening the Upright Qi (a treatment approach known as 'Fu Zheng').

Cancer chemotherapy: comments from a Chinese medicine perspective

Chemotherapy and radiotherapy tend to cause preferential death of cancerous tissue, but also lead to damage and inflammation of healthy tissues. Rapidly growing tissues such as hair follicles, mucous linings and sex cells are damaged. The potential adverse effects include redness and heat of tissues in the short term, and dryness, scarring and infertility in the long term. This suggests that these treatments are intensely Heating, and exert their effects by 'burning' the cancerous mass. In doing so they would risk depleting Yin and Kidney Essence. For this reason complementary treatments prescribed to support chemotherapy are often focused on nourishing Yin and Essence.

Bleeding resulting from damage to blood vessels is a common first symptom of cancer, and can be so severe as to be life-threatening (see Q2.3a-3).

The conventional treatment of cancer

Cancer can clearly lead to distressing symptoms. The ideal cancer treatment would relieve symptoms by total removal of the cancerous growth. However, when the cancer is so advanced that cure is not possible, the main aim of treatment is symptom relief. Treatment that is directed at symptom relief is called 'palliative care'. The provision of palliative care is now considered to be a medical speciality in itself.

Treatment of the cancerous growth

There are three main approaches to treatment aimed at removing or inhibiting the cancerous growth:

- surgery (removal of cancerous tissue)
- chemotherapy (treatment by means of drugs)
- radiotherapy (treatment by substances that emit radiation).

Surgery

The main principle underlying the surgical treatment of cancer is to remove all the cancer cells or, if this ideal is not attainable, to remove as much cancer tissue as possible. Even if total cure is not possible, debulking surgical treatment may be performed to militate against the deleterious pressure effects of tumours.

Cure may be possible if a malignant growth is diagnosed before secondary spread has occurred. The surgical ideal is to cut out (excise) the growth and the normal tissue surrounding it to a certain depth. This may mean that a lot of normal tissue is removed, such as the whole breast in a mastectomy for breast cancer, or a large circle of skin and underlying flesh when a melanoma is excised. The tissue that has been removed can then be examined under the microscope to ensure that all the apparent boundaries of the cancer have been completely excised.

In practice it is never possible to ensure that an excised malignant growth has not already led to tiny secondary metastases. For tumours that are known to spread easily, such as breast, cervical and bowel cancer, a patient who has had surgery may also be offered treatment with radiotherapy and chemotherapy, which is intended to shrink tumours and kill or hinder the growth of any possible remaining cancer cells. This additional supportive treatment is called 'neoadjuvant therapy' if used prior to surgery and 'adjuvant therapy' if used after surgery.

If a cancer is in such a position that it cannot be removed fully by surgery it is described as 'inoperable'. This term applies to very large spreading tumours, or those that are growing into vital structures such as the major blood vessels.

Chemotherapy

Chemotherapy in its broadest sense literally refers to any form of medical treatment that employs chemical substances (drugs). However, the term is most commonly used to describe the drug treatments used in cases of cancer. Chemotherapy in cancer can involve treatments that are intended to target and kill all cancer cells. This is known as 'cytotoxic treatment'. Other forms of chemotherapy have been introduced that aim either to modulate the immune response to the tumour or to affect the way in which it responds to hormones.

The major problem with chemotherapy is that all classes of cancer drug have powerful side-effects (drug-induced disease). The science of cancer chemotherapy is very complex and continually changing in response to the rapidly increasing understanding of the genetics and pathology of cancer. For this reason, its use is usually overseen in clinical practice by hospital specialists. Cancer specialists are known as 'oncologists'.

Cancer chemotherapy: the cytotoxic drugs

Cytotoxic drugs are the group of drugs most commonly used to inhibit the growth of cancer cells. These drugs are preferentially absorbed by rapidly growing cells and lead to their death by inhibiting the replication of the DNA within them. Because of their rapid growth, cancer cells in particular are affected by cytotoxic drugs. However, normal tissues are also affected, largely depending on how rapidly the cells divide in those tissues. The rapidly dividing cells of the lining of the bowel, bladder and lungs, the sex organs, the bone marrow and the hair are particularly affected by the cytotoxics. Common side-effects include inflammation of tissues around the site of injection, sore mouth, nausea and vomiting, hair loss, suppression of blood-cell production in the bone marrow and impaired fertility.

Different cytotoxic drugs affect different aspects of cancer growth, and so are commonly given in combination. This practice also reduces the risk of the tumour developing resistance to the chemotherapeutic agents, an unfortunate consequence of ongoing mutations in cancer tissue.

The alkylating cytotoxics include drugs such as cyclophosphamide, chlorambucil, busulfan and carmustine. These all act by causing damage to DNA. With prolonged use they are very toxic to sex cells (in particular the sperm), and also carry a risk of causing a form of leukaemia.

The anthracyclines, which include doxorubicin, daunorubicin, bleomycin and mitomycin, are antibiotic-like drugs. These tend to inhibit DNA repair in multiplying cells and so lead to cell damage. Their effects seem to be similar to those of radiotherapy, and some of the side-effects include strong inflammatory reactions, including inflammation of tissues at the site of infusion and red skin eruptions.

The antimetabolites, including methotrexate, cytarabine and fluorouracil, block the synthesis of DNA in dividing cells.

The vinca alkaloids, originally derived from the periwinkle plant, block the action of the spindle that separates the two nuclei in dividing cells, and so inhibit cell division. This class of drugs includes vincristine and vinblastine.

The taxanes, such as paclitaxel, are derived from the bark of the yew, and these also interfere with the formation of the spindle in mitosis.

Finally, the platinum-containing cytotoxic drugs tend to cause damaging cross-links between strands of DNA. Drugs of this type include cisplatin and carboplatin.

Cancer chemotherapy: the corticosteroids

Corticosteroids are commonly used in cancer chemotherapy for their anti-inflammatory effects. They have antitumour effects in leukaemia and lymphoma and are frequently included as part of the well-established treatment regimens for these conditions. They are also used to minimise the effects of inflammation, and improve appetite and well-being in advanced malignant disease.

Cancer chemotherapy: biological therapy

The biological agents are all complex protein compounds that are designed to interfere with the growth and development of the cancer tissue. Some, such as interferon-alpha and interleukin-2, are genetically engineered copies of naturally occurring substances important in the control of the immune response. These both hinder cell proliferation and promote the action of the lymphocytes.

An increasing number of genetically engineered antibodies are available that target and cause the destruction of the protein growth factors produced by tumours. These include trastuzumab (Herceptin), which was designed to counteract a growth factor known as Her2. Her2 plays a role in the maintenance of metastatic breast cancer.

Other antibody products have been designed to target cancer cells directly, for example rituximab, which can cause the death of cells in B-cell lymphoma.

Cancer chemotherapy: endocrine therapy

Some breast, prostate and womb (endometrial) cancers are dependent on sex hormones for their continued growth. In these cases, if the hormones are prevented from exerting their effects the cancer will shrink and may even disappear. Endocrine therapy involves treatments that affect the balance of the sex hormones for those forms of cancer that are recognised to be hormone dependent.

For example, approximately one-third of breast cancers will grow more rapidly in the presence of the female sex hormone, oestrogen, as a result of protein oestrogen receptors on the surface of the cancer cells. The male sex hormone, testosterone, likewise stimulates the growth of prostate cancer.

The growth of hormone-dependent tumours may, therefore, be hindered by means of drugs that counteract the effect of the hormones, drugs that inhibit the release of these hormones, or by surgical removal of the ovaries (oophorectomy) or testes (orchidectomy).

Drugs that counteract the effect of oestrogen are commonly used in the treatment of breast cancers. Tamoxifen is a drug that blocks oestrogen receptors and so prevents circulating oestrogen from having an effect on breast cancer cells. Tamoxifen is prescribed in the form of a tablet to be taken daily for life. Anastrozole is an example of a drug that prevents the manufacture of oestrogen in cancer cells from other steroid hormones, and may be more useful in the treatment of hormone-dependent breast cancer in postmenopausal women. Goserelin is an example of a drug that acts at the pituitary gland to reduce the release of a hormone (known as luteinising hormone (LH)), the function of which is to stimulate the hormone production by the ovaries and testes. This drug may be prescribed in both breast cancer and prostate cancer.

The principles of chemotherapy

The smaller the tumour, the more likely it is that cytotoxic drugs can cause sufficient damage to the cancer cells and so completely eliminate the tumour. The dose of the cytotoxic drug has to be moderated by the potential damage it may cause to normal tissues. This is one reason why cytotoxic drugs are given in combination with immunosuppressant drugs and in repeated cycles over the course of a few days or weeks. The immunosuppressant drugs hinder the growth of the tumour, and so keep it small during the course of the treatment. The time allowed between repeated cycles is intended to permit normal tissues to recover before another dose of cytotoxic drugs is given to target the cancer cells.

If, after a course of chemotherapy, all cancer cells seem to have disappeared, the patient is said to be 'in remission'. This is not the same as cure, as there may still be a few tiny clusters of cancer cells remaining that may lead to recurrent tumours in the future. However, the longer patients are in remission, the greater the likelihood is that they have achieved full cure.

Radiotherapy

Certain tumours appear to shrink rapidly in response to radiation treatment. This can be given to the patient either in the form of concentrated X-radiation or gamma radiation emitted by an external machine (external beam radiotherapy), or from an implant of a radioactive substance surgically inserted or injected into the body close to the tumour for a short period of time (brachytherapy). The effect of the radiation is to induce breaks in the DNA and to induce apoptosis (programmed cell death) of dividing cells.

The principles of treatment and risks of radiotherapy are remarkably similar to those of chemotherapy. The aim is to kill all rapidly dividing cells, but normal dividing cells can be damaged at the same time. Radiotherapy, therefore, is also given in cycles of treatment over the course of a few weeks. The primary tumours that may respond well to radiotherapy include brain tumours and tumours of the eye, skin cancer, cancers of the mouth, larynx and oesophagus, cancer of the cervix and vagina, cancer of the prostate and lymphoma. Radiotherapy can also be used as an adjuvant therapy after surgical removal of a primary tumour. For example, patients with cancer of the breast, lung, uterus, bladder, rectum or testis may be treated with radiotherapy after the cancer has been excised.

The risks of radiotherapy are of inflammation and long-term scarring of normal tissue in the area exposed to the radiation, and also of future cancers as a result of the carcinogenic effects of the treatment.

Staging and prediction of benefit

In general, the chances of cure are considered greater when treatment is given to cancer at an earlier stage of progression than one that is more advanced. Complex systems of quantifying exactly how advanced a cancer has become have been developed for most cancer types. This quantification is called 'staging'. It is considered important to stage a cancer accurately before a prediction of outcome can be made. This is why patients with cancer may have to undergo many tests such as biopsies and scans before they begin treatment. Patients may then be given statistical figures to express the chances they have of cure with a particular treatment. These figures will have been derived from clinical studies of the treatment given to patients with the same type of cancer at the same stage of progression.

For example, a patient with a form of testicular cancer may be told that they have a 90% chance of survival. This means that nine in every ten people who received the treatment for that sort of cancer at the same stage of progression in clinical studies recovered completely. Another example is that a patient with oesophageal cancer may be told that they can expect to live for 12 months. This means that in studies of that form of cancer at the same stage the average length of time from diagnosis to death was 12 months.

Another way of expressing outcome is in terms of years of survival. The chemotherapy used for a form of cancer of the ovary may be said to lead to a 70% 5-year survival rate, and a 10% 10-year survival rate. This means that at 5 years after the treatment 70% of patients are still alive, but after 10 years many more have died, leaving only 10% of the original patients alive.

The problem with all these figures is that they are derived statistically from clinical studies involving large groups of people. The patient with cancer is an individual and may or may not be typical of the majority of people in the experimental group. It is impossible to be confident that the statistics are relevant to an individual person. There may be a number of variables, including positive outlook and use of complementary therapies, which may alter dramatically the outcome of that individual's treatment and so make the statistics meaningless in the context of their particular situation.

Palliative treatments in cancer

Surgery, chemotherapy and radiotherapy

The three treatment modalities of surgery, chemotherapy and radiotherapy may also be used in advanced cancer to alleviate symptoms, even when there is no hope of cure. This is because they all tend to remove the bulk of the tumour, and so can temporarily alleviate distressing symptoms.

In palliative treatment, the discomfort of the side-effects has always to be balanced against the amount of relief that can be expected to result from the treatment. This is not always easy to do, and often the patient is left with a difficult decision about whether or not to accept treatment. In recent years the most debilitating side-effect of nausea has been treated effectively with powerful medications (e.g. ondansetron) in 75% of patients on chemotherapy. Advances such as this are likely to increase the proportion of patients with an incurable cancer who are offered chemotherapy or radiotherapy.

It is recognised that many patients may not realise that such invasive treatment is not intended to produce cure, even when every attempt has been made to explain the reality of their poor prognosis. This may lead them to accept treatment while holding false hopes that their cancer will be defeated.

Painkillers

Painkilling (analgesic) medication may be prescribed liberally in cases of advanced cancer. It is considered good practice to maintain a steady dose of painkiller so that distressing pain never 'breaks through'. Ideally, combinations of different classes of painkilling drugs are prescribed, which may act in different and complementary ways to reduce pain. These include the simple painkillers (anti-inflammatory drugs, such as ibuprofen and paracetamol) and opiate drugs, which are related to morphine.

The most important classes of painkillers are discussed in detail in Chapter 4.2c.

Opiate drugs

The opiate drugs fall into a class of medication that is used widely for symptom relief in serious disease in conventional medicine. The most commonly used opiate medications include morphine, diamorphine (heroin) and pethidine. Small amounts of opiate drugs are found in combination with simple painkillers in preparations such as Cocodamol and Codydramol.

Opiates (opioids) are the most powerful painkillers available. Their side-effects include drowsiness, suppressed respiration, constipation and nausea. They also can promote a sense of profound well-being, thus explaining why opioids are also used as illegal recreational drugs. The effects of the opiate drugs wear off rapidly, and this can lead to recurrence of symptoms and a drop in mood. They induce dependency because they reduce the body's response to its naturally produced opiates.

Patients using opiates for pain relief often require gradually increasing doses to keep their symptoms under control. It is not uncommon for a cancer patient eventually to be able to tolerate a dose of opiates that would be lethal to a healthy person.

Constipation almost always complicates the prescription of strong opiates such as morphine or diamorphine. Therefore, most patients will be prescribed a laxative such as dantron as a matter of course.

Non-steroidal anti-inflammatory drugs (NSAIDs)

The NSAIDS are very effective painkillers for pain that has inflammation or bone disease as its cause. Very often, NSAIDs may be prescribed in combination with opiates in the treatment of chronic pain. As NSAIDs carry a high risk of inducing irritation and bleeding of the stomach lining, they are often prescribed together with an acid-suppressing medication such as omeprazole.

Tricyclic antidepressants for pain

Antidepressants such as amitriptyline may be prescribed for their ability to alleviate certain types of chronic pain. They have the additional benefits of mood elevation and sleep promotion.

Drugs for nausea

Nausea is a common side-effect of chemotherapy and painkillers, and can also occur as a result of the cancer alone. It can be a very debilitating side-effect, and affects over 60% of terminally ill cancer patients.

Anti-nausea drugs include metaclopramide which is most effective if the cause of the nausea is gastrointestinal in origin. If the cause is more likely to be a result of some sort of central brain disturbance (as a consequence of metabolic imbalance), then cyclizine, which is used for travel sickness, may be more effective. Major tranquilliser drugs such as prochlorperazine and haloperidol are also effective in reducing central nausea.

To prevent the nausea that results from cancer chemotherapy the $5HT_3$ antagonists such as ondansetron and intravenous corticosteroids may be prescribed in the hospital ward prior to and during treatment. Some centres recommend that during chemotherapy their patients wear "Sea-bands", which put pressure at the wrist on the acupoint Neiguan PC-6.

Treatment for depression

The emotional burden on a patient with cancer has many components. Factors such as fear of dying, regrets about past events, inability to express negative emotions, discomfort from side-effects, changing body image and disempowerment in hospital can all contribute to the development of a disabling depression. It is now recognised that patients require support to enable them to express these issues, and to be given as much dignity and freedom as possible. The ideal is to enable a cancer patient to remain at home for as long as possible.

The more 'holistic' approach to palliative care, which involves counselling, alternative therapies, spiritual support and support of relatives, is intended to help patients deal with the development of distressing symptoms and reduce depression.

The SSRI antidepressants, such as paroxetine and sertraline, are also prescribed very readily in palliative care. They take 2–4 weeks to exert a therapeutic effect.

Red flags of serious disease

From this point on in the text those symptoms and signs of disease (syndromes) that are indicative of potential serious disease will be introduced systematically. Because they should alert the practitioner to a change in management to one that is highly focused on maximising safety, these warning syndromes are called 'red flags'. The presence of a red flag does not necessarily mean that serious disease is present. In this text the term "red flag" will be used to relate to any syndrome that may indicate that the patient would benefit from a referral to a conventional medical practitioner.

At the end of each chapter relating to the description of diseases, red flag syndromes are presented, as they are below, in the form of a table. Each table summarises those red flags that pertain to the diseases that have been just discussed in the chapter. The red flag tables will also provide you with some explanatory information about why the red flag syndrome merits the consideration of referral.

A summary of all the red flags is given in Appendix III, together with guidance about the appropriate response should they be encountered in clinical practice. The red flags in the summary are graded according to the degree of urgency with which they need to be handled.

The red flags of cancer

The red flag syndromes that might indicate the presence of cancer are summarised in Table 2.3a-II, the first of the red flag tables. This table forms part of the summary on red flags given in Appendix III, which also gives advice on the degree of urgency of referral for each of the red flag conditions listed.

Table 2.3a-II Red Flags 1 – cancer

Red Flag	Description	Reasoning
1.1	**Progressive** unexplained **symptoms** over weeks to months: **e.g. weight loss,** recurrent **sweats** (especially at night)**, fevers** and poor **appetite**	Symptoms that progress (i.e. gradually worsen rather than fluctuate in intensity) over this sort of time period are strongly suggestive of cancer
1.2	An unexplained **lump:** characteristically **hard, irregular, fixed and painless**	Cancerous lumps are usually irregular, may be fixed to associated tissues, and often are painless unless they obstruct viscera, cause pressure on other structures, grow into bone or grow into nerve roots
1.3	Unexplained **bleeding:** either from the surface of the skin, or emerging from an internal organ such as the bowel, bladder or uterus	Cancerous tissue is poorly organised, and bleeding may easily be provoked from the surface of an epithelial tumour (e.g. of breast, skin, lung, mouth, stomach, bowel, bladder or uterus)
1.4	**Features of bone marrow failure**: severe progressive **anaemia** (see Chapter 3.4c), recurrent progressive **infections** or **bruising, purpura** and **bleeding**	Secondary cancer and cancer of the blood cells often infiltrate the bone marrow and prevent it from performing its role of producing healthy red and white blood cells and platelets Purpura is pinpoint bruising that appears like a rash of flat purplish spots, and is one of the signs of a low platelet count See also Red Flags 20 – Lymphoma and leukaemia (Table 3.4e-I)

Continued

Table 2.3a-II Red Flags 1 – cancer—Cont'd

Red Flag	Description	Reasoning
1.5	**Multiple enlarged lymph nodes** (greater than 1 cm in diameter) but painless, with no other obvious cause (e.g. known glandular fever infection)	Groups of lymph nodes can be found in the cervical region, in the armpits (axillary nodes) and in the inguinal creases (groin). In health, lymph nodes are usually soft impalpable masses of soft tissue, but these can enlarge and become more palpable when the node is active in fighting an infection, or if It is infiltrated by tumour cells. If a number of nodes are enlarged (to more than 1 cm in diameter) this may signify a generalised infectious disease such as glandular fever or HIV/AIDS The other important cause of widespread lymph node enlargement (lymphadenopathy) is disseminated cancer, and in particular the cancers of the white blood cells, leukaemia and lymphoma If multiple enlarged lymph nodes are found it is best to refer for a diagnosis, and as a high priority if the patient is unwell with other symptoms
1.6	**A single markedly enlarged lymph node** (greater than 2 cm in diameter) with no other obvious cause	Even in the situation of infection it is unusual for a lymph node to become very enlarged. Cancerous infiltration can lead to a firm grossly enlarged lymph node, which may be painless. This is particularly typical of lymphoma
1.7	**Ascites: painless abdominal swelling** due to fluid accumulation	Abdominal epithelial malignancies such as colon cancer, stomach cancer and ovarian cancer may lead to the accumulation of fluid within the abdominal cavity, which initially may be painless. This sign is known as ascites. Ascites is a sign that the cancer has metastasised and so carries a poor prognosis. Other causes of ascites include chronic congestive cardiac failure, liver failure and kidney disease

Self-test 2.3a

Cancer

1. Consider the way a cancer cell forms and develops into a tumour. What are the conventionally accepted
   (i) internal factors, and
   (ii) external factors
   that may lead to the development of cancer?
2. A lipoma is a rounded mass of fatty calls that can be felt a soft painless lump under the skin. It can often be freely moved when palpated. It is often discovered for the first time by the patient when it is quite large (3–5 cm in diameter). It is never associated with enlarged lymph nodes. When surgically removed, the fatty cells are found to be typical or normal fatty cells, and the borders of the lump are clearly defined from adjacent tissue.

   A melanoma is a form of mole found on the skin. Its characteristics are that it may have an irregular border, irregular patches of often dark black pigmentation, and may be raised in an irregular way. It may be first noticed when it changes or enlarges in some way. It can be prone to bleeding when slightly damaged. Enlarged lymph nodes are occasionally associated with a melanoma. What are the characteristics of these tumours that indicate that the lipoma is benign and the melanoma is malignant?
3. Name:
   (i) three approaches to the removal of cancerous tissue
   (ii) three methods of relieving symptoms in the treatment of cancer.
4. What is the conventional understanding about how chemotherapy and radiotherapy may cure cancer (answer this in three sentences only)?
5. List four symptoms/signs that may indicate a diagnosis of cancer in a patient (i.e. name four red flags of cancer).

Answers

1. (i) Internal factors include an inherited tendency to increased mutation. A depleted immune system is another internal factor that can be either inherited or arise due to emotional and physical stresses and ageing.
   (ii) External factors are the carcinogens that promote increased mutation (e.g. cigarette smoke and radiation) and anything external that depletes the immune system (e.g. toxins or HIV infection).
2. The features of a *lipoma* that indicate that it is benign are:
   - smooth borders (rounded), softness, movability, normal cells that do not invade the surrounding tissue, and no association with spread to lymph nodes
   - the fact the lipoma is discovered when it is large does not mean that it is necessarily fast growing – often such lumps are not noticed for years before they are suddenly discovered by the patient
   - painlessness is not a reassuring feature – many malignant lumps are initially painless because they do not have a normal nerve supply

   The features of a *melanoma* that suggest it is malignant are:
   - irregular shape, rapid change, irregular pigmentation, tendency to bleed, and association with spread to lymph nodes
   - a melanoma is usually painless, and when examined under the microscope irregular uncharacteristic (dysplastic) cells are seen that invade local tissues.
3. (i) Surgery, chemotherapy, radiotherapy.
   (ii) Painkillers, antisickness medication, tranquillisers, laxatives, counselling and all three approaches listed in (i).
4. Both treatments are toxic to rapidly dividing cells. They therefore preferentially kill cancer cells. They are given in cycles to allow recovery of normal tissues in between the 'attacks' on the vulnerable cancer tissue.
5. The red flags of cancer are:
   - short history of weeks to months
   - progressive symptoms
   - a lump
   - unexplained bleeding
   - unexplained swelling of the abdomen (ascites).

Infectious disease

2.4

Chapter 2.4a Principles of infectious disease

LEARNING POINTS

At the end of this chapter you will be able to:
- define infectious disease and list the different types of infectious agent
- recognise how the impact of infectious disease in a population depends on its general level of health
- list the different mechanisms by which infections can cause damage to human tissues
- define the concept of herd immunity
- describe how new infections can emerge.

Estimated time for chapter: 75 minutes.

Introduction to the systematic study of disease

The first three sections of Stage 2 introduced the principles of susceptibility to disease and the pathological processes of disease. It was explained how some of the processes of disease, such as the disorders of excessive clotting and cancer, are considered as diseases in their own right. However, in most diseases the name of the condition does not necessarily indicate the underlying processes of disease. From this point onwards, the information given about diseases is structured according either to the pathological agent (e.g. infectious diseases), the physiological system affected (e.g. diseases of the cardiovascular system) or the type of patients affected (e.g. child) rather than according to the process of disease.

As practitioners of complementary medicine, it is of course not necessary to be fully conversant with all the different conventionally described diseases and their treatments. However, it is of great value to be practised in an approach to researching information about a disease and its treatments when it becomes relevant to the management of a particular clinical case. This approach first requires a basic understanding of the physiology of the various systems of the body and the processes of disease as described in the earlier sections of this text. It is also important to be familiar with how information about diseases is presented systematically in medical texts and websites. For this reason, the disease-specific information presented in the following sections of this text is written in language chosen to be accessible to non-medically trained practitioners, but ordered in the way that information is structured in conventional texts. It is intended that these sections of the text will provide a conceptual bridge for the understanding of more in-depth technical descriptions of disease and therapeutics found in other sources of medical information.

Introduction to the study of infectious diseases

This chapter introduces the study of the infectious diseases. Diseases can be broadly classified into infectious and non-infectious disease. Infectious diseases, also termed 'communicable diseases', result from damage to the body following infection or infestation by an external infectious agent. Infection may lead to a range of processes of disease and may affect one or more of the physiological systems.

The infectious agents are summarised in Table 2.4a-I. They may be microscopic, in which case they are called 'microbes'. If a microbe is a bacterium or a single-celled animal such as an amoeba, the term 'microorganism' may also be used, denoting that the microbe is a life form. Viruses are non-living microbes. Most infectious diseases are caused by microbes, but larger creatures such as worms can also cause infectious diseases. When the infectious agents are arthropods (insects and mites) the term 'infestation' may be used to describe the disease process.

Table 2.4a-I The different types of infectious agent

Agent	Description
Microbes	
Viruses and prions	Non-living particles capable of replication; prions are made of protein alone, and viruses of a combination of protein and genetic material
Bacteria	The smallest life form; bacteria consist of single cells, but are more simple in structure than the generalised cell described In Chapter 1.1b
Fungi	Yeasts and moulds; like bacteria, these are composed of very simple cellular units
Protozoa	Single-celled animals such as the amoeba; the cells of protozoa contain all the organelles of the simple cell described in Chapter 1.1b
Larger organisms	
Roundworms, flukes and tapeworms	E.g. threadworm
Mites	E.g. head and body lice
Insects	E.g. fleas

The definition of infectious disease

Infectious diseases are so termed because they are contracted by transmission of the infectious agent from a person, animal or even an inanimate object (termed the 'carrier'). This also explains the use of the term 'communicable'.

Not all infections can be classified as infectious diseases. For example, an infection can arise when a person succumbs to microorganisms that naturally live within the body, but which do not usually cause disease in a state of healthy balance. A bladder infection, also called 'cystitis', is an example of such a disease, in that the bacteria which cause a person to develop cystitis usually originate from the person's own natural bowel bacteria.

The impact of infectious disease

The description of infectious disease can often be found to be the subject of one of the first chapters in general textbooks about pathology and clinical medicine. This is a reflection of the importance of infectious disease. In terms of causation of disability and death, infections are the single most important cause of disease worldwide. However, in developed countries, infections do not cause as much death and disability as they do in developing countries. In the developed world the most important causes of death and disability are now the non-communicable diseases, and most importantly disease of the cardiovascular system, cancer and, in young people, accidents (see Q.2.4a-1).

The modern developments of vaccination and drug treatment for infections are widely acknowledged in conventional medicine to have led to the decline in infectious disease in developed populations. However, it is increasingly understood that the provision of basic needs, such as clean water and removal of sewage (sanitation), good housing and adequate diet, are also important factors which account for the reduction in infectious disease. The provision of these basic needs contributes to the attainment of a basic level of health, and in health the body is better able both to withstand contracting some infections, and also to overcome those infections that do develop.

The study of the epidemiology of diseases such as tuberculosis, rheumatic fever and diphtheria supports this theory that healthy populations resist infectious disease. All these diseases have declined dramatically in well-nourished western populations, and yet are major causes of ill-health in developing countries. For all three, the decline preceded the introduction of vaccinations or antibiotic treatment, and relates more to improvements in nourishment and sanitation. The reports that tuberculosis is on the increase again in western countries reflect an increase largely confined to marginalised groups, such as the homeless, who do not have access to good nutrition and housing.

Measles is an infectious disease from which most well-nourished children make a full recovery, with less than 0.1% developing long-term serious consequences. However, measles is still one of the major causes of infant death and blindness in developing countries, causing death in up to 30% of infants who contract it in some impoverished localities. This illustrates the fact that infectious disease has much more impact in populations who are more susceptible as a result of malnutrition and poor living conditions.

Nevertheless, there are many infections that cause serious disease within healthy populations. Examples of such diseases include bacterial meningitis, certain types of pneumonia, certain types of food poisoning (including *Escherichia coli* serotype O157), human immunodeficiency virus (HIV) infection and many of the tropical diseases (e.g. malaria and typhoid). Although it is true that these diseases often tend to have a greater impact on those who are more susceptible, such as the very young and the elderly, these infections are nevertheless also well recognised to be the cause of significant ill-health and mortality in previously fit young people. This is an indication that some infections can 'take hold' and cause damage even when the individual does not appear obviously to be particularly susceptible to a severe illness.

Immunity and infectious disease

The topic of immunity was introduced in Chapter 2.1d. The general level of immunity to a disease in a population is another major factor that affects the impact of the disease. Diseases that are very common in a population are termed 'endemic'. Chickenpox and the common cold are diseases that are endemic in the UK, whereas malaria is endemic in a tropical country such as Uganda. It is common for a population in a locality which has been exposed from birth to an endemic disease to have less marked reactions to that disease than visitors to that locality. This is why travellers to foreign countries frequently succumb to infections that do not seem to affect the locals, leading to symptoms such as fevers and food poisoning.

The resistance of a population to an endemic disease is attributed in part to 'herd immunity'. This term describes the immunity that results from the fact that a large proportion of the population have already encountered that infection, often in early life. For this reason, they will not thereafter easily contract the disease. If herd immunity exists, the disease is less likely to take hold in the population because there are fewer people to whom it can be passed on. This is one of the principles of vaccination campaigns which aim to ensure that a large proportion of the population is immune. The end result of a successful vaccination campaign is an increase in the herd immunity to a specific disease such as measles.

However, acquired herd immunity is not the whole story. Local people who have not yet experienced endemic diseases still generally appear to be able to fight off these infections when they do experience them more efficiently than travellers to the area. A striking example of this is the impact that was made by minor infections taken by the first explorers to the New World. Diseases such as the common cold and chickenpox caused serious consequences in communities to whom they were totally new infections. It seems as if the immune system of a person in a locality is prepared in some way to deal with an endemic disease, but is seriously challenged by one that is not a normal part of the local pattern of infections. This extra level of protection may possibly be the result of a genetic adaptation of the local population over generations of exposure to endemic diseases (an example of 'natural selection').

If a disease suddenly appears to be on the increase in a population, then the term 'epidemic' is used. An epidemic disease is not necessarily severe, but is occurring much more often than expected. Epidemics occur either because a new type of infectious agent has emerged for which there is no pre-existing herd immunity, or because over the course of time the herd immunity has diminished so that the disease can rapidly take hold once again.

The pathology of infectious disease

There are two properties of infectious agents that result in them being able to cause harm. The first is that they have the ability to penetrate the normal barriers to disease, and the second is that, having penetrated, they are able to damage the body tissues.

An example of these two stages is the damage caused as a result of flea infestation. The flea can penetrate the barrier of the skin because it is able to puncture it by biting. Damage is due to substances in the flea's saliva, which enter the deep layers (dermis) of the skin. These substances are irritating to the cells in the dermis, and so cause inflammation at the site of the puncture. This leads to the small red and itchy bump of the flea bite. In some people these chemicals behave as antigens and provoke a pronounced immune response. This leads to the site of the bite becoming firmer and larger and even blistered over the course of a few days (see Q2.4a-2).

The infectious diseases can lead to damage that results from one or more of the seven processes of disease described in Chapter 2.2a. The flea bite is an example of how an infectious agent can give rise to inflammation, which is the most common disease process to result from infectious disease. However, infectious agents can also lead to disease by causing problems in the immune system, including cancerous change, and by causing degeneration.

The following descriptions of infectious diseases illustrate the diversity of the disease processes involved.

Tonsillitis

The tonsils are masses of lymphoid tissue (like lymph nodes) that sit at the entrance to the pharynx (they can be seen in most people at the back of the mouth just behind the arch formed by the palate). Tonsillitis can be passed on from one person to another by the inhalation of droplets of infected fluid, following a cough for example. However, tonsillitis is not always contagious. Tonsillitis can also occur when a person becomes susceptible to relatively harmless bacteria that they have been harbouring on their tonsils for some time. This explains why some people get recurrent bouts of tonsillitis whenever they are run down.

The symptoms of tonsillitis are primarily due to inflammation of the tonsils. The bacteria and viruses that cause tonsillitis are able to attach to the epithelial cells of the surface of the tonsil by means of chemicals (proteins) on their coating. Damage is caused partly because the microbes can kill tonsil cells by first attaching to them, and as a result they stimulate inflammation. Some bacteria encourage the excessive production of pus, consisting of dead phagocytic leukocytes. The chemicals released during the immune response and inflammation give rise to the general feelings of malaise that are common in tonsillitis. In most cases the immune response is sufficient to hinder the spread of infection so that it settles down within a few days.

The rare complications of glomerulonephritis and rheumatic fever can follow tonsillitis resulting from a bacterium called *Streptococcus*. In these conditions, the antibodies that develop in the immune response to the bacteria do not just target the bacteria, but also proteins in the kidney and heart valves, respectively. This is a type II hypersensitivity reaction. The kidney and valvular diseases that result are, therefore, autoimmune diseases, but ones that are triggered by an infection.

Cold sores

The herpes simplex virus is passed on through intimate contact such as kissing. The virus is present in the saliva of the carrier, and from there penetrates into the cells of the lining of the mouth, where it initially, in a quasi-parasitic way, uses the cell's supply of nutrients to replicate itself. It also penetrates the ends of nerve cells in the connective tissue of the lining of the mouth, and this leads to the characteristic tingling sensation. Eventually, the infected cells will rupture and die, and cause inflammation, which is the cause of the redness and scabbing. Each ruptured cell will release thousands of new viruses into the saliva of the person with the cold sore.

Intense pain can result as an effect of the infection of the nerve cells. When the infection has healed, some viruses remain 'latent' within some of the nerve cells, but these are prevented from replicating by the immune system. When the person becomes run down, this hidden source of infection can emerge as another cold sore.

AIDS

The human immunodeficiency virus (HIV) is carried in body fluids. Close contact with the infected body fluids together with a break in the normal barrier of the skin is necessary for HIV to be transmitted. Sexual contact and childbirth provide these conditions, as does transmission of human fluids by a hypodermic needle.

The presence of the virus in the blood stream leads to an immune response that then causes the flu-like syndrome characteristic of many viral infections. Although antibodies are formed, they are usually unable to clear the HIV from the body. This is because the virus is able to penetrate into leukocytes and in this way hide from the immune response. In this intracellular state the HIV remains, dividing with the leukocytes over a period of years, until gradually the function of those cells becomes impaired. Therefore, the major consequences of HIV infection are not primarily due to inflammation, but instead to a disorder of the immune system. This disorder leads to the combined problems of opportunistic infections and cancer.

In advanced disease, the nerve cells of the brain are also penetrated by the virus and become damaged, leading to a form of dementia. AIDS is, therefore, an example of an infection causing degeneration as well as inflammation and a disorder of the immune system.

These diverse examples illustrate how infections cause disease by various mechanisms. Although inflammation is the most common damaging consequence of infections, autoimmune disease, immunodeficiency, cancer and degeneration can also be caused by infections. Infections can also cause congenital disease in the embryo and fetus if contracted during pregnancy (e.g. congenital rubella syndrome, which results from a German measles infection during the firsttrimester).

Transmission of disease

The three examples of infectious diseases described above also illustrate the diversity of ways in which infections can be transmitted. Tonsillitis is transmitted by inhalation of droplets, the cold sore virus through infected saliva penetrating the mucous membranes of the mouth, and HIV is transmitted via infected body fluids (commonly blood and semen) penetrating the usual skin barriers (see Q2.4a-3).

There is an enormous number of possible routes of infection, illustrating the complex ways by which infectious agents have adapted themselves to find their way into their human hosts. Modes of transmission can be broadly considered in two categories: person-to-person spread and animal-to-person spread. Examples of these are listed in Table 2.4a-II.

Table 2.4a-II The different modes of transmission of infectious agents

Person-to-person spread
• Infection in the gastrointestinal tract passed on through contact with human faeces (usually indirectly by eating contaminated food or water), e.g. typhoid and cholera • Infestations passed on through clothing and bedding, e.g. body lice
Animal-to-person spread
• Infection carried by insects and mites passed on through bites, e.g. malaria • Infection passed on through contact with animal faeces, e.g. food poisoning due to bacteria such as *Salmonella* and *E. coli* originating from poorly cooked contaminated meat and eggs • Infection passed on through eating meat containing parasites, e.g. tapeworm • Infection carried in rat urine that penetrates the skin via contaminated water, e.g. Weil's disease

Emerging infections

For each of the known infections, the causative infectious agent has adapted to target particular human tissues and causes damage in a characteristic way. The conventional view is that such adaptation is the consequence of evolution over the course of many years. Evolution is believed to be the result of mutation that is 'beneficial' to the infectious agent. As a species of microbe replicates, occasionally mutation leads to daughter microbes that are better able to reproduce than are their parents. In the case of infectious disease, this successful adaptation is often one that leads the daughter microbes to be more efficient at infecting human cells. This is because it is through infection that microbes obtain the nutrients necessary for survival and replication.

Evolution in complex species such as humans is believed to occur very gradually over many thousands of years. However, evolution of simple species such as viruses and other microbes may lead to a dramatic change in a species over a much shorter time. This is because the microbes replicate at a very rapid rate.

HIV is an example of an infection that seemed to emerge, probably originally in Africa, within the last 50 years, before which time it was completely unknown. HIV currently appears to be perfectly adapted to thrive in the human body through having a protein on its coat that connects exactly with the proteins on the human leukocyte. One theory is that HIV previously existed as a monkey virus, and through chance mutation acquired this protein that enables it to survive and replicate in humans.

It is now recognised that new microbes are emerging in this way all the time, as they change in form through replication. Over the past quarter of a century, more than 30 new or newly recognised infections have been identified around the world (see Q2.4a-4). The newly emerging infectious diseases include hepatitis C and E viruses, Lyme disease, staphylococcal toxic shock syndrome, H5N1 avian influenza (bird flu), SARS (sudden adult respiratory distress syndrome) virus and nvCJD (new variant Creutzfeldt–Jakob disease) virus.

Mutation does not only give rise to new species of infectious organism; it also can lead to subtle changes in existing organisms. These changes, which lead to new 'strains', can mean that the organism is no longer recognised by the immune system of someone who had previously had immunity to that disease.

This type of mutation appears to occur more readily in some infectious organisms than others. For example, the influenza virus rapidly changes its characteristic coat through mutation. This gives rise to the frequent epidemics of influenza that are experienced in the UK. Each influenza epidemic reflects a wave of infections by a new strain of the virus. This explains why people can contract influenza repeatedly during their life, and why a new vaccine for influenza needs to be developed on an annual basis.

In contrast, the chickenpox virus appears not to mutate significantly, reflected in the fact that most people retain their immunity to chickenpox for life.

Chapter 2.4b The different types of infectious disease

LEARNING POINTS

At the end of this chapter you will be able to:

- understand how the different types of infectious agent can cause disease.

Estimated time for chapter: 100 minutes.

Infectious organisms

The main groups of infectious agents were introduced in the last chapter and summarised in Table 2.4a-I. Each one of these groups is in this chapter considered in turn, together with some of the diseases that they can cause.

Diseases caused by viruses

Viruses and prions are so small that, unlike bacteria and human cells, they cannot be seen using a simple microscope. Instead, a more powerful microscope, called an 'electron microscope', is required to produce images of these particles. Figures 2.4b-I and 2.4b-II show electron micrographs of two different viruses: the envelope-bounded DNA herpes simplex virus, and the icosohedral (20-sided) RNA rotavirus. The size of these viruses is measured in nanometres (nm), which are an unimaginable one-billionth of a metre (1×10^{-9} m) in size. These viruses are 160 and 80 nm in diameter, respectively.

Viruses contain some genetic material that is similar in structure to that found within human chromosomes, together with additional proteins that form a surrounding coat. Prions are composed of a single complex protein alone. Because of their simplicity, viruses and prions often have a structure that resembles a geometric crystal. This is in contrast to the complex and unique rounded structures found in each living cell.

Viruses cause damage because they have adapted to be able to penetrate living cells, and then to utilise the nutrients within those cells to replicate. Viruses cannot replicate, obtain nutrients or respond to environmental changes without living

Self-test 2.4a

Principles of infectious disease

1. How might you define infectious disease?
2. Name the processes of disease that you think might result from an infection (and which then lead to the various symptoms of infectious diseases).
3. What do you think are possible reasons why infectious disease causes such problems in refugee camps? Think broadly about the health of the population in the camp, and how infections are transmitted.
4. From your own knowledge, what do you think are the modes of transmission for the following infections:
   - rabies
   - head lice
   - the common cold
   - traveller's diarrhoea?

Answers

1. Infectious disease is disease resulting from damage by infectious agents. The infectious agent has been transmitted by contact with an infected carrier, which can be either animate or inanimate.
2. Infectious disease may cause damage to human tissue through the processes of inflammation, disturbance of the immune system, development of cancer or degeneration. Inflammation is the most important of these four processes in terms of impact on human health.
3. Infectious disease is a particular problem in refugee camps, mostly because sanitation is poor and diseases such as cholera and typhoid can spread via water contaminated with human faeces.

   The close contact between people in a crowded camp will also increase the incidence of infections that are transmitted by person-to-person spread.

   An additional factor is the increased susceptibility of refugees that results from malnutrition, exhaustion and emotional stress. All these factors will lead to a depleted immune system and an inability to fight infections efficiently.

   If the refugees are located far from their usual homes, they may also be exposed to diseases for which there is no 'herd immunity'. This will mean that relatively minor local diseases such as colds and influenza may have serious consequences.
4. - Rabies is transmitted following an animal bite. The virus is present in the saliva of the infected animal and penetrates the barrier of the skin via the puncture wound of a bite.
   - Head lice are transmitted by close contact with people with head lice. This allows the lice in the hair of one person to move into the hair of another. Children tend to make more close contact with each other than adults, which is why head lice are such a problem in schools.
   - The common cold is transmitted, like tonsillitis, through the spread of infected droplets from the nose and mouth of an infected person. The cold virus stimulates the excessive production of fluid from the nose. This is an adaptation that helps it to spread very effectively.
   - Traveller's diarrhoea is generally contracted after drinking local water, or food prepared using local water in an area that is new to the traveller. The water contains small numbers of microbes originating from human faeces, to which the local people are generally immune but which cause an illness when they enter the digestive system of a traveller.

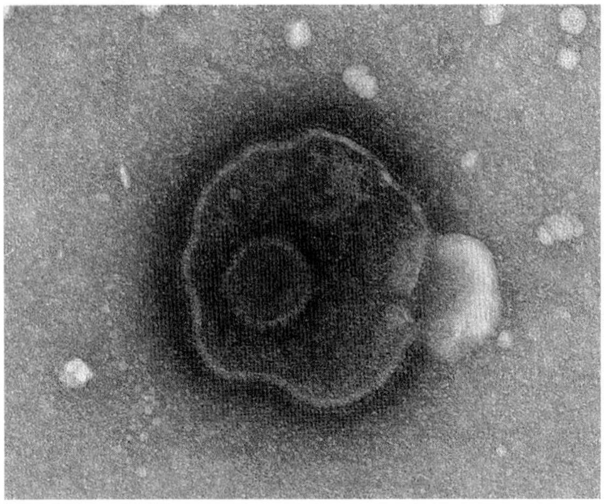

Figure 2.4b-I • Electron micrograph of the herpes simplex virus.

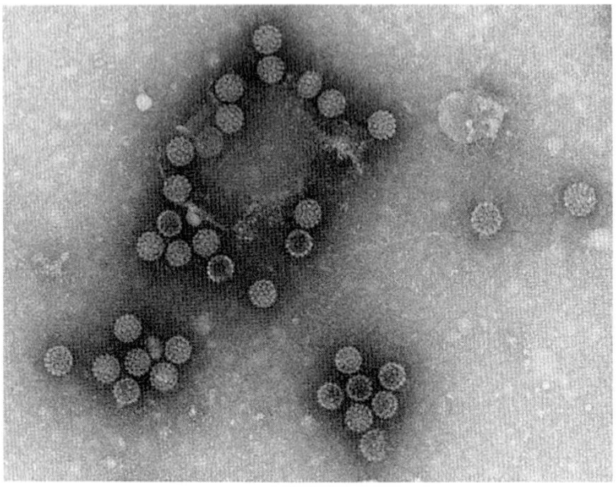

Figure 2.4b-II • Electron micrograph of the human rotavirus.

cells, and so cannot, by definition, be considered a life form. Viruses cause disease both because they damage living cells, and also because they trigger an immune response. The high temperature, rash, aches and malaise characteristic of many viral infections are manifestations of the immune response generated against viruses circulating in the blood stream.

Viruses can damage human cells in different ways: some simply cause cell death, as for example does the cold sore virus. This can have many consequences, depending on which tissue is affected. The death of human cells and release of cellular contents leads to inflammation, so the familiar features of redness, heat, swelling and pain are commonly found when a part of the body is affected by a virus.

Other consequences include:

- disturbance of cell replication, leading to benign growths (e.g. wart virus)
- cancer, as a result of interfering with the proto-oncogene function in a cell (e.g. genital wart virus, which can be a trigger for cervical cancer)
- disturbance of the development of the fetus, leading to congenital malformation (e.g. rubellavirus) if the infection occurs in pregnancy.

An excessive immune response to viruses can also be damaging. Possible consequences include:

- bleeding within tissues (e.g. the viral haemorrhagic disease Lassa fever)
- delayed immune damage to the nervous system, which can manifest as numbness, weakness and mood changes (e.g. Guillain–Barré syndrome).

The much reported 'postviral syndrome', which describes depression and exhaustion following a viral infection, has also been attributed to delayed immune damage to the nervous system following a viral infection.

Viruses are classified into groups (families and subfamilies) according to their structure. Some of the major families of viruses are listed in Table 2.4b-I, and some of the diverse diseases that result from viral infections are listed in Table 2.4b-II (see Q2.4b-1).

Diseases caused by prions

Prions have only recently been discovered and described as infectious agents. They are known to be even more simple in structure than a virus in that they consist of a single protein. Prions are believed to cause disease by mimicking the structure of essential proteins in the nervous system of their animal hosts. They seem to induce an irreversible change of these proteins into more prion proteins. This leads the host cells to degenerate, and enables the prion to increase in quantity. Creutzfeldt–Jakob disease (CJD) and the new variant form (nvCJD) are two prion diseases that have been shown to affect humans. As far as it is known, prion diseases can only be transmitted when infected animal tissue or blood enters the body of another animal, either by the ingestion of infected flesh, or through surgery and possibly through blood transfusion.

Table 2.4b-I Some different families of virus

Class of virus	Description
Adenoviruses	A large group of DNA-containing viruses that commonly cause minor upper respiratory infections
Herpesviruses	DNA viruses responsible for cold sores, chickenpox and glandular fever. All are capable of causing latent infections that can reappear at a later date
Poxviruses	DNA viruses causing crusting diseases such as smallpox, cowpox, monkey pox and orf
Picornaviruses	Small RNA viruses causing diseases including poliomyelitis, viral meningitis and the common cold
Reoviruses	Small RNA viruses responsible for epidemics of infectious diarrhoea and mild respiratory symptoms
Retroviruses	Viruses that are able to replicate by inserting a protein called 'reverse transcriptase' into a cell. Includes the human immunodeficiency virus (HIV)

Table 2.4b-II Various viral diseases

Disease	Causative virus
Pharyngitis (sore throat)	Adenovirus
Cold sores	Herpes simplex
Genital herpes	Herpes simplex
Chickenpox	Varicella zoster
Viral encephalitis	Measles, mumps, herpes simplex
Viral meningitis	Coxsackie virus, measles, mumps
Rabies	Rabies
Croup	Respiratory syncytial virus
Glandular fever	Epstein–Barr virus
Kaposi's sarcoma	Epstein–Barr virus
Smallpox	Variola
Poliomyelitis	Poliovirus
Mumps	Mumps virus
Lassa fever	Lassa virus
Viral pneumonia	Measles, varicella zoster,
Diarrhoea	Rotavirus, noravirus, adenovirus
Rubella (German measles)	Rubella
Yellow fever	Yellow fever
Influenza	Influenza
Measles	Measles
Common cold	Rhinovirus

Diseases caused by bacteria

Bacteria (singular is bacterium) are microorganisms that consist of a single simple cell. The structure is far less complex than the typical animal cell described in Chapter 1.1b. Bacteria do not have nuclei or mitochondria, for example, but instead the copying of the genetic material and the energy-generating processes all take place around large molecules that are situated free within the cell cytoplasm. Nevertheless, the bacterium still uses basic nutrients and reproduces in a similar way. For this reason a bacterium is considered a life form. Bacteria are, on average, about one-tenth of the size of human cells, but can be seen through a simple microscope.

Figure 2.4b-III shows a simplified drawing of a rod-shaped bacterium, *Escherichia coli* (*E. coli*). The size of bacteria is generally measured in micrometres (μm), which are one-millionth of a metre (1×10^{-6} m) in size. An *E. coli* bacterium is 3 μm in length, which is 20 times longer than the diameter of the complex herpes simplex virus.

If a bacterial disease is suspected, a doctor might take a 'swab' of the infected site, for example an inflamed tonsil. The swab is taken to the laboratory, where it is swept across

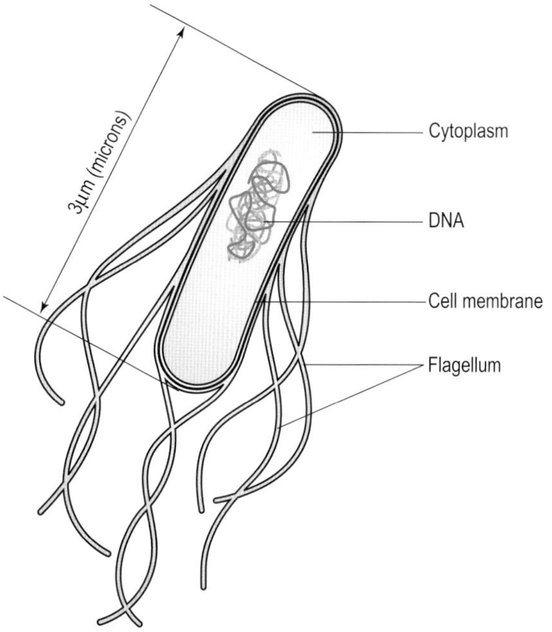

Figure 2.4b-III • Simplified diagram of a coliform bacterium (*E. coli*).

a glass slide, stained with a dye that is absorbed by bacteria, and the 'smear' then viewed through a microscope.

In the examination of a smear from an inflamed tonsil resulting, for example, from infection by the *Streptococcus* bacterium, the microscope might reveal clumps of large epithelial cells from the tonsil, and chains of tiny darkly stained circular forms, the streptococcal bacteria (also known as 'streptococci').

Bacteria are classified according to their shape, ability to absorb stains, and other properties that can be tested in the laboratory, and have been given Latin names that often reflect these characteristics. Very often bacteria are classified as Gram-negative or Gram-positive. This simply indicates the way that a bacterium reacts to a stain first used by an early pathologist called Gram, and is a reflection of the nature of the protective coat around the bacterium. More recently, bacteria have been classified according to their genetic makeup. This has led to reclassification of some groups, because genetic analysis reveals similarities and differences that are not apparent from their morphological characteristics.

Bacteria may also be classified according to their morphology. The two broad categories of cocci (spherical cells) and bacilli (rod shaped cells) are morphological categories.

Important Gram-positive bacteria include species of *Staphylococcus*, *Streptococcus*, *Bacillus*, *Clostridium* (including tetanus), *Mycobacterium* (including tuberculosis), *Corynebacterium* (including diphtheria) and *Listeria*.

Important Gram-negative bacteria include species of *Chlamydia*, *Escherichia* (e.g. *E. coli*), *Salmonella*, *Vibrio* (e.g. cholera), *Helicobacter*, *Neisseria* (e.g. gonorrhoea and meningococcus), *Bordetella* (e.g. whooping cough), *Legionella* (e.g. Legionnaire's disease) and *Treponema* (e.g. syphilis) (see Q2.4b-2).

Some infectious diseases, for example tonsillitis and pharyngitis, can be caused by both bacteria and viruses. Other examples include meningitis, encephalitis, pericarditis, bronchitis and pneumonia. Although in these conditions there are various possible infectious agents, the end result of the infection is similar in terms of the development of inflammation within a particular organ (see Q2.4b-3).

Many infectious diseases are described by terms that end with the suffix '-itis'. However, this suffix refers only to the fact that an organ is inflamed, but not what the cause might be. This is true also for the term 'pneumonia'. In fact, some inflammatory conditions, including bronchitis, pneumonia, cystitis, pericarditis and meningitis, can also be the result of damage by chemicals, radiation and autoimmune disease. They are, therefore, not always infectious diseases.

Diseases caused by protozoa, flukes and worms

Protozoa are single-celled animals and they share all the characteristics of the typical animal cell. Protozoa multiply by simple binary fission (mitosis).

Flukes, tapeworms and worms are more complex multicellular animals that possess a rudimentary nervous system and gut. They multiply by producing eggs that develop through an immature stage to the adult form. Often an additional animal host to the human is required for the life cycle to complete itself. For instance, the eggs of the pork tapeworm have to mature in the flesh of pigs before the parasite can be passed on to humans (as a result of eating infected meat).

Collectively, protozoa, flukes, tapeworms and worms are considered to be parasites when they infect human beings. The scientific definition of a parasite is a plant or an animal that lives in or on another animal and lives at the expense of that animal. In medical usage this term does not apply to bacteria or viruses. Nevertheless, the damage done by parasites is similar to that wreaked by infection with bacteria and viruses, including inflammation and an excessive immune response.

Protozoal diseases include giardiasis and amoebiasis (both causes of diarrhoea), malaria and sleeping sickness (tropical disease), and *Trichomonas* infection (a sexually transmitted disease). Most worm and fluke infections are tropical diseases, although threadworms and toxocariasis are worm infections that can be contracted in the UK.

Diseases caused by fungi

Fungi are a large class of life forms that includes the familiar mushrooms and toadstools, but also moulds and yeasts. Strictly speaking, they are classified as part of the plant kingdom.

Fungi are different from all other plants in that they do not contain the green pigment called 'chlorophyll'. Because of this they cannot use sunlight to manufacture energy. Instead, fungi require living or rotting animal and plant tissue to survive. Therefore, many have evolved to be parasites, obtaining nutrients from other living organisms, including humans.

In general, fungi do not cause serious disease in humans unless there is depletion of the immune system. In people with immunodeficiency, fungal disease can become a significant and sometimes life-threatening problem. However, minor fungal skin and mucous-membrane infections are very common in healthy people. These include athlete's foot, ringworm and thrush.

Athlete's foot is generally a mild fungal infection that targets damp skin. The most common site for the infection to start is the skin between the fourth and fifth toes. It rarely spreads beyond this area, although it can affect the growing nails, resulting in thickening and discolouration.

Ringworm is a fungal skin infection that forms an itchy, spreading ring of redness and scaling on the skin in a way that can be compared to the 'fairy ring' produced by some mushrooms. This mild but very contagious rash is often contracted from handling animals.

Thrush is due to a yeast called *Candida albicans*, which is a natural resident (commensal) of the bowel and genital tract of healthy human beings. It becomes problematic when the natural balance of the microorganisms in the body becomes disturbed. The *Candida* then becomes too dominant, akin to overgrowth of one plant species in a poorly tended garden. Excessive *Candida* leads to thick white patches and discharge, and can cause inflammation of the mucous membranes of the genital tract and the mouth.

Candida syndrome is recognised by some complementary health practitioners as a complex constellation of symptoms that include digestive problems, such as diarrhoea, irritable bowel syndrome and bloating, other fungal problems, such as athlete's foot, and mental problems, such as exhaustion and depression. Thrush may or may not be present in Candida syndrome. The symptoms of chronic fatigue syndrome (also known as 'myalgic encephalomyelitis' (ME)) have also been attributed to *Candida*. Excessive sugars and yeasts in the diet are claimed to be one of the causes of the Candida syndrome, and so the treatment involves a strict diet and the use of antifungal preparations. The use of preparations of the natural bacterium *Lactobacillus acidophilus* is recommended to help regain a healthy natural balance of microorganisms.

Candida syndrome is not recognised in conventional medicine. For this reason, patients who believe that they have Candida syndrome will not routinely be offered antifungal treatment by conventional doctors unless they have the white discharge, soreness and itching characteristic of thrush. The clinical evidence supporting the benefits of *Lactobacillus* supplementation in chronic fatigue and minor digestive disturbance is also not believed to be strong. Nevertheless, many doctors will recommend *Lactobacillus* supplementation to treat depletion of these bacteria resulting from antibiotic treatment or for the treatment of thrush.

Fungal infections are very problematic for someone with immunodeficiency. For example, patients with AIDS commonly experience severe thrush, which can affect the whole oesophagus and mouth as well as the genital mucous membranes. In severe immunodeficiency, *Candida* can spread to invade the lining of the bowel and other deep parts of body, and this can be life-threatening. Many AIDS patients develop a skin condition called 'seborrhoeic dermatitis', which is also due to overgrowth of a usually harmless skin fungus. Unusual fungal infections, such as cryptococcosis and histoplasmosis, are common causes of death in patients with immunodeficiency syndromes such as AIDS.

Infestations

Infestations by arthropods such as lice, scabies and fleas are different in nature to the other infectious diseases, as it is generally the surface of the body only that is affected. Biting and burrowing by these creatures causes damage to skin tissue and allergic responses, which then give rise to itching and discomfort.

Although the itch and discomfort can cause moderate distress, infestations are a cause of serious disease because arthropods can carry other diseases that are transmitted through bites. The 'plague', which caused thousands of deaths in Europe in past centuries, is such a disease, transmitted through the bite of the rat flea. Other arthropod-borne infections include typhus (tick-borne) and malaria (mosquito-borne). Many other less well-known tropical diseases are also transmitted via insect bites.

Beneficial (commensal) microorganisms

It is important to recognise that, in the healthy human being, as in all other large animals, there are thousands of bacteria and fungi 'resident' throughout the body. Microorganisms can be found on all epithelia that are in contact with the outside world, including the skin and the epithelial linings of the lung, bowel and genital organs. A person starts to inherit these 'guests' from the moment he or she is born and comes into close contact with caregivers. Newborn infants are very prone to episodes of oral thrush, possibly an indication that the delicate balance of fungi and bacteria has yet to become established.

Each human being can be considered as a distinct 'ecosystem', in which the human host and its microorganisms live in harmony. It is known that the health of the human depends in part on the balance of these microorganisms. For example, some bacteria in the bowel assist with the digestion of food. It is noteworthy that the medical term for these healthy bacteria is 'commensal', literally meaning that they share the same dining table as their hosts. Also, a healthy balance of microorganisms will prevent the development of infection by less desirable infectious agents. The use of antibiotics and excessive washing (e.g. of the genital areas) can alter this balance, and this is why these practices may lead to problems such as diarrhoea, thrush and soreness.

There is a current trend for supplementing the friendly commensal bacteria of the body with dietary products containing bacteria such as the *Lactobacillus* species (the family of Gram-positive, rod-shaped bacteria, which include those responsible for the conversion of milk to yoghourt). It is recognised that oral supplementation with preparations of live *Lactobacillus* sp. will not only encourage the colonisation of the bowel with these bacteria, but also the external genitalia and the vagina. *Lactobacillus* sp. are recognised to increase the acidity of their environment and also to reduce the overgrowth of yeast-like organisms such as *Candida*, the cause of thrush.

Studying infectious diseases

A knowledge of the classification of infectious agents and their modes of transmission, together with an understanding of how infectious agents can lead to processes of disease is invaluable in the study of infectious diseases. Moreover, it can help in understanding how the different broad groups of infectious agent can each lead to some characteristic manifestations of disease. Table 2.4b-III illustrates some features of diseases that can point to a particular type of infectious agent, but there are many exceptions to these 'rules'.

Information on infectious diseases is often presented in medical textbooks in a structured way. It is usually possible from such texts to access information that is ordered within the following categories:

- causative agent
- mode of transmission
- clinical features
- complications (if any)
- treatment.

Table 2.4b-III The characteristics of disease caused by infectious agents

Infectious agent	Features of disease that are characteristic of the agent
Viruses	Can cause a syndrome of malaise, joint aches, mild fever and slight rash as infection takes hold Lead to watery discharges more commonly than pus Rarely, can lead to cancerous change or benign tumours Infections may be followed by a syndrome of prolonged exhaustion, depression, muscle weakness and numbness
Prions	Transmitted by insertion of infected tissue into the body either by eating or by medical procedures Lead to degeneration of nervous tissue
Bacteria	Pus formation, such as abscesses and boils, may occur The most common disease process in bacterial disease is inflammation. May also trigger autoimmune responses
Protozoa, flukes, and worms	A common cause of tropical intestinal disease. Eggs of parasites often enter the bowel from contaminated food and water Allergic reactions, such as itch and cough, may also occur
Fungi	A cause of relatively mild skin problems in healthy people A major problem in patients with immune deficiency
Infestations	A cause of irritating skin problems, but do not in themselves affect deeper tissues May lead to serious disease by transmission of other infectious agents

For example, a textbook description of the infectious disease measles might give the following information:

- Causative agent: a virus from the family of paramyxoviruses. This tells us that the cause of measles is a viral infection.
- Mode of transmission: the spread is by droplets (infected fluid particles from the nose and throat of a carrier). A person is infectious for a total of 6 days. The infectious period begins 4 days before the rash develops to 2 days after it begins.
- Clinical features: these occur after an 'incubation period' of 8–14 days. This means that the disease will only manifest 8–14 days after contact with a carrier. First, malaise, fever, runny nose (rhinorrhoea), cough and redness of eyes (conjunctival suffusion) occur. This is when the patient is infectious. After 2 days of this, grey spots (Koplik spots) develop in the inside of the mouth. These are diagnostic of measles infection. On day 4, a rapidly spreading maculopapular (spotty, slightly raised) rash moves from the face to include the whole body.
- Complications: measles is generally a mild infection in well-nourished people. However, complications are common in poorly nourished people, and include pneumonia, bronchitis, ear infection and bowel infections. A serious long-term brain infection is a very rare complication in infections in infants less than 18 months old. Measles, when caught in pregnancy, can lead to loss of the pregnancy, but not to fetal abnormalities.
- Treatment: there is no direct treatment of the infection available. Measles in a healthy person generally requires only supportive treatment. However, if the patient is vulnerable because of immunodeficiency or malnutrition, or if neurological or respiratory signs develop, hospital admission and intravenous nutrition may be necessary.

Information about infectious diseases structured under these five headings encapsulates the essential facts required for an understanding of how a disease will impact on the life of a patient. Awareness of these headings can help structure information for the purposes of the study of infectious diseases (see Q2.4b-4).

Self-test 2.4b

The different types of infectious disease

1. What type of infectious agent is the cause of the following infectious diseases:
   (i) shingles
   (ii) scarlet fever
   (iii) impetigo
   (iv) rabies
   (v) typhoid fever
   (vi) meningococcal meningitis?
2. What are the features of the following infectious diseases that are characteristic of the infectious agent? (For example, the muscle aches, malaise and prolonged exhaustion of influenza are characteristic of a viral infection.)
   (i) Common warts (infection by human papilloma virus).
   (ii) Quinsy (very swollen tonsil following a bacterial infection).
   (iii) Threadworm infection.
   (iv) Headlice infestation.
   (v) The common cold (infection by a rhinovirus).

Answers

1. (i) Virus infection (varicella zoster virus).
   (ii) Bacterial infection (*Streptococcus* type A).
   (iii) Bacterial infection (usually *Staphylococcus*; rarely *Streptococcus* type A).
   (iv) Virus infection (rabies virus)
   (v) Bacterial infection (*Salmonella typhi*).
   (vi) Bacterial infection (*Neisseria meningitidis*).
2. (i) Common warts are characteristic of a virus infection because they are a form of benign tumour of the infected skin cells. Viruses are the only form of infectious agent that are recognised to stimulate the development of tumours.
   (ii) Quinsy is characteristic of a bacterial infection because it results from the formation of an abscess (containing pus) in the tonsil.
   (iii) Threadworm infection is characteristic of a worm infection because it is contracted by eating food contaminated with threadworm eggs, it manifests in the bowel, and causes itch in the anal area.
   (iv) Headlice infestation is characteristic of an arthropod infestation because it leads to irritating skin itch, but does not in itself lead to deeper disease.
   (v) The common cold is characteristic of a virus infection in that it leads to the production of profuse watery mucus. (Any phlegm that contains pus following a common cold is more likely to be due to a secondary bacterial infection of the damaged epithelial lining of the nose and throat.)
   The common cold can be also associated with muscle aches, mild fever and malaise.

Chapter 2.4c The red flags of serious infectious disease

LEARNING POINTS

At the end of this chapter you will be able to:
- recognise the red flags of serious infectious disease.

Estimated time for chapter: 40 minutes.

This chapter considers some of those general features of infectious diseases that might point to the possibility of serious underlying disease. These 'red flags' should prompt consideration of making a referral to a medical practitioner.

Some of the most important infectious diseases are described in detail in later chapters according to the system that they predominantly affect. For example, pneumonia is a topic explored in Section 3.3 on the respiratory system. Red flags specific to these important conditions are listed in these later chapters.

Naturally, there will be some overlap between the information given in this chapter and that in the later chapters concerning the infections that affect the various systems. All the information about the various red flags of infectious disease is brought together and reviewed in Chapter 6.3a and summarised in Appendix III.

Vulnerable groups and infectious disease

Infections related to the following categories need to be treated with caution. Although not all these infections will be serious, if there is any uncertainty it is wise to refer for a second opinion (Tables 2.4c-I and 2.4c-II).

Fever, dehydration and confusion

Infections may be accompanied by fever, dehydration and confusion. These three complications of infections are not specific to any particular infectious agent. All three can carry the risk of serious consequences to the patient.

Fever

Fever (by definition a body temperature over 37.5°C) is believed from a conventional medicine perspective to have a positive effect on the course of infection. Fever is a result of the inflammatory and immune responses that occur in infections, but potentially dangerous if the body temperature becomes very high, particularly in young children.

The distinction between a moderate and a high fever is somewhat arbitrary. However, for the purposes of clarity, in this chapter a body temperature of 37.5–38.5°C is classified as a moderate fever, and a temperature greater than 38.5°C is classed as a high fever.

Treatment of all high fevers should start with removal of excess clothing and sponging of the body with tepid water in a draught-free environment.

Conventional advice is to give a maximum dose of paracetamol or aspirin to adults. Aspirin should never be given to children under 12 years old. Instead, paracetamol is available in suspension form for young children. Alternatively, the non-steroidal anti-inflammatory drug ibuprofen may be prescribed in suspension form to children for its antipyretic effects.

From a homeopathic perspective these medications would be described as suppressive in nature, but to prevent serious complications need to be considered for the treatment of a high fever if complementary medical approaches are not effective within 1–2 hours, especially in the case of children.

Dehydration

Infectious diseases can lead to dehydration of the body as a result of prolonged fever with sweating, and also insufficient intake of fluids. Prolonged dehydration and loss of salts can be damaging to the kidneys, and should be prevented if at all possible.

Patients suffering from an infectious disease need to be encouraged to drink plenty of fluids. This is particularly important for young children and the elderly. Ideally, salts need to be replaced as well as water. For most illnesses, diluted fruit juices or squash contain sufficient salts to meet the body's needs. If it is not possible to maintain hydration, the patient should be referred to a hospital setting where they can be administered fluids intravenously ('by drip').

Table 2.4c-I Red Flags 2 – infectious diseases – vulnerable groups

Red Flag	Description	Reasoning
Treat anyone from the following vulnerable groups with caution if they are displaying features of an infectious disease (e.g. **fever**, **confusion**, **diarrhoea and vomiting**, **spreading areas of inflammation** or **yellowish discharges**)		
2.1	**Infants** (especially if less than 3 months old)	Infections in infants can become serious conditions very quickly because of their immature immune system, poor temperature control and small size. Infections lead easily to high fever and dehydration. The infant is at increased risk of convulsions and circulatory collapse However, in this age group fever is common, and usually is **not** serious
2.2	The **elderly**	Infections can take hold rapidly in the elderly because of a weakened immune system. Serious disease can 'hide' behind mild-appearing symptoms
2.3	The **immunocompromised**	The immunocompromised are particularly vulnerable to severe overwhelming infections, in particular of the respiratory and gastrointestinal systems
2.4	In **pregnancy**	Certain infections can directly damage the embryo/fetus or lead to miscarriage. Others may be transmitted to the baby during labour. Prolonged high fever may induce miscarriage or early labour
2.5	Anyone with a **recent history of travel** to a tropical country (within the past month)	Certain tropical diseases (including malaria) can become rapidly overwhelming and may present up to 4 weeks after return from the tropical country

Table 2.4c-II Red Flags 3 –infectious diseases – fever, dehydration and confusion

Red Flag	Description	Reasoning
Definitions Normal body temperature: 36.8°C ± 0.7°C) Fever: body temperature >37.5°C Moderate fever: 37.5–38.5°C High fever: body temperature >38.5°C		
3.1	**High fever in a child (<8 years old)** that does not respond to treatment within 2 hours	High fevers can promote infantile convulsions in young children. Treatment to bring the temperature down includes keeping the environment cool, tepid sponging, and gentle medical approaches such as acupuncture or homeopathy. If all else fails, antipyretic medication such as paracetamol or ibuprofen suspension could be considered
3.2	**High fever in an older child or adult** that does not respond to treatment within 48 hours	Although risk of convulsions is low in this group of patients, a high fever is very depleting and can lead to dehydration. A high fever that does not respond to treatment in 2 days suggests the possibility of a serious condition that merits further investigations
3.3	**Any fever** that persists for or recurs over >2 weeks	Most mild infectious diseases have run their course within a week; a prolonged fever suggests either a chronic inflammatory or infectious condition, or cancer, all of which merit further investigations
3.4	**Dehydration in an infant**: signs include **dry mouth and skin**, **loss of skin turgor** (firmness), **drowsiness**, **sunken fontanelle** (soft spot on the crown of the head in the region of acupoint Du-24 Shenting) and **dry nappies**	A dehydrated infant is at high risk of circulatory collapse because of his or her small size and immature homeostatic mechanisms. Infants who are dehydrated may lose the desire to drink, and so the condition can deteriorate rapidly
3.5	**Dehydration in older children and adults** if severe or prolonged for more than 48 hours: signs include **dry mouth and skin, loss of skin turgor**, **low blood pressure**, **dizziness on standing** and **poor urine output**	Although not as unstable as an infant, a dehydrated child or adult still needs hydration to prevent damage to the kidneys. Referral should be made if the patient is unable to take fluids or if the dehydration persists for more than 48 hours. Refer elderly people immediately, as their ability to take in fluids is often reduced and the kidneys and brain are more vulnerable to damage
3.6	**Confusion in older children and adults with fever**	Confusion is common and benign in young children (<8 years old) and elderly frail people when a fever develops. However, it is not usual in healthy adults. and these should be referred to exclude central nervous system involvement (e.g. meningitis or brain abscess). Refer in all cases if the confusion might pose a risk to the patient or to others.
3.7	**Febrile convulsion in children**: ongoing	Refer as an emergency a child in whom the convulsion is not settling within 2 minutes. Ensure the child is kept in a safe place and in the recovery position while waiting for help to arrive
3.8	**Febrile convulsion in children**: recovered	Refer any child who has just suffered a febrile convulsion (the parents need advice on how to manage future fits, and the child should be examined by a doctor)

Confusion

Confusion is one of the responses of the brain to extreme metabolic disturbance. When exposed to extremes of heat or cold, or imbalances in levels of salts, nutrients and toxins, the function of the brain is impaired and the patient may become confused. Often confusion is accompanied by physical agitation, fearfulness and visual hallucinations.

Extreme fever can induce confusion. However, this is rare in a robust adult, and in this case may indicate a more serious underlying condition such as meningitis. However, children very readily enter a confusional state and this is not necessarily a serious sign. Similarly, elderly people can easily become confused, even in the situation of a mild illness such as a bladder infection. In themselves, confusional states in children and the elderly are not serious. However, they may need to be treated with seriousness and the patient referred if, as a result of the confused state, he or she poses a risk to themselves or others.

Febrile convulsion

High fever can induce a fit in a small child (usually under the age of 6 years), which if prolonged can carry the risk of asphyxiation or permanent brain damage. A febrile convulsion is known to occur in 3% of children. In 2–4% of these cases a febrile convulsion is the first symptom of one of the forms of childhood epilepsy. An ongoing febrile convulsion requires emergency management. If the convulsion has ceased, the child must be referred as a high priority to exclude serious underlying infectious disease such as meningitis and to receive advice on how to prevent a recurrence.

Self-test 2.4c

The red flags of serious infectious disease

For each of the following case histories, state whether you think the patient requires referral to a conventional medical practitioner.

1. You have been called on a home visit to see Jack who is 3 years old and who has been feverish with a temperature of 38°C all night. Although he appears not to be dehydrated, he is now a bit confused and rambling in his speech. His mother has called you because his temperature is now 40°C. He has so far had no medical treatment.
2. The mother of a 16-year-old boy calls to see if you would visit to treat for high fever. The boy has been unwell with headache and flu-like symptoms for a few hours, but now has a very high fever of 40.5°C and appears to be moving in and out of a confusional state. He is convinced he can see ants crawling on his bedclothes and is becoming quite panicky.
3. Barbara is 65 years old and has been experiencing night sweats for the past 3 weeks. She thought she was having another menopause, but has noticed that at times her temperature has been up with these sweats, sometimes as high as 38°C. She has not been feeling herself now for a few weeks, and thinks she may have lost some weight since all this has been going on.
4. Mr Edwards is 85 years old and has called you about feeling very tired and sweaty. He has a fever of 37.8°C and a slight cough. When you visit you notice that his mouth is very dry and his skin turgor low. He cannot remember when he last urinated, and feels too weak to stand up.

Answers

1. Although alarming to the mother, Jack's symptoms are consistent with a viral infection and are not likely to be serious. Although his temperature is high, you should only be concerned if it does not come down to less than 38.5°C with treatment, which should start with tepid sponging.

   If Jack's temperature does not come down at all within 2 hours after tepid sponging, alternative treatments and, finally, paracetamol, you should consider referring Jack to his GP for a home visit. The GP will examine for any obvious treatable causes of high fever, such as a middle-ear infection.
2. This is a different situation. Confusion is not usual with fever in teenagers and adults, and may signify a serious infection. By all means you can go to visit to treat with acupuncture, but make sure the mother calls the GP for advice and/or a home visit as soon as possible.
3. Recurrent fever suggests underlying infection, inflammation or cancer, and merits referral for further investigations.
4. The fact that Mr Edwards is 85 years old should make you concerned that his infection does not progress to a serious condition. An elderly person is in a vulnerable group, in that infections can easily progress.

   However, there are features of dehydration, which mean that Mr Edwards should be referred for assessment by a medical practitioner as soon as possible. In addition, the fact that he is too weak to stand means he is unable to care for himself at home, and if there are no friends or family available this alone is a reason for a high-priority referral.

Chapter 2.4d Diagnosis, prevention and treatment of infectious disease

LEARNING POINTS

At the end of this chapter you will:

- be able to describe the types of tests used to diagnose infectious disease
- be able to explain the principles of prevention of infectious disease
- be familiar with the conventional medicine rationale for vaccination
- be able to recognise the main groups of drugs used to treat infectious disease
- be familiar with the problems that are known to result from inappropriate and excessive prescribing of these drugs.

Estimated time for chapter: 120 minutes.

Introduction

This chapter concludes the study of the conventional approach to infectious disease by exploring how infectious diseases are diagnosed, and then how they are managed (prevention and treatment).

Diagnosis of infectious disease

It was explained in Chapter 1.2a that diagnosis involves the three stages of questioning, examination and investigation. In the diagnosis of infectious disease, questioning and examination are performed to look for characteristic features of the different diseases. Many infectious diseases (e.g. tonsillitis, mumps, threadworm, headlice infestation) have their own distinct pattern of symptoms and signs and can be diagnosed effectively using these two approaches alone.

Additional information can be provided from investigations, which can be broadly categorised as:

- tests to look for the presence of the infectious agent (examination of body fluids and tissue samples)
- tests to look for evidence of characteristic processes of disease (blood tests and imaging techniques such as X-ray imaging)
- tests to examine for a current or previous immune response to the infectious agent (mostly blood tests looking for antibodies).

Tests to look for the presence of the infectious agent

The most straightforward tests for the presence of an infectious agent involve examining specimens of fluids or tissues taken from the body. The simple microscope is necessary to examine for bacteria, protozoa, fungi and the small immature forms of larger parasites (see Q2.4d-1).

The choice of specimen depends on the nature of the disease. If a particular organ is involved, specimens of fluid of tissue from that organ will be sought. Examples include:

- swab from tonsil/throat/nose, and sputum sample in upper respiratory infections
- urine sample in urinary infections
- faeces sample in gastrointestinal infections
- skin swab in skin infections
- scrapings of skin and nail clippings in fungal skin infections
- swab/sample of pus leaking from an abscess/boil.

Obtaining each of the samples listed above involves a relatively non-invasive procedure, but sometimes the search for infection has to be more penetrating. Examples of invasive investigations include:

- blood samples to look for bacteria in the blood (blood culture)
- surgical removal of a sample of deep organ tissue (biopsy), e.g. liver, bone marrow and even brain.

The samples of body fluid or tissue have to be processed in different ways in order to allow an infectious agent to be diagnosed. Often, part of the processing involves allowing the microbe to grow for a few days (culture) before there are sufficient quantities for accurate diagnosis. This is why some tests take some time before the results are ready.

The next stage of processing is to detect the agent in the specimen. This can involve the use of chemical dyes, such as the Gram stain, which show up certain bacteria. More recently, the detection of infection has become an increasingly complex but very precise science with the use of DNA and RNA 'probes'.

Tests to look for evidence of characteristic processes of disease

Some investigations involve examination not for the infectious agent but for the signs that it has caused damage to the body. For example, a sample of the blood can be examined to see if the leukocytes are changed in shape or number in any way. Different diseases lead to different types of change in these white blood cells. The test that is performed is called a 'full blood count'.

Blood tests called the 'erythrocyte sedimentation rate' (ESR) and 'C-reactive protein' (CRP) are commonly performed when it is uncertain whether or not an infection has occurred. The ESR and CRP are both raised when the inflammatory response has been triggered in the body. A common example when these tests might be used is when someone complains of feeling tired all the time, a complaint which very often has no measurable physical cause. The doctor might take blood for an ESR or CRP to exclude the possibility of an infective or other inflammatory reason for the symptoms.

The following five imaging techniques are commonly used in the investigation of infectious diseases:

- chest X-ray
- ultrasound scan
- computerised axial tomography (CT) scan
- magnetic resonance imaging (MRI)
- radionuclide scan.

The chest X-ray differentiates between dense tissue, such as bone, and air- filled tissues, such as the lungs. Patches of infection (fluid) show up as shadows in the lung area. The X-ray image is not able to show up much detail in most body parts, and is most useful for examining bones and the chest. It is acknowledged that excessive exposure to X-rays may cause cancer, but that the exposure from a single X-ray investigation is very unlikely to be damaging.

An ultrasound scan utilises ultrasound waves to produce images of those soft tissue parts of the body that cannot be imaged using X-radiation. The ultrasound scan can show up collections of pus within deep organs. The technique is considered to be very safe compared to X-ray imaging.

The computerised axial tomography (CT) scan uses computer processing of a series of X-ray images to produce an image of a 'slice' of the body. The image produced by a CT scan gives far more detail than an X-ray image, but involves the patient in a prolonged and uncomfortable procedure, and also exposes the patient to more radiation. In infectious disease the CT scan can expose collections of pus in body spaces and patches of infection in the lungs.

The magnetic resonance imaging (MRI) scan produces similar images to the CT scan, although it seems to give better definition of nervous tissue. MRI involves the use of a powerful magnetic field and is thought to be less harmful than X-radiation.

Radionuclide scanning involves first giving the patient a radioactive substance, either by mouth or by injection, and then scanning the body to see the location of the substance in the body. In an infection of unknown source, radioactive leukocytes or antibiotics may be given to the patient. These will concentrate at the site of infection, and a scan will therefore show up the site as an area of increased radioactivity. The radioactivity wears off very rapidly, and the procedure, like X-ray imaging, is considered to be relatively safe to the patient (see Q2.4d-2).

Tests to examine for a current or previous immune response to the infectious agent

The use of tests to examine for a current or previous immune response is also known as 'immunodiagnosis'. This group of investigations focuses on testing for whether the body has started to produce antibodies to a particular infection. The presence of the antibody shows that the body has encountered that infection. The type of antibody found will indicate whether or not the infection is current or whether it occurred in the past. The same tests are performed to check whether somebody is already resistant to a disease, whether they require a vaccination, and also whether a vaccination has induced a sufficient immune response to protect against disease (see Q2.4d-3).

Prevention of infectious disease

Prevention of death and disability from infection is arguably the area in which conventional medicine has had the most impact on health. The death rates from many of the infectious diseases, which were major killers (e.g. diphtheria, tuberculosis, poliomyelitis, cholera, typhoid, leprosy, the plague, smallpox) in the past, have declined so dramatically that these diseases have been virtually eradicated in developed countries. In fact, smallpox is believed to have been entirely eradicated worldwide, with the last case recorded in 1977. The increase in life expectancy that has occurred over the past two centuries can be largely attributed to the reduction in deaths from infections. Although much of this reduction in death and disability from infectious diseases can be attributed to improvements in the general health and well-being of the populations of developed countries, undoubtedly medical approaches to the prevention of infectious disease have also had a significant impact.

In conventional medicine there are four main aspects to the prevention of disease:

- maximising hygiene and the health of the population
- immunisation (vaccination)
- having an active approach to detecting and monitoring new cases of disease ('surveillance')
- rapid isolation and treatment of new cases of disease so that spread is reduced.

Maximising hygiene and the health of the population

There is no doubt that the largest part of the change in life expectancy can be attributed to improved hygiene and health of the population. The beneficial effects of good nutrition, housing and sanitation were introduced in Chapter 2.4a. Many of the world's most deadly diseases cannot take hold in a population that has a good basic level of health and sanitation. Nevertheless, as is described in Chapter 2.4a, some diseases (e.g. meningitis) can have devastating effects even in a seemingly healthy population.

Immunisation

Conventional medicine recognises immunisation as a very powerful weapon in its armoury for the prevention of disease. The principles of immunisation were described in Chapter 2.1d.

There are two main strategies behind the practice of immunisation. The first is to target a vaccine at 'at-risk individuals' so that the personal risk of developing disease is reduced. A well-known example of this approach is the use of certain vaccines for protection against tropical diseases such as hepatitis A, typhoid and yellow fever. Another example is the use of vaccine against influenza in elderly people and those who have particular health problems such as heart disease.

The second strategy is to eradicate or significantly reduce the occurrence of a disease in a population. For this an 'immunisation campaign' is necessary, because a sufficiently large proportion of the population has to be immunised to mimic the situation of 'herd immunity'. It is known that if a large proportion of the population is immune to a disease, epidemics of that disease are unlikely to occur, and the disease may even die out.

This is the rationale behind the childhood programme of immunisations, which involvcs giving vaccines and booster doses for some of the childhood diseases. The UK childhood immunisation schedule aims to protect all children against the following preventable childhood infections:

- diphtheria
- tetanus
- pertussis (whooping cough)
- *Haemophilus influenzae* type b (Hib)
- polio
- meningococcal serogroup C (MenC)
- pneumococcus (*Streptococcus pneumoniae*)
- measles
- mumps
- rubella
- human papilloma virus (HPV)

The timing of the vaccinations in the UK immunisation schedule is summarised in Table 2.4d-I.

In addition to the immunisations listed in the table, the immunisation against tuberculosis (TB), known as the 'BCG', is now offered as part of a risk-based programme. This means it is

Table 2.4d-I The timing of the vaccinations in the UK immunisation schedule

Age at immunisation	Vaccines given	Mode of administration
2, 3 and 4 months	Diphtheria, tetanus and pertussis (whooping cough, polio) and Hib (DTP-Hib)	One combined injection
	Pneumococcus (PCV) at 2 and 4 months	One injection
	Meningitis C (Men C) at 3 and 4 months	One injection
Around 12 months	Hib and Meningitis C	One combined injection
Around 13 months	Measles, mumps, rubella (MMR) and pneumococcus (PCV)	Two separate injections
3–5 years (pre school)	Diphtheria, tetanus and pertussis and polio (DTP/polio)	One combined injection
	Measles, mumps and rubella (MMR)	One combined injection
13 years for girls only	Human papilloma virus (HPV)	3 injections given over the course of 6 months
10–14 years	Tetanus and diphtheria (Td)	One combined injection
	Polio	one combined injection By mouth

targeted at those children most at risk of exposure to TB, such as newborns from immigrant families and recently immigrated children. The national schools programme that offered BCG to all 14-year-old children in the UK was stopped in 2005 because of the declining incidence of the disease in the general population.

The immunisation strategy requires a high coverage of the population to be successful. This is important because most vaccinations have an efficacy of only 90–95% and thus leave 5–10% of those vaccinated still vulnerable to disease. If more than 10% of a population remains unvaccinated, this could mean that 20% of the population is unprotected, giving a herd immunity of less than 80%. The lower the herd immunity is, the greater the risk that an epidemic of the disease could spread within the unprotected minority. The risks of epidemics are greatly reduced if herd immunity can be raised to above 80%. In the UK, the Department of Health coordinates a process of public health education to encourage uptake of vaccination, including internet-based information such as the NHS Choices web resource. In addition, the provision of childhood immunisation is a required service as part of the General Medical Services contract that UK general medical practices have with their local primary care organisation (PCO). This means that UK general practices have developed rigorous reminder-and-recall systems to ensure children do not slip through the immunisation net. As a result of these factors, in recent years national vaccine coverage has been well over 90% of eligible children.

There is good statistical evidence to show that immunisation does reduce the incidence of the immunisable diseases. Although health and hygiene have had by far the most powerful impact in reducing the number of cases for most diseases, including TB and diphtheria, immunisations have been clearly shown to contribute to this reduction.

The statistics that the medical establishment use to support the use of immunisation to prevent disease are the result of long-term, well-conducted studies of immunised and non-immunised populations. It is difficult to refute the results of such high-quality studies and to argue against the suggestion that immunisation reduces the risk of an individual contracting a particular disease and reduces the incidence of the disease in the population.

In conventional medicine terms it is appreciated that vaccinations carry risks of adverse reactions in a small number of people who receive them. However, it is always the case that it is understood for any medically recommended immunisation that the risks to the population as a whole from having the vaccine are far less than the risks to the population as a whole of contracting the disease.

It is not commonly appreciated that vaccines are available for only a few diseases. To date, vaccines have been developed for some viral and bacterial infections, but not for fungal or parasitic diseases or infestations. Despite much research, it has not yet been possible to mimic some diseases, such as the common cold, malaria and HIV, successfully in the form of a vaccine. Vaccines, therefore, can form only a part of the approach to the prevention of infectious diseases.

Surveillance

Most developed countries have a system of disease surveillance in place. Through these systems, cases of important diseases are reported by health professionals, and are recorded and monitored by means of a central database.

The surveillance system in the UK relies largely on notifications of disease from doctors. It is one of the duties of doctors in the UK to submit a notification in writing of every case of a 'notifiable disease' that they treat. Notifiable diseases are those infections that are considered to have the potential to impact significantly on the health of the community (Table 2.4d-II). The list of notifiable diseases includes conditions such as food poisoning, meningitis, most tropical diseases and all the immunisable diseases. HIV infection is not notifiable because of issues relating to confidentiality.

Surveillance depends on the accurate and complete notification of disease. This, of course, can never be fully attained, as doctors are overworked, and may fail to notify or accurately diagnose many cases of infectious disease. Nevertheless, the figures on notified diseases are of sufficiently good quality to produce useful local and national reports of the incidence of these diseases. These reports can demonstrate whether the disease is on the increase, or whether it is declining.

It is this information that has shown the marked reduction in diseases such as measles following the institution of immunisation campaigns. This evidence is the basis on which conventional medicine argues for the continuation of immunisation programmes or for the cessation of an immunisation programme (e.g. the school BCG vaccination programme for TB was stopped in the UK 2005 on this basis). It can lead to a campaign being stepped up (e.g. the pre-school booster dose of MMR vaccine was introduced in 1996 in the UK when it was found that too many children who had only a single dose of vaccine were developing measles). Surveillance can also detect a cluster of cases of an unusual disease (e.g. meningitis or food poisoning) which may highlight the need for a focused local campaign of treatment. This is relevant to the final aspect of prevention of disease – isolation and treatment.

Rapid isolation and treatment of new cases

It is accepted within conventional medicine that improved health and hygiene and a thorough vaccination campaign contributed to the eradication of smallpox. However, there was a fourth approach to prevention that was a vital additional factor. This approach was a worldwide surveillance programme, which involved the rapid reporting and treatment of any patient who developed smallpox. Patients with the disease were nursed in isolation so that the disease could not spread. This programme prevented the development of epidemics of the disease, and gradually the disease became extinct.

This approach of rapid isolation and treatment is considered essential in cases such as bacterial meningitis and food poisoning. In these cases, patients are treated rapidly and possible contacts are actively traced and advised on how to recognise symptoms of the condition, and what to do if they occur. This is a powerful approach to minimising the spread of the disease (see Q2.4d-4).

Prevention, of course, can be seen to overlap with treatment; particularly when treatment involves isolation of cases

Table 2.4d-II Notifiable diseases

Notification of a number of specified infectious diseases is required of doctors in the UK as a 'statutory duty' under the UK Public Health (Infectious Diseases) 1988 Act and the Public Health (Control of Diseases) 1988 Act.	
The UK Health Protection Agency (HPA) Centre for Infections collates details of each case of each disease that has been notified. This allows analyses of local and national trends.	
This is one example of a situation in which there is a legal requirement for a doctor to breach patient confidentiality.	
Diseases which are notifiable include:	
acute encephalitis	plague
acute poliomyelitis	rabies
anthrax	relapsing fever
cholera	rubella
diphtheria	scarlet fever
dysentery	smallpox
food poisoning	tetanus
leptospirosis	tuberculosis
malaria	typhoid fever
measles	typhus fever
meningitis (bacterial and viral forms)	viral haemorrhagic fever
meningococcal septicaemia (without meningitis)	viral hepatitis (including hepatitis a, b and c)
mumps	whooping cough
ophthalmia neonatorum	yellow fever
paratyphoid fever	

of a disease and treatment of contacts who have not yet developed the disease.

Treatment of infectious disease

The ideal treatment option for infectious diseases is the use of a therapy that targets the infectious agent, but which has a minimal effect on the person with the infection. This can be compared to the action of a weedkiller used on a lawn that is specific in its action on the unwanted weeds, while leaving the grass unharmed.

In conventional medicine the main therapy used to treat infections is chemical drugs, either taken internally or applied externally. It is in the drug therapy for infections that the distinction between the different types of infectious agent becomes relevant, as a drug that will damage a bacterium will not necessarily damage a flea, and vice versa. Drugs are developed to target weak spots, which are usually particular to one class of infectious agent only.

Historically, the first drug to target bacterial infections was discovered by serendipity by a scientist called Fleming. In 1928, Fleming discovered that the seemingly harmless *Penicillium notatum* mould, an accidental contaminant of one of his experiments, caused the death of the bacterial cultures that he was trying to grow in his laboratory. In this discovery was the potential for an ideal therapy. This particular mould killed bacteria but was relatively non-toxic to humans. Since Fleming's discovery, a rapidly increasing number of drugs have been developed that have this selective property of targeting an infectious agent. Many of these are closely related in chemical structure to natural substances such as moulds.

Increasingly, 'designer' drugs have been created using the detailed knowledge that there now is about the life cycle of the various infectious agents. The new drugs used to slow down the progression of HIV infection (the highly active antiretroviral therapy (HAART) drugs) are an example of this. These are compounds that have been designed to interfere specifically with the replication of the HIV virus.

In formularies of prescription medications such as the British National Formulary (BNF) or the United States Pharmacopoeia – National Formulary (USP-NF) drugs intended to target infections are usually categorised under the following five headings:

- antibacterial drugs (counteract bacteria)
- antifungal drugs (counteract fungi)
- antiviral drugs (counteract viruses)
- antiprotozoal drugs (counteract single-celled animals)
- antihelminthic drugs (counteract worms, tapeworms and flukes, which are collectively known as 'helminths').

Within these five categories, drugs are then subclassified according to their chemical nature and the specific type of bacterium, virus, fungus or animal parasite that they affect.

Side-effects

As noted earlier, the ideal antimicrobial drug targets the microbe but leaves the human host untouched. Unfortunately, this ideal is never perfectly attained. All antimicrobials can result in side-effects in the person taking them, as well as damage to the infectious agent. Serious side-effects for most antibiotics are not common, but they can be very severe in a small, often unpredictable, proportion of people. The most common side-effects of antimicrobial treatment are allergic reactions such as rash and itch, and gastrointestinal disturbance. The latter often occur because the healthy commensal bacteria in the bowel are affected by the drug.

Drug formularies usually list side-effects in an order that reflects their frequency, with the most common being listed first. For example, the side-effects of a commonly prescribed antibiotic, tetracycline, are listed in the BNF as nausea, vomiting, diarrhoea (antibiotic-associated colitis reported occasionally), dysphagia, and oesophageal irritation. Also, other rare side-effects are listed as including hepatotoxicity, pancreatitis, blood disorders, light sensitivity of the skin, and hypersensitivity reactions (including rash, exfoliative dermatitis, Stevens–Johnson syndrome, urticaria, angioedema, anaphylaxis and pericarditis). In addition, benign intracranial hypertension in adults and bulging fontanelles in infants have been reported.

In the case of tetracycline, the common side-effects of nausea, vomiting and diarrhoea will still not affect the majority of people using the drug, and more rare side-effects such as hepatotoxicity are rare indeed, affecting one in 10,000 patients who take the medication.

Most people who take a drug such as tetracycline will not experience any side-effects, but doctors need to bear the potential risks in mind when prescribing drugs such as this. Some antibiotics may be prescribed for up to months at a time for relatively minor health problems, as is tetracycline, a commonly prescribed treatment for acne, so doctors need to warn patients to be vigilant about the emergence of side-effects.

The conventional view is that antimicrobials are generally seen as harmless to the individual except in the few cases in which side-effects develop. A medical practitioner who freely prescribes repeated doses of antibiotics to a young child with eczema and asthma will not think that the antibiotics will be causing any harm to that child. Likewise, a prolonged course of tetracycline might be prescribed to a fit teenager with acne without any concern that there might be any problem in taking these drugs for such a long time. In cases such as this, the doctor is likely to be prescribing in a way that is in keeping with the values and beliefs of the medical profession. In contrast to the concern with which antibiotics may be held within some complementary health disciplines, in conventional medicine it is simply not believed that antimicrobials, if apparently well tolerated, could in the majority of cases cause long-term problems for the individual.

However, it is certainly the conventional medical view that inappropriate prescribing of antimicrobial drugs can be very harmful to the health of the population, in that it might lead to the development of drug resistance in the microbes endemic in the community. This important concept of drug resistance is discussed in the following section of this chapter.

Principles of treatment with antimicrobials

There is professional concern about the levels of prescribing of antimicrobial drugs. In the UK in 1998, a House of Lords Select Committee produced a detailed report on how the use of antimicrobials in agriculture, as well as in healthcare, should be controlled. The major concern that promoted this inquiry was of the development of antimicrobial resistance.

Chapter 2.4a introduced the concept of emerging infections, and how 'beneficial mutations' can allow microbes to adapt to their environment. Since the widespread use of penicillin, new strains of bacteria have emerged that are no longer killed by penicillin. Some particularly common strains of bacteria now have adapted to produce substances called 'beta lactamases' (including penicillinase), which can destroy penicillin.

It is now widely appreciated that the more an antibiotic is used the more likely it is that these 'resistant' strains will develop. This is not only a product of excessive prescribing for health reasons. There is increasing concern that drug-resistant microbes are developing in farm animals, which are given high doses of antibiotics to promote growth. These bacteria then get passed on to humans through the food chain.

It is also known that an infection that is treated inadequately may also encourage the expansion of drug-resistant mutations. This is particularly likely to occur if the dose of antibiotic is too low to kill the microbe completely, or if the drug is taken on an irregular basis, thus allowing a few remaining bacteria to multiply in the presence of low concentrations of the drug.

The current advice to doctors in choosing a drug to prescribe is as follows:

Do not prescribe in minor infections

It is recognised that in minor infections the majority of prescriptions of antibiotics do not lead to any significant health benefit. In some infections, such as bacterial otitis media (infection of the middle ear) and tonsillitis, the most an antibiotic seems to do is reduce the length of the infection by 1–2 days. It is probably true that for many prescriptions in the community the patient might well have got better without the prescription. Doctors are now being encouraged to think very carefully before prescribing in such cases.

Make sure the correct type and dose of antibiotic is chosen

The best way to ensure that the correct antibiotic is chosen is to take a specimen for diagnosis before treatment is started. This might be a urine sample in a urinary infection or a throat swab in tonsillitis. This specimen has to be cultured in the laboratory. The pathologist dealing with the specimen can then test to see which antibiotics are best to target that particular infection. Often it is necessary to 'treat blind', which means choosing an antibiotic without knowing for sure that the infection is sensitive to that drug. Ideally, the specimen should still be tested, so that if after 2–3 days the result shows that the antibiotic should be changed, this can be done.

In reality, in general practice this process is rarely followed through. Often prescriptions are for minor illness and for short periods (3–5 days). Doctors in these circumstances may choose to treat blind and use an antibiotic that has a very broad action rather than one that targets the particular infection. However, the use of broad-spectrum antibiotics, such as amoxicillin, is known to be more likely to promote the development of drug resistance.

Many people will have recovered from their symptoms in this period, and will not wish to commence (or pay for) a second prescription. To take a test is inconvenient to the patient, and costly to the health service. Many doctors will choose to use the prescription as the test of whether the antibiotic is appropriate, and will only perform tests if the patient does not get better. This could be described as bad practice, but is understandable in the context of a very heavy workload.

Complete the full course of treatment, without skipping doses

For the reasons mentioned earlier, it is important to maintain a high concentration of antibiotic in the blood stream throughout the time required to kill the infectious agent. Some infections are very sensitive and require only a single dose of antibiotic, but others may require months of continuous therapy (e.g. tuberculosis, fungal nail infections, HIV).

It is actually very difficult for most people to maintain a strict regimen of tablet taking when it is required that one dose be taken three times a day for more than 2–3 days. It is no wonder that some of the conditions that require such a regimen to be successful are very difficult to treat. This problem of poor 'compliance' or 'concordance' with the demands of a prescription can have severe consequences. For example, it is believed that the haphazard use of therapy for TB is responsible for the appearance of a multiple-drug-resistant strain. This has led to increasing cases of untreatable, and therefore fatal, TB in the developing world.

Nevertheless, despite the problems of side-effects and drug resistance, there is no doubt that antimicrobial drugs do play an important part in the reduction of disability and death from serious infectious disease. Although it is increasingly clear that many prescriptions of antibiotics for minor conditions are not justifiable clinically, it has to be accepted that antimicrobial therapy can play a vital role in the prevention of and recovery from serious infectious disease (see Q2.4d-5).

Self-test 2.4d

Diagnosis, prevention and treatment of infectious disease

1. What tests might Elisabeth, a 30-year-old housewife with swollen glands and fever, have to undergo to exclude glandular fever (also known as 'infectious mononucleosis')?
2. What are the ways in which the threat to health from tuberculosis (TB) has been reduced in the UK?
3. For each of the following infectious diseases
   - glandular fever
   - vaginal thrush (*Candida*)
   - *Giardia*
   - *Escherichia coli* food poisoning (a form of gastroenteritis)

use the BNF to answer the following questions:

(i) In what section of the BNF, Chapter 5, might you find a suitable antimicrobial drug to treat the disease?

(ii) What would be a possible choice of drug?

(iii) How long would be required to treat the condition?

Answers

1. Glandular fever, which is due to an infection with the Epstein–Barr virus (EBV), usually presents with fever, aches and widespread enlargement of lymph glands, including the tonsils. It may be confused with tonsillitis. This is particularly important as patients with glandular fever can develop a widespread rash if given the penicillin-related antibiotics, which are the treatment for tonsillitis.

   Elisabeth may be subjected to two separate blood tests: a *full blood count* to examine for unusual leukocytes known as 'glandular fever cells'; and a *serological test* that must be performed about a week after symptoms develop (Monospot or Paul Bunnell tests). A *throat swab* may also be taken to exclude bacterial tonsillitis.

2. The major factor that has led to the reduction in the number of cases of TB is *improved health and hygiene*, and in particular *improved nutrition*.

   Other important factors are *vaccination*, *surveillance* and *rapid treatment and isolation of cases* and protection (*prophylaxis*) of close contacts.

   The use of the *BCG vaccine* was introduced as a national programme in 1954. This has been attributed to a further reduction in the number of cases of TB.

   Surveillance for TB is effective in the UK, as new cases are referred to hospital for *isolation and treatment*. Within days of treatment, infectivity is reduced.

   Vulnerable close contacts may be offered drug treatment to prevent the development of disease (*prophylaxis*).

3. The following are the most common choices of treatment for the following diseases.

   Glandular fever:
   (i) antiviral drugs
   (ii) there is no suitable drug, so no treatment is usually given.

   Vaginal thrush:
   (i) antifungal drugs
   (ii) clotrimazole in pessary form (inserted vaginally)
   (iii) usual course is for 3–14 days.

   Giardia:
   (i) antiprotozoal drugs
   (ii) metronidazole (also used as an antibacterial drug)
   (iii) high dose for 3 days or lower dose for 5 days.

   E. coli food poisoning:
   (i) antibacterial drugs
   (ii) no treatment advised in mild cases; ciprofloxacin or gentamicin may be given in severe cases
   (iii) treatment is usually for 7 days.

Information Box 2.4d-I

Infectious disease: comments from a Chinese medicine perspective

These comments relate to Chapter 2.4 and are presented together, rather than as separate paragraphs as in other chapters, because the theory requires greater elaboration of the statements made.

The Chinese medicine interpretation of infectious disease

Two important concepts underpin the Chinese medicine view of conditions that equate to the conventional medicine categories of infectious disease. In significant ways these are alternative descriptions of the same signs and symptoms, but towards the end of these comments the value of their complementary perspectives will become apparent.

The two concepts are:

- *The origin of the Pathogenic Factor*. Chinese medicine describes how the Pathogenic Factor that is manifested in an infectious disease (e.g. Wind Heat) can originate from outside the body

Continued

Information Box 2.4d-I—Cont'd

(i.e. externally; e.g. climatic Wind Heat) or from within the body (i.e. internally; e.g. Wind Heat from stagnation of emotions), or can be a combination of the two.

- *The depth of the Pathogenic Factor.*[1] According to Chinese medicine, the Pathogenic Factor may be situated either on the Exterior of the body or at a deeper level in the Interior. However, the depth of the pathogenic factor does not tell us about its origin. The depth of the pathogenic factor is an important aspect of identification of patterns according to the Eight Principles.[2]

It is important to be very clear about the distinction between the origin of a Pathogenic Factor (External/Internal) and its location/depth (Exterior/Interior). It is also important not to conclude, because of the poetic nature of Chinese descriptions such as 'Wind Heat has invaded the body and caused disease', that the pathogenic factor is synonymous with an infectious agent. This is not the case. The Pathogenic Factor is actually a description of the clinical picture (e.g. redness, fever and pain indicate Heat; rapidly changing symptoms indicate Wind).

The reverse is also true; microbes are not synonymous with the Chinese medicine Pathogenic Factors. However, according to an integrated view of infection, microbes can and do give rise to manifestations (invasion) that are taken to be evidence of Pathogenic Factors. This means that the typical signs and symptoms of infectious diseases from a conventional viewpoint have some close correlations with the Chinese medicine view of Pathogenic Factors and can inform a Chinese medicine diagnosis.

The origin of the pathogenic factor

In the case of an infectious disease interpreted in Chinese medicine terms, the actual origin (cause) of a Pathogenic Factor may be Internal or External, depending on the situation. For example:

- *Pathogenic Factor of External origin*. When the Pathogenic Factor has an External origin, the manifestation of the Pathogenic Factor can be put down purely to the energetic effects of the infectious agent, together with other environmental factors such as climate and diet. For example, a virus infection and exposure to a cold wind may together lead to the manifestation of Wind Cold on the Exterior in an otherwise healthy person.
- *Pathogenic Factor of Internal origin*. When the Pathogenic Factor has an Internal origin, the manifestation of an infection is an appearance of a deeper imbalance (such as pre-existing Damp Heat), and therefore has not been caused by the infectious agent. The infectious agent has simply allowed the expression of the imbalance at a more superficial (Exterior) level. An example of this might be the appearance of cystitis (Damp Heat in the Bladder) in someone who has pre-existing Damp Heat and Kidney Deficiency.

The crucial difference between these two categories is that, in the former, an infectious agent (akin to a 'strong Pathogen') has contributed to the generation of an imbalance, and in the latter the infection appears as a manifestation of an underlying deep imbalance for which the infectious agent is not the trigger. In all probability, the symptoms of most infections are a result of a combination of the two, in that the energetic property of the infectious agent triggers the manifestation of a Pathogenic Factor in a person who already has some degree of underlying imbalance.

The three energetic interpretations of infection are clarified further below.

Pathogenic factor of external origin

Even the healthiest person will succumb to diseases. Despite there being no pre-existing major imbalance, a person with strong Upright Qi may experience strong symptoms when coming into contact with an infectious agent in a sufficiently high concentration, such as the bacteria that can multiply in unclean food.

In a case of vomiting and diarrhoea in a healthy person after eating contaminated food, the Chinese medicine interpretation might be Invasion of Damp Heat in the Intestines. This describes the manifestation of the condition. In this case, the origin of the Pathogenic Factor is External and the development of the syndrome has been triggered by the toxins produced by the bacteria in the contaminated food.

Another example of an infectious disease leading to the appearance of a Pathogenic Factor in this way would be any one of the contagious infestations such as scabies and head lice, which can affect very healthy people who come into contact with them. The itch and rash associated with these diseases are symptoms of Heat, but follow the damage to the skin by mites. In both these infestations, the mites are very irritating to the skin, and based on the signs and symptoms it would be appropriate to describe their bites and burrowing as having led to an invasion of a Pathogenic Factor (in this case Wind Damp Heat).

Pathogenic factor of internal origin

This category tends primarily to be reflected in infectious diseases that affect only people with a particular pre-existing imbalance. In such cases the infection is a consequence of that pre-existing imbalance – the result and not the cause of the imbalance.

Recurrent urinary infections or thrush in people with Damp Heat in the Lower Jiao are good examples. These conditions are far less likely to occur in healthy individuals. Instead, according to Chinese medicine theory, they will affect those with a pre-existing imbalance of Damp Heat and/or Deficiency of Kidney Qi.

In both cases, the infectious agent in conventional medicine terms is usually a microbe that normally forms part of the 'human ecosystem' and which has multiplied out of its usual state of balance to lead to the symptoms of inflammation. If the person regained their healthy state of balance the manifestations would disappear.

Pathogenic factor of mixed origin (external and internal)

This more complicated pattern can explain why it is that conditions such as the fungal infection of athlete's foot are very contagious, and lead to a characteristic collection of symptoms, but at the same time are more likely to occur in people with a pre-existing imbalance such as Internal Damp Heat.

The athlete's foot fungus thrives in damp conditions, and infection often occurs in situations in which external climatic damp is prominent (e.g. swimming pools). This suggests that the Pathogenic Factor in athlete's foot is at least partly of External origin, and anyone who visits a pool may suffer a short-term and easily treatable infection.

However, it does seem that those people who suffer from persistent attacks of athlete's foot often have a pre-existing internal imbalance such as Spleen Qi Deficiency leading to Damp. In these

Information Box 2.4d-I—Cont'd

people the infection has become a trigger for the external and frequent expression of the internal imbalance.

The distinction between these three categories is of fundamental importance in using the classifications of conventional medicine to inform a Chinese medicine diagnosis.

The depth of the pathogenic factor

Over the centuries, the Chinese medicine interpretation of those diseases that involve fever evolved into theories that acknowledge that a Pathogenic Factor can manifest at various levels in the energetic body. Three of these theories identify patterns of disease according to 'The Six Stages', 'The Four Levels' and 'The Three Burners', respectively.[3] According to these interpretations, it is possible to be more precise about how deeply the Pathogenic Factor is manifested in the Interior.

These patterns of differentiation often reflect how diseases progress in a conventional medicine perspective.

The energetics of two common infectious diseases

When interpreting the energetics of infectious disease, the important questions that need to be addressed are:

- What Pathogenic Factors are manifesting (consider symptoms and signs)?
- Are the pathogenic factors manifesting on the Interior (organs) or Exterior (skin and muscles – the domain of the Jing-Luo)?
- What is the origin of the Pathogenic Factor (has it come from without, or has it been generated internally)?

There are several important guidelines to bear in mind. These are:

- Infection will *always* represent the presence of a **Pathogenic Factor**.
- The person who develops the disease may already have a degree of depletion of **Blood**, **Qi**, **Yin** or **Yang**. A Pathogenic Factor such as **Damp** or **Heat** may also be complicating this deficiency. This will affect how the symptoms of disease manifest.
- Characteristics which suggest that the manifestation of the Pathogenic Factor results from an energetic property of the infectious agent (**External origin**) include a *high level of infectiousness* and symptoms that are *strongly characteristic* of a particular type of infectious agent.
- Infections that result from exposure to extremes of climate, or other miscellaneous causes of disease (e.g. unclean food), also suggest a **Pathogenic Factor of External origin**.
- Infections that are not easily contagious but which recur in the same person over and over again suggest a **Pathogenic Factor of Internal origin**.
- **Wind** is often present in infectious disease, and is suggested by any symptoms that change rapidly and move around the body.
- Redness, and fever reflect **Heat**.
- Discharges often reflect **Damp** – yellow/green if **Damp Heat** and white/watery if **Damp Cold**.
- Nasal secretions may simply reflect **Wind** preventing the descent of Lung Qi (as in the common cold or allergies).
- Pus and swellings (including lymph nodes) may represent **Phlegm** or **Damp**.
- Susceptibility to infection reflects depletion of vital substances (**Blood**, **Qi**, **Yin** or **Yang**).
- Susceptibility to infections that manifest on the exterior may reflect depletion of **Wei Qi** in particular (but it is important to remember that the Kidneys (Essence) are the root of Wei Qi[4]).

The common cold

In the case of a familiar example, the common cold, the symptoms are conventionally attributed to infection by any one of a number of viruses. The common cold is unusual in that it is an infectious disease that is neatly described by a basic Organ syndrome, i.e. either Wind/Heat or Wind/Cold invading the Lungs. This makes it a good example to use for an interpretation of energetics.

The common cold gives rise to symptoms such as runny nose, cough, sneezing and slight fever. Often it begins with discomfort in the throat or nose, and then the symptoms change over the course of 2–5 days before the patient gets better.

From a Chinese Medicine perspective:

- **Wind** is present because the symptoms start suddenly, change rapidly and move to different part of the body.
- **Cold** may predominate if secretions are watery and the patient feels cold.
- **Heat** may predominate if secretions are yellowish and fever is marked.
- Profuse secretions suggest impairment of **Descent of Lung Qi** due to **Wind**.

The pathogenic factors manifesting in the common cold

The Pathogenic Factors usually manifest on the **Exterior**. Exterior features are slight fever and sweating, headaches, sneezing and runny nose. There are often no features of a deeper Pathogenic Factor in a simple cold.

Occasionally, symptoms such as diarrhoea accompany a cold. This might suggest possible involvement of the **Interior** with **Depletion of Spleen Qi**.

The origin of the pathogenic factors in the common cold

Most features are suggestive of an **External origin**. The common cold is highly infectious. Often, a particular type of cold that is 'going around' will have a characteristic pattern of symptoms which will be experienced by most people who catch it. This suggests that the cold virus has a characteristic energetic property, and that the Pathogenic Factor is, at least in part, of external origin.

In addition, many people report that their symptoms follow exposure to particular extremes of climate such as cold wind. This suggests that climatic factors can also contribute to the nature of the Pathogenic Factor that is manifested.

Some features, however, may be suggestive of an **Internal origin**. Some people report that they benefit from having an occasional cold, particularly if the symptoms have been quite pronounced, but short lived. This suggests that the infection has enabled clearance of existing internal imbalances, which may be seen as contributing to the severity of the symptoms. However, other people suffer from frequent or chronic cold symptoms that they are never able to shake off. They may suffer from colds even when one is not 'going around', and in energetic terms this suggests that it may have become a lingering Pathogenic Factor of Internal origin.

Integrated energetic interpretation of the common cold

The above considerations can be summarised as follows:

- The different strains of the cold virus seem to have a characteristic energetic property that leads to manifestation of Wind/Heat or Wind/Cold on the Exterior and impairment of the Descent of Lung Qi.
- Deficiency of Wei Qi predisposes to development of the common cold. External climatic factors can contribute to the way in which the pathogenic factors are manifested.
- In health, the development of a cold may permit clearance of an internal imbalance, leaving the person in a more balanced state on recovery.

Continued

Information Box 2.4d-I—Cont'd

Cellulitis

The condition of cellulitis, offers a slightly different perspective from that of the common cold. Cellulitis is an infection of the subcutaneous tissues that usually follows a wound to the skin. It can cause a hot, red swelling of the skin, often around an abrasion on the leg or face and which can spread. The patient feels unwell and feverish. The spread of the infection is often rapid and can lead to a red line tracking up the course of a lymphatic vessel. Lymph nodes draining the infected area are often swollen and tender.

If untreated, cellulitis can become severe, and in some cases life-threatening, as infection leads to local death of tissues and septicaemia (infection in the bloodstream). The cause of cellulitis is a bacterium called *Streptococcus*. However, the *Streptococcus* bacterium can live harmlessly on the skin in healthy people.

Cellulitis is more common in elderly people and in people with chronic conditions such as diabetes.

From a Chinese Medicine perspective:

- **Wind** is present because the symptoms start suddenly, change rapidly and move to different parts of the body.
- Redness, tenderness and fever all indicate that **Heat** is present.

The pathogenic factors manifesting in cellulitis

In cellulitis **Wind Heat** initially manifests on the **Exterior**, as indicated by an enlarging red area on the skin.

Symptoms such as lymphatic vessel involvement and malaise suggest that the infection has moved to a deeper level. As the cellulitis progresses, this suggests a progressively deeper level of pathology into the **Interior**.

The origin of the pathogenic factors in cellulitis

A wound is required to permit 'entry' of the pathogenic factor, and this is suggestive of an **External origin**.

Other features are suggestive of **Internal origin**. Cellulitis is not a contagious disease. It is more likely to occur in people with depleted energy, such as elderly people and diabetics. It is believed to be due to increased susceptibility to a bacterium that can live harmlessly on the skin of healthy people.

Integrated energetic interpretation of cellulitis

The above considerations can be summarised as follows:

- Cellulitis is due to a spreading infection by the *Streptococcus* bacterium. It has features of Wind Heat invasion of the Exterior, but can progress to involve deeper levels in some people.
- Its features are predominantly those of a Pathogenic Factor of Internal origin, which suggests that a person who develops cellulitis is susceptible because they already have deficiency of Vital Substances such as Blood and Qi and Yin, together with Internal Heat. The fact that a break in the skin often triggers cellulitis suggests that a pathogenic factor of External origin is also required to trigger the manifestation of the Internal Heat.

Summary

The Chinese medicine interpretation of what conventional medicine would describe as infectious diseases demonstrates very effectively how the symptoms that form a bridge between the two viewpoints can ultimately enrich an understanding of the pathological processes at play.

[1]Maciocia (1989, p. 293) makes the point that, in practice, the origin of the pathogenic factor is far less relevant than the depth at which it is located in the body.
[2]For a summary of the identification of patterns according to the Eight Principles, see Maciocia (1989, p. 176).
[3]It is not within the scope of this text to explore these theories in detail. If you would like to learn more, see Maciocia (1989, pp 177–178 and 479–483).
[4]See Maciocia (1989, p. 40).

Gastrointestinal disease

3.1

Chapter 3.1a The physiology of the gastrointestinal system

LEARNING POINTS

At the end of this chapter you will be able to:

- list the basic nutrients found in food
- explain the basic structure of the digestive tract
- recognise how each part of the digestive tract is adapted for its particular role in the digestive process
- understand the concepts of metabolism, anabolism and catabolism
- make comparisons between this conventional medicine view and the Chinese medicine interpretation of digestion.

Estimated time for chapter: Part I, 60 minutes; Part II, 60 minutes.

Introduction

This is the first chapter that will examine the physiology and diseases of a particular physiological system, in this case the digestive or gastrointestinal system. This chapter is concerned with the function of the digestive system in health, and provides a foundation for the study of the investigation and treatment of digestive diseases that is described in the next four chapters of this section.

Because of its length, this chapter is divided into Parts I and II. If you are using this book as a study course, then you are advised to work through the two sections of this chapter in separate study sessions.

PART I – From our food to the stomach

The digestive system and digestion

The function of the digestive system is to ensure that the water and nutrients present in the diet are absorbed adequately by the body and extraneous waste products are eliminated effectively. It also has a protective function in that it minimises damage from toxins and microbes in the diet. Digestion takes place along the length of a tube known variously as the 'gastrointestinal tract' or 'digestive tract', the 'gut' or the 'alimentary canal'. All these terms are used in medical language and are interchangeable.

Through the process of digestion, the complex contents of food are broken down to release nutrients in a form that can pass easily through the lining of the digestive tract and thence into the blood stream. Water taken in with the diet is absorbed into the blood stream at the same time. Not all of our food has value as a source of nutrients, and not all the water within it is absorbed. Some is left within the digestive tract to become waste material. This waste food material and water travels down the length of the digestive tract to be expelled in the form of faeces (see Q3.1a-1).

The nutrients in our diet

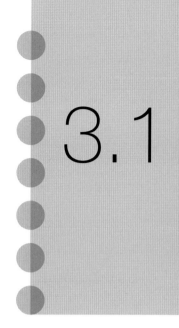

A nutrient is any substance that can be used by the body either to produce energy or to enable other vital chemical processes to take place. There are six basic nutrients: carbohydrates, fats, proteins, mineral salts, vitamins and water. A healthy diet should contain an ideal balance of these nutrients. In addition to these nutrients, a healthy diet also should provide 'fibre'. Fibre is indigestible cellulose from plant-derived foods. Fibre enables healthy transit and elimination of waste, as it provides bulk and water-retaining properties to the faeces.

A healthy diet will consist largely of starchy foods such as bread, rice, pasta and cereals, and fruit and vegetables. Current UK guidelines for the public are that about 60% of the energy value of food (calories) should come from starchy foods and that additional energy should come from at least five portions of fruit or vegetables a day. In addition, there should be some food containing protein, either from the meat/eggs/pulses food group or from the milk/cheese food group. Foods containing fats and sugars should be kept to a minimum. The UK Food Standards Agency 'eat well plate' summarises this advice in pictorial form as shown in Figure 3.1a-I.

Carbohydrates

Starchy foods and fruit and vegetables together provide the carbohydrates that the body needs. Carbohydrates contain the elements carbon, hydrogen and oxygen. These are the foods that, once broken down, provide the basic fuel for the energy-producing process of internal respiration (see Chapter 1.1b). Internal respiration takes place in the mitochondria of all living cells, where simple sugars react with oxygen to produce cellular energy. Carbon dioxide and water are the waste products. The energy produced is stored partly in the form of the 'charged' molecule adenosine triphosphate (ATP), and is partly released as heat.

The most simple carbohydrates are the monosaccharides, or simple sugars, such as glucose and fructose. These are in a perfect form to be utilised by the mitochondria, and so provide the most rapidly accessible form of energy. Monosaccharides taste sweet.

The molecules of the monosaccharides also occur bound in pairs in our food in the form of sweet-tasting disaccharides. Sucrose and lactose (the sugar in milk) are examples of disaccharides. The monosaccharides are also found in the form of chains known as 'polysaccharides', of which starch is an example. These do not immediately taste sweet, but can be broken down in the digestive tract to release the monosaccharides. Starches are, therefore, a form of slow-release energy for the body. Cellulose, which forms the fibrous parts of fruit and vegetables, is also a polysaccharide, but cannot be readily utilised by the human digestive tract. This is why it can perform its role as fibre. Grass-eating animals, however, do have the capability of breaking down cellulose and extracting its valuable food energy.

If carbohydrates are in excess in the diet, superfluous monosaccharides can be converted within the liver to a polysaccharide called 'glycogen'. Glycogen is held in the liver so that when blood sugar levels are low it can readily be converted back to accessible glucose. Any excess carbohydrate after this process has taken place is converted to fat for long-term energy storage.

Fats

Fats are non-soluble oily substances found in diverse foods in our diet, including meat, nuts, eggs, milk and some vegetables. Most fats consist of two components joined together: a fatty acid and glycerol. When broken down by the body, the fatty acids and glycerol are released to provide energy for the bodily processes.

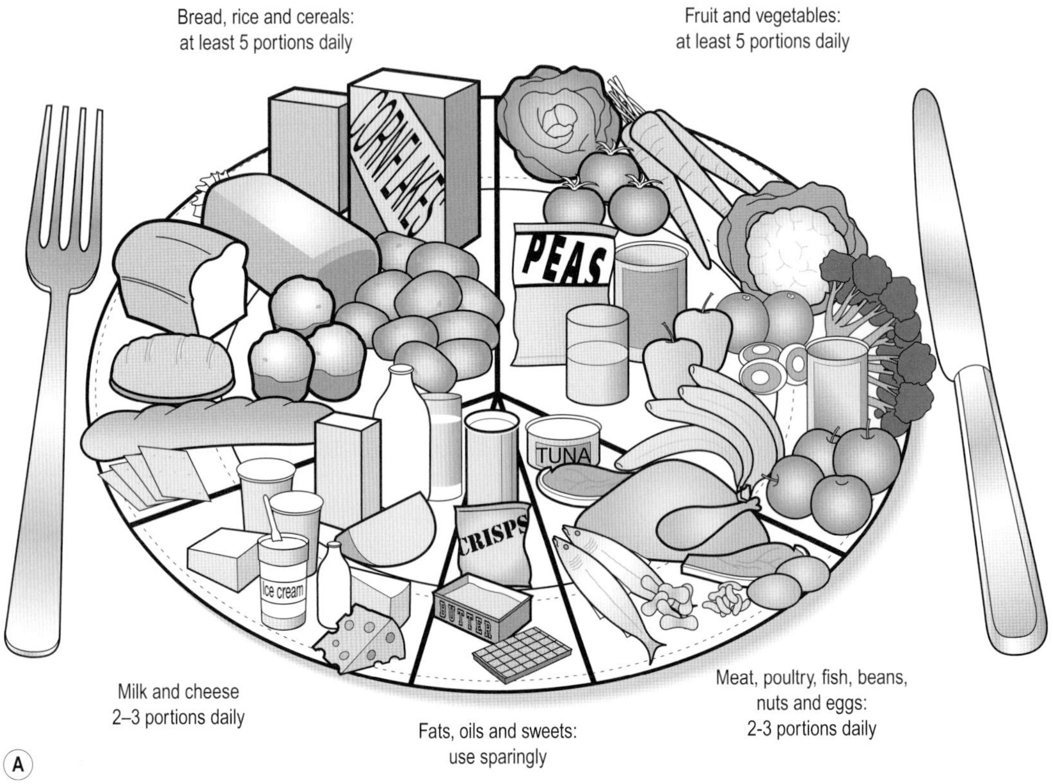

Figure 3.1a-I • The balance of good health.

Saturated fat is so called because of the nature of the chemical bonds in the fat molecules. It consists of molecules containing a saturated fatty acid and a glycerol. Saturated fat tends to form into a solid more readily than unsaturated fat. Lard from meat and butter are both largely saturated fats. Saturated fat is a good source of energy for the body, but an excess in the diet will cause cholesterol to be carried in the blood in the more unhealthy form of low-density lipoprotein and triglycerides (LDL and TGs).

Unsaturated fat is generally derived from vegetable matter, and tends to form a clear oil rather than a solid fat. It consists of molecules containing an unsaturated fatty acid and a glycerol. The omega-3, omega-6 and omega-9 fatty acids are all unsaturated fatty acids derived from unsaturated fats. These polyunsaturated fatty acids are essential components for cellular and intercellular communication processes and the building of cellular structures.

Vegetable, nut and olive oils contain unsaturated fat that provides omega-6 and omega-9 fatty acids. Fish oils contain unsaturated fat that provides omega-3 fatty acids. Most vegetable oils are made of polyunsaturated fats, but olive oil, canola oil and avocados contain a particular form of unsaturated fat known as a 'monounsaturated fat' (this contains omega-9 fatty acids).

Unsaturated fats and monosaturated fats in particular, seem to have the property of reducing the amount of cholesterol that is carried in the blood in the more unhealthy LDL form. For this reason, it is now considered important for a healthy diet that these forms of fats predominate over the saturated fats, and that monounsaturated fats predominate over polyunsaturated fats (as is found in the 'Mediterranean diet'). Unsaturated fats may protect against cardiovascular disease by providing more membrane fluidity than the more solid saturated fats.

Cholesterol is another oily substance that is particularly important for making hormones, including the steroids. Cholesterol is found in dairy products, meat and eggs. It can also be synthesised in the body, particularly in the liver, from more simple molecules. Cholesterol is carried in the blood in the form of complex molecules called LDL, very low-density lipoprotein (VLDL) and high-density lipoprotein (HDL). These structures package the cholesterol so that it is readily accessible to the cells. As mentioned, LDL (and VLDL) is associated with vascular ill-health, but HDL appears to be protective against vascular damage. The balance of these structures in the blood seems to be less affected by the amount of cholesterol in the diet than by the relative amounts of saturated and unsaturated fats (see above).

Trans fatty acids are only found in traces in a natural diet. However, they make up a significant proportion of many western diets because they are found in vegetable oils that have been processed (hydrogenated) to preserve their longevity for foods such as margarines, cakes and biscuits. The American Food and Drugs Administration (US FDA) has estimated that the average American eats 5.8 g of trans fatty acids a day. It is known that trans fatty acids alter the balance of cholesterol in the blood to an unhealthy state (they increase levels of LDL at the expense of the more healthy HDL). In some European states (e.g. Denmark and Switzerland) the use of trans fatty acids in food manufacturing has been banned. Many other countries now have policies whereby the proportion of trans fatty acids has to be described in food labelling.

Proteins

Proteins are complex chain-like structures that are made up of simple molecules called 'amino acids'. All amino acids contain the element nitrogen as well as carbon, hydrogen and oxygen. Some also contain trace minerals such as zinc, iron and copper. There are about 20 different amino acids, which can be combined in potentially infinite permutations to form protein chains. Proteins are made in animal and plant cells at the ribosomes as a result of decoding instructions held on the cellular DNA (see Chapter 1.1b). The ribosome is the site at which amino acids are linked together to form a unique and characteristic protein chain, after which the particular makeup of the protein chain encourages the structure to fold in a characteristic way. This means that proteins are large molecules that have a unique shape. The shape and form of a particular protein might give it special structural properties (e.g. the collagen in skin and hair) or make it soluble in water (e.g. the albumen found in blood and in egg white). In other proteins the shape is essential for communication, and this is the basis of how cell-membrane proteins 'recognise' the external stimulants, such as hormones, that bring about internal change in the cell itself. Antibody–antigen recognition also depends on the antibody having a unique shape that 'fits' the shape of the antigen.

Protein in food is found in meat, eggs, fish, cereals, nuts and pulses. All the essential amino acids can be derived from the complete proteins in meat, fish, eggs, milk and soya. Without soya products, a vegetarian will need to eat combinations of nuts, cereals and pulses to ensure that all amino acids are obtained from the diet.

Protein is converted to amino acids in the body, and these circulate dissolved in the blood so that they reach all the tissues. The ribosomes of the cells utilise amino acids to produce their own proteins so that they can reproduce and continue performing their unique functions. Proteins are used to make cellular and extracellular structures (such as the contractile fibres in muscle cells and the connective tissue fibres in cartilage), plasma proteins (such as the clotting factors and albumen), antibodies, enzymes and also some hormones.

In a state of starvation, proteins are broken down by the cellular mitochondria to produce energy. The by-products of this process include chemicals called 'ketones'. When excess ketones are produced, the body is said to be in a state of 'ketosis'.

Mineral salts

Mineral salts are simple inorganic substances that are required in small quantities to maintain bodily processes. Unlike carbohydrates, fats and proteins, they are not a source of energy. Essential minerals include calcium, sodium, potassium, iodine, phosphate, iron, chromium, zinc, selenium, magnesium and manganese. Certain minerals, such as calcium and phosphate (in bone) and sodium (as dissolved salt in the body fluids), constitute a significant proportion of the body mass, whereas others are required only in trace amounts.

Vitamins

Vitamins are more complex compounds than minerals, and are also essential for bodily processes. They are essential dietary components because either they cannot be made by the body at all or they cannot be made in sufficient quantities to sustain health. Vitamins are now broadly grouped into the four fat-soluble vitamins A, D, E and K, and the nine water-soluble vitamins B1–B8 and C. The lettering system approximately relates to the order in which the vitamins were discovered (beginning with vitamin A in 1909). Those substances initially called F–J were either reclassified as B vitamins or were subsequently deemed not to qualify as vitamins at all. The B vitamins are now recognised to be linked because they are all vital in the production of energy from nutrients by the mitochondria. The food sources and the functions of the 13 vitamins are summarised in Table 3.1a-I.

Water

Water is an essential part of the diet because the body is continually losing water through the urine, faeces, sweat and in exhaled air. About 60% of the adult body mass is water, and all the essential bodily processes take place in a watery milieu. Water has to be lost as it is the vehicle through which waste chemicals (in urine and sweat) and also waste food materials (in the faeces) are carried for expulsion from the body. It is also lost through the breath and sweat to aid with cooling of the body.

On average, about 2.5 litres of water need to be replaced by the diet every day. Much of this is contained in food, and so a human being can survive on about 1.5 litres of water in drinks per day. Any water excess to requirements is passed out of the body in the form of dilute urine. If insufficient water is drunk, the kidneys make dark concentrated urine from the fluid in the plasma, and the water required for excretion of wastes is drawn from the tissues, which then become dehydrated.

Information Box 3.1a-I

The nutrients: comments from a Chinese medicine perspective

In Chinese medicine, each food has a characteristic energetic property and also a tendency to affect a particular bodily substance or organ. For this reason, food can be used as medicine, whereby a diet is recommended to suit the needs of the patient. The taste and the consistency of the food bear an important relationship to its energetic properties. Moreover, the freshness and the method of cooking can have a bearing on the value of the food.

For example, fresh grapes are recognised to Tonify the Qi and Blood, and affect the Lungs, Spleen and Kidneys. Beef is recognised to Tonify Yin and Qi and Blood, and affect the Large Intestine, Stomach and Spleen. Some foods, such as pears, are Cool, and so may be useful in moderation in Hot conditions, and some are Warm in nature, such as chicken liver, and so are used to in Cold conditions.

Despite the fact that most foods contain a complex array and unique balance of nutrients, these distinctions are not made in conventional medicine, in which rather broad statements are made about the six types of nutrients found in food groups. Furthermore, very little emphasis is also placed on how the food is prepared, apart from avoidance of overcooking, in that this might inactivate the vitamin C in fruits and vegetables.

Table 3.1a-I The 13 vitamins, their main food sources and their functions in the body

Vitamin	Food sources	Use in the body
A (retinol)	Green vegetables, milk, liver	Pigments in eye and health of skin
D (calciferol)	Milk, eggs, cod liver oil; ultraviolet light	Calcium absorption and bone formation
E (tocopherol)	Margarine, seeds, green leafy vegetables	Antioxidant: protects fatty acids and cell membranes from damaging oxidation
K (phylloquinone)	Green leafy vegetables	Formation of certain clotting factors
B_1 (thiamine)	Meats (pork), grains, legumes	Carbohydrate metabolism; also nerve and heart function
B_2 (riboflavin)	Milk, liver, eggs, grains, legumes	Energy metabolism
B_3 (niacin or nicotinic acid)	Liver, lean meats, grains, legumes	Energy metabolism
B_5 (pantothenic acid)	Milk, liver, eggs, grains, legumes	Energy metabolism
B_6 (pyridoxine)	Wholegrain cereals, vegetables, meats	Amino acid metabolism
B_7 (biotin)	Meats, vegetables, legumes	Fat synthesis and amino acid metabolism
B_9 (folic acid)	Wholewheat foods, green vegetables, legumes	Nucleic acid metabolism
B_{12} (cobalamin)	Red meats, eggs, dairy products	Nucleic acid production
C (ascorbic acid)	Citrus fruits, green leafy vegetables, tomatoes	Collagen formation in teeth, bone, and connective tissue of blood vessels; may help in resisting infection

A significant state of dehydration will be reflected in a loss of body weight of more than 2–3%. Because the sensitive tissues of the body are not able to withstand the state of dehydration for more than a few days, water is essential for life. Loss of more than 10% of the body weight through dehydration is usually not compatible with life (see Q3.1a-2-Q3.1a-6).

The structure of the digestive tract

The digestive tract is a tube that begins at the mouth and ends at the anus. At both these orifices there is a junction between the tough and dry keratinised epithelium of the skin and the soft and moist mucous epithelium that lines the whole of the digestive tract. This junction can be easily examined in the mouth where the two lips meet. At the junction, the dry, slightly ridged keratinised skin of the external lip becomes moist and smooth mucous epithelium on the inside of the lip.

The tube of the digestive tract has a basic structure that can be found in slightly different forms along its length. The tube has four distinct layers (Figure 3.1a-II):

- The adventitia is the outer layer of the digestive tract. Below the diaphragm, the adventitia forms the peritoneum which is a serous membrane (i.e. it secretes watery fluid). This protects and lubricates the digestive tract so that it can move easily within the abdominal cavity.
- The muscle layer consists of two layers of smooth muscle. The longitudinal and circular fibres contract in coordinated waves to propel the contents of the food down the length of the tract. This motion is called 'peristalsis'.
- The submucous layer is a layer of connective tissue that contains blood vessels, collections of lymph nodes, lymphatic vessels and networks (plexuses) of nerves.

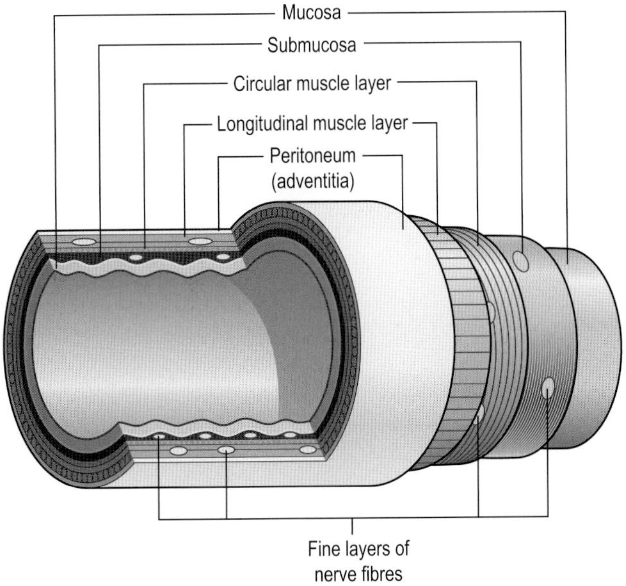

Figure 3.1a-II • The general structure of the digestive tract.

- The mucosa consists of a mucous (epithelial) membrane (see Chapter 1.1d), with its combined functions of protection, secretion and absorption, and two supportive layers beneath this. The mucous membrane secretes mucus for further protection and lubrication. Other specialised cells in the mucous epithelium are sensitive to changes in the contents of the digestive tract. These secrete hormones into the blood stream within the submucous layer.

The mouth is the only section of the digestive tract that does not have this general structure.

The tube of the digestive tract has 'accessory organs', which open out or project into the hollow of the tube. These organs are the tongue, salivary glands, liver, gallbladder, pancreas and appendix.

The structure of the tube itself changes throughout its length according to the function required. The mouth, oesophagus, stomach, duodenum, small intestine, large intestine (colon), rectum and anus are described in more detail below.

The salivary glands open via tubes (ducts) into the mouth, the pancreas, liver and gallbladder all open via ducts into the duodenum, and the appendix opens directly into the beginning of the colon. Figure 3.1a-III illustrates the position of the organs associated with the digestive tract, and how, with the exception of the mouth and the oesophagus, the main part of the digestive tract is situated below the diaphragm.

The mouth

The mouth is where the process of digestion begins. The teeth, tongue and the muscles of chewing are adapted to grind up food into a paste with saliva.

Saliva is produced by six exocrine salivary glands that open into the mouth. The size and extent of these important glands is illustrated in Figure 3.1a-IV.

Saliva is produced is response to the action of eating, and also in response to the anticipation of food. Certain flavours, such as the sourness of lemons, are particularly powerful in inducing a good flow of saliva. About 1.5 litres of saliva is produced a day, and the moisture is very important to help maintain the health of the mouth and to assist with chewing. The moisture is also essential for enjoyment of food, as it enables food to be tasted. Saliva also contains protective substances such as mucus and antibodies, together with the protein lyzozyme, all of which protect the digestive tract from damage by microorganisms and toxins.

The salivary glands also produce the first digestive enzyme that the eaten food will encounter, and thus begins the breakdown of the nutrients into the building blocks that are absorbed into the blood stream. An enzyme is a biological substance that encourages a chemical reaction. In this case the enzyme is called 'salivary amylase', and in its presence the chains of complex polysaccharides in carbohydrate come apart to form disaccharides. This reaction only occurs in the mouth, as the acid contents of the stomach stop the amylase from working. This is why it is important to chew thoroughly (see Q3.1a-7).

The tongue is a muscular structure adapted for two distinct functions: eating (taste, chewing and swallowing) and speech. It is covered with little bumps called 'papillae', which are sensitive

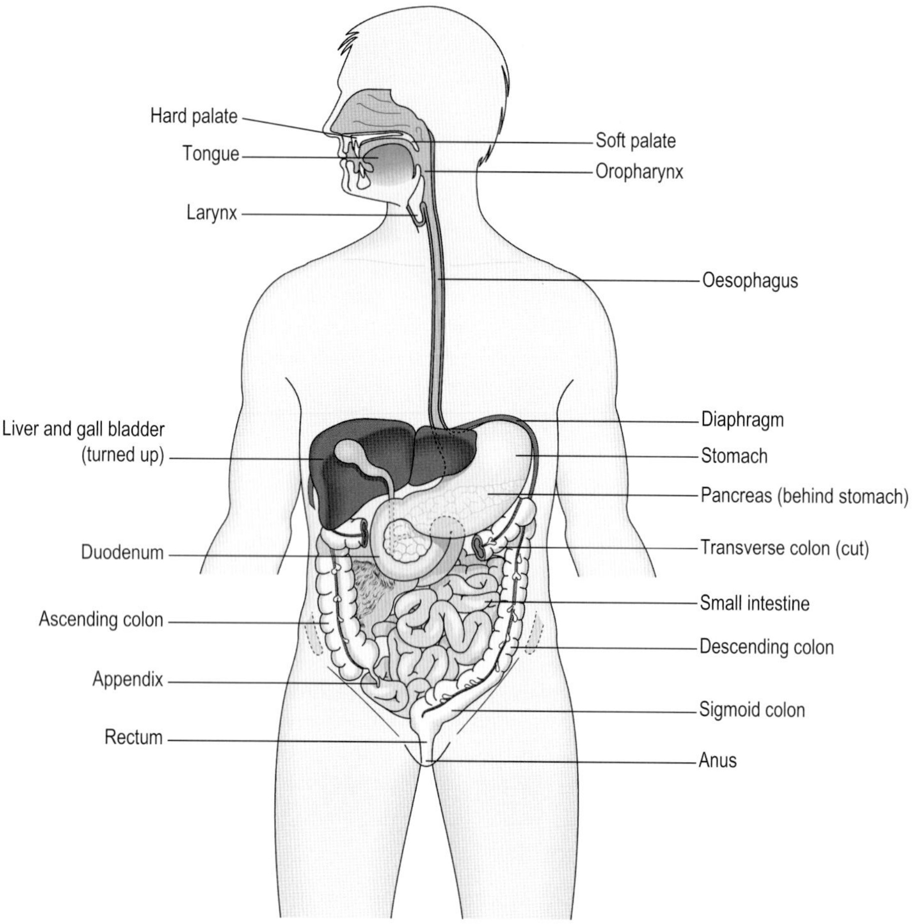

Figure 3.1a-III • The organs of the digestive system.

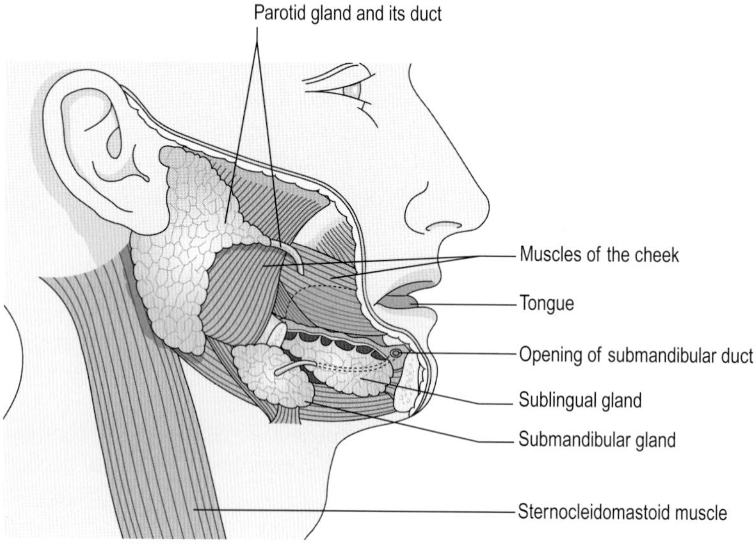

Figure 3.1a-IV • The position of the salivary glands.

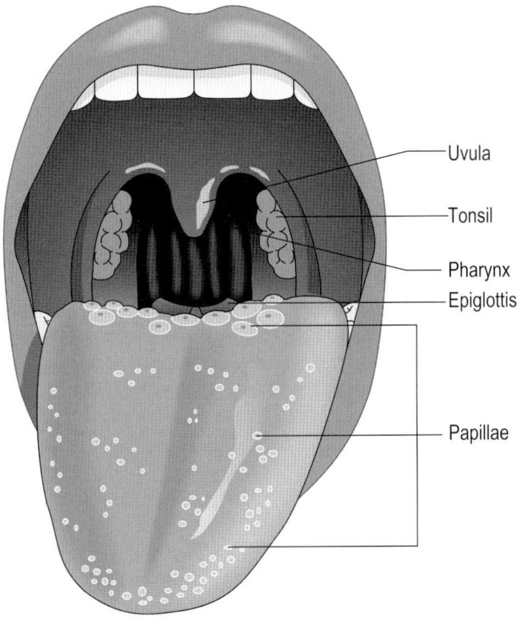

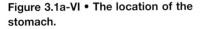

Figure 3.1a-V • The papillae of the tongue.

to the four main tastes: salt, sweet, sour and bitter. The subtleties of taste are also dependent on a healthy sense of smell, as anyone who has a heavy cold will recognise. Figure 3.1a-V illustrates the position of the different sorts of papillae.

The oesophagus

The oesophagus runs from the pharynx at the back of the mouth to the opening of the stomach. The oesophagus runs posterior to the airways which lead to the lungs. A muscle ring (sphincter) at the end of the pharynx prevents air entering the oesophagus during breathing in. The opening of the stomach coincides with the position where the oesophagus passes through the diaphragm. The muscles of the diaphragm act as a sphincter to prevent stomach contents from returning into the oesophagus. This muscle ring is also known as the 'cardiac sphincter', because it lies just below the heart. The cardiac sphincter is situated at the level of the xiphisternal joint (the location of acupoint Ren-16 Zhongting).

The stomach

The stomach is a stretchy expansion of the tube of the digestive tract, but still retains the four layers. Figure 3.1a-VI illustrates that the stomach is bounded by the cardiac sphincter above and the pyloric sphincter below. These muscle rings keep food contents within the stomach for up to 6 hours to enable the beginning of a thorough digestion process. The stomach muscles enable the muscle to churn the food contents stored within it to aid digestion.

Gastric (the term coming from the Greek for 'stomach') juices are secreted by specialised glands that open into the stomach. These juices consist of water, acid and an enzyme called 'pepsin', which enables the breakdown of protein into amino acids. The acid is produced by specialised proteins in the cell walls of the gastric glandular cells known as 'proton pumps'. The stomach lining also secretes copious mucus to protect its own cells from the acid produced by the proton-pump cells.

In the stomach, the food is churned with the fluid of the gastric juice to form a liquid soup known as 'chyme'. The pepsin and the acid work together to break down the protein in the food into amino acids. The smell of this process is the familiar smell of vomit. Very little of the diet is absorbed through the lining of the stomach, but water and alcohol are two exceptions. This explains why drinking alcohol on an empty stomach can have such a rapid effect.

The stomach is also the source of a protein called 'intrinsic factor', which has an attraction for vitamin B_{12} (cobalamin). This attraction is important, as each molecule of this essential vitamin can only be later absorbed if it is bound to a molecule of intrinsic factor (see Q3.1a-8).

Figure 3.1a-VI • The location of the stomach.

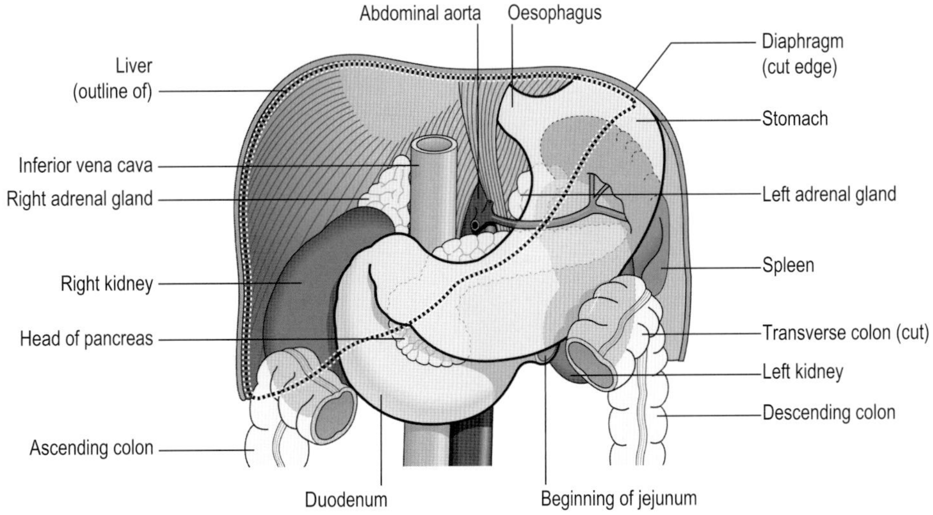

PART II – From the duodenum to the outside world

The duodenum (the first part of the small intestine)

The duodenum is the tubular receptacle for the partly digested food that descends from the stomach. It is into the duodenum that bile from the gallbladder and pancreatic juices from the pancreas enter the digestive tract and mix with the food. Both these fluids are extremely important in the final stages of the digestion of food.

Information Box 3.1a-II

The duodenum: comments from a Chinese medicine perspective

It is interesting to note that the duodenum, the entry point for the pancreatic digestive juices, is situated at the level of the origin of 12th thoracic vertebra, the level of the Back-Shu point of the Spleen (Bl 20; Pishu).

The pancreas

The pancreas is a gland with two distinct roles, one is endocrine and the other is exocrine. (For a reminder of the difference between these two categories of epithelial structure, see Chapter 1.1d.)

The endocrine role of the pancreas is to secrete the hormones insulin and glucagon directly into the blood stream. Both these hormones are important for ensuring that the concentration of glucose in the blood remains at the optimum level for the function of the cells of the body.

Information Box 3.1a-III

The endocrine pancreas: comments from a Chinese medicine perspective

The endocrine role of the pancreas is to allow the accessibility of glucose to the cells, an essential prerequisite for the production of cellular energy in the process of internal respiration. Although this function is not directly related to digestion, it could be interpreted as broadly parallel with the wider Transforming and Transporting function that the Spleen Organ has on Gu (food) Qi.

The exocrine role of the pancreas is to secrete a diverse array of digestive enzymes into the duodenum via the pancreatic duct. The enzymes can digest all three of the complex food components (carbohydrates, proteins and fats), and therefore will complete the work started by the salivary glands and the gastric juices.

Figure 3.1a-VII illustrates how the C-shaped loop of the duodenum hugs the pancreas. The spleen, kidneys, liver and transverse colon are all situated at this level of the abdomen.

The gallbladder

This hollow organ is a store for the fluid called 'bile', which is manufactured in the liver. Bile is dark green and very bitter tasting. It contains substances called 'bile salts', which aid the digestion of fats.

Bile also contains some of the body's waste products that have been processed by the liver. These will pass eventually into the faeces. These by-products of the liver's detoxification

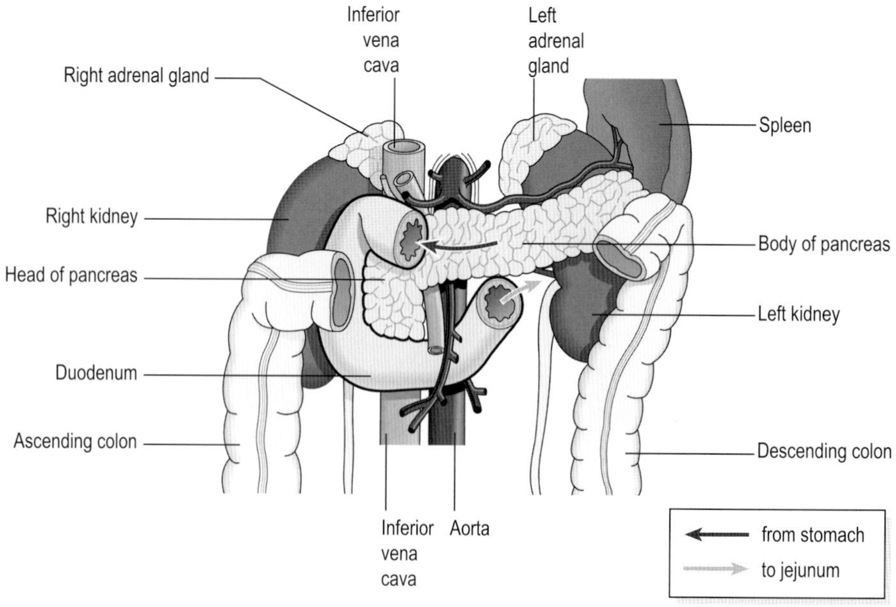

Figure 3.1a-VII • The duodenum and associated structures.

Information Box 3.1a-IV

The anatomy of the organs associated with the duodenum: comments from a Chinese medicine perspective

Note from Figure 3.1a-VII that the spleen lies at the same level as the pancreas. It is possible that the ancient Chinese assumed that the pancreas and spleen were one anatomical organ, as the pancreas is never directly referred to in the classics of Chinese medicine. Anatomically the two organs are very closely related and share a common blood supply. This may explain why digestive functions were attributed to the Spleen. However, the spleen is conventionally considered to have its main role in the lymphatic system, with absolutely no part to play in the digestion of food. It is also interesting to see that the kidneys are also at this level in the body, and very close by are the liver, gallbladder, and loops of the large and small intestines.

Yuan Qi from the Kidneys in Chinese medicine is not only the motive force for all the Organs, but also a catalyst for the conversion of Gu (Food) Qi to Blood.

In the light of this, it makes sense that the physiological kidneys sit at the centre of a cluster of so many organs, and in particular are located very close to those that deal with digestion.

include a deeply hued chemical called 'stercobilin' (derived from the breakdown of haemoglobin), which gives the faeces their characteristic brown colour.

When food enters the duodenum, the cells of its lining respond to the change by releasing hormones, including a substance called cholecystokin (CCK), into the bloodstream. These 'messengers' travel to the gallbladder and stimulate it to contract and release bile when it is most needed. Similarly, other duodenal hormones stimulate the pancreas to release pancreatic juices.

The small intestine

The small intestine is simply a continuation of the duodenum. It receives the fluid mixture of partly digested food and digestive enzymes from the duodenum, powered by the wave-like muscular contractions of peristalsis.

The small intestine is about 5 metres long, and its lining is thrown into folds. Microscopic peaks of mucosa project from these folds, and appear, when greatly magnified, like a vast mountain range. These peaks are called 'villi'. Furthermore, each cell of the mucosa has tiny projections called 'microvilli'. This unique structure greatly increases the area of the mucosa that is in contact with the fluid contents of the digestive tract, an adaptation that maximises absorption. Figure 3.1a-VIII illustrates the microscopic structure of a villus, including the tiny microvilli on each cell, and also the way the blood and lymph supply of the digestive-tract lining project into the centre of the villus.

As the digestive process continues along the length of the small intestine, the saccharides, amino acids, glycerol, water-soluble vitamins, and salts resulting from digestion are taken up (usually by facilitated diffusion) into the mucosal cells.

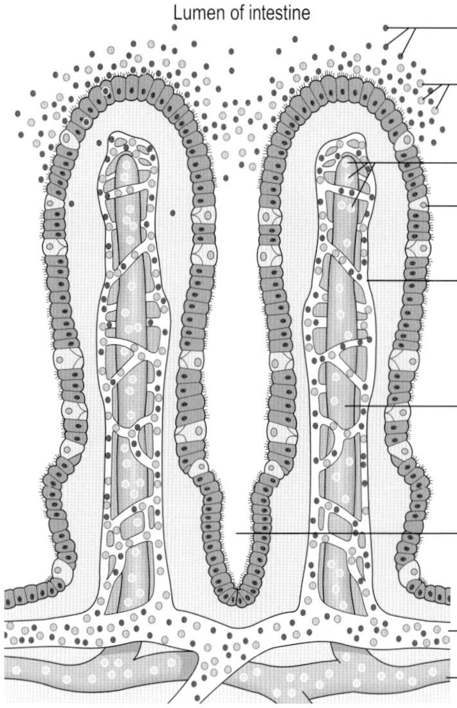

Figure 3.1a-VIII • One complete villus in the small intestine.

From here they pass into the bloodstream. Numerous collections of tiny lymph nodes in the submucosal tissues protect the bloodstream from any infectious agents that may have been present in the diet.

Fatty acids and the vitamin B_{12}–intrinsic factor complex are absorbed by the very end segment of the small intestine (the 'terminal ileum'). The bile acids, which aid the digestion of fats, are also reabsorbed here and circulate in the bloodstream back to the liver, from where they can be used again in the bile. Vitamins A, D, E and K are soluble in fats, and so are also absorbed at this end of the small intestine. Fatty acids, glycerol and these vitamins pass directly into the lymphatic system rather than the bloodstream. The small intestine also reabsorbs over 8 litres of water a day from the fluid contents that initially enter the duodenum. This leaves a semi-solid residue to enter the large intestine. This residue consists of fibre, waste from the bile, and many thousands of dead mucosal cells and intestinal bacteria, which have been shed along the digestive journey (see Q3.1a-9 and Q3.1a-10).

The large intestine

The large intestine, or colon, receives the residue of digestion from the small intestine. The first few centimetres of the colon are called the 'caecum', which literally means 'blind ending'. This is because it is above the caecum that the end of the small intestine opens into the colon, with the result that the caecum is like a cul-de-sac opening out from the passage. At the end of this cul-de-sac is the narrow tube of the appendix. The parts of the large intestine are illustrated in Figure 3.1a-IX. Note how the horizontal stretch of the

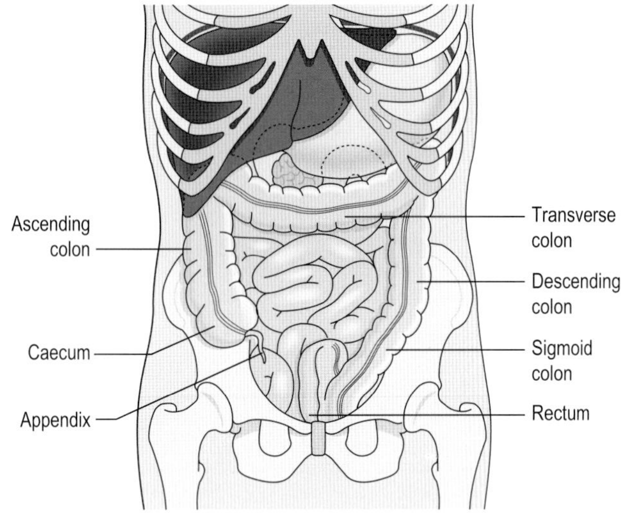

Figure 3.1a-IX • The parts of the large intestine.

transverse colon overlies the duodenum and pancreas at the level of the T12 thoracic vertebra.

The large intestine is the home for most of the 'healthy' bacteria and yeasts which were first described in Chapter 2.4b. The food residue that enters the large intestine is digested further by these 'healthy' organisms. The by-product of this digestion is gas, which is eventually passed out of the anus. Some necessary vitamins are made as by-products of this process, which can then be absorbed into the bloodstream.

In animals that live on a diet of grass, such as sheep, the caecum and appendix are much longer than those in humans and contain many bacteria. Here, the bacteria can digest further the cellulose fibre in grass to release more saccharides, which can be used by the sheep. It is believed that the appendix in humans is simply a vestige of this larger organ found in vegetarian animals. Cellulose cannot be digested by humans, and instead provides an important role as the bulking agent known as 'dietary fibre'.

The muscular contractions of the colon are slow and infrequent. The contractions cause the food residue to move gradually along the length of the colon before entering a storage region called the 'rectum'. The rectum is closed at its bottom end by the muscular sphincter of the anus. When the rectum is filled, there is the sensation of needing to open the bowels. However, the act of emptying the rectum is voluntary, and usually can be delayed to a convenient time. About two-thirds of the fluid that enters the large intestine is reabsorbed, so that the substance that enters the rectum has the familiar consistency of faeces. Mucus secreted along the length of the colon lubricates the passage of the semi-solid faeces (see Q3.1a-11).

The liver

The structure and function of this important organ have been left to last because many of the functions of the liver are not directly related to the process of breakdown of food into basic nutrients. Instead, most of the important functions of the liver are about the processing of these nutrients to make them useful to the cells of the body.

The liver is the largest organ in the body and sits under the diaphragm on the right-hand side. If the palm of the right hand is rested on the lower section of the front of the right-hand half of the rib cage so that the little finger runs along the bottom edge of the rib cage, then the hand will be resting over the liver.

The liver receives all the blood that has passed through the digestive tract, so that it is the first 'stop' for all the nutrients, and also toxins, that have been absorbed during the process of digestion. This nutrient-rich blood passes through tiny channels in the liver called 'sinusoids', so that all the liver cells can come into close contact with it. This means that, at any one time, the liver is holding a large volume of blood within its tissue. This link between the blood leaving the digestive tract and the tissue of the liver is the physical basis for the liver's two distinct roles in the digestive process.

The first role is to act as a filter for toxins and other harmful substances such as drugs and alcohol. The liver cells are able to first absorb and then destroy or change some of these substances which have entered the bloodstream from the diet before they can affect other tissues of the body. This is the reason why many drugs and toxins, if in excess, may damage the liver (e.g. paracetamol and alcohol). There are also many phagocytic white cells (macrophages) lining the sinusoids. One of their functions is to clear away any microbes that may have entered the bloodstream from the diet.

The second role is to begin processing some of the nutrients into a useful form for the cells, or into a form in which they can be stored for later use. Glucose, for example, is stored in the stable form of glycogen within the liver, from which it can be obtained at a later time if sugar supplies are needed quickly. Amino acids are processed so that they can be used by the cells to build new proteins. A similar process occurs for fats. Many vitamins and iron are also stored for later use in the liver. This is why liver is considered to be so nutritious as a food.

Other roles of the liver include:

- The use of amino acids to make the proteins carried within the plasma (including the clotting factors).
- The removal of worn-out red blood cells. The spleen has the main responsibility for this function (see Chapter 3.4a), but is assisted in this task by the liver. Phagocytic white blood cells in the spleen and the liver digest the old red blood cells and then release many of the by-products of digestion into the blood for reuse by the body. The waste product of this process is bilirubin, the green-yellow coloured substance that is excreted into the bile.
- To be a source of heat. The liver is such an active organ that it is one of the most important sources of heat for the body.

The last role to be described here is that of the secretion of bile. In addition to the diverse functions already listed, all the liver cells are able to produce bile and secrete it into tiny tubules in the liver. From here, the bile drains into a duct that leaves the liver and enters the duodenum. The gallbladder also opens into this duct, so that the bile collects here rather than passing directly into the duodenum (Figure 3.1a-X).

Information Box 3.1a-V

The liver: comments from a Chinese medicine perspective

The vascular spaces formed by the liver sinusoids are receptacles for all the blood that drains from the digestive tract. Here, the blood is cleansed and refreshed before travelling on to nourish other tissues. This is in keeping with the Chinese medicine observation that the Liver 'stores Blood' and that this function is necessary for replenishing the Qi.

The liver is also responsible for ensuring that a steady clean supply of useful nutrients is available to the cells. This would very much be in accord with the Chinese medicine function of the Liver of ensuring the smooth flow of Qi. It would also suggest that the liver plays a part in the processes described in Chinese medicine as the Transformation and Transportation of Gu (food) Qi.

However, there is no obvious conventional link between the function of the liver and the function of tendons and the sinews, or indeed in the ability to plan, which are other functions of the Liver Organ in Chinese medicine. The concept of the Hun, or the ethereal soul, has no counterpart in conventional medicine.

Interestingly, however, chronic liver disease can be conventionally recognised to cause changes in the nails, as the deficiency of plasma protein that results leads to characteristically white nails. Similarly, although there is no conventional link between the liver and the eyes in conventional medicine, in chronic liver disease the white of the eyes is the first place in which jaundice becomes apparent.

For more detail on the correspondences between the functions of the liver and gallbladder as described in conventional medicine and the Liver and Gallbladder Organs in Chinese medicine, see Appendix I.

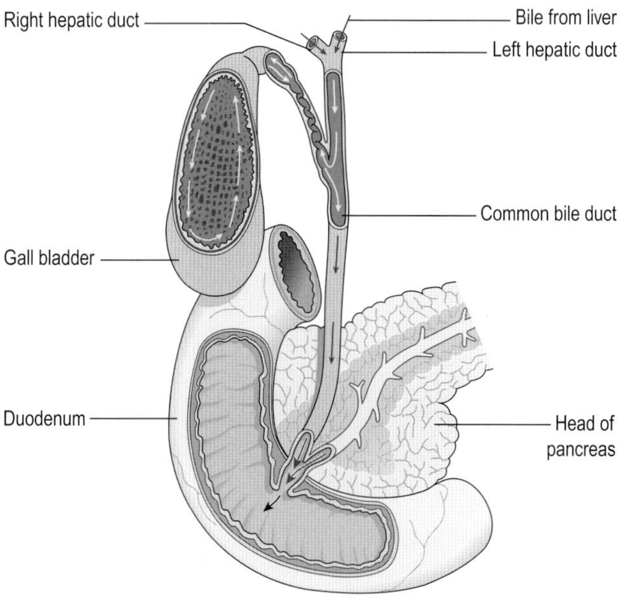

Figure 3.1a-X • The direction of the flow of bile from the liver to the duodenum.

Figure 3.1a-X helps to illustrate how the gallbladder can be surgically removed without disturbing the free flow of bile from the liver. The function of the gallbladder is simply to delay the entry of bile into the duodenum until the best time for digestion of fats. Removal of the gallbladder results in a constant trickle of bile into the duodenum. This is not ideal for perfect digestion of fats, but is not conventionally considered to be a problem for overnourished western people.

The metabolism

This last section of this chapter touches on the metabolism, which can be seen as the end result of the digestive process. 'Metabolism' simply means all the chemical processes that take place in the body. These processes require basic nutrients, oxygen and water to occur.

Metabolism can be broadly considered in two categories:

- *Anabolism* includes all those reactions that lead to the building up of new substances for cellular growth or function (this might be described as a Yin process in Chinese medicine language).
- *Catabolism* includes all those reactions that lead to the breakdown of the complex structures of the cell, and often leads to the release of energy (this might be described as a Yang process in Chinese medicine language).

In health, the anabolic and catabolic processes generally balance each other. This leads to a constant process of turnover of the old substances in the body for replacement with the new. It is this balance that allows for adaptation to change. In times of growth and development the anabolic processes are more prominent, and in times of illness and ageing the catabolic processes are more prominent.

Healthy metabolism is dependent on an adequate supply of 'fuel' – the basic nutrients and oxygen. If either of these is lacking, fuel has to be obtained from within the body. Initially, the glucose store in the liver is drawn upon, but very soon after this body fat and muscle protein is broken down. This is a state in which catabolism is in excess, and is not a healthy state if prolonged. Nevertheless, it is the state that people who diet 'successfully' put themselves into by choice. Conversely, if there is excess fuel, or if the metabolism is sluggish, then a state in which anabolism is in excess results. If there are no demands for the body to grow or develop, then the excess nutrients are laid down as fat.

Information Box 3.1a-VI

The metabolism: comments from a Chinese medicine perspective

Signs and symptoms of disorders of metabolism suggest that the overall control of the metabolism might be broadly equated with the Spleen Organ, as Spleen Deficiency can lead to both weakness and inability to gain weight, and conversely to Accumulation of Damp and weight gain.

Self-test 3.1a

The physiology of the gastrointestinal system

1. What are the six basic nutrients to be found in our diet?
2. What are the essential basic nutrients that are transported, *after* digestion, from the digestive tract to the cells?
3. What components in the diet are digested in the stretch of digestive tract from the mouth to the stomach?
4. How do pancreatic juice and bile contribute to the process of digestion of the food?
5. How is the small intestine adapted to its function of the absorption of food?
6. What nutrients are absorbed from the colon?
7. List six main functions of the liver.
8. Define the term 'metabolism'.

Answers

1. Carbohydrates, proteins, fats, vitamins, mineral salts and water.
2. The essential nutrients that are transported to the cells after digestion are:
   - saccharides (sugars), derived from dietary carbohydrates
   - amino acids, derived from dietary proteins
   - fatty acids, glycerol and cholesterol, derived from dietary fats
   - vitamins, mineral salts and water, unchanged from their state in the diet.
3. Carbohydrates are broken down to saccharides by the enzymes in saliva, and proteins are broken down to amino acids in the stomach. The chewing of food and the churning action of the stomach turn the solid diet into a fluid ready for further digestion in the small intestine.
4. Pancreatic juice contains enzymes, which further break down carbohydrates into saccharides and proteins into amino acids. These enzymes also digest some fats (not including cholesterol, which is absorbed unchanged) into fatty acids, and glycerol. Bile salts in the bile aid the digestion of fatty acids.
5. The small intestine is adapted to maximise absorption by being very long and in the structure of its mucosa, which has folds, villi and microvilli to increase the surface area further. The blood and lymphatic supply of the small intestine is very rich and is arranged so that a blood vessel and a lymphatic vessel project into each of the thousands of villi on the mucosa.
6. The colon absorbs about two-thirds of the water that enters it, and also some essential vitamins that are the by-products of digestion by colonic microorganisms.
7. The functions of the liver include:
   - to store and process the basic nutrients for all the tissues of the body
   - to remove toxins and microbes form the bloodstream of the digestive tract
   - to manufacture the proteins that form part of the plasma of the blood
   - to break down worn-out red blood cells
   - to be a source of heat
   - to secrete bile.

Chapter 3.1b The investigation of the gastrointestinal system

LEARNING POINTS

At the end of this chapter you will be able to:
- recognise the main investigations for gastrointestinal disease
- understand what it means for a patient to undergo these investigations

Estimated study time: 30 minutes.

Introduction

Patients with suspected disease of the gastrointestinal system may be referred for further investigation by their GP either to a gastroenterologist (a hospital physician who specialises in the medical management of digestive disease) or to a surgeon who specialises in surgery of the bowel.

Investigation of the gastrointestinal system

Once referred to any hospital specialist, patients may be offered a series of tests chosen to exclude a wide range of possible diagnoses that may affect the gastrointestinal system. This may mean that the patient may undergo some tests that are not strictly necessary in their particular case, but it is considered good practice to be thorough in the investigation. Some tests might involve the patient in considerable inconvenience or discomfort, but are performed because it is believed that it is best to be as informed as possible about the health of the system before treatment is chosen.

The investigations that are most likely to reveal information about the digestive tract include:

- a thorough physical examination
- blood tests
- examination of faeces
- tests to 'visualise' the inside of the gastrointestinal tract and the accessory organs, including endoscopy, X-ray studies with barium contrast, and ultrasound and computed tomography (CT) scans
- tests to remove samples of tissue for examination (biopsy).

These tests are considered briefly below in turn.

Physical examination of the gastrointestinal system

The physical examination of the gastrointestinal involves the stages listed in Table 3.1b-I. For the purposes of physical examination of a supine patient, the accessible region of abdomen is considered to occupy the approximately hexagonal region that is bounded by the ribs above and the inguinal ligaments and pubic bone below.

Table 3.1b-I The stages of physical examination of the gastrointestinal system

- General examination for signs of severe disease of the gastrointestinal system, such as pale nails, pallor, wasting and oedema
- Visual examination of the lips, mouth and tongue for features of gastrointestinal disease
- Palpation of the cervical (neck) lymph nodes (indicating disease in the mouth and upper oesophagus)
- Palpation of the supraclavicular lymph nodes (indicating disease, in particular cancer, of the lower oesophagus, stomach and duodenum)
- General palpation of the abdomen for tenderness and masses
- Examination of the lower rectum and anal canal by means of insertion of a gloved finger

As Figure 3.1b-I illustrates, many important organs are situated underneath the nine named regions of the abdomen. A lump felt in the suprapubic area, for example, might suggest a problem of the bladder or the uterus, whereas pain in the left iliac fossa would suggest a problem of the colon or left ureter. The names for these nine regions of the abdomen are frequently used in medical texts for the description of abdominal conditions, so it is useful to be familiar with them.

Blood tests

The two most common tests are:

- Full blood count (see Chapter 2.4d). This is the test used to exclude the anaemia that can result from long-term bleeding in conditions such as a chronic stomach ulcer.
- Serum sample. Proteins in the serum of the blood are examined to look for features of liver disease (a test known as the 'liver function test' (LFT)). In addition to the LFT there is a wide range of other less commonly performed serum tests that are used to help diagnose particular digestive diseases.

Examination of faeces (stool sample)

Examination of the faeces may reveal the presence of blood. Culture of the stool is performed to look for infectious agents. The presence of undigested nutrients in the stool, such as fat or sugars, may indicate a problem with digestion known as 'malabsorption'.

Visualisation of the digestive tract

The most efficient way of visualising the oesophagus, stomach and duodenum is by means of a slim, flexible tubular telescope called an 'endoscope'. In upper gastrointestinal endoscopy a heavily sedated patient is encouraged to swallow the tube. As the fibre-optic end of the endoscope descends, images of the lining of the upper digestive tract can be seen by the examining doctor on a screen. This procedure does not use X-rays.

X-ray studies are also used in the investigation of digestive disease. Because the soft tissue of the bowel is not clearly exposed by X-ray imaging, a liquid mixture containing the salt barium sulphate is used to provide 'contrast' between the hollow space within the bowel and the surrounding soft tissues (as the metal of barium shows up as white on X-ray images). In the procedure called 'barium swallow', the patient is requested to drink a liquid containing barium sulphate. As the liquid lines the upper digestive tract, X-ray images will reveal its outline and show up areas of muscle spasm, ulcers or tumours. Figure 3.1b-II is a clear barium-swallow X-ray image, in this case depicting an oesophageal cancer. The white area shows the internal shape of the oesophagus, and the arrows indicate the narrowing caused by the tumour.

The endoscope can also be used to pass a fine tube into the pancreatic duct and bile ducts. Barium can be injected up this tube so that X-ray images can show up the delicate internal structure of the pancreas and the gallbladder. This procedure is known as 'endoscopic retrograde cholangiopancreatography'

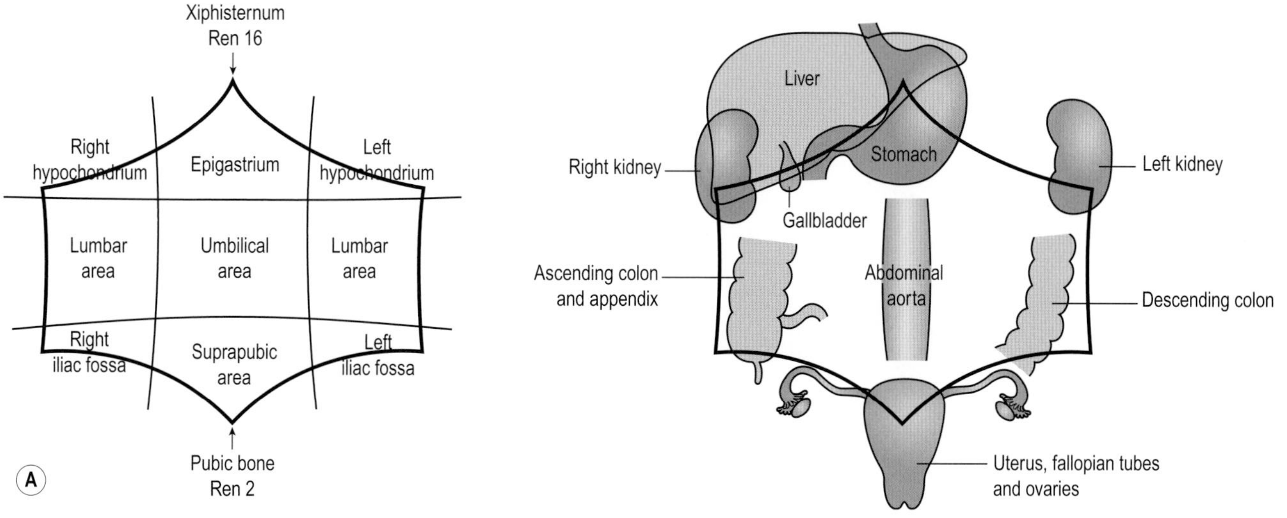

Figure 3.1b-I • The regions of the abdomen and the underlying major organs.

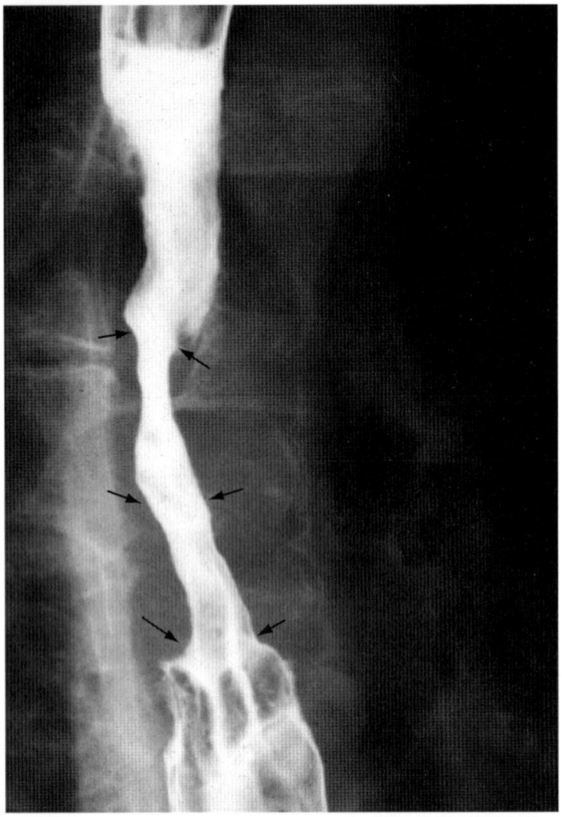

Figure 3.1b-II • A barium-swallow image, showing a carcinoma of the oesophagus (narrowing by tumour indicated by arrows).

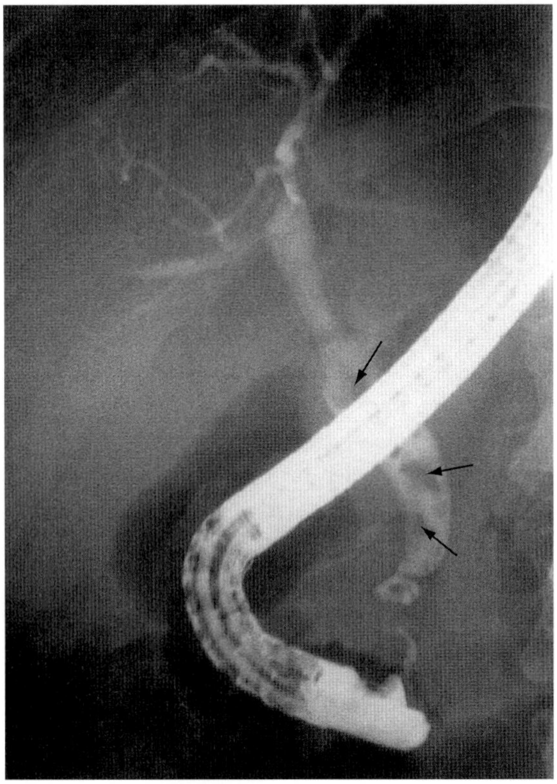

Figure 3.1b-III • An ERCP image from a patient with gallstones • Several stones can be seen within the dilated common bile duct (arrows).

(ERCP). Figure 3.1b-III illustrates an image taken during an ERCP. The thick white curved tube in this image is the end of the endoscope.

To investigate the lower digestive tract, a form of endoscope called a 'colonoscope' is directed into the anal canal and thence into the rectum and colon. To investigate the lower part of the colon (sigmoid colon) and the rectum, a rigid telescope-like instrument called a 'sigmoidoscope' may be used. This is slightly less invasive than a colonoscopy.

A 'barium enema' is a procedure for visualising the lining of the bowel. In this investigation, barium sulphate liquid is injected into the colon via the anus. This is an uncomfortable procedure and may require a night in hospital to 'prepare the bowel' by means of the administration of a strong laxative.

Ultrasound scans, magnetic resonance imaging (MRI) scans and computerised tomography (CT) scans are all useful investigations for diseases of the digestive tract, as these all can reveal the presence of soft-tissue masses, fluid and stones. Ultrasound is the least invasive of these investigations. MRI exposes the patient to strong magnetic and

Self-test 3.1b

The investigation of the gastrointestinal system

1. A patient of yours is seen by a gastroenterologist who suspects possible stomach cancer. What investigations do you think this patient might have to undergo?
2. A patient has epigastric pain. Which organs might be involved?
3. A patient has a swelling in the right iliac fossa. Which organs might be involved?

Answer

1. The patient will first have to undergo a physical examination. If the patient has stomach cancer, the examining doctor might find the following signs:
   - pallor and bodily wasting on general examination
   - an enlarged supraclavicular lymph node
   - an irregular mass in the epigastric area
   - an enlarged irregular liver, indicating secondary cancer in the liver
   - blood tests may reveal anaemia due to long-standing blood loss from the tumour and disturbance of liver function due to secondary cancer
   - the faeces will be tested for the presence of blood
   - an endoscopy may reveal a tumour of the stomach wall; a biopsy would be taken from this tumour at the same time as the endoscopy for examination for cancer cells
   - a barium swallow would probably not be necessary if the results of the endoscopy are negative
   - a CT or ultrasound scan would be performed to look for evidence of secondary spread to the liver and lymph nodes deep in the abdomen.
2. Epigastric pain could signify a problem with the lower oesophagus, stomach, duodenum, pancreas or heart.
3. A lump in the right iliac fossa could signify a possible problem in the appendix, ureter, caecum, fallopian tube or ovary.

radiofrequency fields, but these currently are considered to carry little risk. However, an abdominal CT scan exposes the patient to over 50 times the amount of radiation associated with a chest X-ray, and so its use has to be guided on the basis that the potential benefits of the information outweigh the risks of carcinogenesis (cancer formation) from radiation exposure.

Biopsy of the gastrointestinal tract

'Biopsy' literally means 'examination of a living sample'. In the investigation of digestive disorders, a sample of the bowel lining can be obtained by use of the endoscope tube. Delicate instruments at the end of the tube can be manipulated to pinch off a section of tissue, which can then be removed and examined under a microscope.

Biopsy is a very informative investigation in liver disease. The biopsy of the liver is taken through a small incision in the skin overlying the ribs.

Chapter 3.1c Diseases of the mouth, oesophagus, stomach and duodenum

LEARNING POINTS

At the end of this chapter you will be able to:

- recognise the main features of the most important diseases of the upper gastrointestinal tract
- understand the principles of treatment of a few of the most common diseases
- recognise the red flags of severe disease of the upper gastrointestinal tract.

Estimated study time: 90 minutes.

Introduction

This chapter looks at the most important diseases of the upper digestive tract. The diseases described are those that are important either because they are common, or because they have serious consequences for the patient. These diseases are:

- Diseases of the mouth and salivary glands:
  - mouth ulcers
  - cold sores
  - thrush
  - leukoplakia
  - gingivitis
  - salivary gland infections
  - salivary gland stones
  - salivary gland tumours.
- Diseases of the oesophagus:
  - hiatus hernia and reflux disease
  - stricture of the oesophagus
  - cancer of the oesophagus
  - globus hystericus.
- Diseases of the stomach and duodenum:
  - gastroenteritis
  - cancer of the stomach
  - pyloric stenosis
  - pernicious anaemia
  - gastritis and peptic ulcer.

To help with progression along this journey of diseases of each part of the gastrointestinal tract, it may be useful to be reminded first of the physiological descriptions to be found in the relevant sections in Chapter 3.1a (see Q3.1c-1).

Important diseases of the mouth and salivary glands

Mouth ulcers

The term 'ulcer' describes 'a break in the epithelium'. This term is used for conditions of the gastrointestinal system in which the protective mucosal layer has become damaged for some reason.

Mouth ulcers are usually isolated, small, painful, whitened breaches in the mouth lining, and often have no obvious precipitating cause. They tend to be more common in some people than others. In most cases the sufferer is otherwise well, although occasionally a vitamin deficiency might be found. False or sharp teeth occasionally trigger ulcers. A small mouth ulcer will usually heal within 1–3 days.

A crop of very painful, reddened ulcers points to a viral infection. The very first encounter with the cold sore virus (herpes simplex) can cause such a condition. This is most common in young children, and can be so severe that hospital admission is necessary to give fluids by intravenous drip, as severe inflammation of the mouth prevents eating and drinking for a few days.

Less commonly, mouth ulcers may be part of a more severe digestive condition. The lower gastrointestinal diseases of Crohn's disease, ulcerative colitis and coeliac disease are all associated with mouth ulceration. These conditions are studied in more detail in Chapter 3.1e.

> Information Box 3.1c-I
>
> **Mouth ulcers: comments from a Chinese medicine perspective**
>
> In Chinese medicine, ulcers in the mouth suggest Heat in the Stomach, whereas ulcers on the tongue suggest Heat in the organ suggested by the site of the ulcer on the tongue (commonly Liver and Heart).

Cold sores

The nature of infection by the herpes simplex virus (HSV) in the causation of cold sores was introduced in Chapter 2.4a by means of an example of the pathology of infectious diseases. First infection by HSV may cause a crop of painful ulcers. After this the virus remains 'latent' in a nerve cell, and characteristic symptoms of the painful crusting and weeping cold sore may reoccur at times of stress or exposure to extreme sunlight.

The same virus may also cause genital herpes infections. Oral sex can lead to the transmission of an oral cold sore to the genitalia of the sexual partner (for more detail on genital herpes; see Chapter 5.2d).

Patients may be recommended by their doctor or pharmacist to apply a drug called aciclovir in the form of a cream to the affected area at the onset of a cold sore. Aciclovir prevents the replication of viruses and does seem to shorten or abort the attack, although it does not prevent future recurrences.

Information Box 3.1c-II

Cold sores: comments from a Chinese medicine perspective

In Chinese medicine, cold sores are often described as an invasion of Wind Heat and Damp. Aciclovir, which reduces the inflammation and crusting, is therefore Cooling in its action. As Aciclovir does not treat any underlying Heat and Damp that may have been expressed in the form of the cold sore, it may be described as energetically suppressive in its action.

Oral thrush (candidiasis)

Overgrowth of the *Candida* yeast (thrush) is described in Chapter 2.4b. Overgrowth of the *Candida* yeast in the mouth (oral thrush) appears as white patches on the tongue and lining of the mouth, and may or may not be painful. Thrush of the oesophagus can result in difficult and painful swallowing. Thrush of the oesophagus is a common first feature of the progression of human immunodeficiency virus (HIV) infection to acquired immune deficiency syndrome (AIDS).

Except in the case of newborns, in whom oral thrush is common, thrush in the mouth should be taken as an indication of possible depletion of the immune system. It is seen most commonly in frail elderly people, diabetics and people with HIV infection.

The medical treatment of thrush is by means of antifungal drugs in the form of drops or of lozenges to suck. Nystatin and amphotericin are the two most common preparations.

Leukoplakia

'Leukoplakia' literally means 'white plaques', and appears as a dense, painless immovable white area on the side of the tongue or inside of the mouth.

Information Box 3.1c-III

Oral thrush: comments from a Chinese medicine perspective

In Chinese medicine, thrush would be viewed as a sign of internal Damp or Damp Heat. Nystatin and amphotericin appear to clear Damp. Their action is likely to be suppressive in nature, dealing as they do with only the outward expression of a deeper internal weakness.

Leukoplakia is important as it may reflect early cancerous changes. It is more common in smokers and those who drink alcohol in excess. A patient with leukoplakia should be referred, because an early diagnosis of cancer of the tongue can be life-saving.

Information Box 3.1c-IV

Leukoplakia: comments from a Chinese medicine perspective

In Chinese medicine, the signs and symptoms of leukoplakia would normally represent Damp Cold or Phlegm.

Gingivitis

'Gingivitis' literally means 'inflammation of the gums', and is the common condition that causes bleeding of the gums on brushing. Gingivitis is due to inflammation of the gum in contact with plaque on the teeth, and is encouraged by poor dental hygiene. Gingivitis results from an overgrowth of 'healthy bacteria', which normally reside harmlessly in the mouth. It is very common in pregnancy and is more common in smokers.

Occasionally, gingivitis will flare up to lead to an acutely painful ulcerated gum and tenderness in the associated teeth. This is a common reason for an 'urgent' visit to the dentist. The treatment of this condition which may or may not involve a collection of pus around the roots of tooth (dental abscess) is a 3–7 day course of an antibiotic (usually metronidazole or amoxicilin) and antiseptic mouthwashes. This acute form of severe gingivitis is much more common in smokers. The conventional explanation for the vulnerability to gum disease in smokers is that the toxins in smoke impair the natural immune barriers to infection in the mouth (the mucosa and saliva).

Information Box 3.1c-V

Gingivitis: comments from a Chinese medicine perspective

In Chinese medicine, the signs and symptoms of gingivitis would be described as Heat in the Stomach. Antibiotics in this case are therefore, Cooling in their action.

Salivary gland infections (sialadenitis)

There are three pairs of major salivary glands (see Chapter 3.1a). The parotid glands hug the posterior border of the masseter muscle on the face, the submandibular glands sit under the inferior edge of the lower jaw bone (mandible), and the sublingual glands sit under the tongue. All are exocrine glands and release their secretions via ducts into the mouth cavity.

These glands can become inflamed as a result of infection. The mumps virus is probably the most common cause of this in otherwise healthy people, although this disease is much less common since the introduction of widespread vaccination of children. The 'hamster face' seen in children with mumps is due to inflammation and swelling of the parotid glands.

Bacteria can cause infections in the salivary glands, although this should be seen, like thrush, as a sign of immune depletion. Underlying causes can include dehydration, alcoholism and diabetes. The symptoms include tender painful swollen salivary glands and fever. Eating, which causes salivation, is painful. The cause is an overgrowth of 'healthy' oral bacteria.

Information Box 3.1c-VI

Salivary gland infection: comments from a Chinese medicine perspective

In Chinese medicine, swelling of glands from infection commonly reflects Damp Heat. Salivary gland infections might reflect Damp Heat on a background of Stomach Yin deficiency.

In Chinese medicine, the rapid development of the symptoms of mumps is consistent with an invasion of Wind Heat.

Salivary gland stones

A 'stone' (calculus) forms in a salivary gland when secretions dry up and accumulate to form a hard solid mass. If a stone develops it may periodically block the flow of saliva, most commonly in a single parotid gland. The patient might complain of pain and swelling of the cheek after eating, and may be more at risk of bacterial infections of the salivary glands.

Salivary gland stones that cause persistent problems can be removed by means of a minor surgical procedure.

Information Box 3.1c-VII

Salivary gland stones: comments from a Chinese medicine perspective

In Chinese medicine, the drying of secretions to form a mass suggests Phlegm. Salivary gland stones could be seen as a manifestation of Phlegm in the Stomach on a background of Stomach Yin Deficiency.

Salivary gland tumours

Tumours of the salivary glands are not uncommon. They are most frequently found in the parotid glands of elderly people. They usually give rise to a firm, irregular painless swelling of one cheek. 85% of these tumours are benign and can be removed by surgery. Features that suggest a malignant tumour include rapid irregular growth, lymph-node involvement and weakness of the muscles of the mouth on the same side as the swelling (a result of cancerous infiltration of the facial nerve) (see Q3.1c-2).

Information Box 3.1c-VIII

Salivary gland tumours: comments from a Chinese medicine perspective

The Chinese medicine interpretation of these tumours might be Phlegm and/or Blood Stagnation in the Stomach on a background of severe depletion; possibly Stomach and Kidney Yin Deficiency.

The red flags of diseases of the mouth

Some patients with diseases of the mouth will benefit from referral to a conventional doctor for assessment and/or treatment. Red flags are those symptoms and signs that indicate that referral is to be considered. The red flags of the diseases of the mouth are described in Table 3.1c-I. This table forms part of the summary on red flags given in Appendix III, which also gives advice on the degree of urgency of referral for each of the red flag conditions listed.

Important diseases of the oesophagus

Hiatus hernia and gastro-oesophageal reflux disease (GORD)

The hiatus is the medical name for the gap in the diaphragm through which the oesophagus passes to meet the stomach. The cardiac sphincter of the stomach is situated at the hiatus of the diaphragm.

'Hernia' is the medical term used to describe the movement of an internal organ outside its usual anatomical position through an area of weakness of the surrounding supportive tissue. A hiatus hernia is, therefore, a condition in which part of the stomach has moved upwards through the hiatus so that it sits in the cavity above the diaphragm. This means that the cardiac sphincter has been stretched to permit the stomach to move upwards.

A hiatus hernia is in itself a very common occurrence, and is known to be present in about one-third of people aged over 50 years. In most cases a hiatus hernia is a consequence of a western sedentary lifestyle. In such cases, long-term obesity

Table 3.1c-I Red Flags 4 – diseases of the mouth

Red Flag	Description	Reasoning
4.1	**Persistent oral thrush (candidiasis)** (appearing as a thick, white coating on the tongue or palate)	Although common in the newborn, oral thrush in children and adults is not a normal finding, and merits referral to exclude an underlying cause. Common causes include corticosteroid use (including asthma inhalers), diabetes, immunodeficiency (including HIV/AIDS) and cancer. Dentures in elderly people can also predispose to oral thrush
4.2	**Persistent painless white plaque (leukoplakia)** (appearing as a coat that appears to sit on the surface of the sides of the tongue)	Leukoplakia is a precancerous change that signifies an increased risk of mouth cancer. It is more common in smokers and in those with a high alcohol intake. A particular form of leukoplakia is also associated with HIV/AIDS Early treatment of leukoplakia can prevent invasive mouth cancer, so referral is merited
4.3	**Painless enlargement of a salivary gland** over weeks to months	This needs referral to exclude salivary gland cancer, which is most common in people over the age of 60 years
4.4	**Painful or painless enlargement of a salivary gland** immediately after eating	This suggests a salivary gland stone or obstruction from dried secretions. Early treatment is to maximise hydration by encouraging drinking, and to encourage salivation (e.g. with lemon juice). If the problem is persistent, referral is recommended, as surgical removal of the stone may be necessary
4.5	**Tender or inflamed gums or salivary glands** which do not respond within days to your treatment	May be accompanied by fever or malaise. These symptoms suggest dental abscess or infection of a salivary gland, and if they persist indicate a need for referral for antibiotic treatment to prevent inflammatory damage to the dental roots or salivary glands
4.6	**Ulceration of the mouth** if persistent (for more than one week) or if preventing proper hydration	The most common cause of painful ulceration of the mouth is herpes simplex. This can be so severe as to inhibit drinking in a child. If this is the case, the child may need to be hospitalised for rehydration If ulceration persists for over 2 weeks this might suggest an underlying inflammatory condition (e.g. Crohn's disease) or mouth cancer, which will require further investigation Rarely, severe mouth ulceration can be the first sign of bone marrow failure (see Red Flags A1, in Appenix III), and in this case results from a very low white blood cell count

or habitual straining to open the bowels gives rise to years of increased pressure below the diaphragm. This puts strain on the muscles of the diaphragm that form the cardiac sphincter at the top of the stomach. Gradually, this sphincter is stretched and the top of the stomach is pushed up above the diaphragm. The tight sphincter is then no longer there to prevent stomach contents from 'refluxing' back up into the bottom end of the oesophagus.

It should be easy to understand how pregnancy may cause a temporary hiatus hernia, as the enlarging uterus pushes the abdominal contents up against the diaphragm. This physical effect is compounded by the fact that the hormone of pregnancy, progesterone, exerts a softening and relaxing effect on muscles and ligaments, and likewise affects the cardiac sphincter.

Even if a hiatus hernia is not physically manifest, the function of the cardiac sphincter in containing the stomach contents may be relatively weak. The incompetence of a weak sphincter has the same effect as a hiatus hernia in allowing upwards reflux of the stomach contents. Reflux of acid above the level of the cardiac sphincter can lead to a cluster of symptoms collectively known as 'gastro-oesophageal reflux disease' (GORD) (see Q3.1c-3).

The most important symptom of a hiatus hernia or incompetent cardiac sphincter is heartburn. This is a sensation that ranges from mild burning to intense crushing pain felt in the area of the epigastrium. The pain or burning may also be experienced rising up the sternum from this site towards the middle of the chest, and may even lead to discomfort in the throat area.

Heartburn is a result of the acidic stomach contents passing through the overly lax cardiac sphincter and then irritating the lining of the oesophagus. If prolonged, the lining of the oesophagus can become permanently inflamed, leading to redness, swelling and pain. This is called 'oesophagitis'.

Heartburn may be triggered by leaning forward or lying down, and by anything that makes the stomach contents more irritating, such as alcohol, spicy food, chocolate and coffee. Overeating, smoking and stress are all exacerbating factors.

The pain of heartburn can be so severe that it mimics the pain of a heart attack. Sometimes the only way to distinguish between the two is for the patient to undergo urgent hospital tests. All patients who suffer severe, crushing central chest pain should be referred to a hospital emergency department as a matter of urgency.

Another common unpleasant symptom is for the patient to belch acid fluid into the mouth. This is known as 'waterbrash'.

It has also been increasingly recognised that reflux of tiny amounts of acid, particularly at night, may irritate the vocal cords and respiratory pathways, and result in hoarseness, chronic cough and asthma. These symptoms may develop in the absence of significant heartburn.

In terms of treatment of the symptoms of hiatus hernia and reflux, the best treatment approach is prevention. Loss of weight, treatment of constipation and dietary moderation can reverse the problem entirely in some people. Cutting down on smoking, hot foods and alcohol can markedly reduce symptoms. Simple advice, such as raising the head of the bed, can help night-time symptoms.

Antacid medication (to reduce the acidity of the stomach) is commonly prescribed, and this includes the proton-pump inhibitor group of medications such as omeprazole and the alginates. Alginates may also be prescribed in cases of unexplained hoarseness, chronic cough and asthma to deal with the possibility that acid reflux may be the cause of the condition. Alginates are currently considered to be superior to proton-pump inhibitors in these situations. Both these types of preparation are described in more detail in relation to the treatment of stomach and duodenal ulcers.

Drugs that promote the downward movement of peristalsis can also help in GORD. These include, metoclopramide and cisapride.

In severe cases, surgery to tighten the hiatus can be performed.

Information Box 3.1c-IX

Hiatus hernia and GORD: comments from a Chinese medicine perspective

In Chinese medicine, a hiatus hernia and GORD could be seen as the result of a long-term deficiency of the holding power of Spleen Qi. The rising burning sensation and acid in the mouth could be attributed to Heat in the Stomach, with Stomach Qi rebelling upwards. Intense pain would suggest additional Blood Stagnation, possibly a result of the Heat.

Most drug treatments for reflux reduce the intensity of the acidity. In this way they are energetically Cooling. However, none of them address the root cause of the problem, and therefore they are suppressive in action.

The treatments to enhance peristalsis appear to promote the descent of Stomach Qi and move Stagnation.

Oesophagitis and oesophageal stricture

If the oesophagus becomes very inflamed by refluxed stomach contents, the pain that results locates behind the sternum and can be intense and crushing in nature. This condition is called ‘oesophagitis’. Long-term inflammation of any body part may lead to scarring. Scarring resulting from oesophagitis can lead to narrowing of the width of the lumen (stricture). This is most common in elderly people.

A stricture can lead to a sensation of difficulty in swallowing, known as ‘dysphagia’. The term dysphagia comes from the Greek for ‘difficulty in eating’. (Note that this is different to the term ‘dysphasia’, which comes from the Greek for ‘difficulty in speaking’. Dysphasia describes any problem in producing clear speech. These terms are commonly confused with each other, but mean very different things.)

Dysphagia can have a range of causes, but the characteristic that suggests a problem of a physical blockage is that solid foods are much harder to swallow than liquids. A patient with a stricture might locate the problem low down under the sternum.

A stricture is treated by surgery to stretch the scarred area.

Information Box 3.1c-X

Oesophageal stricture: comments from a Chinese medicine perspective

In Chinese medicine, the symptoms of a stricture could be attributed to Liver Qi Stagnation, giving rise to Qi Phlegm (‘plumstone in the throat’), although if a stricture were to lead to weight loss and malaise then additional more severe imbalances would also be part of the diagnostic picture.

Oesophageal cancer

Oesophageal cancer most commonly develops in the lower two-thirds of the oesophagus and is usually seen in people 55–70 years. In many cases, cancer of the oesophagus has been preceded by long-term acid reflux and oesophagitis, as cancerous change is another complication of chronic inflammation. As well as reflux, obesity, heavy alcohol intake and smoking increase the risk of this fairly common cancer.

The first symptom is almost always dysphagia for solids, which becomes increasingly worse over a period of weeks to months. This symptom means that the cancer is quite advanced. By the time of diagnosis about half of all patients have cancerous spread to their lymph nodes.

The main treatment for early disease is surgical removal of a length of the affected oesophagus. This is a major operation and is only offered to those without lymph-node spread. Overall, nine out of ten patients with this cancer will have died of the disease within 5 years of diagnosis.

Palliative treatment involves the passage of a firm tube into the blocked oesophagus to permit swallowing to continue. This can relieve the distressing dysphagia in terminally ill patients. In selected patients chemotherapy might be offered to help control symptoms.

Information Box 3.1c-XI

Oesophageal cancer: comments from a Chinese medicine perspective

The Chinese medicine interpretation of cancer is Phlegm and/or Qi and Blood Stagnation on a long-term background of depletion of Yin or Yang. In the case of oesophageal cancer, the long-term depletion is likely to be of Stomach and Spleen Yin, with a resulting build up of Heat and Liver Qi Stagnation.

Globus hystericus

This Latin term means 'imagined lump', and is the name used for the common functional symptom described by the ancient Chinese as 'plumstone in the throat'. There is a sensation of a blockage, often at the level of the voice box, and a perception of difficulty in swallowing. Globus hystericus is often seen as an emotional problem in conventional medicine, although it is increasingly recognised as a symptom of gastro-oesophageal reflux disease (GORD).

The key difference between the dysphagia in this condition and between that due to physical obstruction is that the difficulty usually affects liquids and solids equally, and the discomfort is present even when not swallowing. There will be no associated weight loss in globus hystericus.

The main medical treatment for globus hystericus is explanation and reassurance. If GORD is suspected, then alginates or proton pump inhibitors such as omeprazole may be prescribed (see Q3.1c-4).

Information Box 3.1c-XII

Globus hystericus: comments from a Chinese medicine perspective

In Chinese medicine, the symptoms of globus hystericus may readily be attributed to Stagnation of Liver Qi.

Red flags of the diseases of the oesophagus

Some patients with diseases of the oesophagus will benefit from referral to a conventional doctor for assessment and/or treatment. Red flags are those symptoms and signs that indicate that referral is to be considered. The red flags of the diseases of the oesophagus are described in Table 3.1c-II. This table forms part of the summary on red flags given in Appendix III, which also gives advice on the degree of urgency of referral for each of the red flag conditions listed.

Important diseases of the stomach and duodenum

Gastroenteritis

The term 'gastroenteritis' literally means 'inflammation of the stomach and intestines'. In practice, this description is given to infections of the digestive tract that lead to symptoms which include nausea, vomiting, diarrhoea, blood in the stools and abdominal pain. The inflammation of the digestive lining prevents absorption of fluid, and excess fluid in the bowel is what leads to the diarrhoea and vomiting.

A common serious consequence of gastroenteritis is dehydration, which can be life-threatening, particularly in vulnerable individuals such as infants and frail elderly people. The symptoms of early dehydration are dry mouth, and sparse and concentrated urine. Later on the patient may feel faint and confused, the eyes appear sunken, and the skin lacks its usual bouncy quality and will appear dry. In infants, the fontanelle, which is the 'soft spot' in the skull, sinks inwards, and the child becomes floppy and listless. This state can develop alarmingly quickly in vulnerable individuals, and there is a risk of kidney failure. The treatment is urgent administration of fluids, and by intravenous drip if fluids cannot be tolerated by mouth.

Most causes of gastroenteritis in the UK are due to a virus or bacterial infection. Protozoa such as amoeba and *Giardia* are additional causes of cases contracted overseas. Many cases are 'caught' from contact with another person who is excreting the infectious agent in their stools. Contaminated food causes the form of gastroenteritis commonly referred to as 'food poisoning'. Water can also be a source of infection, but this is rare in the UK. Food poisoning is a notifiable disease in the UK, so patients should be advised to report any suspected case to their GP.

Escherichia coli and *Salmonella*, *Cholera*, *Campylobacter* and *Giardia* species are some of the bacterial organisms that can cause gastroenteritis. Norovirus (Norwalk virus) and

Table 3.1c-II Red Flags 5 – diseases of the oesophagus

Red Flag	Description	Reasoning
5.1	**Difficulty swallowing (dysphagia) which is worse with solids** (in particular if progressive over days to weeks)	A sensation of difficultly in swallowing or a lump in the throat is a common and often benign symptom that may fluctuate with emotional stress (in this case known as 'globus hystericus'). Usually swallowing of food is still possible with this form of dysphagia However, if there is a physical obstruction in the oesophagus, which may be the result of cancer or stricture (scarring), then there may be progressive difficulty in swallowing stiff foods, and this will be accompanied by weight loss. This needs prompt referral
5.2	**Difficulty swallowing (dysphagia) associated with enlarged lymph nodes in the neck**	See the notes above. Dysphagia associated with enlarged lymph nodes raises the possibility of a malignant or inflammatory cause, and merits referral
5.3	**Swallowing associated with central chest pain (behind the sternum)**	Swallowing associated with a delayed pain behind the sternum suggests oesophagitis or structural damage to the oesophagus (e.g. a tear or puncture by a fishbone). Refer if the condition is not settling within 24 hours, or sooner if pain is severe

rotavirus are the most common viral causes, and these often become apparent in winter epidemics.

The best treatment is prevention. In addition to provision of clean water and efficient sanitation, personal hygiene practice such as scrupulous hand-washing after going to the toilet is important to minimise spread of infectious viruses and bacteria. This is of particular importance in food handlers.

As bacteria are commonly found on raw meat and in raw eggs, insufficient cooking can lead to contaminated food. Contaminated food left at room temperature is even more risky, as this provides ideal conditions for bacteria to multiply. Any food that has been in contact with raw meat or eggs (such as might occur when using a common chopping board) should also be treated as contaminated.

In established infections, the best treatment is to avoid eating and drink plenty of fluids, and allow the infection to take its course. In healthy people most cases, although unpleasant, get better on their own in 2–5 days. Even alarming symptoms such as blood in the stools should settle down naturally.

Doctors might prescribe a sugar and salt preparation known as 'oral rehydration therapy' or ORT to dissolve in water. This replaces mineral salts that are lost through vomiting and diarrhoea.

Antibiotics are usually used only in those cases in which the symptoms are not settling within a few days. It is not considered good practice to prescribe antibiotics in simple cases of gastroenteritis.

Frail patients with dehydration and anyone with severe dehydration should be nursed in hospital.

Antibiotic use can induce a form of gastroenteritis, partly as a result of reducing the 'healthy' commensal bacteria of the bowel. In most cases this gives rise to mild self-limiting diarrhoea, and recovery may be aided by supplementing the diet with live yoghurt (to restore the balance of healthy bacteria). In vulnerable people, and particularly in a hospital setting where this infection is more likely to be contracted, the bacterium *Clostridium difficile* can take hold in the digestive system. This can lead to a potentially devastating form of gastroenteritis. The treatment for this antibiotic-induced infection is administration of even more powerful antibiotics. This treatment is problematic, as antibiotic resistance is increasingly prevalent.

Information Box 3.1c-XIII

Gastroenteritis: comments from a Chinese medicine perspective

A Chinese medicine interpretation of gastroenteritis would vary according to the symptom picture. Diarrhoea and blood suggest Damp Heat in the Intestines, whereas the other symptoms of nausea, vomiting and cramps suggest Liver Qi Stagnation invading the Stomach and Spleen. Dehydration could be described as Stomach Yin Deficiency leading to Kidney Yin Deficiency.

Dyspepsia, gastritis and peptic ulcers

'Indigestion' is a commonly used term that may be applied to the symptoms of any one of the three conditions of dyspepsia, gastritis and peptic ulcer. Together these conditions account for one of the heaviest cost burdens on the UK National Health Service budget resulting from prescribed medication for a single disease group. This is because most people will have at some point experienced 'indigestion', and many will seek prescribed medication for their symptoms (see Q3.1c-5).

Dyspepsia, like dysphagia, is a symptom and not a disease. The term, which is derived from the Greek meaning 'bad digestion', is used to describe any discomfort arising from the process of digestion in the stomach. The common equivalent of this term is 'indigestion', although this word is notorious amongst doctors for being used by patients to describe any sort of discomfort from the chest to the groin. It is important that practitioners obtain a precise description of symptoms from their patients rather than simply accepting a complaint of 'indigestion' to be the same as their own understanding of the term.

Typically, dyspepsia involves discomfort in the epigastric region, which often has a burning or gripy quality. It is usually related to eating, being triggered either by hot, spicy foods, alcohol and caffeine, or by leaving too long a space between meals. The symptoms of dyspepsia and heartburn can overlap.

Gastritis is inflammation of the stomach lining. The lining becomes reddened and thickened, and may bleed in places. It can only be definitely diagnosed by using an endoscope. The symptoms are of a mild to severe dyspepsia. Gastritis can be caused by overeating, spicy foods, alcohol and caffeine. Aspirin, and the painkillers known as 'non-steroidal anti-inflammatory drugs' (e.g. ibuprofen or diclofenac) are known to cause slight gastritis in most people who take them. In some people this can become a severe situation.

Stress is a known cause of inflammation of the stomach lining. A shock resulting from a car accident or a surgical operation can cause sufficient stress to lead to an acute flare up of gastritis.

Mild gastritis may have no symptoms or may give rise to dyspepsia. Severe gastritis may lead to epigastric pain and vomiting, and, at worst, bleeding into the stomach. The patient may vomit blood, which appears like black gravel (due to the action of the stomach acid on the blood), or may pass altered blood in stools, which then look like black tar. A severe haemorrhage can be life-threatening and so is a medical emergency.

It is now known that many people who suffer with gastritis have the *Helicobacter pylori* bacterium in their stomach. This is an initially silent infection, which is contracted in early adult life and which in some people gives rise to long-term inflammation of the stomach. In fact, over 60% of the population may be carrying this organism, many of whom contracted it during childhood, but not all of these will develop symptoms.

The presence of *H. pylori* can be diagnosed by means of a breath test in which the patient blows a breath sample after drinking a formulated drink. Alternatively, it can be diagnosed by means of faeces analysis or by a blood test which looks for antibodies to the bacterium. It is now considered good practice to aim to eradicate *H. pylori* by means of a short-term course of two high-dose antibiotics combined with a proton-pump inhibitor ('triple therapy'), because chronic infection with this bacterium is associated with an increased risk of stomach cancer.

'Peptic ulcer' is the term used to describe a breakdown of the mucosal lining of either the stomach or the duodenum. The terms 'gastric ulcer' and 'duodenal ulcer' are used to describe the site of the peptic ulcer.

Peptic ulcer disease (PUD) can be seen as a progression of gastritis or inflammation of the duodenum (duodenitis). The causation of a peptic ulcer is generally the same as that for gastritis, and it tends to run in families. The *H. pylori* bacterium is strongly linked to PUD.

Gastric and duodenal ulcers tend to have slightly different characteristics in terms of causation and symptoms, but in practice are often difficult to distinguish without performing an endoscopy.

Dyspepsia is the main symptom of peptic ulcer, and often pain is present. The patient may describe a gnawing hunger pain, but sometimes the pain can be intense and stabbing. Often the patient can point to a particular site in the epigastrium where they locate the pain. This 'pointing sign' is believed to be highly suggestive of an ulcer. If the ulcer is on the posterior wall of the stomach or the duodenum, the pain may also be felt in the mid-back.

A gastric ulcer is more likely to lead to nausea and loss of appetite. Eating makes the symptoms worse, so the patient may lose weight. It is less common than duodenal ulcer.

A duodenal ulcer is more likely to lead to hunger pains, and certain foods such as milk may relieve the discomfort. The pain is worse when the duodenum is empty, and it may therefore occur at night. The patient may put on weight. Duodenal ulcer is common. It is estimated that about 15% of the population may suffer from a duodenal ulcer at some point in their lives.

Many peptic ulcers will heal spontaneously, like mouth ulcers, although there may well be a recurrence when the person is exposed to a trigger such as overeating, an alcohol binge or stress. Some ulcers become 'chronic', meaning that the patient suffers from long-term digestive discomfort and recurrent pain. The two serious, but rare, complications are haemorrhage and perforation.

Haemorrhage results from stomach acid eroding the exposed area of stomach lining and damaging the blood vessels in the deeper layers. A slight, but persistent, haemorrhage can lead to loss of iron and the development of anaemia. The blood loss might not be noticed by the patient, as it can be hidden in the stools. However, a severe haemorrhage can be life-threatening and can lead to shock (for more explanation of the syndrome of shock see Chapter 3.4d).

Perforation means that the full thickness of the stomach wall has been breached so that the stomach contents leak out into the surrounding peritoneal cavity. This situation leads to acute abdominal pain resulting from an inflammation of the peritoneum (peritonitis). This is almost invariably fatal unless treated as a surgical emergency. The symptoms are those of the 'acute abdomen'. This important syndrome is described in detail in Chapter 3.1d.

Dyspepsia, gastritis and peptic ulcer disease should all respond dramatically to lifestyle changes, and these are similar to those recommended for gastro-oesophageal reflux disease. However, many western patients find these changes hard to make.

Nowadays, the main treatment of these conditions is by means of drugs rather than surgery. All the drugs used can also be used to treat oesophageal reflux.

Self-medication with antacids is extremely common. Drugs such as Rennie and Remegel counteract the acid in the stomach and can relieve the burning discomfort of dyspepsia and heartburn. There is now a very wide range of antacid medications that can be bought by patients over the counter at a pharmacy. As a result of powerful advertising, many of these brands are household names. Patients may even forget that these are medications, and this is worth bearing in mind when taking a medication history to ask specifically about antacid use.

The UK National Institute of Health and Clinical Excellence (NICE) guideline on dyspepsia suggests that, in most cases, medical treatment can be instituted without the need for diagnostic endoscopy. The exceptions are those cases in which there might be alarm symptoms of progressive disease (cancer) or of imminent or ongoing bleeding or perforation. These alarm symptoms include new onset of symptoms after the age of 55 years, weight loss, unexplained iron-deficiency anaemia and severe pain.

If there are no alarm symptoms, the recommended medical approach is first to test for *H. pylori* infection, and if this is present to treat the infection with triple therapy. This might be sufficient to resolve the symptoms. If *H. pylori* infection is not present, then the patient may be prescribed a proton-pump inhibitor (such as omeprazole). These drugs prevent the formation of gastric acid by the parietal cells in the stomach lining. In the majority of patients one of these two medical approaches will resolve the symptoms. The H_2 blockers (e.g. ranitidine or cimetidine) are a less commonly prescribed alternative to the proton-pump inhibitors. These also reduce gastric acid secretion, but seem to be less effective than the proton-pump inhibitors. Because of recurrence of symptoms on withdrawal from H_2 blockers or proton-pump inhibitors, some patients remain on a regular dose of these drugs for months to years. It is now recognised that withdrawal from these medications results in a temporary state of excessive acid production, which means that it is all the more likely that a patient will be reluctant to withdraw from them.

Even in the case of haemorrhage, most bleeding peptic ulcers respond to drug treatment alone. It is only in rare cases that patients who suffer from either a severe haemorrhage or a perforation will require emergency surgery.

Pyloric stenosis

Pyloric stenosis is a condition in which there is a stricture of the outflow of the stomach, the pyloric sphincter. In adults, just as in oesophageal stricture, the cause is usually scarring following the inflammation of an ulcer or gastritis. Occasionally, cancer is a cause.

The main symptom of pyloric stenosis is vomiting without pain. Often the vomiting is forceful or 'projectile'. The patient can rapidly develop dehydration.

Information Box 3.1c-XIV

Peptic ulcer: comments from a Chinese medicine perspective

In Chinese medicine, the symptoms of dyspepsia, gastritis and peptic ulcer disease would be classified as manifestations of Stomach Heat (Fire) on a background of Stomach Yin Deficiency. The pain of an ulcer signifies Liver Qi invading the Stomach and/or Stagnation of Blood in the Stomach.

The antacids and anti-ulcer drugs are Cooling. They do not cure the underlying condition, and therefore are suppressive. Anti-ulcer drugs are powerful in their action and have many possible side-effects, which include gastrointestinal and liver disturbance. This implies that they tend to deplete the Spleen Qi and Stagnate Liver Qi.

Antibiotic treatment has a more long-term effect. The clearance of *H. pylori* suggests that this treatment can actually clear the Heat pathogen from the stomach. The antibiotics themselves are energetically Cold and Damp, and so side-effects such as thrush and loose stools may occur.

Pyloric stenosis can be an inherited condition, in which case it becomes apparent in the first few weeks of life. The newborn infant will also develop projectile vomiting and is at great risk of dehydration.

The only treatment for this congenital condition is surgery.

Stomach cancer (gastric carcinoma)

Stomach cancer is a common form of cancer in the west. It now seems to be strongly linked with *H. pylori* infection, presumably as a result of the long-term inflammation that this infection causes. It is also believed that components of the western diet (e.g. salt and nitrates, and nitrosamines from overcooked meat) may also increase the risk of cancer.

The main symptoms of stomach cancer are pain and dyspepsia. As the cancer may have developed in someone who had tended to experience indigestion for years, the early symptoms may be ignored. For this reason stomach cancer is often diagnosed late, with up to 30% of people having metastases (usually in the liver) at the time of diagnosis. If pain and dyspepsia develop for the first time in someone over the age of 55 years it is reasonable to consider referral for investigations to exclude stomach cancer.

A minority of patients with stomach cancer have a small enough tumour for it to be totally removed with surgery, but in most cases the cancer is inoperable. For these patients chemotherapy may be offered, to prolong life but not to cure.

Information Box 3.1c-XV

Stomach cancer: comments from a Chinese medicine perspective

In Chinese medicine, cancer is understood to be the result of either Phlegm and/or Blood Stagnation. These together account for the mass and the pain. These effects often develop on a background of long-term depletion of Stomach Qi or Yin.

Only one in ten of people diagnosed with stomach cancer will be alive 5 years after diagnosis.

Pernicious anaemia

This is a type of anaemia that results from an inability to absorb vitamin B_{12} from the diet. Before it can be absorbed from the small intestine, vitamin B_{12} needs to be linked with a bodily-produced substance called 'intrinsic factor' (see Chapter 3.1a). Intrinsic factor is manufactured by cells in the stomach lining. In pernicious anaemia these cells are progressively destroyed by an autoimmune process, and the person is no longer able to absorb vitamin B_{12}.

Vitamin B_{12} is necessary for the healthy formation of red blood cells, and also for the functioning of the nervous system. Therefore, in untreated pernicious anaemia the patient gradually develops anaemia and eventually a severe form of irreversible disease that leads to paralysis and dementia.

This autoimmune condition is not uncommon in elderly women, affecting about 1 in 8,000 of the population over the age of 60 years. It used to be fatal, hence the term 'pernicious'. Nowadays, if the condition is diagnosed and treated early with regular vitamin B_{12} injections, the symptoms disappear totally.

Pernicious anaemia is associated with other autoimmune conditions such as thyroid disease, Addison's disease and vitiligo (patchy depigmentation of the skin), and so these conditions may coexist in the same patient (see Q3.1c-6).

Information Box 3.1c-XVI

Pernicious anaemia: comments from a Chinese medicine perspective

In Chinese medicine, the impaired digestive function in pernicious anaemia, in which there is insufficient production of gastric acid, sore mouth and lemon yellow skin coloration, might be described in terms of depletion of Stomach and Spleen Qi. Anaemia is a manifestation of Blood and Qi Deficiency. The development of the paralysis and dementia is due to malnourishment of the nervous system. These symptoms suggest that vitamin B_{12} also nourishes Kidney Essence (Jing), so untreated pernicious anaemia can lead to Jing Deficiency.

Vitamin B_{12} injections could, therefore, be seen as a replacement treatment that nourishes Blood, Qi and Jing. The treatment does not address the underlying Stomach and Spleen imbalances, but is not according to the definition made in this text suppressive, because the underlying imbalances are irreversible and supplementation brings the body to an improved state of balance.

Red flags of the diseases of the stomach

Some patients with diseases of the stomach will benefit from referral to a conventional doctor for assessment and/or treatment. Red flags are those symptoms and signs that indicate that referral is to be considered. The red flags of the diseases of the stomach are described in Table 3.1c-III. This table forms part of the summary on red flags given in Appendix III, which also gives advice on the degree of urgency of referral for each of the red flag conditions listed.

Table 3.1c-III Red Flags 6 – diseases of the stomach

Red Flag	Description	Reasoning
6.1	**Severe diarrhoea and vomiting** if lasting more than 24 hours in infants or the elderly	In most cases diarrhoea and vomiting is self-limiting and will need no medical intervention. However, infants and the elderly are vulnerable to dehydration and should be referred for assessment if symptoms continue for more than 24 hours
6.2	**Diarrhoea and vomiting** if continuing for more than 5 days in otherwise healthy adults	See the notes above. If symptoms persist for more than 5 days this is unusual and merits referral for investigation of a possible infectious or inflammatory cause Food poisoning is the consequence of eating food that is contaminated with infectious organisms, commonly a result of poor food hygiene together with insufficient cooking Food poisoning and dysentery (bloody diarrhoea resulting from *Shigella* infection) are notifiable diseases[1]
6.3	**Diarrhoea and vomiting** associated with features of dehydration (see Table 2.4c-II)	If features of dehydration: (low blood pressure, dry mouth, concentrated urine, poor skin turgor, confusion) are apparent, then refer as a matter of high priority, and urgently in infants and the elderly, as continuing vomiting will exacerbate an already unstable situation Food poisoning is the consequence of eating food that is contaminated with infectious organisms, commonly a result of poor food hygiene together with insufficient cooking Food poisoning and dysentery (bloody diarrhoea resulting from *Shigella* infection) are notifiable diseases[1]
6.4	**Vomiting of fresh blood or altered blood** (looks like dark gravel or coffee grounds)	The appearance of blood in the vomit is always of concern, as it is not possible to gauge the severity of bleeding and whether or not the internal bleeding is continuing Refer if more than about a tablespoon of blood appears in the vomit (small amounts may simply be the result of a tear of the oesophagus lining during vomiting) The blood may originate from the stomach or the duodenum, and may indicate peptic ulcer disease or stomach cancer
6.5	**Projectile vomiting** persisting for more than 2 days	Projectile vomiting (vomit appears at a higher speed than usual) suggests a high obstruction to the outflow of the stomach and should be referred as there is high risk of loss of fluids and salts. Refer straightaway if this is suspected in a baby (a sign of the congenital deformity of pyloric stenosis)
6.6	**Epigastric pain** or **dyspepsia** for the first time in someone over the age of 55 years or if resistant to treatment after 3 months	Pain from the stomach or duodenum typically radiates to the epigastric region. If the stomach is inflamed, this area can be tender on palpation and may be accompanied by a sensation of acidity or fullness (dyspepsia). However, these symptoms are very common and can respond well to dietary modification and complementary therapies. Only refer if the patient is not responding to treatment within 3 months or if the symptoms are presenting for the first time in someone over the age of 55 years (as the risk of cancer is more common in older age groups)
6.7	**Altered blood in stools (melaena).** Stools look like black tar	Altered blood in stools (stools look tarry and have an unusual metallic smell) indicates bleeding from the more proximal aspects of the digestive tract including the stomach. If melaena is apparent in the stools, bleeding is significant and merits prompt referral
6.8	**Onset of severe abdominal pain with collapse (acute abdomen).** The pain can be constant or colicky (coming in waves) Rigidity, guarding and rebound tenderness are serious signs	'Acute abdomen' is a term that refers to the combination of severe abdominal pain together with an inability to continue with day-to-day activities ('collapse'). This syndrome can have benign causes such as irritable bowel syndrome, dysmenorrhoea and ovulation pain Referral is necessary to exclude more serious possibilities. including appendicitis, perforated ulcer, peritonitis, obstructed bowel, pelvic inflammatory disease and gallstones Colicky pain indicates obstruction of a viscus (hollow organ) Rigidity of the abdomen, guarding (reflex protective spasm of the abdominal muscles) and rebound tenderness (pain felt elsewhere in abdomen when the pressure of the palpating hand is released) all suggest inflammation or perforation of a viscus

[1]Notifiable diseases: notification of a number of specified infectious diseases is required of doctors in the UK as a statutory duty under the Public Health (Infectious Diseases) 1988 Act and the Public Health (Control of Diseases) 1988 Act. The UK Health Protection Agency (HPA) Centre for Infections collates details of each case of each disease that has been notified. This allows analyses of local and national trends. This is one example of a situation in which there is a legal requirement for a doctor to breach patient confidentiality.
Diseases that are notifiable include: acute encephalitis, acute poliomyelitis, anthrax, cholera, diphtheria, dysentery, food poisoning, leptospirosis, malaria, measles, meningitis (bacterial and viral forms), meningococcal septicaemia (without meningitis), mumps, ophthalmia neonatorum, paratyphoid fever, plague, rabies, relapsing fever, rubella, scarlet fever, smallpox, tetanus, tuberculosis, typhoid fever, typhus fever, viral haemorrhagic fever, viral hepatitis (including hepatitis A, B and C), whooping cough, yellow fever.

Self-test 3.1c

Diseases of the mouth, oesophagus, stomach and duodenum

1. On examining the tongue of an elderly patient, you notice a thickened white area along one side that seems very much part of the tongue tissue. What condition might your patient have and how would you manage this situation?
2. A patient of yours, a 45-year-old businessman, explains that he has been taking Gaviscon (alginate) tablets from the chemist for years, but has just found that Zantac (ranitidine) tablets, although expensive, keep his heartburn totally at bay. How might you discuss his situation with him?
3. Another elderly patient of yours has not been well for some weeks. He tells you that his digestion has not been right, and he has lost over a stone in weight. Recently, he has had some pain in the upper abdomen, and for the last 2 days has been vomiting so powerfully that he did not have time to get to the toilet. What conditions do you suspect, and how might you manage this situation?

Answer

1. Your patient might have the precancerous condition, leukoplakia. The best response is to refer your patient to his GP with a letter explaining that you suspect the diagnosis of leukoplakia and you would be grateful for his opinion.
2. The issue here is that your patient has been taking suppressive medication for symptoms that might well respond to a combination of a change in lifestyle and complementary medicine. How you deal with this depends on the rapport you have with the patient. Ideally, you can explain why suppressive treatment is undesirable, and that reduction in weight, alcohol intake, smoking, hot foods and stressful eating patterns, together with acupuncture and herbs, may well reduce the symptoms.
   Note that, in this case, 'heartburn' is your patient's description, and the cause of this symptom may actually be oesophageal reflux, gastritis or peptic ulcer. The exact diagnosis does not matter to you, as the management should be the same. He has no red-flag symptoms or signs at this stage so there is no need to refer.
3. The history of progressive symptoms is suggestive of stomach cancer. The recent vomiting may indicate pyloric stenosis (outflow obstruction) due to tumour. In this case it is not important for you to know the precise diagnosis; what you should be clear about is that this patient needs a high priority referral to his GP. It might be easier to try to speak to the GP on the phone about this patient rather than communicate by letter.

Chapter 3.1d Diseases of the pancreas, liver and gallbladder

LEARNING POINTS

At the end of this chapter you will be:
- able to name the main features of the most important diseases of the accessory organs of the gastrointestinal tract
- able to recognise the features of the acute abdomen
- able to understand the principles of treatment of a few of the most common diseases
- recognise the red flags of serious diseases of the pancreas, liver and gallbladder.

Estimated time for chapter: 90 minutes.

Introduction

This chapter focuses on the important diseases of the main accessory organs of the gastrointestinal tract: the pancreas, liver and gallbladder. These are:

- Diseases of the pancreas:
  - acute pancreatitis
  - chronic pancreatitis
  - cancer of the pancreas
  - (cystic fibrosis, studied in Section 3.3)
  - (diabetes mellitus, studied in Section 5.1).
- Diseases of the liver:
  - acute hepatitis
  - chronic hepatitis
  - cancer of the liver
  - cirrhosis of the liver
  - primary biliary cirrhosis.
- Diseases of the gallbladder:
  - gallstones
  - acute cholecystitis
  - chronic cholecystitis.

Before the individual diseases are described in turn, it is important to first introduce a syndrome (i.e. a condition with a characteristic constellation of symptoms and signs) that can result from a number of severe intra-abdominal diseases, the 'acute abdomen' (see Q3.1d-1).

The acute abdomen

The 'acute abdomen' is the general term used to describe a syndrome in which a patient becomes acutely ill and has symptoms and signs that are related to the abdomen. It can be caused by severe disease of any of the abdominal organs. The patient characteristically has severe abdominal pain, which has come on rapidly, and may be unable to move easily because of pain. The pain may be constant or intermittent. The syndrome is important as it is a common reason for an urgent admission to a hospital emergency department.

Not all diseases that cause an acute abdomen are serious (e.g. constipation and ovulation pain can occasionally lead to this syndrome), but if it occurs it should be taken seriously as it can be the result of one of a few life-threatening conditions.

Any patient with this syndrome is usually assessed in a hospital emergency department by a surgeon, who will make an examination and perform tests to exclude any serious causes that may need urgent surgery.

Tables 3.1d-I and 3.1d-II list the important causes of the acute abdomen (note that not all the conditions are gastrointestinal). All these conditions are studied in detail in this and later chapters.

The acute abdomen has some characteristic signs that can be felt by an examining doctor. These are rigidity, guarding and rebound tenderness, which develop because a serious problem in the abdominal cavity causes the abdominal muscles and the bowel to go into spasm. The abdomen feels rock hard or 'rigid'. The patient involuntarily protects the area by further muscle tension (guarding), and pain is particularly severe when an examining hand is lifted suddenly from the skin (rebound tenderness).

Sometimes these features are found only in a localised area. For example, in womb infections pelvic inflammatory disease, rigidity, guarding and rebound tenderness are found in the suprapubic area and right and left iliac fossae only. If the features are more generalised and the pain is worst centrally, this implies a more generalised problem such as peritonitis.

If a patient is developing the features of an acute abdomen they require urgent medical assessment, or direct admission to a hospital emergency department if very unwell or frail.

Information Box 3.1d-I

The acute abdomen: comments from a Chinese medicine perspective

In Chinese medicine, the acute abdomen would be viewed as a Full Condition (aggravated by pressure), which could be attributed to a range of syndromes according to the site of pain and exact pattern of symptoms.

These include Stasis of Blood in the Stomach, Liver Qi Stagnation invading the Spleen, Small Intestine Qi Pain, Small Intestine Qi Tied, Cold in the Intestines, Damp Heat in the Liver and Gallbladder, Damp Heat in the Intestines, Heat obstructing the Large Intestine, and Blood and Qi Stagnation in the Lower Jiao. Sometimes it is difficult to distinguish between these syndromes, but this is not so important in practice as the treatment principles and points used often overlap.

Table 3.1d-I Serious causes of the acute abdomen

- **Perforation** of the stomach, small and large intestines
- **Rupture** of a major organ (e.g. spleen, or fallopian tube in ectopic pregnancy)
- **Inflammation** of an organ (e.g. pancreas, appendix, gallbladder)
- **Inflammation** of the lining of the bowel (**peritonitis**)
- **Obstruction** of the bowel
- **Stones** in the bile ducts or ureter

Table 3.1d-II Less serious causes of the acute abdomen

- Menorrhagia, ovulation pain and infections of the womb
- Inflammatory bowel disease
- Irritable bowel disease
- Constipation

The diseases of the three major accessory organs are now to be considered. For a reminder of the physiology of these organs, see Chapter 3.1a.

Important diseases of the pancreas

Acute pancreatitis

As described in Chapter 3.1a, one important function of the pancreas is to release powerful enzymes of digestion via the pancreatic duct into the duodenum. In acute pancreatitis the pancreas is inflamed, and this inflammation causes the enzymes to be released within the pancreas tissue. This leads to a vicious cycle, in which the enzymes start digesting the pancreas itself, which in turn becomes more inflamed.

The most common known causes of acute pancreatitis are acute alcohol abuse, infection by the mumps virus and blockage of the pancreatic duct by a gallstone. However, in many cases no obvious cause can be found.

The condition of acute pancreatitis is extremely severe. The inflammation of the pancreas leads to intense abdominal pain, nausea and vomiting, and fever. The pain also tends to be felt in the centre of the back.

The pancreatic enzymes can penetrate into the peritoneal cavity, which causes generalised inflammation of the peritoneum, the lining of all the organs of the gastrointestinal tract. This condition is peritonitis, which has already been introduced as a possible outcome of perforation of a peptic ulcer. Pancreatitis, therefore, is a cause of the acute abdomen syndrome.

The treatment of pancreatitis involves urgent admission to hospital. The digestive system is rested by ensuring the patient stays 'nil by mouth', and fluids are given to the patient by intravenous drip. Mild cases can respond very quickly to this treatment, and many patients achieve full recovery.

In severe cases many patients will die (the mortality from acute pancreatitis is 12%) because the damage to the important organs of the gastrointestinal tract is too great to allow recovery. In those who recover, the pancreas may be permanently damaged, leading to the condition of chronic pancreatitis.

Chronic pancreatitis

Chronic pancreatitis can result from the permanent damage resulting from an acute attack, or may develop gradually over the course of a few years. In this condition the pancreas is damaged and is unable to produce sufficient digestive enzymes (exocrine function), and in some cases may not be able to produce sufficient insulin (endocrine function).

The most common cause of chronic pancreatitis is long-term (10 years or more) high alcohol intake, but there are other rare causes, including cystic fibrosis and a congenital susceptibility.

Initially, the main symptom is abdominal pain, which can be severe and can be felt in the epigastrium and the centre of the back. Patients may need to take regular doses of very strong morphine-related painkillers. This can lead to problems with addiction.

The lack of digestive enzymes will lead to the nutrients in the diet not being adequately absorbed. Instead, they are left in the bowel to become part of the stools, which become loose and foul smelling. This state is called 'malabsorption', and the patient will lose weight and suffer from vitamin deficiencies. If insulin production is affected, diabetes may develop (see Section 5.1).

The treatment of this condition is usually supportive only. The patient is urged to stop drinking alcohol and is given drugs for the pain. Synthetic pancreatic enzymes can be taken by mouth with meals for those with malabsorption. These assist in the digestion of food. Patients with diabetes are treated with insulin to control their blood sugar level.

Occasionally, surgery to remove part of the damaged pancreas may be performed for pain relief. This is a major operation, and does not always make a great difference to the symptoms, particularly if the patient continues to drink alcohol.

> **Information Box 3.1d-II**
>
> **Pancreatitis: comments from a Chinese medicine perspective**
>
> In Chinese medicine, the intense acute symptoms of pancreatitis would correspond to syndromes that include Small Intestine Qi Tied and Stagnation of Blood in the Intestines.
>
> The chronic severe pain of pancreatitis suggests Blood Stagnation. The failure of digestion, with loose, foul-smelling stools, suggests Spleen Qi Deficiency and possibly Damp Heat invading the Spleen. This would fit with the history of alcohol abuse. Diabetes is called the 'Thirsting and Wasting Disease' and corresponds to Internal Heat leading to Yin Deficiency.
>
> Because pancreatic enzymes support the digestive process, and treat the diarrhoea resulting from malabsorption, their action in Chinese medicine could be described in terms of nourishing Spleen Qi.

Pancreatic cancer

Pancreatic cancer is usually a disease of elderly people. As the pancreas is not contained in a tight anatomical space, this means that significant growth can occur before symptoms become apparent. Common first symptoms include back and abdominal pain, as the mass extends backwards to infiltrate local tissues, or jaundice, as the mass obstructs the flow of bile into the duodenum. The backlog of bile leads to jaundice because the breakdown product of red blood cells, bilirubin, starts to build up in the bloodstream (for an explanation of the physiology, see Chapter 3.1a). Jaundice is a condition in which there is a yellow discoloration of the skin, and particularly the whites of the eyes. Bilirubin in the skin causes itch, which can be extremely distressing. Excess bilirubin in the urine turns the urine dark, whereas the lack of bile in the stools means that stools become pale. Other symptoms include loss of appetite and loss of weight. Very rarely, the first symptoms will be those of the acute abdomen, as the tumour can trigger an episode of acute pancreatitis.

The diagnosis of pancreatic cancer is a very serious one, as very few patients with this diagnosis (less than 2%) survive for more than 2 years. This is because, by the time the tumour is picked up, it has usually grown to such a size as to be inoperable. It does not respond well to chemotherapy or radiotherapy. Very rarely, a major operation can be performed on small tumours, which can improve the chances of survival.

The treatment is, therefore, usually palliative. Morphine-based painkillers are considered essential in advanced disease. As jaundice can lead to uncomfortable itch and malaise, the blocked bile duct can be unblocked by inserting a thin tube, known as a 'stent', by means of an endoscope (see Q3.1d-2).

> **Information Box 3.1d-III**
>
> **Pancreatic cancer: comments from a Chinese medicine perspective**
>
> In Chinese medicine, the type of pain associated with pancreatic cancer is usually a feature of Blood Stagnation. The growing mass suggests Phlegm. This fits with the fact that this cancer is considered more likely in those who smoke and have a high-fat diet. As always in cancer, there is an underlying severe deficiency, which in this case would most likely embrace Spleen Qi Deficiency/ Stomach Yin Deficiency.

Red flags of the diseases of the pancreas

Some patients with diseases of the pancreas will benefit from referral to a conventional doctor for assessment and/or treatment. Red flags are those symptoms and signs that indicate that referral is to be considered. The red flags of the diseases of the pancreas are described in Table 3.1d-III. This table forms part of the summary on red flags given in Appendix III, which also gives advice on the degree of urgency of referral for each of the red flag conditions listed.

Important diseases of the liver

Acute hepatitis

'Hepatitis' literally means 'inflammation of the liver', and the acute form can have a wide range of possible causes. The most well-known cause is infection by the hepatitis virus, of which

Table 3.1d-III Red Flags 7 – diseases of the pancreas

Red Flag	Description	Reasoning
7.1	**Symptoms of acute pancreatitis** (acute abdomen (see Table 3.1c-III), with severe central abdominal and back pain, vomiting and dehydration)	Pancreatitis is a serious inflammatory condition of the pancreas that may develop for no obvious reason, but can be associated with high alcohol consumption or gallstone obstruction. The patient needs to be 'nil by mouth' and urgently referred for supportive hospital care
7.2	**Symptoms of chronic pancreatitis** (central abdominal and back pain, weight loss and loose stools over weeks to months)	Chronic pancreatitis may result from long-term alcohol abuse; episodes of acute pancreatitis may be due to an inherited tendency. The scarred pancreas can generate deep chronic pain, and the lack of digestive enzymes can lead to the syndrome of malabsorption. There is a risk of diabetes
7.3	**Malabsorption syndrome** (loose pale stools and malnutrition; weight loss, thin hair, dry skin, cracked lips and peeled tongue) Will present as failure to thrive in children	The malabsorption syndrome results when there is an inability to absorb the nutrients in the diet, and weight loss and mineral and vitamin deficiencies result. Loose stools are the result of the presence of unabsorbed fat. Chronic pancreatitis is one of the causes of malabsorption syndrome
7.4	**Jaundice** (yellowish skin, yellow whites of the eyes and maybe dark urine and pale stools). Itch may be a prominent symptom	Jaundice results from a problem in the production of the bile by the liver, or an obstruction to its outflow via the gallbladder into the duodenum. Pancreatic cancer may cause jaundice by growing to obstruct the outflow of the bile via the bile duct Jaundice always merits referral for investigation of its cause

there are a number of types. Hepatitis A, B and C are the most important in terms of rates of significant infections. These viruses result in distinct disease syndromes, which will be summarised in more detail presently.

Other common causes of inflammation of the liver are other types of infectious agents, alcohol abuse and reactions to prescribed drugs. Many drugs in overdose, most famously paracetamol, can cause severe inflammation of the liver.

Hepatitis has characteristic symptoms, irrespective of the cause. The inflamed liver leads to pain situated under the right side of the ribs (right hypochondrium). The inflammation affects the ability of the liver to clear toxins and also to clear the bilirubin from the bloodstream to make bile. The consequences of this are that the patient with hepatitis feels very unwell, and the build up of bilirubin in the bloodstream leads to jaundice which is indicated by the signs of yellow skin discoloration, dark urine and pale stools.

If the inflammation is very severe, acute hepatitis can lead to acute liver failure, which is life-threatening because the essential functions of maintaining adequate blood sugar levels and clearing toxins are totally lost. A patient with acute liver failure will rapidly fall into a coma if the condition is not reversed.

Treatment of hepatitis primarily involves the removal of any factors that may be causing further liver damage (e.g. prescription drugs) and to support the patient through recovery. In the case of paracetamol overdose medication (acetylcysteine) can be given that reverses the toxic effect of the paracetamol if the patient can be treated early enough. Patients with acute liver failure will need specialised nursing, with administration of intravenous fluids and nutrients. In rare cases, liver transplantation can save the life of a patient with acute liver failure (see later in this chapter for more detail on liver transplantation).

Viral hepatitis

The three most common hepatitis viruses each lead to a form of hepatitis with characteristic features.

Hepatitis A (infectious hepatitis) is the commonest form of hepatitis worldwide, and is contracted from contaminated food and water. Jaundice develops within 2–6 weeks of initial infection, during which time the patient is infectious. In most cases, after 2–3 weeks of feeling unwell, the patient makes a recovery. Most patients feel unwell for some time after this, and may remain unable to tolerate alcohol and fatty food for many months afterwards. Acute liver failure and death are very rare complications of hepatitis A. It is only in these very severe situations that the medication interferon-alpha may be given to reduce inflammation. The hepatitis vaccine that is offered to many travellers abroad is to protect against hepatitis A. A single dose gives immunity for one year, which is increased to 10 years if a booster dose is given 6 months later.

Hepatitis B is a very different condition to hepatitis A, although it also leads to acute hepatitis. One major difference is that, even after recovery, the virus can persist in the blood of some people. These 'carriers' of hepatitis B remain in a lifelong infectious state. Infection with the virus does not necessarily lead to inflammation of the liver, and may pass unnoticed. Therefore, not all carriers will be aware that they have had hepatitis. This is in contrast to hepatitis A, in which patients are no longer infectious after recovery.

The hepatitis B virus can only be transmitted through infected body fluids such as semen or blood. In this way it is comparable to HIV infection. People at risk of contracting hepatitis B include healthcare workers who deal with body fluids, drug users who share needles, those who have unprotected sex with virus carriers and babies born to mothers who carry the virus. Hepatitis B carriage is rare in western populations, but in parts of Africa and the Far East up to 10–15% of the population may carry the virus. It is very important to make travellers to these parts of the world aware of this fact.

In those people who develop acute hepatitis, the disease is more severe than for hepatitis A. The incubation period is longer, with symptoms appearing 1–6 months after exposure. The hepatitis lasts for longer, and requires a longer recovery period. About 1% of patients with hepatitis B die from acute liver failure. A further 10% never fully recover, and instead develop a long-term condition called 'chronic hepatitis'. In this condition the function of the liver gradually deteriorates until the terminal condition of cirrhosis develops (see later). These patients are also at particular risk of developing liver cancer. It is these long-term problems that make hepatitis B such a dreaded disease. Figure 3.1d-I illustrates the possible outcomes of acute hepatitis B infection.

Treatment for acute hepatitis B is generally supportive, although interferon-alpha and other antiviral drugs may be prescribed in cases of chronic disease.

The vaccine for hepatitis B is usually only offered in the UK to healthcare workers, newborn babies of mothers who carry the virus and those who have close contact with at-risk people (e.g. prison officers).

Hepatitis C causes a condition in which most patients do not develop the symptoms of acute hepatitis, but many continue to carry the virus. This has the serious long-term consequence of chronic hepatitis in up to 85% of those infected. In these patients there is particular risk of cirrhosis (develops in 20–30%) and liver cancer.

Hepatitis C was only identified in 1988, and it has been discovered to be the cause of thousands of cases of hepatitis resulting from blood transfusion prior to that date. Up to 80% of haemophiliacs are estimated to have been infected

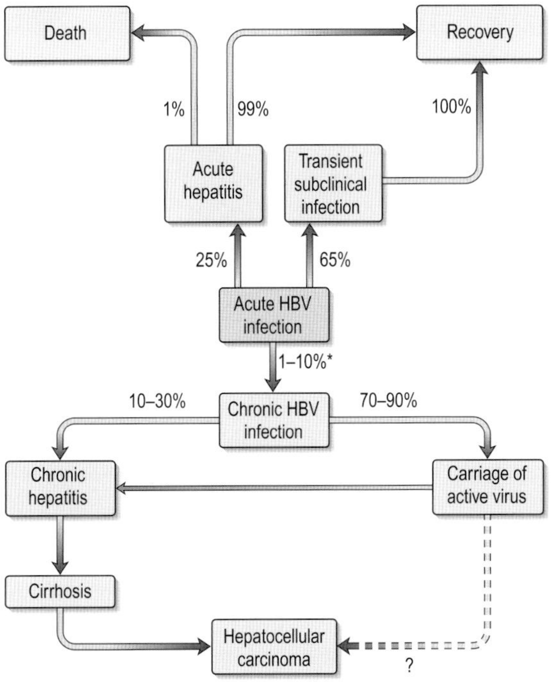

Figure 3.1d-I • The clinical course of hepatitis B infection.

with hepatitis C prior to 1988. Nowadays, donated blood is tested for hepatitis C.

Hepatitis C is very common in the intravenous-drug-using community, and is particularly virulent in those who have untreated HIV infection.

If hepatitis C is demonstrated by liver biopsy to be causing a moderate to severe form of liver fibrosis, then long-term treatment with interferon-alpha and the antiviral drug ribavarin is recommended. This treatment needs to be maintained for at least 6 months, and is a cause of malaise and depression whilst it is ongoing. Nevertheless, this therapy gives a good chance of total clearance of infection in certain patient groups. In the UK, the decision to treat a case of hepatitis C in this way is always made by a specialist.

Chronic hepatitis

This long-term condition of inflammation of the liver has already been mentioned as a possible outcome of infection with hepatitis B and C. It can also be an outcome of an autoimmune process (see Chapter 2.2c).

The initial changes of chronic hepatitis will only be revealed by means of the 'liver function' serum blood test. Over the course of time, the damage to the liver cells revealed by this test worsens. An inexorable rise in the serum levels of liver enzymes such as aspartate transaminase signifies progressive damage to liver cells.

Corticosteroid drugs and immunosuppressant medication (such as azathioprine) are given to slow the progression of autoimmune chronic hepatitis. These drugs often have to be maintained long term to keep the disease at bay, and therefore patients will suffer from the side-effects of long-term steroid treatment (see Chapter 2.2c). However, drug treatment is successful in inducing remission in 80% of cases.

Untreated or unresponsive chronic hepatitis eventually leads to damage of a substantial proportion of the liver cells, with areas of scarring within the liver substance. When scarring has occurred, there is little hope of recovery of the function of the organ. This condition is called *cirrhosis* of the liver. If the disease progresses to cirrhosis then this means irreversible damage has occurred and the only option the patient has for survival is liver transplantation.

Cirrhosis of the liver

The term 'cirrhosis' is derived from the Greek root for 'yellow', a reflection of the jaundice that can develop in advanced cases. The most common causes of this state of cell damage and scarring to the liver are long-term alcohol abuse and viral hepatitis (B and C) infections. There are a number of much less common causes, including autoimmune hepatitis (described above) and biliary cirrhosis (described below). The conditions haemochromatosis, Wilson's disease and alpha-1-antitrypsin deficiency are rare genetically transmitted causes.

Serious chronic damage to the liver has a number of long-term effects. There are two main consequences of severe liver damage:

- gradual loss of the important functions of the liver due to loss of the liver cells
- increasing restriction of the usually free flow of blood through the liver due to the scarring.

These consequences are described below.

Loss of the functions of the liver

Progressive damage to the liver cells means that the sex hormones and blood proteins (including clotting factors) are not manufactured. In addition, bilirubin builds up in the bloodstream, toxins are not cleared from the body and the blood sugar level becomes unstable. This can lead to progressive symptoms and signs of bruising and bleeding, jaundice, itching, illness and confusion. The nails become pale because of reduced proteins in the bloodstream. Pubic hair can become thin, and men may develop breast tissue and shrunken testicles due to problems in the manufacture of the sex hormones. Increasing confusion and the onset of a coma due to toxins is the most common cause of death in cirrhosis.

Another characteristic feature of chronic liver disease, which can be found on examination of the skin, is the presence more than five small (2–6 mm diameter) 'stars' of broken veins on the face, arms or hands. These are known as 'spider naevi' because of their shape.

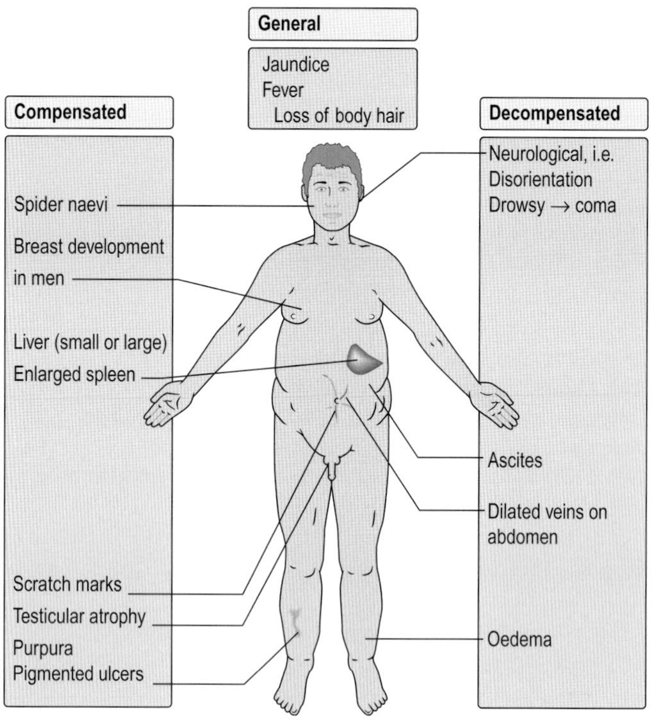

Figure 3.1d-II • The physical signs seen in cirrhosis of the liver.

Restriction of the blood flow through the liver

Scarring around the blood vessels that drain blood from the digestive tract through the liver leads to a build up of pressure within the blood vessels of the digestive tract. This can lead to stretching of these veins under pressure, which then become dilated (varicose). The most serious consequence of this is that varicose veins in the oesophagus can spontaneously rupture, leading to severe haemorrhage into the stomach. This often comes without any warning symptoms or signs. The patient will suddenly start to vomit darkened blood, and may collapse due to extreme blood loss. This is also a common cause of death in cirrhosis.

A combination of increased pressure in the digestive circulation and low blood protein leads to the movement of fluid from the bloodstream out into the tissues (oedema). This occurs particularly in the peritoneal area surrounding the lower digestive organs, so that the abdomen noticeably swells with the fluid. Fluid accumulating in the peritoneal space is called 'ascites'. Ankles and calves may also become swollen.

A final complication of cirrhosis is that it increases the risk of liver cancer, presumably as a result of chronic damage to the liver tissue.

A sinister aspect of cirrhosis is that it tends to develop silently, and symptoms generally only become apparent once the disease process is very advanced. The complexity of the features of chronic liver disease/cirrhosis is illustrated in Figure 3.1d-II.

Treatment for cirrhosis is limited. Patients with cirrhosis from alcohol abuse are urged strongly to stop drinking, but in those with an alcohol problem this often comes much too late in their habit to be able to make changes. If ascites has developed, then a low-salt diet may be recommended and diuretics prescribed.

Oesophageal haemorrhage is a medical emergency from which one in five patients dies. The endoscope is used to visualise and treat the bleeding veins. However, for those who survive this, the risk of a rebleed within the next 2 years is very high.

The only potential cure for cirrhosis is to transplant the liver. Patients receive a liver from a donor who has died no more than 20 hours earlier. The recipient has to remain on lifelong immunosuppressant drug treatment (see Chapter 2.2c) to suppress the immune system and prevent the body from rejecting the foreign liver. This means that the patient will suffer from the side-effects of these powerful drugs, and will be at increased risk of opportunistic infections. The immunosuppressants are commonly prescribed in combination, and include tacrolimus, ciclosporin, azathioprine and corticosteroids.

Nevertheless, liver transplantation is one of the most successful transplant procedures, with over 75% of recipients surviving to at least 5 years following the operation. Most centres do not offer the possibility of this operation to those who cannot abstain from alcohol.

Primary biliary cirrhosis

Primary biliary cirrhosis (PBC) is a rare autoimmune condition in which damage occurs to the tiny bile ducts in the liver. It predominantly affects women around the age of 50 years, and is commonly associated with other autoimmune conditions such as thyroid disease, rheumatoid arthritis and glomerulonephritis.

The first symptoms include itch and malaise and the progressive development of jaundice. Diarrhoea can develop because of poor fat absorption. The condition is diagnosed by means of a rise in alkaline phosphatase on serum testing of liver function and the presence of characteristic antimitochondrial antibodies (AMA). Definitive diagnosis is by liver biopsy.

> **Information Box 3.1d-IV**
>
> **Hepatitis: comments from a Chinese medicine perspective**
>
> In Chinese medicine, the symptoms of acute hepatitis correspond to Damp Heat in the Liver and Gallbladder, and possibly the Spleen, depending on the balance of symptoms. Acute liver failure may be interpreted as depletion of Liver Yin.
>
> Chronic hepatitis and cirrhosis are the long-term consequence of Damp Heat in the Liver and Gallbladder, which in turn leads to a complex state of energetic depletion. The tendency to profuse bleeds, itching and broken veins on the face reflects the presence of Internal Heat. The loss of the substance of the liver organ suggests depletion of Liver Yin, presumably as a consequence of the Heat. Oedema in advanced liver disease is a result of low blood albumin and also excessive constriction of the portal venous system. The oedema develops slowly, is located in dependent parts of the body and is pitting in nature. In the absence of signs of Heat or Wind, in Chinese medicine all these would be attributed to depletion of either Spleen or Kidney Yang. Tendency to cancer and the end-stage occurrence of confusion and coma may be a reflection of insubstantial Phlegm, a consequence of long-standing Damp Heat and Stagnation.

Treatments can be given to relieve itch (cholestyramine) and diarrhoea (codeine). One drug, ursodeoxycholic acid, may slow progression of disease, but in most cases the outlook is very poor, particularly once jaundice has developed. There is a risk of recurrence of the disease in a transplanted liver, but this is the only treatment that offers any chance of a cure.

Liver cancer

Cancer in the liver is very common, but in 90% of cases is due to secondary spread of a cancer originating elsewhere. The most common primary sites for secondary liver cancer are the digestive tract, the breast and the lung. Once cancer has spread to the liver it is very rare for the person to be cured.

Primary cancer arising in the liver is much less common. It is most common in those who are carrying the hepatitis B or C virus, or in those who have cirrhosis of the liver. The only possibly treatment is surgery, including liver transplantation in certain cases, but the cancer is only rarely operable. Most people with this cancer die within 6 months of diagnosis.

Both types of cancer can present with symptoms and signs of an enlarged liver, pain in the right hypochondrium, with weight loss and loss of appetite (see Q3.1d-3).

> **Information Box 3.1d-V**
>
> **Liver cancer: comments from a Chinese medicine perspective**
>
> In Chinese medicine, both primary and secondary cancer of the liver may correspond to Blood Stagnation or Phlegm on a background of longstanding deficiency of Yin, Yang, Qi or Blood. The pain and swelling in the right hypochondrium is characteristic of Liver Blood and Qi Stagnation.

Red flags of the diseases of the liver

Some patients with diseases of the liver will benefit from referral to a conventional doctor for assessment and/or treatment. Red flags are those symptoms and signs that indicate that referral is to be considered. The red flags of the diseases of the liver are described in Table 3.1d-IV. This table forms part of the summary on red flags given in Appendix III, which also gives advice on the degree of urgency of referral for each of the red flag conditions listed.

Important diseases of the gallbladder

Gallstones

As is described in Chapter 3.1a, the gallbladder is a storage vessel for the bile, which is manufactured in the liver. Bile consists of some waste products, including bilirubin, and also chemicals called 'bile salts', which are essential for the digestion of fats. In addition, bile contains the fatty substance cholesterol.

In some people the composition of this rich mixture in the gallbladder becomes unbalanced, so that some of the substances come out of solution and form solid masses. This is more likely to occur if cholesterol is present in excess in the bloodstream, a result, in part, of the rich western diet. These masses, which can range in size from that of lead shot to large marbles, are known as 'gallstones'.

Gallstones, which tend to rest in the gallbladder, very often cause no problem. It is estimated that up to one-fifth of adults in the west have gallstones. They are twice as common a finding in women as in men, and seem particularly common in overweight western women of late childbearing age.

> **Information Box 3.1d-VI**
>
> **Gallstones: comments from a Chinese medicine perspective**
>
> In Chinese medicine, the condensation of the fluid bile to form masses would be seen as formation of Phlegm. This fits with the observation that a fatty diet predisposes to gallstones.

Acute cholecystitis

The term 'cholecystitis' comes from the Greek roots 'chole' for bile and 'cystis' for bladder. It is a common condition involving acute inflammation of the gallbladder due to gallstones blocking the free flow of bile. Figure 3.1d-III is a diagrammatic representation of the liver and gallbladder. It illustrates three of the problems that can result from gallstones: the stones can leave the gallbladder and become lodged in either the neck of the gallbladder or the cystic duct, or in the common bile duct, which leads into the duodenum, or finally in the pancreatic duct.

Table 3.1d-IV Red Flags 8 –of diseases of the liver

Red Flag	Description	Reasoning
8.1	**Jaundice** (yellowish skin, yellow whites of the eyes, and maybe dark urine and pale stools). Itch may be a prominent symptom	Jaundice results from a problem in the production of the bile by the liver or an obstruction to its outflow via the gallbladder into the duodenum Jaundice may result from inflammation of the liver (hepatitis) or from liver cancer. Hepatitis can be a result of infection (e.g. hepatitis A, B or C, or glandular fever), but can also result from the negative effects of certain prescription medications and excess alcohol on the liver tissue Jaundice always merits referral for investigation of its cause Viral hepatitis of any form is a notifiable disease[1]
8.2	**Right hypochondriac pain** (pain under the right ribs) **with malaise** for more than 3 days	This suggests liver or gallbladder pathology and should be considered for investigation even in the absence of jaundice if persisting for more than 3 days
8.3	**Vomiting of fresh blood or altered blood** (looks like dark gravel or coffee grounds)	The appearance of blood in the vomit is always of concern, as it is not possible to gauge the severity of bleeding and whether or not the bleeding is continuing Refer if more than about a tablespoon of blood appears in the vomit (small amounts may simply be the result of a tear the oesophagus lining during vomiting) There can be profuse bleeding from the base of the oesophagus in chronic liver disease, as distended varicose veins (varices) can rupture in this site. The patient in this situation can easily go into shock (see Red Flag Table A17 in Appendix III) and needs to be treated as an emergency
8.4	The syndrome of **oedema**, **bruising** and **confusion** in someone with known liver disease	Liver disease may remain in a stable state for months to years, but the patient may become suddenly much more unwell once a certain point of progression of the disease has passed. This is the point at which the liver is no longer able to perform its function of manufacture of blood proteins and detoxification. Bruising, oedema and confusion can result. This syndrome requires urgent medical management

[1]Notifiable diseases: notification of a number of specified infectious diseases is required of doctors in the UK as a statutory duty under the Public Health (Infectious Diseases) 1988 Act and the Public Health (Control of Diseases) 1988 Act. The UK Health Protection Agency (HPA) Centre for Infections collates details of each case of each disease that has been notified. This allows analyses of local and national trends. This is one example of a situation in which there is a legal requirement for a doctor to breach patient confidentiality. Diseases that are notifiable include: acute encephalitis, acute poliomyelitis, anthrax, cholera, diphtheria, dysentery, food poisoning, leptospirosis, malaria, measles, meningitis (bacterial and viral forms), meningococcal septicaemia (without meningitis), mumps, ophthalmia neonatorum, paratyphoid fever, plague, rabies, relapsing fever, rubella, scarlet fever, smallpox, tetanus, tuberculosis, typhoid fever, typhus fever, viral haemorrhagic fever, viral hepatitis (including hepatitis A, B and C), whooping cough, yellow fever.

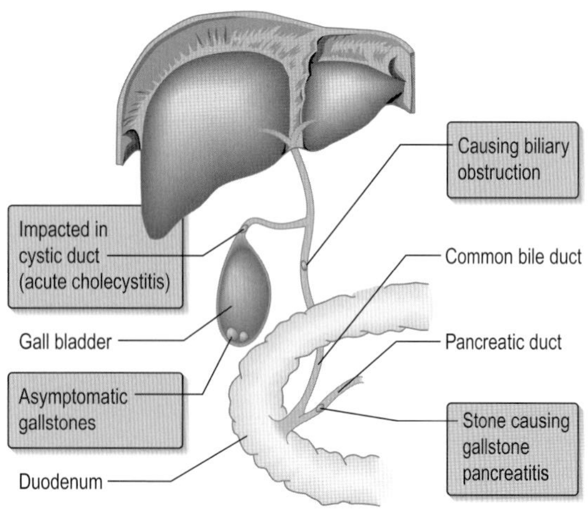

Figure 3.1d-III • The three important clinical outcomes of gallstones.

Stones in the neck of the gallbladder or cystic duct obstruct the outward flow of bile. The gallbladder contracts against a resistance, which causes intense pain. Because the contractions occur in waves, the intense pain also comes in waves. At its peak the pain can be so severe as to cause the patient to writhe, sweat and vomit. Pain that fluctuates in intensity like this is conventionally termed 'colic'. This pain is therefore known as 'biliary colic'. Biliary colic may be brought on after a fatty meal, because it is the presence of fat in the duodenum that stimulates the contraction of the gallbladder.

Often the stone drops back into the gallbladder, and the attack will subside. Sometimes the stone becomes impacted. This means that the bile in the gallbladder becomes stagnant, and eventually infection will develop. The gallbladder becomes very inflamed and the patient becomes acutely unwell. The features of the 'acute abdomen' develop, and the condition needs urgent treatment to relieve the blockage before the infection leads to peritonitis.

Stones in the common bile duct will not only cause colic as the fine duct contracts to release bile into the duodenum, but will also prevent the free flow of bile from the liver. This means that, as was described for pancreatic cancer, bilirubin cannot be cleared from the blood by the liver. It therefore starts building up in the blood, and the patient becomes jaundiced.

Sometimes, a stone becomes lodged at the far end of the common bile duct at the 'sphincter of Oddi', where the pancreatic duct opens into the duodenum (see Figure 3.1d-III). This is how gallstones can cause pancreatitis, as a stone at this site will block the free outflow of pancreatic enzymes (see Q3.1d-4).

The simple-non-invasive ultrasound scan is used to distinguish acute cholecystitis from the other abdominal conditions. In the case of cholecystitis this will reveal gallstones in a thickened and distended gallbladder. If diagnosis is uncertain, a test called a 'hepatobiliary imino-diacetic acid (HIDA) scan may be performed; this scan, which involves the injection of a radioactively marked precursor chemical, tracks the flow of bile from the liver and will expose whether or not bile is entering the gallbladder. Increasingly, a non invasive MRI scan called 'magnetic resonance cholangiopancreatography '(MRCP) may be used, as this produces clear three-dimensional images of the biliary ducts and gallbladder, together with associated structures.

The pain of an acute attack of cholecystits is treated with powerful opiate painkillers given by injection. These not only relieve the colic, but may allow the gallbladder and ducts to relax so that the stone either drops back into the gallbladder or is passed into the duodenum. Opiate painkillers are studied in more detail in Chapter 4.2c. Many patients with an attack settle down if they are kept 'nil by mouth', as this will remove the stimulation of the gallbladder to contract. Strong antibiotics are given because it is assumed infection of the stagnant bile in the gallbladder is also part of the condition.

Most people who have had an acute attack will be offered a cholecystectomy to remove the gallbladder. This is because it is very common for attacks of acute cholecystitis to recur. This is considered the best treatment for this condition. It is now performed by means of a flexible telescope (the laparoscope) through a tiny 'keyhole' incision in the right hypochondrium, and patients recover quickly from the operation. In fit people the operation can be performed whilst they are in hospital within 2–3 days of the acute attack, while in the less fit the attack is allowed to settle down so that the patient can be in the best possible physical state for a planned ('elective') operation.

The conventional understanding is that the loss of the gallbladder has no ill effects in most people. It is, however, recognised that some people suffer from long-term uncomfortable symptoms after the surgery. A recurrence of pain similar to biliary colic in the months to years after gallbladder removal is known as the 'postcholecystectomy syndrome'. In many cases this is attributed to excessive bowel spasm, but in a few the problem may be the result of a retained gallstone or to spasm of the sphincter of Oddi, problems that can be relieved by another minor operation.

If stones are blocked in the common bile duct they can be removed at the same time as a visualisation procedure using an endoscope; this is known as 'endoscopic retrograde cholangiopancreatography' (ERCP). The endoscope is passed into the duodenum, from where a fine tube is inserted into the opening of the common bile duct. Contrast medium is injected up the common bile duct so that X-ray images can be taken of the biliary tree. Guided by X-rays, an instrument is passed through this tube to 'net' the lodged stone and drag it into the duodenum. If ERCP-guided removal of stones fails, open surgery is necessary.

Patients who opt not to have the operation after their acute attack can help their condition by cutting down on the amount of cholesterol in their diet. Drugs (including the synthetic bile salts, e.g. ursodeoxycholic acid, and the statins, e.g. simvastatin) can be prescribed that encourage the gallstones to dissolve back into the bile. Another option is to break up the stones using an ultrasound technique called 'lithotripsy'. This does not require an operation, but is only likely to be successful if the stones are greater than 10 mm in diameter.

Although removal of stones by endoscopy, drugs or 'shock waves' can be effective, the stones may recur because the root cause has not been dealt with.

Chronic cholecystitis

'Chronic cholecystitis' is the term given to a condition in which there are recurrent bouts of griping right-sided hypochondrial pain together with an intolerance of fatty food. The patient may complain of 'wind' or 'indigestion', and may take antacids in an attempt to relieve the symptoms.

It used to be believed that the symptoms were due to a chronically inflamed gallbladder. This was because in some (but not all) people an ultrasound scan showed a shrunken gallbladder with stones. However, it was found that removal of the gallbladder often did not necessarily remove the symptoms. It is now considered that chronic cholecystitis is a 'functional' condition, in that the symptoms do not seem to be related to a specific gallbladder problem. Chronic cholecystitis is therefore seen as a condition very like irritable bowel syndrome (see Chapter 3.1e). There is no satisfactory medical treatment for these symptoms.

It is important to recognise that conventional medicine does not address the root cause of gallbladder disease. For this reason, lifestyle changes and Chinese medicine may have a lot to offer a patient who suffers from gallstones. It would be reasonable to counsel a patient who suffers from acute cholecystitis to accept urgent pain relief if your treatment has not helped, but to consider delaying a decision to have surgery while they see if alternative treatment approaches are of benefit (see Q3.1d-5).

Red flags of the diseases of the gallbladder

Some patients with diseases of the gallbladder will benefit from referral to a conventional doctor for assessment and/or treatment. Red flags are those symptoms and signs that indicate that referral is to be considered. The red flags of the diseases of the gallbladder are described in Table 3.1d-V. This table forms part of the summary on red flags given in Appendix III, which also gives advice on the degree of urgency of referral for each of the red flag conditions listed.

Information Box 3.1d-VII

Cholecystitis: comments from a Chinese medicine perspective

In Chinese medicine, the acute attack of acute cholecystitis corresponds to Damp Heat in the Liver and Gallbladder, with underlying Phlegm. The intense pain of biliary colic suggests that Blood Stagnation is present also, possibly as a consequence of Heat and Qi Stagnation.

Damp Heat in the Liver and Gallbladder can be attributed, in part, to Damp and Hot foods in the diet or climatic factors. In addition, a major factor in its causation is considered to be suppressed frustration, leading to Stagnation of Liver Qi. This emotional component is not recognised in conventional medicine.

The symptoms of chronic cholecystitis fit with Liver Qi Stagnation invading the Spleen, or Damp Heat in the Liver and Gallbladder.

A gallstone may be interpreted as a manifestation of Insubstantial Phlegm, a result of the 'steaming and brewing' of Phlegm by Heat. Therefore, treatments that allow the passage of a stone may be described in terms of expelling this accumulated Phlegm. However, these do not address the root cause of the problem, and thus are energetically suppressive in nature. Likewise, removal of the gallbladder does not address the root cause, and possibly leaves the person with more depletion of Liver and Gallbladder Qi than before. The underlying causes of Damp Heat in the Liver and Gallbladder have not been addressed, and this could explain why some people suffer from persistent symptoms.

Table 3.1d-V Red Flags 9 – diseases of the gallbladder

Red Flag	Description	Reasoning
9.1	**Jaundice** (yellowish skin, yellow whites of the eyes, and maybe dark urine and pale stools). Itch may be a prominent symptom	Jaundice results from a problem in the production of the bile by the liver, or an obstruction to its outflow via the gallbladder into the duodenum Jaundice may result from sudden obstruction of the flow of bile by a gallstone. In this case it is usually accompanied by severe colicky pain. It can also develop gradually as a result of gradual obstruction by a tumour of the gallbladder or duct Jaundice always merits referral for investigation of its cause
9.2	**Right hypochondriac pain** (pain under the right ribs) **with malaise** for more than 3 days	This suggests liver or gallbladder pathology and should be considered for investigation even in the absence of jaundice if persisting for more than 3 days
9.3	**Right hypochondriac pain** that is very intense and comes in waves. May be associated with fever and vomiting May be associated with **jaundice** This is one of the manifestations of the **acute abdomen** (see Red Flag Table A6 in Appendix III)	Obstruction of a bile duct by gallstones causes waves of intense pain as the duct attempts to contract against the obstruction. Fever and malaise can develop as the obstructed gallbladder becomes inflamed

Self-test 3.1d

Diseases of the pancreas, liver and gallbladder

1. What is the meaning of the term 'colic'?
2. Why is chronic cholecystitis believed by some doctors to be a functional disease?
3. How might you manage the situation of a 35-year-old, teetotal female patient who describes herself as suffering from three bouts of severe gripy pain in the right hypochondrium lasting a few hours each in the past 2 months?
4. You notice that an elderly patient of yours who has been generally stable over the past few months is jaundiced (whites of the eyes are yellow, and a generally dark hint to the skin). The patient says that they feel much the same as ever.
   (i) What conventional diagnoses might you be thinking about?
   (ii) How would you manage this patient?
5. A stressed, 45-year-old teacher comes to you for treatment of abdominal pain. He admits that he uses the occasional alcohol drink to calm him down in the evening. The pain he describes is fairly constant and generally located in the epigastric area. When you question him about his digestion he admits that his stools are quite loose and foul smelling at the moment. On examination he is quite thin and is tender deep in the epigastric and right hypochondrial areas.
   (i) What conventional diagnoses might you be thinking about?
   (ii) How would you manage this patient?

Answer

1. Colic is the term used to describe the fluctuating nature of pain that results from distension of a hollow organ such as the gallbladder or bowel. Every time the organ contracts, the pain reaches a crescendo before dying down again. The pain at its peak can be excruciating.

2. A functional disease is one in which there are symptoms, but no definite underlying physical cause can be found. For this reason, only the symptoms can be treated as opposed to an underlying cause. Chronic cholecystitis is now considered to be a functional disease, as the symptoms are not always related to definite disease of the gallbladder, and removal of the gallbladder does not usually help the condition.
3. Gripy, right-sided hypochondrial pain, particularly if severe, is most likely to be caused by gallstones in this patient, although the syndrome of chronic cholecystitis is a possibility. Other possibilities include irritable bowel syndrome and hepatitis, although the latter would be most unlikely without jaundice or obvious risk factors such as alcohol abuse.

   It would be reasonable to discuss your diagnosis with the patient, explaining that a possible diagnosis for these symptoms is gallstones, for which the conventional treatment is cholecystectomy. You may suggest that she goes to her GP so that an ultrasound scan can be organised to confirm the diagnosis. Assuming the diagnosis is confirmed as gallstones, as this patient is not currently in acute pain, you could suggest that she defers a decision about the operation until she has tried lifestyle changes (focusing on reduction of Damp Hot foods and stuck emotions) and Chinese medicine.
4. Silent onset of jaundice in an elderly person is highly suggestive of pancreatic or liver cancer (cancer of the gallbladder is another rare possibility). You should refer your patient as a high priority to his GP for investigation of the jaundice.
5. Chronic epigastric pain and the possibility of a regular high alcohol intake suggests either a peptic ulcer or chronic pancreatitis. The development of the loose stools suggests the latter. Whatever the diagnosis, you need to achieve sufficient rapport with your patient to discuss the possible diagnoses and their relationship with alcohol. You should refer the patient so that he can be investigated fully to exclude alcohol-related chronic pancreatitis, because the associated complications of diabetes and malabsorption can both benefit from conventional treatment.

   Ideally, you would continue to treat your patient with Chinese medicine to support him in the process of dealing with his symptoms, and to help him overcome the underlying stress and alcohol problem.

Chapter 3.1e Diseases of the small intestine and colon

LEARNING POINTS

At the end of this chapter you will:

- be able to name the main features of the most important diseases of the lower digestive tract
- understand the principles of treatment of a few of the most common diseases
- recognise the red flags of serious diseases of the small intestine and colon.

Estimated time for chapter: 90 minutes.

Introduction

This chapter describes the important diseases of the lower digestive tract; i.e. the small intestine and colon (including the rectum and anus). These are:

- Diseases of the small intestine:
  - malabsorption syndrome
  - coeliac disease
  - intestinal obstruction and abdominal hernias
  - inflammatory bowel disease (Crohn's disease).
- Diseases of the large intestine:
  - irritable bowel syndrome
  - inflammatory bowel disease (Crohn's disease and ulcerative colitis)
  - appendicitis
  - diverticulitis
  - constipation
  - cancer of the colon and rectum.
- Diseases of the anus:
  - haemorrhoids
  - rectal prolapse
  - anal fissure (see Q3.1e-1).

Important diseases of the small intestine

Malabsorption syndrome

The concept of malabsorption was introduced when chronic pancreatitis was described in Chapter 3.1d. In chronic pancreatitis, the essential nutrients that should be obtained from the diet cannot be absorbed because the pancreatic enzymes are lacking and the food cannot be fully digested in the small intestine.

In small intestinal disease, malabsorption occurs for a different reason. In this case, although the pancreatic enzymes have fully digested the food into small molecules, the lining of the intestine is diseased, and this prevents their absorption.

There are a number of intestinal diseases that can lead to malabsorption, the most common being coeliac disease and Crohn's disease (discussed below). All these diseases have features in common, all resulting from the fact that lack of absorbed nutrients leads to malnutrition. The patient with malabsorption will lose weight and their muscles will waste. Anaemia occurs due to deficiencies of iron, vitamin B_{12} and folic acid. A wide range of other symptoms can occur due to other vitamin deficiencies.

The excess nutrients, including undigested fat, pass into the colon. These lead to loose, foul-smelling stools with excess gas. The patient may suffer from abdominal distension and vague abdominal pain.

Malabsorption is diagnosed by detecting fat and nutrients in the stools. Blood tests will reveal anaemia and features of other vitamin deficiencies. Endoscopy, barium contrast X-ray studies and biopsy are used to examine the lining of the small intestine.

The treatment of malabsorption is to treat the cause. Without this, oral vitamin and nutrient supplements cannot be of help because these too will not be absorbed. While the cause is being treated, it may be necessary to administer nourishment by means of intravenous drip (total parenteral nutrition) if the patient is extremely undernourished.

> **Information Box 3.1e-I**
>
> **Malabsorption: comments from a Chinese medicine perspective**
>
> In Chinese medicine, the symptoms and signs of malabsorption correspond to Spleen Qi or Yang deficiency. The anaemia corresponds to the Blood Deficiency which occurs as a result.

Coeliac disease

This term originates from the Greek word 'koelia', meaning 'belly'. In coeliac disease the lining of the small intestine is damaged as a result of a sensitivity to gluten, a component of wheat, barley, rye and oats. Gluten sensitivity is relatively common, affecting just less than one in 1000 people. It appears to run in families.

Coeliac disease may never be diagnosed because the sensitivity is not always very severe. In some people, slight digestive problems may be the only consequence of having the condition.

In severe cases the condition becomes apparent in childhood. Affected children will not put on weight or grow adequately after weaning. Sometimes diagnosis is delayed until adulthood, when for some reason the sensitivity worsens and the patient starts to lose weight and develop abdominal discomfort and diarrhoea.

Gluten sensitivity can be diagnosed by means of detecting particular antibodies or digestive enzymes that are present in the blood 95% of people with coeliac disease. A reversible flattened appearance to the intestinal lining is seen if a biopsy is taken from the duodenum, and this more invasive investigation is the definitive test.

The treatment of the condition is total lifelong avoidance of gluten. This leads to a dramatic reversal of symptoms in most people. In some patients any slight 'lapse', such as eating a piece of cake, can lead to recurrence of symptoms.

> **Information Box 3.1e-II**
>
> **Coeliac disease: comments from a Chinese medicine perspective**
>
> In Chinese medicine, coeliac disease corresponds to Spleen Qi or Yang deficiency. The Spleen in patients with coeliac disease appears to be vulnerable to the Damp nature of gluten-rich foods.

Inflammatory bowel disease – Crohn's disease

The term 'inflammatory bowel disease' is used to embrace two conditions: Crohn's disease and ulcerative colitis. These have some features in common and may be very difficult to distinguish between in practice.

Crohn's disease is a condition that can affect any portion of the digestive tract, but most commonly leads to disease of the small intestine and the colon. The cause of Crohn's disease is unknown, although it is recognised to be more common in smokers and those who eat a high-sugar, low-fibre diet. Claims that it has a relationship to measles infection or vaccine have not been proven conventionally. The disease does tend to run in families.

Ulcerative colitis is a condition that is confined to the colon. For this reason it is described in more detail later this chapter.

In Crohn's disease, the bowel spontaneously becomes inflamed and thickened. Deep ulcers form in the lining of the affected bowel. This leads to malabsorption if the small bowel is affected, and diarrhoea with profuse pus and mucus if the colon is affected. Often blood can be found mixed in the stools. In both cases, the abdominal pain is gripy and can be severe. Commonly mouth ulcers occur, and the patient feels generally unwell.

The inflamed bowel can adhere to other structures in the abdominal cavity, and sometimes the ulcers erode through to another organ forming a fistula (see Chapter 2.2b). Faeces, pus and mucus can then pass through the fistula to different sites, such as the bladder, or even out onto the skin.

The condition tends to come on for the first time in adulthood, often at a time of stress. Symptoms tend to become manifest in bouts called 'relapses'. The diarrhoea and pain can be so severe as to fit the syndrome of the acute abdomen, and so can result in emergency hospital admission.

The treatment is to rest the bowel by making the patient 'nil by mouth'. Sometimes this is sufficient to allow the attack to settle down and the patient to resume normal life for a while. In more severe cases, corticosteroids or other immunosuppressant drugs are given (see Chapter 2.2c), sometimes for weeks on end. A very simple diet (elemental diet) can be prescribed, which helps healing, but a return to a normal diet can cause a relapse.

The symptoms in some patients do not settle even with powerful drug treatment. Persistent diarrhoea and inflammation can lead to loss of essential nutrients and salts. In these patients emergency surgery is performed to remove the affected length of bowel. Most patients (50–80%) with Crohn's disease will eventually have to have surgery for their condition. In some cases the problems caused by the acute attack are so severe that the patient dies.

A relatively minor surgical treatment for Crohn's disease is the formation of a 'defunctioning ileostomy'. In this operation the small intestine is opened out onto the skin of the right iliac fossa. This means the fluid contents of the small intestine pass out of this opening and allow the colon to be rested. This can help the inflammation to settle down, and immediately relieves the symptom of diarrhoea. At a later date the ileostomy is surgically repaired and normal bowel function can be resumed.

Sometimes, because of widespread inflammation, it is necessary to remove the whole of the colon and rectum and a portion of the small intestine. The end of the remaining small intestine is opened to form an ileostomy (from the medical term for the small intestine; the 'ileum'), and in this case the ileostomy is permanent. The faeces that normally enter the colon are discharged out of the ileostomy and into a bag placed over the opening. Unlike faeces, the discharge is much more fluid and continuous, so the bag has to be emptied frequently.

Surgery is also necessary if fistulas form between the digestive tract and another organ or the skin. Fistulas occur in 10% of cases.

Crohn's disease is a serious condition, which can seriously affect quality of life, and which may lead to premature death.

> **Information Box 3.1e-III**
>
> **Crohn's disease: comments from a Chinese medicine perspective**
>
> In Chinese medicine, the symptoms of Crohn's disease correspond to a combination of Liver Qi Stagnation invading the Spleen, Spleen Yang deficiency and Damp Heat in the Large Intestines.

Intestinal obstruction

The passage through the small intestine and colon can become blocked for a variety of reasons. These include the inflammation of Crohn's disease, and diverticulitis and cancerous growths. Also, a loop of the bowel can become pinched as it penetrates into the small opening of a hernia (see below) or by the scarring that can follow surgery (adhesions).

A blockage of the bowel has comparable effects to the blockage of the bile ducts. As the bowel contracts against the blockage, the patient experiences waves of colicky pain. A blockage in the small intestine will rapidly lead to vomiting and dehydration as the contents of the digestive tract are forced backwards by the contractions. A blockage of the colon is more likely to lead to distension as gas and fluid accumulates in the small intestine. Eventually, vomiting will also occur. If the blockage is persistent, whether in the small intestine or colon, it will lead sooner or later to the acute abdomen syndrome, and require urgent surgical attention.

The patient is treated by being kept 'nil by mouth', and open surgery is used to excise the affected segment of bowel. The two remaining ends of the bowel are usually sewn back together.

If the colon is obstructed close to the rectum, a colostomy may have to be formed, which may or may not be possible to reverse at a later date. A colostomy looks similar to an ileostomy, but the faeces that are passed into the bag have a normal consistency. A colostomy is, therefore, generally easier for the patient to manage than an ileostomy.

Abdominal hernias

'Hernia' is the term used to describe the situation when the contents of a body cavity become displaced outside of the cavity through a breach in the cavity wall. An example already described in Chapter 3.1c is the hiatus hernia, where a part of the stomach has become displaced above the diaphragm through a breach in the muscular cardiac sphincter.

In abdominal hernias some of the soft and moveable intra-abdominal contents of loops of bowel, associated fat and blood vessels become displaced outside the muscular abdominal wall. Breaches can develop in the abdominal wall either as a result of congenital weakness, or because of the excessive intra-abdominal pressure that can result from coughing, straining, obesity and pregnancy. Common sites for abdominal hernias to develop include the region of the umbilicus, the linea alba (which separates the two bands of the rectus abdominis muscle), the inguinal canal (through which the spermatic cord passes to reach the testicles), and the femoral canal (through which the femoral artery, vein and nerve pass to reach the front of the thigh). Inguinal and femoral hernias appear as smooth bulges in the groin.

In their early stages, hernias tend to appear when the person is standing, or when the intra-abdominal pressure is raised, for example when they cough. The hernia appears as a bulge and may be associated with a dragging discomfort. In most cases the hernia will disappear if the patient lies down. If the hernia does not reduce easily on lying down or with firm pressure, then it is said to be 'incarcerated'.

Minor hernias may be simply left untreated if not causing too much discomfort, or alternatively may be made more comfortable by the application of pressure. For example, an inguinal truss may be worn to support the region of an inguinal hernia. However, surgical repair of hernias is usually a straightforward operation and is usually recommended. In many cases it can be performed as a laparoscopic (keyhole) day-case procedure and has a relatively rapid recovery time (return to work and driving in less than 2 weeks).

The reason why surgical repair of a hernia is often recommended is that there is a risk with hernias that loops of bowel and their associated blood supply can become trapped and pinched in the hernial sac. This can then lead to the syndrome of intestinal obstruction or even death of bowel tissue. In this case, the patient will experience the symptoms of intestinal obstruction, including intense colicky abdominal pain, abdominal distension and vomiting. An experienced surgeon may be able to reduce the trapped hernia manually, but in most cases emergency surgery is required to treat an obstructed hernia (see Q3.1e-2).

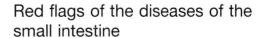

Red flags of the diseases of the small intestine

Some patients with diseases of the small intestine will benefit from referral to a conventional doctor for assessment and/or treatment. Red flags are those symptoms and signs that indicate that referral is to be considered. The red flags of the diseases of the small intestine are described in Table 3.1e-I. This table forms part of the summary on red flags given in Appendix III, which also gives advice on the degree of urgency of referral for each of the red flag conditions listed.

Information Box 3.1e-IV

Intestinal obstruction: comments from a Chinese medicine perspective

In Chinese medicine, the pain of obstruction would correspond to Small Intestine Qi Tied and/or Liver Qi Stagnation invading the Spleen. Vomiting in intestinal obstruction is the result of reversed waves of peristalsis. It is vigorous in nature and would be described as a Full condition. Reversed peristalsis might be described in terms of Stomach Qi rebelling upwards.

A region of herniation suggests deficiency in the holding power of the Spleen Qi.

Important diseases of the colon and rectum

Irritable bowel syndrome

Irritable bowel disease (IBS) is also known as 'spastic colon' and 'functional bowel disease'. The term 'functional' means that the symptoms have no physically measurable cause, and so treatment can only be targeted at the symptoms. In IBS the bowel tends to contract overforcefully. This tight contraction is called 'spasm'.

Table 3.1e-I Red Flags 10a – diseases of the small intestine

Red Flag	Description	Reasoning
10.1	**Malabsorption syndrome** (loose, pale stools and malnutrition; weight loss, thin hair, dry skin, cracked lips and peeled tongue). Will present as failure to thrive in children	The malabsorption syndrome results when there is inability to absorb the nutrients in the diet, leading to weight loss and mineral and vitamin deficiencies. Loose stools are the result of the presence of unabsorbed fat Disease of the small intestine (most commonly coeliac disease and Crohn's disease) can result in the malabsorption syndrome
10.2	**Diarrhoea** with **mucus and gripy pain** if not responding to treatment within a week	Persistent diarrhoea with mucus suggests either a serious episode of bowel infection or an episode of inflammatory bowel disease (Crohn's disease or ulcerative colitis) Both causes merit prompt referral for treatment
10.3	**Onset of severe abdominal pain with collapse ("the acute abdomen)**. The pain can be constant or colicky (coming in waves). Rigidity, guarding and rebound tenderness are serious signs.	The 'acute abdomen' refers to the combination of severe abdominal pain together with an inability to continue with day-to-day activities (collapse). This syndrome can have benign causes, such as irritable bowel syndrome, dysmenorrhoea and ovulation pain. You should refer to exclude more serious possibilities, including appendicitis, perforated ulcer, peritonitis, obstructed bowel, pelvic inflammatory disease and gallstones Colicky pain indicates obstruction of a viscus (hollow organ) Rigidity of the abdomen, guarding (reflex protective spasm of the abdominal muscles) and rebound tenderness (pain felt elsewhere in abdomen when the pressure of the palpating hand is released) all suggest inflammation or perforation of a viscus Features of abdominal pain in children that suggest a more benign (functional) cause include mild pain that is worse in the morning, location around the umbilicus, and pain that is worse with anxiety
10.4	Any episode of **blood mixed in with stools**	Red blood mixed in with stools suggests bleeding from the lower part of the small intestine, the large intestine or rectum. Possible causes are bowel infections, diverticulitis, inflammatory bowel disease (Crohn's disease or ulcerative colitis) and bowel cancer. All merit referral for investigation and treatment
10.5	**Signs of an inguinal hernia: swelling in groin which is more pronounced on standing**, especially if uncomfortable	An inguinal hernia is the result of a weakness in the abdominal wall in the region of the inguinal crease (the groin). The abdominal contents can bulge into a narrow necked passageway formed by this weakness, and this can be very uncomfortable. An inguinal hernia carries a risk of being the site at which the loop of bowel can become obstructed and then there is a risk of strangulation of that portion of the bowel. The patient should be referred for a surgical assessment of the risk of complications Refer as a high priority if a hernia has become acutely painful

Symptoms of IBS include constipation and diarrhoea, which can alternate, and gripy abdominal pain. The stools in IBS are often described as like sheep or rabbit droppings or like ribbons. Mucus may be passed with the stools. Weight loss, blood in the stools and late age at onset (after the age of 40 years) are not characteristic features and suggest a more sinister cause, such as bowel cancer.

The patient may also experience dyspepsia and symptoms of chronic cholecystitis. Bloating and excess wind are common, and symptoms are characteristically brought on by stress or by eating certain foods, and helped by lying down. Unlike the symptoms of Crohn's disease, IBS rarely causes a problem at night-time. Occasionally, an attack of IBS can be so severe as to present in a hospital emergency department as an acute abdomen.

All investigations have normal results, as is usually the case in functional conditions. In some clinical studies, up to 80% of patients with IBS were found to meet the criteria for a concurrent psychiatric diagnosis such as anxiety or depression.

Conventional treatment is often unsatisfactory. Lifestyle changes focused on stress management are likely to be most effective. In some people, dietary changes such as cutting out dairy products can help. A drug called mebeverine anxiety or depression is commonly prescribed. This tends to relax spasm of the bowel and can relieve symptoms. A preparation made from a plant called ispaghula is prescribed to provide dietary fibre. This can help those patients with IBS who tend to constipation. Loperamide may be prescribed in those cases in which diarrhoea predominates.

Increasingly, doctors are recognising that targeting mental emotional imbalances may be helpful in IBS, and so may prescribe antidepressants, refer the patient for counselling or psychotherapy, or recommend hypnotherapy.

> **Information Box 3.1e-V**
>
> **Irritable bowel syndrome: comments from a Chinese medicine perspective**
>
> In Chinese medicine, the symptoms of IBS correspond to Liver Qi Stagnation invading the Spleen and/or Stomach. Mebeverine would appear to smooth Liver Qi, but is suppressive in nature because it does not attend to the root cause of Spleen Qi deficiency. Fybogel would appear also to smooth Liver Qi. It also does not treat the root cause of the problem.

Constipation

Like the term 'indigestion', 'constipation' describes a symptom and has a very different meaning to different individuals. Many people would say that they were constipated if their bowels did not open every day, but another common use of the term is to describe difficulty opening the bowels irrespective of frequency. This is another example of when it is important to get a very clear description of precise symptoms from the patient. The medical definition of constipation is either in terms of low frequency of opening the bowels (less than three times a week) or the subjective experience of difficulty in passing faeces, including the experiencing of straining (this is not a healthy aspect of opening the bowels) or discomfort.

The conventional medicine understanding is that constipation is a result of eating a refined western diet and a sedentary lifestyle. It is a particular problem for elderly people. It is recognised that constipation is not a problem in developing countries in which the diet contains a lot of fibre from vegetables and whole grains.

Some prescribed drugs can cause constipation, in particular those that contain opiates such as morphine, some antidepressants and iron preparations. Occasionally, constipation may be the consequence of a medical condition such as hypothyroidism, spinal nerve injury or high calcium levels, and it is important that these conditions are first excluded before the symptoms are managed.

The initial problem with constipation is that it can cause discomfort and a feeling of ill-health. However, persistent straining over the years, can lead to conditions such as hiatus hernia, diverticulitis and haemorrhoids (piles).

It is conventionally recognised that medication for constipation can lead to dependence on the prescribed drugs. Therefore, initial medical advice is to supplement the diet with fruit and other sources of fibre, such as bran, and to exercise more often.

Preparations that contain natural fibre (e.g. ispaghula husk) are commonly used. If these are not helpful, then drugs that stimulate the bowel, such as senna haemorrhoids (piles), may be chosen. An alternative approach is to use a preparation that encourages fluid to stay within the faeces. These are called 'osmotic laxatives', and include lactulose. The problem with all these preparations is that the patient commonly becomes unable to stop taking them without the constipation returning, often in a more severe form.

In severe cases of constipation, a gradual form of intestinal obstruction can develop. This is most likely in the elderly and infirm, in whom symptoms of bloating, abdominal pain and, eventually, vomiting may develop. Severe chronic constipation is both prevented and treated by means of an enema. This is a technique in which fluid is passed into the colon through a tube passed into the anus. This can have the effect of loosening and flushing out blocked stools. Laxative preparations can also be inserted in the form of an enema.

> **Information Box 3.1e-VI**
>
> **Constipation: comments from a Chinese medicine perspective**
>
> In Chinese medicine, constipation can be a Full condition due to Heat in the Large Intestine. It can also be attributed to Dryness of the Large Intestine due to Blood or Yin Deficiency.
>
> All laxatives are suppressive in that they do not attend to the root of the problem, and may even worsen the underlying condition in that when they are withdrawn the bowel may be even more sluggish. It is recognised that the bowel movements can become dependent on the action of stimulant laxatives in particular.

Appendicitis

As its name implies, appendicitis is a condition in which the appendix becomes inflamed. It is the most common cause of the acute abdomen that requires surgical attention, affecting 6% of the UK population at some point in their lifetime. Despite it commonly being considered a disease of childhood, appendicitis can occur at any age.

The cause generally appears to be blockage of the hollow of the appendicitis with solidified faeces. This means the contents of the blind end of the appendix become stagnant. Just as when the neck of the gallbladder becomes blocked, this stagnation leads to infection, which in turn causes inflammation. The appendix contains a lot of lymphoid (immune) tissue, which readily swells when infection develops, and this contributes to the tendency for the passageway (the lumen) in the appendix to become blocked.

The pain of the appendix starts centrally and is vague. The patient may first lose their appetite, and occasionally may vomit. Over the next few hours, as the outside of the appendix becomes inflamed, the site of the tenderness becomes much more localised at a point in the right iliac fossa. The signs of rigidity, guarding and rebound tenderness (see Chapter 3.1d under Acute abdomen) are present in this area. If the appendix becomes very inflamed it may perforate, releasing its irritating contents into the peritoneal cavity. If generalised peritonitis occurs, the signs of guarding, rigidity and tenderness spread to include the whole abdomen, and the patient becomes much more unwell. In peritonitis the infection can spread rapidly throughout the whole abdominal cavity, and is a life-threatening condition (see Q3.1e-3).

Appendicitis is diagnosed primarily clinically on the basis of the characteristic history with additional features such as migration of pain to the right iliac fossa, guarding tenderness and rigidity, and a raised white cell count being very suggestive. Ultrasound and CT scans are increasingly used to refine the diagnostic process, although they may cause a dangerous delay in treatment in a more advanced case.

It is very common for cases of irritable bowel syndrome, dysmenorrhoea, ovulation pain, ruptured ovarian cyst and ectopic pregnancy to be misdiagnosed as appendicitis, but medical wisdom is that in a case where there is uncertainty it is better to operate, and find that the working diagnosis was wrong, than delay a life-saving operation because of the uncertainty (see Q3.1e-4).

Removal of the appendix can be performed through a keyhole incision, so that if appendicitis is diagnosed early there is rapid recovery. Treatment of established peritonitis involves an open abdominal operation to remove the infected tissue and wash the cavity to remove the pus. The patient is given strong antibiotic injections for at least a week after the operation.

Information Box 3.1e-VII

Appendicitis: comments from a Chinese medicine perspective

In Chinese medicine, appendicitis is viewed as one or more of Damp Heat in the Large Intestine, Stagnation of Qi and Blood, or Accumulation of Toxic Heat. It is sometimes considered to be a condition treatable by means of acupuncture, which if mild need not always require surgery. This is in contrast to the conventional medicine view.

Diverticulitis (diverticular disease)

Diverticulitis is a condition of the last stretch of the colon, the sigmoid colon, which is situated in the left iliac fossa.

A diverticulum (plural: diverticula) is a little pouch extending from the wall of the bowel, like the bulging out of a weak area in an inflated balloon. These pouches can become multiple in older people, particularly in those who have been prone to constipation as a result of a refined western diet. It is estimated that diverticula have developed in 30% of western people by the age of 60 years. However, in 90% of people, they cause no problem at all. The problem for the remaining 10% with diverticula is that, like the appendix, they provide a cul-de-sac for the passage of faeces. Faeces can collect in the pouches and become stagnant. The pouches then become inflamed. This condition is called diverticulitis.

Figure 3.1e-I shows two different images of diverticula. The barium enema (a) shows the lining of the sigmoid colon and the hollows of the pouches coated with barium (black in this image). The colonoscopy (b) shows the pink interior of the bowel, with the openings of the pouches leading off from this.

If inflammation is mild, then diverticulitis can grumble on, with symptoms of bouts of pain in the left iliac fossa, slight fever and occasional blood in the stools. Often there is alternating constipation and diarrhoea (the condition can overlap with IBS). These mild attacks can be treated by prescriptions of oral antibiotics such as co-amoxiclav or metronidazole.

Long-term slight blood loss can lead to anaemia. Sometimes the bleeding from an inflamed diverticulum can be profuse and require emergency treatment.

Occasionally, the inflammation is severe and the condition becomes very similar to appendicitis. The patient may then require emergency surgery to prevent peritonitis.

The symptoms of diverticulitis are indistinguishable from colon or rectal cancer, and so patients with blood mixed in the stools and pain in the left iliac fossa should always be referred for investigation.

Information Box 3.1e-VIII

Diverticulitis: comments from a Chinese medicine perspective

In Chinese medicine, the symptoms of diverticulitis can be equated with Liver Qi Stagnation invading the Spleen either with Damp Heat in the Large Intestine or Accumulation of Toxic Heat.

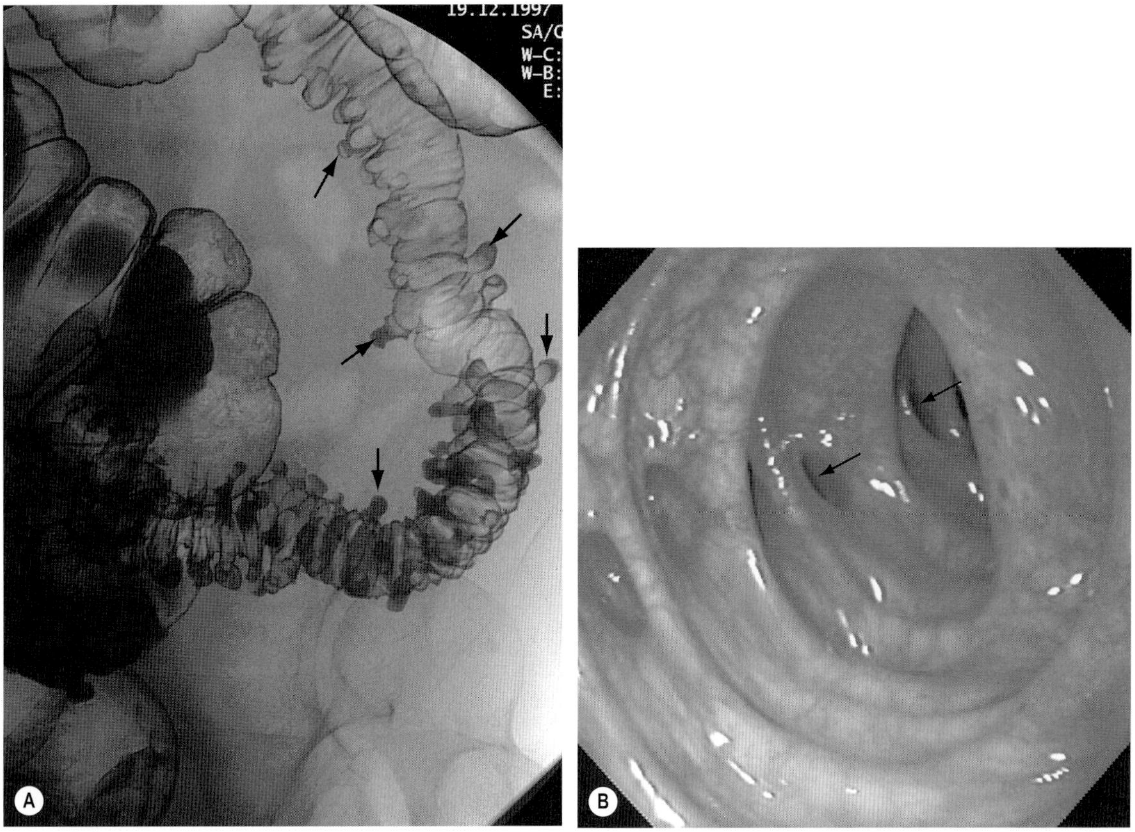

Figure 3.1e-I • (a) Barium enema image showing diverticula (arrows). (b) Colonoscopy showing openings to diverticula (arrows).

Inflammatory bowel disease – ulcerative colitis

Inflammatory bowel disease was introduced earlier in this chapter, with Crohn's disease as one possible manifestation. Ulcerative colitis is in many ways a similar disease, so much so that in about 10% of patients with inflammatory bowel disease it is difficult to distinguish between the two.

There are important differences, however, which means that the outcome of the two conditions can be quite different. In ulcerative colitis the inflammation of the bowel is less extensive in that it usually affects only the lining of the colon. However, ulcerative colitis results in much larger bleeding areas of ulceration. In Crohn's disease the inflammation can extend throughout the thickness of the bowel wall and can affect anywhere in the digestive tract.

In contrast to Crohn's disease, in ulcerative colitis malabsorption and fistulas do not occur. The main symptoms in common with Crohn's disease are bouts of profuse diarrhoea and mucus with gripy pain, all associated with fever and malaise. Blood in the stools is an additional marked symptom in ulcerative colitis, which is less common in Crohn's disease.

Some people with ulcerative colitis may have rare isolated attacks, but otherwise lead a normal life. In others, life can become dominated by frequent relapses and persistent bowel symptoms. Also, in contrast to Crohn's disease, ulcerative colitis is more common in non-smokers than smokers, and stopping smoking may actually trigger a worsening of symptoms.

As with Crohn's disease, in a severe attack the patient may be very unwell and require hospital admission. There is a small risk of perforation of the bowel in an acute attack, and this can lead to life-threatening peritonitis.

Most patients with ulcerative colitis are prescribed a drug that is known to reduce the risk of relapse. Sulphasalazine, mesalazine and olsalazine are three of the most commonly prescribed preparations. The immunosuppressant azathioprine may also be prescribed. These are all powerful drugs and have a number of possible serious side-effects, including digestive disturbance, kidney damage, hepatitis and bone marrow failure. Nevertheless, these drugs can very much improve the quality of life for people with ulcerative colitis.

Corticosteroids may be given by mouth and by enema during an acute attack. Severe attacks require hospital admission and additional immunosuppressant drugs such as ciclosporin, tacrolimus and infliximab.

If there is a very severe attack, or the symptoms are very unpleasant and persistent, the surgical option of total removal of the colon may be chosen (colectomy). It may be possible to do this without the need for a colostomy, although this may be necessary in many cases. If colostomy is necessary, it may be possible to reverse this at a later date by linking the end of the shortened bowel to the anus (ileoanal pouch). Colectomy will effectively 'cure' ulcerative colitis, as the condition only affects the colon. In those who do not have this operation there remains an increased risk of colonic cancer which relates to the extent and length of time for which the bowel has been inflamed.

Information Box 3.1e-IX

Ulcerative colitis: comments from a Chinese medicine perspective

In Chinese medicine, the symptoms of ulcerative colitis, like Crohn's disease, would equate to combination of Liver Qi Stagnation invading the Spleen, Spleen Yang deficiency and Damp Heat in the Large Intestines.

Sulphasalazine, mesalazine and olsalazine would appear to move Liver Qi and Clear Heat, but the side-effect of organ failure suggests that they can severely deplete Yin in the long term. They are suppressive, as are the corticosteroids used in ulcerative colitis.

Cancer of the colon and rectum

Tumours developing from the wall of the colon are common in the west. It is estimated that up to one-tenth of the population will develop a benign tumour of the bowel, otherwise known as a 'polyp', although this is a rare occurrence in people from developing countries. Polyps usually do not cause any problem, and most people are unaware of having them. Occasionally, they can bleed and cause anaemia.

In some cases polyps can become malignant. The more polyps there are, the more likely this is. There is one condition that runs in families (familial polyposis coli) in which hundreds of polyps develop in the colon in later life. There is definitely an increased risk of colon cancer in this condition. Patients with this condition who have too many polyps to be removed surgically may be advised to have the entire colon removed in order to prevent the risk of developing cancer.

Malignant tumours of the colon and rectum are common. They will affect just under one in 30 of the population, most commonly being diagnosed at age 60–65 years, and are the second most common cause of death from cancer. It is recognised that there is a link between colon cancer and polyps and a diet high in meat and animal fat and low in fibre. There is also a recognised increased risk of colon cancer in people who have ulcerative colitis. Colon cancer tends to run in families.

Half of cases of colon cancer occur close to or inside the rectum. These tumours commonly bleed and lead to the warning symptoms of a change in bowel habit and blood mixed in with the stools. If a change in bowel habit occurs anew in someone older than 50 years the person should be referred for investigation. Blood mixed in with the stools should always be referred for further investigation.

Other problems that can lead to the diagnosis of colon cancer include the development of anaemia from long-standing, low-grade blood loss, and an acute abdomen syndrome resulting from intestinal obstruction.

If a tumour is found, the affected segment of the bowel is removed and, if possible, the ends stitched back together again. With rectal tumours this is often not possible, and the patient is left with a colostomy.

The outcome of the operation depends on the stage of progression of the tumour. Colonic carcinomas are graded according to the Dukes system. Dukes grade A means that the tumour is confined to the lining layer of the bowel, the mucosa. If this is the case, then after surgical removal there is a very high cure rate, with no need for chemotherapy or radiotherapy. Dukes grade B means that the tumour is confined to the bowel but has penetrated to deeper levels. The risk of recurrence after surgery is moderate, and some doctors prefer to prescribe chemotherapy after surgery to reduce the risk of recurrence. Dukes grade C means that the tumour has spread to the lymph nodes, and in this case risk of recurrence is high. Chemotherapy is often used in this situation. Dukes grade D cancers are those that have metastasised to other parts of the body. They are unlikely to be cured, but surgery and chemotherapy may be used for palliation.

Information Box 3.1e-X

Bowel polyps and tumours: comments from a Chinese medicine perspective

In Chinese medicine, the development of polyps, and cancer within polyps, suggests Damp and Phlegm. This fits with the link between colon cancer and a high-fat diet. The sluggish bowel movements, which are common in western people, are a reflection of Stagnation of Qi, which of course can promote the accumulation of Phlegm. As is common in cases of cancer, the patient will have some long-term underlying deficiency, such as deficiency of Qi of the Spleen or Large Intestine.

Important diseases of the anus

Haemorrhoids (piles)

Haemorrhoids are fleshy swellings of the highly vascular mucous lining of the anal canal. Initially, the swellings are hidden in the anal canal (first-degree haemorrhoids) but they can enlarge and start to prolapse outside the anal margin where they are felt as soft painless fleshy protuberances. If these protuberances can easily retract back into the anal canal they are known as second-degree haemorrhoids, and if the patient has to push them back in they are classified as third-degree. Fourth-degree haemorrhoids remain permanently prolapsed and are the form most likely to require surgical repair.

Any condition that increases the pressure in the abdomen can lead to the blood vessels in the anal margin becoming distended and the loose fleshy tissue in this area swelling as a consequence. Obesity, pregnancy and a habit of straining on defecation are all contributory factors in the development of haemorrhoids.

Initially, when the bulging tissue is hidden within the anus it may not cause any problems. The most common complication of this hidden swelling is that defecation can cause the surface of the tissue to bleed, particularly if the stool is hard and difficult to pass. This leads to fresh blood dropping from the anus after a bowel motion, although the stool itself has no blood within it. Although this can be distressing for the patient, this bleeding is not a serious sign, in contrast to the sign of blood mixed in with the stools, which points to more serious diagnoses such as inflammatory bowel disease or cancer.

Prolapsing haemorrhoids (second- and third-degree) cause problems because they can be difficult to clean, and so itching can be a problematic symptom. Sometimes, small loose flaps of skin known as 'skin tags' develop close to the region of the haemorrhoid, and these can cause the same problems. Anal itch can be a very distressing problem in some patients, and may be relieved by proprietary creams which contain soothing agents, local anaesthetics and corticosteroids.

Most haemorrhoids respond to increasing dietary fibre, which ensures that the stools remain soft, and by avoidance of straining. Haemorrhoids of pregnancy usually resolve once the baby is born.

Conventional surgical treatments include injection of sclerosant chemicals to cause the excessive soft tissue to scar and shrivel, freezing and infrared coagulation of the haemorrhoid, and pinching off of regions of the haemorrhoid with rubber bands (banding). All these treatments may be performed by a specialist as outpatient procedures. In the case of fourth-degree haemorrhoids, excision surgery may be the only effective treatment option.

Occasionally, one of the blood vessels in the haemorrhoid fills with clotted blood, usually as a result of trauma. This appears as a tense, sometimes exquisitely painful purple lump at the anal margin. In most cases the intense pain caused by this thrombosed external haemorrhoid (also known as a 'perianal haematoma') will settle down, with bed rest and application of ice, within 2 weeks. In severe cases, a minor surgical operation to remove the clot will bring immediate relief.

Information Box 3.1e-XI

Haemorrhoids: comments from a Chinese medicine perspective

In Chinese medicine, haemorrhoids can be viewed as the consequence of Spleen Qi Sinking. The profuse fresh blood and itching also suggest that Heat can be a factor in their development.

Anal fissure

In contrast to haemorrhoids, which are usually painless, anal fissue is a very painful and sometimes chronic anal condition. A fissure is a crack in the anal skin that initially forms when the patient strains to pass a bowel motion. Once formed, the crack is very painful, and may not get the chance to heal because the action of opening the bowels tears it open again.

An anal fissure can result in a small amount of blood appearing after the bowel has opened. Again there is no blood mixed in with the stool.

Many fissures will heal if the patient is encouraged to make sure that the stool is softened. Laxatives can help with healing. Sometimes a minor surgical operation is required to stretch the anal sphincter muscle. This, paradoxically, can help the fissure to heal.

Information Box 3.1e-XII

Anal fissure: comments from a Chinese medicine perspective

The intense pain of a fissure suggests local Blood and Qi stagnation. Bleeding suggests the presence of Heat. There is the possibility of underlying Blood/Yin deficiency, which has caused the dry anal skin and constipated bowels.

Rectal prolapse

In rectal prolapse, the mucous lining of the rectum drops out of the anus, causing a soft moist mass to appear at the anus. This is usually a problem of frail elderly people who have poor muscle tone. It can also occur in young children.

Often the condition is temporary, but may require surgical repair because of mucus discharge and incontinence, and the tendency of the soft rectal lining to become damaged and ulcerated (see Q3.1e-5).

Information Box 3.1e-XIII

Rectal prolapse: comments from a Chinese medicine perspective

In Chinese medicine, rectal prolapse might be understood to be the result of Spleen Qi Sinking.

Red flags of the diseases of the large intestine and anus

Some patients with diseases of the large intestine and anus will benefit from referral to a conventional doctor for assessment and/or treatment. Red flags are those symptoms and signs that indicate that referral is to be considered. The red flags of the diseases of the large intestine and anus are described in Table 3.1e-II. This table forms part of the summary on red flags given in Appendix III, which also gives advice on the degree of urgency of referral for each of the red flag conditions listed.

Table 3.1e-II Red Flags 10b – diseases of the colon and anus

Red Flag	Description	Reasoning
10.2	**Diarrhoea** with **mucus and gripy pain** if not responding to treatment within a week	Persistent diarrhoea with mucus suggests either a serious episode of bowel infection or an episode of inflammatory bowel disease (Crohn's disease or ulcerative colitis) Both causes merit prompt referral for treatment
10.3	**Onset of severe abdominal pain with collapse (the acute abdomen)**. The pain can be constant or colicky (coming in waves). Rigidity, guarding and rebound tenderness are serious signs	The 'acute abdomen' refers to the combination of severe abdominal pain together with inability to continue with day-to-day activities (collapse). This syndrome can have benign causes, such as irritable bowel syndrome, dysmenorrhoea and ovulation pain. You should refer to exclude more serious possibilities, including appendicitis, perforated ulcer, peritonitis, obstructed bowel, pelvic inflammatory disease and gallstones Colicky pain indicates obstruction of a viscus (hollow organ) Rigidity of the abdomen, guarding (reflex protective spasm of the abdominal muscles) and rebound tenderness (pain felt elsewhere in the abdomen when the pressure of the palpating hand is released) all suggest inflammation or perforation of a viscus Features of abdominal pain in children that suggest a more benign (functional) cause include mild pain that is worse in the morning, location around the umbilicus, and pain that is worse with anxiety
10.4	Any episode of **blood mixed in with stools**	Red blood mixed in with stools suggests bleeding from the lower part of the small intestine, the large intestine or rectum. Possible causes are bowel infections, diverticulitis, inflammatory bowel disease (Crohn's disease or ulcerative colitis) and bowel cancer. All merit referral for investigation and treatment Blood that drips from the anus after defecation is common and is usually the result of haemorrhoids (piles). If the blood is not mixed in with the stools there is no need to refer straight away
10.6	**Altered bowel habit lasting for over 3 weeks** in someone over 50 years of age	Most people have a predictable pattern of defecation. A change in this pattern for more than 3 weeks may be a warning sign of inflammatory bowel disease or cancer. Consider referral in all those over 50 years old who develop this symptom because of the high risk of bowel cancer in this age group
10.9	**Painless lump felt in anus**	This could be a skin tag or anal warts, and possibly an anal carcinoma. Refer for diagnosis if the lump persists for more than 2 weeks
10.10	**Painful lump felt in anus**	This could be a prolapsed haemorrhoid (could be serious if the blood supply is pinched off), a perianal haematoma (benign) or an anal carcinoma. It needs referral for diagnosis if pain is severe

Self-test 3.1e

Diseases of the small intestine and colon

1. (i) What is the meaning of the term 'malabsorption'?
   (ii) What are the consequences for the patient who has malabsorption?
2. What are the general symptoms and signs of inflammatory bowel disease (i.e. those features that are common to Crohn's disease and ulcerative colitis)?
3. A patient of yours makes an urgent appointment for abdominal pain that started yesterday. When you see her she is distracted by the pain and wants to lie still. She describes the pain as coming in waves every few minutes or so. She has been sick this morning, but has had no diarrhoea. She is very reluctant for you to touch her abdomen, which feels to you unusually firm. How do you manage this situation?
4. A 45- year-old female patient has noticed gripy abdominal pain in the left iliac fossa for the past month or so. She has not previously had problems with her bowels. She describes sometimes having to rush to the toilet and sometimes being constipated. There has been no blood in the stools. She generally

feels a bit unwell, has lost a few pounds in weight, and is not making much progress with your treatment. How would you manage this case?

Answer

1. (i) Malabsorption means that the nutrients in the food cannot be absorbed via the small intestine into the bloodstream. There are a number of causes of malabsorption.
   (ii) The patient may suffer from weight loss and diarrhoea. Abdominal discomfort and bloating can occur. Anaemia will develop, as well as other signs of vitamin deficiencies.
2. The general symptoms and signs of inflammatory bowel disease result from inflammation of the bowel: the patient may feel unwell and will have profuse diarrhoea, with mucus, and gripy abdominal pain that can be so severe as to merit hospital admission. Blood can be mixed in with the stools, and the patient can become dehydrated. These symptoms may occur in bouts called 'relapses', in between which the patient can be relatively well.
3. Irrespective of the precise diagnosis, this patient has an acute abdomen, indicated by the sudden onset and severity of the pain. Her reluctance to be examined is a sign of guarding, and the abdominal firmness could reflect rigidity. You should discuss the situation with her GP on the phone straight away, or consider arranging for an ambulance. It is still reasonable to give your patient an emergency treatment whilst awaiting conventional medical help if this is feasible.
4. You should be concerned about the change in bowel habit relatively late in life. This is not typical of irritable bowel syndrome, and other possible causes, such as cancer of the colon and early inflammatory bowel disease, should be thought of. In view of the lack of response to treatment, and the fact that the patient feels unwell and has lost some weight, it would be wise to refer her with a letter to her GP so that she can have some conventional medical investigations.

3.2

The cardiovascular system

Chapter 3.2a The physiology of the cardiovascular system

LEARNING POINTS

At the end of this chapter you will be able to:

- describe the role of the cardiovascular system
- understand the structure of the heart and blood vessels
- understand the concept of blood pressure
- compare and contrast some conventional and Chinese medicine interpretations of the functions of the vessels, the heart and the pericardium.

Estimated time for chapter: Part I, 60 minutes; Part II, 60 minutes.

Introduction

This section of Stage 3 focuses on the cardiovascular system, also known as the 'circulatory system'. Like Chapter 3.1a, this chapter is divided into two parts. If you are using this book as a study course, then, because of its length, you are advised to work through the two sections of this chapter in separate study sessions.

Part I – The vessels and the heart organ

The cardiovascular system consists of all those structures that have the role of transporting the blood to all parts of the body. The cardiovascular system enables the blood to perform its roles of protection, providing nutrients, and removal of toxins for all the body tissues.

The cardiovascular system can be considered in terms of two main parts, the blood vessels and the heart, and these are explored in turn in this chapter. The vessels are the channels through which the blood flows. The three main types of blood vessel are the arteries, the veins and the capillaries. The heart is the pump that provides the power to create the flow of blood through the vessels.

Sometimes the lymphatic system first referred to in Chapter 2.1d, is also included as part of the cardiovascular system. However, in this book, for the sake of clarity, the lymphatic system is treated as a separate system.

The blood (haematological system) is not conventionally considered to be a part of the cardiovascular system. The blood is described in Section 3.4.

Very simplistically speaking, a typical conventional practitioner might view the cardiovascular system as a fleshy pump, albeit a rather complex one, which is linked up to a series of soft-tissue pipes. Although emotions, and stress in particular, are recognised in modern medicine to have a bearing on the function of the cardiovascular system, the heart and vessels do not have any of the deep emotional correlations that they are ascribed in Chinese medicine and other holistic complementary medical disciplines. For example, a modern heart surgeon may not necessarily consider the part that love plays in the life of a patient to have anything to do with the task of improving the function of that patient's heart. In contrast, a holistic practitioner is much more likely to be interested in how a person's relationships and zest for life are linked to the health and function of the Heart Organ.

The blood vessels

The 'vascular system' is the term used to describe the vessels alone. It consists of a network of tubes lined with endothelium (a form of epithelial tissue). These tubes are at their widest as they leave the heart, and then divide, like the branches of a tree, to form thousands of tiny capillaries within the tissues. The capillaries then meet up again to form wider and wider tubes, which return the blood back to the heart.

Blood vessels that lead blood away from the heart are called 'arteries' and those that lead blood back again to the heart from the tissues are called 'veins'. 'Arterioles' and 'venules' are the names given to the smallest types of arteries and veins.

Arteries

One major characteristic of arteries is that they contain muscle and an elastic material called 'elastin' in their wall, which means that they have the capacity to contract and expand. As a result of the muscle in the arterial walls, arteries can alter the flow of blood to an area of the body by altering in width. This is a very important concept to grasp in preparation for learning about blood pressure later in this chapter.

The blood in arteries is under high pressure because it has just been pumped from the heart. This is why a severed artery will spurt blood in pulses. It is from the arteries, and not the veins, that a Chinese medical practitioner can sense the state of Blood and Qi when 'taking the pulse'.

One important disease of arteries, arterial thrombosis, has already been described in this text (Chapter 2.2d).

Veins

An important feature of veins is that they contain valves. The blood within the veins is under much lower pressure than that in the arteries, and the valves ensure that the flow of blood back to the heart remains one-way. Veins rely on the pumping action of the muscles to aid in the movement of blood back to the heart. This is partly why sedentary people may develop swollen ankles at the end of the day, as fluid accumulates in the tissues of the lower parts of the body.

One important potentially life-threatening venous disease, deep vein thrombosis, has already been described (Chapter 2.2d). The more common and benign condition of varicose veins is described later in this section (Chapter 3.2d).

Capillaries

Capillaries are minute vessels with walls that are only one cell thick. A significant characteristic of capillaries is that they enable the rapid transfer of nutrients, gases and waste products to and from the blood across their very thin walls.

Capillaries were introduced in Chapter 2.2b, where inflammation was described. In inflammation, the gaps between the cells in the capillary wall widen, making the capillaries leaky (see Q3.2a-1).

The transfer of nutrients from capillaries to the tissues

Healthy blood that has just passed through the digestive system will contain a high concentration of basic nutrients, including simple sugars, cholesterol, triglycerides, fatty acids, amino acids from proteins, vitamins and minerals (see Chapter 3.1a for a reminder of the origin of the basic nutrients and how they are processed by the digestive system). Once the blood has passed through the capillaries of the lungs, it will also contain a high concentration of oxygen. Chapter 1.1b explained how oxygen is one of the essential ingredients which, together with glucose and other simple nutrients, is used by the mitochondria of every cell in the body to produce the energy required for many vital cellular processes.

The body relies on the transport processes of diffusion, osmosis and active transport for nutrients and oxygen to enter the bloodstream from the tissues of the digestive system and the lung. These processes are described in detail in Chapter 1.1c.

Oxygen, simple sugars, fatty acids, vitamins and minerals all pass with ease through the single-celled wall of the capillary by diffusion. The movement is particularly rapid when it is from a region in which these nutrients are in high concentration to one in which there is a low concentration. For both oxygen in the lungs and nutrients in the tissues of the digestive system this movement occurs so that these substances readily enter the circulating fluid component of the blood, the plasma.

Conversely, when the nutrient and oxygen rich plasma reaches other tissues in which the concentration of nutrients and oxygen may be relatively low, the nutrients and oxygen tend to move out of the blood and into the tissues. This transfer of nutrients from digested food in the intestines and of air from the lungs into the tissues happens within a few seconds. Because diffusion is a spontaneous process, this transfer is incredibly energy efficient, requiring no extra energy over that required by the heart to pump the blood.

In addition to this energy-efficient transfer of oxygen and nutrients into the tissues, another wonderful aspect of the process of diffusion is that it underpins the movement of waste products out of the tissues. As waste products, such as urea from protein metabolism and carbon dioxide from respiration, build up in the tissues, the tendency is for them to move back into the bloodstream, where they are kept at a relatively low concentration. The waste products can then be carried to the liver, kidneys, sweat glands and lungs, each of which is specially adapted to remove otherwise toxic by-products from the body (see Q3.2a-2).

Similarly, water moves into and out of the plasma with ease. In this case, the process is called 'osmosis'. This is the term used to describe the movement of water from a region in which it is part of a dilute solution to one in which it is part of a more concentrated solution. This is the means by which water will move from a vase into a wilted (dehydrated) flower stem. In the same way, by osmosis, water will enter the plasma from the tissues if the plasma is more concentrated than the tissue fluid. Conversely, If the plasma is relatively well hydrated, water will move out of the plasma into the tissues. This is another very energy-efficient mechanism, and it ensures that water is transported from the digestive system to the tissues that need it.

The 'desire' for water to move from a region of low concentration to one of high concentration is described in scientific terms as 'osmotic pressure'. This pressure relates directly to the difference in concentration between two regions, and so to the tendency that water will have to move between these regions. When the osmotic pressure is high (e.g. in a dehydrated plant stem), a lot of water can be encouraged to move (in this case against the downward pull of gravity and into the stem). Thus, in the body, if a dehydrated person drinks some water, there will be a rapid movement of water from the digestive system, through the plasma and into the dehydrated tissues, all under the 'pull' of the increased osmotic pressure of the concentrated tissue fluids.

One other factor needs to be considered in this description of the movement of nutrients into and out of the bloodstream, and this is the effect of the physical pressure of fluid in the vessels. Just as air in an inflated tyre is under a measurable degree of pressure (which is what makes the tyre feel inflated), so is the blood in a blood vessel under a degree of pressure. In the blood vessels the internal pressure varies according to the proximity to the heart. Arteries close to the heart contain blood that is being pumped by muscular contractions of the heart, and this blood is therefore under significant pressure. As the arteries branch into more and more numerous smaller vessels the pressure within them gradually decreases, so that at the start of the capillary bed the pressure is much lower. Nevertheless, at the arterial end of the capillaries the pressure is still sufficient to force some fluid through the gaps between the cells of the capillary walls and into the tissues. This can be compared visually to squeezing an inflated bicycle tube punctured with numerous tiny holes; the greater the pressure applied, the more air that is able to escape through the holes. However, unlike the air escaping from a squeezed and punctured bicycle tube, the tendency for water to move out of the blood vessels by physical pressure is countered by the tendency of fluid to stay in the blood vessels under osmotic pressure. In health, a delicate balance between the two forces is established, ensuring that the tissues remain perfectly hydrated, becoming neither too dry nor too waterlogged.

It is worth remembering for the present that just under half of the volume of the blood is made up of blood cells that are too large to move between the gaps in the capillaries. A good proportion of the composition of the remaining plasma consists of dissolved protein molecules, which are also too large to pass through the gaps in the capillaries. Therefore, the movement of fluid across capillary membranes is selective for the remaining small molecules, such as water itself, salt and sugars. This is the property of semipermeability, as first described in Chapter 1.1c.

An understanding of these forces that affect the movement of fluid between the blood and the tissues is a helpful foundation for the study of the important condition of oedema, which is described in Chapter 3.2f (see Q3.2a-3).

To summarise, the balance of these forces is such that the net movement of fluid is out of the capillaries at the arterial end and into the capillaries at the venous end. This is ideal to suit the body's needs. It means that nutrients and oxygen tend to move out into the tissue fluid from the arterial end, and wastes and carbon dioxide tend to move into the venous end of the capillaries. This is how the blood 'deposits' its nutrients into the cells that need them and transports away the wastes from the tissues at the capillaries (see Q3.2a-4 and Q3.2a-5).

The pathway of the arteries

Figure 3.2a-I illustrates the pathway of the major arteries that lead away from the heart. The diagram shows how the blood is directed from the heart to all parts of the body. The arch of the largest blood vessel in the body, the aorta, is shown leaving the top of the heart and then descending to run deep in the body, through the diaphragm to the pelvis. Here, it splits into two main branches, which supply blood to each leg.

Information Box 3.2a-I

The vessels: comments from a Chinese medicine perspective

Maciocia (1989) states that, in *The Simple Questions* (*Suwen*), the vessels are said to be controlled by the Heart, but adds that the Lungs also control circulation of Blood in the vessels because of their role in Governing the circulation of Qi throughout the body.

One of the Chinese medicine functions of the Lungs is to inhale 'pure Qi' and to exhale 'dirty Qi '. The pure Clear Qi (air) combines with Gu Qi (food) to form Gathering (Zong) Qi in the chest. True (Zhen) Qi is a further refinement of Gathering Qi and Original Qi, which also arises in the chest. The Lung then enables the dispersion of this Qi in its dual form of Nutritive (Ying) Qi and Defensive (Wei) Qi to the whole of the body. Therefore, the Lungs are important for the generation of essential energy throughout the whole of the body.

This makes an interesting comparison with the conventional medicine interpretation that the vessels permit the transportation of nutrients and oxygen to all the tissues and thus facilitate the production of cellular energy from these 'ingredients' in the mitochondria present in all cells of the body. This is very much in keeping with the Chinese medicine association of the vessels with the Lung Organ.

Figure 3.2a.II shows how the major branches of the aorta in the neck, the common carotid arteries, branch to supply blood to the head. One branch, the internal carotid artery, divides to enter the skull and supply the brain with blood (see Q3.2a-6).

Now turn back to Figure 3.2a-I, which shows how arterial branches from the aorta divide down each limb to take blood to the hands and the feet. Compare this with Figure 3.2a-III, which shows the pathways of the veins that return the blood to the heart, ending in two major vessels called the 'superior vena cava' and 'inferior vena cava'. Note how the basic pathways of the veins mirror those of the arteries. This is the pattern for almost all parts of the body, in that an artery delivering blood to a body part runs very close to the vein that is draining the blood away from that part.

The main difference between the positions of arteries and veins is that some veins tend to run closer to the surface of the body, whereas arteries generally lie much deeper. The veins that run close to the surface are called 'superficial veins'. All the blue-coloured vessels that can be seen through the skin in areas such as the back of the hand, the crooks of the elbows and the neck are superficial veins, not arteries. If these vessels are palpated, no pulse will be felt, and it will be found that they are very easy to compress.

In addition to superficial veins, there is also a system of 'deep veins'. The blood draining from the surface of the body runs first into the superficial veins, and then enters the deep veins through vessels that penetrate the deeper tissues called 'perforators'. It is important to be clear about the distinction between superficial and deep veins in order to understand the pathology of the condition of varicose veins, described in Chapter 3.2c.

Figure 3.2a-I • The pathway of the arteries from the heart.

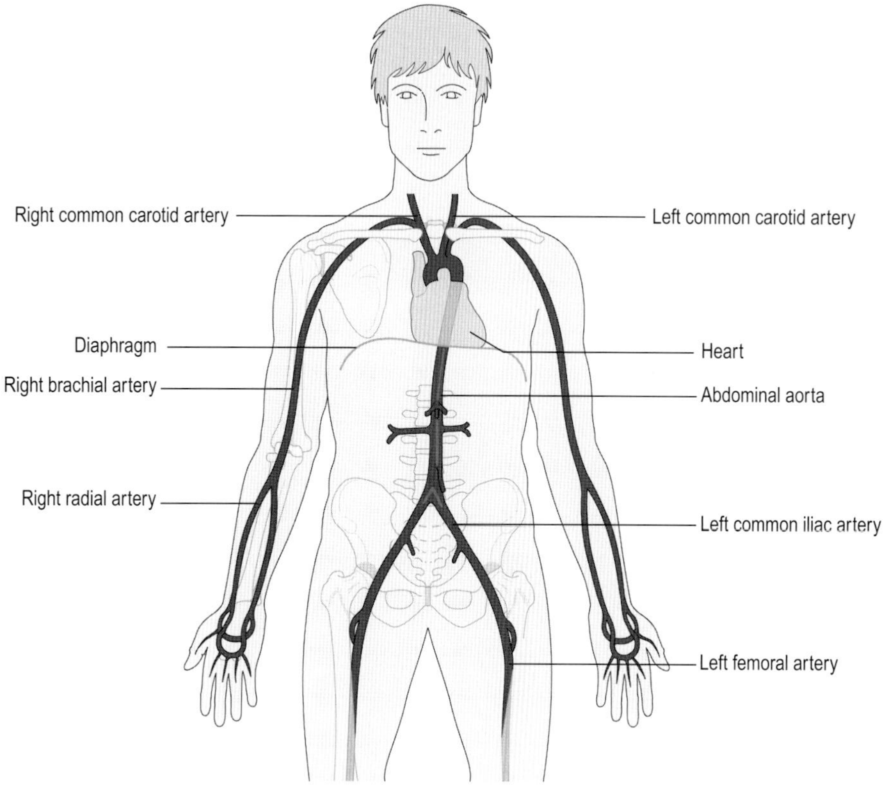

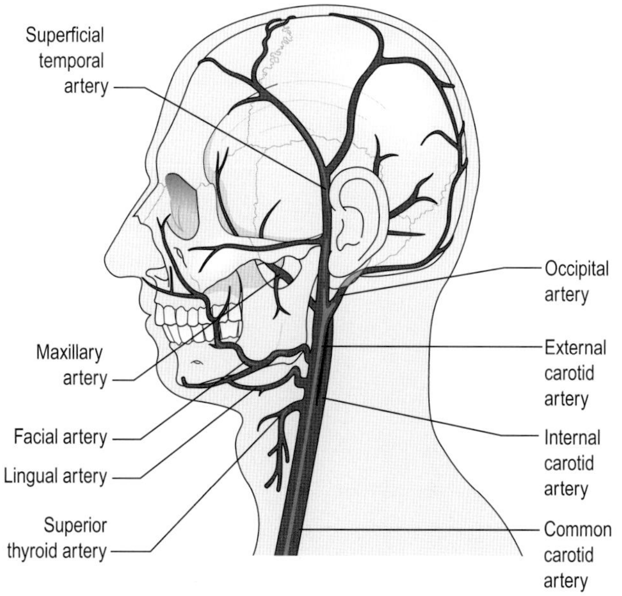

Figure 3.2a-II • The pathway of the left common carotid artery.

The structure of the heart

The heart is a fist-sized organ that sits just to the left of midline in the chest (see Figure 3.2a-I). It is situated between the two lungs, and together these organs fill the space that overlies the diaphragm (the thoracic cavity; Figure 3.2a-IV). These organs are so closely related that the inside surfaces of the lungs bears the impression of the shape of the heart upon them.

The heart is largely made up of cardiac muscle (the myocardium), and is divided into four chambers. It might be helpful now to turn back to the description of the tissue types given in Chapter 1.2d for a reminder of the characteristics of cardiac muscle, and how the cardiac muscle cells communicate with each other through specialised 'joints' (see Q3.2a-7).

The healthy heart is lined with endocardium, a smooth epithelial tissue lining that is continuous with the lining of the blood vessels. The outside of the heart is protected by a tough fibrous sac called the 'pericardium'. In between the pericardium and the heart organ is a very small space containing fluid. This fluid lubricates the movement between the heart and the pericardium, and contains immune cells. The remainder of the organ consists of the naturally contractile myocardium (see Q3.2a-8).

To understand the action and some of the structural disorders of the heart, it is important to understand that the heart is divided into two halves: the right half deals with the flow of the blood from the body and to the lungs, and the left half deals with the flow of the blood from the lungs and to the body. Each half has two chambers known as the 'atria' (plural of 'atrium') and the 'ventricles', and together these form the four chambers of the heart. There are two valves situated in each half of the heart. Their function is to ensure that the blood flow is always one way. Figure 3.2a-V illustrates the position and shape of the four chambers and the valves of the heart, and the direction of blood flow through the two halves of the heart.

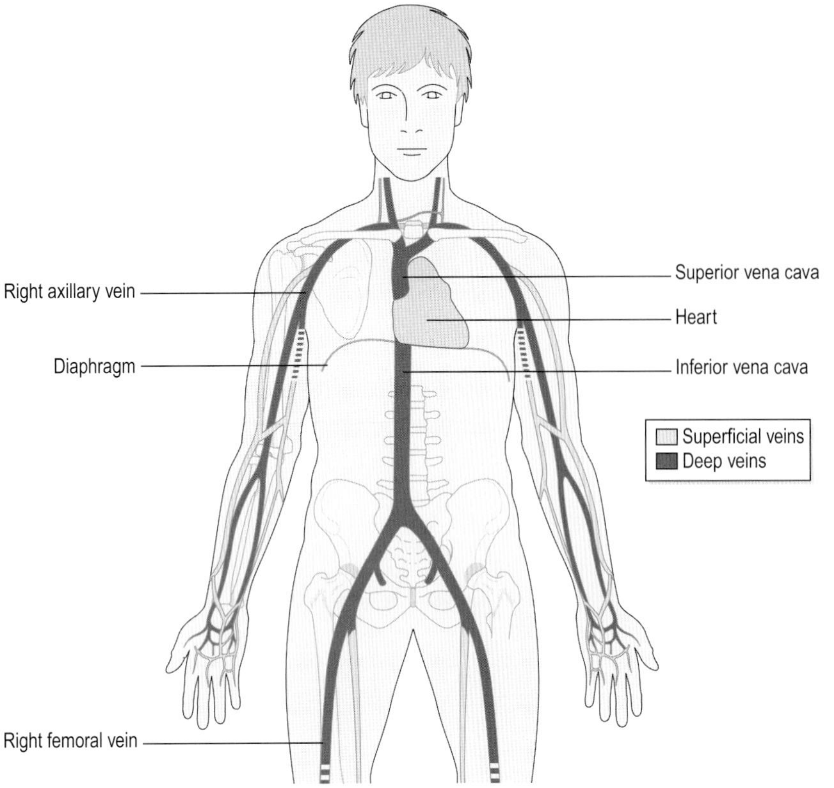

Figure 3.2a-III • The pathway of the veins leading back to the heart.

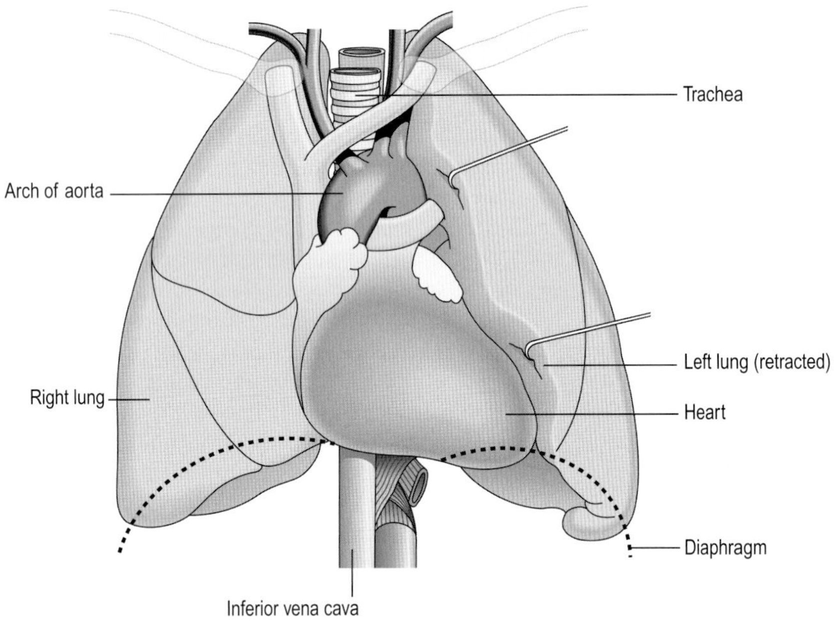

Figure 3.2a-IV • The organs associated with the heart in the thoracic cavity.

The flow of blood through the heart

The double structure of the heart means that blood can flow through the heart twice in each full circulation of the body. It might help when reading the following description of the flow of the blood to use Figure 3.2a-V to visually trace the pathway the blood takes.

The flow of blood through the right side of the heart

Blood returning from most of the tissues of the body enters the right atrium of the heart from the two large veins, the superior and inferior vena cavae. This blood has given up its oxygen and is carrying relatively high levels of waste products

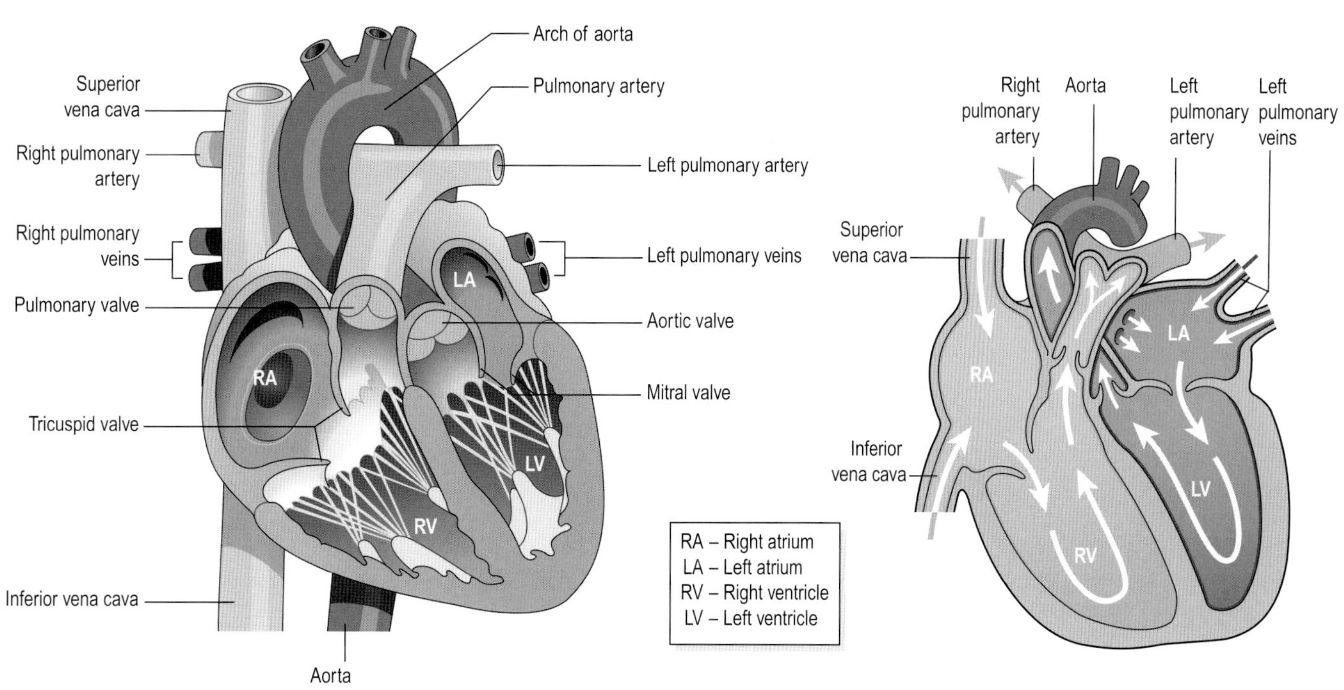

Figure 3.2a-V • The interior of the heart and its blood flow.

such as carbon dioxide and urea. The right atrium contracts to forces the blood through the tricuspid valve, and thus into the right ventricle. The right ventricle then contracts, and this forces the blood through the pulmonary valve into the pulmonary artery. The pressure of blood in the contracting right ventricle closes the tricuspid valve, making a very subtle clapping noise. The blood rushing into the pulmonary artery does not flow back into the right ventricle when it finishes its contraction as the pulmonary valve also closes in turn, making its own clapping noise as it does so. The blood entering the pulmonary artery then passes into a concentrated network of capillaries within the tissue of the lungs.

The flow of blood through the left side of the heart

When blood has passed though the capillary network of the lungs, it has given up its carbon dioxide and is rich in oxygen, all through the effortless process of diffusion (see Chapter 3.3a for more detail about the structure of the blood vessels in the lungs). This oxygen-rich blood is a brighter shade of red than the darker venous blood. It flows through the pulmonary vein and into the left atrium of the heart. The left atrium contracts to force the blood through the mitral valve, and thus into the muscular left ventricle. The left ventricle then contracts, and this forces the blood through the aortic valve into the arch of the aorta, the widest part of the widest blood vessel in the body. The pressure of the blood in the contracting right ventricle closes the mitral valve, also making a subtle clapping noise. Just as was described for blood leaving the right ventricle, blood rushing into the aorta does not flow back into the left ventricle when it finishes its contraction. This is because the aortic valve also closes in turn, making its own clapping noise as it does so.

It might be appreciated from this description that the flow of the blood in the body can be compared to a figure-of-eight, with the heart situated at the crossing point of the lines of the eight. In this delicate but powerful pumping system, both the right and the left heart contract together in a single heartbeat. This results in a double pumping action, which means that the pulse of flow of blood within the lungs and body occurs at exactly the same time, and the clapping of the four valves closing in turn makes the heart sounds that are audible by means of a stethoscope.

In summary, it is important to understand that the route of the flow of blood through the two halves of the heart is as follows:

- oxygenated blood from the lungs enters the left heart
- the left heart pumps oxygenated blood to all the tissues of the body
- tissues absorb oxygen so that the blood becomes deoxygenated
- deoxygenated blood from the body returns to the right heart
- the right heart pumps deoxygenated blood to the lungs
- blood absorbs oxygen from the lungs so that it becomes oxygenated
- oxygenated blood from the lungs enters the left heart ... and so on (see Q3.2a-9).

The blood supply to the heart

It might appear surprising that the heart itself requires a blood supply. However, the heart muscle is working continuously for a full lifetime and requires a consistent supply of oxygen and nutrients. These high demands cannot be met by the blood flowing through the chambers of the heart alone.

Figure 3.2a-VI illustrates how vessels, known as the 'coronary arteries' ('cor' is the Latin root meaning 'heart'), branch

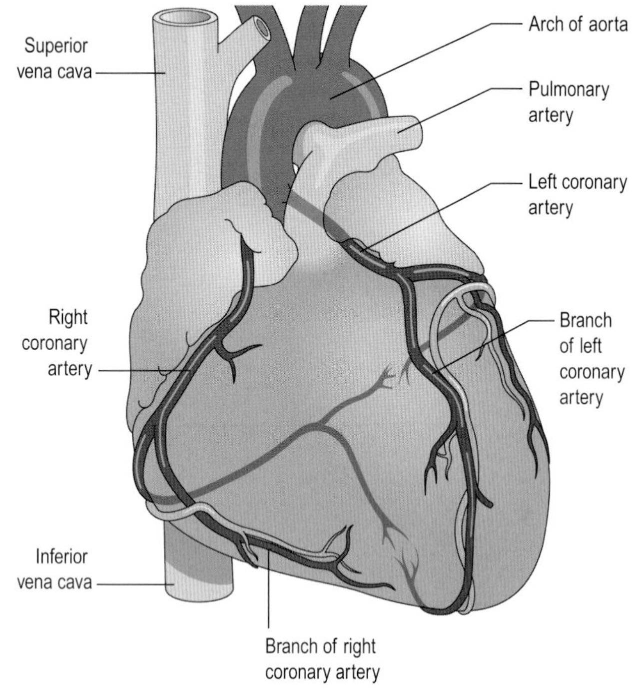

Figure 3.2a-VI • The blood supply to the heart.

from their origin at the aorta to wrap around the heart muscle. An understanding of this blood supply will be good preparation for the study of coronary heart disease (Chapter 3.2e) which is the most important cause of death, after cancer, in developed countries.

The conduction system of the heart

The conduction system of the heart is what enables the heart to contract in such a way that a wave of contraction moves from the top of the heart to the tip (apex). This means that the blood within the heart is pumped smoothly through the two chambers of the two sides.

The conduction system consists of strands of specialised cardiac muscle cells, which run from a specialised 'node' situated in the wall between the atria in the upper part of the heart. These cells branch out from this region to connect to all parts of the heart muscle. This node (more specifically known as the 'sinoatrial node') is the heart's own 'pacemaker'. The cells of this pacemaker have an internal rhythm, giving them the property of being able to contract at a rate of just over once every second. Because of the joints between cardiac cells, the contraction of the cells in the pacemaker can stimulate the contraction of neighbouring cells in the conduction system, and so on until the whole heart muscle has contracted.

Various factors can affect the rate at which the pacemaker cells contract, which explains why people can be aware of changes in their heart rate from time to time. The most important factor is the nerve supply to the heart. The nerve supply to the heart is part of the autonomic nervous system (described in more detail in Stage 4.1). The autonomic nervous system plays an essential role in the maintenance of homeostasis in the body, and very probably in the mechanism of many of the effects of acupuncture. For the time being, all that need be understood about this system is that it deals with the control of the involuntary aspects of the function of the body, such as breathing, digestion and sweating. It is conventionally seen as two opposing systems; the sympathetic nervous system (SNS) and the parasympathetic nervous system (PNS). Most parts of the body are under the influence of both these systems.

In the heart, the sympathetic nerves cause the pacemaker to contract more rapidly, and the heart muscle to contract more forcefully (in Chinese medicine this would be interpreted as a Yang response). The parasympathetic nerves cause the pacemaker to contract more slowly, and the heart muscle to contract less forcefully (a Yin response) (see Q3.2a-10).

Emotional states, such as fear and anxiety, and exercise all lead to an increased heart rate as a result of activation of the sympathetic nervous system. Other factors that contribute to a relatively increased heart rate include body temperature, being female and young age (infancy and childhood).

The generation of the pulse

The pulse wave, which is of interest to practitioners both of Chinese medicine and conventional medicine, is a direct consequence of the rhythmic pumping of the heart. As blood is forced through the chambers of the heart by the wave of contraction from the base to the apex of the heart, the arteries that leave the heart bulge with the increased amount of blood that has been forced into them, and this distension is propagated down the length of the major arteries. Arteries are elastic vessels that can stretch, but are not flaccid. This bulging is felt on palpation at any artery as a pushing outward of the vessel wall, known as the 'pulse'.

When conventional medicine practitioners assess the pulse they use quite firm pressure. In this way they can feel the physical force of the blood in the artery. Practitioners of Chinese medicine apply very little pressure to assess the pulse. This is because they are less concerned with the physical force of the blood and more with the energetics of the vital substances of Blood and Qi, which move with the physical blood (see Q3.2a-11).

The heart sounds

Practitioners of conventional medicine use a stethoscope to listen to the heart sounds. In a healthy person, the heart sounds are like the familiar repeated 'lub-dub' used so often to heighten emotion in televised hospital dramas. As mentioned previously, the heart sounds are produced by the heart valves closing as the blood is forced through them. In each chamber, one valve closes before the other, thus producing the 'lub-dub' sound.

Different conditions of the heart lead to very subtle changes in these sounds. A valve that does not close properly will give a muffled sound as blood leaks through it, and this is known as a 'murmur'. In conventional medicine, the ability to use a stethoscope to interpret these changes in detail is considered a skill that requires many years of practice.

Part II – The blood pressure and the Chinese medical view

The blood pressure

The blood pressure is simply a measure of the force that the bulge of blood in the arteries exerts on the walls of the arteries. Blood pressure can be assessed approximately by palpation of the artery. An artery that feels very tense during the pulse can reflect a high blood pressure, whereas a weak, flaccid pulse can reflect a low blood pressure.

The blood pressure oscillates up and down during the heartbeat. When the heart reaches the peak of contraction, the blood pressure also reaches a peak, and this is called the 'systolic blood pressure'. When the heart relaxes after its contraction, the blood pressure drops down to its lowest point, the 'diastolic blood pressure'. When a conventional doctor palpates the force of the pulse, information about the difference between systolic (peak) and diastolic (trough) pressure can also be obtained.

Adequate blood pressure is essential to ensure a steady flow of nutrients to all parts of the body. In times of physical stress the blood pressure rises, but this is appropriate to the body's needs. It is only if the blood pressure remains at too high a level for the body's requirements for too long that long-term damage to the circulatory system can occur. The condition of high blood pressure (hypertension) is explored in more detail in Chapter 3.2d.

Two important factors combine to affect the blood pressure. The first is the amount of blood being pumped by the heart at any one time. A rapid and forceful heartbeat will lead to a higher blood pressure than a slow and relaxed heartbeat. A frightening experience or strenuous exercise will both temporarily put up the blood pressure, as they both lead to an increased and more forceful heart rate.

The second factor that increases the blood pressure is the amount of tension in the muscles of the artery walls. If the artery walls are tightly constricted, then the pressure of the blood being forced through them will be raised. There are many factors that cause the artery walls to constrict. One familiar cause is extreme cold, which causes the small arteries in the skin to constrict. This leads to cold flesh, numbness and a bluish discoloration. This is an important reflex in the body, because it means that the heat of the blood is not lost so readily from the skin, and is kept deep in the interior where it is vital for the effective function of the organs.

It is important for homeostasis that the blood pressure remains generally within a certain range. It has been found that most healthy individuals have comparable ranges of blood pressure. Young people tend to have lower blood pressures than older people, and women tend to have lower blood pressures than men.

Control of blood pressure

It now might be appreciated that the blood pressure has to be responsive to a wide range of conditions, which include emotional stress, exercise, pain and blood volume.

As with the heart rate, the most important system that controls the blood pressure is the autonomic nervous system. The muscles within the small artery walls are supplied by sympathetic nerves, and thus it is the sympathetic nervous system (SNS) that deals with increasing the heart rate. In the small blood vessels, the sympathetic nerves, when activated, lead to constriction. Conditions such as emotional stress, exercise, pain and loss of blood volume activate the SNS and lead to constriction of the vessels (see Q3.2a-12).

Two of the many chemicals that are integral to the activation of the SNS are the hormones adrenaline and noradrenaline. A release of adrenaline from the adrenal glands will lead to an increased heart rate, constriction of the artery walls and an increase in blood pressure. This is explained in more detail in Section 5.1 (see Q3.2a-13).

When the SNS is not activated, the action of the parasympathetic nervous system (PNS) becomes dominant. In this situation, the heart rate slows down, the blood vessels relax and the blood pressure drops. A faint often occurs as a result of a strong emotional response to a shock (different to fear) or even to excessive joy. This has the effect of activating the PNS. The result of this is that the heart rate suddenly slows and the blood pressure drops. This leads to a sudden drop in the supply of blood and nutrients to the brain, and the person will feel dizzy and may very briefly lose consciousness. However, the act of fainting, and the drop in blood pressure that accompanies it, then stimulates the SNS, which immediately reverses the situation. A hallmark of a faint is that the person very quickly begins to regain consciousness (within seconds) as the blood pressure rises and the blood supply returns to the brain.

This is also what occurs when a person receiving acupuncture experiences needle shock, which very occasionally occurs during a first treatment. Although alarming for the practitioner, this type of faint is usually nothing to worry about, as long as the patient starts to regain consciousness immediately.

Measurement of blood pressure

Although blood pressure can be roughly assessed by palpation of the pulse, the way to obtain a reliable numerical measure of the blood pressure is by means of an instrument called the 'sphygmomanometer'. This consists of an inflatable fabric cuff, which is wrapped around a limb, usually the upper arm, and a device to measure the pressure within the cuff.

The pressure can be assessed by a simple manually operated pressure gauge, similar to those used to measure car-tyre pressure, in which case the equipment is called an 'aneroid sphygmomanometer'. Increasingly, in medical settings an 'oscillometric' assessment is made, which involves a digitally processed result drawn from the mean arterial pressure. This requires an automated digital sphygmomanometer. The British Hypertension Society currently recommends a wide range of oscillometric models for reliable assessment of blood pressure.

However, for accurate measurement, many doctors still consider the bulky mercury-containing sphygmomanometer to provide the gold standard for measurement. For this reason, the numerical value of blood pressure is conventionally expressed in millimetres of mercury (mmHg). A normal systolic pressure falls within the range 100–140 mmHg, and a normal diastolic pressure falls within the range 65–90 mmHg. The blood pressure is expressed as a combination of these two values. For example, a blood pressure of 120/80 mmHg ('120 over 80') would be considered to be a normal blood pressure, and one of 150/105 mmHg would be considered to be a high (albeit only moderately raised) blood pressure.

In blood pressure assessment the cuff is inflated to a pressure high enough to totally compress the arteries within the limb. This will be equivalent to a pressure higher than the systolic pressure, and can be in the range of 200–250 mmHg. At this pressure the compression of the artery leads to a total cessation of blood flow through the artery, and the pulse can no longer be felt or picked up by an oscillometer. This stage is often uncomfortable for the patient, but this level of pressure should be maintained only for a moment.

In aneroid assessment, a stethoscope is placed over the artery that is distal to the cuff. This is usually at the brachial artery, the pulse of which can be palpated at the elbow (in the region of the acupoint Quze PC-3). The pressure in the cuff is then gradually reduced. As the pressure in the cuff falls to that of the systolic pressure, squirts of blood can be forced through the now partially compressed artery. This is heard as a pulsatile rushing noise through the stethoscope. The systolic pressure is recorded as the pressure of the cuff when the rushing noises are first heard.

As the pressure in the cuff is reduced further to close to the diastolic pressure, more and more blood can pass through the brachial artery. As the blood flows more easily, the rushing noises become increasingly soft. When the pressure in the cuff reaches the diastolic pressure, all the blood can pass freely through the vessel and the sounds disappear altogether. The diastolic pressure is recorded as the pressure of the cuff when the rushing noises stop altogether.

The British Hypertension Society has written guidelines for health professionals on how to take accurate blood pressure measurements and how to treat high blood pressure. These guidelines ask for careful repeated measurements, although this ideal may be rarely achieved in real practice because of time constraints. However, this is not a trivial issue; an inaccurate measurement will lead to a false assumption about the true level of blood pressure, and can lead to inappropriate treatment.

The 2004 British Hypertension Society Guideline (IV) states that the patient should be seated and should be relaxed. The arm should be resting on a surface so that it is at the level of the heart. The cuff pressure should be deflated very slowly (no more than 2 mmHg per second) so that the rushing sounds can be accurately matched with the cuff pressure. The blood pressure measurement should be repeated after 1–2 minutes and the first reading discarded. If more readings are taken then the mean of these readings should be calculated to give the final measurement.

This description of blood pressure assessment has been given in detail because many complementary therapists routinely assess the blood pressure of their patients.

Information Box 3.2a-II

The heart and pericardium: comments from a Chinese medicine perspective

In Chinese medicine, the Heart and Pericardium are Organs to which specific functions are ascribed, and which are represented on the exterior of the body by the Heart and Pericardium channels, respectively.

Maciocia (1989) again quotes *The Simple Questions* (*Suwen*) when outlining the Chinese medicine view that the Heart is 'like the Monarch and it governs the mind'. He lists the six functions of the Heart Organ, which are to:

- govern Blood
- control the blood vessels
- manifest in the complexion
- house the mind (Shen)
- open into the tongue
- control sweat.

For those who may be familiar with Chinese medicine categorisation, it can help develop clarity of thought to consider each of these in turn, and reflect how the Chinese view compares with a conventional medicine perspective.

First, in this categorisation government of Blood refers to two aspects: the transformation of Food (Gu Qi) into Blood, and also the healthy circulation of Blood. By contrast, in conventional medicine the manufacture of blood from basic nutrients takes place largely in the bone marrow, although the healthy circulation of blood is, of course, recognised as the domain of the cardiovascular system.

As explained earlier, control of the blood vessels is linked to two organs in Chinese medicine:, the Heart and the Lungs. This partly refers to maintenance of healthy vessels, and is a reflection of healthy Gathering (Zong) Qi made by the Lung Organ from food (Gu Qi) and 'air'. In conventional medicine terms, the health of the blood vessels results from a healthy cardiovascular system, and does not obviously relate to the lungs. However, it is interesting to reflect that arteriosclerosis, a major cause of vascular (vessel) disease in the western world, is the result of an activity that directly damages the lungs, namely smoking.

The complexion is conventionally considered to be a reflection of the health of the skin rather than the heart. However, in conventional medicine it is recognised that certain cardiovascular conditions can cause signs that appear on the face. Malar flush, the pink coloration of the cheekbone area, is one example. This finding, considered an indication of Yin Deficiency in Chinese medicine, is, in a florid form, a medically recognised sign of the valvular heart disease known as mitral stenosis.

The mind/spirit is not associated with the cardiovascular system at all in conventional medicine. However, the English language reveals that in western culture a deep connection has been made between the heart and the emotions. Phrases such as 'my heart isn't in it', 'to be heartbroken', 'he was heartless' and 'have a heart!' (to name only a very few) are evidence of this connection. In many older cultures the heart is integral to the concept of mind and thought.

The tongue and speech are also not associated with the cardiovascular system in conventional medicine, although one of the signs of severe heart disease is recognised to be cyanosis, in which a bluish discoloration is seen on the lips and tongue. There is also some recognition that aphasia is a frequent component of shock, which can manifest in other heart-related symptoms.

Sweating is not directly linked to the cardiovascular system from a conventional medicine perspective.

The functions of the Heart according to a conventional and Chinese perspective can be summarised in the form of a correspondence table (for an introduction to the Organ correspondence tables, see Appendix I). This table illustrates the idea that the functions of the fleshy pump, which conventional medicine calls the heart, may be the domain of not only the Heart Organ in Chinese Medicine, but also the Kidney and Liver Organs. It will follow from this that diseases of the conventionally viewed cardiovascular system may manifest in Chinese medicine syndromes involving the Heart, Kidney and Liver Organs.

Correspondence table for the functions of the Heart as described by conventional and Chinese medicine

Functions of the heart

- Acts as a pulsatile pump to enable circulation of the blood (**Heart and Liver Organs**)
- The origin of the heart muscle impulse (the pacemaker) (**Heart Organ**)
- Contributes to the maintenance of blood pressure (**Heart Organ and Kidney Yang**)
- Will respond to bodily requirements by an alteration in the strength and rate of pumping (**Heart Organ and Kidney Yang**)

Functions of the Heart Organ[1]

'The Heart is like the monarch and it governs the mind'

- It governs blood (**bone marrow, heart, blood vessels**)
- It controls the blood vessels (**blood vessels, adrenal glands, autonomic nervous system**)
- It manifests in the complexion (**heart, blood vessels, blood, skin**)
- It houses the mind (**brain**)
- It opens into the tongue (**digestive system**)
- It controls sweat (**skin, autonomic nervous system**)

[1]Maciocia G 1989 The foundations of Chinese medicine. Churchill Livingstone, Edinburgh.

The Pericardium Organ in the Chinese medicine tradition is loosely associated with the more superficial layers of the heart organ, the fibrous pericardium and the myocardium (Larre et al 1986). The function of the Pericardium (Heart Protector) is similar to that of the Heart, but it also has the particular function of protection of the Heart against external pathogenic influences. This has some overlap with the conventional medicine view in which the pericardium and the fluid which that lies between it and the myocardium are very much seen as providing mechanical and immunological protection. In addition, there is the broader role, together with the Kidneys and Triple Burner Organs, of being associated with the Gate of Vitality (Ming Men). The Pericardium has been linked to the role of the sympathetic nervous system.

Correspondence table for the functions of the Pericardium as described by conventional and Chinese medicine

Functions of the pericardium

- It is a fibrous membrane that surrounds the heart and allows its free movement. It also protects from mechanical injury. The serous fluid it encloses contains protective antibodies and immune cells (**Heart, Liver and Kidney Organs**)

Functions of the Pericardium[1]

'The Pericardium is an ambassador and from it joy and happiness derive'

- Like the Heart it governs blood (**bone marrow, heart, blood vessels**)
- Like the Heart it houses the mind (**brain**)
- Together with the Kidneys and Triple Burner Organs it has been associated with the Gate of Vitality (Ming Men) (possibly the healthy function of the **metabolic processes** that go on in all the cells and particularly the **sympathetic nervous system**)

[1]Maciocia G 1989 The foundations of Chinese medicine. Churchill Livingstone, Edinburgh.

Self-test 3.2a

The physiology of the cardiovascular system

1. What are the broad differences between arteries and veins?
2. How does the structure of capillaries suit their function?
3. Why do you think the circulation flows as a figure-of-eight, with the heart at the cross of the eight shape?
4. What do you think might be the result if one of the three major coronary arteries suddenly becomes blocked by a thrombosis?
5. How do you think a coronary artery thrombosis might affect the conduction system of the heart?
6. Why is it recommended to take the blood pressure in a patient who has been resting for at least 5 minutes?

Answers

1. Arteries are the vessels that carry blood away from the heart. They contain muscle and elastin in their walls and carry blood under high pressure. They can alter in width to control the blood flow within them. They tend to run at a deeper level than veins.
   Veins are the vessels that return blood to the heart. They carry blood under low pressure, and require valves to ensure that the flow of blood is one way. Veins tend to run more superficially in the body than do arteries.
2. Capillaries have a single-celled endothelial wall that permits ready exchange of substances by diffusion. This allows the passage of nutrients, such as oxygen, saccharides and amino acids, from the blood into the tissues, and the passage of wastes, such as carbon dioxide, from the tissues back into the blood. The complex branched structure of capillaries enables blood to be circulated very close to the diverse cells throughout the body.
3. The figure-of-eight shape has two loops: one loop is the circulation through the lungs, also known as the pulmonary circulation. The other is the circulation through the rest of the body, also known as the systemic circulation. The double pumping action of the heart ensures that blood flows evenly through this double loop. In this way, all deoxygenated blood arriving at the heart from the body is passed through the lungs to be reoxygenated before it returns to the body tissues.
4. A sudden occlusion of a coronary artery will lead to an infarction of the heart muscle supplied by that artery. Because the heart has a high demand for nutrients and oxygen, an infarction can develop rapidly within a few hours, but will have the red flags of severe cramping pain developing seconds after the occlusion. This of course is the mechanism of a heart attack (also known as a 'myocardial infarction').
5. The infarction due to a coronary thrombosis can lead to disturbance or death of the cardiac muscle fibres, which are central to the conduction system of the heart. If this occurs, a patient having a heart attack may suffer from an irregular heartbeat, or even cardiac arrest (cessation of adequate pumping action of the heart).
6. It is known that both exercise and emotional stress can cause the blood pressure to be raised. If this is a temporary response, as long as the pressure not too high, then it is considered an appropriate bodily response. Taking the blood pressure under these conditions might give a misleadingly high reading.

Chapter 3.2b The investigation of the cardiovascular system

LEARNING POINTS

At the end of this chapter you will be able to:
- recognise the main investigations for cardiovascular disease
- understand what it means for a patient to undergo these investigations.

Estimated time for chapter: 30 minutes

Introduction

The investigations and treatments for a patient with cardiovascular disease are usually managed within one of three hospital specialities: vascular surgery, cardiology and cardiothoracic surgery.

In the UK, patients who have a problem primarily with their blood vessels will usually be referred by their GP to a surgeon who specialises in disease of the vessels (a vascular surgeon). This is because the treatments for severe vascular disease very often involve a surgical operation.

In contrast, most patients with a suspected heart problem will be referred in the first instance to a physician who specialises in heart disease (a cardiologist). If the cardiologist decides that the heart requires a surgical operation, he or she will then refer the patient to a cardiothoracic surgeon.

The investigation of the vessels and circulation

The investigation of the vessels and circulation includes:

- a thorough physical examination
- Doppler assessment of the blood flow in the vessels
- blood tests
- tests such as a Doppler ultrasound scan and angiography to visualise the vessels in the thorax, abdomen, pelvis and legs.

These investigations are now considered briefly in turn.

Physical examination of the vessels and circulation

The physical examination of the vessels and circulation involves the stages listed in Table 3.2b-I (see Q3.2b-1).

Table 3.2b-I The stages of the physical examination of the blood vessels and circulation

- General examination for signs of poor circulation
- Palpation of the pulses (radial, brachial, femoral, popliteal and foot pulses)
- Assessment of specific regions of the body for dilated blood vessels (aneurysms)

General examination of the skin

The examination of the skin is focused on looking for evidence of poor circulation. Signs of this include weak or impalpable pulses, dry, shiny or itchy skin, reduction in body hair, and purplish discoloration. If the reduction in the circulation is very severe, areas in which the skin has broken down (ulcers) may be seen. The finding of blackened patches of gangrenous skin is a grave sign of advanced vascular disease.

Measurement of the blood pressure in the upper and lower limbs

This is an essential part of the physical examination of the vascular system. A device called a 'Doppler probe' is used to assist this. The same sort of probe is used by midwives to 'listen' to the heartbeat of the fetus through the mother's abdomen. In this case the probe is picking up the movement of blood within the fetal circulation, so that the 'heartbeat' is made audible as a rapid pulsatile rushing noise.

The Doppler probe makes use of ultrasound waves to measure the flow rate of blood. A simple hand-held Doppler probe can be placed against a blood vessel, and will produce an audible rushing noise corresponding to the flow in the artery. If an artery is constricted, this sound will be absent.

The Doppler probe is very commonly used instead of a stethoscope when measuring the blood pressure in the lower limb. A comparison is made between the pressure measured at the brachial artery and that measured at the ankle artery (assessed using a blood pressure cuff wrapped around the thigh). In health, the ankle artery pressure should be slightly higher than that in the arm. However, in disease of the vessels, the major arteries that lead to the leg from the aorta can become severely constricted, which in turn reduces the pressure of blood within them. In this situation, the blood pressure measured in the leg will be lower than that measured at the brachial artery. In severe vascular disease the ankle artery measurement can be less than half the brachial artery blood pressure.

Physical examination of the deep arteries

The examining surgeon will palpate the central abdomen and the pelvis to assess the width of the deep arteries, the aorta and the common iliac arteries. In vascular disease, as the vessel walls become damaged, the major vessels may be come distorted and dilated, and be at risk of rupturing. A dilated artery or aneurysm may be felt on abdominal palpation as a pulsatile mass.

Blood tests

Blood tests can be performed to exclude certain conditions that can contribute to disease of the vessels. The most common tests to be performed are serum tests to check for raised blood lipids (such as cholesterol) and glucose (indicative of diabetes). The erythrocyte sedimentation rate (ESR) or C-reactive protein (CRP) (see Chapter 2.4d) may be measured to exclude the rare inflammatory conditions that may affect the blood vessels. A full blood count (FBC) is performed to exclude anaemia, because in anaemia the oxygen-carrying capacity of the blood is markedly reduced and this can worsen the symptoms of vascular disease. For this reason, it is important to diagnose and treat anaemia in someone with disease of the blood vessels.

Tests to visualise the deep vessels in the thorax, abdomen and pelvis

Non-invasive tests, such as an ultrasound scan or magnetic resonance imaging (MRI), may be performed to examine the structure of the deep arteries such as the aorta and its lower abdominal branches. Ultrasound images, which are combined by computer processing with information obtained using a Doppler probe, can give very good information about the state of the blood flow within these blood vessels.

Increasingly, the Doppler ultrasound scan is taking the place of a more invasive method of investigation called 'angiography'. The angiogram is a very accurate method for getting good pictorial information about the arteries to the lower limbs, but is more invasive and carries more risks of arterial damage than an ultrasound scan. To obtain an angiogram, a fine, flexible tube is passed into a limb artery, such as the femoral artery at the groin skin crease. The tube is then threaded 'upstream', with guidance from x-ray pictures, to the part of the circulation to be studied. A dye that shows up on X-ray images (known as a contrast medium) is then released from the tip of the tube, and its flow is captured on X-ray films. These pictures will show the tree-like branching of the blood vessels in the area examined (Figure 3.2b-I).

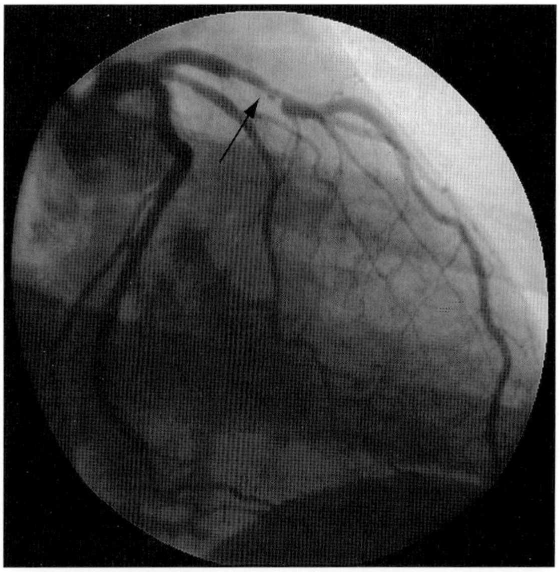

Figure 3.2b-I • An angiogram showing the three major blood vessels of the heart (left coronary angiogram) • The image shows contrast medium filling the coronary vessels. The arrow points to the left anterior descending artery. The path of the artery is partly blocked by an irregular defect. This is a region of atheromatous plaque, and is likely to be the cause of chest pain in this person (see Chapter 3.2e).

An angiogram will demonstrate areas in which the circulation is absent or depleted, and can, as in Figure 3.2b-I, expose areas of narrowing in vessels. It will also show up the dilatation in vessels known as 'aneurysms'.

Angiography carries a small risk of damage to the major blood vessels, which in some cases can have very severe consequences such as haemorrhage, thrombosis or embolism. For this reason, the angiogram is only performed in those situations in which the result of the test is believed to have an important bearing on the subsequent treatment of the patient (e.g. to clarify a decision on whether or not to go ahead with surgery). Increasingly, angiography is performed in combination with MRI or computed tomography (CT) scanning, and this technique permits a detailed three-dimensional study of the path and patency of the blood vessels.

Increasingly, a test known as 'ambulatory blood-pressure monitoring' is used in addition to resting brachial blood pressure assessment to give more information about how the blood pressure varies from day to day outside the clinic situation. It is well known that some people find clinic situations very stressful. This can lead to a marked rise in a usually normal blood pressure to abnormal levels (a phenomenon known as 'white-coat hypertension'). In ambulatory blood-pressure assessment the patient is fitted with an automatic pressure-testing device, which self-inflates to assess blood pressure at intervals during the day and night. Patients are encouraged to record their day-to-day activities to see if there are specific situations that provoke any measured rises in blood pressure (Figure 3.2b-II).

The investigation of the heart

The investigation of the heart includes:

- a thorough physical examination
- blood tests
- electrocardiography (ECG) at rest and during exercise
- chest X-ray
- tests to visualise the heart muscle (in particular echocardiography)
- tests to assess the pressure of blood within the heart
- tests to visualise the coronary arteries (angiography).

These are considered briefly in turn below.

The physical examination of the heart

The physical examination of the heart involves the stages listed in Table 3.2b-II.

A thorough physical examination of the heart can pick up gross abnormalities of the heart rhythm, strength of heartbeat and integrity of the heart valves. However, physical examination can reveal very little about the health of the coronary arteries, unless coronary artery disease has already caused significant damage to the heart muscle itself. This is important to realise, as a 'clean bill of health' from an examining doctor does not necessarily exclude severe underlying heart disease.

Table 3.2b-II The stages of physical examination of the heart

• General inspection for signs of severe disease of the cardiovascular system, such as cyanosis, oedema and enlarged liver
• Palpation of the radial pulse (rate, rhythm, volume and shape)
• Visual assessment of the pulse wave in the jugular veins at the neck
• Palpation of the impulse of the heart beat at the fifth intercostal space below the left nipple, and at other specific areas over the chest
• Auscultation of the heart sounds and murmurs using the stethoscope
• Assessment of brachial artery blood pressure

Blood tests

Blood tests are used to exclude conditions that may affect the heart, such as high blood cholesterol (hypercholesterolaemia) and diabetes. Note that these are also the conditions tested for in the investigation of vascular disease.

When the heart has been acutely damaged by a heart attack, the dying heart-muscle cells release substances known as 'cardiac enzymes' into the bloodstream over the next few days. A serum sample can reveal the presence of these enzymes and thus aid the diagnosis of a heart attack. The cardiac enzymes that are currently tested for include troponin, creatinine kinase, aspartate transaminase and lactate dehydrogenase. The levels of these markers all rise and fall at slightly different times in the few days after a heart attack. They are very useful for defining the time and also the severity of the heart attack.

Apart from the situation of a very recent heart attack, blood tests cannot be used to diagnose any of the other common forms of heart disease, such as valvular heart disease, most forms of cardiomyopathy and congenital heart disease.

Electrocardiography (ECG) at rest

Electrocardiography (ECG) is a non-invasive technique that assesses the electrical activity of the heart as measured by electrodes on the surface of the skin. The electrodes are placed on the skin of the wrists, the ankles and at six points on the chest. The electrical activity on the skin originates from the electrical discharge in the conduction system of the heart. The information from these skin sites can be processed to produce a graphical readout that indicates the electrical activity of the heart.

The ECG trace can give information on the health of the conduction system of the heart. As the conduction system consists of cardiac-muscle cells, the ECG will also give information on the health of the cardiac muscle. It cannot give information on the health of the coronary arteries, unless this is directly affecting the function of the heart conduction system (such as might occur during an attack of angina – see Chapter 3.2e). Often, the information from an ECG is difficult to interpret. Therefore, an ECG recording has to be interpreted in the context of the results of other tests done at the same time.

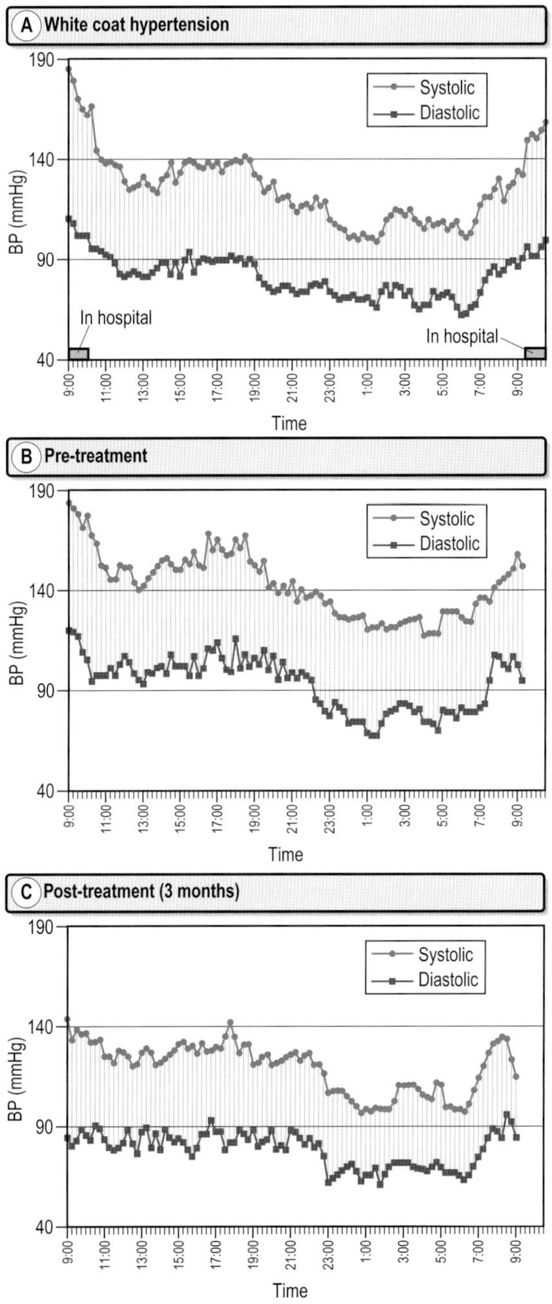

Figure 3.2b-II Results of 24-hour ambulatory blood-pressure monitoring • (a) White coat hypertension in one patient (normal blood pressure is 140 mmHg systolic and 90 mmHg diastolic; indicated by the thin black lines). Note that the blood pressure is in the normal range except for the time during and shortly after the patient is in hospital • (b) The plot for another patient who is hypertensive for most of the day • (c) The plot of the same patient as in (b) after 3 months on medication for high blood pressure.

ECG recording carries absolutely no risk to the patient, as the electrodes are simply detectors of electrical activity, and do not have any influence on the physiology of the patient.

24-hour ECG

This is a technique in which the aim is to 'capture' an episode of a heart condition that has not been found on simple ECG testing. In 24-hour ECG recording, the patient is wired up to a small ECG recorder that they carry strapped to their body for the next day. The tape is subsequently removed and analysed. 24-hour ECG recording is primarily used to investigate episodic irregularities in heart rhythm (arrhythmias).

Like the resting ECG, the 24-hour tape recording carries no risk to the patient.

Exercise ECG

In this test, a patient is 'wired up' as for an ECG, but is asked to walk on a treadmill while the recording is taken. The work required of the patient is gradually increased while the ECG reading is observed. In some patients, exercise might bring on an episode of an irregular heartbeat or of chest pain, and the ECG in such circumstances can confirm the diagnosis.

Unlike the resting ECG, the exercise ECG carries a risk for some patients. The aim of this test is only to take the patient to a level of exercise that will enable a diagnosis to be made, but not to such a level that might promote a serious attack of their condition. However, very occasionally, an attack of the condition is provoked by the physical exertion. Exercise ECG is, therefore, always performed under medical supervision.

Chest x-ray

Although the chest X-ray is commonly associated with the lungs, it can also be very useful in revealing features of some heart conditions. This is because the x-ray picture gives an outline of the heart and of the major vessels that leave the heart (aorta, vena cavae and pulmonary vessels) (Figure 3.2b-III).

A chest x-ray can show up the enlargement of the heart and blood vessels that may occur in heart failure (see Chapter 3.2f). Valvular disease of the heart can also give a characteristic X-ray picture. X-ray images cannot be used to diagnose coronary artery disease.

Tests to visualise the heart muscle

Echocardiography

Echocardiography is an extremely valuable non-invasive test for looking at the structure of the heart. It uses ultrasound scans to produce images of the heart that not only reveal the outline, but also show the four chambers of the heart, the valves, and the speed of flow and pressure of blood within the heart. Blood flow and pressure are assessed using the same principle as with the Doppler probe.

This investigation is considered to be totally harmless. In addition, it usually does not involve the patient in any discomfort, as the probe is placed against the chest wall. Very occasionally, it is necessary to place the Doppler probe in the oesophagus to obtain a good image of the posterior aspect of the heart. This requires the patient to be sedated, but is nevertheless still a very safe procedure.

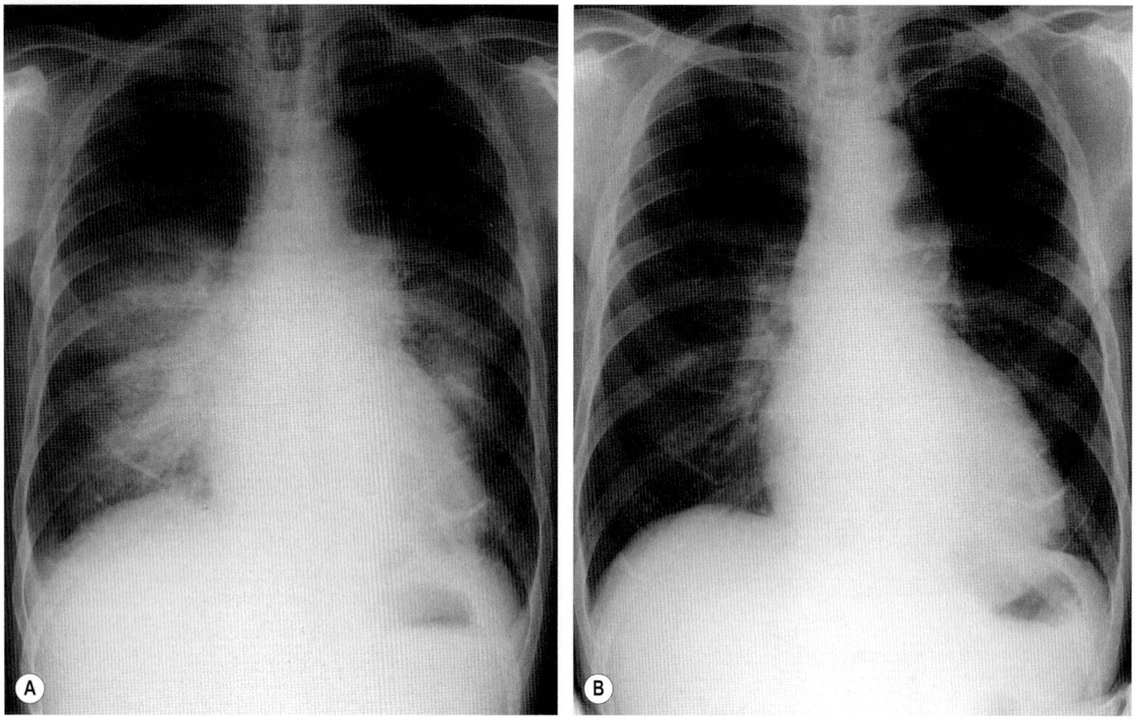

Figure 3.2b-III Chest x-ray images before and after treatment for pulmonary oedema • These images illustrate the value of the chest x-ray in investigating heart disease. In both images the very dark areas with a faint horizontal striping across them are the images of the air-filled lungs and overlying ribs. The white shadow between the lungs is the central mass of soft tissue, which includes the oesophagus and trachea. The heart is the lower part of this shadow, which projects slightly more to the right of the picture (to the left side of the patient) • (a) The abnormal cloudiness of the lung fields that occurs when fluid accumulates in them as a result of weakened pumping of the heart • (b) The same lungs after medical treatment. The lung fields now appear 'clear', a sign that treatment has been successful.

Echocardiography has become an essential tool for the precise assessment of valvular conditions, heart muscle problems and heart failure (see Chapters 3.2f and 3.2g). However, it cannot give information about the condition of the coronary arteries.

Nuclear imaging

Nuclear imaging describes a number of techniques that involve the intravenous injection of a radioactive 'dye', which can then be detected by a machine called a 'gamma camera'. The dyes most commonly used incorporate the radioactive heavy metals technetium and thallium attached to biological compounds which are naturally concentrated in healthy areas of heart muscle and bloodstream, respectively. Images of the healthy parts of the heart and the chambers of the heart can thus be produced.

Magnetic resonance imaging (MRI)

The MRI scan is another method for producing a clear image of the structure of the heart. The images can be synchronised with the ECG to provide pictures of the heart during different stages of the pumping cycle (Figure 3.2b-IV).

Tests to assess the pressure of blood within the heart

Although the ECG can give approximate estimates of the pressure of the blood in the four chambers of the heart, the most accurate method is cardiac catheterisation. Cardiac catheterisation is an invasive investigation. Catheterisation of the right side of the heart involves the passing a fine tube into a vein (usually the jugular vein of the neck or the femoral vein in the groin) and thence to the vena cava and right atrium. To investigate the left side of the heart, a fine tube is usually inserted into the femoral artery in the groin and then directed via the aorta to the left atrium.

This important test is used to diagnose the seriousness of valvular disease and heart failure. It is uncomfortable and is usually carried out under anaesthetic. Catheterisation of the heart carries a small risk of thrombosis, embolism and haemorrhage.

Tests to visualise the coronary arteries (angiography)

Angiography is considered to be the most accurate test for visualising the internal state of the coronary arteries. Coronary angiography involves the same procedure as described for the investigation of vascular disease. It is usually performed as an extension of left-sided cardiac catheterisation.

Once the catheter has reached the aorta, its tip is directed into the openings of the three coronary arteries (see Figure 3.2a-VI for a reminder of how the coronary vessels leave the aorta). A contrast-medium 'dye' is injected into the three arteries. X-ray images can then show up the flow of

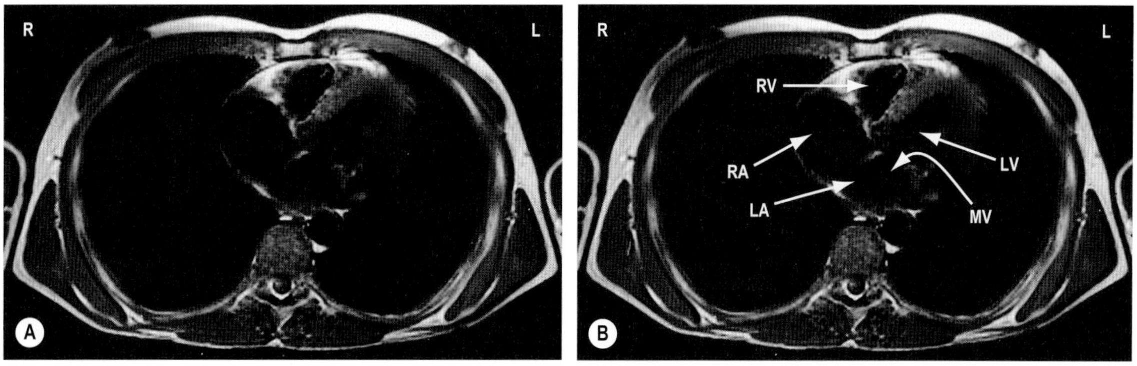

Figure 3.2b-IV • MRI scan of a cross-section of the lungs and heart at the level of the mid-thorax • These images illustrate the level of detail that can be obtained by means of MRI scanning (compare with the coarse detail seen in the X-rays in Figure 3.2b-III) • (a) A computer-generated 'slice' through the chest of a patient, presented as if the patient were lying on his back with his feet pointing in the direction of the observer. The white portions at the periphery of the image represent the bony ribs and scapulae, and the black areas the airspaces of the lungs. In the middle a section through a thoracic vertebra can be seen, and above this the heart • (b) The four chambers of the heart, the right and left atria (RA and LA), and the right and left ventricles (RV and LV). MV indicates the mitral valve sits between the left atrium and the left ventricle.

blood within these vessels, and also any obstructions to the normal pattern of flow. A clear image taken by means of a coronary angiogram is shown in Figure 3.2b-I.

Coronary angiography is performed in cases of severe angina (see Chapter 3.2e) to determine whether or not a surgical operation (angioplasty or coronary artery bypass graft) might be of benefit to the patient.

Even more so than for cardiac catheterisation, coronary angiography carries some risk to the patient (just under 1 in 1,000 procedures results in a fatal complication).

Self-test 3.2b

The investigation of the cardiovascular system

1. Ron is a 60-year-old smoker who goes to his physician complaining of severe cramp in his left calf whenever he walks more than a few yards. The pain also comes on in bed at night. The doctor suspects that the circulation to Ron's left lower leg has been severely impaired as a consequence of smoking, and refers him to a vascular surgeon. What investigations might Ron expect to undergo?
2. Elsie is 57 years old and is concerned about bouts of racing in her heartbeat, which seem to come on for no reason a few times a day. When the attack comes on, she has to sit still and rest until it is over. Her doctor suspects that the problem lies in the conduction system to Elsie's heart. What investigations do you think Elsie might undergo should she be referred to a cardiologist?

Answers

1. The vascular surgeon will want to perform a thorough physical examination of Ron's vascular system. All the pulses will be palpated and the limbs will be examined for any signs of long-term poor circulation (in particular, cold feet, shiny hairless skin, ulcers or gangrene). The surgeon may also palpate Ron's abdomen to check that there are no palpable aneurysms of the deep arteries.

   The blood pressure in the lower limbs will be compared to the brachial blood pressure with the aid of a Doppler probe.

   Blood tests will be performed to exclude diabetes and high blood lipids, both of which can lead to impaired circulation.

   The condition of the blood vessels to the lower limb may then be examined with the use of ultrasound scans and angiography, with or without MRI scanning. Ron might expect to undergo one or more of these tests, but possibly these would be scheduled for another occasion.
2. A cardiologist would first make a thorough physical examination of Elsie's cardiovascular system. This would involve examination of the radial pulse rate, rhythm and character, and examination of the heart by visual examination of the pulse in the veins at the neck, palpation of the heart impulse and by use of the stethoscope. The stethoscope would also be used to listen to the lungs, as heart failure (see Chapter 3.2f) can cause accumulation of fluid in the lungs.

   A blood pressure measurement would be taken.

   An ECG recording would be made. Elsie might be requested to wear an ECG monitor at home so that the episodes of racing heartbeat can be recorded for later examination. If there was any concern about coronary heart disease, Elsie might be asked to have an ECG exercise stress test to see how her heart responds during exercise.

   Blood tests would be taken to exclude diabetes and high blood lipids.

   An ultrasound scan might be performed to examine the structure of the heart and the effectiveness of its pumping action. However, the more invasive tests of nuclear imaging and angiography would only be performed in Elsie's case if the cardiologist strongly suspected a problem with coronary artery blood flow.

Chapter 3.2c Diseases of the blood vessels

LEARNING POINTS

At the end of this chapter you will be able to:

- recognise the main features of the most important diseases of the blood vessels
- understand the principles of treatment of a few of the most common diseases
- recognise the red flags of severe disease of the blood vessels.

Estimated time for chapter: 100 minutes.

Introduction

This chapter introduces the most important diseases of the blood vessels. The diseases studied are:

- Diseases of the arteries:
  - arteriosclerosis
  - vasculitis
  - atherosclerosis.
- Diseases of the veins:
  - varicose veins
  - ischaemia of the legs
  - aneurysms
  - thrombophlebitis (phlebitis)
  - Raynaud's disease
  - deep vein (venous) thrombosis.

For a reminder of the physiology of the arteries and veins, see Chapter 3.2a (see Q3.2c-1).

Important diseases of the arteries

Arteriosclerosis (hardening of the arteries)

Arteriosclerosis is the loss of flexible compliance in the vessel walls. A degree of arteriosclerosis is a normal aspect of ageing, but in some people this process is accelerated and then becomes an important cause of premature ill health.

As described in Chapter 3.2a, the arteries normally have an ability to be responsive to the body's needs by expansion or contraction. This responsiveness is a result of the elastic structure of the artery walls. With ageing, the elastic tissue is gradually replaced by firmer connective tissue, which in some instances can accumulate calcium. This firm and sometimes calcified connective tissue is unable to contract and expand, and the vessels become hardened.

One of the important causes of premature arteriosclerosis is high blood pressure (hypertension). It is believed that the body responds to the increased pressure within the vessels by laying down more connective tissue in the vessel walls. However, in the larger vessels, the stiffened walls contribute to the further development of hypertension, because the vessels become less compliant. As hypertension is actually a cause of arteriosclerosis, this means a vicious circle is set up in which the arteriosclerosis worsens.

Smoking is also recognised to lead to arteriosclerosis, because it both reduces the oxygen delivery to the vessel linings and increases the levels of damaging and highly reactive 'free radicals' in the body.

The stiffened large vessels also are at risk of becoming distorted, particularly if the blood pressure is high. Distorted vessels can suddenly rupture and cause a life-threatening haemorrhage. A distorted and dilated blood vessel is called an 'aneurysm'. This condition is described later in this chapter.

Stiff connective tissue can also cause the inside of smaller arteries to become narrowed. A narrowed and stiff vessel will not permit sufficient blood flow to the organs and to other tissues supplied by the small arteries. Depending on the arteries affected, conditions such as kidney failure, dementia and skin ulcers can be serious consequences of arteriosclerosis.

> **Information Box 3.2c-I**
>
> **Arteriosclerosis: comments from a Chinese medicine perspective**
>
> In Chinese medicine hardening and stiffening are generally suggestive of Qi Deficiency and Stagnation, as the responsiveness and springiness characteristic of healthy living tissue is seen as a reflection of freely moving Qi. We might, therefore, expect to see other symptoms and signs of Qi Deficiency and Stagnation when arteriosclerosis has developed.
>
> The fact that vessels are controlled by the Heart and the Lungs in Chinese medicine could suggest that it is a deficiency of the Qi of the chest, Zong Qi in particular, which may underlie the development of arteriosclerosis. This accords with the fact that smoking, a known causative agent in arteriosclerosis, is also recognised in Chinese medicine to damage Zong Qi.

Atherosclerosis

Atherosclerosis is a condition that can affect the larger arteries in middle to later life. It commonly coexists with the changes of arteriosclerosis.

Atherosclerosis also involves a hardening of the arteries, but in this case the hardening is due to the accumulation of a fatty deposit on the lining of the vessels known as 'atheroma'. Atheroma is recognised to begin to develop in the form of 'fatty streaks' on the inner lining of blood vessels from as early as the teenage years. Atheroma contains cholesterol and other fatty substances, and with time can become hardened by connective-tissue cells and calcium. In addition to causing stiffening and distortion of the larger vessels, atheroma causes other problems because it narrows the inside of the large vessels and reduces blood flow. It also causes the affected blood vessels to have an irregular and fragile lining (Figure 3.2c-I).

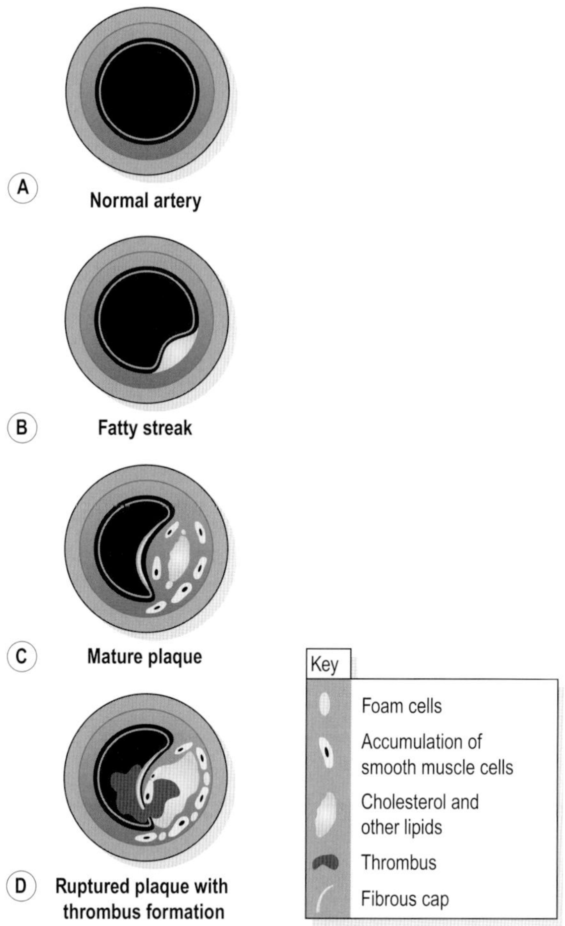

Figure 3.2c-I • The stages in the development of an atheromatous plaque in an artery.

The irregular lining of vessels affected by atherosclerosis can stimulate the clotting process of the blood, so that small blood clots can develop at sites where atheroma is present. This process will be all the more likely if the fragile lining of the atheromatous plaque ruptures and leaks irritating substances into the affected blood vessel. These processes can lead to the conditions of thrombosis and embolism (see Chapter 2.2d). Atherosclerosis can, therefore, lead to infarction of tissues (i.e. tissue death resulting from a suddenly reduced blood supply).

Conditions such as heart attack (myocardial infarction) and stroke (cerebral infarction) are very common severe consequences of atherosclerosis, and it is believed that in many cases it is the rupture of an atheromatous plaque that is a trigger for these devastating conditions.

It is known that low levels of physical exercise, a fatty diet and smoking are all powerful contributors to the development of atheroma. High levels of certain blood lipids (fats) also increase the tendency of atheroma to develop. Diabetes is another cause of long-term adverse changes to the lining of the blood vessels, in this case because raised blood glucose alters the microscopic structure of the lining of the vessels. The causes of atheroma are explored in greater detail in Chapter 3.2e on coronary heart disease (see Q3.2c-2).

Information Box 3.2c-II

Atherosclerosis: comments from a Chinese medicine perspective

The build up of a fatty deposit within the vessels is suggestive of the Chinese medicine concept of 'Phlegm without a form' or 'non-substantial Phlegm'. This term is used to describe conditions in which painless lumps and growths develop. Phlegm is usually generated by the action of Heat on Damp, so the lifestyle factors of 'Damp forming' diet and excess Heat are contributory factors. This again seems to match with the conventional medicine understanding that both a fatty diet (Damp forming) and smoking (Heat inducing) can contribute to atheroma.

Phlegm may also develop in conditions in which Qi is Stagnant, and treatments to move Qi are usually integral to the treatment of Phlegm. It has already been suggested that Qi Deficiency might underlie hardening of the arteries (arteriosclerosis), and so atherosclerosis, which commonly coexists with arteriosclerosis, may well also indicate the same.

Moreover, the impaired blood flow and clotting that can develop from atheroma can easily lead to symptoms of Blood Stagnation (intense fixed pain and purplish discoloration), which in Chinese medicine is often seen to result from both Phlegm and Qi deficiency.

Ischaemia of the legs

As noted in Chapter 2.2d, 'ischaemia' literally means 'poor blood supply'. Ischaemia of the legs is a consequence of a poor blood supply to the lower half of the body. Depending on whether or not the ischaemia is of sudden or gradual onset, there are two distinct syndromes relating to leg ischaemia. These are known as 'acute leg ischaemia' and 'chronic leg ischaemia'.

The most common cause of both types of leg ischaemia is atherosclerosis of the lower aorta and also of the vessels that branch from the aorta in the lower abdomen to enter the pelvis and to supply the legs. Figure 3.2a-I illustrates the pathway of the aorta and shows how it divides just above the pelvis to form the common iliac arteries. These are the vessels that, in turn, provide arterial branches that supply the deep tissues of the pelvis and the legs.

Leg ischaemia can also result from atherosclerosis of the vessels of the thigh and the lower leg. Arteriosclerosis in the smaller vessels that supply the skin and muscles of the leg often coexists with atherosclerosis of the larger vessels, and this worsens the condition.

In acute leg ischaemia, a major vessel that supplies the leg becomes blocked by thrombosis. The thrombosis is usually the consequence of atherosclerosis on the inside of the vessel. The sudden reduction in blood supply leads to a rapid onset of intense cramping pain in the calf, and the limb becomes cold, pale and mottled. This condition is a surgical emergency, and requires removal of the clot before irreparable damage to the tissues of the leg can occur. If the clot is extensive, a surgical operation may be necessary, in which the vessel is cut open to remove the clot. However, some patients can be helped by drug treatment to dissolve the clot. This medical approach, called 'thrombolysis', is discussed in more detail in the next two chapters in the description of heart attack in Chapters 3.2d and 3.2e. If the treatment is ineffective or comes too late, amputation may the only option for the patient.

Information Box 3.2c-iii

Acute leg ischaemia: comments from a Chinese medicine perspective

A sudden onset of severe pain, with cold and mottling, the consequence of acute leg ischaemia, would be indicative in Chinese medicine of Cold Painful Obstruction Syndrome, with predomination of Blood Stagnation. Treatment would be to expel Cold and to Move Stagnant Blood and Qi.

Chronic leg ischaemia is a condition resulting from a gradual reduction in the ability of sufficient blood to flow to the lower legs. The main symptom is cramp-like pain (known as 'claudication', a word derived from the Latin term for 'limping') in one or both calves. This pain may be provoked by exercise, when there is an increased demand for a good blood supply to the calf muscle. Pain can also come on in bed at night, when it can be helped by dropping the lower leg over the side of the bed. This is to be distinguished from the common symptom of benign night-time cramp, which is a much more intense pain associated with contraction of the muscles of the calf, and is not helped by lowering the leg.

The physical signs of poor circulation to the legs which can be found by an examining doctor have been described in Chapter 3.2b. Typically, the feet are cold and without palpable pulses. The skin of the feet may be shiny and purplish, and body hair absent. The blood pressure in the leg will be much lower than expected.

In severe cases of chronic leg ischaemia, skin ulcers or patches of blackened skin (gangrene) may be seen on the skin of the heel or toes; a sign that long-term poor circulation has led to death of these tissues. These areas can be very painful.

A patient with the symptoms of chronic leg ischaemia will undergo a Doppler ultrasound scan or an angiogram to visualise the condition of the deep blood vessels in the lower abdomen and leg. In this way the severity of the condition can be assessed.

Some patients may respond rapidly to simple measures such as stopping smoking, treatment of hypertension and a gentle exercise programme. Regular low-dose aspirin is given because it prevents clotting by preventing platelet adhesion (see Chapter 2.2d).

Those who are found to have only a short region of narrowing of a blood vessel may be treated by means of balloon angioplasty. In this operation the patient is sedated and a catheter inserted into the affected vessel. The end of the catheter (the 'balloon') is then gently inflated when situated in the region of the narrowing. The inflated end compresses the atheroma against the vessel walls, and so, in most cases, widens the narrowing. There is a small risk with this procedure of damage to the vessel or rupture of the atheromatous plaque with further narrowing, but in the majority of patients it provides a relatively non-invasive answer to their symptoms.

Patients with more extensive disease respond very well to surgical 'bypass' of the affected vessels. In this operation the affected aorta and iliac vessels are bypassed by the insertion of either a manmade length of tubing (commonly made of an inert material such as Teflon) or a length of a wide vein taken from the thigh of the patient during the same operation. The blood can then flow freely through this new passageway to the legs. This operation carries a small risk of thrombosis and haemorrhage at the site of the replaced 'vessel'.

Unfortunately, not all patients can benefit from this operation, either because their health is so poor due to atherosclerosis elsewhere, or because the smaller vessels of the legs are so badly affected that the operation would not be of help to them.

In severe inoperable cases, the only answer may be amputation of the affected lower leg. This is always undertaken when gangrene has set in, and when the circulation cannot be improved sufficiently for it to heal. Smokers and people with diabetes are the two categories of patients who are most likely to have to undergo amputation for leg ischaemia.

Information Box 3.2c-IV

Chronic leg ischaemia: comments from a Chinese medicine perspective

The symptoms and signs of ischaemia of the lower legs are deep cramping pain on exercise and poorly nourished tissues. These symptoms suggest Stagnation of Blood and Qi, with underlying Qi deficiency. The presence of atheroma in the vessels suggests that the development of Phlegm may be a contributory factor to the Stagnation, and this may also be manifested in the pulse and tongue of the patient.

By preventing the clotting of blood, Aspirin would appear to have the energetic effect of Moving Qi and Blood, which could be interpreted as a Warming or Heating action. If so, this is in keeping with its known side-effects of inflammation of the stomach lining and gastric haemorrhage.

Aneurysms

'Aneurysm' is the medical term used to describe a dilated artery. This is most likely to occur in an artery affected by arteriosclerosis or atherosclerosis, although there are other rare causes of aneurysms.

The aorta is a common site for the development of an aneurysm (Figure 3.2c-II). This is because the aorta carries blood under high pressure, and is also commonly affected by arteriosclerosis and atherosclerosis.

Aortic aneurysms can be detected by abdominal palpation, and their presence confirmed by means of abdominal ultrasound scans. They are a relatively common finding in elderly people, in particular men. Usually they are relatively small

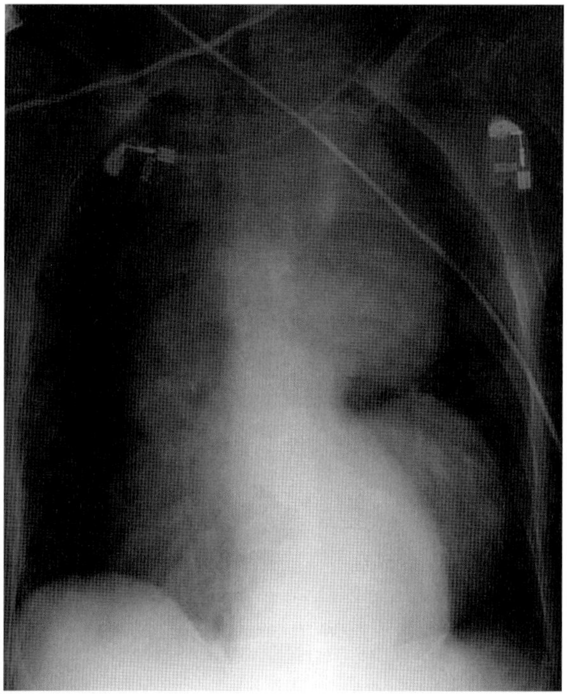

Figure 3.2c-II • X-ray image of the chest, showing an aneurysm of the arch of the aorta • This image demonstrates a sizeable aneurysm of the aorta; compare this with the normal x-ray image shown in Figure 3.2b-III.

(less than 5 centimetres in diameter) and are unlikely to lead to any immediate problems. However, larger aneurysms can press onto adjacent organs and may lead to back and abdominal pain. It is known that the larger the aneurysm, the more likely it is to rupture.

If an aortic aneurysm spontaneously ruptures, the patient is likely to collapse because of severe internal bleeding, and may have intense back and abdominal pain. As this event is most likely to occur in a frail elderly person, there is a high risk of sudden death.

Surgical treatment of an aneurysm involves a bypass of the affected aorta with an artificial length of vessel, by a similar method as described for leg ischaemia. This is a major operation, requiring the patient to recover in intensive care, and of course carries risks. If the operation is carried out as an emergency the operative mortality is very high (about half of patients who are operated on for a ruptured aortic aneurysm will not survive the operation). However, if the operation is performed as a precaution against rupture in a stable patient the success rate is far higher. For this reason, if an aneurysm of over 5 centimetres is detected, surgery may be offered even if the patient is otherwise healthy and has no symptoms.

Another fairly common site for aneurysms is around the vessels that enter the base of the brain. Because of their size and shape, these are known as berry aneurysms. In contrast to aortic aneurysms, these aneurysms are usually present from birth, and are not related to arteriosclerosis or atherosclerosis. However, there is a risk that these too will spontaneously rupture, even in young people. If this occurs, a haemorrhage in the area around the base of the brain is the result. This is called a subarachnoid haemorrhage. This life-threatening event is described in more detail in Section 4.1.

Information Box 3.2c-V

Aneurysms: comments from a Chinese medicine perspective

As the health of the vessels in Chinese medicine is underpinned by healthy Zong Qi, this might suggest that the weakness and dilatation of an aneurysm reflects Deficiency of Zong Qi. However, the reported pain and rupture resulting from an aneurysm is more suggestive of Qi and Blood Stagnation of the Chest or Abdomen. The affected patient would be in a state of collapse, with cold extremities and thready pulses, both of which might be described in Chinese medicine as Collapse of Yang.

Vasculitis

'Vasculitis' is a general term used to describe any inflammation of blood vessels. Most cases of vasculitis are the result of the disordered immune process that occurs in many of the multisystem (rheumatic) autoimmune disorders (see Chapter 2.2c). The inflammatory diseases that can involve the blood vessels include temporal arteritis (large vessels affected), polyarteritis nodosa, Kawasaki disease (medium-sized vessels affected), systemic lupus erythematosus (SLE), Wegener's granulomatosis and rheumatoid arthritis (small vessels affected).

In many of these disorders, although many tissues may be affected, it is the damage to arteries that leads to the most serious consequences of the disease. In these conditions, antibodies attach to the artery wall, and this leads to inflammation. Long-term inflammation leads to thickening of the artery and thus narrowing of the inside of the vessel. This can result in impaired blood supply. In a few of these conditions, the inflammation can occasionally cause an aneurysm and rupture of the vessel.

The consequences of vasculitis depend on the size and site of the vessel involved. Typical features of autoimmune vasculitis are summarised in Table 3.2c-I. No single autoimmune disease will lead to all these features, each type of autoimmune disease having its own characteristic pattern of how the blood vessels are affected. For example, SLE most commonly involves the facial skin and joints, but in severe cases will characteristically involve the brain and kidneys.

Some infectious conditions can lead to a vasculitis. For example, the purpuric rash that is found in a severe case of meningococcal meningitis is due to widespread infection in the bloodstream causing patches of vasculitis. The affected small vessels rupture, which leads to a bruising rash that does not fade when pressure is applied to the skin (unlike most skin rashes). Vasculitis is also a recognised consequence of hepatitis B and C.

Table 3.2c-I The local effects of vasculitis

Site of vasculitis	Possible features
Skin	Red rashes, itchy lumps, purpura and bruises
Brain	Headache, stroke or mental symptoms
Kidney	Kidney failure
Eye	Sudden or gradual loss of sight
Nerves	Numbness and weakness
Gastrointestinal system	Pain and haemorrhage
Cardiovascular system	Angina and heart attack
Joints and muscles	Arthritis, muscular pain and weakness
General features	Fever, malaise and weight loss

Information Box 3.2c-VI

Vasculitis: comments from a Chinese medicine perspective

The inflammation and thickening of vessels and the resulting impaired blood supply in vasculitis might suggest the Chinese pathogenic factors of Heat and Phlegm and Stagnation. The involvement of vessels, in particular, suggests a background of Zong Qi deficiency, and the fact that the immune system is disordered suggests weakness of Kidney Qi. Very often these conditions tend to run in families, which supports the view that the inherited weakness is rooted in weak Kidney Essence (Jing).

Patients with immune-related inflammatory vasculitis may demonstrate symptoms and signs that confirm these imbalances: rashes and fevers suggest Heat, nodules and joint deformities suggest Phlegm, and intense pain from joints or angina would suggest Stagnation. The lungs are frequently involved in these conditions, with breathlessness resulting from fibrosis, which again may suggest Zong Qi deficiency. The kidneys are also often affected, with kidney failure being a very common cause of serious ill health and death in these patients (Kidney Qi Deficiency).

Raynaud's disease

'Raynaud's disease' is the medical term for a common condition in which the muscular wall of the small vessels of the fingers spontaneously tighten (go into 'spasm'). The condition can occasionally also affect the toes. The spasm cuts off the blood supply, with the result that the affected fingers go initially purple or blue, and then white. The fingers feel numb and cold, and can be very painful.

Most people feel more pain as the condition reverses and the blood flow is restored. The fingers recovering from such an attack may appear temporarily reddened before returning to normal. An attack can last for up to a few hours.

The cause of uncomplicated Raynaud's disease is unknown, but it is recognised to be more common in slim young women. Undereating can lead to a propensity to the condition. Cold, anxiety and vibration to the hands are triggers for an attack.

If attacks of Raynaud's disease are prolonged and frequent, the impaired blood supply can cause damage to the tissues of the fingers. The skin can become dry and thickened and, in some rare cases, patches of gangrene can develop.

Occasionally, Raynaud's disease has vasculitis as an underlying cause, when it appears as part of a multisystem autoimmune disease. In this case, the impaired blood supply results from inflammation-mediated muscular spasm. Other symptoms of a generalised autoimmune disease may be present, and blood tests such as the ESR and CRP may indicate active inflammation.

Patients with Raynaud's disease are advised to avoid the triggers of attacks by keeping their hands warm and by stopping smoking. In severe cases, the drug nifedipine is prescribed. Nifedipine is one of a family of drugs (the calcium-channel blockers) that block the entry of calcium into smooth muscle and cardiac muscle cells and have the effect of dilating blood vessels. The most common side-effects of nifedipine as listed in the *British National Formulary* (BNF) are flushing and headaches. These develop as a result of dilatation of blood vessels in the face, scalp and brain.

Rarely, a surgical approach called 'sympathectomy' may be employed, in which the nerves that cause constriction of blood vessels are damaged by injection at the site in the neck from where they leave the spinal cord.

Information Box 3.2c-VII

Raynaud's disease: comments from a Chinese medicine perspective

The symptoms of cold and poor circulation to the fingers suggest Yang Deficiency and Deficiency of Zong Qi, as it is Zong Qi that is responsible for circulation to the extremities. The intense pain and purplish discoloration that can accompany the condition could well be interpreted as Cold and Qi deficiency leading to Blood Stagnation.

Nifedipine, by relieving these symptoms, could be viewed as Heating in nature, and the facial flushing and headaches that are common side-effects support this supposition. The flushing and headaches are commonly full-type symptoms, and this might correspond to Stomach Heat or Liver Fire Blazing. Other side-effects include rapid heart rate, rashes, itch, eye pain, muscle aches and jaundice, and together these suggest that the predominant action of nifedipine is one of creating Heat in the Liver and Heart.

Important diseases of the veins

Varicose veins

Varicose veins are veins that have become distended and distorted as a consequence of prolonged increased pressure of blood flow within them (see Q3.2c-3). The tendency to develop varicose veins runs in families. It is a combination of congenital susceptibility and increased pressure on the veins that leads to their development.

The most well-recognised site for the development of varicose veins is the lower leg (for a description of the deep and superficial veins in the leg, see Chapter 3.2a). Varicose veins is a condition that affects the superficial leg veins only; the veins that run deep in the leg muscle are not affected. In contrast, it is the deep veins and not the superficial veins that are affected by deep vein thrombosis (DVT).

It is believed that factors such as prolonged standing, obesity and pregnancy contribute to the development of varicose veins in the legs. Standing leads to high pressure in the deep veins of the lower leg as a result of the columns of blood pooling within them. As the superficial veins feed into the deep veins through 'perforator' veins, the pressure in these superficial veins is likewise increased when a person stands. The pressure is increased further if the person is obese and there is excess fatty tissue around the veins. When a person walks or runs, the pressure in the leg veins is reduced because the muscular contractions of the calf and thigh help keep the blood flow moving up out of the deep veins and towards the heart, and this can then allow the drainage of the superficial veins. In pregnancy, the enlarged uterus can compress the deep veins in the pelvis, and leads to increased pressure of blood in the deep leg veins.

In prolonged standing, obesity and pregnancy, prolonged increased pressure within the deep veins in the leg can act to distort the structure of the valves in the perforator veins that connect the deep veins to the superficial veins. As the valves distort they can no longer close properly, so that the smooth flow of blood out of the superficial veins is impaired, and the superficial veins become distended with blood.

One common consequence of the distension of blood through superficial varicose veins is a build up of fluid in the tissues of the lower leg, which can cause the ankles to swell slightly. The medical term for excess fluid in the tissues is 'oedema'. Varicose veins are, therefore, one of the many causes of oedema, although in this case it is not usually a serious condition. It is generally mild (i.e. it does not extend to above the malleoli of the ankles) and is worse only after standing or at the end of the day.

The most commonly experienced problem of varicose veins is that they are considered unsightly. The poor blood flow to the skin around varicose veins can lead to purplish, thread-like 'broken veins' appearing on the skin, and the oedema compounds this problem. This is a cause of distress for some people.

Less commonly, the veins can ache, and this can be to such a degree as to impair a person's quality of life. The skin around the vein can itch, and can develop patches of eczema.

The three serious conditions that can result from varicose veins are ulceration of the skin of the calf, haemorrhage and thrombophlebitis. Skin ulceration can occur near long-standing varicose veins because of the long-term effect that the impaired circulation and build-up of oedema has on the skin. The skin becomes thin, dry and vulnerable to injury, and after injury the healing of the skin is impaired due to the poor circulation. The most common sites for a varicose skin ulcer to develop are on the inside aspect of the ankle and the lower calf (Figure 3.2c-III).

Haemorrhage can occur if an injury breaks the skin and damages the vein. Instead of the usual ooze of blood, a gush of dark blood can occur due to the increased pressure of blood flow within the vein. This will usually settle down with the prompt application of firm pressure, but recovery may be complicated by poor healing.

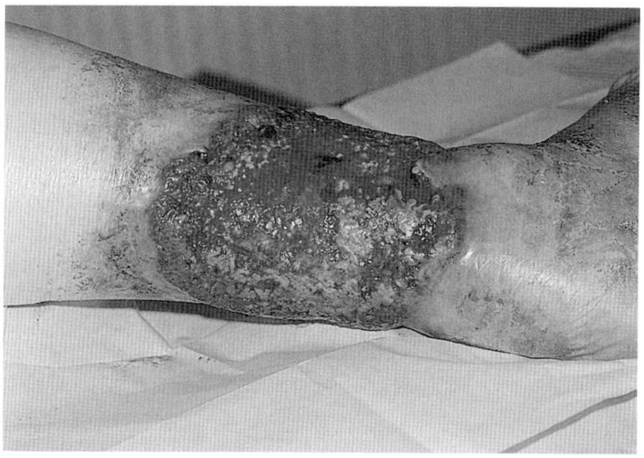

Figure 3.2c-III • Varicose ulcer of the inner aspect of the lower leg • This picture shows a very severe case of ulceration in which a large area of the skin has lost its integrity as a result of long-term poor venous blood flow.

Thrombophlebitis is described in the next section of this chapter.

When assessing a person with varicose veins, a vascular surgeon will check the extent to which the local skin has been compromised by poor circulation and will assess the back flow of blood through the venous valves by means of Doppler probes. Ideally, surgery for varicose veins is only performed for reasons of bleeding, pain, ulceration, thrombophlebitis or a severe impact on the quality of life. This, strictly speaking, means that surgery is not generally advised for purely cosmetic reasons. This approach is reasonable, because in most cases surgery will not reduce the unsightly broken thread veins and discoloration resulting from varicose veins.

Before surgery is contemplated, most patients are advised initially to try lifestyle changes such as losing weight, walking more and putting their feet up when resting. Support stockings can improve the return of the blood from the superficial to the deep veins of the leg.

Mildly affected veins, and especially those below the knee, may be injected with a chemical that causes them to close up completely (sclerotherapy). This is considered to be a minor treatment. The remaining superficial veins of the leg readily enlarge to take over the role of the injected veins. One downside of sclerotherapy is that the varicose veins fairly commonly recur some time after the treatment, particularly if the underlying causes have not been dealt with.

Surgery for varicose veins involves either removing a length of affected vein through a small incision in the skin, or tying off the connections that the superficial vein had with the deep veins via perforating veins with a surgical stitch, or both. These operations carry small risks of infection of the wounds, haemorrhage from the cut veins and thrombophlebitis (see below). The recurrence rate of varicose veins after surgery is high, but not as high as for sclerotherapy. The problem returns in about one in ten people who have the operation. After both these treatments the patient is advised to wear a support bandage for a few weeks, to lose weight if relevant, and do as much walking as possible.

Information Box 3.2c-Viii

Varicose veins: comments from a Chinese medicine perspective

As veins are vessels, a weakness in the structure of veins could reflect a deficiency in Zong Qi. Outward prolapse of the veins, both in the legs and particularly in the gastrointestinal tract, as is the case for oesophageal varices and piles, suggests weak Spleen Qi not 'holding' these vessels in place. Varicose veins are commonly seen on the inner aspect of the calf, the course of the Spleen channel.

The problem of poor blood flow through the veins suggests Qi and Blood Stagnation. The pain and purplish discoloration of varicose veins are symptoms that fit with these patterns. The itch that can affect the skin close to a varicose vein might be explained by Heat resulting from Stagnation.

Sclerotherapy and surgery both treat at the level of the manifestation rather than the root of the problem, and are therefore suppressive in nature. This means that the imbalances of Qi deficiency and Blood and Qi Stagnation are not likely to be improved by these treatments, as witnessed by the tendency for the problem to return after these procedures. The advice to walk more and lose weight by eating a healthy diet would help to move Qi and to Nourish Spleen Qi, and so deal more directly with the underlying energetic imbalances.

Information Box 3.2c-ix

Thrombophlebitis: comments from a Chinese medicine perspective

The localised pain, heat and redness of thrombophlebitis might suggest a Chinese medicine diagnosis of local Blood Stagnation with Heat. In the absence of external injury, these imbalances may be considered to be the result of internal factors. The location of the inflammation in relation to specific channels would be relevant to a Chinese practitioner. For example, thrombophlebitis in the distribution of the Stomach channel might be a superficial manifestation of Stomach Heat. The symptomatic benefit of aspirin or NSAID medication may point to their ability to move Qi and Blood.

Thrombophlebitis

'Thrombophlebitis' literally means 'inflammation and clotting in a vein'. It is a condition of the superficial veins in which the blood within the vein forms small clots and the lining of the wall of the vessel becomes inflamed.

Thrombophlebitis of the superficial veins in the legs manifests in very painful, hot and red patches on the leg, but is rarely serious. In contrast to the dangerous condition of thrombosis of the deep veins of the leg (DVT), the blood clots in superficial veins can usually not send emboli to the deep veins of the pelvis and thence to the heart and the lungs.

The most common underlying problem in a case of thrombophlebitis is varicosities of the veins. The distorted lining of varicose veins can stimulate the clotting cascade, and the clotting leads to inflammation of the veins.

The advice to the patient with thrombophlebitis is to rest the limb and to take aspirin or non-steroidal anti-inflammatory medications such as ibuprofen for their painkilling and clot-preventing effects. These different medications should not be taken together, as together the risks of dangerous side-effects such as kidney damage and bleeding become significant.

Rarely, a case of thrombophlebitis can spread to involve the deep veins of the leg and can result in deep vein thrombosis, which is a much more serious condition.

Deep vein (venous) thrombosis (DVT)

DVT was explored briefly in Chapter 2.2d. The most common site for DVT to occur is within the deep veins of the calf. This is a serious condition, because the deep veins of the calf have a direct communication with the deep veins of the pelvis, and thence to the heart and lungs. A clot (thrombosis) of the deep veins of the leg can, therefore, spread upward to involve the pelvic veins, or can produce fragments (emboli) that can travel up through the right side of the heart to lodge in the arterial tree of lungs (pulmonary embolus).

A clot in the deep vein of the leg is most likely to occur if the circulation is sluggish. This situation can develop from a combination of factors, including inactivity, obesity, old age, recent surgery, pregnancy, and factors that lead to an increased tendency for the blood to clot, such as an inherited tendency to clotting, the oral contraceptive pill, smoking or serious illness.

A clot in the deep veins of the leg leads to an acutely swollen, purplish, tender and hot calf. The pain is increased if the patient flexes the foot upwards, but they should not be asked to do this because of the risk of dislodging emboli.

Diagnosis of a DVT may be made by injecting contrast-medium 'dye' into the vein, which can then be visualised by means of x-rays (venogram). Increasingly, a confident diagnosis can be made by means of a Doppler ultrasound scan, which can show up clots in the larger vessels of the thigh. A blood test for by-products of clotting (D-dimer test) can also help to confirm the diagnosis in uncertain cases, thus making the more invasive venogram unnecessary.

A patient who has had a DVT is started on oral warfarin tablets (see Chapter 2.2d) as soon as possible, and is advised to remain on this drug for between 12 weeks and 6 months. Warfarin counteracts the formation of some of the clotting factors in the liver, and so reduces the tendency of the blood to clot. As warfarin takes some days to have an effect in the body, for the first few days all patients also receive by injection the fast-acting drug heparin. Both these treatments reduce the risk of the development of pulmonary emboli, and can contribute to the dissolution of the clot.

The patient with a DVT is advised to rest the limb totally for the first couple of days. Support stockings that have been designed to keep the deep veins as open as possible are also prescribed for the first few days after the thrombosis.

Even when the risk of emboli has passed (within a few weeks), many patients who have suffered a DVT continue to have problems. These patients are at greater risk of developing oedema, varicose veins and varicose ulcers because the free flow of blood through the leg may be permanently impaired (see Q3.2c-4).

Information Box 3.2c-X

Deep vein thrombosis: comments from a Chinese medicine perspective

The swollen, purplish, painful and hot leg resulting from a DVT might be diagnosed primarily as Blood and Qi Stagnation with Heat. The Chinese medicine interpretation of the action of warfarin is described more fully in Chapter 2.2.

Red flags of diseases of the blood vessels

Some patients with diseases of the blood vessels will benefit from referral to a conventional doctor for assessment and/or treatment. Red flags are those symptoms and signs that indicate that referral is to be considered. The red flags of the diseases of the blood vessels are described in Table 3.2c-II. This table forms part of the summary on red flags given in Appendix III, which also gives advice on the degree of urgency of referral for each of the red flag conditions listed.

Table 3.2c-II Red Flags 11 – diseases of the blood vessels

Red Flag	Description	Reasoning
11.1	**Features of limb infarction** (suddenly extremely pale, painful, mottled and cold limb). If infarction is severe, the limb may feel more numb than painful	Infarction results from the sudden obstruction of arterial blood supply to a limb, usually by blood clot. The patient requires urgent referral for surgical removal of the obstruction
11.2	**Features of severely compromised circulation to the extremities:** • pain in the calf that is related to exercise and relieved by rest • pain in the calf in bed at night, relieved by hanging the leg out of bed (i.e. not cramp) • cold, purplish shiny skin • areas of blackened skin (gangrene)	If obstruction to the arterial circulation is gradual and/or partial, pain will only appear when oxygen demands are higher than normal. Pain may appear during exercise and when in bed, and there will be changes on the skin of the affected limb that suggest chronic (long-standing) poor circulation. There is a high risk of infarction and also progressive gangrene, which could lead to the need for amputation. These symptoms require referral for assessment, lifestyle advice (especially stopping smoking) and consideration for vascular surgery
11.3	**Features of an aortic aneurysm:** • pulsatile mass in abdomen greater than 5 cm in diameter (Usually affects people over the age of 50 years and is associated with the degenerative changes of atherosclerosis)	The aorta is palpable in the abdomen as a pulsatile tube of about 2 cm in diameter. In the case of aneurysm the width of this tube is increased, and a palpable width of greater than 5cm merits assessment by ultrasonography so that risk of rupture can be formally assessed Early treatment of high-risk cases is life-saving Refer urgently if abdominal pain or central back pain develops with a coexistent aortic aneurysm (see Red Flag 11.4)
11.4	**Features of a ruptured aortic aneurysm:** acute abdominal or back pain with collapse; features of shock may be coexistent This is one of the manifestations of the acute abdomen (see Red Flag Table A6 in Appendix III)	A rupture of an aortic aneurysm is a medical emergency and the patient needs urgent surgical treatment A rupture may be presaged by abdominal discomfort or back pain, so if these symptoms develop in the presence of a suspected aneurysm refer as a matter of high priority/urgency
11.5	**Features of meningococcal septicaemia:** acute onset of a purpuric rash, possibly accompanied by headache, vomiting and fever	The purpuric rash in meningococcal septicaemia is a result of vasculitis (inflammation of the blood vessels). This is a serious warning sign of a devastating disease process and the patient requires urgent referral for antibiotic treatment Meningococcal septicaemia is a notifiable disease[1]
11.6	**Features of severe consequences of varicose veins:** broken or itchy skin close to the veins indicate a risk of varicose ulcer	Varicose veins are usually benign, but can reduce the effectiveness of the drainage of blood from the affected area. This can result in weakened, dry and itchy (eczematous) skin. A break in the skin can easily develop into an ulcer, and this situation would merit referral for assessment and nursing care Thrombophlebitis (inflammation of a length of a varicose vein) need not be referred if localised and superficial

Continued

Table 3.2c-II Red Flags 11 – diseases of the blood vessels—Cont'd

Red Flag	Description	Reasoning
11.7	**Features of a deep vein thrombosis (DVT):** a hot, swollen, tender calf; can be accompanied by fever and malaise There is an increased risk after air travel and surgery, and in pregnancy, cancer and if taking the oral contraceptive pill	DVT develops slowly and needs to be distinguished from gastrocnemius muscle strain (redness would be minimal and no fever) and thrombophlebitis (redness localised to the path of a varicose vein) A suspected DVT merits high-priority referral, as without anticoagulant treatment there is a risk of pulmonary embolism (blood clot breaking off to lodge in the arterial circulation of the lungs) The patient should be advised to refrain from unnecessary exercise until they have been medically assessed

[1]Notifiable diseases: notification of a number of specified infectious diseases is required of doctors in the UK as a statutory duty under the Public Health (Infectious Diseases) 1988 Act and the Public Health (Control of Diseases) 1988 Act. The UK Health Protection Agency (HPA) Centre for Infections collates details of each case of each disease that has been notified. This allows analyses of local and national trends. This is one example of a situation in which there is a legal requirement for a doctor to breach patient confidentiality.

Diseases that are notifiable include: acute encephalitis, acute poliomyelitis, anthrax, cholera, diphtheria, dysentery, food poisoning, leptospirosis, malaria, measles, meningitis (bacterial and viral forms), meningococcal septicaemia (without meningitis), mumps, ophthalmia neonatorum, paratyphoid fever, plague, rabies, relapsing fever, rubella, scarlet fever, smallpox, tetanus, tuberculosis, typhoid fever, typhus fever, viral haemorrhagic fever, viral hepatitis (including hepatitis A, B and C), whooping cough, yellow fever.

Self-test 3.2c

Diseases of the blood vessels

1. An elderly male patient describes a pain that he gets in his calf on walking as 'gripping'. When you question him further, he also mentions that he occasionally gets the same pain in bed at night. On examination his feet are cool, purplish and the skin is shiny and hairless.
   (i) What condition do you suspect?
   (ii) Do you think you should refer this gentleman for a conventional medicine opinion?
2. You have a 24-year-old female patient who is a model. She is currently troubled by poor circulation to her hands and feet. She is so sensitive to cold weather that her fingers can suddenly turn white and numb, and when the warmth returns they become very painful. On examination, the skin of the hands is dry and the fingers are slightly reddened.
   (i) What condition do you suspect?
   (ii) Do you think you should refer this woman for a conventional medicine opinion?
3. A 45-year-old patient who is slightly overweight is concerned about her varicose veins. They ache if she has been standing too long, and at the end of the day her ankles are slightly swollen. On examination there are raised irregular bluish veins running along the inside of both calves, but the skin overlying them appears healthy. The veins are slightly tender to touch. Do you think you should refer this woman for a conventional medicine opinion?

Answers

1. (i) The symptoms and signs point to a diagnosis of chronic leg ischaemia (also known as 'leg claudication').
   (ii) It would be advisable to refer this patient because he has features to suggest that the circulation to his feet is severely impaired. A medical investigation would exclude other serious conditions such as diabetes and atherosclerosis affecting the coronary vessels of the heart. Prescription of low-dose aspirin is a very simple and low-risk method of reducing his risks of serious complications. Angiography may reveal that your patient could benefit from angioplasty or surgery.
2. (i) The symptoms and signs point to a diagnosis of Raynaud's disease.
   (ii) Your patient has no features to suggest that the circulation to her fingers has been severely impaired. It is therefore not necessary to refer for an immediate opinion, as the condition may well respond quickly to simple lifestyle advice and complementary approaches.
3. Although the varicose veins are uncomfortable, it does not appear that your patient is at immediate risk of developing a varicose ulcer. You therefore do not need to consider immediate referral. The symptoms of pain and swelling of the ankles may respond to complementary approaches, particularly if you can support your patient in losing some weight.

   If the patient is unable to lose weight, it is unlikely that any complementary therapy can have much impact on the damage to the internal structure of the veins, and therefore may not change their appearance. If your patient is really distressed about the cosmetic aspect of the veins, you could inform her that surgery is an option, but has the risk of complications and recurrence of the varicose veins.

Chapter 3.2d Hypertension

LEARNING POINTS

At the end of this chapter you will:
- be familiar with the definition of hypertension and how it is believed to affect health
- understand the principles of treatment of hypertension
- be able to recognise the red flags of hypertension.

Estimated time for chapter: 90 minutes.

Introduction

This chapter explores the conditions that can result from uncontrolled hypertension, and the medical approach to the management of hypertension.

What is hypertension and how is it caused?

For a reminder of the physiology of the blood pressure and the principles of its measurement, see Chapter 3.2a.

What is hypertension?

As described in Chapter 3.2a, hypertension is a state in which the blood pressure is maintained at a level that is too high for the body's requirements. Hypertension, as defined by the World Health Organization International Society for Hypertension (WHO/ISH) is blood pressure above 140/90 mmHg (millimetres of mercury). By this definition, the state of hypertension is extremely common. One population-based study in 2003 showed that 28% of North American adults and 44% of European adults in the age range 18–74 years could be classed as hypertensive.

Although the upper range of normal for blood pressure is defined in modern medicine as 140/90 mmHg, the optimal level of blood pressure is considered by the WHO/ISH to be less than 140/85 mmHg.

The level of the blood pressure is important for health because, as demonstrated from studies of large populations, the higher a person's blood pressure, the greater the risk that person has of developing cardiovascular conditions such as stroke, heart attack and heart failure.

It is important to recognise that a person with optimal blood pressure is still at risk of these conditions, because they are all a result of the normal process of ageing. However, as the blood pressure of an individual increases, so does the risk of developing these conditions. There is no sudden increase in risk as the blood pressure starts to exceed the normal range. Instead, the risk rises gradually. This can be compared to having a motorway speed limit for safe driving being set at a fixed level such as 70 miles per hour. Although it is obvious that driving at 75 miles per hour is more risky than driving at 65 miles per hour, it does not mean that driving above 70 miles per hour is suddenly much more dangerous. So it is with blood pressure.

Moreover, the risks of having an accident at 75 miles per hour vary from individual to individual, depending on other factors such as driving skills, reaction times, the nature of the road and the quality of the car. It might be appreciated that skilled drivers who just exceed the speed limit are unlikely to have an accident, whereas a distracted or drunk driver might be at high risk of an accident even when driving well below the speed limit. The combined effect of other factors on the risk of adverse outcomes is similar with hypertension. Someone whose blood pressure is high at 150/95 mmHg, but who has a healthy diet, is a non-smoker and in a physically active occupation may well have a much lower risk of cardiovascular disease than someone with normal blood pressure who is a smoking and fast-food-eating office worker.

The current teaching in medicine is that a diagnosis of hypertension should be put into context with a person's lifestyle. Not all cases of hypertension need be treated with medication. Instead, a change in lifestyle may be sufficient. A diagnosis of hypertension may cause a lot of anxiety for a patient, but actually in many cases the patient can be reassured that there is a lot they might be able to do for themselves to ensure their risk of adverse outcomes is reduced to an insignificant level.

The causes of hypertension

Up to nine out of ten people who are diagnosed with hypertension will have no recognised medical cause for this 'problem'. The medical term for high blood pressure of unknown cause is 'essential hypertension'. It is believed that a range of factors act together to give rise to essential hypertension. These include family history, ethnic origin, dietary factors, nicotine and alcohol intake, obesity, levels of activity and emotional factors. Recent studies suggest that the level of nutrition of the fetus in the womb may also have a bearing on the level of blood pressure in later life. Low birthweight appears to be linked with hypertension in adulthood.

A small rise in blood pressure resulting from arteriosclerosis is a very normal part of ageing. However, as discussed in the previous chapter, the development of arteriosclerosis can lead to a vicious circle, in which essential hypertension worsens.

About 10% of people with hypertension have an underlying physical cause. This is known as 'secondary hypertension'. About half of the people with secondary hypertension have kidney damage, a consequence of the fact that the kidney is the source of hormones that are crucial in the control of blood pressure. Hypertension and the kidneys will be discussed in more detail later in this chapter. Other medical conditions that can lead to hypertension include endocrine diseases (such as Cushing's disease) and an inherited narrowing (coarctation) of the aorta. Drugs such as corticosteroids and the contraceptive pill can also lead to a rise in the blood pressure.

Hypertension and disease

Hypertension and the circulatory system

It has already been explained how a prolonged state of hypertension leads to arteriosclerosis of the small blood vessels and how this tends to increase the blood pressure further. Arteriosclerosis can also lead to ischaemia of essential organs and other body parts, such as the tissues of the lower limbs. This explains why the risk of chronic leg ischaemia in a person with hypertension is two times that of a person with normal blood pressure.

Hypertension also appears to contribute- to the development of atherosclerosis of the larger vessels. This can also lead to ischaemia, and increases the risk of thrombosis, embolism and infarction.

A common serious complication of sustained hypertension is impaired blood supply to the brain. Thrombosis and haemorrhage of the vessels of the brain are two consequences of hypertension, and when significant they manifest in stroke. The risk of a stroke in a person with high blood pressure is six times that of a person with normal blood pressure. This condition is discussed in more detail in Section 4.1.

Another common serious complication is impairment of the blood supply to the heart, leading to all the manifestations of coronary heart disease (CHD), including angina and heart attack (coronary thrombosis). The risk of death from CHD, including heart attack and angina, in a person with high blood pressure is three times that of a person with normal blood pressure. CHD is discussed in more detail in Chapter 3.2e.

Sustained hypertension will also affect the heart muscle. Years of pumping blood within a system at high pressure puts strain on the heart. One response of the heart to this pressure is to enlarge, rather like an exercised biceps muscle. Although this may sound like a healthy response, an enlarged heart above a certain size cannot pump as efficiently, and it simply cannot cope with shifting the volume of blood that is required of it. This means that fluid starts to accumulate at the venous side of the heart, in both the bodily tissues and the lungs. This condition is known as 'heart failure', which term simply means that the heart is failing to pump as efficiently. It can be a mild condition, and does not mean that the heart is going to stop (contrary to a common misunderstanding of the term). Heart failure is discussed in more detail in the next Chapter, 3.2e.

Hypertension and the kidneys

As stated previously, kidney disease can lead to hypertension. Conversely, sustained hypertension can damage the delicate structure of the kidneys. But, a damaged kidney can in itself lead to hypertension, so here is another vicious circle in which hypertension leads to a condition that in itself worsens the hypertension. For this reason, control of blood pressure is vital for patients with kidney disease, as a high blood pressure can lead to a rapid deterioration of their condition. Kidney disease is explored in more detail in Chapter 4.3c.

The kidneys are particularly vulnerable to further damage in people with diabetes and those who are pregnant. For this reason a rise in blood pressure is treated with great seriousness in both these conditions, and medical treatment is likely to be commenced at an earlier stage than for other patients (blood pressure in diabetes and pregnancy is explored further in Sections 5.1 and 5.3).

Malignant hypertension

If the blood pressure becomes very high, the risks of serious complications are very much increased. A diastolic pressure of greater than 120–140 mmHg may lead to severe damage to small blood vessels in the kidneys, which then rapidly leads to increased blood pressure. This is a vicious circle in which there is a high risk of death due to a stroke. This condition is understandably termed 'malignant hypertension'.

Although mild hypertension usually does not give rise to symptoms, in malignant hypertension the rapid cycle of progressive damage will lead to symptoms such as severe headache and blurring of vision. This condition requires urgent medical attention, and is treated in hospital with strong antihypertensive medication (see Q3.2d-1).

Prevention and treatment of hypertension

The approach to prevention and treatment of hypertension depends very much on the level of the measured hypertension. As mentioned in Chapter 3.2a, the British Hypertension Society recommend that the average of two readings is taken when the blood pressure is measured and, unless very high, the measurement should be repeated on three separate occasions before treatment decisions are made. Once a reliable measurement has been established, the level of hypertension is graded as 'mild', 'moderate' or 'severe'. Table 3.2d-I shows the ranges of systolic and diastolic pressure that fall into these categories.

Categorisation of severity of blood pressure

If either the systolic or diastolic pressure is in a higher category than the other, the overall category of the blood pressure is given that of the highest reading. For example, a blood pressure of 160/85 is classified as moderate hypertension, even though the diastolic reading is in the normal range. These are the categories that have been used in the guidelines written in 2004 by the British Hypertension Society for the treatment of hypertension.

Table 3.2d-I The categorisation of hypertension according to severity

	Mild hypertension	Moderate hypertension	Severe hypertension
Systolic pressure (mmHg)	140–159	160–199	200 or more
Diastolic pressure (mmHg)	90–99	100–109	110 or more

These guidelines are summarised in an accessible form in Chapter 2.5 of the British National Formulary (BNF).

The current advice in the British Hypertension Society guidelines is that all hypertensive patients with mild to moderate hypertension should follow advice about lifestyle changes before any other treatment is considered. These lifestyle changes are described below in the section entitled Prevention of Hypertension.

Medical treatment of hypertension

Treatment of mild hypertension

The guidance is that patients whose blood pressure is mildly elevated need not be treated with drugs unless other risk factors such as coronary heart disease, diabetes or damage to organs such as the kidney or brain, are present. Heavy smoking or high blood cholesterol are risk factors that are also taken into account.

Mathematical formulae are now used by doctors to calculate the combined effect of risk factors and to produce an estimate of 'coronary risk'. If coronary risk is calculated as 'low', then treatment is not considered to be necessary for mild hypertension. If the other risk factors are present, advice to improve lifestyle factors is given and drug treatment is prescribed only if the blood pressure remains high after 3 months of monitoring.

Treatment of moderate hypertension

If no other risk factors are present, weekly measurement of blood pressure for 1–3 months is advised before considering drug treatment. Patients with sustained moderate hypertension, and any of the risk factors listed above will be given drug treatment after a shorter period of 3–4 weeks of monitoring.

Treatment of severe hypertension

All patients with severe hypertension will be prescribed medication if the blood pressure levels remain high after 1–2 weeks of monitoring. People whose blood pressure exceeds 220 mmHg systolic or 120 mmHg diastolic will be treated immediately.

Any features of malignant hypertension will be referred for urgent hospital treatment.

The message to take home from this description of the British Hypertension Society guidance to doctors on when to treat hypertension is that not all patients with mild to moderate hypertension will require drug treatment, particularly if they have a good response to lifestyle changes, such as increasing levels of exercise, cessation of smoking and a focus on healthy eating and weight loss.

Prevention of hypertension

In terms of the prevention of hypertension, there are some factors, such as age, family history and ethnic origin, that of course cannot be changed, but there are many modifiable risk factors for hypertension. Table 3.2d-II summarises the various lifestyle changes that can have a positive impact on reducing blood pressure (see Q3.2d-2).

Drug treatment of hypertension

For those patients who have sustained mild hypertension and other risk factors for disease, or for those with sustained moderate to severe hypertension who do not respond to lifestyle changes, drug treatment is recommended. There is a wide range of different types of medication that can be used to reduce blood pressure. The most important of these can be found in Sections 2.2, 2.5 and 2.6 of the BNF.

Although patients should initially be started on a single drug, many patients will require two or more drugs in combination to reduce the blood pressure to within the normal range. Because each drug has its action on a different part of the circulatory system, when used in combination drugs can have a more powerful effect than a single drug alone.

Table 3.2d-II Lifestyle factors that have an impact on blood pressure

Lifestyle factor	Explanation for effect on blood pressure
Loss of weight	It is known that the blood pressure rises as weight is gained, and drops again if the weight is lost. Excess weight puts strain on the cardiovascular system
Restricting salt	Salt in the diet increases the blood pressure. It has been shown that simply not adding salt to food in cooking or at the table, without making any other dietary changes, can reduce the blood pressure by up to 5 mmHg
Reduction in alcohol intake	Cutting down to less than 4 units of alcohol a day will lead to a reduction in blood pressure in heavy drinkers
Stopping smoking;	Each cigarette causes a temporary rise in blood pressure and contributes to the development of arteriosclerosis. Stopping smoking will halt this process. If stopping occurs early enough in life, the changes of early arteriosclerosis may reverse
Increased physical activity	Although physical exertion temporarily increases the blood pressure, the long-term benefit to the circulation is that the blood pressure is reduced, as long as the exercise is regular and not too excessive
Reducing stress	Although the link between chronic stress and hypertension is difficult to study, some studies have shown that practices such as meditation and Tai Chi can reduce the blood pressure in the short term. Although it is not of proven benefit, it would make sense to encourage hypertensive patients to make lifestyle changes that could reduce the stress that they experience in life
Maintaining health in pregnancy	Focusing on a healthy lifestyle during pregnancy with the aim of benefiting the health of the baby in much later life. Hypertension in adult life has been linked to low birthweight

The three recommended types of drugs used in the initial treatment of hypertension are the diuretics (BNF Section 2.2), the angiotensin-converting enzyme inhibitors (ACE inhibitors) and angiotensin II receptor antagonists (BNF Section 2.5), and the calcium-channel blockers (BNF Section 2.6).

Beta blockers used to be widely prescribed for the treatment of hypertension, but these are no longer considered to carry the greatest benefits for patients in terms of overall risk reduction. Nevertheless, they may still be prescribed as an additional drug when the action of one or two others is not sufficient, or if side-effects prevent the use of the other three types of medication.

Because these drugs are so commonly prescribed, they are described below in turn.

Diuretics

The term 'diuretics' applies to a range of drugs that promote the production of an increased volume of urine by the kidneys. They reduce the pressure in the circulatory system by reducing the volume of circulating blood. This could be compared to letting excess air out of an overinflated tyre.

A patient on diuretics will have to urinate more frequently, and will feel thirsty. The diuretics will reduce any fluid accumulation in the tissues and can reduce swollen ankles. For the same reason these drugs will also lead to dry skin. A potentially serious but common side-effect is that the reduced blood pressure can lead to dizziness on standing (postural hypotension). Falls in the elderly are a known adverse consequence of the prescribing of diuretics.

Most people tolerate the drugs for years on end, but serious side-effects are well recognised. These include loss of essential minerals, such as sodium, potassium and magnesium in the urine. These losses can be life-threatening if not detected. Conversely, diuretics can produce an undesirable rise in blood sugar and lipids (including cholesterol), and for this reason their use should be avoided in diabetic people. Rare side-effects include gout (an acute condition of hot, swollen joints), rashes and damage to the blood cells.

Commonly prescribed diuretics for hypertension that are listed in the BNF include bendroflumethiazide and cyclopenthiazide, and chlortalidone. These are all from the thiazide family of diuretics.

ACE inhibitors

ACE inhibitors act at the lungs to reduce the production of the hormone angiotensin II. Angiotensin has two main functions. The first is to increase the tone of the blood vessels and thus maintain blood pressure. The second is to stimulate the kidneys to produce the hormone aldosterone, which promotes fluid retention, again to maintain blood pressure. ACE inhibitors therefore have a double action of causing relaxation of blood vessels and excretion of fluid by the kidneys.

ACE inhibitors are protective in patients with heart failure, and can prevent worsening kidney damage in patients with diabetes. They are, therefore, the first choice of drug for these groups of people.

Important side-effects include fainting or dizziness due to a sudden drop in blood pressure, and this is most likely on initiation of treatment.

ACE inhibitors can lead to reduced blood flow to the kidneys, and so are dangerous in people who have a poor blood supply to their kidneys. As this condition may be undiagnosed, regular blood tests should be done on patients starting on ACE inhibitors to check their kidney function.

Another common, although not serious, side-effect is persistent cough and weak voice. Others include nausea, diarrhoea, headache and rashes.

Commonly prescribed ACE inhibitors that are listed in the BNF include captopril, lisinopril, ramipril and perindopril.

Angiotensin II antagonists

The angiotensin II antagonists are newer drugs that have a similar action to ACE inhibitors but may offer fewer side-effects in some people. They have been less widely studied and so are usually reserved for situations in which ACE inhibitors cannot be tolerated.

Commonly prescribed angiotensin II antagonists that are listed in the BNF include candesartan, losartan and telmisartan.

Calcium-channel blockers

These drugs prevent the entry of the mineral calcium into heart muscle and blood vessel cells, and so reduce the strength of the contraction of these tissues. The reduced force of pumping and the relaxation of the blood vessels that results both contribute to a drop in blood pressure.

Side-effects of these drugs include flushing and headaches, due to dilation of blood vessels in the face and scalp, irregularities of the heartbeat and worsening of heart failure, and ankle swelling.

Commonly prescribed calcium-channel blockers that are listed in the BNF include nifedipine, felodipine, diltiazem and verapamil.

Beta blockers

The term 'beta blocker' applies to drugs that counteract the effect of adrenaline in the body. Adrenaline raises the blood pressure by increasing the heart rate and increasing the force of the heartbeat. It also causes an emotional sensation of urgency, anxiety or fear.

Beta blockers reduce the blood pressure by slowing down the heart and reducing the strength of its contractions. They also reduce drive and anxiety levels. This effect improves the quality of life for some people, but can manifest as tiredness, depression, coldness and impotence in others.

Other important side-effects of beta blockers include worsening of asthma (as adrenaline prevents constriction of the small airways of the lungs) and worsening of heart failure (due to reduced effectiveness of the pumping of the heart). They should, therefore, be avoided in people with these conditions.

However, beta blockers are now frequently prescribed for people who have suffered from a heart attack, as clinical studies have demonstrated that by reducing the work of the heart they can improve the prognosis for these people.

Commonly prescribed beta blockers that are listed in the BNF include atenolol and propranolol (see Q3.2d-3 and Q3.2d-4).

Information Box 3.2d-I

The development of hypertension: comments from a Chinese medicine perspective

The main symptoms of hypertension often suggest underlying patterns of either Kidney Yang or Kidney Yin deficiency in Chinese medicine. The failure of blood vessels to relax, a contributory factor in hypertension, could readily be ascribed to a Deficiency of Kidney Yang allowing Deficient Yin to accumulate and affect relaxation.

Deficiency of Yin would also fail to nourish Liver Yin, in turn leading to Hyperactivity of Liver Yang. The resulting Rising Liver Yang and Liver Wind are clearly suggested by the more full symptoms and signs of blood pressure, including headaches and stroke.

Hyperactivity of Liver Yang might also be thought of as corresponding to the effects of excessive adrenaline. Although adrenaline originates from the adrenal glands, which sit close to the kidneys, part of its function is to prepare and equip the body for dynamic change, a characteristic of the Liver Organ. Adrenaline is certainly Yang in nature, as it increases heart rate, muscle strength and metabolic rate, and slows down the more Yin functions such as digestion. The bodily changes brought about by adrenaline, if excessively secreted, are indicative of Liver Yang Rising, and eventually of Liver Fire.

The fatty diet, physical inactivity and smoking that contribute to the development of hypertension are conventionally interpreted as the cause of the excessive fatty deposit (atheroma) that coats the inside of the large arteries of some hypertensive people. The coating is suggestive of Phlegm Damp in Chinese medicine. This makes sense, as a fatty diet will contribute to accumulation of Damp, and the heat from smoking can be interpreted as causing transformation of Damp into Phlegm. Lack of exercise can contribute to stagnation and accumulation of fluids and so can exacerbate the development of Phlegm Damp.

The conventional medicine observation that hypertension can become more pronounced with age is consistent with the Chinese medicine view that Liver and Kidney Yin Deficiency are a significant part of the depletion that comes with old age The lack of compliance of the hardened blood vessels in arteriosclerosis, an important precursor to the hypertension of old age, suggests Yin deficiency, as Yin describes a condition of softness and the ability to yield.

It is interesting to consider that the Depletion of the Kidneys is very much integral to the understanding of hypertension in Chinese medicine, and to compare this with the conventional understanding that kidney function is very closely associated with the control of blood pressure.

Information Box 3.2d-II

The treatment of hypertension: comments from a Chinese medicine perspective

The four classes of drugs used in the treatment of hypertension have different modes of action and different side-effect profiles. This suggests that the interpretations of their actions according to Chinese medicine theory will also be different.

The following interpretations have been made by means of the systematic approach introduced in in Chapter 1.3b and which is illustrated further in Appendix II.

Diuretics: a Chinese energetic interpretation

Diuretics promote urination and lead to reduced body fluids, dry mouth and thirst. The loss of fluids directly reduces the pressure in the circulatory system. This would normally be interpreted in terms of Clearance of Damp (or Transformation of Water) a process which relies on Kidney Yang. However, the side-effects include excessive urination, dizziness on standing, a rise in blood lipids and glucose, gout, dry skin, rashes and imbalance in the levels of sodium, potassium and magnesium in the blood. These suggest additional energetic imbalances. These will be considered in turn:.

Excessive urination might correspond to Boosting of Kidney Yang, but the depletion of fluids to Subduing of Kidney Yin. As explained in Chapter 1.3b, it is suggested that drug-induced "boosting" of a substance such as Kidney Yang will come at the cost of long tem depletion of the same substance, and so depletion of Kidney Yang also might be expected in the long tem. Dizziness on standing might correspond to a depletion of Kidney Yang. A rise in blood lipids might correspond to accumulation of Phlegm Damp (as, in extreme cases, high blood lipid levels lead to external manifestations of Damp/Phlegm, the xanthelasmata). An increase of blood sugar might correspond to Subduing of Spleen Yang, as it represents an inability to make full use of the Qi obtained from food. Gout is a deforming inflammatory arthritis, and as such might be diagnosed as a manifestation of Heat and Phlegm (Hot and Bony Bi Syndrome).

Other side-effects that might correspond to a Subduing of Yin include dry skin and mouth, rashes and damage to the blood cells. Excessive loss of the minerals magnesium and potassium from the kidneys can lead to irritability, fits and instability of the heartbeat, all suggesting damage to the Yin.

If diuretics are withdrawn, the blood pressure will rise again. This suggests that the mode of action is suppressive.

In summary, according to this method of energetic interpretation, diuretics appear to Transform Damp but seem to have a deleterious effect on the Kidney in terms of Boosting Kidney Yang at the expense of Subduing and Depleting deep reserves of Kidney Yin and Yang. The side-effects of these drugs also suggest that there may be concomitant accumulation of Phlegm Damp and Heat, together with the Subduing of Spleen Qi/Yang.

Beta blockers: a Chinese energetic interpretation

These slow the heart rate and reduce the force of the heartbeat, both of which actions reduce blood pressure. The side-effects include depression, impotence, feelings of cold, asthma and heart failure.

A slower and less forceful heartbeat could suggest a Subduing of Heart Yang.

The side-effects of depression, impotence and feelings of cold all suggest that the depletion caused by beta blockers Subdues Kidney Yang. The accumulation of fluid that can result from worsening of heart failure is perhaps another manifestation of this. The asthma caused by beta blockers could be described in Chinese medicine as failure of the Kidneys to receive Lung Qi, and this would fit with the interpretation of Subduing of Kidney Yang.

For the same reason as for diuretics, the mode of action of beta blockers is suppressive.

In summary, according to this method of energetic interpretation, beta blockers tend to Subdue the functions of Heart and Kidney Yang. This suggests that they are Cold in nature.

ACE inhibitors: a Chinese energetic interpretation

These act by reducing the action of the hormone angiotensin on the blood vessels and the kidney. Angiotensin is produced in the lungs.

Continued

Information Box 3.2d-II—cont'd

The other action of angiotensin is at the kidneys to promote fluid retention. By counteracting this effect, ACE inhibitors promote the excretion of fluid. Postural hypotension is a common side-effect of treatment. Other side-effects include cough, weak voice, rashes and kidney damage.

The action of the ACE inhibitors in promoting urination is consistent with clearance of Damp, and the action on the blood vessels could possibly be associated with Subduing of Zong Qi, the Qi that supports the blood vessels. This fits with the very common side-effects of persistent dry cough and weak voice.

There is no doubt that in most forms of kidney disease and in diabetes ACE inhibitors have a protective effect on the kidneys and can arrest or slow down the progressive damage to the kidneys in hypertensive disease. This might be interpreted in terms of Boosting Kidney Yin. Postural hypotension and increased urination suggest, however, that this might be at the expense of Subduing or Depletion of Kidney Yang.

The common side-effects of nausea, diarrhoea and headache suggest additional drug-induced disease, possibly due to Subduing of Spleen Qi and/or Stagnation of Liver Qi.

The mode of action of ACE inhibitors is suppressive.

In summary, according to this method of energetic interpretation, ACE inhibitors tend to Subdue the functions of Kidney Yang and Zong Qi. They also appear to Boost Kidney Qi. Their energetic effects appear to be directed primarily towards the Lungs and Kidneys.

Calcium-channel blockers: a Chinese energetic interpretation

Calcium channel blockers reduce the force of contraction of the heartbeat and also promote relaxation of the tone of the blood vessels. Their most prominent side-effects include flushing and headaches, and heart failure. Other less common symptoms include rash, itching, eye pain and visual disturbances, muscle aches and jaundice.

The effect on the heart and blood vessels suggests Subduing of Heart Yang, together with Subduing of Zong Qi, a component of Heart Yang. The accumulation of fluid that can occur in worsening of heart failure could be seen as a manifestation of Subduing of Kidney Yang.

Flushing and headaches are symptoms of Full Heat, and may suggest Liver Yang Rising or Liver Fire Blazing. The other less common side-effects also suggest that these drugs cause Liver Qi Stagnation and/or Heat.

The mode of action of calcium-channel blockers is suppressive.

In summary, calcium channel blockers appear to reduce the Blood Pressure by Subduing Heart and Kidney Yang and Zong Qi. They also seem to cause Heat and Liver disharmony, and appear to act primarily at the Heart, Kidneys and Liver.

Summary of the Chinese energetic interpretation

In summary, all these antihypertensive drugs appear to affect the Kidneys. In particular, all Subdue Kidney Yang in addition to other imbalances characteristic of the type of drug.

However, there seems to be a paradox here. Depletion of the Kidneys, including depletion of Kidney Yang, is considered in Chinese medicine to be a primary cause of hypertension, and yet drugs that Subdue Kidney Yang seem to reduce hypertension. To understand this it is important to reconsider the factors that contribute to a normal blood pressure level.

The blood pressure is maintained firstly by a forceful and lively heartbeat, and good tone of the blood vessels. These are all Yang in nature. Adequate retention of fluid in the circulation by the kidneys is also necessary. This is Yin in nature. The drugs tend to counteract these normally healthy aspects of the Yang and Yin in the body. However, in doing so, the suppression that these drugs produce, dealing with the symptoms but not the underlying cause, may lead to a deepening imbalance.

In reaching this conclusion, it is important to emphasise that conventional medication may still be the best possible option for a patient with hypertension. In many situations, suppression of symptoms is literally vital for the patient when their symptoms threaten to bring about a catastrophic event such as a stroke or heart attack. In discerning the true benefit of a medication it is necessary to weigh up the current risk to the patient of deteriorating health from the hypertension, against how much and how quickly other more gentle treatment can redress the energetic imbalance. This is not always an easy assessment to make.

However, if it is clear that the patient's condition is unstable and the risk is high (according to the British Hypertension Society guidelines summarised earlier in this chapter), suppressive medication may be a necessary option to help regain some stability. This will buy time to enable more gentle complementary medical treatment, together with appropriate lifestyle changes, to be directed at the energetic root of the problem.

The red flags of hypertension

Some patients with hypertension will benefit from referral to a conventional doctor for assessment and/or treatment. Red flags are those symptoms and signs that indicate that referral is to be considered. The red flags of hypertension are described in Table 3.2d-III. This table forms part of the summary on red flags given in Appendix III, which also gives advice on the degree of urgency of referral for each of the red flag conditions listed.

Note that referral is not synonymous with asking for medical treatment. The British Hypertension Society guidelines are clear about the fact that, if coronary risk is low, medication is not necessary. Referral in the situation of mild and moderate hypertension is primarily so that the patient's coronary risk can be assessed accurately.

Chapter 3.2e Coronary heart disease

LEARNING POINTS

At the end of this chapter you will:
- be able to recognise the risk factors for coronary heart disease
- be familiar with the way in which coronary heart disease can affect the heart and the circulatory system
- be able to understand the principles of treatment of coronary heart disease
- be able to recognise the red flags of severe coronary heart disease.

Estimated time for chapter: 100 minutes.

Table 3.2d-III Red Flags 12 – hypertension

Red Flag	Description	Reasoning
12.1	**Features of malignant hypertension:** diastolic hypertension >120 mmHg with symptoms, including recently worsening headaches, blurred vision, chest pain	At a certain level hypertension leads to a negative cycle of increasing vascular damage and worsening hypertension. This is malignant hypertension, which carries a high risk of stroke and other cardiovascular events. Visual disturbances and headaches are serious signs
12.2	**Seriously high hypertension:** systolic pressure ≥220 mmHg; diastolic pressure ≥120 mmHg; no symptoms	Refer immediately; current medical guidelines[1] suggest that immediate medical management is required to prevent stroke or other cardiovascular events
12.3	**Severe hypertension:** systolic pressure ≥180 mmHg; diastolic pressure ≥ 110 mmHg	Refer for treatment if not responding to your treatment in 2 weeks, or straight away if major risk factors[2] are present Current medical guidelines[1] recommend medical treatment if there is no improvement in the blood pressure within 2 weeks
12.4	**Moderate hypertension:** systolic pressure ≥160 mmHg and <180 mmHg; diastolic pressure ≥100 mmHg and <110 mmHg	Refer for treatment if not responding to your treatment within 4 weeks, or straight away for medical assessment if major risk factors[1] are present Current medical guidelines[2] recommend medical management if not improving over 4–12 weeks, and within 4 weeks if risk factors are present In people over the age of 80 years the threshold for treatment if no risk factors are present is less stringent: treatment is advised if blood pressure exceeds 160/90 mmHg, and has been sustained for 3–6 months
12.5	**Mild hypertension:** systolic pressure ≥140 mmHg and <160 mmHg; diastolic pressure ≥90 mmHg and <100 mmHg	Refer for treatment if major risk factors[1] are present and if there is no improvement within 3 months If no major risk factors are present, refer for treatment only if you suspect cardiovascular risk is increased because of the presence of other risk factors such as smoking or hyperlipidaemia In people over the age of 80 years the threshold for treatment if no risk factors are present is less stringent: treatment is advised if blood pressure exceeds 160/90 mmHg, and has been sustained for 3–6 months
12.6	**Hypertension of any level with diabetes**	Always refer for medical management, as the wisdom is that blood pressure should be maintained below 130/80 mmHg in people with diabetes because of the much greater risk of vascular and renal complications
12.7	**Hypertension of any level with established kidney disease**	Always refer for medical management, as the wisdom is that blood pressure should be maintained below 130/80 mmHg in people with kidney disease because of the much greater risk of worsening kidney damage
12.8	**Hypertension of any level in pregnancy**	Always refer because of the increased risk of pre-eclampsia and placental damage.

[1]Advice in this section is based on the chapter on cardiovascular diseases in the 2008 version of the British National Formulary (RSPG), and this takes into account the recommendations of the Joint British Societies (JBS2: British Societies' guidelines on prevention of cardiovascular disease in clinical practice. *Heart* 2005; 91(Suppl V): v1–v52).

[2]In this case major risk factors are features that are known to be associated with an increased risk of a cardiovascular event in the presence of hypertension; these include diabetes, past history of heart disease, chronic leg ischaemia and kidney disease.

Medical doctors now use risk-factor calculation tables to more accurately predict statistical risk in an individual case, and this can help with decision-making about whether or not medication is appropriate. Other risk factors, such as sex, age, smoking status and lipid levels, are taken into account in these calculations. Medication is considered advisable in those for whom the 10-year risk of a cardiovascular event is predicted to be over 20%. For this reason, referral is advised for risk assessment if any of the risk factors mentioned above are present or suspected to be present. For example, if lipid levels are not known, referral should be considered. Risk calculation can help a patient make a more informed decision about the potential benefits of medication, and may also help them make the decision to adjust their lifestyle to improve their risk status.

In line with current medical wisdom, all patients with hypertension may benefit from advice on lifestyle changes to reduce blood pressure or cardiovascular risk; these include smoking cessation, weight reduction, reduction of excessive intake of alcohol, reduction of dietary salt, reduction of total and saturated fat, increasing exercise, and increasing fruit and vegetable intake.

Self-test 3.2d

Hypertension

1. Andrea is a 45-year-old housewife. She neither smokes nor drinks. She is having acupuncture to help her lose weight, but when you take her blood pressure, you find that it is 150/105 mmHg. This is the average of two readings. When you repeat the measurement one week later it is 145/100 mmHg.
   (i) How would you grade this level of hypertension?
   (ii) What lifestyle advice would you give to Andrea?
   (iii) When, if at all, would you consider referring Andrea for a medical opinion?
2. Jack is a 70-year-old gardener of slim build. He has diabetes, which is well controlled with diet and acupuncture alone. Since he was diagnosed as diabetic, he has stopped smoking and cut down his drinking to half a pint of beer a day. His blood pressure has averaged 155/95 mmHg on two separate occasions.
   (i) How would you grade this level of hypertension?
   (ii) What lifestyle advice would you give to Jack?
   (iii) When, if at all, would you consider referring Jack for a medical opinion?

Answers

1. (i) Although the systolic readings are consistent with mild hypertension, the diastolic readings fall into the moderate class. Andrea's hypertension should therefore be classed as moderate.
   (ii) As the contributory factors of smoking and alcohol are not an issue for Andrea, your lifestyle advice should include the following:
   - continue to aim to normalise your weight
   - do not add salt to your food, and try to use only unprocessed foods that have no salt added
   - try to include some regular physical activity in your daily life (ideally, give specific advice on what sort of exercise and for how long and when this could incorporated)
   - advice to help reduce stress appropriate to Andrea's situation.

   (iii) As long as Andrea has no other cardiovascular risk factors, it would be safe to continue to treat her with acupuncture to see if her blood pressure can be reduced to a normal level over a 3-month period. If her blood pressure reduces over this period to a mild level it would be safe to continue to treat her for longer (probably no more than 3 months) before considering referral. If there is no reduction in blood pressure, it is advisable to refer her for a medical opinion.

   However, you do not know Andrea's blood lipid levels, and for this reason you do not know if this is a hidden risk factor. For this reason, Andrea needs to be referred so that her lipid levels can be assessed and her cardiovascular risk score calculated.

2. (i) Jack's hypertension should be classified as mild.
   (ii) As Jack is slim, has attended to the contributory factor of smoking, and is likely to be getting sufficient physical activity appropriate to his age through gardening, your lifestyle advice could include the following:
   - do not add salt to your food, and try to use only unprocessed foods that have no salt added
   - the amount of beer that you drink will not be doing you any harm, as long as it does not increase above this level
   - advice to help reduce stress appropriate to Jack's situation.

   (iii) Jack's diabetes is a very significant cardiovascular risk factor. Moreover, his blood pressure is well above the target range of less than 130/80 mmHg. For this reason he needs to be referred for assessment for medical treatment. The ideal medication for hypertension in diabetes is an ACE inhibitor, as this is recognised to have a protective effect on the vulnerable kidneys.

Introduction

This chapter focuses on two of the conditions that can result from disease of the coronary arteries. These conditions are embraced by the term 'coronary heart disease' (CHD). The two other major conditions that can result from CHD are heart failure and irregularities of the heart rhythm (arrhythmias). These two conditions have other causes in addition to CHD, and are discussed in Chapter 3.2f. CHD is also known as 'ischaemic heart disease' (IHD) and 'coronary artery disease' (CAD).

The causes of coronary heart disease

The study of CHD as described in this chapter will be supported by turning back to Chapter 3.2a to revise the physiology of the blood flow to the heart muscle, and also to Chapter 3.2c to read about the pathology of atheroma and atherosclerosis.

CHD is the term applied to the conditions that can result from the 'furring up' of the coronary arteries by atheroma. As described in Chapter 3.2c, atheroma in the coronary vessels reduces the blood flow and increases the risk of thrombosis in these vessels.

It is believed that a wide range of risk factors and protective factors work together to affect an individual's risk of developing CHD. These can be broadly categorised into unmodifiable factors and lifestyle factors (which can be modified).

Unmodifiable risk factors

The most important unmodifiable risk factors are age, gender and family history. Obviously, these risk factors cannot be altered by attention to advice or through medical treatment.

Age

The risk of developing CHD increases with age, as development of atheroma is part of the ageing process.

Gender

The risk of developing CHD is greater in men, although the difference in the risk between the sexes evens out after the menopause. It is believed that physiological levels of the female hormone oestrogen are protective against CHD.

Family history

The risk of developing CHD in an individual is greater if the person's close relatives have had CHD. The risk is also higher in some ethnic groups, irrespective of lifestyle. This means that susceptibility to the condition can be inherited.

Lifestyle factors

The three most important lifestyle factors that contribute to the development of CHD are a high level of blood lipids, smoking and lack of physical exercise.

Blood lipids

'Blood lipids' is a term that refers to the fats that circulate in the bloodstream. These lipids are essential for health, but if their levels become too high or out of balance, they can contribute to the fatty deposit of atheroma. The lipids are found in four important forms in the blood known as high-density, low-density and very-low-density lipoprotein (HDL, LDL and VLDL) and triglycerides.

HDL, LDL and VLDL contain cholesterol and contribute to the total cholesterol level, which is commonly the figure that patients will be told about by their doctor. Ideally, the total cholesterol level should be less than 5.0 mmol/l (millimoles per litre), although, as is also the case for blood pressure, it is well known that a significant proportion of people in western populations have a cholesterol level that exceeds this upper limit of normal.

HDL is one form of cholesterol that does not seem to contribute to coronary risk, and instead it may even be protective. HDL levels seem to increase with exercise. For this reason the ratio between total cholesterol and HDL is used for the calculation of coronary risk. This ratio will be lower in value the higher the level of HDL, and so it accounts for the protective effect of HDL. Triglycerides are usually not of concern for most people, but may become adversely high in people with diabetes and in certain family groups.

It is known that some people are more prone to developing adversely high blood lipids than others, and this trait runs very strongly in families. If this inherited problem is marked, it is diagnosed as 'hyperlipidaemia'. CHD is much more common in people with hyperlipidaemia than in the general population.

It is now known that certain types of fats in the diet directly increase the levels of the unhealthy LDL and VLDL in the bloodstream. The fats known as 'saturated' fats (found in dairy products and meat), and 'trans fatty acids' (found in cheap margarines, biscuits and cakes) appear to increase the levels of undesirable lipids.

In contrast, the fats known as 'polyunsaturated' fats and 'monounsaturated' fats (found in vegetable oils and olive oil, respectively) appear to reduce the levels of LDL and VLDL, and may also instead increase levels of the protective HDL. Fish oils also appear to be beneficial.

A typical western diet, which is high in dairy produce, fatty meats, cakes and biscuits, is therefore a lifestyle factor that can, over the years, contribute to the development of atheroma.

Smoking

Smoking increases the development of arteriosclerosis and atherosclerosis and also can increase the tendency of the blood to clot. Contrary to popular understanding, the greatest health impact of smoking comes from the fact that it causes CHD rather than from its undeniably adverse effect on the lungs.

Studies of large populations indicate that the increased risk of CHD in a smoker drops to become the same as that of a non-smoker within 5 years of stopping smoking.

Lack of physical exercise

Other studies of large populations indicate that those who are physically active are half as likely to develop CHD as those who are inactive. This is comparable to the difference in risk between smokers and non-smokers. Physical exercise improves the blood supply to the heart and improves the balance of healthy to unhealthy blood lipids. It is now believed that regular moderate exercise such as brisk walking or cycling is more beneficial than less frequent strenuous exercise such as playing squash or running.

Conventional healthy-living advice to all people therefore includes attention to the fats in the diet, quitting smoking and taking up regular physical activity. If all three of these factors can be attended to, the risk of developing atheroma and CHD drops dramatically. In addition to these three most important lifestyle factors there are numerous other factors that are conventionally believed to affect the development of atheroma.

Other dietary factors

It is now believed that there are other components of the diet, in addition to the healthy fats such as vegetable, olive and fish oils, which are actually protective against CHD. Foods that provide the vitamins A, C and E (the 'antioxidant' vitamins), such as fresh fruit and vegetables, and garlic have been shown in some studies to reduce the risk of CHD. Flavonoids, another component of fruit and vegetables, also appear to be beneficial. These are also present in tea, and green tea in particular.

Alcohol up to an amount of 2–3 units a day also appears to be protective. The risk of CHD in moderate drinkers actually appears to be less than in those who do not drink alcohol at all. Red wine has recently been considered to be of particular benefit, possibly because it contains flavonoids as well as alcohol. However, consumption of more than 3–4 units of alcohol a day is detrimental. This is because above this level the alcohol contributes to hypertension and produces an unhealthy rise in blood lipids.

Salt can be harmful because it increases the blood pressure in some people, and this in turn promotes the development of atherosclerosis.

All the beneficial dietary factors can be found in the widely acclaimed 'Mediterranean' diet. Populations who eat a diet rich in fresh fruit, vegetables and fish, plenty of garlic and olive oil, moderate amounts of wine and moderate amounts of meat, but little other saturated fat, demonstrate a relatively low prevalence of CHD.

Diabetes

People with diabetes mellitus (see Chapter 5.1d) and poorly controlled blood sugar levels are more prone to both atherosclerosis and arteriosclerosis. This is, in part, due to the effect of the high sugar levels on the walls of the blood vessels, and partly due to the fact that diabetics are prone to raised blood lipids. For this reason, diabetic people are advised to be very attentive to modifying their dietary, exercise and smoking habits to minimise their overall risk of CHD.

It has been confirmed by clinical studies that good control of blood sugar through diet and drugs will also reduce the risk of damage to the blood vessels in some diabetics.

Table 3.2e-I Important factors in the aetiology of coronary heart disease

Unmodifiable risk factors	Lifestyle risk factors	Lifestyle protective factors
• Age	• High levels of saturated fats and trans fatty acids in the diet	• Polyunsaturated and monounsaturated fats
• Gender	• Smoking	• Fish oils
• Family history	• Low level of physical activity	• Vitamins A, C and E as part of a healthy diet (not in the form of supplements)
	• Excess salt in diet	• Flavonoids
	• Alcohol intake greater than 4 units/day	• Garlic
	• Diabetes mellitus	• Regular moderate physical activity
	• Hyperlipidaemia	• Moderate alcohol intake
	• Social causes of stress	
	• Hypertension	

Hyperlipidaemia

This is the condition in which the blood lipids are raised above a healthy level. It can be assessed by means of the fasting lipids blood test. The term 'hyperlipidaemia' is generally reserved for people who have total fasting levels of cholesterol of over 6.5 mmol/l or triglycerides greater than 3.0 mmol/l. Because of the high risk of CHD, people with hyperlipidaemia are advised to be very careful about fat in their diet, and may be prescribed lipid-lowering medication such as a statin or a fibrate.

People who have had symptoms of CHD may be advised to take lipid-lowering medication, even if their blood lipids are not very high. This is because clinical studies have shown that such treatment can reduce the risk of subsequent deaths from CHD. The energetics of lipid-lowering medication is explored later in this chapter.

Hypertension

The link between hypertension and CHD has been explored in detail in Chapter 3.2d.

Social effects and stress

There is good evidence to show that people in low socioeconomic groups and in populations subjected to great stress have increased rates of CHD. These increased rates cannot be accounted for solely by poor access to good diet, high levels of smoking and alcohol intake. The current theory is that the stress that arises from being in a low social class or in a nation in turmoil directly affects the development of CHD. Although this factor is recognised in conventional medicine, the mechanism of how stress leads to CHD has not yet been fully explained.

Other factors

Other factors that have more recently been linked with an increased risk of CHD include increased tendencies to blood clotting, increased levels of an amino acid called 'homocysteine', and increased inflammation, possibly linked to the gastric bacterium *Helicobacter pylori*. At present, none of these factors has been sufficiently established by research evidence to be reflected in wide-scale public health advice for the prevention of CHD.

The important factors that affect the development of CHD are summarised in Table 3.2e-I. An awareness of these factors can inform the approach of complementary therapists to giving lifestyle advice to patients with CHD.

The manifestations of coronary heart disease

The heart is supplied with blood by means of the coronary arteries. The damage to the blood supply of the heart resulting from coronary atheroma has four major manifestations: angina, heart attack, heart failure and disorders of the heartbeat (arrhythmias). Angina and heart attack are discussed in some detail in this chapter because of their importance in terms of their frequency and their impact on health.

Angina

If one or more of the coronary vessels becomes 'furred up' by atheroma, the amount of blood that can be supplied to the heart muscle decreases. When the heart muscle is required

Information Box 3.2e-I

The causes of atheroma: comments from a Chinese medicine perspective

As suggested in Chapter 3.2c, the substantial fatty deposit of atheroma could possibly be an internal manifestation of non-substantial Phlegm. The hardened non-compliant vessels that result from a combination of atheroma deposition and arteriosclerosis suggest that Qi Deficiency, and in particular deficiency of Zong Qi, the Qi that supports the health of the vessels, might also be factors.

It was also suggested that high levels of lipids in the bloodstream might be interpreted as a manifestation of Phlegm Damp. In people who have very high level blood lipid levels, the serum of the blood actually looks cloudy instead of clear, and this fits with the interpretation.

Smoking leads to Zong Qi Deficiency, Heat and Phlegm. Low levels of physical activity can lead to Qi Stagnation. This might explain why these risk factors are so important in the development of atheroma.

The protective effect of vitamins, flavonoids and the vegetable and fish oils may be a result of the ways in which these foods can Nourish Spleen Qi and so help to transform Damp.

Alcohol in moderate doses is Warming, and therefore can Move Qi and Blood, but in excess is a source of Damp-Heat. This may explain why alcohol can be protective, but is damaging when taken to excess.

Garlic is known to be Warming and Pungent, and also helps to Clear Damp and Phlegm through moving Qi and Warming the Stomach and Spleen. This is in accordance with the conventional medicine observation that garlic can reduce levels of blood lipids.

Social stresses may Deplete and Stagnate Qi. Loss and emotional isolation are two emotional states that may be particularly important. As these emotions tend to affect the Heart and Lungs, these will both tend to deplete Zong Qi, the Qi of the chest, and so have a negative effect on the health of the vessels.

to do work with an insufficient blood supply, the muscle becomes 'ischaemic'. This leads to intense cramping pain, in the same way as is experienced in chronic leg ischaemia. Ischaemic pain of the heart is called 'angina pectoris' (angina).

Initially, angina may come on only in situations of extreme exercise, but as narrowing of the coronary vessels worsens the pain will occur at progressively lower levels of exertion. It can also occur whilst eating or when the patient is exposed to the cold. Severe angina can be extremely disabling. In stable angina the pain gets better if the patient rests.

The pain is characteristically described as 'heavy' or 'tight', and is not usually described as 'stabbing' (contrary to what is frequently said in Chinese medicine textbooks; possibly a result of mistranslation of a Chinese term). The pain is felt in the centre of the chest (rather than to the left), and may radiate up to the neck and down one or both arms.

In some people, particularly the elderly, painless angina may occur. Sometimes all the patient experiences is a feeling of tightness in the chest or breathlessness. However, it is important to recognise that in elderly people serious conditions may produce relatively few symptoms.

If the obstruction of the coronary arteries becomes very severe, angina may come on spontaneously when the patient is at rest. This is a serious symptom, and is described as 'unstable angina'. The rest pain of unstable angina is a warning symptom of impending heart attack.

Angina is initially diagnosed from the patient's symptoms, but as chest pain can have a wide range of possible causes the diagnosis is confirmed through hospital investigations. Most patients with angina will undergo a resting ECG and an exercise ECG (treadmill) assessment. If surgery is a possibility, coronary angiography and other imaging tests of the heart muscle may be performed (see Chapter 3.2b).

The treatment of angina: prevention of progression

The treatments used to prevent the worsening of angina have a lot in common with the treatments used to prevent all types of CHD. First, the patient is encouraged to attend to lifestyle changes, as discussed earlier in this chapter. Dietary advice is given and the patient is counselled about taking gentle exercise and stopping smoking.

All patients with CHD will be prescribed low-dose aspirin (75 mg) to be taken on a daily basis. Aspirin reduces the tendency of the blood to clot, and in this way reduces the risk of a coronary thrombosis (heart attack). If hypertension and diabetes are present they are controlled as much as possible in order to minimise coronary risk.

Many patients will also be prescribed a drug to reduce the level of blood lipids. The most commonly prescribed group of lipid-lowering drugs is the statins (see BNF, Chapter 2.12).

Statins

The statins affect the liver to reduce its production of cholesterol. The main side-effects are digestive disturbances and headaches, although rarely inflammation of muscles and severe liver disturbance can occur. Commonly prescribed statins include simvastatin and pravastatin.

Treatment of the symptoms of angina

The symptoms of angina can be treated by three classes of drugs, which in severe angina may be used in combination. These are the nitrates, calcium-channel blockers and beta blockers.

Nitrates

Nitrates are the first type of drug chosen for patients with angina. Glyceryl nitrate (GTN) is a preparation that can be taken under the tongue (sublingually), by tablet or by aerosol spray, from where it is rapidly absorbed to lead to a reduction in symptoms. Other preparations of long acting nitrates are taken by mouth on a regular basis to prevent symptoms.

Nitrates act by dilating large blood vessels. They therefore dilate the coronary vessels, and in this way counteract the narrowing in these vessels that has led to the symptoms of angina. The common side-effects of flushing, headache and feeling faint on standing are all results of the dilatation of blood vessels elsewhere in the body.

Commonly prescribed long acting nitrates include isosorbide dinitrate and isosorbide mononitrate.

Calcium channel blockers and beta blockers

The remaining two classes of drugs used for angina are the same as those used for hypertension (the action of these is described Chapter 3.2d) (see Q3.2e-1).

If a patient has an acute attack of unstable angina that does not settle rapidly, he or she is initially treated as an emergency in hospital, with bed rest, opiate painkillers, and oral nitrates. The painkillers and nitrates are intended to minimise the stress and anxiety resulting from pain. There is currently debate over whether administration of oxygen is beneficial in unstable angina, although until very recently it used to be a mainstay of treatment in the acute situation. Aspirin and a beta blocker are given by mouth, and an infusion of the anticoagulant heparin is administered. If chest pain continues despite all these treatments, intravenous nitrate drugs are also given.

Surgical treatment of angina

If the pain is still not settling and the ECG indicates that the heart is suffering from poor blood supply, the patient is considered for one of the two surgical approaches to treating obstructed coronary arteries: percutaneous transluminal coronary angioplasty (PTCA) and coronary artery bypass graft (CABG). Ideally, these procedures are performed in a stable patient to prevent worsening of angina, but in this situation will be carried out as an emergency.

Angioplasty (PTCA)

Prior to emergency angioplasty, an infusion of a drug that inhibits platelet adhesion (tirofiban) may be commenced. This can further reduce the risk of thrombosis while the patient is prepared for the operation. Angioplasty is always preceded by an angiography (see Chapter 3.2b). After the angiography has exposed which coronary vessels are most blocked by atheroma, the tube that has been used to perform the angiography is left in place at the entrance to the coronary vessels. A skilled operator can then direct a finer tube from this point to actually enter the coronary vessel. When situated at the point of greatest narrowing, the end of the tube is inflated slightly. This compresses the atheroma flat against the wall of the vessel, and widens the passageway for the flow of blood (Figure 3.2e-I). In some cases, a small tube (stent) is left situated in the vessel to keep it open. Although angioplasty is a surgical procedure, in the UK it is performed by a physician (i.e. a cardiologist) rather than a surgeon.

The advantage of angioplasty is that it can provide immediate relief from the symptoms of angina, and involves the patient in relatively little discomfort. Angioplasty carries a small risk of triggering thrombosis of the coronary vessel at the time of the procedure, and, although it may relieve symptoms temporarily, it does not seem significantly affect the long-term prognosis for the patient.

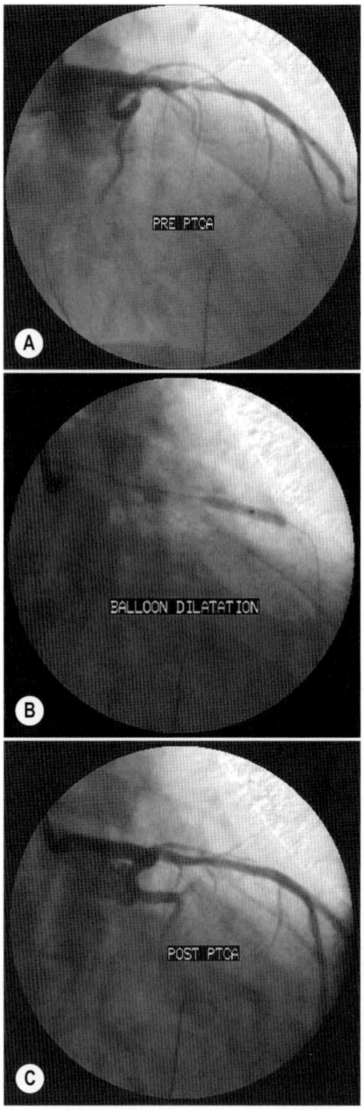

Figure 3.2e-I • The dilatation of a coronary artery by means of angioplasty (PTCA) • (a) A narrowed coronary artery during angiography. (b) The same artery with a tubular balloon inflated in the narrowed portion. (c) The same artery after angioplasty; the narrowing has disappeared.

Because angioplasty actually may damage the coronary vessel rather than clear the blockage, approximately 2% of patients have to proceed to emergency heart surgery (CABG) after an angioplasty.

Coronary artery bypass graft (CABG)

In this operation one or more of the three coronary arteries are bypassed using either lengths of veins taken from the thigh or lengths of arteries taken from the wall of the chest. This is a major operation, requiring an incision down the midline of the chest and a period of recovery in an intensive care unit.

The success rate in terms of symptom relief is higher for some patients than for angioplasty. In some patients CABG may also reduce the risk of future heart attacks or other deaths from CHD.

CABG carries the risks that come with all major operations. In addition, there are risks that the patient can suffer a heart attack or a stroke. For these reasons, the operation is restricted to those people who are relatively fit, and who thus have a good chance of benefiting from the procedure.

Treatment of angina: summary

The treatment for the prevention of worsening of angina involves:

- lifestyle advice
- daily low-dose aspirin
- a lipid-lowering drug in those with high blood lipids
- medical management of hypertension and diabetes, if present.

The treatment for the symptoms of angina involves:

- painkillers
- oxygen
- anticoagulants, including aspirin and heparin
- nitrates
- calcium-channel blockers
- beta blockers
- angioplasty (PTCA)
- coronary artery bypass graft (CABG).

> **Information Box 3.2e-II**
>
> **Angina: comments from a Chinese medicine perspective**
>
> In Chinese medicine, the symptom of the intense pain of angina would be diagnosed as Heart Blood Stagnation. The recognition that atheroma very frequently underlies angina would suggest that the patient would demonstrate other symptoms and signs of Phlegm and Zong Qi Deficiency.
>
> Cold, Phlegm and Heart Blood/Qi Deficiency are the factors that are considered to promote the development of Stagnation of Blood of the Heart. The emotions of sadness and anger would be particularly important in the aetiology of this syndrome.
>
> Aspirin is Warming, and in this way tends to Clear Cold and Move Blood.
>
> By lowering the blood lipid level, the statins appear to Clear Damp Phlegm. However, side-effects of muscle aches, headache and digestive disturbance suggest they also cause disharmony of the Liver and Spleen.
>
> Nitrates increase the blood flow to the heart, and this can be interpreted as Heat moving Stagnation. The side-effects of flushing and throbbing headache suggest Full Heat (Stomach or Liver).
>
> All these treatments are suppressive in nature.

Heart attack

Heart attack (also known as 'myocardial infarction') is a result of a sudden blockage of the coronary arteries, usually as a result of a blood clot (coronary thrombosis). This leads to infarction of the heart muscle (the myocardium). Although this can occur on a background of a history of worsening angina, it can also occur out of the blue.

The sudden loss of blood supply to part of the heart is a great shock to the muscle cells. Some of these cells will die, and the resulting damage leads to severe pain, which can be described as 'crushing' or like a 'tight band around the chest'. The quality of the pain is the same as that of angina, which means that in practice it is often difficult to distinguish a heart attack from unstable angina. The pain of the heart attack is often associated with a cold sweat and an emotional sense of deep fear, sometimes described as 'a sense of impending doom'. The patient can be restless and may vomit.

Just as with angina, the symptoms of heart attack may be much less prominent in elderly people. An episode of tiredness, a 'funny turn' or some unexplained breathlessness may be all that an elderly person experiences. In fact, ECG tests occasionally demonstrate the changes characteristic of a previous heart attack, but the patient is unable to describe any past episode that could explain these changes. These painless heart attacks are termed 'silent infarctions'.

Heart attacks can have a number of serious consequences. Up to half of all patients die within the first few hours because damage to the pacemaker cells of the heart causes the heart to stop beating. This is called 'cardiac arrest', and although this may be reversed by emergency treatment, if it occurs in a situation where there is no experienced first aider on hand it is rapidly fatal.

After a heart attack, some patients may continue to suffer from instability of the pacemaker system of the heart. This means they are at particular risk of cardiac arrest within the first few days after a heart attack. A patient who has recently had a heart attack may therefore experience palpitations. These irregularities of the heart rhythm are called 'arrhythmias'. This is why patients who have suffered a heart attack are initially nursed under close observation.

In other patients, the damage to the heart muscle recovers to some extent, but the muscle is never as strong as it was. This leads to inefficiency of the pumping action of the heart, which can manifest as the condition of chronic heart (cardiac) failure. In some patients the damage to the heart muscle is so great that the pumping action of the heart suddenly becomes very weak. This results in the condition of acute heart failure, and the patient experiences severe breathlessness. The conditions of arrhythmia, chronic heart failure and acute heart failure are explored in more detail in Chapter 3.2f.

Some patients make a full recovery from a heart attack as the damaged muscle heals and new blood vessels form. However, the underlying problem of atheroma will not heal unless the factors causing atheroma are removed. This means that these patients are at high risk of a recurrence unless they can attend to making significant changes in their lifestyle. This is the reason why only about half of those patients who survive a heart attack will still be alive 10 years later.

The treatment of acute heart attack

The immediate risks of a heart attack are cardiac arrest and permanent damage to the heart muscle. The prevention and treatment of these complications are discussed below.

Treatment of cardiac arrest

Cardiac arrest can occur at any time, but occurs particularly within the first 48 hours of the attack, so the patient should be under intensive medical supervision. If cardiac arrest occurs, the circulation ideally should be sustained by cardiopulmonary respiration (CPR) until medical treatment is available.

For those patients who have suffered cardiac arrest, initial medical treatment involves applying an electric shock to the chest (cardioversion), and this can be sufficient to restart the failing pacemaker of the heart. Various drugs, including adrenaline, may be injected to stimulate the heartbeat.

The combination of CPR and cardioversion for cardiac arrest is known to be life-saving. However, access to these treatments is not always available, and without them a cardiac arrest will rapidly become a fatal condition.

Treatment to reduce permanent heart-muscle damage

For those patients who have not suffered cardiac arrest, the initial treatment is to encourage the patient to be as calm as possible. As for unstable angina, aspirin is given orally. Nitrates may be given, and a strong painkiller (diamorphine (heroin)) is injected intravenously to reduce the pain and induce calm. Clopidogrel, a drug which, like aspirin, prevents clumping of platelets, may also be given at this stage.

It is important that an acute heart attack is differentiated from unstable angina, as the two conditions require different treatments. An ECG recording and the results of blood tests for cardiac enzymes are crucial in helping to differentiate between the two syndromes. Once the diagnosis has been confirmed, and if there no reasons why it would be contraindicated, a 'clot-busting medication is given. The medical term for a 'clot-busting' drug is 'fibrinolytic', because such drugs reverse the stage in the clotting cascade that involves the formation of fibrin. If given within the first 24 hours, fibrinolytics can totally dissolve, or at least reduce the size of some coronary thromboses, and, together with aspirin, are known to be life-saving. Streptokinase and tissue plasminogen activator (tPA) are the most commonly used fibrinolytics in the UK.

A beta blocker is often given by injection at this stage, as these drugs reduce the workload on the heart. Clinical studies have demonstrated that beta blockers provide additional survival benefit, although they cannot be given if the patient is suffering from severe heart failure or asthma.

However, if the patient is found to be suffering from a degree of heart failure, an ACE inhibitor can be given to reduce the workload of the heart. These drugs were described in some detail in Chapter 3.2d.

A statin is also prescribed if the total cholesterol is greater than 4.0 mmol/l, which it will be in the majority of patients. This too is recognised to improve the chances of long-term survival after a heart attack.

Long-term treatment of heart attack

A patient who has suffered an uncomplicated heart attack is usually discharged from hospital within 3–5 days of the attack. Treatment from this stage on is aimed at preventing a recurrence, and the lifestyle aspect of this is similar to what is recommended for patients with angina. However, after a heart attack, a patient may also be recommended to continue taking quite a few new medications. A typical 'cocktail would include aspirin, clopidogrel, a beta blocker, an ACE inhibitor and a statin. All five of these medications are prescribed to reduce the risk of recurrence, and, with the exception of clopidogrel, which is prescribed for one year only, most may be continued for life.

Increasingly, heart attack patients are referred for 'cardiac rehabilitation' sessions, in which they are given a structured programme of gentle exercises, guidance about lifestyle change and access to a support group. It is believed that the exercise component of these sessions in particular may help to encourage new growth of coronary vessels and so prevent recurrence of the heart attack.

On discharge from hospital, the patient is advised to increase daily activities very gradually. They are advised not to drive for 4 weeks, the time during which the risk of arrhythmias is significant. Most patients can return to normal activities by 2 months.

Treatment of heart attack: summary

The treatment for acute heart attack involves (see Q3.2e-2):

- emergency management of cardiac arrest
- aspirin and clopidogrel
- oxygen
- strong painkillers (diamorphine or morphine) and nitrates
- fibrinolytic (clot-busting) medication
- beta blockers
- ACE inhibitors
- statins.

The treatment for the recovery period involves:

- lifestyle advice and a graded return to daily activities
- aspirin and clopidogrel
- statins
- beta blockers and ACE inhibitors.

The red flags of angina and heart attack

All patients with angina and heart attack will benefit from referral to a conventional doctor for assessment and/or treatment. Red flags are those symptoms and signs that indicate that referral is to be considered. The red flags of angina and heart attack are described in Table 3.2e-II. This table forms part of the summary on red flags given in Appendix III, which also gives advice on the degree of urgency of referral for each of the red flag conditions listed.

Information Box 3.2e-III

Heart attack: comments from a Chinese medicine perspective

In Chinese medicine, the pain of the heart attack would usually be diagnosed, as is the case for angina, as Heart Blood Stagnation. Similarly, a background of Phlegm and Zong Qi Deficiency may be apparent. However, the severity of the condition in some cases, with cold sweating and high risk of cardiac arrest, implies that Heart Yang has been severely damaged, and is at risk of Collapse.

Aspirin and clopidogrel, because they encourage the free movement of blood, may be considered as Warming in nature, and in this way they can move Heart Blood Stagnation.

Adrenaline will also stimulate Heart Yang, but in doing so is likely to draw on reserves of Yin.

By dissolving a clot and allowing the clot to move, fibrinolytic drugs can be interpreted as Heating, and so will move Heart Blood Stagnation. However, they can give rise to the side-effect of serious haemorrhage, which is an adverse manifestation of Heat.

The energetics of the ACE inhibitors and beta blockers are more complex, as they both have a tendency to deplete Yang (see energetic descriptions in Chapter 3.2d), which would seem detrimental. What both these drugs do is reduce the immediate workload of the heart, so that the muscle is under less strain and is able to be better nourished by the blood in the coronary arteries. This would imply that they have the ability to Boost Heart Qi and Blood, but this energetic benefit is at the cost of overall depletion. So, in the long term, this action, which is suppressive in nature, is possibly depleting, but in the short term can prevent further Heart Blood Stagnation, and therefore can be life-saving.

Self-test 3.2e

Coronary heart disease

1. Jack is a 70-year-old gardener with diabetes and mild hypertension. In recent weeks he has not been feeling too good. He describes episodes of 'feeling queer' when he has been at work in the garden in the recent cold weather. During these episodes he feels dizzy and finds it difficult to catch his breath, but feels much better again after a few minutes when he goes indoors for a rest and a cup of tea.
   (i) What is a possible serious cause of Jack's recent symptoms?
   (ii) What are other possible diagnoses?
   (iii) Would you consider referral in this case?
2. Dave is a 25-year-old student. He has quite a reckless lifestyle, partying to the early hours, with smoking and drinking. He uses cannabis frequently. He is preoccupied with the symptoms he can experience in his body, and in particular with some episodes of chest pain that come on out of the blue and feel like a knife going into the left side of the chest. The pain can be felt goes down his arm. He feels breathless and his heart starts racing when this happens. His dad has recently had to have a heart bypass operation at the age of 65 years for severe angina.
   (i) What is a possible serious cause of Dave's recent symptoms?
   (ii) What are other possible diagnoses?
   (iii) Would you consider referral in this case?

Answers

1. (i) It is possible that Jack is suffering from episodes of angina. Although he feels no chest pain, this is well recognised in angina in elderly people, and in particular in those who suffer from diabetes. His age, hypertension and diabetes are all risk factors for coronary heart disease (CHD).
   (ii) Other possible explanations include simple overexertion, irregularities of the heart rhythm and transient ischaemic attacks (these last two are also serious, and are discussed in Chapter 3.2f).
   (iii) It would be wise to refer Jack, as the history is highly suggestive of early angina, which is a red flag for a risk of a future heart attack.
2. (i) It is also possible that Dave is suffering from angina, although this diagnosis is most unusual in someone of his age. The stabbing, left-sided chest pain is not characteristic of CHD. Although he is a smoker, it is unlikely that smoking will have caused sufficient damage to the coronary vessels by the age of 25 years, in the absence of other risk factors. He does have a family history of CHD, but age of onset of symptoms also runs in families, and Dave's father's angina started at a much later age.
   (ii) The most likely conventional medicine diagnosis is episodes of anxiety leading to panic attacks. Palpitations and increased anxiety are very characteristic of panic. The use of cannabis can in some people lead to excessive awareness and fear about bodily symptoms.
   (iii) Your decision to refer depends upon your confidence about the diagnosis. If you have any uncertainty you should refer to exclude the diagnosis of CHD.

   A referral may also be helpful, even if you are sure that Dave is suffering purely from panic attacks, as a 'clean bill of health' from the doctor may help him deal with his symptoms. This decision has to be made with care, as some people with anxiety about bodily symptoms may be more disturbed rather than reassured by the process of having medical tests, even if the results are normal.

Table 3.2e-II Red Flags 13 – angina and heart attack

Red Flag	Description	Reasoning
13.1	**Features of stable angina:** central chest pain related to exertion, eating or the cold, which improves with rest. Pain is heavy and gripping (rather than sharp or stabbing), and can radiate down the neck and arms Beware: can present as episodes of breathlessness/chest tightness, but without pain, in the elderly	Chest pain is a common anxiety symptom and is also a common feature of peptic ulcer disease, hiatus hernia and oesophagitis. Stable angina is distinguished from these syndromes by being predictably related to exertion, and generally develops in those over 35 years of age. It is far more likely to develop in older people and those with cardiovascular risk factors (see notes to Red Flags Table A12 in Appendix III) However, if there is any doubt, it is advisable to refer for medical assessment, as angina carries a high risk of heart attack and other cardiovascular events
13.2	**Features of unstable angina or heart attack**: sustained intense chest pain associated with fear or dread; palpitations and breathlessness may be present; the patient may vomit or develop a cold sweat Beware: can present as sudden onset of breathlessness, palpitations or confusion, but without pain, in the elderly	Very intense and heavy chest pain that tends to radiate to the left shoulder and arm is suggestive of cardiac pain. If sustained, this is a situation in which there is a high risk of cardiac arrest or worsening cardiovascular damage. Keep the patient calm, upright and still while waiting for help to arrive Under UK Health and Safety Executive guidance,[1] qualified first aiders are permitted to administer aspirin in the situation of suspected heart attack. There is very strong clinical evidence to support the benefits of aspirin in reducing the risk of fatal complications, and this effect is more powerful the sooner the aspirin is given The patient should be offered one 300-mg tablet to be chewed or swallowed. Aspirin is contraindicated in children under the age of 12 years, in pregnancy, if the patient has a bleeding disorder or is on anticoagulant medication, and in cases where there is a known allergy to aspirin or aspirin-induced asthma NB: Chest pain is a common anxiety symptom and is also a common feature of peptic ulcer disease, hiatus hernia and oesophagitis. If associated with anxiety, the pain is more likely to be centrally located and be sharp in quality
13.3	**Sudden-onset, tearing chest pain with radiation to back:** features of shock may be present (faintness, low blood pressure, rapid pulse)	This intense acute form of chest pain is suggestive of a dissecting aortic aneurysm. In this case urgent referral is required, but aspirin should not be given, as it promotes bleeding

[1]For the UK Health and Safety Executive guidance on first aid at work and the administration of aspirin, go to http://www.hse.gov.uk/firstaid/faqs.htm

Chapter 3.2f Heart failure and arrhythmias

LEARNING POINTS

At the end of this chapter you will be able to:
- understand the meaning of the terms ‘acute’ and ‘chronic’ heart failure
- differentiate between benign and more serious arrhythmias
- understand the treatment of heart failure and arrhythmias
- recognise the red flags of severe heart failure and arrhythmias.

Estimated time for chapter: 120 minutes.

Introduction

This chapter introduces the two other conditions that can result from CHD: heart failure and abnormalities of the heart rhythm (arrhythmias). Both these conditions can have other causes, which are also described in this chapter.

The conditions studied in this chapter are:

- Heart failure:
  - acute heart failure
  - chronic heart failure.
- Arrhythmias:
  - tachycardia and bradycardia
  - atrial fibrillation
  - supraventricular tachycardia
  - ectopic beats
  - ventricular fibrillation
  - heart block.

Heart failure

Heart failure is the inability of the heart to pump blood efficiently through the circulatory system. It affects about 10% of people over the age of 65 years.

In heart failure, because the pumping action is not sufficiently powerful to deal with all the blood arriving at the heart, blood accumulates in the vessels that lead to both sides of the heart. These vessels are the pulmonary veins, which transport blood from the lungs into the left side of the heart, and the systemic (bodily) veins, which transport blood from all the other tissues of the body to the right side of the heart. Figure 3.2f-I illustrates how the blood flows in a figure-of-eight pathway between the lungs and the body, and through the two sides of the heart.

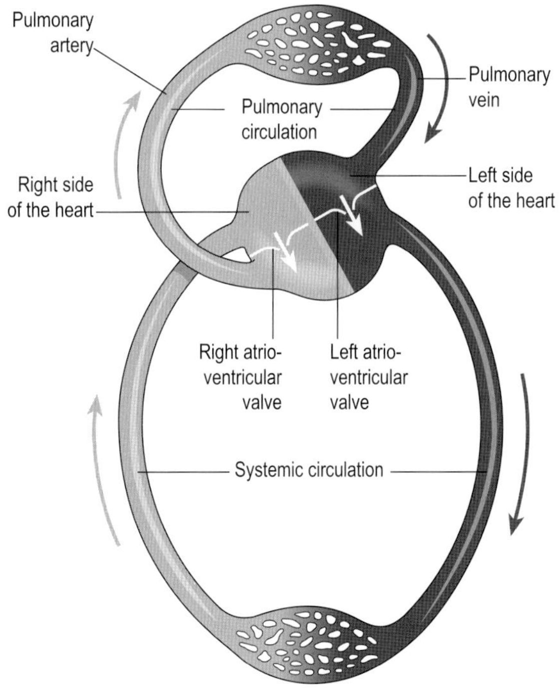

Figure 3.2f-I • The relationship between the pulmonary (involving the lungs) and systemic (bodily) circulations.

In heart failure, the heart is continually under strain. This strain can cause further weakening of the heart's pumping function, which means that the condition, if left untreated, can deteriorate rapidly. For this reason, only half of those who are diagnosed with heart failure will still be alive after 5 years. However, in recent years it has been shown that certain medical treatments can prolong life expectancy in heart failure, and for this reason it is important that early stages of heart failure are diagnosed and treated appropriately.

Heart failure can be categorised as acute or chronic, according to the rate at which the condition develops.

Acute heart failure

Acute heart failure is a serious condition. It occurs when the heart suddenly loses its pumping efficiency, and most commonly occurs as a result of a heart attack. In acute heart failure, the weakened heart muscle is suddenly faced with a large volume of blood that it is unable to pump. This has the most profound effects in the tissue of the lungs.

The sudden accumulation of blood in the pulmonary veins in the lungs leads to increased blood pressure within the lung capillaries. The increased pressure forces excess fluid from the capillaries into the tissue of the lungs. This fluid accumulates in the air spaces of the lungs, and severely impairs the ability of the lungs to take in oxygen. Oedema is the term given to excessive fluid in the tissues (see Chapter 3.2a), and this condition is therefore called 'pulmonary oedema'.

A patient with acute heart failure will experience a sudden onset of breathlessness. Some patients will cough up frothy fluid in an attempt to clear the air spaces in the lungs. In severe cases, the lips and the tongue will appear blue, as oxygen fails to reach the blood because of the fluid in the lungs. The patient has to sit upright and may feel panic stricken. Without medical treatment to reverse the situation many patients with acute heart failure will die.

Treatment of acute heart failure

Patients with acute heart failure are treated as an emergency. Oxygen is given to assist breathing and improve the ability of the heart to pump. Diamorphine (heroin), a powerful painkiller is also given, to relieve the panic and to treat the pulmonary oedema, as this drug tends to decrease the blood pressure in the veins of the body.

In addition, a powerful diuretic (furosemide or bumetanide) is given intravenously. This leads to a rapid shift of fluid from the circulation through the kidneys to the bladder. Diuretics are also used in the treatment of hypertension to encourage the kidneys to excrete fluid from the circulation (see Chapter 3.2d).

Information Box 3.2f-I

Pulmonary oedema: comments from a Chinese medicine perspective

In Chinese medicine, the symptoms of the condition of pulmonary oedema in acute heart failure would usually be diagnosed as Kidney Yang Deficiency with Water Overflowing to the Lungs and the Heart. One reason given for the Water Overflowing is that when Kidney Yang is deficient there is insufficient Fire of Ming Men. With insufficient Fire of Ming Men, the Yang of the Heart cannot be warmed, and fluid accumulates in the Lungs and Heart. The condition can progress to Heart Yang Collapse.

Diamorphine relieves pain, relaxes the blood vessels and can induce a state of euphoria and mental detachment. In excessive doses, diamorphine can induce confusion, coma and death as a result of depression of breathing. Side-effects are nausea, constipation, drowsiness and reduced depth of breathing. It can also cause pinpoint pupils, dry mouth, sweating and difficulty in urination. It is powerfully addictive.

The pain relief, euphoria (joy) and mental detachment suggest that diamorphine acts by in some way obstructing the Orifices of the Heart. The Pathological Factors that have this property include Phlegm, Full Heat and Blood Stagnation. Of these three, it would seem most likely that the numbness and later confusion and drowsiness associated with opiates is most fittingly attributed to Phlegm. The nausea could also be attributed to Phlegm obstructing the chest. Therefore, diamorphine might be described as Phlegm Inducing.

The initial beneficial effect on the blood vessels in the lungs could represent Boosting of Lung (or Zong) Qi, but with the long-term consequence of depletion of Lung Qi, reflected in the long-term effects of depression of breathing and constipation.

Dry mouth, sweating and difficulty in urinating suggest Subduing of Kidney Yin. Kidneys and Lungs are closely related, and it seems that diamorphine exerts much of its influence on the Kidney–Lung axis. Interestingly, the pupils are related to the Kidneys in Chinese medicine.

By stimulating urination, strong diuretics such as furosemide could be described as Clearing Damp (Transformation of Water) by Boosting Kidney Yang. Diuretics like furosemide are conventionally recognised to be toxic to the kidneys, and so their powerful action (Yang in nature) might ultimately be seen as depleting of Kidney Yin and Yang.

Sometimes nitrates are administered in the emergency situation (see Chapter 3.2e), as these also have the ability to cause dilatation of blood vessels and so may relieve the strain on the failing heart.

The combination of these treatments, although not always successful, can bring rapid relief to the patient, and can reverse a condition that otherwise could be fatal. After this emergency treatment, the patient requires intensive nursing care and treatment of the underlying cause of the acute heart failure.

Chronic heart failure

Chronic heart failure is the result of a much more gradual deterioration of the heart's ability to pump. A slight degree of heart failure is so common that it can almost be considered to be a normal part of ageing.

Coronary heart disease is probably the most common cause of chronic heart failure. Other causes include factors that increase the effort required of the heart, such as scarred heart valves, long-standing lung disease or persistent hypertension. Anaemia and thyroid disease are conditions in which the heart has to work harder than usual and can also lead to heart failure. Irregularities of heart rhythm (arrhythmias) that impair the smooth pumping action of the heart are another common cause.

In contrast to acute heart failure, in chronic heart failure, the body has a chance to adapt to the gradual build up of pressure within the veins leading to the heart. The response to the increased pressure in these veins is that fluid moves out gradually into the tissues of the body as well as into the lung tissue.

Failure of the right side of the heart to pump efficiently leads to a build up of fluid (oedema) in the tissues of the body. This initially is most marked in the areas of the body affected most by gravity, namely the feet and ankles. However, in severe chronic heart failure, the fluid can accumulate in other important tissues, including the liver and the bowel. This can have the serious consequence of damage to the function of these vital organs.

Failure of the left side of the heart to pump efficiently leads to a build up of fluid within the lungs. As this build up is gradual, the patient will experience increasing breathlessness on exertion and possibly a recurrent cough.

A patient with mild chronic heart failure may suffer from slight swelling of the ankles and shortness of breath on exertion, whereas a patient with severe chronic heart failure may have marked leg and ankle swelling, liver and digestive disorders, and experience exhaustion and disabling breathlessness.

Chronic heart failure can be diagnosed by physical examination of the heart, lungs and those areas where oedema is likely to develop (e.g. the ankles).

A chest X-ray image and an ECG might show characteristic changes of heart failure, but the most informative non-invasive method of investigation of heart failure is recognised to be echocardiography (cardiac ultrasound scan) (see Chapter 3.2b). Ideally, all patients should receive this test before treatment is started, so that a firm diagnosis can be made.

Treatment of chronic heart failure

The treatment of chronic heart failure should always include treatment of the underlying cause. If coronary heart disease is the cause, reduction of risk factors is essential. Hypertension should be treated (see Chapter 3.2d), valvular problems corrected by surgery (see Chapter 3.2g) and arrhythmias treated (see later in this chapter).

Reduction of dietary salt should be advised, as salt encourages retention of water. Alcohol can impair the pumping action of the heart further, so this also should be avoided.

Recent advances in the drug treatment of heart failure have led to the introduction of a wide range of potentially useful drugs. The most commonly prescribed drugs are the diuretics and ACE inhibitors, but increasingly patients may be prescribed one or more of the following: vasodilators, nitrates, digoxin, beta blockers or alpha blockers. All these classes of drugs are listed in Chapter 2 of the BNF.

Diuretics include the thiazide diuretics, such as bendroflumethiazide, which are prescribed also for hypertension, and the more powerful loop diuretics, such as furosemide, which are given in acute heart failure. Both these drugs act at the kidney in different ways to promote urination, and therefore help to shift accumulating fluid from the circulation. The patient will notice a reduction in ankle oedema and relief of breathlessness within a few days of taking diuretics. However, there is no evidence that diuretics increase life expectancy in heart failure.

The action of ACE inhibitors in hypertension is described in Chapter 3.2d. ACE inhibitors both reduce the tone of the small arteries and promote urination. The relaxed blood vessels and reduction of fluid in the circulation reduces the load on the heart. Clinical studies have demonstrated that patients with heart failure who are prescribed ACE inhibitors and diuretics have an increased life expectancy compared to those prescribed diuretics alone (see Q3.2f-1).

Beta blockers can be helpful in heart failure as they reduce the pressure against which the struggling heart muscle has to work. Increasingly beta blockers are being introduced to patients early in the course of their condition as it has become recognised recently that, like ACE inhibitors, that they reduce mortality in heart failure.

Arrhythmias

'Arrhythmia' is the medical term used to describe a range of abnormalities of heart rhythm. The basic problem in arrhythmias is either rooted in the function of the pacemaker at the centre of the heart, or in that of the conducting fibres that transmit the regular electrical impulse from the pacemaker to the rest of the heart so that it contracts in a controlled and efficient way.

It may help to turn back to Chapter 3.2a to read about the conduction system of the heart in preparation for the study of arrhythmias (see Q3.2f-2).

Causes of arrhythmias

As described above, a heart attack can lead to arrhythmias, as the damage resulting from infarction can involve either the pacemaker or the conducting fibres in the heart. The degeneration resulting from coronary heart disease, even without the sudden damage of a heart attack, is probably the most important cause of the arrhythmias found in elderly people. In CHD the pacemaker and conducting fibres of the heart can degenerate as a result of chronic poor blood supply and so become more vulnerable to triggering arrhythmias.

Arrhythmias can occur for reasons other than CHD. In particular, some can result from a congenital abnormality of the pacemaker system. Other causes of arrhythmias include damage of the heart muscle by drugs (e.g. digoxin) and alcohol, infections of the heart and pericardium (e.g. pericarditis), and strain on the heart muscle, which can result from scarred heart valves. The latter two causes are discussed in Chapter 3.2g.

Disorders of rate (benign arrhythmias)

Arrhythmias can be classified as a benign finding. This means that the disorder does not indicate a fundamental problem with the pacemaker system of the heart. Benign arrhythmias are always disorders of rate rather than rhythm. In conventional medicine, a rapid pulse (tachycardia) is defined as a rate of above 100 beats/minute in an adult, and a slow pulse (bradycardia) as a rate of less than 60 beats/minute.

Benign (sinus) tachycardia

Common non-cardiac causes of a rapid but regular heart rate include anxiety, exercise, pregnancy and fever. Anaemia and thyroid disease are two diseases that can lead to a rapid heart rate.

This tachycardia is not always so benign. If very rapid, the racing heart cannot pump efficiently, and heart failure may develop. This is a known consequence of conditions such as severe anaemia and an overactive thyroid gland. The tachycardia can lead a patient with coronary atheroma to experience angina because the coronary vessels are unable to meet the heart's increased demand for oxygen and nutrients.

Benign (sinus) bradycardia

Common non-cardiac causes of a slow pulse rate include cardiovascular fitness (a very common finding in athletes) and extreme cold (hypothermia).

Deficiency of thyroid hormone can also lead to a slow pulse. Some drugs, most commonly beta blockers, can lead to a bradycardia.

Again the bradycardia is not always so benign. If the pulse rate is very slow the patient may experience episodes of dizziness or fainting.

Information Box 3.2f-II

Benign arrhythmias: comments from a Chinese medicine perspective

In Chinese medicine, a benign tachycardia is experienced as a Rapid Pulse, indicating Full or Empty Heat, and a benign bradycardia is experienced as a Slow Pulse, indicating Full or Empty Cold. Although a slow pulse may be interpreted as a marker of fitness from a western perspective, from a Chinese medicine perspective the slowness would suggest that excessive exercise has led to some depletion of Yang.

All the other arrhythmias to be studied in this section involve a disorder of the conduction system of the heart itself. The investigations and treatment of these arrhythmias have features in common, so these shall be discussed first.

The investigation of arrhythmias

Arrhythmias can, of course, be detected at the pulse, but can only be diagnosed accurately by means of an ECG recording (see Chapter 3.2b). The ECG can help distinguish between arrhythmias that have similar pulse patterns but different underlying causes. Sometimes a 24-hour ECG is required to capture the irregularity of rhythm when it is intermittent.

Most patients with an arrhythmia will also undergo echocardiography (see Chapter 3.2b) to exclude valvular and other structural problems, and to assess whether or not there is any degree of heart failure.

Treatment of arrhythmias

Symptomatic or life-threatening arrhythmias are treated medically by a range of different types of drugs collectively termed the 'antiarrhythmic drugs'. All these drugs are conventionally recognised as suppressive rather than curative, as withdrawal of the drug usually results in recurrence of the problem.

The drugs include digoxin (see BNF, Chapter 2.1), verapamil, a calcium-channel blocker (see BNF, Chapter 2.6.2), beta blockers (see BNF, Chapter 2.4) and a range of drugs listed in the BNF as antiarrhythmic drugs (see BNF, Chapter 2.3). The latter include drugs such as amiodarone and disopyramide.

These different drugs act at different parts of the conducting system of the heart, and so the energetic interpretation of each type is different. Only digoxin, the most commonly prescribed antiarrhythmic drug, is discussed in detail in this chapter. The calcium-channel blockers and beta blockers have been described in detail in Chapter 3.2d.

Planned cardioversion by electric shock is a useful technique for some patients. This is described below under the heading Atrial Fibrillation.

Many patients benefit from the surgical insertion of an artificial pacemaker. This is a small, battery-powered unit that is inserted under the skin of the upper chest. Wires lead from the unit and pass via the blood vessels to rest against the inside wall of the heart. Most pacemakers are now dual-chamber units, which means they can stimulate both the atria and the ventricles, and so simulate a natural heartbeat.

The pacemaker unit contains a sensor that can detect deficiencies in the heart rhythm. When an absent or irregular heartbeat is detected, an electrical impulse is sent to the heart to override the failing conducting system, and a regular rhythm is thus reinstated. Some advanced pacemakers can appropriately alter the rate of the heart according to activity or respiration. The programming of the pacemaker can be performed remotely once it has been inserted, so adjustments to its function can be made if necessary.

Some patients may benefit from a surgical operation to remove (by means of radio waves) an abnormal part of the conducting system of the heart. This surgery is called 'ablation therapy'. It is considered a relatively minor intervention, as it is performed as part of a cardiac catheterisation procedure (see Chapter 3.2b). Sometimes, if this involves necessary damage to the natural pacemaker, an artificial pacemaker is inserted to thereafter provide a regular electrical stimulus to the heart (so-called 'ablate and pace' treatment).

Implantable defibrillators (ICDs) are increasingly used to prevent sudden death. These devices (Figure 3.2f-II) are similar in size to a pacemaker, but are programmed to deliver an electric shock to the heart should the sensor detect a burst of chaotic ventricular rhythm. Clinical trials have shown that in certain groups ICDs significantly reduce the risk of sudden cardiac death.

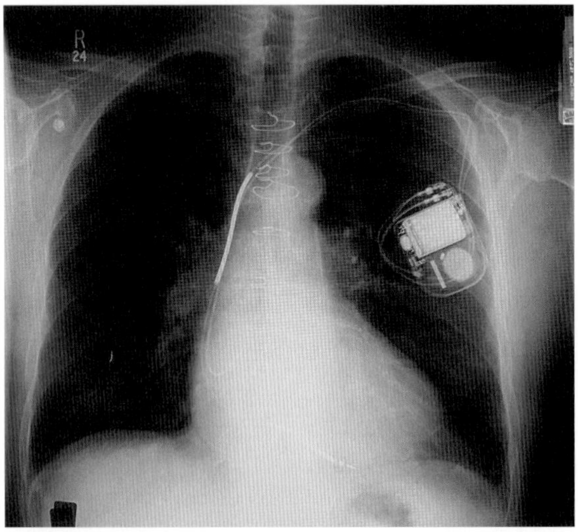

Figure 3.2f-II • Chest x-ray image showing the location of an ICD • As with the pacemaker, the ICD is located just superior to the pectoral muscles. The image illustrates the pathway of the leads through the subclavian vein and the superior vena cava, and thence to the right side of the heart.

In summary, the treatment of arrhythmias includes:

- treatment of the underlying cause
- antiarrhythmic drugs
- cardioversion by electric shock
- insertion of an artificial pacemaker
- surgical ablation therapy
- implantable defibrillators (ICDs).

Ectopic beats

The most common disorder of rhythm (rather than rate) is called an 'ectopic beat'. This is felt as a single beat that is out of time with the regular rhythm of the normal heartbeats. The patient may experience a palpitation at the time of the ectopic beat, or may be totally unaware of it.

Ectopic beats are more frequent when at rest and in the elderly. On their own, unless very frequent (more than one every 10 beats) or accompanied by symptoms, they are not conventionally considered to be a cause for concern.

However, the development of frequent ectopic beats is considered to be a sign of degeneration of the pacemaker system of the heart. A patient with frequent ectopic beats may be investigated for heart disease, and may be offered antiarrhythmic drugs.

Information Box 3.2f-III

Ectopic beats: a Chinese medicine perspective

Ectopic beats would possibly be diagnosed by a Chinese practitioner as a Knotted pulse, as the pulse rate is basically regular but has pauses at irregular intervals. However, a Knotted pulse is also classically a slow pulse. This is not always the case with ectopic beats, which can occur with a pulse of normal or rapid rate. Nevertheless, whatever the pulse rate, the occasional dropped beats probably would represent a degree of depletion of Heart Qi or Yang, as it is Heart Yang that dominates the function of the Heart.

Atrial fibrillation

Atrial fibrillation (AF) is a very common arrhythmia in old age, and may not be noticed by the patient. Although CHD is the most common cause of AF, other common causes include narrowing of the heart valves, thyroid disease and excessive alcohol intake.

The cause of AF is a degeneration of the pacemaker of the heart, which can then no longer transmit a regular impulse to the atria, the upper chambers of the heart. For this reason, the contraction of the atrial muscle fibres is uncoordinated (the fibres are said to be in 'fibrillation'). Heart muscle in fibrillation cannot perform a pumping function.

However, in AF, a second pacemaker deeper in the heart takes over and transmits irregular impulses to the ventricles, the lower chamber of the heart. The ventricles can often take almost the full load of the pumping function of the atria, which is why some patients may be unaware of their AF. However, other patients can suffer palpitations and breathlessness, because the second pacemaker is too fast and irregular, and the inefficient pumping leads to a degree of heart failure.

The pulse of a patient with AF is said to be 'irregularly irregular' in rhythm. This means that there is no pattern to the heartbeat. The pulse varies in both volume and rate from beat to beat. The pulse rate can also be very rapid. In some people, the condition is paroxysmal, meaning that the arrhythmia occurs in episodes separated by periods of normal rhythm.

Apart from causing an inefficient heart pumping action, the fibrillation of the atria has another severe consequence, which is that the turbulent blood within the chambers can clot and form emboli. Although tiny, these particles of clot can travel in the circulation to the brain to cause significant damage. The emboli can lodge in cerebral arteries and lead to areas of infarction. Infarction in the brain leads to the clinical syndrome of stroke.

Sometimes the emboli in the brain are so small that they can break up and the effect on the brain is only temporary. In this case the patient will experience repeated episodes of temporary brain disturbance, such as loss of vision, confusion or dizziness, which last for a few minutes only. These episodes are called 'transient ischaemic attacks' (TIAs). Although temporary, TIAs need to be recognised as red flags that a permanent stroke may follow shortly. For this reason, the treatment of AF, particularly if there is a history of TIAs, is taken very seriously.

There are three considerations in the treatment of AF:

- control of the rate, which is important if the rate is too fast
- control of the rhythm
- prevention of the formation of emboli (anticoagulation).

In elderly people and in those in whom the pacemaker is likely to be permanently damaged, control of rate becomes the most important aspect of treatment. In most people, rate can be controlled by one or more of three types of drug: digoxin-like drugs, calcium-channel blockers and beta blockers.

Digoxin (also known as 'digitalis'), which is a derivative of the foxglove (*Digitalis lanata*), is a very toxic substance if taken to excess, which means that the dose has to be controlled very carefully, and may need to be checked by means of blood tests. Digoxin increases the force of the heartbeat and tends to steady the irregularity in AF. In this way it can reverse the heart failure of AF. If digoxin reaches toxic levels it can cause nausea and vomiting, visual disturbance and severe life-threatening arrhythmias. The actions of calcium-channel blockers and beta blockers are described in Chapter 3.2d.

However, drug treatment of heart rate does not reduce the risk of thromboembolism in AF. For this reason, patients with sustained AF are prescribed either aspirin or warfarin (see Chapter 2.2d) to reduce the tendency of the blood to clot in the atria. Because of the increased risk of blood-clot formation, warfarin is prescribed to most people over the age of 75 years and anyone with previous stroke, impaired heart function or diabetes. Warfarin treatment requires the clotting ability of the patient's blood to be assessed regularly by means of blood tests. The aim of the treatment is to increase the time for clotting to fall within the range of between 2 and 3 times that of normal clotting (i.e. to have an international normalised ratio (INR) between 2 and 3). Aspirin is reserved for younger people who are deemed to have no other obvious risks for vascular disease.

Increasingly, patients who develop AF may be offered treatment for the underlying rhythmic disturbance. In those whose pacemaker is not fully degenerated, electric shock (cardioversion) can reinstate regular rhythm. This approach is used particularly in young people and in those who are suffering severe symptoms due to a rapid heart rate. The shock is administered while the patient is under anaesthetic and in some people can totally reverse the arrhythmia.

Other patients may be given a high dose of one of the powerful antiarrhythmic drugs (e.g. amiodarone) by injection. This can have the same effect as an electric shock cardioversion.

Rarely, surgery to the heart may be performed to remove the area of the pacemaker system that is considered to be causing the problem, and then an artificial pacemaker is inserted ('ablate and pace' treatment).

Information Box 3.2f-IV

Atrial fibrillation: a Chinese medicine perspective

Depending on the actual rate and type of irregularity, the pulse in atrial fibrillation (AF) might be described as Choppy, Hasty or Knotted by a Chinese medicine practitioner. These pulse findings represent severe Blood Deficiency, Heart Qi or Yin Deficiency with Heat, or Cold with Heart Qi or Yang Deficiency, respectively. All of these suggest severe depletion of the Heart. In AF, the quivering of the fibrillating atrial muscles, and the paroxysmal nature of the condition, might also suggest the presence of Wind.

The breathlessness and palpitations that can accompany AF also suggest severe Heart Qi/Yang Deficiency. This can progress to a state of heart failure in which fluid accumulates in the lungs and body tissues. This would be described as Kidney and Heart Yang Deficiency, with Water overflowing to the Heart and Lungs.

By improving contractility and normalising the heart rate, digoxin appears to boost Heart Yang, but in excess can cause severe and rapid arrhythmias, possibly because this benefit is at the cost of damage to Heart Yin and the Heat that is associated with this. The digestive and visual disturbances that digoxin can cause suggest that in excess it is harmful to the Spleen and Liver.

The electric shock administered in cardioversion normalises the heart rate and rhythm and thus boosts Heart Yang.

Ventricular arrhythmias

In contrast to atrial fibrillation, which may not seriously impair the pumping action of the heart, if fibrillation of the ventricles occurs, the heart cannot pump at all. A patient in ventricular fibrillation will rapidly lose consciousness and die without emergency treatment. Ventricular fibrillation is, in fact, the main cause of cardiac arrest following a heart attack. If an infarcted area of muscle incorporates the conducting system of the heart, the heart muscle fibres go into uncoordinated movement, leading to a quivering mass of tissue that cannot pump.

Ventricular tachycardia describes episodes of a rapid ventricular rate, which in most people leads to dizziness or collapse because of inefficient pumping. Ventricular tachycardia is a red flag for ventricular fibrillation, and is thus treated very seriously.

The first emergency treatment that should be given in ventricular fibrillation is CPR. This does not necessarily reverse the fibrillation, but will provide a temporary pumping action for the body until electric-shock treatment (cardioversion) can be given. In some people, simply the physical pressure on the chest can reverse the fibrillation. However, most people require the electric shock of cardioversion, and possibly drugs such as adrenaline to enable a normal pacemaker action to be restored. If the damage to the heart from the infarction is too great, these treatments cannot be successful.

After a successful reversal of ventricular fibrillation, an ECG may reveal changes that show bursts of ventricular tachycardia or a continued instability of the heartbeat. This means that a repeated episode of fibrillation is more likely to occur. In this case a powerful antiarrhythmic drug is given intravenously to stabilise the pacemaker system. Some people with continued instability of the heartbeat may be prescribed an antiarrhythmic drug long term, or alternatively might be offered the implantation of a defibrillator device (ICD, described earlier in this chapter).

Information Box 3.2f-V

Ventricular arrhythmias: a Chinese medicine perspective

In Chinese medicine, the fibrillation of the ventricles again suggests Wind. In the case of heart attack, this Wind has possibly been generated as a response to Heart Blood Stagnation and Phlegm (which were both suggested earlier as components of the aetiology of coronary heart disease). The consequence of this is Heart Yang Collapse.

Electric shocks, by restoring normal heart function, could be described as Stimulating Heart Yang. A strengthened Heart Yang will permit movement, and thus the clearance of the internally generated Wind.

Supraventricular tachycardia

A supraventricular tachycardia (SVT) is a disorder of rapid heart rate. It is not classified as benign, as during the arrhythmia the electric impulse travels to the ventricles either from a site other than the atrioventricular node or via an unusual pathway of the conducting system.

The patient, who is often a young adult on first presentation, experiences a sudden onset of palpitations. This may come on out of the blue, but sometimes is provoked by coffee or exertion. The pulse rate can be very rapid (140–280 beats/minute). Additional symptoms include dizziness, breathlessness and sometimes chest pains. In some cases the episode stops spontaneously within minutes to hours of onset.

The most common condition that can mimic an SVT is a panic attack, in which anxiety causes the heart to race. One differentiating feature, apart from the level of the associated anxiety, is the rate of the pulse. In a panic attack the pulse rarely exceeds 140 beats/minute.

The simplest treatment for an attack of SVT is for the patient or a practitioner to massage the area that overlies the carotid arteries in the neck (in the region of acupoint Stomach-9; Renying). Ideally, the patient should be lying supine during this manoeuvre. The pressure in this area sets up a reflex that causes the heart rate to slow down. Other techniques include immersing the face in cold water and rapid squatting. In a significant proportion of episodes these simple techniques will stop the tachycardia.

If non-medical approaches are not successful, antiarrhythmic drugs are given intravenously to stop the SVT. The most common drug now given is adenosine. This is a very rapid-acting drug that can cause a temporary block in the pacemaker and so can abort the arrhythmia. This drug has to be given under medical observation just in case a serious arrhythmia results from treatment.

A long-term prescription of an antiarrhythmic drug may be given to prevent future attacks. Beta blockers or calcium-channel blockers are commonly prescribed. Currently, many patients with SVT are offered surgical ablation therapy to remove the abnormal part of the conducting system. This is not considered to be a major operation, as it can be performed by a similar approach as used for cardiac catheterisation (see earlier in this chapter). This procedure is successful in over 95% of cases.

Information Box 3.2f-VI

Supraventricular tachycardia: a Chinese medicine perspective

The very rapid rate of the pulse in supraventricular tachycardia (SVT) suggests Empty or Full Heat. This would accord with the observation that coffee, which is Heating, through depleting the Kidneys and aggravating the Liver, can trigger attacks of SVT. The rapid onset and abrupt end of an episode of SVT suggests that Wind might also be an additional factor.

The physiological cause of SVT is an area of abnormal heart tissue, which in many cases can be successfully ablated to cure the problem. Ablative surgery could possibly enable Clearance of underlying Pathological Factors which may have been present since before birth. Although physically damaging, this treatment might engender an energetic cure.

Heart block

This rather alarming term describes an arrhythmia that results from an impairment of the smooth passage of an electrical impulse through the conducting system of the heart. It is almost as if there is a literal block in the way. In most cases the 'block' is due to an area of damaged heart muscle resulting from CHD. Like AF, heart block is an arrhythmia that can be a common incidental finding in elderly people.

The result of partial heart block is that one or more impulses fail to 'get through' the conduction system, and this can lead to a regular pulse with missed beats at regular intervals. If no impulses 'get through' from the node to the rest of the heart, a second pacemaker can set up a regular rhythm from the ventricles. This leads to a very slow regular heart rate of about 40–50 beats/minute. This is called 'complete heart block'. Heart block, even when complete, may give rise to no symptoms, but can lead to breathlessness, palpitations and, in the case of complete heart block, blackouts. Blackouts resulting from complete heart block are called 'Stokes–Adams attacks'. A patient recovering from a Stokes–Adams attack may be aware of rapid palpitations and facial flushing.

The concern about heart block is that it may herald a more serious arrhythmia, and so, if diagnosed, it may be treated with insertion of an artificial pacemaker.

From the point of view of a complementary therapist, as a simple rule of thumb, if the presence of either heart failure or the pulse irregularity of a non-benign arrhythmia is suspected, referral should be considered. A medical diagnosis can help with an assessment of the seriousness of the underlying condition. If the diagnosis suggests a life-threatening condition, medical treatment, although suppressive in nature, needs to be offered to the patient (see Q3.2f-3).

Information Box 3.2f-VII

Heart block: a Chinese medicine perspective

The pulse of partial heart block would be described as Intermittent, signifying in Chinese medicine a serious imbalance of one of the Yin organs. Complete heart block gives rise to a pulse that would be described as Slow. Heart block can be interpreted as a Deficiency of Heart Qi/Yang (with Internal Cold if there is complete heart block).

A pacemaker stimulates Heart Yang, and in this way counteracts the fundamental imbalance of Yang underlying heart block.

The red flags of heart failure and arrhythmias

Most patients with heart failure and arrhythmias will benefit from referral to a conventional doctor for assessment and/or treatment. Red flags are those symptoms and signs that indicate that referral is to be considered. The red flags of heart failure and arrhythmias are described in Table 3.2f-I. This table forms part of the summary on red flags given in Appendix III, which also gives advice on the degree of urgency of referral for each of the red flag conditions listed.

Table 3.2f-I Red Flags 14 – heart failure and arrhythmias

Red Flag	Description	Reasoning
14.1	**Features of mild chronic heart failure:** slight swelling of ankles, slight breathlessness on exertion and when lying flat, cough, and with no palpitations or chest pain **Dry cough** may be the only symptom in sedentary elderly people	Chronic heart failure refers to a condition in which the pumping ability of the heart is reduced, and this results in accumulation of tissue fluid in the lungs (breathlessness) and ankles (oedema). It may remain undiagnosed if mild, but it is associated with increased risk of worsening damage to the heart. Current medical guidance is that all patients will benefit in terms of symptoms and life expectancy from medical treatment of heart failure, and referral is recommended for assessment by electrocardiography (ECG) and echocardiography
14.2	**Features of severe chronic heart failure: marked swelling of ankles and lower legs, disabling breathlessness and exhaustion**	Severe chronic heart failure is a serious condition associated with a high mortality. It will benefit from medical management, and this is associated with an improved life expectancy
14.3	**Features of acute heart failure:** sudden onset of disabling breathlessness, and watery cough	Acute heart failure results from a sudden loss in the ability of the heart to pump effectively, and most commonly results from heart attack, arrhythmia or valvular damage. The patient requires emergency treatment and needs to be kept calm and sitting upright until help arrives
14.5	A pulse that is obviously **irregularly irregular (atrial fibrillation)**	An irregularly irregular (totally unpredictable) pulse is a feature of atrial fibrillation. This arrhythmia carries a risk of the production of tiny blood clots within the chaotically contracting atria of the heart. These clots may then be dispersed (as emboli) to lodge in the circulation of the brain, and so carry a risk of transient ischaemic attack and stroke Refer as a high priority if features of heart failure or angina are also present, or if there is a history of blackouts or neurological symptoms
14.6	A very rapid pulse of 140-250 beats/minute (most likely to be supraventricular tachycardia or atrial fibrillation)	Episodes of tachycardia (very rapid pulse) can be exhausting for the patient and may progress to a more serious arrhythmia or lead to the symptoms of acute heart failure If the attack is not settling in 5 minutes refer urgently for medical management. If the attack settles refer as a high priority so that the cause can be investigated

Continued

Table 3.2f-I Red Flags 14 – heart failure and arrhythmias—Cont'd

Red Flag	Description	Reasoning
14.7	A very slow pulse of **40-**50 beats/minute (**complete heart block**) that is either of recent onset or is associated with features such as **dizziness, lightheadedness** or **fainting**	Some healthy individuals have a naturally slow heart rate, particularly if they have trained as athletes. However, if the rate suddenly drops to 40–50 beats/minute this is characteristic of complete heart block, wherein the natural pacemaker of the heart has become unable to transmit a more frequent impulse to the ventricles. In this case the patient will start to feel dizzy and breathless and may pass out (Stokes–Adams attack). Refer urgently if ongoing, and as a high priority if the attack has settled down. The patient will need assessment for an implanted pacemaker system
14.8	A pulse that is **regular** but **skips beats at regular intervals** (i.e. one out of every 3–5 beats is missing) (incomplete **heart block**)	The occasional missed beat (ventricular ectopic beat) is not a worrying finding. It is more likely to occur in older people However, if the beat is missed at a regular and frequent rate (more often than one in every five beats) this suggests the conduction defect of incomplete heart block. As this carries a risk of progression to a more serious arrhythmia, it merits referral for cardiological assessment If the patient is well and was unaware of the problem until you found it, refer non-urgently
14.9	**Unexplained falls or faints** in an elderly person may be the result of an arrhythmia (**cardiac syncope**)	A temporary cardiac arrhythmia may result in a dizzy spell or sudden loss of consciousness from which an elderly person may recover very quickly. These episodes may account for unexplained falls. Consider referral if a patient reports a fall but cannot remember how it happened
14.10	**Cardiac arrest:** collapse with no palpable pulse	Cardiac arrest results from the arrhythmia known as ventricular fibrillation. The most common cause is heart attack, but it can also occur spontaneously as a result of degenerative damage to the conducting system of the heart. It may also result from electric shock In contrast to atrial fibrillation, in which the heart continues to pump fairly efficiently, when the ventricles of the heart go into chaotic rhythm the pumping function of the heart is totally lost and there is immediate circulatory collapse. Once help has been called, the patient requires urgent cardiopulmonary resuscitation from a qualified first aider

Self-test 3.2f

Heart failure and arrhythmias

1. Moira is 77 years old and has mild hypertension, for which she has been treated with a beta blocker, atenolol. Recently, she has noticed that her ankles have started to swell and she is not feeling at all herself. She is tired, and walking is much more of an effort. She is finding that if she lies flat in bed she is breathless, so she uses four pillows to prop herself up. She is sure that her tablets do not agree with her.
   (i) What condition do you suspect that Moira has developed?
   (ii) Do you think Moira is correct in assuming that the tablets may have caused her symptoms?
   (iii) Would you refer Moira for a conventional medicine opinion?
2. Amy, a 47-year-old woman, is wanting acupuncture for very heavy periods. She feels exhausted all the time, and her friends tell her she looks white as a ghost. She says that she notices her heartbeat racing after the slightest exertion and she needs to rest often. When you examine her, the pulse rate is 100 beats/minute but is regular.
   (i) What sort of arrhythmia is this in conventional medicine terms?
   (ii) What is a possible cause of the arrhythmia?
   (iii) Would you refer Amy for conventional medical treatment?
3. Mr Williams is an 80-year-old patient who comes to you for regular treatment to keep in him 'in balance'. At his most recent appointment you notice that his usually regular pulse is irregularly irregular, but the rate is not too high at 84 beats/minute. When you question Mr Williams, he admits he has not felt too good recently, he has felt more tired and breathless, and occasionally has felt palpitations.
   (i) What conventional medicine diagnosis does the pulse indicate?
   (ii) What complication might explain Mr Williams' breathlessness?
   (iii) What are the reasons why you might refer him for conventional medicine diagnosis and treatment?

Answers

1. (i) Moira has developed symptoms that suggest mild chronic heart failure.
   (ii) Moira could have developed heart failure as a consequence of ageing and longstanding hypertension. However, she may be correct in assuming that the beta blockers have made the condition more apparent. Beta blockers act by reducing the force of contraction of the heart muscle (they deplete Heart Yang in Chinese medicine terms). This can be sufficient to precipitate the appearance of symptoms of heart failure in someone whose heart is already under strain. However, when prescribed with ACE inhibitors Beta blockers are known to be a valuable treatment for heart failure.
   (iii) In an uncomplicated case of mild chronic heart failure it can be safe to delay referral to see how the patient responds to your treatment. However, in Moira's case you should consider referral to ensure she receives full investigations and a review of medication. The most appropriate choice of medication for

Moira would be an ACE inhibitor and diuretic, as these treat both hypertension and heart failure. She may find that she is offered Beta blocker therapy once again when she has stabilised on these medications.

2. (i) The rapid but regular pulse rate is characteristic of a benign tachycardia.
   (ii) Although there are other possibilities, severe anaemia due to longstanding blood loss may be the cause of the tachycardia in Amy's case. This would also explain her tiredness and pallor.
   (iii) Anaemia can respond to dietary changes and complementary therapy, but the response is likely to be slow. However, the response to treatment (such as with acupuncture) of menorrhagia can be more rapid. As Amy is suffering such marked symptoms you should consider referral for assessment of the anaemia and treatment of iron deficiency. If Amy is concerned about taking conventional medication you could advise her that iron supplements are energetically appropriate for her condition. (She could instead buy a more naturally produced alternative, such as Floradix, although these preparations are less powerful in their effect.)
3. (i) The irregularly irregular pulse indicates that Mr Williams has atrial fibrillation.
   (ii) The breathlessness suggests that the arrhythmia has led to a degree of chronic heart failure.
   (iii) You should consider referral for a confirmation of the diagnosis and an assessment of the degree of heart failure and need for treatment. Treatment in atrial fibrillation is important because of the risk of worsening heart failure, transient ischaemic attacks and stroke. The risk is particularly high in people over the age of 75 years.

Chapter 3.2g Diseases of the heart muscle, pericardium and heart valves, and congenital heart disease

LEARNING POINTS

At the end of this chapter you will be able to:

- recognise the diseases of the heart muscle and pericardium
- understand the problems that can result from disorders of the heart valves
- understand the principles of treatment of these conditions
- recognise the ways in which the heart can be affected in congenital heart disease
- understand the principles of correction of congenital heart disease.

Estimated study time: 90 minutes.

Introduction

This final chapter on the cardiovascular system focuses on the conditions that affect the structural components of the heart – the heart muscle, the pericardium and the heart valves. The inborn structural problems of the heart, which include 'hole in the heart' and 'blue baby' syndrome, are also described. These problems are collectively termed 'congenital heart disease'. Prior to reading this chapter it might be helpful to turn back to Chapter 3.2a for a simple reminder of the structure of the heart chambers and valves.

The conditions studied in this chapter are:

- Diseases of the heart muscle:
  - myocarditis
  - cardiomyopathy.
- Diseases of the pericardium:
  - acute and chronic (constrictive) pericarditis.
- Diseases of the heart valves:
  - incompetent (leaking) valves
  - stenosed (constricted) valves
  - endocarditis
  - congenital heart disease.

Diseases of the heart muscle

Myocarditis

As might be understood from the name, myocarditis refers to inflammation of the heart muscle (myocardium). The most common causes of this inflammation are infections by viruses, bacteria and protozoa, and adverse reactions to drugs. The viruses that cause myocarditis may be the same as those that usually cause colds and flu in most people, suggesting that the patient with myocarditis has a pre-existing susceptibility. The inflammation may be due in part to direct toxicity of the causative agent, and later because the effect of the agent on the cardiac cells is to stimulate an autoimmune response against the myocardium.

The inflammation affects the pumping action of the heart, and so patients will have fever, a rapid pulse and, in severe cases, features of heart failure (see Q 3.2g-1).

Because of the rapid onset, the inability of the inflamed heart to pump efficiently leads to breathlessness as a result of pulmonary oedema (see Chapter 3.2f). The patient is treated with bed rest to rest the heart, and antimicrobial drugs if appropriate. The heart failure is controlled by means of diuretics, ACE inhibitors, beta blockers and/or digoxin until the inflammation settles down.

It is considered important for the patient to refrain from athletic activities for 6 months to allow full healing after an episode of myocarditis. Most patients who survive the acute inflammation get completely better, although some are left with a permanent impairment of the heart muscle known as 'cardiomyopathy'. This condition is discussed presently.

Cardiomyopathy

'Cardiomyopathy' is a general term used to describe any impairment in the ability of the heart muscle to perform its pumping action. As stated above, inflammation in myocarditis can leave the patient with a permanent cardiomyopathy. Other causes include damage from drugs and alcohol, and rare inherited conditions. CHD can lead to a form of cardiomyopathy that results from the long-standing state of impaired nourishment of the heart muscle.

Information Box 3.2g-I

Myocarditis: comments from a Chinese medicine perspective

A rapid onset of fever and tachycardia could be diagnosed in Chinese medicine as an invasion of Wind Heat. This would be in keeping with a condition that results commonly from an external agent such as a virus. However, damage to the cardiac muscle cells and the resulting inflammation is suggestive of the more profound imbalance of Heart Yin Deficiency, and this is evidence that the Heat has penetrated to a deep level to cause this imbalance. It would make sense from a Chinese medicine perspective that a pre-existing imbalance of Heart Yin would predispose a person to be vulnerable to this condition. The development of pulmonary oedema would be diagnosed as Deficiency of Heart and Kidney Yang, with Water Overflowing to the Heart and Lungs, and this would make sense in that a severe depletion of Yin (substance) is usually accompanied by a deficiency of Yang (function).

Information Box 3.2g-II

Cardiomyopathy: comments from a Chinese medicine perspective

The reduced ability of the heart to pump efficiently and the resulting oedema would be diagnosed as Heart and Kidney Yang with Water Overflowing. However, the fundamental root of the problem is in the substance of the heart muscle, which is impaired due either to a genetic weakness or to damage by toxins or infectious agents. This would constitute Depletion of Heart Yin. Stiffened, dilated or scarred myocardium could be described in terms of Blood Stasis or Phlegm (resulting from depletion of Yin and Yang). Sudden unexpected death from ventricular fibrillation suggests Invasion of Wind and Yang Collapse. In contrast to acute myocarditis, in which deficient Yin and Heat are the prominent imbalances, in cardiomyopathy it is deficient Yang that predominates.

By replacing a failing, distorted heart muscle with a healthy functional one, heart transplantation literally replenishes Yin and Yang, but comes at a cost. The foreign antigens (which can possibly be likened to Pathogenic Factors) induce autoimmune damage that has to be kept in check by immunosuppressant medication. Degenerative change suggestive of Blood Stasis and Phlegm (atheroma and hyperlipidaemia) is an unfortunate consequence of a partly suppressed immune response to a foreign heart.

The main problem in cardiomyopathy is that the heart cannot pump efficiently, and so the state of heart failure develops. In contrast to acute myocarditis, because of the gradual onset in cardiomyopathy this is usually chronic heart failure. The damage to the heart muscle may also affect the pacemaker system, so arrhythmias, which can sometimes be life-threatening, may also develop (see Q3.2g-2).

Cardiomyopathy is one possible cause of sudden death in apparently healthy young people. These deaths commonly occur when the person has been engaged in strenuous activity. It seems that in these tragic cases an undiagnosed cardiomyopathy has led to ventricular fibrillation and thus to cardiac arrest. Another cause of sudden cardiac death is undiagnosed coronary heart disease or congenital heart disease (see later in this chapter).

In cardiomyopathy, the damage to the heart muscle has been done, and treatment is therefore aimed at reducing heart failure and the risk of arrhythmias by means of the approaches discussed in Chapter 3.2f. In some cases the deterioration in the function of the heart is so severe that life expectancy is assessed to be less than 6 months. In these cases cardiac transplantation is the only available option.

Heart transplant certainly improves life-expectancy in many people, as 75% of patients who have received a new heart will be alive 5 years after the operation. However, the risks and complications of this operation, and the life-long immunosuppressive treatment (see Chapter 2.2c) that has to follow it, are significant. Atherosclerosis of the coronary arteries in the transplanted heart is a particular problem, which seems to be in part a response of immune rejection of the foreign vascular tissue, and in part a result of the hypertension and hyperlipidaemia that can also be a response to transplantation. Nevertheless, the immediate result of a successful cardiac transplantation is a huge improvement in quality of life.

Diseases of the pericardium

Pericarditis

'Pericarditis' refers to inflammation of the pericardium, the fibrous protective lining of the heart muscle. The condition can be acute or chronic in its development.

Acute pericarditis is usually due to infection or to the inflammation that follows the damage caused by a heart attack. As in myocarditis, the most usual infectious agents are the viruses that cause colds and flu. In the few days after heart attack it is probably inflammatory agents released from infarcted myocardial cells that trigger inflammation. If the pericarditis develops over a week after the heart attack it may be the result of an abnormal immune reaction to the damaged heart-muscle lining (Dressler's syndrome).

Acute viral pericarditis commonly affects young adults. It is usually a less severe condition than myocarditis, although it can have severe complications. Nevertheless, from a holistic perspective, the development of pericarditis also suggests that the patient has a pre-existing susceptibility in terms of depletion of Heart energy. Pericarditis is increasingly diagnosed in people who have human immunodeficiency virus (HIV) infection.

The symptoms of acute pericarditis include a sharp pain in the centre of the chest, which can be felt in the region of acupoint Ren-17 (Shanzhong). The pain can go up to the neck and is worse on movement, lying down and breathing in. Fever and a rapid heart rate are usually present.

The medical treatment is rest in bed and non-steroidal anti-inflammatory drugs (NSAIDs) such as ibuprofen (except in the case of heart attack, when these drugs should be avoided).

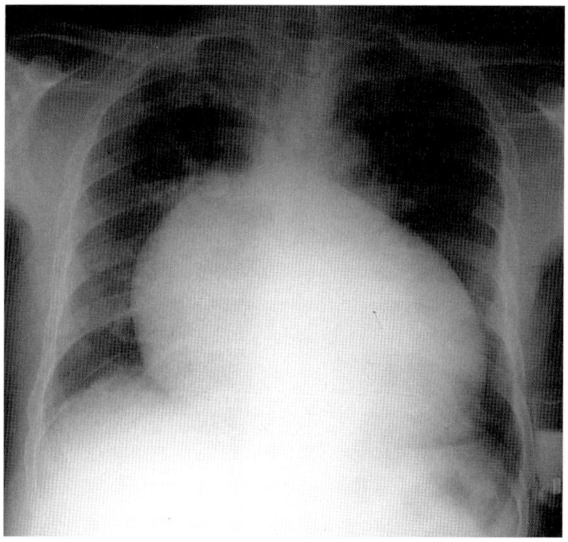

Figure 3.2g-I • Chest x-ray image showing the appearance of a large pericardial effusion • The heart appears globular, and the cardiac shadow is almost double the width of that seen in a normal chest x-ray image.

Information Box 3.2g-III

Acute pericarditis: comments from a Chinese medicine perspective

The stabbing pain of acute pericarditis would be interpreted as Heart Blood Stagnation. The fever and rapid pulse rate suggest Full or Empty Heat. As is the case with myocarditis, viral infection may have led to an invasion of External Wind Heat, which has penetrated to the interior to damage Heart Yin and thus led to the Blood Stagnation. In other cases (e.g. following a heart attack) the depleted Heart Yang may have contributed to the development of Blood Stagnation.

The impaired action of the heart in constrictive pericarditis and pericardial effusion suggests that the initial acute condition has led to marked depletion of the Heart function, in particular of Heart Yang. The thickened stiff pericardium or fluid-based effusion both suggest that Phlegm or Damp, in addition to Blood Stagnation and Yang Deficiency, are contributing to the symptoms. The patient will develop the features of Heart and Kidney Yang Deficiency with Water Overflowing as heart failure ensues.

Most people will fully recover from an episode of pericarditis, although a small proportion may suffer from recurrent episodes.

In more severe cases, the inflammation affects the function of the heart, and arrhythmias or heart failure can develop. In some cases, excess fluid builds up between the two lining layers of the pericardium, forming a pericardial effusion (Figure 3.2g-I). This can be so extensive as to constrict the heart function and thus lead to heart failure. In these cases, the patient requires more intensive medical observation, as the condition may worsen or life-threatening arrhythmias may occur.

In a small minority of cases the inflammation does not settle and a long-standing condition called chronic pericarditis develops. One of the consequences of long-standing inflammation is scarring or fibrosis (see Chapter 2.2b). The scarred pericardium becomes thickened, irregular and tight, and can physically restrict the pumping of the heart, when it is known as constrictive pericarditis, which can lead to severe chronic heart failure.

Recurrent attacks of pericarditis may be kept at bay by means of immunosuppressant medication (e.g. colchicine and azathioprine).

The main treatment for constrictive pericarditis is surgical removal of a section of the damaged pericardium. This permits the heart to pump more freely. Many patients continue to suffer from impairment of heart function after this operation.

Diseases of the heart valves

The diseases of the heart valves have some features in common – they all tend to lead to a degree of heart failure and also may lead to arrhythmias (see Chapter 3.2f).

The symptoms can initially be treated with drugs but, if severe, surgical treatment of the damaged valve may be necessary. Patients with valvular disease are susceptible to a very severe infectious condition of the valves called endocarditis (discussed later in this chapter).

For simplicity, the diverse problems are listed below in two categories: incompetent valves and stenosed valves.

Incompetent (regurgitating) valves

As explained in Chapter 3.2a, heart valves are essential to ensure a one-way flow of blood through the two sides of the heart. Some conditions of the heart valves cause them to become leaky or 'incompetent'. The other term used to describe this phenomenon of leaky valves is 'regurgitation'.

The name given to a particular condition relates to the exact site of the leak. For example, mitral incompetence (or regurgitation) refers to a leaky mitral (left atrioventricular) valve.

The main consequence of a leaky valve is that, during contraction of the heart, blood is forced the wrong way, with the result that blood dams up at the venous side of the heart (see Q 3.2g-3).

Heart failure is an important consequence of valve incompetence. The symptoms of the heart failure depend on the side of the heart affected. In mitral incompetence, it is the left side, and so blood dams up in the pulmonary veins of the lung and causes pulmonary oedema. This is known as 'left-sided heart failure'. In tricuspid incompetence it is the right side that is affected, and the symptoms that result from bodily oedema are most prominent. This is known as 'right-sided heart failure'.

Other symptoms of valve incompetence include arrhythmias and exhaustion.

Incompetent valves in elderly people commonly are the consequence of what used to be a common and severe childhood illness, rheumatic fever. Rheumatic fever is a bacterial infection that primarily causes an inflammation of the joints, but can progress to lead to an antibody-mediated inflammation of the heart and valves. The way in which rheumatic fever affects the joints is described in Chapter 4.2f. People who recover from rheumatic fever are commonly left with scarring or weakening of the heart valves. Sometimes the damage to the valves only becomes apparent in later life. This cause of valve incompetence is much less common in younger people because over the past few decades rheumatic fever has become a very rare disease in developed countries. It is, however, still a significant cause of ill-health in the developing world.

Other causes of valve incompetence include damage to the structure of the heart from coronary heart disease and myocarditis. It can also be an inherited condition.

Valve incompetence may be diagnosed initially by the detection of a 'murmur' through the stethoscope. The structure of the damaged valve can then be assessed by means of echocardiography (cardiac ultrasound scan). A patient with severe valvular disease may also require cardiac catheterisation in order to assess accurately the degree of heart failure.

The initial treatment of valve incompetence depends on the severity of the symptoms. If progressive heart failure is developing and is not responding to drugs, surgical replacement of the heart-valve is the best treatment (see below).

Stenosed valves

The other major problem that can occur with the heart valves is that they can become scarred and tightened. This is called 'valve stenosis'. A tightened (stenotic) valve will restrict the passage of blood through the heart. This puts the heart muscle under strain, and reduces the amount of blood that can exit the heart to go to the rest of the body. Stenosis will also cause blood to dam up on the venous side of the heart and is thus also a cause of right or left heart failure.

The condition is named after the affected valve. The two most common forms of stenotic valvular disease are mitral stenosis and aortic stenosis.

The symptoms include those of left- or right-sided heart failure. Because of the severely reduced amount of blood leaving the heart, blackouts can occur. The strain on the heart muscle can lead to palpitations due to arrhythmias. Mitral stenosis is particularly associated with atrial fibrillation, and in severe cases there is a risk of sudden death.

The most common cause of valve stenosis in elderly people is childhood rheumatic fever. The tightening can get progressively worse over a period of years. Stenosis can also be due to a congenital defect. In the elderly it can be a degenerative condition, as over the years degeneration and the deposition of calcium in the valves has led them to harden and narrow.

The investigations of valve stenosis are the same as those for valve incompetence.

Valve stenosis may be improved by a simple operation (which may be performed as an extension of a cardiac catheterisation) to stretch or cut the tightened valve. Otherwise, a valve replacement is necessary.

Valve replacement

This surgical procedure can transform the lives of people who would otherwise be severely disabled by valvular disease. The replaced valve is either a mechanical structure, or is fashioned from a pig valve, or a human valve taken from the body of someone who had chosen to donate organs after death.

Foreign heart valves do not seem to stimulate an immune response and so, unlike the cardiac transplant, the patient does not need to take immunosuppressive medication because there is no risk of 'rejection' of the valve.

The problem with mechanical valves is that their clumsy structure can stimulate clotting and the formation of emboli within the heart. For this reason, the patient with a mechanical valve will have to take a high dose of warfarin continually for the rest of their life.

Both types of valve may wear out and require replacement within about 10 years, although a mechanical valve generally has a longer life than a tissue valve.

Implanted valves are at risk of becoming infected, and this leads to the very serious condition of endocarditis (discussed below).

Information Box 3.2g-IV

Valvular disease: comments from a Chinese medicine perspective

In Chinese medicine, the symptoms of valvular disease suggest a Deficiency of Heart Yin. Interestingly, one of the conventionally recognised features of mitral stenosis is a malar flush (reddening of the upper aspect of the cheeks), which in Chinese medicine is a recognised marker for Yin Deficiency. The symptom of palpitations, common in valvular heart disease, is consistent with this interpretation.

The development of heart failure would suggest additional depletion of Yang, with Water Overflowing to the Heart and the Lungs.

The thickened tightened valves in stenosis and the risk of embolism suggest that Phlegm and Blood Stagnation are also a contributory factor.

Endocarditis

Endocarditis is inflammation of the endocardium, the lining epithelium of the heart, and is usually the result of a bacterial infection. Often the infectious agent is found to be one of the usually 'healthy' types of bacteria that normally reside in the patient's throat or bowel.

People who have damaged heart valves or a heart-valve replacement are more at risk of endocarditis. Any procedure that increases the risk of surface bacteria entering the bloodstream (including dental and surgical operations) may cause endocarditis in at-risk groups. Intravenous drug users are also at high risk from the injection of contaminated material into the bloodstream.

This infection is very relevant to the practice of acupuncture, as endocarditis is one of the serious recognised complications of acupuncture treatment worldwide. However, this complication of acupuncture is very rare in the UK, as a result of good attention to sterile needling procedures.

The infectious agent travels to the heart via the bloodstream, and causes damage after settling on the lining of the heart muscle and valves. The bacteria colonise at the edge of valves and can lead to progressive damage to their structure. The inflammation leads to the formation of clumps of platelets and other debris, which can break off from the valves to form emboli.

A patient with endocarditis will initially suffer from a prolonged state of malaise, with intermittent fever, flitting joint pains, night sweats and tiredness. At this stage it may be difficult to diagnose the cause of the illness. After some weeks the progressive valve damage gives rise to features of heart failure or emboli in the circulation. The patient may develop syndromes of thrombosis and infarction in the diverse tissues of the body, including the kidneys and brain.

The condition is diagnosed by means of echocardiography, and samples of blood are taken to culture the infectious organism. Because diagnosis is often delayed, the patient can become very unwell. Also, significant damage to the heart may have occurred before appropriate antimicrobial treatment can be given.

Powerful antibiotics in combination are given intravenously for 2 weeks. Antibiotics in tablet form are then continued for a few more weeks.

Severe valvular damage requires emergency valve replacement. This operation carries great risks because the patient is already in such an unstable state. Overall, 30% of patients who have endocarditis will either die or suffer long-term disability as a result of the condition.

Information Box 3.2g-V

Endocarditis: comments from a Chinese medicine perspective

In Chinese medicine, the features of intermittent fever and solid clumps of infection on the heart valves can be interpreted as Wind Damp Heat Invasion. Flitting joint aches and joint swelling reflect Bi Syndrome due to Wind Damp Heat.

The Heat damages the Yin of the Heart, leading to the night sweats and damaged structure of the valves. Eventually, the Heart and Kidney Yang are also damaged, leading to Water Overflowing to the Heart and Lungs. Thrombosis and embolism would be diagnosed in terms of Blood Stagnation.

Prophylaxis of endocarditis

Because endocarditis is a particular risk for people with damaged or replaced heart valves, until recently people with those conditions were advised to take precautionary measures whenever there was a high probability of bacterial infection entering the bloodstream. The medical term for precautionary measures is 'prophylaxis'.

In particular, patients with valvular problems and who had to undergo significant dental treatment or invasive medical investigations such as endoscopy were advised to take antibiotics during the course of the procedure. However, in 2008 the National Institute of Health and Clinical Excellence (NICE) published a guideline and review of evidence for prophylaxis against endocarditis. The conclusion of this guideline is that antibiotic prophylaxis may in fact carry more risks than benefits, and so should no longer be offered to patients. This is, as the guideline states, 'a paradigm shift', and as such it may take many years for the advice to filter down to current medical practice.

However, prophylaxis has never been considered necessary for minor procedures such as taking blood, because the risk of infection by the insertion of a sterile needle is considered to be low. Although recent critics of acupuncture have suggested that antibiotic prophylaxis should be given to acupuncture patients with heart-valve problems, this is inconsistent with current medical thinking about the risks of introducing infection by means of a needle. Moreover, taking into account the current NICE guidance, it need not be a concern at all, as long as single-use, non-indwelling needles are used.

Having said this, it is the responsibility of acupuncturists to be very familiar with the features of endocarditis, so that if a patient develops early symptoms he or she can be referred for early treatment. The main red flag of endocarditis is intermittent unexplained fever for more than 2 weeks.

Congenital heart disease

'Congenital heart disease' is the term used to describe a range of defects of the heart and valves that may develop in the growing fetus. Some of these defects are minor, but some can be very severe, leading to cyanosis (blue baby syndrome) and heart failure in the first few weeks of life. Others do not seem to produce significant problems in early life (like some of the valvular diseases) but can progress as the child gets older. If undetected, these defects can lead to severe and sometimes fatal heart disease.

The cause of most cases of congenital heart disease is unknown. However, factors that are known to increase the chances of a congenital defect include maternal rubella (German measles) infection, high maternal alcohol intake, and maternal exposure to certain drugs and radiation in pregnancy. There is a slightly increased risk of congenital heart disease in children born to parents who have a heart defect.

Defects of the chromosomes that cause conditions such as Down syndrome also commonly give rise to heart defects in affected babies.

In most cases, the defect only causes a problem after birth; prior to this the oxygenation of the blood takes place via the placenta. However, with the increasing use of ultrasound scanning in midpregnancy, the defects are often detected before birth. This helps to avoid the situation of defects only becoming apparent in later life when irreparable damage has been done to the circulatory system.

Congenital heart disease is common, affecting approximately one in 100 babies. In many of these cases, the defect is a minor one, and may be detected at an early health check by means of the characteristic murmur heard via the stethoscope. In such cases, after investigation by echocardiography, parents can be reassured that the defect will resolve itself as the child's heart grows.

Hole in the heart

The most common severe defects involve a gap in the muscle wall that separates the two sides of the heart, which is commonly called a 'hole in the heart' and in conventional medicine is termed a 'septal defect'. If a large septal defect is detected early, the gap in the muscle is repaired surgically. The operation is often straightforward and can have very good results.

However, a septal defect is one of the conditions that can go undetected in early childhood, and over the ensuing years can lead to progressive strain on the heart and the circulatory system. Affected adults may develop recurrent chest infections and breathlessness on exertion as first symptoms. If not diagnosed early and surgically repaired, it may not be possible to reverse the damage done to the circulatory system and so may result in death in early adulthood from heart failure.

Narrowing of the aorta or aortic valve

These defects, also known as 'aortic coarctation' (narrowing of the vessel) or 'aortic stenosis' (narrowing of the valve) severely impair the ability of the heart to pump blood into the bodily circulation and can lead to heart failure very shortly after birth. The affected baby is breathless and is unable to feed. If less severe, the defect may appear only later in childhood, with dizziness, fainting and chest pains.

The treatment is surgical correction of the narrowed valve or aorta.

Cyanotic heart disease

In cyanotic heart disease, a complex defect is present that causes some of the deoxygenated blood arriving at the heart not to be directed to the lungs as it should be. Instead it is redirected straight back into the bodily circulation. This means that the body does not receive the full amount of oxygen it requires.

As deoxygenated blood is blue in colour, the child will have a bluish tinge to the lips and tongue (cyanosis), particularly after exercise. A characteristic sign is that the child is breathless and may need to squat to rest after exercise. This is another condition that may get diagnosed only later in childhood. The treatment is by means of a complex operation, which should be performed as early as possible.

Long-term consequences of corrected congenital heart disease

This is still an area in which there is incomplete knowledge, as it is only over the past 30–40 years or so that some of the most complex of the life-preserving surgical techniques have been developed. It is not yet fully known how the history of congenital heart disease and its surgical correction will affect the lives of affected individuals in the future.

The structure of the heart will never be perfect after surgical correction. It is now becoming apparent that some of the young adults who have undergone the more major forms of surgery may suffer from arrhythmias due to the impairments in the structure of the heart muscle. They are also at an increased risk of cardiomyopathy and sudden cardiac death (see Q3.2g-4).

Information Box 3.2g-VI

Congenital heart disease: comments from a Chinese medicine perspective

According to Chinese medicine, congenital defects are often rooted in a Deficiency of Essence (Jing). The defective heart structure and resulting weakened function correspond to Deficient Heart Yin and Yang. Heart failure is Water Overflowing to Heart and Lungs secondary to Heart Yang deficiency. The bluish colour seen in children in cyanotic heart disease suggests that Qi or Blood Stagnation has developed as a consequence of severe Heart Deficiency.

The red flags of diseases of the heart muscle, pericardium and valves

Red flags are those symptoms and signs that indicate that referral is to be considered. The red flags of most of the conditions discussed in this chapter have already been described, because severe myocarditis, cardiomyopathy and congenital heart disease in adults all present first with symptoms either of arrhythmias or of heart failure (see Table 3.2f-I).

Table 3.2g-I Red Flags 15 – pericarditis

Red Flag	Description	Reasoning
15.1	**Features of uncomplicated pericarditis:** sharp central chest pain which is worse on leaning forward and lying down. Fever should be slight and pulse rate no more than 100 beats/minute **Complications include**: • features of **heart failure (breathlessness and oedema)** • features of **arrhythmia (tachycardia)** • symptoms of **heart attack/unstable angina**	Pericarditis can result from a viral infection or as part of a complex metabolic illness such as renal failure, and can complicate recovery from a heart attack In its uncomplicated form, the patient will have central chest pain that is affected by posture and other chest movements. If pericarditis is suspected it is advisable to refer the patient for further cardiac investigations in hospital as the condition can deteriorate and affect the rhythm or pumping capacity of the heart Refer urgently if complications are apparent

The red flag of endocarditis is intermittent unexplained fever lasting for more than 2 weeks, which is one of the red flags for infectious diseases in general. The red flags for congenital heart disease in young children have a lot of similarities to those for many childhood chronic illnesses (see Section 5.4).

Thus the only additional red flags listed here are those for pericarditis, and these are described in Table 3.2g-I. This table forms part of the summary on red flags given in Appendix III, which also gives advice on the degree of urgency of referral for each of the red flag conditions listed.

Self-test 3.2g

Diseases of the heart muscle, pericardium and heart valves, and congenital heart disease

1. Jason is 25 years old and has been using the homeopathy you prescribe for general well-being for 3 years now. He now complains of a chest infection, but when you question him he describes a sharp pain in the centre of his chest that is worse on breathing in. He has no cough or breathlessness, but does have a slight fever. On examination his pulse is 100 beats/minute.
   (i) What conventional medicine diagnosis do you suspect?
   (ii) Would you consider referral to a conventional medicine practitioner?
2. Harry is a 65-year-old patient and had a valve replacement 5 years ago. His problem had been a tight mitral valve (mitral stenosis) that developed after a childhood attack of rheumatic fever. He has had a metal valve inserted and feels generally very well since the operation. He wants acupuncture for an aching knee.
   What are the two reasons why Harry may be more at risk of an adverse reaction to acupuncture than other people?

Answers

1. (i) Jason's symptoms suggest a diagnosis of pericarditis rather than a chest infection. One other possibility is pleurisy, which you will study in Chapter 3.3e.
   (ii) In general, the symptoms are those of mild pericarditis. The pulse rate is rather high, but in the absence of any irregularity there is no need to refer urgently on the basis of this finding alone. However, although symptoms are mild, it would be wise to seek a conventional medicine opinion, as the condition may deteriorate and it would be helpful for the doctor to make an assessment of risk at this stage. Ideally, Jason could be assessed as a high priority (i.e. within the next 1–2 days).
2. (i) Because Harry has a metal valve in place he will be having to take a regular high dose of warfarin to prevent clotting. This means he will be at more risk than other people of bruising and bleeding. You need to explain this to Harry. When treating the knee, in particular, you should consider using fine needles and shallow insertion, and take special care not to penetrate the joint space.
   (ii) Harry is more at risk than other people of endocarditis. The risk from acupuncture treatment with sterile needles is extremely low, but whilst treatment is ongoing you should be alert over the next few weeks for any possible red flags of endocarditis, in particular an unexplained fever of more than 2 weeks duration, long-standing malaise or any features of heart failure.

The respiratory system

3.3

Chapter 3.3a The physiology of the respiratory system

LEARNING POINTS

At the end of this chapter you will be able to:

- describe the role of the respiratory system
- understand the structure of the upper respiratory tract, including the nose, sinuses, pharynx, larynx and trachea
- understand the structure of the lower respiratory tract, including the bronchi, bronchioles, alveoli and other structures of the lungs.

Estimated time for chapter: 100 minutes.

Introduction

This chapter concentrates on the physiology and pathology of the respiratory system, looking at the structure and function of the respiratory system in health.

The role of the respiratory system

The respiratory system is specialised to enable an adequate supply of oxygen to the tissues. As was described in Chapter 1.2b, oxygen is one of the essential ingredients for the process of cellular respiration. It is also the role of the respiratory system to allow carbon dioxide, a waste product of respiration, to be removed from the body.

In common usage, the term 'respiration' refers simply to the act of breathing. However, in physiology there are three aspects to respiration that can be clearly defined. These are external respiration, internal respiration and cellular respiration.

The respiratory system is primarily concerned with external respiration, which is the process of breathing leading to the exchange of gases between the blood and the lungs.

Internal respiration is the exchange of gases between the blood and the cells of all the body tissues, and is one of the functions performed by the circulatory system.

Cellular respiration is the process (described in Chapter 1.2b) by which oxygen and nutrients are converted to cellular energy (adenosine triphosphate (ATP)) and carbon dioxide within the cell itself. It is important to be clear about the distinction between these three processes, as these terms help define the precise roles of the respiratory system.

The respiratory system is conventionally divided into two sections, the upper and lower respiratory tract. A simple representation of the organs of the respiratory tract is given in Figure 3.3a-I. The division between the upper and lower parts occurs at the point at which the trachea splits into the two tubes called 'bronchi'.

The diagram illustrates that this division occurs at a deep level in the chest, just above the position of the heart. The diagram also illustrates the close physical relationship between the heart and the lungs. In fact, if the heart is removed through dissection, an imprint of its shape is seen in the tissue of the lungs.

The upper respiratory tract

The upper respiratory tract leads from the entrance of the respiratory system at the nose to the end of the trachea, the tube which directs the inhaled air into the chest cavity (thorax) towards the lungs.

The function of the upper respiratory tract is to provide a plentiful supply of warm, clean and moist air to the lungs. To help it perform this function it consists of wide air spaces

Figure 3.3a-I • The organs of respiration.

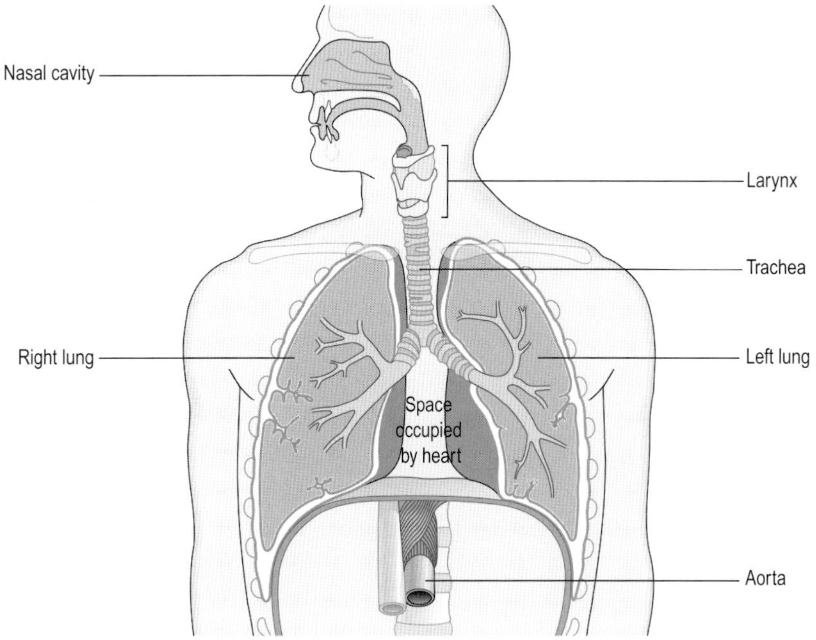

and is lined by a specialised form of epithelium. The respiratory epithelium consists largely of ciliated columnar cells but it also has many mucus-secreting (goblet) cells.

The water-containing mucus moistens the air that rushes through the respiratory tract, and picks up dirt particles and other foreign bodies present in the air. Cilia are structures akin to microscopic hairs on the surface of cells. They are powered by the energetically charged molecule ATP to move in coordinated waves. In the respiratory tract the cilia beat in an upward direction. Their function is to cause an upward movement of the mucus, allowing the foreign material to be moved away from the delicate lung tissue and up to the back of the throat, from where it can be swallowed or expectorated.

The connective-tissue layer below the respiratory epithelium has a number of lymphocytes scattered throughout its length. These respond to foreign antigens by producing antibodies and attracting other immune cells. This is an important aspect of the protection of the respiratory tract from infection.

The important parts of the upper respiratory tract are the nose, the pharynx, the larynx and the trachea.

The nose

In the breathing of a healthy person at rest, all air is drawn in through the nostrils into the nasal cavity. This space has a deeply ridged surface which has a rich blood supply. This means that the current of air comes into contact with a large area of warm epithelium before its descent towards the lungs. In addition to the cilia on the epithelial cells, body hairs are present in the opening of the nose to filter out any large foreign particles.

Opening out into the nasal cavity are the sinuses. These are cavities deep within the facial bones that have narrow passageways leading into the nasal cavity. Their function is to give the voice a resonant quality, the loss of which is apparent in anyone who has suffered from a 'head cold', when the sinuses become filled with thick secretions. A tiny duct leading from each eye also opens into this space. This continually drains away tears from the eyes. The runny nose that accompanies a bout of crying is a result of the excess tears flooding into the nose through this duct.

The nose is the specialised sense organ for smell. To perform this function, delicate nerves originating from the base of the brain penetrate the bone above the nasal cavity to supply the nasal lining. These are sensitive to the chemicals in the incoming air, which become dissolved in the mucus. The sense of smell is also important to enrich the experience of taste. Occasionally, in a head injury, these nerves become permanently severed, even though there may be no other major brain damage. The person may recover fully but be left without a sense of smell and with a highly impaired sense of taste.

Other nerves in the nose are very sensitive to the irritation that can result from foreign particles and from inflammation of the lining of the nose. These nerves can trigger the protective reflex of the sneeze, which is a very effective mechanism for expelling unwanted material from the nasal cavity.

The pharynx

The pharynx is the space at the back of the nose that connects with the throat. The adenoids (nasal tonsils) are two collections of lymph-node tissue situated at the back of this space. The tonsils (palatine tonsils), which are similar collections of lymphoid tissue, are situated a little lower down. The palatine tonsils can be seen in most people on either side of the space behind the arch of the palate, as illustrated in Figure 3.1a-II, whereas the adenoids are hidden up behind the palatoglossal arch.

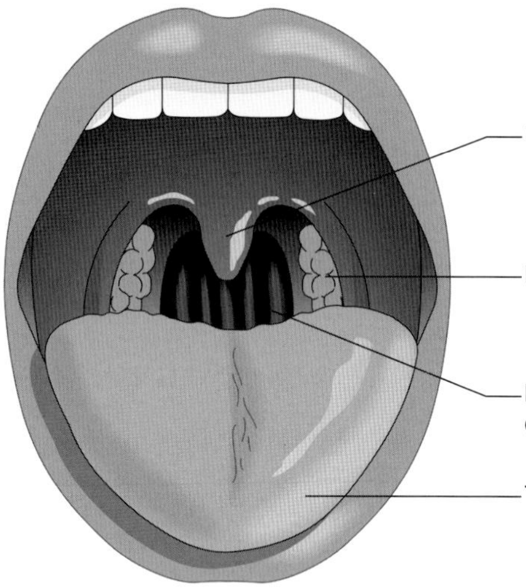

Figure 3.3a-II • The location of the palatine tonsils.

The function of the tonsils is to complement the protective function of the lymphocytes in the respiratory epithelium. Their presence is an indication of the need for the lungs to be protected from foreign material. The adenoids are most active in early childhood, because this is the time when immunity to a wide range of infections has to be rapidly developed. After 5 years of the age, in most people the adenoids shrink to a negligible size, although the palatine tonsils persist into adulthood.

The eustachian tube opens from the middle ear into the pharynx close to the location of the adenoids. The middle ear is also lined with respiratory epithelium, and the eustachian tube allows the drainage of mucus from this enclosed space.

The larynx

The larynx, popularly known as the voice box, is the structure that separates the pharynx from the trachea. Although it is primarily associated with voice production, it also plays a very important protective role. Figure 3.3a-III is a diagrammatic representation of the nasal cavity, pharynx and larynx, which illustrates how these structures relate to each other.

The tube-like larynx has stiff cartilage in its walls which enables it to maintain its shape. The cartilage at the front of the larynx is what can be seen and felt as the 'Adam's apple'. Because the thyroid gland sits close to this structure, the medical term for this is the 'thyroid cartilage'.

The vocal cords are two fine flaps of tissue that are suspended from the surrounding cartilage tube. Figure 3.3a-IV shows a view of the aperture of the larynx. The vocal cords are depicted on either side of the aperture, leaving a triangular space through which the air can pass. Tiny muscles in the larynx contract to change the shape of this triangle between the vocal cords so that the space can vary from being a wide gap to a tiny 'chink'. The tone of the muscles also affects the tightness of the vocal cords. During quiet breathing the gap is wide to allow a free passage of air in and out of the lungs. During speech, the gap narrows and the cords tighten. The expired air causes vibration of the tightened cords, which produces the sound of the voice. The tighter the cords, the higher the pitch of the voice.

The protective reflex of the cough involves a temporary tightening of the vocal cords so that the gap closes altogether. This occurs during a forced expiration of air. The closed gap means that the pressure of air below the vocal cords is suddenly increased. At this point the muscles relax and the

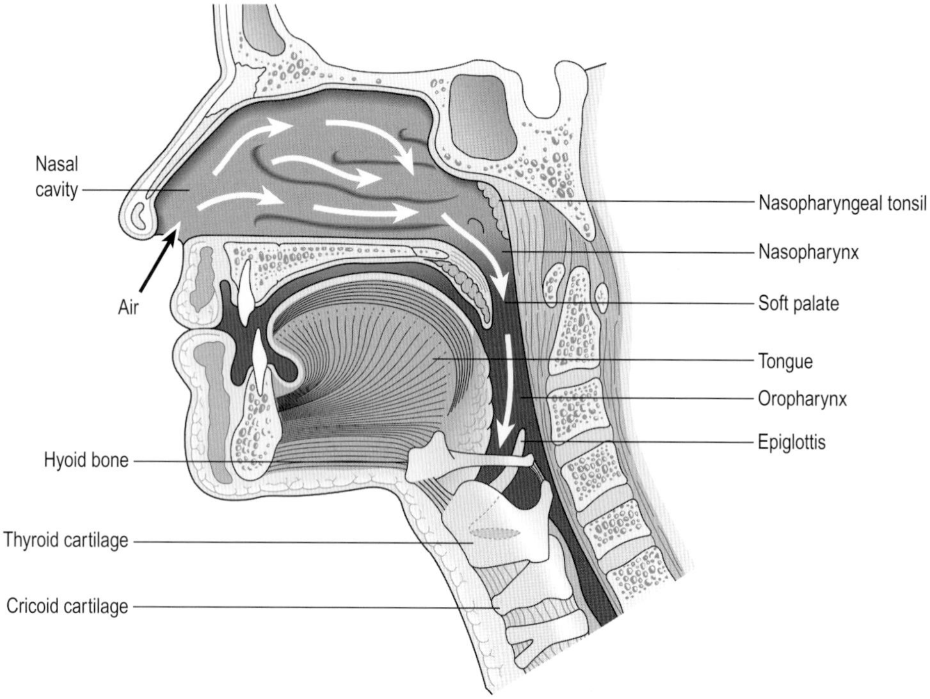

Figure 3.3a-III • The pathway of the air from the nose to the larynx.

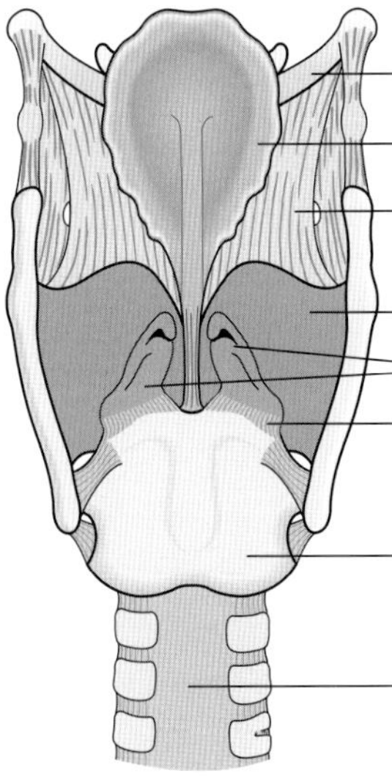

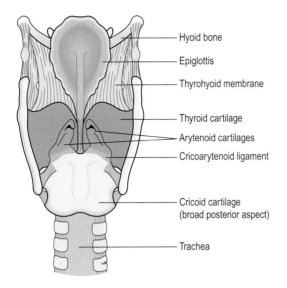

Figure 3.3a-IV • The interior of the larynx, viewed from above.

gap widens. This results in a sudden forceful rush of air accompanied by the familiar sound of the cough. Like the sneeze, the cough is stimulated by the irritation of nerves in the larynx and the tubes that branch from the trachea into the lungs. The cough also has the effect of expelling unwanted material from the trachea, larynx and pharynx out through the open mouth.

The other important protective structure in the larynx is a stiff flap of cartilage-containing tissue called the 'epiglottis', which sits above the larynx. During swallowing this flap descends to completely cover the gap between the vocal cords. This protects against the inhalation of food during swallowing.

The trachea

The trachea is the wide tube that descends from the larynx to the division of the bronchi deep within the thorax. It is held open by rings of cartilage within its walls and is also lined by respiratory epithelium (see Q.3.3.a-1).

The lower respiratory tract

The lower respiratory tract begins where the trachea divides into the two narrower tubes called the *bronchi*. The bronchi further subdivide, like the branches of a tree, to penetrate the tissue of the two lungs.

The bronchi and bronchioles

The bronchi and the smaller tubes into which they divide (the bronchioles) are structurally similar to the trachea, and are also lined with respiratory epithelium. Therefore, they too are concerned with ensuring the air that reaches the depths of the lungs is as warm, moist and as clean as possible.

The width of these air passages varies according to need. During exercise the bronchi and bronchioles widen, so that a large amount of air can enter the lungs in each breath. At rest, they narrow again because the need for a large volume of air is not so necessary, and because the protective mechanism of these tubes is more efficient when they are narrower.

The alveoli

At the end of each of the tiniest branches of the tree-like air passages that penetrate the lung are masses of tiny air sacs only a few cells in diameter. These are known as 'alveoli' (singular 'alveolus'). The lungs are composed of millions of these tiny air spaces packed together, and all connecting with the outside world through the bronchioles and bronchi. The alveoli are lined with only a single layer of flat squamous epithelium, and are supplied by a dense network of fine blood capillaries.

Figure 3.3a-V illustrates how the alveoli branch from the bronchioles, and how a network of capillaries supplies each one.

Exchange of gases in the alveoli

The blood that enters the capillaries surrounding the alveoli has originated from the pulmonary arteries. These large vessels originate from the right ventricle of the heart and carry deoxygenated blood pumped by the right side of the heart. The blood is deoxygenated because the cells of the body tissues have used up all the oxygen in the process of cellular respiration. As well as being deoxygenated, this blood is also carrying a high concentration of carbon dioxide, the by-product of cellular respiration. In contrast, the air inspired into the alveoli is rich in oxygen from the outside air, and carries very little carbon dioxide. Therefore, there is a tendency for the oxygen in the alveoli to move into the deoxygenated blood in the capillaries. This movement occurs readily, as oxygen can

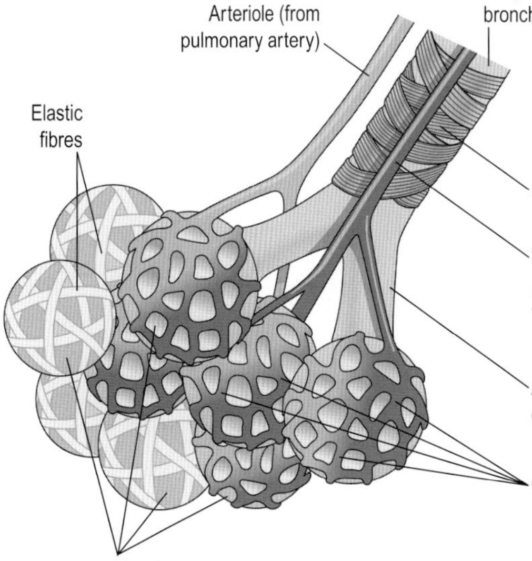

Figure 3.3a-V • An alveolus and its capillary network.

diffuse with no restriction through the cell membranes of the alveolar and capillary walls. At the same time, there is a movement of carbon dioxide out of the capillary blood and into the alveolar air. This exchange of the two gases of respiration occurs very rapidly (see Q 3.3a-2).

The capillaries that leave the alveoli converge to form the pulmonary veins, which return all this blood to the left side of the heart. This blood is now rich in oxygen, and has been cleared of carbon dioxide. The pulmonary veins are the only veins in the body that carry oxygenated blood. All the other veins carry blood away from the body tissues, and this blood is of course deoxygenated.

The air left in the alveolus now contains more carbon dioxide than oxygen, and is expelled to the outside world by the process of expiration, so that the whole process can begin afresh with the next in-breath.

This process of exchange of gases is assisted by the fact that there are millions of alveoli, each with its own rich blood supply. In some conditions, such as emphysema, the delicate structure of the alveoli is damaged and their number is reduced (see Chapter 3.3e). This severely impairs the process of exchange of gases, so that the blood does not get replenished with an adequate amount of oxygen, and carbon dioxide fails to be fully cleared.

The lungs

The lungs consist of the branching air passages of the bronchi and bronchioles, and the thousands of alveoli clustered around the ends of the bronchioles. The lungs are surrounded and supported by elastic connective tissue, which has the tendency to cause the fully expanded lung to contract. The lungs sit within the thorax, which is protected by the rib cage and its supportive muscles, and they rest on the sheet of muscle below known as the 'diaphragm'.

The lungs are surrounded by a double layer of protective fluid-secreting serous membrane called the 'pleura'. In the pleura the secreted fluid forms a thin lubricating layer between the two pleural membranes akin to the fluid that separates the pericardium from the heart. The outer pleural membrane is attached to the inner surface of the rib cage from above and at the sides, and to the diaphragm below. It is this attachment that prevents the elastic lungs from collapsing. Figure 3.3a-VI illustrates the relationship between the pleura and the lungs.

External respiration

External respiration is the process whereby air is drawn into the lung tissue through inspiration and is then expelled through expiration. This process permits the exchange of gases to occur.

Inspiration involves the inflation of the lungs. Like an expanded bellows, the inflated lung naturally draws air into itself. The lungs are inflated by a lifting and expansion of the rib-cage walls and a descent of the diaphragm. This action occurs as a result of contraction of the diaphragm and of the muscles that link the ribs together.

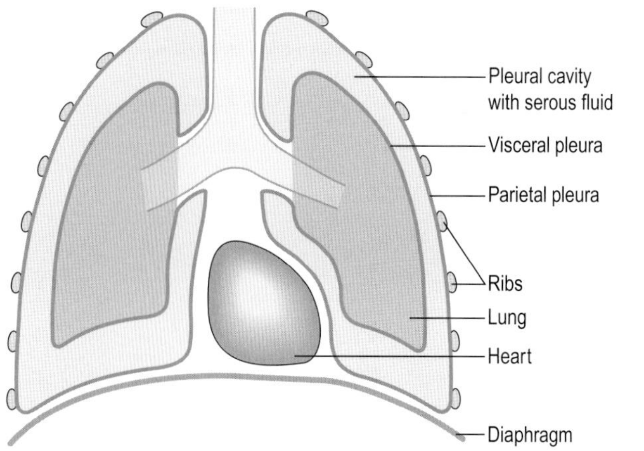

Figure 3.3a-VI • The relationship of the pleura with the lungs.

Expiration involves the deflation of the lungs. This naturally forces air back out of the lungs. In relaxed breathing, expiration requires no muscular effort. A simple relaxation of the rib cage and diaphragm has the effect of reducing the volume of the thorax and thus deflating the lungs.

In normal, quiet breathing the cycle of inspiration and expiration occurs at about 15 times per minute (4 seconds/cycle). There is an automatic reflex that originates from a control centre in the base of the brain that sets this regular rhythm. Nerves travel down from this control centre to stimulate the synchronised and rhythmic muscular contraction of the rib cage and diaphragm (see Q3.3a-3).

All variations in the resting respiratory rate are brought about by changes that take place in the breathing control centre in the brain. The breathing control centre is essential for maintaining homeostasis of the levels of oxygen and carbon dioxide in the arterial blood. The oxygen level must of course be maintained at a high concentration, whereas the level of carbon dioxide must not be allowed to rise too high. To perform this role, the breathing control centre contains cells that are very sensitive to the level of carbon dioxide in the blood. A miniscule rise in the level of carbon dioxide leads to an increase in the breathing rate so that excess carbon dioxide can be 'blown off'. If the level of carbon dioxide drops, so does the rate of breathing, and the levels in the blood can build up again.

The control centre in the brain is also sensitive to drops in the concentration of oxygen in the blood. However, the responsiveness of the control centre to carbon dioxide also indirectly controls the homeostasis of oxygen in the blood, as increased external respiration will increase oxygen levels, and reduced external respiration will reduce oxygen levels.

Any voluntary wish to modulate the breathing, such as for speech, singing or laughing, generates nerve impulses from other parts of the brain (the cerebral hemispheres) to the control centre of breathing, which then alters the breathing rate accordingly. The sneeze and cough reflexes involve a direct link between the irritated nerve endings and the control centre.

The way in which the brain is responsible for the voluntary and involuntary control of body functions is described in more detail in Chapter 4.1 on the nervous system (see Q3.3a-4).

Information Box 3.3a-I

The lungs: comments from a Chinese medicine perspective

The functions of the Lungs are to:

- govern Qi and respiration
- control channels and blood vessels
- control dispersing and descending
- regulate the Water passages
- control skin and body hair
- open into the nose
- house the corporeal soul (Po).

Government of Qi and respiration refers to two aspects, as described below.

Government of Qi

The Government of Qi refers to the conversion of Gu (food) Qi and Heavenly (Clear) Qi in the Lungs to produce Zong (Gathering) Qi. Zong Qi is important for supporting the Lungs, the Heart and the circulation. It also gives strength to the voice.

The Lungs are seen as the site of the combination of Gu Qi and Heavenly Qi into a readily available source of energy (Zong Qi) for the organs of the Upper Jiao, as well as for the circulation and the voice.

In conventional medicine no distinction is made between different sorts of energy as there is in Chinese medicine with the various type of Qi. There is also no idea that the Lungs play any role in the production of energy over and above their function in external respiration, which is to draw oxygen into the body.

However, conventional medicine recognises that a weak voice might be a product of weak expiration, as it is the force of the out-breath that controls the strength of the voice.

Government of respiration

Government of respiration refers to external respiration. Here is a direct parallel with the understanding of conventional medicine. Strictly speaking, the role of the breathing control centre in the brain would also be seen in Chinese medicine as part of the Lung functions, as it plays an important part of the control of external respiration.

Control of channels and blood vessels

There is no direct correspondence here with conventional medicine, as the channels are not conventional concepts, and the blood vessels are seen as part of the circulatory system.

Control of dispersing and descending

The dispersing function refers to the ability of the Lungs to spread Wei Qi and body fluids to all body parts. This protects the body from external pathogens and keeps the skin and muscles moist and warm. It is also important for the control of sweating. The lungs are not seen to have this sort of function in conventional medicine. Instead, the defensive and warming roles would be attributed to the immune system and circulatory system, respectively. Conventionally, the skin is seen as the organ that deals with sweating.

The descending function refers to the descent of Qi, which is important to enable clearance of fluids via the Kidneys and Bladder, and also for defecation. If impaired, the loss of this function may give rise to oedema, retention of urine and constipation.

However, in conventional terms there is no link between the lungs and the kidneys or the large intestine. Although the lungs can become 'waterlogged' in a case of pulmonary oedema, this usually is the result of a condition that primarily affects another part of the body, such as heart failure.

Regulation of the Water passages

This is part of the dispersing function of the lungs (see above).

Control of the skin and body hair

Again there is little correspondence with conventional medicine, as the skin and body hair are not seen as linked to the function of the lungs. Although the common skin condition of eczema is commonly associated in conventional medicine with asthma, these are still seen as separate conditions. The reason they are understood to be linked lies in a deficiency of the immune system, not the lungs.

Opening into the nose

The nose is an organ of the respiratory system, so there is an obvious correspondence here with conventional medicine.

Housing the corporeal soul (Po)

The Po is the most physical aspect of the spiritual body and gives rise to clarity of thought and movement. Its health relies on a healthy rhythm of breathing.

In Chinese medicine it is believed that imbalanced emotions, in particular grief and anxiety will upset the pulsating rhythm of the Po by constraint of free movement of the chest.

Although conventional medicine makes no explicit link between the lungs and emotions or spirit, it is recognised that emotions have an effect, via the breathing control centre in the brain, on the respiratory rate and rhythm.

Summary

In summary, the Lungs in Chinese medicine have a much broader role than their purely physical counterpart in conventional medicine. It seems that the role of the Lungs in Chinese medicine also embraces aspects that would be attributed in conventional medicine to the cardiovascular, urinary, gastrointestinal and immune systems as well as the skin.

The functions of the Lung according to a conventional and Chinese perspective can be summarised in the form of a correspondence table (for an introduction to the Organ correspondence tables, see Appendix I). This table illustrates the idea that the functions of the air-filled sacs, which conventional medicine calls the lungs, may be the domain not only of the Lung Organ in Chinese Medicine, but also of the Kidney and Liver Organs. It will follow from this that diseases of the lungs may manifest in Chinese medicine syndromes involving the Lung, Liver and Kidney Organs.

Continued

Information Box 3.3a-I—Cont'd

Correspondence table for the functions of the Lung as described by conventional and Chinese medicine

Functions of the lung

- Involved in the process of 'external respiration', which enables the exchange of oxygen and carbon dioxide between the circulation and the outside environment (**Lung and Kidney Organs**)
- Helps to maintain a healthy balance of oxygen, carbon dioxide and acidity of the blood (**Lung and Liver Organs**)
- Helps protect the body from noxious substances in the inhaled air (**Lung and Kidney Organs**)
- Enables the production of a hormone (angiotensin) that is important in the maintenance of blood pressure (**Kidney, Spleen and Heart Organs**)
- Very closely linked in structure and function to the heart on which they depend for an adequate supply of blood to oxygenate (**Heart, Kidney and Liver Organs**)
- Provides a steady flow of air to power the production of speech from the larynx (**Lungs, Liver and Heart Organs**)

Functions of the Lung Organ

'The Lungs are like a minister from whom policies are issued'

- Governs Qi and respiration (respiratory system, process of cellular respiration that goes on in the mitochondria of all cells, circulatory system)
- Controls the channels and the blood vessels (**circulatory system**)
- Controls dispersing and descending (**immune system, skin, large intestine, bladder**)
- Regulates the water passages (**circulatory system, kidneys, bladder**)
- Controls skin and (body) hair (**skin, immune system**)
- Opens into the nose (**nose, upper respiratory system**)
- Houses the corporeal soul (**no correspondence to a physiological organ**)

Self-test 3.3a

The physiology of the respiratory system

1. What is the primary role of the respiratory system?
2. List three parts of the respiratory tract that would protect a person from smoke inhalation (NB: There are more than three.) Remember that smoke consists of tiny particles that are very irritating to the respiratory epithelium.
3. What is it that prevents the elastic lungs from collapsing in a healthy person?

Answers

1. The primary role of the respiratory system is external respiration. This involves the drawing in of clean, warm, moist air into the air spaces of the lungs so that the exchange of oxygen and carbon dioxide can take place between the outside air and the blood.
2. The lungs are protected from inhaled smoke by the following factors:
   - mucus produced by the respiratory epithelium
   - the wave-like motion of cilia on the respiratory epithelium
   - hairs in the nose, which trap foreign particles
   - the cough reflex
   - lymphocytes, which phagocytose foreign particles and damaged epithelial cells.
3. The lungs are protected from collapsing because the outer layer of the pleura is firmly attached to the rib cage, muscles and diaphragm, which comprise the inside of the walls of the thorax.

Chapter 3.3b The investigation of the respiratory system

LEARNING POINTS

At the end of this chapter you will be able to:

- recognise the main investigations of the respiratory system
- understand what a patient might experience when undergoing these investigations.

Estimated time for chapter: 30 minutes.

Introduction

The bulk of minor respiratory disease, particularly infectious disease affecting the upper respiratory tract, is managed in the UK entirely by the GP. More severe problems affecting the nose and throat may be referred for the opinion of a specialist in diseases of the ear, nose and throat.

A patient with any other severe respiratory disease will be referred by their GP to a specialist in respiratory medicine. These doctors are commonly known in the UK as chest physicians.

If a surgical operation is necessary, the chest physician will refer the patient to a thoracic surgeon. Very often the thoracic surgeon is also skilled in the surgery of the heart, in which case the proper title is 'cardiothoracic surgeon'.

The investigation of the respiratory system

The most common investigations of the respiratory system include:

- a thorough physical examination
- laryngoscopy to examine the vocal cords
- microscopic examination of the sputum
- lung-function tests to assess the mechanics of the breathing
- blood tests
- chest X-ray imaging, computed tomography (CT) scans and bronchoscopy to visualise the lungs
- biopsy of the lung tissue.

Table 3.3b-I The stages of physical examination of the lungs
• General examination for signs of poor oxygenation of the blood (seen as the bluish discoloration of the lips and tongue known as 'cyanosis') and for the swelling of the base of the nails, known as 'clubbing' (this is a sign of severe lung disease such as cancer and bronchiectasis)
• Visual assessment of the rate and quality of the breathing
• Physical examination of the chest for deformities, with the use of percussion to assess for any abnormal areas of dense tissue (indication of infection, fluid or tumour)
• Auscultation of the breath sounds in all parts of the chest

Physical examination

The physical examination of the respiratory system involves the stages listed in Table 3.3b-I.

Laryngoscopy

This is an examination performed by an ear, nose and throat specialist to examine the vocal cords. It involves the skilled insertion of an instrument, which carries a tiny mirror, into the mouth and thence into the pharynx. Laryngoscopy is usually painless.

Examination of the sputum

A patient with infection or a possible tumour will be requested to produce a sample of phlegm. This can reveal the presence of infectious organisms, and occasionally in cancer can contain cancerous cells. In the case of infection, the sample can be used to test for sensitivity to a range of antibiotics.

Lung-function tests

Lung-function tests are performed when disease of the lower respiratory tract is suspected. These tests require the patient to blow into a machine that measures the force and volume of the out-breath, and detects the changes that are characteristic of the diseases which lead to restricted breathing, such as asthma and emphysema. These tests are straightforward and painless for the patient to perform.

The most simple of these tests is the peak expiratory outflow assessment, which is done using a peak-flow meter. This is a hand-held tool that the patient can be taught to use at home. Its main purpose is to assess the severity of asthma in a patient on ongoing treatment. It does not provide as detailed or helpful information as the more complex tests available in a hospital outpatient department.

Blood tests

Serum samples can be used to examine for antigens of infectious agents and for antibodies to confirm the presence of infection. Certain antibodies can also indicate the tendency to allergy, which is common in asthmatics.

In lower respiratory tract disease, a sample of arterial blood is drawn from the radial artery to measure the concentration of oxygen in the blood.

Chest X-ray imaging

This test is performed on all patients with suspected lower respiratory tract disease. Most serious disease, such as pneumonia, cancer, emphysema and lung fibrosis, will show characteristic changes on a chest X-ray image. However, in asthma, even when severe, the chest X-ray image usually appears normal.

Computed tomography (CT) scan

This test is most commonly used to assess the size and spread of lung cancer. CT will reveal not only the lung tissue, but also the lymph nodes deep within the chest.

Figure 3.3b-I shows a CT scan of the lungs in a patient with advanced lung cancer. This is a 'slice' of the upper chest presented as if the patient is lying on their back with their feet facing the viewer. The white structures are bones, and the sternum, one vertebral body, some ribs and the scapulae are visible. The very black areas are regions of normal air spaces in the lungs. The cancer is clearly seen as a grey shadow invading the normal lung tissue.

The less-invasive technique of magnetic resonance imaging (MRI) is less valuable in imaging of the tissues of the lung because the respiratory movements affect the quality of the images.

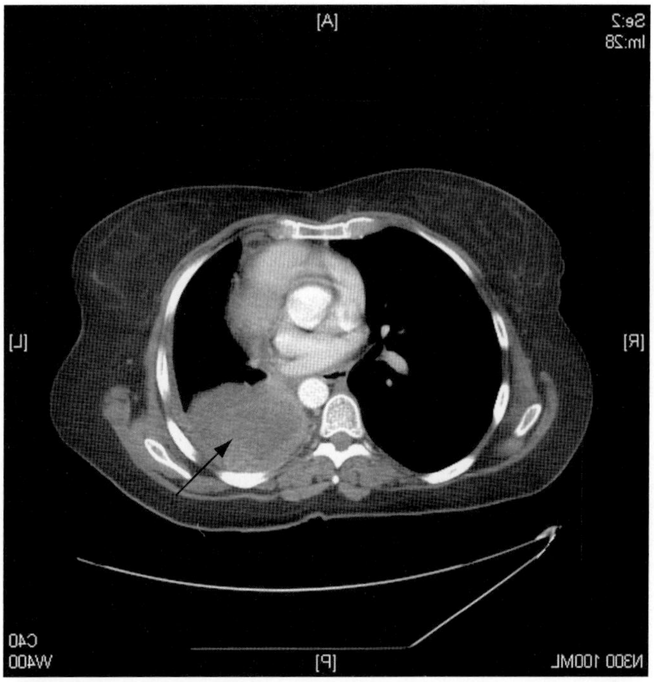

Figure 3.3b-I • A CT scan of the lung indicating a large area of cancerous tissue (arrow).

Bronchoscopy

This invasive test involves the passage of a flexible telescope into the wider air passages of a sedated patient. The tube can be inserted as far as the larger bronchioles. Tumours can be seen directly by means of this technique.

Alternatively, salt water can be squirted down the tip of the tube to retrieve cells from the deeper parts of the lungs in cases of possible infection or cancer when sputum does not reveal any features of disease. This technique is known as 'bronchoalveolar lavage'.

Biopsy of the lung tissue

Biopsy involves the removal of a piece of lung tissue for examination under the microscope. The biopsy can be taken from the bronchi or bronchioles through the bronchoscope. Biopsy of the pleura can be taken through a small incision in the skin overlying a gap between the ribs. Sometimes a thoracic surgeon is required to open up the chest to remove tissue from deep in the chest.

Biopsy is most commonly used to confirm the diagnosis of cancer, but also can be used when infection is suspected, but cannot be detected by any other means.

Fluid can also be drawn from between the pleura by means of a syringe needle inserted between the ribs into the space. This is used only in those conditions that have caused fluid to accumulate in this space, known as pleural effusion. Such conditions include cancer of the bronchus, pneumonia and pulmonary oedema.

Self-test 3.3b

The investigation of the respiratory system

1. Harry is 53 years old and has been smoking all his adult life. Recently he has become more breathless, and over the past 2 weeks has noticed blood in his sputum. His GP is concerned that Harry might have developed cancer and refers him for assessment by a chest physician. What tests do you expect Harry might have to undergo?

Answers

1. Harry will first be given a thorough physical examination. His fingers will be examined for clubbing and his tongue will be checked for cyanosis. The lymph nodes in the neck will be palpated to exclude any enlarged irregular nodes, which may occur in lung cancer. The rate and quality of his breathing will be assessed visually.

   The physician will percuss Harry's chest for areas of dullness, which can signify an underlying mass in the lung tissue. He or she will then use a stethoscope to listen (auscultate) to see if the breath sounds are smooth and symmetrical.

   Harry will be given a chest X-ray and will be requested to produce a sample of sputum.

   If the examination or chest X-ray reveals features suggestive of cancer, Harry will have to undergo a bronchoscopy. A biopsy might be taken at the time of this test of any suspicious looking areas of the bronchi or bronchioles.

   A CT scan will be performed to confirm a diagnosis of cancer and to help stage the progression of the disease.

Chapter 3.3c Diseases of the upper respiratory tract

LEARNING POINTS

At the end of this chapter you will:

- be able to recognise the main features of the most important diseases of the upper respiratory tract
- understand the principles of treatment of a few of the most common diseases
- be able to recognise the red flags of severe disease of the respiratory system.

Estimated time for chapter: 100 minutes.

Introduction

Minor diseases of the upper parts of the respiratory tract such as experience of coughs, colds, and flu, are a well-recognised part of normal life. Conditions that affect the structures progressively further down the respiratory tract, such as the tonsils, larynx and trachea, are seen in conventional medicine as more serious conditions. Nevertheless, on the whole, most acute conditions of the upper half of the respiratory tract are relatively benign.

The conditions of the upper respiratory tract studied in this chapter are:

- Acute infections of the upper respiratory tract:
  - the common cold
  - sinusitis
  - tonsillitis and pharyngitis
  - glandular fever
  - laryngitis, tracheitis and croup
  - epiglottitis
  - influenza.
- Allergic rhinitis.
- Cancer of the larynx (see also Chapter 2.3a) (see Q3.3c-1).

Acute infections of the upper respiratory tract

With the exception of some forms of tonsillitis and pharyngitis and the childhood infection acute epiglottitis, all the common infections of the upper respiratory tract are initially caused by viruses. There is a wide range of viruses that has been identified to affect the respiratory epithelial cells. Viruses tend to enter the upper respiratory tract through inhalation of infected droplets of moisture. The inhaled virus is able to penetrate and damage the cells, and this leads to inflammation (redness and swelling) and the production of sometimes profuse watery secretions. Fever is a common symptom of these infections, although frequently it is mild in nature. Breathlessness (which is significant if respiration rises to over 30 breaths/minute in adults) is not a feature of upper respiratory conditions. Breathlessness suggests a more serious lower respiratory condition or obstruction to the upper airways, and if severe merits same-day referral for a medical opinion.

The different syndromes that result from upper respiratory infection seem to be dependent on the characteristics of the virus. Some primarily affect the throat and the nasal lining, leading to the symptoms of the common cold, whereas others tend to affect lower structures, causing tonsillitis or laryngitis for example. The evidence for this is that a virus that is 'going around' will cause the same sorts of symptoms in most people who contract the infection.

Usually, viral infections of the upper respiratory tract are short lived. In some people the infections can progress to affect further regions of the respiratory system, including the lower respiratory tract. In these cases, it is often believed that a further bacterial infection has arisen in the region of the already damaged respiratory epithelium. Commonly it is one of the 'healthy' bacteria, which usually reside harmlessly in the lining of the upper respiratory tract, that causes these complications. Therefore, these sorts of deeper bacterial infections are not usually contagious. This complication of bacterial infection is recognised to be more likely in people who are susceptible due to some form of chronic ill-health. As long as upper respiratory conditions last for less than 5 days there is usually no need for medical referral, except in the case of infants or frail individuals.

The treatment for all minor viral upper respiratory conditions needs be supportive only, as the antiviral drugs currently available are expensive, carry risks and only shorten rather than eliminate the symptoms of illness in healthy individuals. For this reason, the use of these drugs in the NHS is restricted according to the UK National Institute of Health and Clinical Excellence (NICE) guidance (2009), being given only in cases of influenza in vulnerable individuals. Common treatment approaches recommended by doctors include aspirin and paracetamol to reduce pain and fever, plenty of fluids to counteract fluid loss through fever, keeping warm and letting the body rest.

There is no doubt that smokers are more prone to severe forms of upper respiratory tract infections. It is also recognised that atmospheric pollution results in increased rates of severe respiratory infections. Both these factors reduce the health of the respiratory epithelium so that it is less well equipped to deal with minor infections. Smoking, in particular, is known to damage the action of the cilia in the respiratory epithelium and also to cause a change in the production of the mucus so that it becomes much thicker and thus resistant to clearance from the air passages.

The accumulation of thick and sticky mucus that results when a smoker develops a viral respiratory infection is much more likely to become further infected by bacteria and to result in a persistent phlegmy infection.

The cough and profuse phlegm familiar to people who have recently stopped smoking is a healthy sign. It is a result of the recovery of the cilia, which then are able to clear accumulated toxins and mucus from the lower parts of the respiratory tract.

The common cold

The common cold virus affects the nose and pharynx (throat), leading to sore throat, stuffy and runny nose, and watery eyes. The secretions are usually clear. Fever is slight or absent. Simple treatments for the common cold include vitamin C and zinc preparations and steam inhalations to loosen secretions. Eucalyptus and menthol oils can be a helpful addition to a steam inhalation, and these aromatic compounds are also commonly found in proprietary cough sweets and medicines. Aspirin or paracetamol may be taken to relieve the discomfort of sore throat and to reduce fever.

Decongestant preparations that act by constriction of the blood vessels of the nose are not generally considered to be of great benefit. However, they are freely available as proprietary medications in the form of tablets or nasal sprays containing drugs similar in action to the chemical ephedrine. Decongestants reduce the swelling of the nasal lining and reduce the secretions. However, these are conventionally recognised to be suppressive, and it is recognised that the symptoms may recur in a more pronounced form when the drug wears off. Examples of decongestant medication include Vicks Sinex nasal spray and Sudafed nasal spray.

Some cold preparations available from the chemist contain mild sedatives, which help by allowing the person to rest.

A common cold is not seen to be serious in conventional medicine except in people who have a risk of further infection due to ongoing chronic disease or immunodeficiency.

Sinusitis

Sinusitis is the result of infection of the respiratory epithelium that lines the sinus cavities situated in the facial bones. Although it is commonly triggered by a virus infection, sinusitis can readily become more persistent due to subsequent bacterial infection. This is because the narrow opening of the inflamed sinuses into the nasal cavity easily becomes blocked, and the stagnation of the secretions within predispose to further infection, often by the 'healthy' bacteria that usually reside harmlessly in the nose.

Prolonged sinusitis is more likely to occur in certain susceptible people. Susceptibility can be the result of a congenital structural abnormality sinuses (and so could run in families), a tendency to produce excessive phlegmy secretions, and of smoking.

The symptoms of sinusitis include painful and tender sinuses, with foci of pain over the inner aspect of the eyebrows and in the centre of the cheekbones. In a persistent infection the patient may feel very unwell and feverish, and may have a headache over the forehead. Thick green secretions, indicating bacterial infection, may be produced.

Supportive measures include inhalation of aromatic oils, such as Olbas oil, in steam. Doctors will frequently prescribe antibiotics (most commonly amoxicillin) in a severe case of sinusitis, although increasingly other antibiotics such as doxycycline or erythromycin may have to be chosen because of increasing bacterial resistance to amoxicillin.

In susceptible people, sinusitis, even when treated with antibiotics, can become recurrent. Occasionally it can become

Information Box 3.3c-I

The common cold: comments from a Chinese medicine perspective

In Chinese medicine, the symptoms of the common cold are described as an invasion of Wind Heat or Wind Cold (and occasionally Wind Damp Heat or Wind Dry Heat) on the Exterior. They are believed to occur because of the relative weakness of Wei Qi compared to the strength of the Pathogenic Factor. As such, if treated in its early stages by releasing the Exterior and Clearing Wind, the development of a common cold is believed to be preventable.

According to the Six Stages theory, a common cold due to Wind Cold is at the most superficial Greater Yang (Tai Yang) level. According to the Four Levels theory, a common cold due to Wind Heat is at the most superficial Defensive (Wei) Qi Level.

In contrast to conventional medicine, an Invasion of Wind Heat or Wind Cold is taken very seriously, as there is a risk it may descend to deeper energetic levels and change into Heat unless appropriate care and treatment is given.

From the integrated perspective of infectious disease introduced in Chapter 2.4d, the infectious viruses might be seen as the source of a Pathogenic Factor of external origin, whereas many bacterial complications of these infections would be seen as the result of additional Pathogenic Factors of internal origin. This is comparable to the concept in Chinese medicine that superficial invasions of Wind Heat or Wind Cold can progress to deeper levels in people with depleted Qi, and so fits in with the idea that in these cases the Pathogenic Factor is of internal origin.

For example, the development of a phlegmy bacterial bronchial infection following a minor viral illness, as is common in heavy smokers, could be interpreted in Chinese medicine as the accumulation of Heat and Phlegm at a deeper level than the Exterior. These pathogenic factors are consequences of long-term damage from smoking, and so would be recognised as Internal in origin.

Aspirin may be an appropriate energetic remedy for an invasion of Wind Cold or Wind Heat, in that it is believed to release the exterior and promote sweating. Aspirin is also anti-inflammatory and will temporarily relieve discomfort due to fever, sore throat and aching joints. This suggests a clearing of Heat from the Exterior level and a moving of stagnant Qi. However, the tablet preparation of aspirin is also Heating at a deep level, as evidenced by its causing inflammation of the stomach and increasing the tendency to bleed. This may not be desirable in a patient with Wind Heat invasion. Although aspirin clears Heat at a superficial level, the appearance of Heat at a deeper level suggests this could be, in part, the result of suppression.

Paracetamol also temporarily reduces fever, inflammation and pain. Like aspirin, this represents the clearing of Heat from the Exterior level and moving of stagnant Qi. Although it does not have the Heating properties of aspirin, in overdose it is known to be toxic, to the liver in particular. The temporary effects suggest the mechanism is also suppressive.

Decongestant drugs reduce secretions from the nose and stuffiness. This would correspond to the clearing of Wind Cold. Interestingly, these drugs have a very close relation in Chinese medicine known as ma huang (ephedra), which as a pungent warm herb is recognised to Clear Wind Cold. However, conventionally, decongestants are recognised to be suppressive in action. This suggests that if used without simultaneous attention to the root deficiency, the action of ma huang can also be suppressive.

chronic, with symptoms that never totally go away. In such cases the patient may be referred to an ear, nose and throat specialist for consideration of endoscopic sinus surgery, which is a means of widening and draining the sinus passages.

Information Box 3.3c-II

Sinusitis: comments from a Chinese medicine perspective

In Chinese medicine, sinusitis may simply be a manifestation of Wind Heat or Wind Cold invasion, but more severe cases may indicate other full conditions such as Lung Heat, Liver and Gallbladder Fire or Stomach and Spleen Damp Heat. These conditions occur on a pre-existing deficiency, commonly of the Spleen, which predisposes to accumulation of Damp, Phlegm and Heat.

In sinusitis the tenderness is commonly focused around acupoints Zanzhu Bl-2, Sibai St-2 and Juliao St 3.

If, as in most cases, the problem is a result of an internal imbalance, antibiotic treatment will not be treating the root cause, and due to its Cold and Damp nature may be compounding the problem with additional drug-induced disease. Therefore, the main action of antibiotics in this sort of case is suppressive. This explains why sinusitis can often recur after treatment.

Inhalations of steam benefit the Lung in a case of Lung Heat because they provide moisture. It is also possible that pungent aromatic oils stimulate Lung Qi.

Tonsillitis and pharyngitis

It is very common for a virus infection to affect the back of the throat and/or the tonsils without also affecting the nasal lining. The inflammation that results from this sort of infection is termed 'pharyngitis' (sore throat) or 'tonsillitis', depending on the site of the worst symptoms.

Like the common cold, this sort of viral infection, although uncomfortable, should be mild and short lived. In more severe cases the tonsils can become very inflamed and enlarged, and this can be accompanied by high fever, headache, joint pains and malaise.

Infection with the bacterium *Streptococcus pyogenes* used to be a very common cause of tonsillitis and pharyngitis, although it is now less common. The bacterial tonsillitis is characteristically more severe than that resulting from a viral infection, and yellow areas of pus can often be seen on the tonsil. However, there is no absolute distinction, as some viral tonsillitis can be very severe, and may also generate pus on the tonsil. Bacterial tonsillitis and pharyngitis can be diagnosed by means of a throat swab, although this takes a few days to process.

The treatment for bacterial tonsillitis is penicillin(phenoxymethyl) rather than amoxicillin. Often, a doctor might choose to prescribe penicillin in a severe case of tonsillitis, even when it is uncertain that the cause is bacterial. The delays involved in processing a throat swab and the discomfort for the patient deter many doctors from performing this test. This is an example of 'treating blind' (see Chapter 2.4d). In many cases it may never be known whether the antibiotic helped because the tonsillitis naturally gets better in most people by 3–7 days of onset.

There are two reasons to prescribe antibiotics in tonsillitis. The first is that the symptoms of bacterial infection may be reduced in severity by penicillin. The second, more important, reason is that in some people the *Streptococcus* infection can have more serious complications. These are scarlet fever, rheumatic fever and glomerulonephritis (also known as acute nephritis). However, for reasons that are unclear, these complications are becoming increasingly uncommon, even when the use of antibiotics is accounted for. For this reason current medical guidelines (NICE 2008) recommend that antibiotics are not prescribed in uncomplicated cases of pharyngitis and tonsillitis.

In rare cases, one tonsil can become very inflamed and full of pus. This condition, known as 'quinsy' (peritonsillar abscess), is very debilitating, and is associated with fever. The treatment is with antibiotics and may require urgent surgical drainage of the pus from the tonsil. In some cases the enlarged tonsil may compromise breathing, in which case it becomes a surgical emergency.

In some people, and children in particular, tonsillitis can become recurrent. It used to be common practice to remove the tonsils surgically in such cases. However, surgery is now performed only relatively rarely, as it is recognised to be a risky and traumatic experience for a child, and does not necessarily reduce recurrent attacks of pharyngitis. Tonsillectomy would only currently be considered if attacks of tonsillitis exceeded five a year for at least 2 years.

Glandular fever (infectious mononucleosis)

Glandular fever is one of the more severe forms of viral tonsillitis, and is caused by a virus known as the Epstein–Barr virus (EBV). However, most cases of EBV infection are mild. The evidence for this comes from studies of healthy students, in which blood tests showed that up to 90% of the students had contracted the infection at some point in their lives. Most of these infections had occurred without the students knowing that they had contracted glandular fever.

However, severe cases can be prolonged and draining. The patient can suffer from severe tonsillitis, with fever and joint aches. The lymph nodes in the neck are enlarged. There may be abdominal pain as other lymph tissue in the body, including the spleen, can become enlarged, and the liver may become inflamed. Occasionally, a red, measles-like rash can develop, particularly in patients who have been mistakenly prescribed amoxicillin because a bacterial tonsillitis was suspected. In very rare cases the virus can affect the lining of the brain and cause meningitis.

EBV infection can be diagnosed by a blood test that detects antibodies to the virus in or after the second week of symptoms. Treatment is supportive only. In severe cases, when there is enlargement of the spleen, corticosteroid tablets may be prescribed.

Laryngitis, tracheitis and croup

Some of the other viral infections primarily affect the larynx and the trachea. The result is inflammation of these tissues, leading to one or more of hoarseness, cough and pain felt beneath the sternum. The pain is related to coughing and deep breathing.

Again, these infections may only be short lived except in those who are susceptible, particularly young children and

Information Box 3.3c-IV

Glandular fever: comments from a Chinese medicine perspective

In Chinese medicine, most mild cases of glandular fever would have the same diagnosis as tonsillitis.

In severe cases, the swelling of glands, muscle and joint aches, and disturbance of the liver and spleen suggest that the Pathogenic Factor has penetrated to deeper levels. This suggests either Residual Pathogenic Factor with Damp Heat in the muscles, or the Lesser Yang (Shao Yang) pattern of the Six Stages, or a combination of both.

Information Box 3.3c-III

Tonsillitis: comments from a Chinese medicine perspective

In Chinese medicine, the signs and symptoms of tonsillitis and pharyngitis are usually attributed to Wind Heat invasion. In children in particular, Stomach Heat may be an additional internal source of the Pathogenic Factor. The symptoms of severe tonsillitis correspond to the Chinese medicine condition of Fire Poison, especially with the accumulation of pus and high fever that can occur in such cases. There may be underlying Kidney or Spleen deficiency in cases of Fire poison.

Quinsy is a severe example of Fire Poison, and develops because of underlying deficiency. Antibiotics, although necessary in many cases because of the severity of the condition, are suppressive in action. Surgical drainage is energetically appropriate, as it is simply speeds up the body's tendency to discharge pus, and probably acts by enabling clearance of the Fire Poison (extreme Damp Heat).

Interestingly, Fire Poison has been described in Chinese medicine as one of the causes of acute nephritis. This fits with the conventionally recognised association between streptococcal tonsillitis and acute nephritis.

Antibiotic treatment in tonsillitis may often have either no effect or a simple placebo effect if prescribed in viral infections. However, it may also damage Stomach and Spleen Qi because of its Cold and Damp nature, and so may be less than helpful in the patient with viral tonsillitis. It may be the appropriate energetic remedy in streptococcal infections if the Pathogen is of external origin, however. This is most likely if the case is one of many 'going round'. Often, tonsillitis has an internal component, and is an external manifestation of internal Stomach Heat. If this is the case, antibiotics will be suppressive, and recurrence of the 'infection' is a possibility.

Recurrent tonsillitis always suggests an internal cause. In such cases, treatment with antibiotics and tonsillectomy are suppressive in nature.

smokers. In susceptible people there is a risk that tracheitis can descend to involve the bronchi and cause a much more severe and prolonged infection.

In children under the age of 3 years the swelling of the vocal cords can be so severe as to lead to difficulty in breathing. The affected child will be hoarse, have a rapid respiratory rate and may have a barking cough. If severe, a rasping noise, known as 'stridor', is heard as the child breathes in. In very severe cases the child needs to be nursed in a steam-filled tent in an intensive care unit to allow for safe recovery. The barking cough in such cases is called 'croup', and may persist in a child for weeks.

In some cases laryngitis may persist to give a syndrome of persistently hoarse voice and thick stringy mucus that is difficult to clear. This is known as 'chronic laryngitis'. The patient is otherwise well. This is more common in people who smoke or in those who overuse their voices, such as singers.

The treatment of chronic laryngitis is to rest the voice and avoid smoking. Steam inhalations can soothe the vocal cords and loosen the mucus. However, if the hoarseness persists for more than 3 weeks it is considered good practice for the patient to be referred to an ear, nose and throat specialist. The vocal cords can then be examined by laryngoscopy to exclude the unlikely possibility of a tumour of the vocal cords.

Information Box 3.3c-V

Laryngotracheitis: comments from a Chinese medicine perspective

In Chinese medicine, the symptom of a hoarse voice is usually associated with Wind Heat or Wind Cold invasion. However, the pain and depth of tracheitis suggests that the Pathogen has penetrated to a deeper level than the Exterior. The cough and breathlessness that accompany tracheitis in children in particular is suggestive of Lung Heat (Qi Level according to the Four Levels categorisation). Chronic laryngitis is also consistent with a diagnosis of Lung Heat, although in these cases the likely origin of the Heat is internal, as the condition affects smokers in particular. The dryness resulting from Lung Heat explains why inhalation of steam can be of relief.

Epiglottitis

Acute epiglottitis is a childhood infection by the bacterium *Haemophilus influenzae* B (HiB). This infection in most marked in children under 5 years old. The infection has a rapid onset, with a high fever and difficulty breathing. Inflammation of the epiglottis narrows the aperture of the larynx, and in severe cases this leads to acute stridor and can cause death by asphyxiation. The same bacterium can also cause a form of meningitis.

For this reason, a child with stridor must be treated as an emergency and is nursed in an intensive care unit. It is essential in such cases that the child is not asked to open his or her mouth to show the tongue, as this can precipitate total blockage of the airway. The antibiotics chloramphenicol and cefotaxime are the recommended medical treatments for this infection.

A vaccine is available to protect children against HiB infections, and is given in the first few weeks of life as part of the routine childhood vaccination programme in the UK. There is clear evidence that the introduction of this vaccine in the UK was followed by a marked drop in the reported number of cases of HiB infections.

Information Box 3.3c-VI

Epiglottitis: comments from a Chinese medicine perspective

In Chinese medicine, the symptoms of epiglottitis would be regarded as an Invasion of Wind Heat that has penetrated to the Qi Level to lead to Lung Heat, as is evidenced by the high temperature and the stridor.

Influenza (flu)

Influenza is a result of infection by one of the many strains of the influenza virus. This tends to invade pharyngeal epithelium, but it also gives rise to a much more severe form of general malaise than the common cold. Symptoms include sore throat, dry cough, muscle aches, headache, high fever and exhaustion. A period of up to a few weeks of tiredness and depression is common following recovery.

In susceptible people, particularly the very young and elderly, the virus can also affect the respiratory epithelium of the lower respiratory tract, and this can lead to bacterial infections in the form of bronchitis and pneumonia. In very weak individuals this can be life-threatening.

As with all viral infections, treatment is supportive. Bed rest is recommended, and the patient is advised to take regular doses of aspirin or paracetamol, with plenty of fluids. If bacterial infection of the lower respiratory tract is suspected, antibiotics will be given and hospital admission may be necessary. In susceptible individuals the antiviral drugs zanamivir and oseltamivir may be prescribed to reduce the severity of complications.

In the UK a vaccine is available every autumn/winter that is specific to the currently most virulent and common strain of influenza. This is recommended to be given annually to all elderly people and to any others who may be particularly susceptible because of chronic heart, kidney or lung disease, diabetes or immunosuppression. However, the vaccine is known to protect only about 70% of those who receive it, and it does not protect them from any of the other respiratory viruses. Oseltamivir may be prescribed as a prophylactic medication for individuals at high risk because of susceptibility.

Swine flu is a strain of influenza which reached epidemic proportions in 2009. Because of international concerns about a possible high mortality rate, antiviral prescriptions became a routine aspect of treatment for symptoms of infection in many developed countries. A vaccine specific for the swine flu strain has now been developed, which in UK is now offered to vulnerable groups, including children under the age of 5, pregnant women, elderly people and those with chronic respiratory, cardiac or renal disease.

Allergic rhinitis

'Rhinitis' is the medical term for inflammation of the nose, the symptoms of which are similar to those of the common cold, including a runny and blocked-up nose.

Information Box 3.3c-VII

Influenza: comments from a Chinese medicine perspective

In Chinese medicine, all cases of influenza would be seen as an invasion on the Exterior of Pathogens such as Wind Heat or Wind Cold. In this way, there is no clear distinction made between influenza and the common cold. The severity of the condition in many cases suggests that the Pathogen has descended to the Qi Level to lead to syndromes such as Lung Heat or Stomach Heat. The precise syndrome depends on the symptoms of the patient.

As described in Chapter 2.2c, there are two main types of allergy that affect the nose, hay fever (seasonal rhinitis) and the more chronic condition of perennial rhinitis. In both, the symptoms include runny nose, sneezing, itchy throat and blocked-up nose. In hay fever, itchy and watery eyes are additional common symptoms. Both forms of rhinitis are the result of excessive sensitivity of the immune cells of the respiratory lining to common substances in the atmosphere, such as pollen, house dust and animal dandruff.

In some cases the sinuses can also become inflamed, and this can predispose to bouts of sinusitis, with tender sinuses, headaches and thick yellow discharge from the nose.

Patients who have a long history of allergic rhinitis may develop permanent fleshy swellings of the nasal lining called 'nasal polyps'. 'Polyp' is the term given to a growth, either benign or malignant, that has a stalk as its attachment to the flesh from which it grows. Nasal polyps are benign swellings but may be the cause of a permanently blocked up nose.

Medical treatment of rhinitis includes avoidance of the allergen, regular antihistamine medication (including cetirizine, loratidine and fexofenadine) and anti-inflammatory medication (e.g. sodium cromoglicate) in the form of a nasal spray or eye drops. Decongestant medication (e.g. xylometolazine), some formulations of which can be bought without the need for a prescription, may also be used by the patient. A corticosteroid nasal spray (beclometasone or fluticasone) may be very effective in suppressing symptoms. In severe cases, oral corticosteroids may be prescribed.

A course of oral corticosteroids may help nasal polyps to subside, but if there is no response to medical treatment the only satisfactory treatment is surgical removal.

Information Box 3.3c-VIII

Allergic rhinitis: comments from a Chinese medicine perspective

In Chinese medicine, both types of allergic rhinitis could be seen as invasion of Wind Heat or Wind Cold on a background of deficiency of Wei Qi. The development of sinusitis suggests a Pathogen at a deeper level, such as Liver and Gallbladder Heat, Lung Heat or Spleen Heat. In these cases, as sinusitis is a chronic condition, the origin of the Pathogen is internal.

Nasal polyps are fleshy swellings that might be interpreted as accumulations of Phlegm.

Cancer of the larynx

Laryngeal cancer predominantly affects male smokers, and commonly develops between the ages of 55 and 65 years. The cancer develops on the larynx as a result of long-term irritation from cigarette smoke. The first symptoms often occur early in the disease, as the delicate structure of the vocal cords is frequently affected and unexplained hoarseness develops. If other parts of the voice box are affected the tumour may grow for some time until the patient notices symptoms or swollen lymph nodes in the neck.

The diagnosis is made by laryngoscopy and removal of tissue for a biopsy, and MRI is used to stage the progression of the disease. If caught early, there is a high cure rate with radiotherapy to the larynx alone. In these cases, speech is preserved, although the voice may remain hoarse. If the tumour is extensive the whole of the larynx has to be removed, and the trachea is opened into the neck in an operation known as tracheotomy. An artificial opening with a valve, also known as a tracheostomy, is inserted into the hole in the neck to keep it open and to protect it from foreign bodies.

The patient has to breathe through this opening, and can no longer speak. Some patients learn to speak by using air swallowed first into the stomach, but this is not always possible. The risk of infections of the lower respiratory tract is high in patients with a tracheostomy because the defence mechanisms of all the upper respiratory tract have been removed.

It is a sad fact that 10% of the people who have been 'cured' of laryngeal cancer develop lung cancer at a later stage in their life. This second cancer is almost never curable (see Q3.3c-2).

Information Box 3.3c-IX

Cancer of the larynx: comments from a Chinese medicine perspective

In Chinese medicine, the symptoms of cancer of the larynx would reflect Phlegm and Stagnation in the Lungs. The long-standing depletion that underlies this has resulted in most cases at least in part from smoking. Treatment can only be suppressive, and the high recurrence rate of cancer in 'cured' individuals is evidence of this.

The red flags of upper respiratory disease

Some patients with upper respiratory diseases will benefit from referral to a conventional doctor for assessment and/or treatment. Red flags are those symptoms and signs that indicate that referral is to be considered. The red flags of the upper respiratory diseases are described in Table 3.3c-I. This table forms part of the summary on red flags given in Appendix III, which also gives advice on the degree of urgency of referral for each of the red flag conditions listed.

Table 3.3c-I Red Flags 16 – diseases of the upper respiratory tract

Red Flag	Description	Reasoning
16.1	**Features of progressive upper respiratory infection in susceptible people** (e.g. the frail **elderly** and the **immunocompromised** and people with **pre-existing disease of the bronchi and bronchioles**): i.e. **cough and fever** or **new production of yellow/green phlegm** each persisting for more than 3 days	In healthy people an upper respiratory infection (i.e. affects any part of the respiratory tract above and including the bronchi) may be protracted but is not necessarily a serious condition. In most cases, as long as there is no breathlessness, it is safe to treat conservatively and there is no need for antibiotics In healthy people, consider referral if there is no response to treatment within 1–2 weeks In the elderly and the immunocompromised (including those with chronic diseases, such as cancer, kidney failure and AIDS) severe infections can be masked by relatively minor symptoms, and it is advisable to refer any respiratory condition that persists for more than 3 days People with pre-existing lung disease (e.g. asthma. chronic bronchitis, emphysema, lung cancer, cystic fibrosis) are at increased risk of progressive infection and similarly merit early referral
16.2	**Features of progression of infection to the lower respiratory tract: moderate to severe breathlessness**[1] with **malaise** suggests the involvement of the bronchi or lower air passages. Usually accompanied by **cough** and **fever**, but may be the only symptom of an infection in the elderly or immunocompromised	Even in healthy people an infection that descends to below the bronchi is a more serious condition, as the ability of the lungs to exchange carbon dioxide and oxygen will be compromised by the narrowing of the thin airways of the bronchioles and inflammation of the alveoli (air sacs) Breathlessness is a feature of lower respiratory tract narrowing or infection and should be taken seriously, especially in the elderly, the immunocompromised and those with pre-existing lung disease (such as asthma, chronic bronchitis, emphysema, lung cancer, cystic fibrosis) Respiratory rate of more than 30 breaths/minute is a marker of significant breathlessness Consider referral for medical diagnosis and possible antibiotic treatment
16.3	**A single, grossly enlarged tonsil**: if the patient is unwell and feverish and has foul-smelling breath this suggests **quinsy**	Quinsy is the development of an abscess in the tonsil. It carries a serious risk of obstruction of the airways and requires a same-day surgical opinion. Refer urgently if the patient is experiencing any restriction to breathing (stridor may be heard; see Red Flag 16.5)
16.4	**A single, grossly enlarged tonsil**: if the patient appears well, **lymphoma** is a possible diagnosis	If the patient appears well, you need to consider that a single enlarged tonsil in a young person may very rarely result from a lymphoma, and the patient should be referred for exclusion of this diagnosis. However, grossly enlarged tonsils are not an uncommon finding in someone who has suffered recurrent tonsillitis, but in this case the tonsils are usually bilaterally enlarged
16.5	**Stridor** (harsh, noisy breathing heard on both the in-breath and the out-breath)	Stridor suggests an upper airway obstruction. It is a serious warning sign if it develops suddenly. It suggests possible swelling of the air passages due to laryngotracheitis, quinsy or epiglottitis. If restriction to breathing is significant the patient with stridor will be sitting very still. It is important not to ask to see the tongue, as this can affect the position of the epiglottis and may worsen the obstruction. Exposing the patient to steam (from a nearby kettle or running shower) can alleviate swelling while help arrives
16.6	Any new onset of **difficulty breathing** in a small child (<8 years old), including unexplained blockage of a nostril	Always take a new onset of difficulty in breathing in a child seriously and refer for medical assessment to exclude serious disease. Possible common causes include lower respiratory infections, asthma, allergic reactions, inhalation of foreign bodies and congenital heart disease
16.7	An unexplained **persistent blockage of nostril on one side** in an adult (for more than 3 weeks)	One-sided blockage of a nostril is unusual in benign conditions (such as nasal polyposis). It may be the presenting sign of a carcinoma of the nasopharynx. A one-sided bloody discharge is a warning sign of this

[1] *Categorisation of respiratory rate in adults*

- Normal respiratory rate in an adult: 10–20 breaths/minute (one breath is one inhalation and exhalation).
- Moderate breathlessness in an adult: >30 breaths/minute.
- Severe breathlessness in an adult: >60 breaths/minute.

Categorisation of respiratory rate in children

- The normal range for respiratory rate in children varies according to age.
- The following rates indicate moderate to severe breathlessness:

newborn (0–3 months)	>60 breaths/minute
infant (3 months to 2 years)	>50 breaths/minute
young child (2–8 years)	>40 breaths/minute
older child to adult	>30 breaths/minute.

Self-test 3.3c

The diseases of the upper respiratory tract

1. A 30-year-old woman has had a cough for 3 weeks now. It started with a runny nose and sore throat. She also had 1 day of hoarseness, but this is better now. She feels alright, but a bit hot and bothered and run down. However, she is not breathless or feverish. The main problem is the cough; it helps to bring up some phlegm, which is thick and yellowish in colour, but usually the cough is dry. It hurts a bit at the top of her chest when she coughs vigorously.
   (i) What is the conventional medicine diagnosis?
   (ii) How might a conventional doctor treat this patient?
   (iii) Should you refer this patient?
   (iv) What is a possible diagnosis in Chinese medicine?

Answers

1. (i) The beginning of this woman's problem started with what sounds like a common cold due to a virus infection. The virus also affected the vocal cords, causing a brief episode of laryngitis. However, instead of clearing up within 3–5 days, the condition has become more chronic, with the production of some thick yellowish mucus, and persistent inflammation of the trachea (indicated by the pain high up in the chest on coughing). This is most likely due to a complicating infection by bacteria, and we should not be too surprised if we found out that our patient was a smoker or was run down in some way before she contracted the cold. The infection is not severe, but is lingering on.
   (ii) A GP might attempt to clear up the cough with an antibiotic prescription, although increasingly GPs are tending to avoid prescribing of antibiotics in minor respiratory infections.
   Instead the GP might take samples of sputum to look for the offending bacterium, and ask the patient to return in a few days. If after this time the cough is still present, most GPs would then be tempted to prescribe.
   (iii) The patient has no red flags of severe disease and so there is no need to refer in this case, unless you have any reason to suspect immunodeficiency (extremely rare).
   (v) In Chinese medicine the initial diagnosis is invasion of Wind Heat or Wind Cold, but the persistence of the condition suggests that the Pathogen has penetrated to the Qi level. A dry cough, yellowish phlegm, and a sensation of heat in this case is most suggestive of Lung Heat, but could also be due to pre-existing Lung Yin deficiency.

Chapter 3.3d Diseases of the bronchi and bronchioles

LEARNING POINTS

At the end of this chapter you will:
- be able to recognise the main features of the most important diseases of the airways of the lower respiratory tract
- understand the principles of treatment of a few of the most common diseases
- be able to recognise the red flags of severe disease of this part of the respiratory system.

Estimated time for chapter: 100 minutes.

Introduction

This chapter looks at the diseases that affect the airways of the lower respiratory tract, the bronchi and the bronchioles. The conditions studied are:

- Infections of the airways of the lower respiratory tract:
  - acute bronchitis
  - chronic bronchitis
  - bronchiolitis.
- Bronchial asthma.
- Bronchiectasis and cystic fibrosis.
- Cancer of the bronchus (lung cancer) (see Q3.3d-1).

Infections of the airways of the lower respiratory tract

Acute bronchitis

Acute bronchitis is not dissimilar to many of the infections of the upper respiratory tract described in Chapter 3.3c. It is frequently the result of a virus infection, and has symptoms of dry cough, and a sensation of tightness or even pain felt beneath the sternum. However, because the bronchi are relatively narrow tubes, the swelling of their lining from inflammation can cause a marked reduction in the amount of air that can freely travel through them. This can lead to wheezing and shortness of breath, although in uncomplicated viral bronchitis these symptoms should not be severe.

Viral bronchitis can very easily become complicated by bacterial infection. In this case infection is usually due to one of the bacteria that in health reside harmlessly in the respiratory tract. Bacterial infection is particularly likely to occur in smokers or, ironically, in people who have just stopped smoking; in the latter because the production of thick mucus is temporarily increased.

In bacterial bronchitis the cough becomes productive, and sometimes profuse yellow-green phlegm is coughed up. Despite the relatively deep situation of the infection, most people do not feel extremely unwell, and fever may only be slight. Most recover from this infection as they would from infections higher up the respiratory tract.

Some doctors may prescribe antibiotics such as amoxicillin, tetracycline or erythromycin, although these may not be necessary for recovery in healthy people.

Information Box 3.3d-I

Acute bronchitis: comments from a Chinese medicine perspective

In Chinese medicine, the fever, breathlessness and productive cough of acute bronchitis suggest that an invasion of Pathogens such as Wind Cold or Wind Heat has been succeeded by the penetration of Heat to the Qi Level (according to the Six Stages categorisation). The Qi-level syndrome that would fit with bronchitis is Lung Heat.

The symptoms of bacterial infection suggest that Heat and Phlegm are more marked than in viral infection. This development is more likely in those with a degree of pre-existing Lung Yin deficiency, which can result from smoking. In a smoker some of the full Heat and Phlegm may also be of internal origin.

As bacterial infection occurs against a background of Lung deficiency, antibiotics treat only the manifestation of the imbalance, and so the treatment suppressive in nature.

Chronic bronchitis

Chronic bronchitis is a common condition in which a combination of recurrent infections and smoking (or other atmospheric pollutants) has led to long-term (chronic) changes in the lining of the bronchi and bronchioles. There are a number of definitions of chronic bronchitis, all of which describe chronic bronchitis as a prolonged cough that is productive of sputum and that recurs for a number of years in a row. A large proportion of long-term smokers would qualify as having chronic bronchitis according to these definitions.

The main change in chronic bronchitis is that the mucus cells of the respiratory epithelium tend to produce thick, sticky mucus in excess. Because of smoking or pollutants, the cilia are not functioning well, and the mucus cannot be cleared efficiently. These changes in themselves encourage the development of further infections and inflammation of the lining of the air passages. The chronic inflammation leads to swelling of the air passages and thus a reduction in their internal diameter. This restricts easy breathing, and breathing can become laboured or wheezy.

The initial changes in the bronchi and bronchioles are reversible if the patient can stop smoking, but in long-standing cases the airways become permanently scarred as a result of the inflammation, and remain narrowed and irregular.

One problem with chronic bronchitis is that, once established, the patient is more prone to further bouts of acute bronchitis (infections), which then worsen the ongoing inflammation. A vicious cycle of progressive damage is established, particularly if the patient is unable to give up smoking. The damage often goes hand in hand with smoking-related damage deeper in the lung. This deeper condition, known as emphysema, affects the delicate structure of the alveoli (see Chapter 3.3e). Together, chronic bronchitis and emphysema form a disabling syndrome of chronic breathing difficulties known as chronic obstructive pulmonary disease (COPD) (see Chapter 3.3e).

The treatment of chronic bronchitis is to stop smoking and avoid pollutants. Conventional advice is to treat any bacterial infections promptly with antibiotics to minimise further damage to the lining of the air passages.

Information Box 3.3d-II

Chronic bronchitis: comments from a Chinese medicine perspective

In Chinese medicine, depending on the precise symptoms, the symptoms of chronic bronchitis could fit with either one of Damp Phlegm or Phlegm Heat Obstructing the Lungs. Both of these are chronic conditions in which the Pathogens are primarily internally generated.

Stopping smoking will both enable the recovery of damaged Lung Yin and remove a potent source of Phlegm and Heat and is, therefore, an energetically appropriate treatment. Antibiotics tend to be suppressive, but they may be necessary to prevent progressive damage to the lungs in a persistent case of bacterial infection.

Bronchiolitis

This is a viral infection of childhood that tends to affect the small air passages of the lungs, although it often begins with 1–2 days of upper respiratory tract symptoms. The respiratory syncytial virus (RSV) is the most common causative agent. The affected child will suffer from restricted breathing due to the narrowing of the air passages, and will have a rapid and laboured breathing rate. Wheezy noises are heard through the stethoscope. In a proportion of cases the lung tissue also becomes infected, and this, as a form of pneumonia, is a much more severe condition. Treatment of bronchiolitis is initially supportive. Steam inhalation can be very soothing. Severe cases may first be treated with oral steroids, but if they do not respond, may need to be hospitalised. Red flag signs include cyanosis, poor feeding and a rapid respiratory rate (>50 breaths/minute).

Information Box 3.3d-III

Bronchiolitis: comments from a Chinese medicine perspective

In Chinese medicine wheezy rapid breathing called 'Xiao-Chuan', a term that comes from the words meaning 'wheezing' and 'breathlessness', is seen as the result of Phlegm in the Lungs. The origin of the Pathogenic Factor is, in part, external.

Bronchial asthma

Asthma is a condition that affects 5–8% of the population of the UK. In asthma, breathing is impaired due to a narrowing of the airways of the lower respiratory tract. Usually this narrowing is reversible, which means that the difficulty in breathing comes in bouts. The underlying problem in asthma is that the lining of the airways is much too sensitive to a wide range of factors, which, when they occur, lead to a rapid development of inflammation and the production of mucus. This inflammation causes swelling and narrowing of the airways, and the mucus can actually plug up some of the smaller air passages of the bronchioles.

The factors that can trigger an asthma attack include:

- animal dandruff
- faeces of the house dust mite and cockroach
- pollen and moulds
- substances in the diet, such as egg, milk, wheat and fish
- some drugs (especially aspirin, and other non-steroidal anti-inflammatory drugs such as ibuprofen)
- industrial fumes, cigarette smoke and other atmospheric pollution
- cold air and exercise
- respiratory infections
- extremes of emotion.

The external factors such as animal dandruff and house dust are known as allergens because they can provoke an allergic response. The allergens that affect an individual will be specific to that individual. For example, some people will be sensitive to only one or two of the allergens on this list, such as pollen in the summer. In others the sensitivity is so broad that often it may be unclear why an attack of asthma has developed.

It is known that asthmatics have excessive numbers of a certain sort of leukocyte called a 'mast cell' in their lung tissue. The mast cell is very sensitive to noxious substances, and when it comes into contact with them it releases powerful chemicals such as histamine that stimulate inflammation in the bronchial airways. This is meant to be a protective response to enable the lung to clear irritating material, but is excessive in asthma. It is an example of a condition in which the immune system is overactive.

Many people with asthma also have other conditions that result from an overactive immune system, such as eczema and hay fever. The tendency to be 'allergic' in this way to a wide range of substances is known as 'atopy', and seems to run quite strongly in families. In these people the diagnosis of atopy can be confirmed by skin-prick tests, in which a minute amount of a number of different common allergens is inserted into the skin by a shallow injection. Atopic people may show a small area of reddening and swelling around the site of the prick over the next couple of days. This is a confirmation of sensitivity to that allergen. Skin-prick tests can be useful for people with atopy as they can identify which of the common allergens should be avoided. When asthma can be shown to have an external cause in this way it is termed 'extrinsic asthma'.

Atopic people with asthma often have characteristic symptoms of allergy from early childhood. However, some people only develop asthma in later life, and these people seen to be less sensitive to the common allergens. This sort of asthma is termed 'intrinsic asthma'. In practice, the treatment of both types of asthma is similar.

Asthma does seem to be more common in westernised cultures, and its reported incidence, particularly in children, is on the increase. The reasons for this are unclear, although some conventional theories attribute the rise to increases in certain sorts of atmospheric pollutants in industrial countries. This fits with the observation that asthma is a very common finding in some industries in which the workforce is more exposed to certain chemicals in the atmosphere of the workplace.

The symptoms of an asthma attack result from the narrowing and blocking of the airways by inflammation and mucus. The attack may develop within seconds to minutes after exposure to an allergen, to cold or extreme emotion, or may be delayed by a few hours. The person will feel increasing difficulty in breathing. Many people find it hard to say whether it is breathing in or out that is most difficult, but lung-function tests will often demonstrate a much prolonged expiration time. This is an objective measure of difficulty breathing out.

During an asthma attack, the act of breathing becomes hard work, and because not so much oxygen is reaching the lungs the breathing rate increases to make up for this. The sensation of not being able to get air into the chest can induce panic in many people, which can further affect the breathing pattern, as well as worsen the asthma attack itself. A common symptom is the production of a wheezy noise, particularly on breathing out, which results from the air whistling through the narrowed airways. However, dry cough may be the only symptom in mild cases, which may confuse the diagnosis, particularly in children.

In mild cases the attack can settle down in minutes to hours, but often the breathing is affected for a few days afterwards, during which time the lungs are particularly sensitive to further attacks.

In severe cases the breathing never fully settles down to normal. The person with severe asthma can be always wheezy and breathless, and may suffer frequent bouts of worsening breathlessness on top of this. In all cases the symptoms get worse at night. Waking at night with cough or difficulty breathing is an indication that the asthma is quite severe. It is well known that asthma attacks can be at their worst in the early hours of the morning.

In some cases an attack can lead to such an extreme reduction in the width of the airways that the patient is simply unable to inhale sufficient oxygen for their requirements. As the attack worsens, the respiratory rate increases to a severe level (30 breaths/minute or more). A patient in this state will need to hold themselves still and upright and will be reluctant or unable to talk freely. The heart rate becomes rapid (100–130 beats/minute) as a result of the body's response to the stress of not having enough oxygen (adrenaline is released). This extreme condition is unlikely to settle of its own accord and is termed 'status asthmaticus'. All the features described in this paragraph are red flags of severe disease.

The development of status asthmaticus can be so rapid and extreme that the person can die. It requires emergency treatment with oxygen and drugs to reverse the narrowing of the airways. This dangerous form of asthma is most likely to occur in those who have suffered from severe asthma for some time. Occasionally, it can develop out of the blue in someone who has previously had only minor symptoms or even no symptoms at all.

Asthma is diagnosed on the basis of the symptoms and by means of lung-function tests. These tests indicate that the force and length of expiration is abnormal when the patient encounters one or more of the factors that trigger the attacks. A distinguishing feature of asthma is that this abnormality usually improves when the triggers are removed. A chest X-ray image is usually normal in asthma.

The simplest measure of expiration is the 'peak expiratory flow rate', which is measured using a hand-held peak-flow meter. This gives an objective measure of the force with which the person can blow out. The figure obtained has to be adjusted for the patient's size and sex. The patient has to be carefully instructed in how to blow into the meter, or the readings obtained will not be helpful.

The peak-flow meter can demonstrate the hour-to-hour variability in peak-flow rate that is characteristic of asthma. It is used in general practice, and by patients at home, to monitor their current state and response to treatment. Ideally, the peak flow should be in the normal range for the person's size and sex, and should show very little variability at different times of the day.

Figure 3.3d-I shows a graph of the peak-flow readings taken at three times a day by a person with asthma over the course of 2 weeks. It can be seen that in the first few days the peak-flow measurements show great variation, with the lowest readings occurring in the early morning. In this patient, treatment with corticosteroid medication affects this pattern, leading to a general improvement in peak-flow rate and a marked reduction in the variability of the peak flow.

A good measure of successful treatment of asthma is that the hour-to-hour variability of the peak-flow measurements is reduced. This is an important point to be appreciated by complementary therapists when using peak-flow readings to monitor the effects of treatment. For useful monitoring it is necessary to look at measurements taken at different times of the day, over the course of a few days, and this of course requires the patient's help in taking measurements at home.

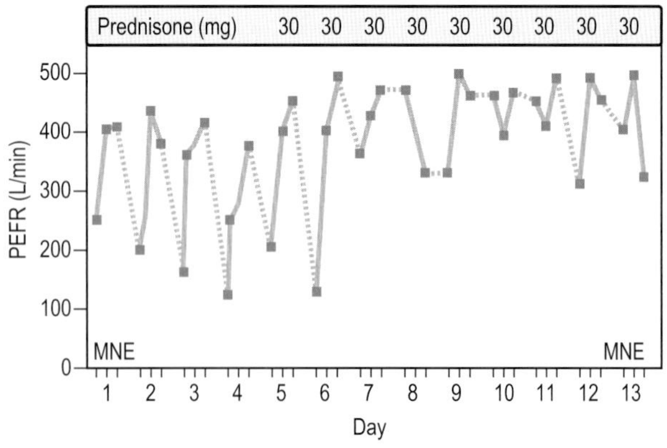

Figure 3.3d-I • The day-to-day variability in peak-flow rate in a patient with asthma and the response to corticosteroid medication (started on day 5). MNE; morning, noon and evening.

The treatment of asthma depends on the severity of the condition. Because it is such an important condition, the British Thoracic Society and Scottish Intercollegiate Guidelines Network have produced guidelines for the management of asthma, which are now highly respected amongst doctors in the UK. These are comparable to the guidelines produced by the British Hypertension Society for the management of hypertension, in that they grade the asthma according to certain features, and then recommend treatment and lifestyle advice for each grade of asthma.

The guidelines advise on a stepwise management of asthma, which is summarised in detail in Section 3.1 of the *British National Formulary*. The general points about the management of asthma that can be distilled from these guidelines are that there are three broad types of treatment:

- avoidance of triggers (including allergens, smoking and family stress)
- use of drugs called 'bronchodilators' to reduce the narrowing of the airways (by inhaler or tablets)
- use of anti-inflammatory drugs, in particular corticosteroids, to reduce the development of inflammation in the airways (by inhaler or tablets).

All patients with even very mild symptoms may be offered a bronchodilator. This type of drug, usually administered by inhaler, rapidly reverses the narrowing of the airways in asthma. The drug most commonly prescribed is salbutamol. The drug is taken whenever breathing becomes limited, although this should not be necessary more than once or twice a day in mild asthma. Salbutamol mimics the effect of adrenaline (the other name for this group of drugs is 'beta stimulant', and their action is thus the opposite of that of the beta blockers), and therefore can have the side-effects of increased heart rate and a sensation of anxiety and sleeplessness, although these would be unusual at a dose of one or two inhaled puffs a day.

In all but the mildest forms of asthma (when salbutamol is required more than twice a week, or more than once at night) the guidance is to add in a regular dose of an anti-inflammatory drug to be used in addition to the bronchodilator. This means that most people with asthma will be prescribed two inhalers, one to be taken when they feel wheezy (the bronchodilator), and one to be taken twice a day (the anti-inflammatory). In adults the most commonly prescribed anti-inflammatory drug is a corticosteroid (e.g. beclomethasone and fluticasone). In children, a drug called sodium cromoglicate may be used first, although many children will eventually be prescribed a steroid inhaler because it seems to work better for them.

Both bronchodilators and anti-inflammatory drugs are taken in mild to moderate cases of asthma by inhaler, because this is known to concentrate the drug in the lungs and thus general side-effects to the rest of the body are minimised.

It is important to recognise that to give a steroid inhaler to people with mild asthma is considered good practice in conventional medicine. This is because use of the steroid in all but the mildest cases has been shown to reduce the severity and frequency of severe attacks. Studies indicate that regular inhaled steroids reduce the numbers of cases of status asthmaticus and deaths from asthma.

Important side-effects from the steroid inhalers include hoarseness of voice due to an effect on the vocal cords, thrush in the mouth and slight growth retardation in children. All these appear to be significant only when very high doses are given.

In more severe cases of asthma the dose and frequency of bronchodilators and anti-inflammatory drugs is increased. The next recommended step is that a long-acting form of beta agonist is prescribed. Oral theophyllines are also recommended as an additional type of bronchodilator. A newer medication that is currently recommended as an adjunct in asthma that has not responded fully to inhaled beta agonists and steroids alone is one of the leukotriene receptor antagonists such as montelukast. If the asthma still fails to settle, oral corticosteroid medication may have to be initiated, and for some patients long-term corticosteroid therapy is a necessity in order to prevent life-threatening exacerbations of the condition.

In an acute bout of asthma, the guidelines suggest that the patient is advised to step up the dose of steroids rapidly in order to control the symptoms, and only to reduce back to the usual dose once the bout has settled down again. In a very severe attack steroids may be given by tablet or even intravenously, and bronchodilators may be given in very high doses via a mask and a machine called a 'nebuliser'. Some patients with severe asthma may have both a nebuliser and access to oxygen at home to deal with sudden severe attacks.

A patient in status asthmaticus is usually treated in hospital with oxygen and intravenous steroids and bronchodilators, and medical care may be offered in the setting of an intensive care unit.

Bronchiectasis

'Bronchiectasis' is the term used to describe a condition in which the airways have become permanently damaged so that they are distorted and dilated, usually as the result of a severe infection. The damaged air passages are unable to be fully cleared of mucus because the cilia on the respiratory epithelium are damaged, and this means that infection is commonly present in these parts of the airways.

A person with bronchiectasis will always produce phlegm, sometimes in large quantities, and is more prone to bouts of acute bronchitis, which of course may worsen the underlying condition. The phlegm predisposes to further infections, but also is the cause of ongoing inflammation and scarring of the airways. Rarely, the affected area can bleed, and the patient will cough up blood. In some cases this bleeding can be so profuse as to be life-threatening.

The most common cause of bronchiectasis used to be whooping cough (pertussis) in childhood, but this has become much less common as the health of western populations has improved and since the introduction of pertussis vaccination. Now the most common cause of this condition is the congenital disease cystic fibrosis, which is discussed in more detail below.

It is very important for the patient with bronchiectasis to clear the excessive mucus that accumulates in the damaged airways. In severe cases, a physiotherapist can help the patient to cough up the phlegm while the patient is in a tipped position ('postural drainage').

It is believed that any infections should be treated rapidly with antibiotics so that further damage to the structure of the airways is prevented.

In very severe progressive cases, the only option for the patient is to have a heart–lung transplant. The heart is removed at the same time as the lungs in this condition because it too is damaged as a result of the long-term strain

Information Box 3.3d-IV

Asthma: comments from a Chinese medicine perspective

In Chinese medicine, asthma is known as 'Xiao-Chuan', a term reflecting the combination of wheezing and breathlessness that occurs in asthma. The differentiation of asthma is complex and depends on the symptoms of the individual.

In most cases, the commonly recognised symptoms point to an underlying deficiency of the Qi of both the Lungs and the Kidney. Kidney Qi deficiency appears to be particularly prominent in atopic individuals. In Chinese medicine, Lung Qi is important for the action of expiration and Kidney Qi for inspiration (the Kidneys are said to grasp Lung Qi in inspiration).

Combined Lung and Kidney Qi deficiency predisposes to invasion of Wind Cold, which can in itself lead to an acute bout of asthma. The rapidity with which some attacks follow exposure to certain allergens is characteristic of Wind invasion. In many cases, mucus and phlegm is a prominent feature, and this would be diagnosed as Accumulation of Phlegm, or Retention of Phlegm Heat. Anger and frustration leading to an asthma attack would be diagnosed as Liver Qi insulting the Lungs.

Bronchodilators allow the relaxation of the tight smooth muscle of the airways and do this by mimicking adrenaline, a hormone released by the adrenal glands. The function of adrenaline is Yang and moving in nature. Bronchodilators therefore boost Kidney Yang and also Move Stagnant Qi. Their action is suppressive in nature because they do not deal with the root cause of the problem, which returns when they wear off. It is possible that frequent use of bronchodilators is depleting to the Kidneys, Lungs and the Heart because they produce excessive stimulation of the functions of these Organs.

Anti-inflammatory drugs Subdue the Heat and Phlegm, which could be interpreted as the result of the inflammation and mucus in asthma. They would appear also to Boost Lung and Kidney Qi, as their use prevents further attacks of asthma. Again, these drugs are suppressive because they do not cure the root problem, which will recur, although sometimes at a much later date, when the drugs are withdrawn. This would imply that the removal of the asthma symptoms is at the cost of accumulation of Heat and Phlegm at deeper levels. Long-term depletion of the Kidneys and Lungs may result, so that a dependence on the drugs is induced.

of pumping blood through scarred lungs (see Chapter 3.2f, where it is described how chronic lung disease is one of the causes of chronic heart failure). As with a heart transplant, a heart-lung transplant is a risky procedure for the patient, and requires long-term immunosuppressive medication after recovery from the operation. Only 70% of patients who have this operation will still be alive 3 years after the operation.

Information Box 3.3d-V

Bronchiectasis: comments from a Chinese medicine perspective

In Chinese medicine, the signs and symptoms of bronchiectasis would correspond to the chronic conditions of Accumulation of Phlegm or Phlegm Heat Obstructing the Lungs. Although the initial damage may have been triggered by an infection and a Pathogen of external origin, the severity of the condition indicates that the Phlegm and Heat is largely of internal origin.

The tendency to Heat and the destruction of the structure of the lungs implies that the underlying deficiency was originally of Lung Yin. Profuse bleeding and profuse discoloured phlegm are both indications of Full Heat.

Postural drainage is an energetically appropriate therapy, as it enables the clearance the Phlegm/Heat, which of course is the natural tendency of the body.

Although antibiotics are known to slow the progression of the condition, they deal only with the manifestation of the problem, and therefore are suppressive in nature. Their energetic nature is Cold and Damp, which can predispose to the formation of more Phlegm by injuring the action of Spleen. However, it is difficult to argue against their use in bronchiectasis, as there is good evidence for benefit in terms of prolonged life expectancy.

Cystic fibrosis

Cystic fibrosis (CF) is a relatively common inherited condition, which usually occurs when a baby inherits a CF gene from each of their parents. This occurs in just under one in 2,000 births. The carriage of this gene is common, with one in 22 Caucasians possessing it. However, most carriers are totally unaware of the fact that they are carriers because the condition is, in genetic terms, a recessive condition. This means that it only manifests if the person carries two CF genes, one from each parent. Because of the nature of the recessive inheritance of the condition, most babies born with CF are not diagnosed for some months to years after birth.

The main problem in CF is that the mucus produced by the body is excessively thick and sticky. This is of particular significance in the lower respiratory tract, where the healthy production of mucus is an important barrier to disease. This means that a baby with CF will have frequent infections of the lower respiratory tract, including bouts of pneumonia. As the child gets older, phlegmy conditions of the nose and throat, such as sinusitis, also become frequent. The inability to clear the thickened secretions in infection means that the permanent and progressive condition of bronchiectasis may develop early in life, particularly if the condition is not diagnosed until relatively late.

The other major physical problem of CF is related to the digestive tract. Thickened secretions in the pancreas can lead to a failure to produce sufficient pancreatic enzymes. This leads to a form of malabsorption, as described in Chapter 3.1e. The management of this complication of CF is by means of artificial pancreatic enzymes, which can be taken by mouth with meals.

CF also causes male infertility, as the underlying problem of CF affects the development of sperm. Although women with CF are technically fertile, the ill-health caused by the condition leads to failure of ovulation in many women.

Diagnosis of CF is by means of sweat analysis, which reveals abnormally high sodium and chloride levels, and genetic screening is likely to reveal one of the common CF gene mutations.

Treatment of CF involves meticulous attention to clearing of phlegm by postural drainage and rapid treatment of infections with antibiotics. This has led to problems of antibiotic resistance in many patients with CF, who by adulthood will be carrying bacteria that are no longer affected by the common antibiotics. This has become so problematic that patients with CF may be advised not to mix with other patients with CF or other chronic lung disease in order to prevent transmission of these resistant 'super-bugs'. This has obvious effects in terms of social isolation, particularly when the patient with CF has to be hospitalised. Drugs that break down mucus (dornase alpha) may be administered by means of a nebuliser with some benefit.

Recently, in-depth knowledge of how the gene defect in CF causes faulty mucus production has led to research into the development of some powerful 'designer drug' therapies. CF is one of the few genetic diseases in which the use of a normal gene, cloned into virus vectors from healthy human cells, has been used to produce some benefit to patients. These treatments are still in the experimental stages, and are not yet widely available.

Even in recent decades, people with CF were not expected to live past their mid-teens, but now most people with the disease live well into adulthood. This is attributed to early recognition of the disease and skilled attention to the excessive phlegmy secretions and frequent infections. However, most tend to die relatively young of progressive lung damage due to bronchiectasis or uncontrollable infection. Heart–lung transplant may be available to those whose life expectancy is less than 18 months.

A genetic test is available that can detect the majority of people who carry a mutated CF gene. It is currently only available to couples planning to have children who have a person with CF in their immediate family.

Information Box 3.3d-VI

Cystic fibrosis: comments from a Chinese medicine perspective

In Chinese medicine, cystic fibrosis would have the same diagnosis as bronchiectasis. The inherited nature of the condition and its effect on fertility suggests that Jing deficiency is an additional factor. Malabsorption due to pancreatic failure could be seen as a manifestation of Spleen Qi deficiency.

Cancer of the bronchus (lung cancer)

Lung cancer accounts for 19% of cancer diagnoses in the UK, and 27% of cancer deaths. In most cases of lung cancer the site of the tumour is in the bronchi or bronchioles. Only 2% of all lung cancers actually originate in an alveolus. This is because the main trigger for lung cancer is of external origin, most commonly being the carcinogens in cigarette smoke. Other important lung carcinogens include asbestos, iron oxides and environmental radon. Because of the protective nature of the lining of the airways of the lower respiratory tract, toxins such as those contained in cigarette smoke are deposited on the walls of the airways before they have a chance to reach the alveoli.

Lung cancer is the third most common cause of death in the UK after heart disease and pneumonia. It used to be a disease that affected men much more than women, but is now known to be increasing in women. This is attributed to the rapid increase in smoking in women, which began in the middle of the 20th century and is continuing, particularly in younger women.

Lung cancer develops from one of the lining cells of the respiratory epithelium. As it grows to obstruct the airway it can cause symptoms such as cough, with or without phlegm, or heavy chest pain. Occasionally, a first symptom is coughing up of small amounts of blood, a symptom referred to as 'haemoptysis'. Less common first symptoms result from quite advanced disease, and include breathlessness, loss of weight, hoarseness and enlarged lymph nodes in the neck. Hoarseness can occur because the nerve that supplies the larynx passes deep within the chest and so can be damaged by a spreading lung cancer.

Advanced lung cancer can compress the other structures in the chest cavity to cause difficulty in swallowing and swelling of the face and neck. In an advanced cases breathlessness might become very severe, because the growing cancer is secreting fluid that accumulates in the pleural space and compresses the lung (pleural effusion). The presence of the obstructing tumour increases the risk of infection, and pneumonia can develop in advanced disease.

The cancer tends to spread first to the lymph nodes deep within the chest and then most commonly to the bones, leading to deep bone pain and risk of fracture. Spread to the liver and the brain is also fairly common.

A chest X-ray image will reveal the presence of a 'shadow' on the lung of many people who have symptoms due to lung cancer. The diagnosis is confirmed by examination of sputum for cancer cells and by means of a bronchoscopy, when a biopsy may be taken for accurate diagnosis of the type of cancer. A CT scan is usually performed to look for evidence of spread to the lymph nodes or the liver. This is important for staging of the cancer.

Most types of lung cancer are known not to respond to chemotherapy, and most of these are too advanced at diagnosis to be removed by surgery. Of the small percentage of patients with cancers that can be removed by surgery, only one-fifth will be still alive after 5 years. If surgery is not possible, high-dose radiotherapy may slow the progression of the disease, but still has a low overall cure rate. The few cancers that are known to respond to chemotherapy (small-cell tumours) do so rapidly and dramatically, but in most cases they tend to recur after a few months. Rarely, chemotherapy can give a few years of remission from the tumour.

In summary, most lung cancers are very resistant to modern cancer treatment. Only 6–8% of all people treated for lung cancer will be alive 5 years after diagnosis. In most people who receive such therapies, the most that can be expected is a few more months of life, with, hopefully, a reduction in distressing symptoms for this period.

Palliative care includes radiotherapy for painful bone tumours and rapidly enlarging tumours in the chest. Corticosteroids and strong morphine-based painkillers can improve mood, appetite and the sensation of breathlessness.

> **Information Box 3.3d-VII**
>
> **Lung cancer: comments from a Chinese medicine perspective**
>
> In Chinese medicine, lung cancer, like most cancers, may be seen as Phlegm and Blood stagnation on a background of long-standing deficiency of Yin and/or Yang. In Lung cancer, which is almost always associated with long-term smoking, the background deficiency is likely to be of Lung Yin. This fits with the recognition that modern treatments, which tend to be Heating and therefore depleting of Yin, are not very successful in lung cancer. All these treatment approaches are, of course, suppressive in nature.

Breathlessness

In contrast to the diseases of the upper respiratory tract, one key feature of diseases of the bronchi and bronchioles is breathlessness. Usually any inflammation above the voice box will not be sufficiently severe as to compromise intake of air to the lungs. Coughs and colds and laryngitis may be uncomfortable, but will not affect the amount of oxygen reaching the lungs. The exception to this rule is the extreme upper respiratory obstruction that might occur in epiglottitis and inhalation of a foreign body (leading to the harsh inspiratory and expiratory noise of stridor).

Inflammation or constriction of the smaller airways will often lead to reduced exchange of oxygen and carbon dioxide because of the restriction to airflow posed by the narrowed air passages. The brainstem responds to the increased carbon dioxide and reduced oxygen levels in the bloodstream that result from poor gas exchange, and stimulates deeper and more rapid breathing. The patient will experience this as breathlessness.

The normal respiratory rate for a healthy adult is 10–20 breaths/minute. In breathlessness, this rate is increased and, particularly if of recent onset, the patient has a sensation of difficulty in breathing. For the purposes of this chapter, a

Table 3.3d-I Categorisation of respiratory rate in adults

Category	Rate[1]
Normal	10–20 breaths/minute
Moderate breathlessness	>30 breaths/minute
Severe breathlessness	> 60 breaths/minute

[1]One breath is one inhalation and exhalation.

Table 3.3d-II Categorisation of respiratory rate in children

Category	Rate[1]
Normal	Varies according to age
Moderate to severe breathlessness:	
newborn (0-3 months)	>60 breaths/minute
infant (3 months to 2 years)	>50 breaths/minute
young child (2–8 years)	>40 breaths/minute
older child to adult	>30 breaths/minute

[1]One breath is one inhalation and exhalation.

respiratory rate of more than 30 breaths/minute is classified as moderate breathlessness, and a rate of 60 breaths/minute is classified as severe breathlessness (see Table 3.3d-I). The corresponding rates for children are higher (see Table 3.3d-II).

Moderate or severe breathlessness of recent onset, and which is also associated with a fever, suggests infection of the lungs themselves (pneumonia) rather than the bronchi (bronchitis). This serious condition is described in Chapter 3.3e (see Q3.3d-2).

The red flags of diseases of the bronchi and bronchioles

Some patients with diseases of the bronchi and bronchioles will benefit from referral to a conventional doctor for assessment and/or treatment. Red flags are those symptoms and signs that indicate that referral is to be considered. The red flags of the diseases of the bronchi and bronchioles are described in Table 3.3d-III. This table forms part of the summary on red flags given in Appendix III, which also gives advice on the degree of urgency of referral for each of the red flag conditions listed.

Table 3.3d-III Red Flags 17a – diseases of the bronchi and bronchioles

Red Flag	Description	Reasoning
17.1	**Features of progressive upper respiratory infection in susceptible people** (e.g. the frail **elderly** and the **immunocompromised** and people with **pre-existing disease of the bronchi and bronchioles**): i.e. cough and fever or new production of yellow-green phlegm, each persisting for more than 3 days	In healthy people an upper respiratory infection (i.e. one that affects any part of the respiratory tract above and including the bronchi) may be protracted but is not necessarily a serious condition. In most cases, as long as there is no breathlessness, it is safe to treat the infection conservatively and there is no need for antibiotics In healthy people, consider referral if there is no response to treatment within 1–2 weeks In the elderly and the immunocompromised (including those with chronic diseases such as cancer, kidney failure and AIDS) severe infections can be masked by relatively minor symptoms, and it is advisable to refer any respiratory condition that persists for more than 3 days People with pre-existing lung disease (e.g. asthma. chronic bronchitis, emphysema, lung cancer, cystic fibrosis) are at increased risk of progressive infection and merit early referral
17.2	Any new onset of **difficulty breathing** in a small child (<8 years old)	Always take a new onset of difficulty in breathing in a child seriously and refer for medical assessment to exclude serious disease. Common causes include lower respiratory infections, asthma, allergic reactions, inhalation of foreign bodies, and congenital heart disease
17.3	**Features of severe asthma**: at least two of the following: • rapidly worsening breathlessness • respiration rate >30 breaths/minute (or more if a child; see footnote[1]) • heart rate >110 breaths/minute • **reluctance to talk** because of breathlessness • **need to sit upright and still** to assist breathing • **cyanosis** is a very serious sign	Severe asthma is a potentially life-threatening condition and may develop in someone with no previous history of severe attacks Urgent referral is required so that medical management of the attack can be instigated. Keep the patient as calm as possible while help arrives Cyanosis describes the blue colouring that appears when the blood is poorly oxygenated. Unlike the blueness from cold, which only affects the extremities, central cyanosis from poor oxygenation can be seen on the tongue It may be very difficult to differentiate an asthma attack from the more benign situation of panic attack (characterised by a feeling of intense fear, racing heart, increased depth of breathing, numbness and tingling of extremities, and mild muscle spasms), and it is possible for the two to coincide, as an experience of breathlessness can

Table 3.3d-III Red Flags 17a – diseases of the bronchi and bronchioles—Cont'd

Red Flag	Description	Reasoning
		trigger a panic reaction. In this situation the key feature is respiratory rate, and if this does not reduce in response to calming measures within a few minutes, and to rebreathing exhaled carbon dioxide (by breathing into a paper bag) within a minute or two, then referral needs to be considered. Central cyanosis would never be apparent in a panic attack, so if present this is an absolute indication for urgent referral
17.4	Any episode of *coughing up* of more than a teaspoon of **blood** (**haemoptysis**)	Blood-streaked sputum is a common and benign occurrence in upper respiratory tract infections, and is not a reason for referral if the infection is self-limiting A larger amount of fresh blood may herald more serious bleeding in those with bronchiectasis. Also it may be the first symptom of lung cancer or tuberculosis. Blood in the sputum also occurs in the case of pulmonary embolism
17.5	**New onset of chronic cough** or **deep persistent chest pain in a smoker**	The most common first symptom of lung cancer is a chronic irritating cough which is different to the clearing of phlegm that characterises the smoker's cough. Rarely, lung cancer can cause deep persistent chest pain, but this is a less usual first symptom
17.6	**Unexplained hoarseness** lasting for more than 3 weeks: may be the first symptom of **laryngeal or lung cancer** (particularly in smokers over 50 years old)	Prolonged hoarseness is usually benign in origin and may be diagnosed as chronic laryngitis. This painless syndrome is commonly the result of misuse or overuse of the vocal cords However, the possibility of laryngeal cancer in smokers over 50 years old needs to be considered. Lung cancer can also be a cause of hoarseness, as the laryngeal nerve, which passes deep in the chest, can be damaged by an infiltrating tumour. Again, smokers over 50 years old are a high-risk group Referral is advised to exclude these less likely possible causes of chronic hoarseness

[1] *Categorisation of respiratory rate in adults*

- Normal respiratory rate in an adult: 10–20 breaths/minute (one breath is one inhalation and exhalation).
- Moderate breathlessness in an adult: >30 breaths/minute.
- Severe breathlessness in an adult: >60 breaths/minute.

Categorisation of respiratory rate in children

- The normal range for respiratory rate in children varies according to age.
- The following rates indicate moderate to severe breathlessness:

newborn (0–3 months)	>60 breaths/minute
infant (3 months to 2 years)	>50 breaths/minute
young child (2–8 years)	>40 breaths/minute
older child to adult	>30 breaths/minute.

Self-test 3.3d

The diseases of the bronchi and bronchioles

1. James is a 10-year-old boy with asthma. His GP has prescribed a salbutamol inhaler to use for his symptoms, which normally only affect him when he does sport at school. Recently, James has become more generally wheezy and has been waking at night occasionally with a dry cough. He has been using his inhaler up to four times a day, when previously there were many days when he did not use it at all. The GP is keen to introduce a steroid inhaler of beclomethasone, which he says James should take twice a day in addition to his salbutamol. His mother is very concerned about this and wants to try acupuncture first.
   (i) Has the GP acted appropriately in James' case?
   (ii) How do you think you should manage the situation in terms of advice on whether James should start using the corticosteroid inhaler?
2. You have a 17-year-old patient who has cystic fibrosis. You have been treating her for some time for deficiency of the Lungs and Kidneys, and with points to clear Phlegm from the Lungs. Recently, she has become more unwell and slightly more breathless, and her phlegm has become more discoloured and profuse. She is very keen not to take another course of antibiotics. How might you advise her?
3. A 58-year-old patient mentions that she has coughed up some phlegm with blood in it. She is a long-term smoker, and is obviously very concerned about the possibility of cancer. She is very reluctant to visit her GP because she is embarrassed about her smoking. She has no other symptoms except for an occasional dry smoker's cough. How would you deal with this situation?

Continued

Self-test 3.3d—Cont'd

Answers

1. (i) In terms of conventional practice, the GP has acted appropriately in advising a step up in treatment to the use of a regular dose of inhaled steroids. This is the advice given in the British Thoracic Society and Scottish Intercollegiate Guidelines Network guidelines on the management of asthma, and is intended to help settle down James' symptoms and reduce the risk of a very severe asthma attack.

   (ii) In this situation you can explain to James' mother that the GP's advice is good practice in conventional medicine. However, James is not acutely unwell, and you could suggest that you could start treatment to see whether or not James has a good response before he tries the steroid inhaler.

   You should monitor the treatment by making a thorough record of James' symptoms both during the day and at night, and can use his need for the salbutamol inhaler as an indication of how his asthma is improving. You might choose to encourage James to record his peak-flow readings at the same time three times a day to check that variability in peak flow is decreasing with your treatment. You could use these objective measures of improvement to feed back the results of the treatment by letter to the GP.

   If James' symptoms do not respond to acupuncture within a couple of weeks, and sooner if there is any worsening, it may be wise to allow him to use the steroid inhaler to control the symptoms, while you continue treatment with the intention of weaning him off the inhaler once he is more stable.

2. It sounds as if this patient has developed a bacterial infection. This is a red flag of severe disease in a patient with cystic fibrosis. What you need to be clear about is that the conventional wisdom is that bacterial infections lead to progressive damage to the lungs in cystic fibrosis, and antibiotics have been shown to prevent this damage.

   You need to be sure that your patient fully understands this before you agree that you will treat her to see if acupuncture can help her recent symptoms. If she is fully aware of the potential risks of a persistent infection to her already weakened lungs then you can go ahead and treat. In such a case it is advisable to offer daily treatment and monitor progression carefully. If there is any deterioration, you should consider advising that she accepts conventional medical treatment.

3. Coughing up of blood out of the blue is a red flag of lung cancer, and so this symptom should be taken very seriously in this woman, who is a smoker. Despite her fears, it is wise to encourage her to see the doctor for further investigations.

Chapter 3.3e Diseases of the alveoli and pleura

LEARNING POINTS

At the end of this chapter you will:

- be able to recognise the main features of the most important diseases that affect the air spaces of the lungs, the alveoli and the pleura (the lining of the lungs)
- understand the principles of treatment of a few of the most common diseases
- be able to recognise the red flags of severe disease of these parts of the respiratory system.

Estimated time for chapter: 100 minutes.

Introduction

This concluding chapter on the respiratory system looks at those diseases that primarily affect the deepest parts of the lung tissue – the tiny air spaces called the alveoli. For completeness, the diseases that can affect the pleural linings are also discussed. The conditions studied in this chapter are:

- Deep infections of the lower respiratory tract:
  - pneumonia
  - pleurisy
  - tuberculosis (TB).
- Emphysema and chronic obstructive pulmonary disease (COPD).
- Fibrosis of the lung and occupational lung disease.
- Pulmonary embolism and infarction.
- Common causes of collapse of the lung (see Q3.3e-1).

Deep infections of the lower respiratory tract

Pneumonia

'Pneumonia' is the term used to describe a deep inflammation of the lung tissue that involves the airspaces or alveoli, and is most commonly a result of infection.

Pneumonia is the second most common cause of death in the UK according to the information obtained from death certificates. This is a slightly misleading statistic, because very commonly an episode of bronchopneumonia is the final event that causes death in elderly people who have become frail for a variety of other underlying reasons such as Alzheimer's disease, cancer or chronic heart failure. For this reason, pneumonia has somewhat cynically been termed 'the old man's friend' because it can lead to a relatively rapid and pain-free death in people who are reaching the end of their natural lives.

However, pneumonia can also be a devastating and depleting illness in children and younger adults, and used to be a dreaded cause of many premature deaths as recently as the earlier decades of the 20th century. In recent years, the improvement in the general health of the population, together with the use of antibiotics, has changed this situation. Nowadays, deaths from acute pneumonia are relatively rare except in those who have some form of immunodeficiency resulting from conditions such as cancer or acquired immune deficiency syndrome (AIDS).

Pneumonia can be caused by a wide range of infectious agents, including viruses, bacteria and fungi. However, in contrast to the other infections of the respiratory tract, which tend to be viral in origin, an episode of pneumonia is more likely to be caused by bacteria, which tend to produce much more severe inflammation and more pus (coughed up as coloured phlegm) than do viruses. This is an indication that pneumonia is a condition that tends to affect those who are already energetically depleted in some way. In healthy people, the defence mechanisms of the respiratory tract are able to prevent the penetration of external infectious agents to the deep parts of the lung. Therefore, it may come as a surprise that the most common forms of bacterial pneumonia are caused by bacteria that can reside harmlessly in the respiratory tract of healthy people (most importantly *Streptococcus pneumoniae* and *Haemophilus influenzae*).

In pneumonia, the inflammation leads to damage to the delicate alveolar lining and accumulation of fluid and cell debris within the air spaces. This causes irritation and a marked reduction in the amount of oxygen that can enter the blood from each in-breath. In the most common form of bacterial infection, the inflammation is confined to a single lobe of one lung. This is termed 'lobar pneumonia'. In other forms of pneumonia the inflammation can be more widespread, with the smaller bronchioles also becoming inflamed. This is called 'bronchopneumonia'.

The primary symptoms of pneumonia are cough (which may be dry or productive of coloured phlegm) and moderate to severe breathlessness. The patient will feel unwell and feverish, although the severity of these symptoms depends on the nature of the infection and the strength of the individual. In some cases the breathlessness can be so severe as to require emergency treatment. The features of severe breathlessness are similar to those of severe asthma. A rapid respiratory rate of 30 breaths/minute or more, needing to sit up and sit still to breathe, and difficulty in talking are serious signs.

A blue discoloration of the tongue and lips, known as 'cyanosis', is a very severe sign indicating that there is insufficient oxygen reaching the blood. At this stage in a severe infection, the patient may be so ill that they do not have the energy to maintain rapid respirations. Breathing may become more shallow and the patient may drift in and out of consciousness. This state, when the level of oxygen in the blood cannot be maintained, is called 'respiratory failure', and the patient requires emergency treatment to prevent death.

In hospitals, the severity of pneumonia is graded according to five parameters (the CURB-65 scoring system). The factors that are recognised to predict a more serious outcome include confusion, raised urea levels, rapid respiratory rate (>30 breaths/minute) and low systolic blood pressure, and age greater than 65 years. A low CURB 65 score helps a doctor to decide that the episode can be safely managed at home.

In all types of pneumonia the investigations and treatment are similar. X-ray images and sputum samples are taken to assess the extent of infection and to diagnose the type of infection. Blood tests can be used to provide evidence either of infectious agents or of a recent immune response, and this can help diagnose the type of infection.

According to the type of infection, appropriate antibiotics are prescribed, initially to be taken by mouth. If breathlessness is severe, the patient is given emergency support in hospital. This may include the administration of oxygen, with antibiotics given intravenously. Oxygen may be administered under a degree of pressure by a close-fitting mask to assist in gaseous exchange (this is known as continuous positive airway pressure (CPAP) or bi-level positive airway pressure (BIPAP)). Occasionally, the patient may have to receive assisted breathing on a mechanical ventilator in an intensive care unit (this is known as 'ventilation').

Lobar pneumonia

Approximately half of all cases of pneumonia are lobar pneumonia, in which the infectious agent is a bacterium called *Streptococcus pneumoniae*. The infection is usually confined to a single lobe of one lung and the overlying pleural linings of that lobe. This infection tends to affect people who are depleted in some way or have pre-existing lung damage. It also may follow on from a viral infection of other parts of the respiratory tract.

In this streptococcal pneumonia there is a rapid onset of very high fever, breathlessness and cough. Pain may be felt on inspiration on one side of the chest. A common sign is the development of a cold sore, which is a well-known response to high fever.

Most cases should respond to benzylpenicillin, amoxicillin or erythromycin, although the full period of recovery from the infection is usually long. After treatment has been completed, the patient is frequently left in a state of exhaustion, which can last for some weeks. Chest X-ray images are used to ensure that the infection has cleared from the chest, and that there are no other underlying problems in the lung, such as cancer, which may have led to the infection in the first place. Full recovery is less likely in the very frail.

Other pneumonias

Most other common forms of pneumonia are usually less severe than lobar pneumonia. The next most common type in the UK is caused by an organism called *Mycoplasma*. This tends to affect younger people, and leads to vague symptoms such as headache, mild fever, tiredness and occasional cough. Because of the vague symptoms, diagnosis may be delayed, but usually the infection responds to antibiotics. Occasionally, a protracted state of exhaustion may also result from this infection. Another severe bacterial pneumonia is caused by the organism *Staphylococcus aureus*, which can reside harmlessly on the skin and in the nose. This organism tends to infect already damaged lungs, and it most commonly occurs when frail individuals develop viral infections such as measles or influenza. Staphylococcal and streptococcal pneumonia account for many of the deaths that occur in epidemics of influenza.

Legionnaire's disease

This is a rare pneumonia that tends to affect older or immunocompromised individuals, but can also occur in outbreaks in institutions in which the showers or cooling systems have become contaminated with the infectious organism *Legionella pneumophila*.

The patient can become very unwell, with high fever and confusion, as well as cough and breathlessness. Up to one-third of elderly people with this infection will die from the pneumonia, although most fit people recover spontaneously. The infection does respond to antibiotics (ideally erythromycin with rifampicin), although sometimes the diagnosis is delayed because this type of pneumonia is relatively rare.

Opportunistic pneumonias

Opportunistic diseases are those that affect individuals with immunodeficiency. Opportunistic pneumonias are a significant cause of ill-health and death in the immunocompromised. Diagnosis may be delayed because these conditions often do not lead to such marked symptoms as other types of pneumonia.

One of the most common types of opportunistic pneumonia in AIDS patients is *Pneumocystis* pneumonia (PCP), caused by a fungus, the spores of which are inhaled from the air. The symptoms may appear gradually over the period of a few weeks, with cough and slight fevers. Without early treatment, the infection can cause severe lung damage, and the patient may eventually require ventilation. This pneumonia responds to antibiotics including cotrimoxazole (Septrin) and pentamidine, although these are most effective if given early in the course of the disease. Patients will then be advised to continue taking low doses of these antibiotics in the long term to prevent relapse of the infection. Pentamidine may be administered by inhalation in mild cases.

Bronchopneumonia

Bronchopneumonia is a form of pneumonia that affects a very depleted patient and can be caused by a range of the infectious agents already described. In this condition the inflammation spreads to involve a diffuse area of the lungs and bronchioles, and often occurs because the patient is unable to cough up the thickened lung secretions that result from inflammation. This is the form of pneumonia that is commonly the actual cause of death in frail patients who are close to the end of their natural lives.

Pleurisy

'Pleurisy' is the term used to describe the pain that develops when the pleural lining of the lung is inflamed. The most common cause of pleurisy is infection, although it can also result from lung cancer and lung infarction from a pulmonary embolus (see later in this chapter).

Lobar pneumonia frequently leads to pleurisy because it usually causes inflammation that extends to the outer margins of the lung tissue. Another less serious cause of pleurisy is a virus infection, which can affect the pleural lining without infecting the lung itself.

In pleurisy the patient experiences a localised, sharp and sometimes severe pain that is worse on deep breathing and twisting movements of the chest. The pain is provoked when the two inflamed pleural linings rub against each other. Often this rubbing can be heard as a scratchy noise through the stethoscope.

The treatment of pleurisy is by treating the underlying cause and giving painkillers for relief of symptoms. This is of particular importance in pneumonia as the pain of pleurisy can be so severe as to inhibit deep breathing and coughing, which are important for the healing of the infection. Viral pleurisy, although very painful, will get better spontaneously within a few days.

> **Information Box 3.3e-I**
>
> **Pneumonia: comments from a Chinese medicine perspective**
>
> In Chinese medicine, an uncomplicated case of pneumonia would correspond to Lung Heat or Lung Phlegm Heat at the Qi Level, according to the Four Levels categorisation. The cough and breathlessness are due to Heat or Phlegm Heat obstructing the descent of Lung Qi.
>
> The rapidity of development of some pneumonias, including lobar pneumonia, is an indication that Invasion of Wind Heat can be an initiating cause. The cold sore that commonly occurs in pneumonia is a manifestation of Wind Damp Heat.
>
> As pneumonia frequently occurs on a background of deficiency, this suggests that there is a pre-existing deficiency of the Lung, probably of Lung Yin, and that the Pathogenic Factors are, at least in part, internally generated as a consequence of the deficiency.
>
> The intense pain of pleurisy would normally be associated with Stagnation of Blood and Qi in the chest. In pneumonia this probably is a result of Heat, and in viral infection may be ascribed to Wind invasion.

Tuberculosis

Tuberculosis (TB) is an infection caused by a bacteria-like organism called *Mycobacterium tuberculosis*. This causes a particular form of deep lung infection that is unlike the other forms of pneumonia already discussed.

TB of the lung develops after inhalation of infected droplets, after which the organism settles usually in the upper part of one lung. In most healthy individuals the immune system deals with this primary infection and the person develops immunity without experiencing any symptoms. The organism can also enter the digestive tract through infected milk, but this does not now occur in the UK because of the two practices of screening of cattle for infection and pasteurisation of milk.

In depleted individuals in particular, the immune response to the primary infection may lead to a prolonged inflammatory reaction at the site of the infection, after which the infection is not necessarily fully cleared. Instead, a firm nodule is left at the site of this infection, which can be seen on a chest X-ray image, together with enlarged lymph nodes at the centre of the chest. In these individuals there might be a vague illness, with fluctuating fever and cough over the course of a few weeks. In some of these cases the inflammation may eventually settle down, but in other cases it can progress over the course of weeks to months to involve more of the lung tissue. This can result in pneumonia and bronchiectasis.

Occasionally, the nodule can break down to release thousands of TB organisms into the rest of the lung and sometimes the bloodstream, which then go on to lead to widespread inflammation in diverse parts of the body, including the bones and the brain. This is known as 'military TB', and is a life-threatening complication of the primary disease.

In the cases in which the inflammation in the nodule of infected tissue has settled down, the problem may recur after many years, when the infection latent in the nodule for all that time becomes active again. This is known as 'post-primary TB'. Post-primary TB usually occurs because the immune system of the person has become deficient in some way. It can occur in old age, or when the person has become ill for another reason, such as cancer or diabetes. For this reason it is often a much more severe infection than the primary infection.

The person with post-primary TB may become gradually more unwell over a period of weeks, with weight loss, exhaustion and night sweats. A persistent productive cough is a very common symptom, and is very significant because the sputum often contains highly infectious TB organisms. At this infectious stage, the diagnosis may not be made for weeks, so the infection may have been spread to many other people before the patient can be treated with antibiotics. Often the symptom that provokes the person to seek medical help is the appearance of blood in the sputum, a common occurrence in established post-primary TB.

Occasionally, the reactivated TB occurs in a different site of the body than the lungs, such as the bowel or the bone, but this is uncommon in the UK.

Diagnosis can be made on the basis of characteristic changes seen on the chest X-ray image, and by examination of the sputum for TB organisms. Sometimes bronchoscopy is necessary to obtain infected tissue for diagnosis and choice of appropriate antibiotics.

Without treatment, some patients with severe primary TB, and many patients with post-primary TB, would die from progressive damage to the lungs and bodily exhaustion. Severe TB used to be known as 'consumption' because of the way people with TB could waste away whilst the disease took hold in their bodies. Common terminal events used to include profuse bleeding from the lungs or pneumonia.

The incidence and seriousness of the disease has markedly declined in the UK since the beginning of the 20th century. This is largely due to improvements in the general health of the population. In addition, the advent of antibiotics has enabled established cases to be controlled rapidly. Vaccination against TB, introduced in the 1950s, has reduced the risk of contracting the infection in many individuals.

Conventional treatment of TB involves a cocktail of antibiotics (including initially all four of rifampicin, isoniazid, pyrazinamide and ethambutol) that has to be taken consistently for 6–12 months to be fully effective. Often the treatment produces relief of symptoms and infectivity in a very short time, and some patients stop taking the medication prematurely. This is more likely to occur in countries in which antibiotics are costly or in short supply. This is a major problem in the treatment of TB. It is known that if the drugs are not taken continuously the infection may recur, and antibiotic-resistant types of organism are encouraged to develop. In some developing countries, antibiotic-resistant strains are leading to epidemics of untreatable TB, such as were seen in this country many decades ago.

The vaccine for TB is known as the BCG, which stands for the French name of the strain of bacterium contained in the vaccine (Bacille Calmette-Guerin). It consists of a strain of organism that is alive but far less virulent than TB. It induces immunity in recipients, leading to a 70% reduced risk of developing TB. BCG is only given to those people who can be shown by a skin-prick test (the 'daisy test') to have not already built up their own immunity to the disease. However, because the incidence of TB is falling generally in the UK to very low levels, in many UK districts the practice of vaccinating teenagers has been stopped. Vaccination is still offered shortly after birth only to those infants who may be at high risk of coming into contact with the disease early in life.

In order to minimise the spread of disease in the UK, any case of TB that does occur is treated with seriousness. The patient is urged to continue with regular medication for the full recommended time period, and all close contacts during the possible time period of infectivity are traced and tested for active TB by X-ray imaging and skin-prick tests.

In the UK, most new cases of TB occur either in the immigrant population, often as cases of reactivated post-primary TB, or in elderly people who contracted the primary infection in childhood. There is a worrying increase of TB in homeless people, a problem that is difficult to control because of difficulties in ensuring adequate completion of antibiotic treatment, thorough contact tracing and treatment of infected contacts.

Patients with AIDS are the other population in whom TB is of increasing concern. Because of the immunodeficiency that develops in AIDS, TB can take rapid hold and may be difficult to clear with antibiotics. The patient requires an even longer period on antibiotic treatment, during which time there is a risk of the development of antibiotic resistance. In developing countries in which TB is endemic, the combination of TB and AIDS is a deadly one, leading to many premature deaths.

Information Box 3.3e-II

Tuberculosis: comments from a Chinese medicine perspective

In Chinese medicine, the swelling and inflammation associated with TB would be seen as Phlegm Heat obstructing the Lungs. The fever and wasting that arise in post-primary infection would be taken as evidence of depletion of Yin and/or Yang. In light of this interpretation, TB may be seen to be energetically comparable to cancer.

TB is essentially a condition that affects people who are already depleted in some way. Because antibiotic therapy does not treat the root cause of the condition, it is suppressive in nature. Nevertheless, there is no doubt that antibiotic therapy is a powerful method of halting the disease.

Emphysema

Emphysema refers to a condition in which the delicate structure of the alveoli and the smallest bronchioles has permanently broken down as a result of inflammation in the deep part of the lungs. In some forms of emphysema the tiny walls that separate the alveoli are destroyed, while in others the terminal bronchioles dilate, and in both the air spaces within become enlarged. The dilatation that can occur in these deep parts of the lung in two types of emphysema are illustrated in Figure 3.3e-I.

Emphysema can severely impair the exchange of gases that should take place between the walls of the alveoli and the blood in the capillaries, which, in health, form a close network around the alveoli. The response of the body to the resulting impaired uptake of oxygen and accumulation of carbon dioxide is to increase the respiratory rate, so that the patient with emphysema is breathless, particularly on exertion.

The most common cause of emphysema is smoking. However, the tendency to emphysema does run in families. In susceptible individuals with an inherited tendency, and in particular that which comes from a recessively inherited genetic disorder, alpha-1-antitrypsin deficiency, the effect of smoking is much more marked. This susceptibility is not that rare, as it is estimated that one in ten people carry a defective alpha-1-antitrypsin gene. The inflammation that results from long-standing asthma can also lead to emphysema.

The changes of emphysema commonly coexist with those of chronic bronchitis, which was described in the Chapter 3.3d. Together, these conditions lead to a syndrome called chronic obstructive pulmonary disease (COPD). (In some texts this is referred to as chronic obstructive airways disease (COAD).) The patient with COPD will therefore have symptoms of cough with phlegm, wheezing and breathlessness that never fully remits. It is not uncommon for patients with COPD also to develop symptoms of asthma, with bouts of increased breathlessness. These can be only partly relieved by bronchodilator and corticosteroid treatments, a characteristic of the reversibility of asthma.

COPD is diagnosed on the basis of impaired results from lung-function studies, which involve the patient blowing into a machine called a 'spirometer'. This assesses the rate of expiration and the capacity of the lungs to expel air, both of which may be reduced in COPD. Similarly, in COPD there will be a reduced peak-flow rate, but usually little of the day-to-day reversibility seen in asthma.

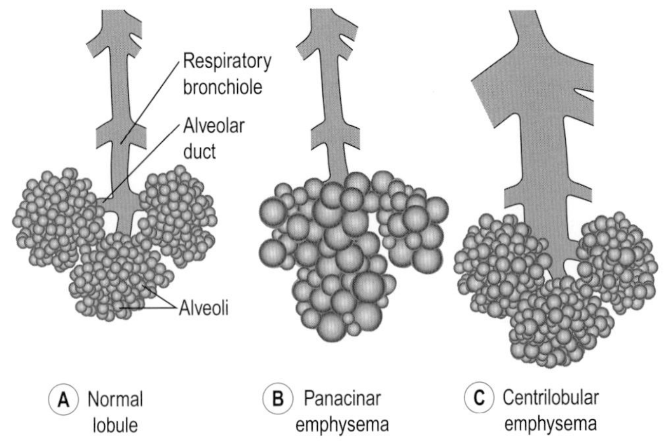

Figure 3.3e-I • Diagram showing the dilatation of the air spaces in two forms of emphysema • (a) Normal alveolae. (b) Dilated alveolar spaces in panacinar emphysema. (c) Dilated bronchioles in centrilobular emphysema.

Emphysema and COPD are progressive conditions that will continue to deteriorate if the patient continues to smoke. In some patients, due to narrowing of the smaller airways by inflammation, air becomes trapped in the dilated alveolar air spaces, which then expand, sometimes to form large air-filled spaces called 'bullae' (singular 'bulla'). The chest of a patient with this problem looks permanently overinflated. Occasionally, a bulla can rupture to release air into the surrounding pleural space. This condition of air in the chest cavity external to the lung is called pneumothorax, and leads to collapse of one of the lungs.

Patients with COPD are prone to bouts of acute bronchitis and pneumonia. Each infection is likely to leave the lungs in a worse condition, so that a vicious circle of infection and damage is set up. For this reason, antibiotics are prescribed readily to patients with COPD.

In very severe disease, the heart comes under strain as it has to pump blood through damaged lungs, and right-sided heart failure with oedema may develop (a condition known as cor pulmonale).

In the end stages of the condition the person with severe COPD may require long-term oxygen therapy (LTOT) to remove the disabling symptom of breathlessness. The patient will need to have oxygen cylinders at home to enable adequate treatment. In many patients, oxygen therapy can prolong life because it helps to relieve some of the pressure on the failing heart muscle. Patients with features of asthma will be prescribed high doses of inhaled bronchodilators and corticosteroids. The usual cause of death in severe COPD is bronchopneumonia.

Information Box 3.3e-III

COPD: comments from a Chinese medicine perspective

In Chinese medicine, the symptoms of COPD would correspond to Accumulation of Phlegm, with Phlegm Heat or Damp Phlegm obstructing the Lungs. The destruction of the lung tissue that occurs in emphysema represents a background of Deficiency of Lung Qi and Yin.

Fibrosis of the lung and occupational lung disease

'Fibrosis' is the medical term used to describe scarring. In lung fibrosis the scarring affects the alveoli and the smallest bronchioles, and leads to narrowing of the airways and loss of elasticity of the lungs. This can severely impair the action of breathing.

Fibrosis is often the end result of a long-standing process of inflammation, which can result from irritation caused by inhaled substances in the form of tiny particles. Many of these substances are found within industrial settings. For example, coal dust, silica from stone and asbestos can lead to impairment in the function of the lungs in people who have jobs such as mining, stonemasonry and ship-building. Allergy to a mould that grows on stored hay can produce a similar sort of scarring reaction in farm workers, in a condition known as 'farmer's lung'. Rarely, the fibrosis can be a result of certain prescribed drugs, and occasionally can develop with no obvious cause (when it is known as 'cryptogenic fibrosing alveolitis').

The main symptom of fibrosis is progressive breathlessness. In farmer's lung the initial symptoms include fever and increased breathlessness after working with hay. In severe cases the patient will have the blue discoloration of the lips and tongue known as 'cyanosis'. In these severe cases the heart is put under strain because it has to pump blood through scarred lung tissue, and this can lead to heart failure with oedema.

Asbestos is a particularly harmful dust because, in addition to causing inflammation and scarring, it is highly carcinogenic. People who have been exposed to asbestos dust have an increased risk of bronchial cancer, and a very high risk of an otherwise rare cancer of the pleural lining of the lung called 'mesothelioma'. Both these types of cancer are resistant to modern treatments.

Apart from eliminating the cause of fibrosis, the treatment is supportive only, as the condition is irreversible. The patient with severe fibrosis will require oxygen therapy to relieve breathlessness and reduce the strain on the heart. Patients in the UK whose fibrosis has resulted from industrial exposure to dusts may be eligible for financial compensation from the government.

Information Box 3.3e-IV

Lung fibrosis: comments from a Chinese medicine perspective

In Chinese medicine, the impaired elasticity and narrowing of the airways of the lungs in fibrosis would correspond to depletion of Lung Qi (Yang) and Yin. The oedema that results from heart failure in chronic lung disease is a form of Kidney and Lung Yang Deficiency. The cyanosis that develops in the end stages of all severe lung disease is a sign of severe Stagnation of Blood due to Yang Deficiency.

Pulmonary embolism and infarction

Pulmonary embolism has been described in Chapter 2.2d, in which the disorders of excessive blood clotting are explored. Pulmonary embolism was described as a possible serious consequence of deep vein thrombosis (DVT).

Pulmonary embolism is the end result of unwanted material, usually in the form of blood clots, entering the blood vessels that lead from the right side of the heart to the lungs. This material lodges in the progressively narrowing blood vessels of the lung, and leads to infarction of the part of lung supplied by those vessels. The wider the vessel that is blocked, the greater the amount of lung which is infarcted.

The small clots that can break off from a DVT are probably the most common cause of pulmonary embolism. However, other causes of excessive clotting in the blood, such as serious chronic disease (including cancer), the contraceptive pill and occasionally pregnancy, can also cause the condition without a prior DVT.

A small pulmonary embolism may affect only a tiny part of the lung close to the pleural lining. This will result in death of that part of the lung and a small area of inflammation. The inflammation may cause a temporary bout of pleurisy, but is likely to heal.

If this event occurs a number of times it can lead to progressive irreversible damage to the lung. Air can enter the lung, but the circulation to the lung has been gradually reduced so that the exchange of gases is impaired. The patient might become increasingly breathless over the course of a few weeks. The heart comes under strain as the free circulation of blood is impaired, and angina or chronic heart failure might develop.

A medium to large pulmonary embolus suddenly cuts off the blood supply to a much larger portion of the lung. This can be so severe as to lead to acute heart failure and sudden death. If less severe, intense chest pain and breathlessness is experienced, and the patient has to be treated as a medical emergency.

Pulmonary embolism is diagnosed definitively by means of CT angiography of the pulmonary arteries, and if this is not available by a scintigram scan, which exposes poorly perfused areas of the lung following an injection of a radioactive tracer chemical (known as a VQ scan). The D-dimer blood test can be used to check to see if thrombosis has occurred (D-dimers are fragments of the clotting protein fibrin, the levels of which are raised shortly after an episode of thrombosis).

In all cases, the aim of treatment is to maximise oxygen transfer, so 100% oxygen is administered by means of a mask. Then, in order to reduce the tendency of the blood to clot. heparin, a rapidly acting anticoagulant medication, is given by intravenous infusion. If the patient is gravely unwell as a result of a massive embolism, a 'clot-busting' drug such as streptokinase or alteplase may be given to unblock the artery in the lung that contains the clot. These drugs work in the same way as when given for a heart attack.

Once the acute symptoms have been controlled, warfarin is prescribed to inhibit the blood clotting in the long term, and is continued for between 6 weeks and 6 months. Patients considered to be at high risk of recurrence of this life-threatening condition may be advised to continue with warfarin therapy for life.

Information Box 3.3e-V

Pulmonary embolism: comments from a Chinese medicine perspective

In Chinese medicine, the symptoms of pulmonary embolism correspond to acute Heart Blood Stagnation, and like a heart attack may lead to Heart Yang Collapse.

Heparin and warfarin reduce the tendency of the blood to clot, and may be described as Heating.

Collapse of the lung

There are a number of conditions in which the tissue of the inflated lung loses its shape, and the open air spaces collapse. As described in Chapter 3.3a, the natural tendency of the elastic tissue of the lung is to collapse down, and this is prevented in health by the integrity of the lining membrane of the pleura, which are normally firmly attached to the walls of the chest cavity.

The most important condition causing lung collapse, of which acupuncturists in particular should be aware, is pneumothorax. In pneumothorax, air comes between the pleural linings and allows the lung to collapse. The rupture of bullae in emphysema is one cause of pneumothorax. However, the most common cause of pneumothorax is when the normal lung is punctured as a result of injury. A broken rib resulting from a traumatic accident can easily puncture the underlying lung, and the air that escapes leads to a pneumothorax.

Pneumothorax is a known, but rare, adverse event arising from acupuncture treatment to the shoulder and chest. The lungs lie only a few millimetres under the skin in some thin people, and so they can easily be reached by even a shallow needle insertion. Usually, a thin needle puncture of lung tissue will not cause a collapse to the lung. However, a rough or repeated insertion may have this unfortunate consequence, particularly in a person affected by a chronic lung disease such as emphysema.

Occasionally, a pneumothorax can occur spontaneously in an otherwise fit young person. This is usually attributed to the presence of a previously undiagnosed bulla that has ruptured because it is much weaker than normal lung tissue. A few bullae can be present from birth in some people, rather akin to the occasional weak area of thin rubber that might be found on the surface of a balloon.

Other causes of collapse of the lung include the accumulation of a large amount of fluid in the space between the pleural membranes. Fluid collecting in this space is called pleural effusion, a term first introduced in this text when pleural effusion was described as a possible complication of lung cancer. In this case, the fluid has been secreted by cancer cells. Other sources of fluid include bleeding from an internal chest injury or inflammatory fluid developing as a result of pneumonia, particularly lobar pneumonia.

Figure 3.3e-II is a diagrammatic representation of a collapsed lung surrounded by a pleural space containing air,

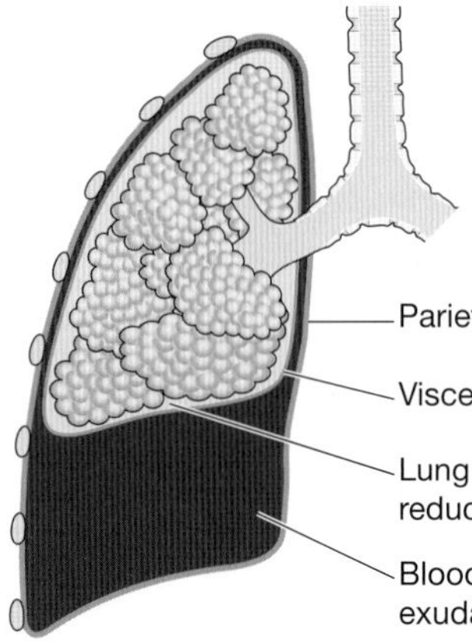

Figure 3.3e-II • A pressure collapse of the lung.

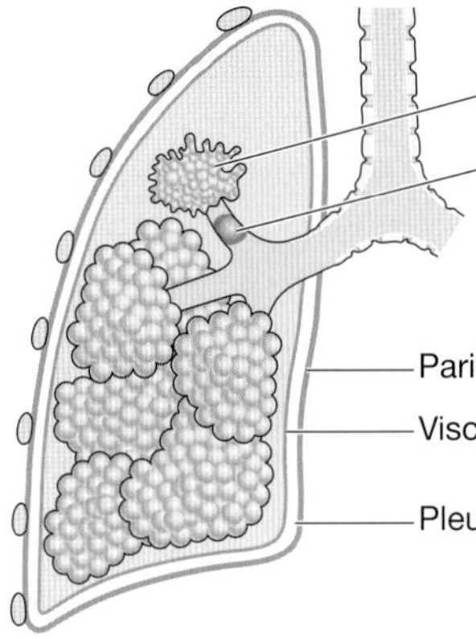

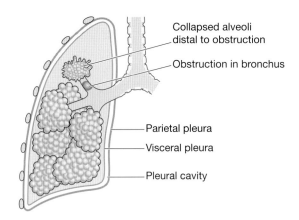

Figure 3.3e-III • An absorption collapse of the lung.

blood or the fluid that results from inflammation (inflammatory exudate). The diagram illustrates how the lung can contract down to a fraction of its normal size if compressed by fluid or air in the pleural space. As the diagram indicates, the common term for this sort of collapse of the lung is 'pressure collapse'.

The other cause of collapse, 'absorption collapse', is illustrated in Figure 3.3e-III. In this case the whole lung, or just part of it, has collapsed because some or all of the airways have become totally blocked due to an infection or tumour. The lung behind (distal to) this obstruction collapses because the air within it gradually becomes absorbed into the blood, and cannot be replaced. The pleural space then fills with tissue fluid (coloured in pale grey in the diagram).

In pressure collapse, such as pneumothorax, the onset of symptoms is usually sudden. The patient experiences a sudden onset of breathlessness, and often the pain of pleurisy. Usually the patient is not in severe distress, but this depends on the degree of collapse. Occasionally, as can occur with tension pneumothorax, the situation becomes a medical emergency, as the exchange of gases is severely impaired and the patient goes into respiratory failure.

The treatment of lung collapse depends on the cause. Pneumothorax, if mild, can resolve spontaneously over the course of a few days, as the puncture in the lung heals. If air continues to leak out of the lung, the excess air can be drained away by means of a tube inserted into the pleural space through a small incision between the ribs. This allows the lung to reinflate, and usually the puncture or rupture can then heal naturally. Occasionally, a surgical operation is necessary to repair the damaged lung.

In a similar fashion, fluid in the pleural space can resolve spontaneously, but may also need to be drained away, particularly if it contains blood. In cancer, the fluid may continue to accumulate, and the pleural effusion may need to be drained repeatedly to keep the patient relatively comfortable.

If the collapse has occurred due to obstruction, again resolution may be possible if the obstruction can be removed. This is not always possible, in which case the lung remains permanently damaged and reduced in capacity (see Q3.3e-2).

The red flags of diseases of the alveoli and pleura

Some patients with diseases of the alveoli and pleura will benefit from referral to a conventional doctor for assessment and/or treatment. Red flags are those symptoms and signs that indicate that referral is to be considered. The red flags of the diseases of the alveoli and pleura are described in Table 3.3e-I. This table forms part of the summary on red flags given in Appendix III, which also gives advice on the degree of urgency of referral for each of the red flag conditions listed.

Information Box 3.3e-VI

Lung collapse: comments from a Chinese medicine perspective

In Chinese medicine, the breathlessness that results from collapse of the lung might correspond to deficiency of either one or both of Lung Yin and Qi (Yang), because the underlying problem is of the integrity of the structure of the lung itself.

The pleurisy that commonly accompanies pneumothorax suggests Blood and/or Qi Stagnation. This may purely be the result of an injury, but may develop from internal deficiency (e.g. the rupture of a weak part of the lungs).

Table 3.3e-I Red Flags 17b – diseases of the alveoli and pleura

Red Flag	Description	Reasoning
17.2	Any new onset of **difficulty breathing** in a small child (<8 years old)	Always take a new onset of difficulty breathing in a child seriously and refer for medical assessment to exclude serious disease. Common causes include lower respiratory infections, asthma, allergic reactions, inhalation of foreign bodies and congenital heart disease
17.4	Any episode of **coughing up** of more than a teaspoon of **blood (haemoptysis)**	Blood-streaked sputum is a common and benign occurrence in upper respiratory tract infections, and is not a reason for referral if the infection is self-limiting A larger amount of fresh blood may herald more serious bleeding in those with bronchiectasis. Also it may be the first symptom of lung cancer or tuberculosis. Blood in the sputum also occurs in the case of pulmonary embolism
17.7	**Features of infection of the alveoli (pneumonia):** these include: • **cough** • **fever** • **malaise** • **respiratory rate** >**30 breaths/minute (or more if a child: see footnote[1])** • **heart rate** >**110 beats/minute** • **reluctance to talk** because of breathlessness • **need to sit upright and still** to assist breathing • **cyanosis** is a very serious sign	Pneumonia means that inflammation (usually as a result of infection) has descended to the level of the air sacs (alveoli) in the lungs. As these sacs are involved in the exchange of gases, breathlessness is always part of the picture of pneumonia. As the infection is so deep the patient can become extremely unwell and may need hospital treatment Use the severity of the symptoms to guide the urgency of the referral
17.8	**Features of pleurisy:** localised chest pain that is associated with inspiration and expiration. Refer if associated with fever and breathlessness, as this is an indication of associated pneumonia	Pleurisy is the syndrome that results when a region of the pleural lining of the lungs becomes inflamed. This leads to a localised region of chest-wall pain that worsens with coughing and on breathing in. Pleurisy may be a complication of the spread of pneumonia to the periphery of a lung, in which case it would be associated with malaise and breathlessness. It may appear without deeper lung damage and may result from a viral infection. It can also result from non-infectious causes, such as pulmonary embolism If there is no breathlessness there is no need for immediate referral
17.9	**Features of tuberculosis infection: chronic productive cough, weight loss, night sweats, blood in sputum** for more than 2 weeks	Tuberculosis is more common in people who have lived in countries where tuberculosis in endemic and in those who live in situations of poverty and in overcrowded damp conditions. It can also develop in people who have close contact with those at high risk. Referral is for isolation, diagnosis and initiation of a prolonged programme of antibiotic therapy. Contacts will be traced and tested for infection if the diagnosis is confirmed. Tuberculosis is a notifiable disease[2]

Continued

Table 3.3e-I Red Flags 17b – diseases of the alveoli and pleura—Cont'd

Red Flag	Description	Reasoning
17.10	**Features of pulmonary embolism:** sudden onset of **pleurisy** with **breathlessness**, **cyanosis**, **collapse**	Pulmonary embolism is the result of a lodging of a blood clot or multiple blood clots (emboli) in the arterial circulation supplying the lungs (pulmonary circulation). If the blood clot is large there can be a sudden reduction in the oxygenation power of the lung, and this can result in collapse and sudden death. In less severe cases the infarction of the lung tissue manifests as pleurisy with breathlessness, and blood may be coughed up in the sputum This syndrome merits urgent referral for anticoagulation (thinning of the blood)
17.11	**Features of sudden lung collapse (pneumothorax):** onset of severe **breathlessness**; may be some **pleurisy** and **collapse** if very severe	Pneumothorax can occur spontaneously, or may be provoked by a puncture of the lungs. It is notorious amongst acupuncturists as a possible complication of needling vulnerable points in the thorax, and practitioners should be vigilant that in extremely rare cases the symptoms can develop gradually up to 24 hours after a needle puncture

[1] *Categorisation of respiratory rate in adults*

- Normal respiratory rate in an adult: 10–20 breaths/minute (one breath is one inhalation and exhalation).
- Moderate breathlessness in an adult: >30 breaths/minute.
- Severe breathlessness in an adult: >60 breaths/minute.

Categorisation of respiratory rate in children

- The normal range for respiratory rate in children varies according to age.
- The following rates indicate moderate to severe breathlessness:

newborn (0–3 months)	>60 breaths/minute
infant (3 months to 2 years)	>50 breaths/minute
young child (2–8 years)	>40 breaths/minute
older child to adult	>30 breaths/minute.

[2] Notifiable diseases: notification of a number of specified infectious diseases is required of doctors in the UK as a statutory duty under the Public Health (Infectious Diseases) 1988 Act and the Public Health (Control of Diseases) 1988 Act. The UK Health Protection Agency (HPA) Centre for Infections collates details of each case of each disease that has been notified. This allows analyses of local and national trends. This is one example of a situation in which there is a legal requirement for a doctor to breach patient confidentiality.

Diseases that are notifiable include: acute encephalitis, acute poliomyelitis, anthrax, cholera, diphtheria, dysentery, food poisoning, leptospirosis, malaria, measles, meningitis (bacterial and viral forms), meningococcal septicaemia (without meningitis), mumps, ophthalmia neonatorum, paratyphoid fever, plague, rabies, relapsing fever, rubella, scarlet fever, smallpox, tetanus, tuberculosis, typhoid fever, typhus fever, viral haemorrhagic fever, viral hepatitis (including hepatitis A, B and C), whooping cough, yellow fever.

Self-test 3.3e

The diseases of the alveoli and pleura

1. A 45-year-old patient has called for a home visit to have acupuncture treatment for pain in his chest. When you arrive you notice that he is slightly breathless and his temperature is raised at 38°C. The pain he is feeling is on one side of his chest. It hurts to breathe deeply, to cough and to move suddenly. However, the ribs overlying the pain are not tender at all. He is suppressing his desire to cough, but when he does cough it is dry.
   (i) What is the name for this sort of pain?
   (ii) What is the range of possible explanations for this sort of pain?
   (iii) What do you think is the most likely explanation in this patient?
   (iv) Would you refer the patient for conventional medical treatment?
2. A 65-year-old new patient is a retired miner. He has a long-standing problem with breathlessness on exertion. He was a heavy smoker, but has recently stopped smoking. When you question him he admits that he is still coughing up phlegm, which is clear in colour, on a daily basis. On examination, his resting respiratory rate is 20 breaths/minute, but this increases as he undresses and gets up on the treatment couch. He says that he has not troubled the doctor about his condition.
   (i) What are the possible causes of this man's breathlessness?
   (ii) Would you consider a referral to a conventional doctor?

Answers

1. (i) Pain of this nature is called pleuritic pain or pleurisy.
   (ii) The most common cause of pleurisy is infection, either resulting from pneumonia or from an isolated viral infection of

Self-test 3.3e—Cont'd

the pleura. Other important causes include pulmonary embolism, pneumothorax and a rare complication of lung cancer. The inflammation that is the cause of the pleurisy in these three conditions can also cause fever in some cases.

(iii) Infection would be the most likely cause in this patient. The patient's high fever is more characteristic of lobar pneumonia than a viral infection.

(iv) Infection can respond to alternative treatment, but is would be wise to refer your patient as you cannot exclude more serious causes such as pulmonary embolism.

Assuming an infective cause in confirmed by medical investigations and if the patient is fairly fit, you can advise that he could defer antibiotic treatment, whilst you give him a trial of treatment. However, if this course of action is chosen you will need to treat this patient and monitor his condition on a daily basis.

You might also consider referral for Chinese herbs, as these are considered to be more efficacious than acupuncture alone in deep conditions of the Lung. Antibiotic treatment is advisable if the patient's condition does not improve rapidly within the first day and certainly if there is any deterioration.

2. (i) The breathlessness occurs at rest, and is quite severe because it worsens with very little physical activity. The most likely causes include COPD as a result of long term smoking. Lung fibrosis is also a possibility because of this man's exposure to coal dust. You should not forget that lung cancer is a possibility, even in the absence of other more specific symptoms and signs.

(ii) As this patient has not been to see a doctor, referral is advisable to get a clear diagnosis of the problem and to exclude lung cancer. This might be of particular importance to this patient, as a diagnosis of lung fibrosis might entitle him to a pension for occupational lung disease.

However, the most likely diagnosis is COPD. In this case, the patient has done the best possible thing for his health by stopping smoking.

Should the patient develop an infection such as acute bronchitis or pneumonia at a later date, it may be wise to refer for antibiotic treatment, as it is known that infection can cause worsening damage in someone with chronic lung disease.

The blood

3.4

Chapter 3.4a The physiology of the blood

LEARNING POINTS

At the end of this chapter you will:

- understand the composition of the blood
- understand the functions of the plasma, red blood cells, white blood cells and platelets
- be able to describe the role of the blood.

Estimated time for chapter: 50 minutes.

Introduction

In this last section of Stage 3 the physiology and pathology of the blood and its associated diseases are explored. Some of the different aspects of the function of the blood have already been described when discussing inflammation, clotting, the immune system and the cardiovascular system.

The composition of the blood

In Chapter 2.1c it was explained that the blood is composed of a fluid called plasma and three types of blood cells: the red blood cells (erythrocytes), the white blood cells (leukocytes) and the platelets (thrombocytes).

The plasma

The plasma forms just over half (55%) of the volume of the blood. Plasma consists of water in which a number of substances are dissolved (see Q.3.4a-1).

Plasma is quite a thick (viscous) fluid, a property resulting from the proteins dissolved in it. One important function of these proteins is to help keep the watery part of the blood within the blood vessels. As the proteins are too large to move out of the blood vessels by diffusion, they maintain a level of concentration in the blood which contributes to its osmotic pressure (see Chapter 1.1c) (see Q3.4a-2).

The most abundant of the plasma proteins is albumin, which is similar in structure to the protein of egg white. Albumin is made by the liver, and its main role is to contribute to osmotic pressure. All the plasma proteins, for example the clotting factors and antibodies, have important functions. The transport proteins are important in that they help carry some salts and hormones that would otherwise be relatively insoluble in plasma.

Plasma is also the vehicle by which the nutrients and oxygen, which are essential for the life of the cells, actually reach the tissues. Although oxygen tends to be concentrated in the red blood cells, it also has to move freely through the plasma so that it can pass from the alveoli to the red blood cells and thence to the tissues.

As the vehicle for the transport of hormones, plasma is also important for communication between one part of the body and another. For example, thyroid hormone is secreted by the thyroid gland into the bloodstream and carried to all the tissues of the body, and so in this way the plasma is essential for the role of the endocrine system (see Stage 5.1).

The blood cells

All three types of blood cell originate from the bone marrow. The bone marrow contains a number of immature cells called 'stem cells', and it is these that are the starting material for all the different subtypes of blood cells, including all the leukocytes, such as macrophages and mast cells, which leave the blood to perform immune functions in the tissues. Figure 3.4a-I gives a diagrammatic representation of how the stem cell is the 'great grandparent' of the red blood cell (the erythrocyte), the platelet and the six different categories of white blood cell (the granulocytes and agranulocytes). It is important to appreciate this process before approaching the study of the condition of leukaemia.

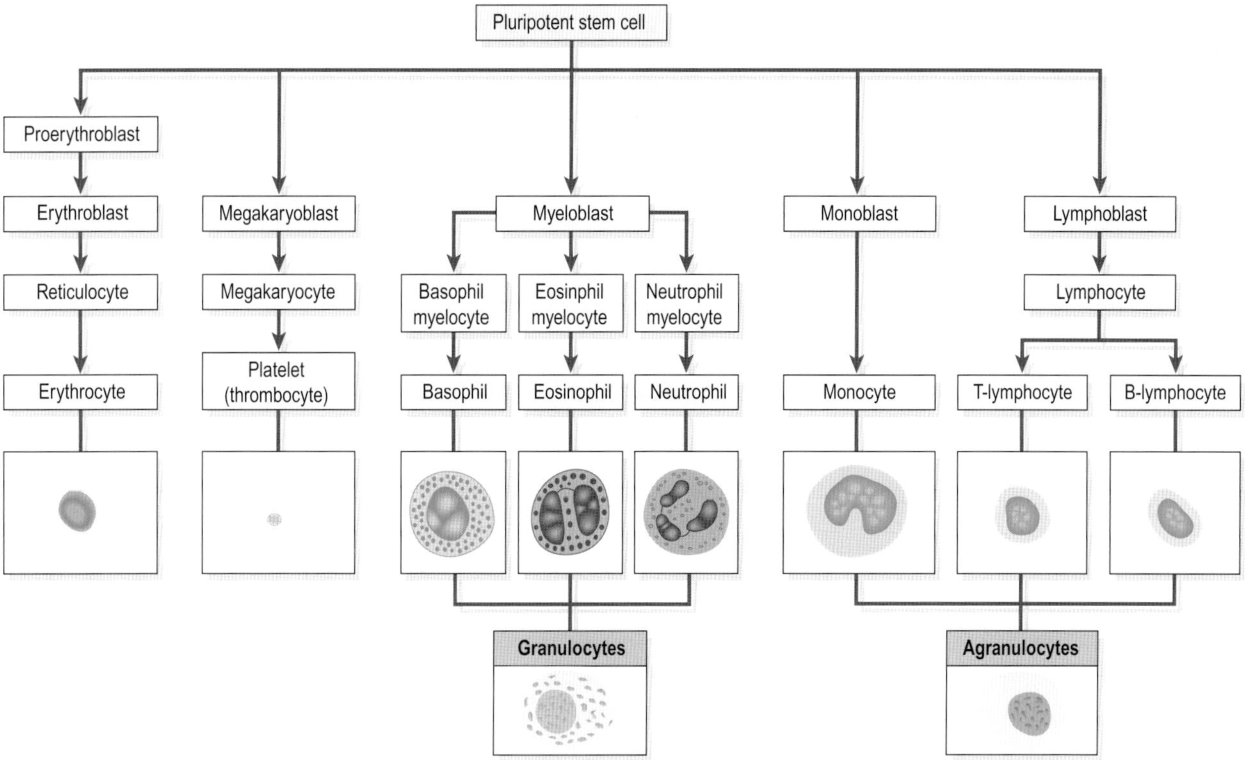

Figure 3.4a-I • The stages in the development of the blood cells.

Red blood cells (erythrocytes)

The primary function of red blood cells is to carry oxygen from the lungs to the tissues. To do this, red blood cells contain an iron-containing protein called 'haemoglobin', which has a strong affinity for oxygen molecules. Because of its haemoglobin, a red blood cell can carry much more oxygen than could be dissolved in an equivalent volume of plasma, and this is essential to enable the blood to carry sufficient oxygen for the body's requirements.

When haemoglobin attracts and holds on to oxygen molecules, it turns bright red, giving the blood its characteristic colour. When it releases oxygen, the colour of the haemoglobin, and therefore the blood, becomes a more purple shade of red. This is why arterial blood in the body circulation is bright red and venous blood is darker.

The haemoglobin is manufactured within the maturing red blood cell in the bone marrow. Iron, obtained from the diet, is an essential ingredient in this process. The vitamins folic acid and vitamin B_{12}, also obtained from the diet, are important factors that enable the production of healthy red blood cells.

The production of red blood cells is stimulated by the hormone erythropoietin, which is released by the kidneys. The hormone is released when the blood fails to perform its role of oxygenation of tissues in the conditions of anaemia and acute blood loss (see Chapters 3.4c and 3.4d).

Before the maturing red blood cell leaves the bone marrow to enter the blood, the nucleus breaks down. The red blood cell then takes on a disc-like shape, which enables it to be flexible enough to move in large numbers through the finest capillaries. Once in the circulation, the life of the red blood cell is about 120 days, after which it is broken down in the spleen, the liver, and parts of the bone marrow by phagocytic white blood cells. In this process, the iron is removed from the haemoglobin and recycled for further use in the body. The by-product of this process is bilirubin, which is a digested form of haemoglobin, and this is taken up by the liver and excreted into the bile (see Chapter 3.1a) (see Q3.4a-3).

The surface of the red blood cells expresses characteristic forms of polysaccharide molecules, and these are the basis for categorising a person into one of the four blood groups, A, B, AB or O, and also as whether they are rhesus (Rh) positive or rhesus negative. This terminology reflects the two important ways in which blood groups are classified: the ABO system and the rhesus system.

The ABO system categorises blood according to the presence or absence of two genetically determined polysaccharides (antigens), known simply as A and B, on the surface of the red blood cell. Group A means that substance A is carried on all the red cells, whereas the red cells of group B carry substance B. The red cells of blood group AB carry both A and B, whereas those of blood group O carry neither.

The rhesus system, at its most simple, categorises blood into whether or not it carries a particular substance called rhesus D. Rhesus-positive people carry rhesus D on their red cells. The rhesus system is independent of the ABO system.

If blood of different blood groups is mixed there is a tendency for the red blood cells to clump together and break down. This is called 'incompatibility', and results from antibodies to 'foreign' blood groups present in the serum of the blood samples. Some combinations of blood groups are much more likely to have this reaction than others. For this reason, before being used in a blood transfusion, donated blood is 'typed' to ensure that the ABO and rhesus D factors are exactly the same as those of the intended recipient.

Platelets (thrombocytes)

The platelets, like the red blood cells, are cells without nuclei that originate from the bone marrow. Their function is to work together with the clotting-factor proteins in the plasma to enable an efficient and controlled clotting reaction (see Chapter 2.1c).

White blood cells (leukocytes)

The diverse functions of the white blood cells were introduced in the description of wound healing, inflammation and the immune system in Sections 2.1 and 2.2.

There are two broad groups of white blood cell, which are categorised according to whether or not the cytoplasm contains granules. These are the granulocytes and agranulocytes (see Figure 3.4a-I).

Granulocytes contain granules, which consist of chemicals (enzymes) that are important for the destruction of unwanted foreign matter and in the generation of inflammation. Some of the granulocytes are able to phagocytose (see Chapter 1.1c) small particles such as damaged bacteria. All the granulocytes can move, like an amoeba, out of the blood vessels and into the tissues when their presence is required.

The agranulocytes, which include the lymphocytes and monocytes, do not contain granules. Lymphocytes are the cells that provide the foundation of the immune response. They secrete antibodies in response to antigens and carry specific antibodies on their surface. Monocytes are cells that are able to phagocytose foreign material and debris from damaged and ageing cells. Macrophages are a type of monocyte that are plentiful in connective tissue for this purpose.

The role of the blood

The blood is a part of the body that is in constant movement, and which by means of the blood vessels reaches all body parts. Its primary role is to transport essential substances from one part of the body to another and to remove waste products.

It is because of the healthy flow of blood that all the cells of the body can have a constant environment. This environment provides water, nutrients, oxygen, protection, the perfect balance of acidity and salts, and warm temperature, and is always cleansed of wastes. In short, blood is a cornerstone of the state of balance called 'homeostasis', and the fact that it is crucial for maintaining balance is of course likely to be of interest to those who hold to a holistic approach to medicine (see Q3.4a-4-Q3.4a-5).

Information Box 3.4a-I

The functions of the blood: comments from a Chinese medicine perspective

To consider the role of the blood in Chinese medicine, it is useful to list the functions of the substances Blood and Qi as they are generally understood.

(i) The functions of Blood are to:
- nourish
- moisturise
- house the Shen.

(ii) The functions of Qi are to:
- transform
- transport
- hold
- raise
- protect
- warm.

There are marked correspondences with the conventional understanding of the function of blood, but the conventional view embraces some of the functions of both Blood and Qi in Chinese medicine. The nourishing and moisturising function of the physical blood is attributed to Blood, whereas the transporting, protecting and warming functions are attributed to Qi. Of course, the close relationship between Blood and Qi is recognised in Chinese medicine in the sayings 'Blood is the mother of Qi' and 'Qi is the commander of Blood'.

As always with these comparisons, there are marked differences. The physical blood has no relationship with the mental, emotional or spiritual aspects corresponding to the Shen, the spiritual aspect of the Blood in Chinese medicine.

Information Box 3.4a-II

The manufacture of blood: comments from a Chinese medicine perspective

In the physiology of Chinese medicine, Blood is made from Gu (food) Qi, which originates from the Spleen. Gu Qi requires the motive force of Lung Qi to reach the Heart, where it is transformed into Blood. This process is aided by Original (Yuan) Qi and Jing (Essence), which produces Marrow.

In this ancient interpretation of how Blood is made there are some clear correspondences with the conventional understanding of the manufacture of blood. The basic materials for the physical blood come from the diet. This includes water, basic nutrients, iron and the vitamins, folic acid and vitamin B_{12}. These can be compared to the Gu Qi made by the Spleen.

The stem cells in the bone marrow are the templates for all the blood cells, and are present in marrow from before birth. These may be comparable to Yuan Qi and Jing. The kidneys also play an important role in the production of blood, in that they secrete the hormone erythropoietin. This could be seen as a physical aspect of Yuan Qi.

The lungs and the heart are important in the circulation of the blood, as they sit at the central point of the circulation. The heart provides the motive force for the blood, and this prevents clotting. The lungs ensure oxygenation of the blood, so that the blood is able to give life to the cells. These organs are essential for maintaining the nature of living blood.

The other Organ that is considered in Chinese medicine to have an important relationship with blood is the Liver. The Liver is considered to be a storehouse for the Blood, particularly when a person is at rest. When the Blood is in the Liver it can be nourished. This is one of the reasons why in Chinese medicine adequate rest is considered to be important for healthy Blood.

In conventional medicine the liver can also be said to store blood, as it holds a large proportion of the circulating blood at any one time. The liver manufactures the plasma proteins and enables an even release of the most basic nutrient, glucose, into the blood. This picture is consistent with the storing and nourishing functions of the Liver Organ.

Despite all these correspondences it is important to be clear when talking to patients that the physical blood and the Chinese medicine energetic concept of Blood are not the same thing. The physical blood is a reflection of some of the aspects of Blood, the Vital Substance, but also carries some of the characteristics of Qi.

Self-test 3.4a

The physiology of the blood

1. (i) What two components of the blood are responsible for ensuring that the cells of the body have an adequate supply of oxygen?
   (ii) How is the blood specialised for this role?
   (iii) What are three substances obtained from the diet which are of particular importance in ensuring that the blood can perform this role?
2. Why is it important to ensure a good 'match' of blood groups before a blood transfusion is given to a patient?
3. How does the function of physical blood relate to the protecting function of Qi?
4. From what part of the body do all blood cells originate?

Answers

1. (i) Oxygen is transported in the blood in two ways: (a) a small amount of oxygen is always dissolved within the plasma; and (b) the red blood cells carry the largest amount of oxygen, bound to a substance called haemoglobin.
   (ii) Blood is specialised for this role by having a large number of red blood cells, which have a flexible shape so that they can pass through the smallest capillaries. Haemoglobin has a particular affinity for oxygen. The presence of haemoglobin in red blood cells means that they are specialised to absorb and transport a large amount of oxygen as they pass through the lung capillaries.
   (iii) Iron, folic acid and vitamin B_{12} are the three substances in the diet that are essential for the healthy development of the red-blood cells. Without sufficient amounts of any one of these three substances, the red cells would be unable to produce sufficient haemoglobin, and therefore could not carry enough oxygen to meet the body's requirements.
2. A mismatch of blood groups is called 'incompatibility'. Incompatible blood cells tend to clump together and break down. This can be life-threatening if it occurs within the blood vessels of a patient receiving a transfusion.
3. The blood performs a protective role in two main ways. First, it contains clotting factors and platelets, which work together to ensure a healthy clotting response in the case of injury to the blood vessels. This would be related in Chinese medicine partly to the role of Spleen Qi in Holding Blood. (The other contributing factor in Chinese medicine in prevention of bleeding is healthy Yin, which is the energetic foundation to the healthy substance of tissue. Bleeding can be a result of the Empty or Full Heat, which can follow on from Yin Deficiency– see Chapter 2.1c.)

   Secondly, the blood carries the leukocytes and antibodies to all the tissues of the body. These are essential for both a healthy inflammatory reaction and the immune response. This can be compared in Chinese medicine to the role of Wei Qi, and the motive force of Lung Qi, which enables the spreading of Wei Qi to all superficial parts of the body.
4. All blood cells originate from the immature stem cells, which are situated in the bone marrow. (In newborns this marrow is situated within all the bones, but in adults the blood-forming marrow is largely confined to the vertebrae, the ribs, the skull bones and the ends of the long bones.)

Chapter 3.4b The investigation of the blood

LEARNING POINTS

At the end of this chapter you will:

- be able to recognise the main investigations used for diseases of the blood
- understand what a patient might experience when undergoing these investigations.

Estimated time for chapter: 30 minutes.

Introduction

Mild forms of the most common non-cancerous diseases of the blood, the anaemias, may be investigated and managed solely by a family physician (GP), who is able to examine the patient and take blood samples to be sent to a laboratory for interpretation.

The investigation of more severe diseases of the blood is carried out by a hospital specialist called a 'haematologist'. A doctor who specialises in haematology has been trained not only in the clinical skills required to examine and treat patients with blood diseases, but also in the examination of samples of blood and bone marrow under the microscope.

The investigation of the diseases of the blood involves:

- a thorough physical examination
- blood tests
- examination of a sample of bone marrow
- biopsy and other tests to visualise the lymph nodes.

Physical examination

The physical examination of a patient with a suspected disease of the blood involves the stages listed in Table 3.4b-I.

Blood tests

A great deal of information can be obtained about the blood from tests that involve the patient in relatively little discomfort. All the tests described below are used in the investigation of a wide range of diseases affecting all the body systems. Because these tests are performed so frequently, they are described in some detail.

The full blood count

The full blood count (FBC) is one of the most commonly performed blood tests. The FBC can give information about all three types of blood cell (red blood cells, white blood cells or leukocytes, and platelets).

To perform a full blood count about 5 millilitres of venous blood is taken by syringe, usually from a vein at the elbow (in the approximate area of acupoint Chize Lung-5). This blood is mixed in a tube with an anticoagulant to prevent clotting, and sent to a laboratory where it is 'examined' using a machine. The machine, called a cell counter, is able to recognise the various blood cells in the sample by their size, and gives a figure for the numbers of the different sorts of blood cell within the sample. The relative numbers of the different sorts of leukocytes can be estimated. The concentration of haemoglobin in the sample and the sizes of the red blood cells can also be measured.

These figures are then compared to the normal range of values found in an average population. Therefore, the FBC can show if there are too many or too few of any one type of blood cell, if the haemoglobin is too low, and if the red cells are abnormal in shape or size.

Blood film

In this examination of the blood, a drop of the blood sample taken for the FBC is placed on a microscope slide and examined by a haematologist. This examination can give more precise information about abnormalities in the shape and structure of the various blood cells.

Erythrocyte sedimentation rate

The erythrocyte sedimentation rate (ESR) and the level of C-reactive protein (CRP) are both measures of an active inflammatory response taking place in the body. The ESR is simply a measure of how rapidly the red blood cells settle out of a shaken sample of blood, like particles of mud might settle out of a sample of river water. The rate at which the cells settle is dependent on the proteins, such as antibodies, in the plasma. The ESR is raised if the body is dealing with an ongoing infection, inflammation, cancer or trauma. The ESR is not very specific, but if raised is a sign that there is an ongoing state of physical imbalance in the body. Another measurement called the 'plasma viscosity' gives similar information.

The C-reactive protein

C-reactive protein (CRP) is one of the plasma proteins, the levels of which rise during inflammation. If the CRP level is raised, the body is dealing with acute inflammation or trauma. This test is therefore a bit more specific than the ESR, but is more expensive to perform.

Serum samples

Serum can be obtained from the blood by allowing venous blood to clot in a test tube. The fluid that separates from the clot is plasma without the clotting factor fibrinogen. This fluid is called serum. A wide range of assays can be performed on the serum sample to investigate diseases that affect the body systems. For example, substances as diverse as vitamin C, insulin, calcium and cannabis can all be detected from serum samples, although a separate blood sample is required for each assay.

Contrary to popular belief, a single blood test cannot reveal information about all these diseases and substances. A single sample of about 7 millilitres of blood can only be used for one or two assays. Alcohol, for example, will only be detected if the alcohol assay has been requested. Even if present, alcohol will not be detected if the doctor has requested that the blood is tested only for thyroid hormone.

In diseases of the blood, some of the most commonly performed serum tests are for iron, vitamin B_{12} and folic acid (also called folate in some texts), all of which are important in the investigation of anaemia.

Table 3.4b-I The stages of physical examination of the blood

- General examination for signs of anaemia: including pale nails, pale creases in the palms of the hands, general pallor of the skin, sore tongue without coating, and cracked lips in severe cases
- Examination of the lymph nodes: to look for the enlargement that can occur in cancers that affect the blood cells
- Examination of the heart and lungs: to exclude the rapid heart rate and pulmonary oedema that can result from severe anaemia (see Chapter 3.3c)
- Examination of the spleen and liver: these can become enlarged in various diseases of the blood

Examination of the bone marrow

In all severe conditions of the blood, including anaemia, examination of the bone marrow can reveal whether there are abnormalities in the development of the blood. The blood-forming marrow is a dense blood-like fluid that can be drawn up into a syringe. The removal of the sample of bone marrow involves the insertion of a large needle into the bone of the iliac crest after the area has been numbed with a local anaesthetic. Despite the anaesthetic this is a much more painful procedure than the simple blood test.

The sample obtained is examined in the same way as the blood film. The bone marrow sample will reveal the shape and structure of the stem cells and the immature forms of the three different types of blood cell.

Biopsy and other tests to visualise the lymph nodes

The two most common forms of cancer that affect the cells of the blood are leukaemia and lymphoma. These diseases are the focus of Chapter 3.4e. In both these conditions the lymph nodes may become engorged with increased numbers of cancerous white blood cells.

In lymphoma, the lymph node is the primary site of the tumour. Surgical removal and examination (biopsy) of an affected superficial node can give valuable information about the tumour. Computed tomography (CT) scans can give more information about the state of lymph nodes deeper in the body. Both these tests can be important for the accurate staging of lymphomas.

Self-test 3.4b

The investigation of the blood

1. You have referred a patient to her GP because you think that her symptoms suggests that she actually may be clinically anaemic. She is pale and tired, but is also very breathless on exertion and experiences frightening palpitations after very little physical effort. These symptoms have responded only a little to your treatment. What can you explain to this patient about the investigations she might have to undergo?

Answer

1. It is likely that your patient's GP will first perform a physical examination to look for signs of anaemia, and this should include examination of the heart and the lungs.

   The GP will also take a blood sample so that a full blood count (FBC) can be performed. A serum sample might also be taken at the same time to check that levels of iron, vitamin B_{12} and folic acid are within the normal range. These tests may be sufficient to clarify a diagnosis.

   If the GP has any doubt about the diagnosis, your patient may be referred to a haematologist who, in addition to the blood test, may also take a sample of bone marrow for examination.

   Your patient may also have to undergo further tests to clarify a possible source of bleeding (e.g. upper gastrointestinal endoscopy) if iron-deficiency anaemia from blood loss is suspected.

Chapter 3.4c Anaemia

LEARNING POINTS

At the end of this chapter you will:
- be able to define the term 'anaemia'
- be able to recognise the range of conditions that might cause the state of anaemia
- understand the principles of treatment of the most common forms of anaemia
- be able to recognise the red flags of severe anaemia.

Estimated time for chapter: 100 minutes.

Introduction

'Anaemia' is a term derived from the Greek words meaning 'no blood', and is used to describe the range of conditions that lead to an impairment in the ability of the red blood cells to transport oxygen to the tissues. In a person with anaemia, the concentration of haemoglobin in the blood is less than that in healthy people.

In Chapter 3.4d the ways in which a sudden loss of a large quantity of blood might affect the body are explored. Although this condition also reduces the ability of the blood to transport oxygen to the tissues, this is not the same as anaemia. In acute blood loss, the red cells and the concentration of haemoglobin are normal, but the volume of the circulating blood is reduced.

It is important at this stage to clarify that the term 'anaemia' does not say anything about the underlying disease process. It simply describes the end result. If doctors are to treat anaemia effectively, the underlying cause of the problem must first be diagnosed.

However, despite the variety of causes of the condition, there are some features that all patients with anaemia have in common.

The clinical features of anaemia

Symptoms of tiredness, breathlessness and feeling faint, together with the sign of pallor are characteristic of anaemia. In addition, palpitations, chest pain and oedema may also be experienced by the patient with severe anaemia. There are also a range of other symptoms that are specific to particular types of anaemia (see Q3.4c-1).

The symptoms of tiredness, breathlessness and depression are a consequence of the cells of the body not receiving the nourishment, in the form of oxygen, that they require. Oxygen is an essential ingredient in the process of cell respiration, and thus it is understandable how an insufficient supply of oxygen to the tissues of the body can lead to these general symptoms of anaemia (see Q3.4c-2).

Information Box 3.4c-I

Anaemia: comments from a Chinese medicine perspective

It is important to be clear that the symptoms of anaemia and the syndrome of Blood Deficiency in Chinese medicine have some close similarities but are not directly equivalent.

According to Chinese medicine, the general features of Blood Deficiency include the symptoms of dizziness, poor memory, numbness, floaters and blurred vision, difficulty in sleeping, depression, anxiety and lack of initiative and the signs of pallor of the face, pale lips and tongue, and dry tongue.

The features that are specific to Heart Blood Deficiency include facial pallor, poor memory, poor sleep and anxiety, and the features that are specific to Liver Blood Deficiency include floaters and blurring of vision, numbness and lack of initiative.

If Blood Deficiency becomes severe it leads to Yin Deficiency. Additional features of Heart Yin Deficiency include palpitations, restlessness, tendency to be easily startled, and dry tongue, and additional features of Liver Yin Deficiency include dry eyes and withered nails.

It is clear from this summary that there are some correspondences between the features of anaemia and the features of Blood Deficiency. Nevertheless, anaemia and Blood Deficiency are not the same thing. The physical blood embodies some characteristics of the energetic Blood, but equally some of Qi. Therefore, symptoms of Qi Deficiency as well as of Blood Deficiency might well be expected in someone with anaemia.

The condition of Blood and Yin Deficiency can exist even when all blood tests show that the level of haemoglobin and the structure and number of the red blood cells are normal. However, it is safe to assume that, if anaemia has been diagnosed, Blood Deficiency, as well as some Yin Deficiency and some Qi Deficiency, will be present.

It may be helpful to think of anaemia as one possible manifestation of Blood and Yin Deficiency. In anaemia, the energetic imbalance of Blood Deficiency has become manifest in a measurable physical change in the haemoglobin levels and red blood cells.

The sign of pallor is due to the reduction in levels of the bright red coloured haemoglobin in the blood.

Palpitations and chest pain occur in severe anaemia because the heart responds to the reduced level of oxygen in the blood by pumping faster. This has the initially beneficial effect of increasing the amount of oxygen that reaches the tissues at any one time, but can place strain on the heart muscle itself. The symptoms of *angina* may result in someone who has a degree of *atherosclerosis*, and occasionally oedema may develop as a result of *heart failure*.

The causes of anaemia

The causes of anaemia are conventionally categorised into two groups:

- anaemia due to impaired production of red blood cells
- anaemia due to increased destruction of red blood cells.

Impaired production of red blood cells

Impaired production of red blood cells most commonly results from a deficiency of the three essential factors required for the healthy development of red blood cells: iron, vitamin B_{12} and folic acid. This leads to an anaemia in which the red blood cells produced in the bone marrow are unable to carry the amount of oxygen that could be carried by normal red blood cells.

Another important cause of reduced production of red blood cells is bone marrow failure. The most common cause of bone marrow failure is cancer. Secondary cancer and blood cancers can form in the marrow spaces in the bones and prevent the healthy growth of bone marrow.

Red blood cells are also underproduced in severe chronic disease such as kidney failure (chronic renal failure) or rheumatoid arthritis. In kidney failure the anaemia results from insufficient production of erythropoietin, which is normally made by the healthy kidneys. In other chronic diseases, the cause for the anaemia is less clearly understood. "Anaemia of chronic disease" (AOCD) may be a mild anaemia, but still can be sufficiently severe to lead to symptoms.

Increased destruction of red blood cells

Red blood cells can become prematurely destroyed either because they have become damaged in some way, or because there is excessive enlargement of the spleen, the main organ responsible for the natural breakdown of the red cells. Again, in these types of anaemia the number of red blood cells in the blood is reduced.

The inherited conditions of sickle cell anaemia and thalassaemia are both conditions in which the red cells are abnormal in shape and are more prone to destruction. Both these conditions are examples of anaemia due to the premature destruction of red cells.

The anaemias resulting from impaired production of red blood cells

Iron-deficiency anaemia

Iron-deficiency anaemia is the most common cause of anaemia in western countries. Moreover, it is one of the most important causes of ill-health worldwide. In developing countries, deficiency of iron in the diet contributes to poor growth and development, and impairs the ability to fight infections. Iron-deficiency anaemia is the underlying cause of millions of premature deaths, especially of women in childbirth, babies and children. Iron deficiency can be compounded in people in tropical countries by the anaemia that can result from malaria and other parasitic infections.

Iron-deficiency anaemia can result either from inadequate amounts of iron-containing foods in the diet, or from excessive loss of the iron contained in the blood. A combination of the two is commonly present.

Iron is initially obtained in infancy from breast milk, although the amount of iron in breast milk is considered to be insufficient as the only source of iron in children over the age of 1 year. For this reason, many milk formulas produced for bottle feeding are supplemented with iron. After weaning, iron is obtained from foods such as meat and fish, eggs, whole grains and dark leafy vegetables. In the west many processed cereal products are fortified with iron.

In the west, despite an abundance of food, many people are at risk of iron deficiency because of an inadequate diet. People who are particularly at risk are small children, people on long-term slimming diets, vegetarians and vegans, and elderly people.

Another group of people who are at risk of iron deficiency are those who cannot absorb iron from the diet because of malabsorption (see Chapter 3.1e).

In health, the body holds a lot of iron in reserve. The bulk of this is held within the haemoglobin of the red cells, and is 'recycled' for further use when the old red cells are broken down by the spleen. The remainder of the body's iron stores are found in the liver and the muscles. The body can withstand a period of weeks of a relatively low intake of dietary iron. However, unless the diet can provide sufficient iron, the stores will eventually run out, as iron is gradually lost through the sweat and urine as well as through bleeding.

Iron stores run out much more quickly if excessive blood is lost on a recurrent basis. As many blood donors might wish to testify, the body can withstand a significant loss of blood as long as sufficient time is allowed for the iron stores to recover before the next episode of blood loss. However, in some situations a steady loss of iron from long-term bleeding may be too great to be recovered from the diet alone. This most commonly results from heavy menstrual bleeding, or in people who are unknowingly losing just a few millilitres of blood a day into their bowel from gastrointestinal conditions such as a stomach ulcer. In these cases, the iron stores gradually run down until the manufacture of red cells is affected, and then anaemia develops.

Pregnancy and the months following childbirth are recognised as times during which the iron stores can become depleted. The pregnant woman loses iron as it passes through the placenta to the developing fetus, and then a large amount of blood can be lost at delivery. The iron stores will be depleted further as the mother breastfeeds.

It is recognised that it is very common for iron stores to be depleted, although not by enough to affect the production of red blood cells and to cause anaemia. This is called 'latent iron deficiency', and is obviously a state in which the body is not in a good state of balance. Latent iron deficiency is not conventionally recognised to be associated with specific symptoms.

When the iron stores are very low, the red cells produced in the bone marrow are small and pale because of the reduced amount of haemoglobin. They are also reduced in number. This pattern is characteristic of iron deficiency, and so a simple FBC can often be all that is needed to confirm the diagnosis. Serum samples will show reduced levels of iron in the blood.

A patient with iron-deficiency anaemia will experience all the general symptoms of anaemia, their severity depending on how much the level of haemoglobin has been reduced. Additional symptoms that are recognised to occur in iron-deficiency anaemia are believed to be a result of deficiency of iron in certain other tissues of the body such as the skin, the mucous membranes and the nails. In severe iron deficiency a patient might have dry skin and a tendency to bruising, concave (spoon-shaped) nails and a sore tongue and cracked lips. The tongue loses its coat and can appear bright red (likened to a beefsteak). It is known that, in very severe cases, the retina at the back of the eye can show areas of swelling and bleeding, and this carries a risk of blindness.

In all cases of iron-deficiency anaemia, the diagnosis alone is not a sufficient basis on which to start treatment. In all cases, the possibility of malabsorption or excessive blood loss should also be excluded, and this may involve the patient in a referral to a gastroenterologist to exclude chronic bowel disease or bleeding from the bowel. A referral to a gynaecologist may be made for the treatment of heavy menstrual bleeding (see Chapter 5.2c).

Dietary causes of anaemia can be rapidly addressed by giving the patient iron supplements in tablet form. Ferrous sulphate and ferrous fumarate are two common preparations. Many iron supplements cause gastrointestinal side-effects such as nausea, acid indigestion and constipation, although more naturally derived preparations are available (not on prescription) which are claimed to have fewer of these side-effects.

Iron supplements are given in pregnancy often in mild cases of anaemia, because of the anticipated further iron losses that might occur during childbirth and breastfeeding. Unfortunately, the side-effects of nausea, indigestion and constipation can be particularly problematic in pregnancy.

It is only in very extreme cases of anaemia, or in cases in which the bowel cannot absorb iron, that iron is given by other means. In these cases iron may be given by intravenous injection, although this carries risks of more severe side-effects.

In anaemia due to malabsorption or blood loss, the cause of the anaemia should be treated in addition to supplementing the iron stores of the body with iron preparations.

Information Box 3.4c-II

Iron-deficiency anaemia: comments from a Chinese medicine perspective

In Chinese medicine, the symptoms of iron-deficiency anaemia closely correspond to the syndromes of Heart and Liver Blood (and Yin) Deficiency with Qi Deficiency.

Iron-containing foods include meat and fish, eggs, whole grains and dark leafy vegetables. All these foods would be considered in Chinese medicine to be 'Blood Forming'.

Latent iron deficiency is not conventionally recognised to lead to any symptoms. However, it is possible that those non-anaemic people who experience the symptoms of Blood Deficiency might have latent iron deficiency. This might explain why it is recognised in Chinese medicine that a diet rich in 'Blood Forming' foods can be of benefit to all people with Blood Deficiency, even if they are not anaemic. The 'Blood Forming' diet will build up the iron stores of people with latent iron deficiency, and so will help these people regain a more balanced energetic state.

Medicinal iron preparations nourish the Blood but are also Heating in nature and can deplete Stomach Yin. They may also Stagnate Liver Qi.

Vitamin B_{12} deficiency and pernicious anaemia

Vitamin B_{12} can be obtained from the diet in foods such as meat, fish and eggs, but not from plants. The liver contains a large store of vitamin B_{12}, which will run out only after 2 years of lack of the dietary vitamin. For this reason dietary causes of vitamin B_{12} deficiency are rare, exception in people on a strict vegan diet.

A healthy stomach is required for the uptake of vitamin B_{12}, because the parietal cells of the stomach lining are the source of a chemical called 'intrinsic factor', which is necessary for the absorption of the vitamin. People who have had their stomach removed by surgery are prone to vitamin B_{12} deficiency for this reason. However, the most common condition to affect the stomach and prevent healthy absorption of vitamin B_{12} is pernicious anaemia. In pernicious anaemia the parietal cells of the stomach lining are gradually damaged by an autoimmune process. This condition is most common in middle-aged and elderly women. It tends to run in families, and this suggests an inherited susceptibility to autoimmune disease.

Lack of vitamin B_{12} leads to impaired development of the red blood cells. The affected cells are larger than normal, but do not contain sufficient haemoglobin for adequate oxygen transport. The general symptoms and signs of anaemia are present, although the pallor may have a slight yellowy tinge. Lack of vitamin B_{12} affects other tissues, and this leads to additional symptoms. As in iron-deficiency anaemia, a sore mouth and tongue can develop. However, the most serious symptoms relate to the nervous system.

In advanced pernicious anaemia the patient develops numbness and weakness of the limbs, impaired vision, and eventually dementia, as the nerves are deprived of this essential vitamin. Before injectable vitamin B_{12} supplements were available, the damage to the nervous system led to permanent disability and sometimes death. This explains why this form of anaemia was described as 'pernicious'.

The FBC shows the enlarged blood cells suggestive of vitamin B_{12} deficiency, but the diagnosis is fully confirmed by means of serum tests for vitamin B_{12} and a specialised urine test to see if the patient is able absorb the vitamin from a capsule of radioactive vitamin B_{12} (the Schilling test). In over 90% of patients antibodies are found to parietal cells and intrinsic factor, and this is usually sufficient to confirm diagnosis without performing a Schilling test.

If the cause is dietary, then vitamin B_{12} supplements in tablet form can be given. However, in pernicious anaemia these cannot be absorbed by the bowel because of the lack of intrinsic factor. However, the symptoms of pernicious anaemia can now be totally reversed by regular injections of vitamin B_{12}. These injections are usually given at 3-month intervals for the rest of the patient's life.

Although in pernicious anaemia the patient does not usually suffer from any gastric symptoms, the autoimmune process affecting the lining cells of the stomach is a form of inflammation. Because of this, in some patients, it can eventually lead to cancer.

Information Box 3.4c-III

Pernicious anaemia: comments from a Chinese medicine perspective

In Chinese medicine, the vitamin B_{12} deficiency may correspond with Heart and Liver Blood and Yin Deficiency. The symptoms of numbness and visual impairment particularly suggest a Deficiency of Liver Blood. The eventual development of dementia suggests that there has been a progression to severe depletion of Kidney Yin.

The underlying destruction of the lining cells of the stomach could correspond to a Deficiency of Spleen and/or Stomach Yin. The yellowish tinge to the pallor also suggests Spleen Deficiency. This fits with the Chinese medicine understanding that a healthy Spleen is necessary for the formation of blood.

Vitamin B_{12} supplements nourish the Blood and Yin, and the Liver in particular. They do not address the underlying cause of the pernicious anaemia. Although this is technically a suppressive treatment, there is no doubt that it is life saving.

Deficiency of folic acid

Like vitamin B_{12}, folic acid (folate) is also important for the healthy development of red blood cells in the bone marrow. Folic acid is found in the diet in meat and in dark green, leafy vegetables. The body does not have very rich reserves of folic acid, so dietary lack can lead to anaemia within a few months. Elderly people and people who are dependent on alcohol are particularly vulnerable to folic acid deficiency.

The body uses folic acid when there is rapid repair or growth of cells, as it is used up during mitosis. Pregnancy is a time when folic acid stores can become depleted, as the vitamin is used up by the developing fetus. Deficiency can also develop when the body is recovering from major trauma, or in a chronic disease, especially in the case of a rapidly growing cancer.

The red blood cells in folic acid deficiency are large, but have too little haemoglobin. These changes are similar to those caused by vitamin B_{12} deficiency.

Folic acid deficiency leads to the general symptoms of anaemia. A sore tongue may also occur, but there are no other additional symptoms. The most serious consequence of folic acid deficiency is on the developing fetus. If the diet in very early pregnancy is inadequate, insufficient folic acid can lead to defective development of the spinal cord in the first few weeks of the life of the fetus, and the condition *spina bifida* can result. This is why all pregnant women are urged to take folic acid supplements for the first 20 weeks of pregnancy. Studies have shown that folic acid supplementation in pregnancy can reduce the frequency of cases of spina bifida.

Diagnosis of folate-deficiency anaemia is confirmed by a FBC and a serum test for folic acid (folate).

Symptoms can be reversed by treatment of any underlying cause, and by folic acid supplementation.

Information Box 3.4c-IV

Folate-deficiency anaemia: comments from a Chinese medicine perspective

In Chinese medicine, anaemia due to folic acid deficiency seems to correspond to Deficiency of Heart and Liver Blood and/or Yin. In addition, folic acid seems to play an important role in nourishing the Jing of the fetus, as its deficiency leads to symptoms that Chinese medicine would ascribe to Jing Deficiency.

Bone marrow failure and aplastic anaemia

Bone marrow failure occurs when the normal bone marrow is prevented from developing. This can be the result of cancer in the bones taking over the marrow spaces. Another cause is when the marrow is damaged by certain drugs and radiation. Unfortunately, the treatments that are given for cancer can also cause bone marrow failure, although this is usually temporary. Occasionally, infections, including tuberculosis and certain viruses, can damage the bone marrow sufficiently to cause failure. In many cases the cause is unknown, but may be attributed to an autoimmune process akin to autoimmune idiopathic thrombocytopenic purpura (AITP) (see Chapter 2.1c).

All three types of blood cell can be depleted in bone marrow failure. This leads to three major problems: thrombocytopenia from insufficient platelets, immune deficiency from insufficient white blood cells, and anaemia from insufficient red blood cells. Occasionally, only one type of developing cell is affected. If only the red blood cell is affected, the condition is termed 'aplastic anaemia'.

A patient with bone marrow failure will suffer from bleeding, opportunistic infections and the severe general symptoms of anaemia. All three of these problems can be life-threatening, and the patient will require nursing in a specialised environment. Blood and platelet transfusions and intravenous antibiotics may be necessary. In some cases of unknown cause, the patient might respond to treatment with corticosteroid drugs. If the cause is irreversible, the patient will eventually die, usually from uncontrollable bleeding or from infection. The one treatment available for severe irreversible cases is bone marrow transplantation. This risky procedure is explained in more detail in Chapter 3.4e.

Information Box 3.4c-V

Bone marrow failure: comments from a Chinese medicine perspective

In Chinese medicine, the symptoms of anaemia due to bone marrow failure point to severe Deficiency of Blood and Yin. The damage to the marrow represents damage to Kidney Yin and Jing.

Anaemia of chronic disease

In a wide range of chronic diseases the patient may develop a form of anaemia that cannot be helped by supplementing iron, vitamin B_{12} or folic acid. This form of anaemia is poorly understood, but possibly is a result of the long-standing depletion that results from the underlying condition. Usually, anaemia of chronic disease is not severe, but will contribute to the general feeling of malaise that accompanies chronic diseases.

In chronic renal failure the anaemia has a more understood cause. The damaged kidney is no longer able to produce the hormone erythropoietin, which stimulates the production of red blood cells. In this case the anaemia can become very severe, as a result of greatly reduced numbers of red blood cells. This problem can be treated by injections of synthetic erythropoietin. Before this genetically engineered treatment was available, the only alternative for patients was to receive repeated blood transfusions.

The anaemias resulting from increased destruction of red blood cells

Inherited anaemias

Some people are born with a problem that affects the shape of the red blood cells. The misshapen cells are more fragile than healthy red blood cells. In some of these conditions the underlying problem lies in the structure of the haemoglobin, resulting from a mutation in the genetic code for haemoglobin.

In health, one function of the spleen is to recognise the ageing red blood cells, which become fragile and misshapen, and to remove them from the circulation. In these inherited disorders the spleen removes and destroys the misshapen cells prematurely, and this is the main cause of the anaemia. Sickle cell anaemia and thalassaemia are two of the most common inherited anaemias worldwide.

Sickle cell anaemia

Sickle cell anaemia is a condition that is particularly common in black Africans. Up to 25% of black Africans carry a mutation in the haemoglobin gene that has been inherited from at least one parent. The condition is only very severe if the child has inherited two mutations, one from each parent. If only one gene has been inherited, this is called 'sickle cell trait', and only rarely causes serious problems.

In sickle cell disease, the haemoglobin has an abnormal shape like a sickle, which becomes most pronounced when there is very little oxygen in the blood. The sickle-shaped cells are very fragile and can be destroyed as they pass through the tiny capillaries of the circulation, and are also removed and destroyed by the spleen. This will occur more often under conditions where the oxygen level in the blood is reduced, such as when the body is using up more oxygen during infection or following trauma, or when the external oxygen levels are low, such during an aeroplane flight.

If many red cells are destroyed at once, this can lead to a very severe situation called a 'sickle crisis'. The broken irregular cells can block up the capillaries and can lead to multiple small areas of infarction. This can affect all body parts, including the bones, the lungs, the brain, the kidney and the skin.

Severe complications of infarction of these body parts include intense bone pain and chronic infections of areas of dead bone, lung infarction with pleurisy, strokes, kidney failure and skin ulcers.

The patient in a sickle crisis needs intensive hospital treatment. Intravenous fluids and oxygen are given to nourish the tissues and to reverse the 'sickling' of the cells, and strong opiate painkillers are required. A blood transfusion may be necessary. Recurrent sickling crises may lead to progressive disability and premature death.

In between sickle crises, the red cells are broken down more rapidly than should occur in health, particularly by the spleen, but the patient is generally well. A blood test will show reduced numbers of red blood cells and the occasional sickle-shaped cell.

A test for sickle cell anaemia is now given in the UK to all newborn babies of African descent as part of the heel-prick test. A drop of blood is all that is required to test for the condition. An early diagnosis will give a child the best possible start in life, as the parents can be made aware about how to act to prevent the development of sickling crises.

Information Box 3.4c-VI

Sickle cell anaemia: comments from a Chinese medicine perspective

In Chinese medicine, the symptoms of sickle cell anaemia would equate to Blood Deficiency and Blood Stagnation, which are worsened under conditions that reduce the availability of oxygen to the tissues. This suggests that the deficient Lung Qi may be part of the root of this condition. Because sickle cell anaemia is inherited, the principal root of the Blood Deficiency would appear to lie in Kidney Jing.

The sickling crisis is an extreme form of Blood Stagnation, which is a consequence of the Blood Deficiency. Oxygen and fluids nourish the Blood, and so help to move Stagnation.

Thalassaemia

The term 'thalassaemia' comes from the Greek meaning 'blood like sea water'. It refers to a number of similar types of an inherited disorder of haemoglobin. Thalassaemia is common in people from the shores of the Mediterranean, from the Middle East, India and Indonesia, and is particularly common in the Greek Cypriot community.

Depending on the nature of the inherited genes, the condition ranges from a mild anaemia to one that causes death in childhood. In severe cases, the abnormal haemoglobin leads to fragility of the red cells and premature destruction of these by the spleen from very early infancy. This leads to a much more severe anaemia than is found in most people with sickle cell disease.

In the baby with severe thalassaemia, the anaemia stimulates the release of erythropoietin from the kidneys, which in turn stimulates the increased production of red blood cells in the marrow. However, this has negative consequences in that the bone marrow expands in the soft developing bones and leads to enlargement and thickening of those bones, and particularly the bones of the skull. Despite this response, the red cells produced are not effective in transporting oxygen, and the child needs repeated blood transfusions. Often the spleen is removed in an older child to reduce the rate at which the red blood cells are destroyed.

Although such intensive treatment may allow the child to reach adulthood, repeated blood transfusions cause long-term problems because the iron contained within them cannot be removed rapidly enough from the body. The excess iron is toxic, and can cause severe damage to the heart, liver and endocrine glands. Many people with severe thalassaemia will suffer from extreme ill-health. Premature death is usual.

In some cases, bone marrow transplantation using marrow taken from a brother or a sister can provide the child with a source of healthy blood cells. This procedure carries great risks, but can reduce disability in early childhood in those children in whom the procedure is successful (see Chapter 3.4e).

Information Box 3.4c-VII

Thalassaemia: comments from a Chinese medicine perspective

In Chinese medicine, thalassaemia could be equated to severe Blood Deficiency. The effect of erythropoietin on the bone marrow suggests an inherited imbalance in the Kidney Qi. The root of the problem would therefore be a Deficiency of Kidney Jing.

Blood transfusion initially nourishes the Blood and Yin, but the toxicity of the excess iron eventually depletes the Yin and Yang of the deep organs.

Other causes of premature destruction of red blood cells

Red blood cells can be prematurely destroyed for reasons other than inherited defects of the red cell. However, all conditions involving premature destruction of cells will lead to a condition known as 'haemolytic anaemia'. If very severe, the accumulation and clumping of damaged red blood cells in the circulation can lead to infarction of tissues.

Another problem results from the excess haemoglobin that is released from damaged red blood cells. This is broken down by the liver and spleen into the yellowish substance called 'bilirubin'. Bilirubin is usually taken up by the liver and excreted as bile. However, the liver cannot cope with this excessive amount of bilirubin, and so it builds up in the bloodstream, leading to jaundice (see Chapters 3.1a and 3.1d).

Occasionally, infections and drugs can damage the red cells, leading to premature haemolysis. Malaria is the most common infection worldwide that has this serious consequence. In a case of severe malaria, the rapid destruction of those red blood cells that have been infected by the malarial parasite can lead to strokes and profound anaemia with jaundice. The excess bilirubin spills over into the urine and makes it dark in colour. This is why another name for severe malaria is 'blackwater fever'.

The other common cause of premature haemolytic damage to red cells is attack by antibodies. This is the fundamental cause of incompatibility of blood in transfusion. A mismatched blood transfusion will lead to damage to the patient's red cells caused by antibodies contained in the transfused blood. In severe cases this can lead to a sudden reduction in the number of red blood cells, fever because of the inflammatory response, and infarctions of diverse body tissues.

Rhesus disease of the newborn

Another time when antibodies can damage red blood cells and lead to haemolysis is when the blood group of a pregnant woman is different to that of her unborn child. This problem is usually only clinically important when the mother is rhesus negative and the child is rhesus positive. Maternal antibodies to the rhesus factor can cross the placenta and damage the rhesus-factor-containing fetal red cells. This can cause severe anaemia, jaundice and sometimes death of the unborn baby.

It is recognised that these antibodies develop particularly in women who have already had a rhesus-positive baby, and seem to form just after the first baby is born. Usually, the blood of the mother and fetus do not mix, but it is believed that a little fetal blood enters the mother's circulation during childbirth, and also during miscarriage. This can be sufficient to stimulate the mother's immune system to produce anti-rhesus antibodies, which are then forever present and can cause problems in subsequent pregnancies.

For this reason, the blood group of all women is tested in early pregnancy. An additional test in rhesus-negative women looks for the presence of antibodies to the rhesus factor, and this test is repeated during the pregnancy.

The development of rhesus antibodies to fetal rhesus-positive blood cells can be prevented. After childbirth or miscarriage, all rhesus-negative women are given an 'immunisation' of an antibody that can destroy any rhesus-positive cells that may have entered their circulation. This allows the removal of the foreign blood cells before the mother can develop an immune memory to the rhesus factor. This immunisation has dramatically reduced the death and disability that can result from rhesus incompatibility in the newborn.

However, not all cases can be prevented. If rhesus incompatibility is suspected in pregnancy, the mother is referred to a specialist in the condition. Advanced techniques can be used to test for anaemia in the fetus and actually to transfuse blood while it is in the womb. The baby may require intensive care after birth and treatment for the jaundice that can result from the damage to its red blood cells (see Section 5.4) (see Q3.4c-3).

Information Box 3.4c-VIII

Haemolytic disease of the newborn: comments from a Chinese medicine perspective

In Chinese medicine, the symptoms associated with rhesus incompatibility might represent Blood Deficiency and Blood Stagnation. Jaundice is usually ascribed to Damp Heat in the Liver and Gallbladder, and may result from the Blood Stagnation.

The underlying root of the problem is an attack of an essentially normal fetus by antibodies present in the mother's blood. This attack will inevitably damage Jing, as it occurs at such a vulnerable time in fetal development.

Information Box 3.4c-IX

The treatment of patients with anaemia: advice for complementary health practitioners

A clinical diagnosis of anaemia suggests that there is a significant imbalance of vital substances (in Chinese medicine this would be framed as Deficiency of Blood and Qi), and so nutritional supplementation and herbal treatments would be appropriate in addition to solely energetically focused treatments such as acupuncture and homeopathy.

In cases of anaemia due to poor diet, medicinal supplements of iron, vitamin B_{12} or folic acid (depending on the underlying cause of the anaemia) may be energetically appropriate remedies. All these are available in naturally produced preparations, and are relatively inexpensive compared to herbs.

To recommend supplements it is essential to be sure of the underlying cause of the anaemia. Therefore, it is wise to refer a patient for a conventional diagnosis so that any underlying problem such as blood loss or malabsorption can be excluded, and so that the appropriate supplements can be recommended. This advice is of particular importance in pernicious anaemia. If folic acid supplements are mistakenly given in pernicious anaemia, these can lead to worsening of the damage that vitamin B_{12} deficiency can cause to the nervous system.

The other advantage of a conventional diagnosis is that a full blood count (FBC) can provide a numerical and objective measure of the degree of anaemia. This can be a useful benchmark against which to assess the benefits of future treatment.

The red flags of anaemia

Some patients with anaemia will benefit from referral to a conventional doctor for assessment and/or treatment. Red flags are those symptoms and signs that indicate that referral is to be considered. The red flags of anaemia are described in Table 3.4c-I. This table forms part of the summary on red flags given in Appendix III, which also gives advice on the degree of urgency of referral for each of the red flag conditions listed.

Table 3.4c-I Red Flags 18 – anaemia

Red Flag	Description	Reasoning
18.1	**Features of long-standing anaemia**: any of the general symptoms of anaemia should be considered as a reason for referral so that serious treatable causes can be excluded. For example, **pallor**, **tiredness**, **breathlessness on exertion**, feeling of **faintness**, **depression**, **sore mouth** and **tongue**	'Anaemia' is the term that refers to a reduced level of haemoglobin (the iron-containing pigment that enables red blood cells to carry high concentrations of oxygen to the tissues) in the blood. When haemoglobin levels are low, the tissues experience a relative lack of oxygen. The cardiovascular system responds by increasing the heart rate, and the respiratory rate increases. Iron stores in the body become low as iron is utilised to the maximum, and the tissue cells suffer, meaning that the person suffers malaise and sore mouth and tongue Referral is important to establish the cause of the anaemia. Causes include increased blood loss (particularly from menstruation and bleeding from the stomach or bowel, and prolonged use of aspirin or non-steroidal anti-inflammatory drugs), reduced production of blood in the marrow (due to poor diet, malabsorption of iron, vitamin B_{12} or folic acid from the diet, and bone marrow disease) and chronic illness Mild anaemia is common in pregnancy
18.2	**Features of severe anaemia**. The following suggest that the anaemia is very severe: **extreme tiredness and breathlessness on exertion**, **excessive bruising** and **severe visual disturbances**. There may also be features of strain on the **cardiovascular system**: **chest pain on exertion**, features of **tachycardia** and increasing **oedema**	See above If the anaemia is severe, this puts extra strain on the heart as it attempts to increase oxygen delivery to the tissues by increasing cardiac output. This can lead to cardiac failure and angina
18.3	**Features of pernicious anaemia: tiredness**, **lemon-yellow pallor** and gradual onset of **neurological symptoms (numbness, weakness)**	Pernicious anaemia is a form of anaemia that results from an impaired ability to absorb vitamin B_{12} from the digestive tract. The underlying cause is an autoimmune disease that affects the production of a protein called intrinsic factor from the stomach. Intrinsic factor needs to bind to vitamin B_{12} before the vitamin can be absorbed As vitamin B_{12} is also vital to the health of the nervous system, neurological symptoms can develop if deficiency is prolonged. Treatment involves regular and lifelong injections of vitamin B_{12}

Self-test 3.4c

Anaemia

1. A 32-year-old patient is complaining of the symptoms that might be diagnosed in Chinese medicine as Heart and Liver Blood Deficiency. She feels tired all the time and her memory is poor. She is anxious and jumpy and has poor sleep. Her periods are scanty and her skin is dry. She has floaters in her vision and itchy eyes. You notice that she is remarkably pale, her tongue is dry with a red tip, and her pulse is very fine. You suspect that she may have clinical anaemia. When you question her further you find that she is a Buddhist and has been a strict vegan for a few years.
   (i) What are the most likely conventional diagnoses in this patient?
   (ii) Would you refer her for a conventional opinion? If so, why?
2. Carol is 55 years old and has advanced breast cancer. She has recently completed a series of chemotherapy treatments, and has become very pale and tired over the last couple of weeks. You are concerned that she has developed a few bruises at the sites of needle insertions during the last treatment, which is unusual for her.
   (i) What are the possible medical explanations for Carol's recent symptoms?
   (ii) How would you deal with this situation?

Answers

1. (i) The most likely diagnosis from the information you are given is anaemia due to dietary deficiency. In particular, both iron and vitamin B_{12} deficiency can result from a strict vegan diet. It is possible that there are other underlying physical causes, but you need to question the patient further to exclude these.
   (ii) From a Chinese medical perspective you could treat this patient with acupuncture to see if her symptoms improve. A discussion about her diet may be of help if you can encourage her to increase her intake of Blood Forming foods. However, it sounds like her Blood Deficiency is quite severe, and a referral for Chinese Herbs may be a helpful option to treat her immediate deficiency.
   You should also refer her to her GP for a conventional diagnosis, as this may only involve a simple blood test, and will give you an objective measure of the degree of deficiency from which to start treatment. A diagnosis will also be of help should you choose to advise your patient to take iron or vitamin supplements.
2. (i) It seems that your patient might be becoming anaemic. She may also have a problem with blood clotting, as evidenced by increasing bruising from needle insertions.
   Possible causes of anaemia in a patient with advanced cancer include folic acid deficiency, anaemia of chronic disease, and bone marrow failure, either due to cancer treatment or because the marrow has been taken over by cancer cells. Bone marrow failure will also lead to impairment of the clotting function due to thrombocytopenia.
   (ii) The best course of action in this situation is to refer Carol to her GP for tests to diagnose the type of anaemia and to exclude the most serious diagnosis of bone marrow failure. It would be wise to avoid any needling until you are assured that there is no problem in the clotting function.

Chapter 3.4d Acute blood loss, transfusion and disorders of the spleen

LEARNING POINTS

At the end of this chapter you will:
- understand the meaning of the medical term 'shock'
- be familiar with the conditions in which transfusion of blood or one of its component parts may be used
- be able to recognise the conditions that result from disorders of the spleen.
- be able to recognise the red flags acute blood loss

Estimated time for chapter: 90 minutes.

Introduction

This chapter begins by summarising the ways in which the sudden loss of a large volume of blood can affect the body. Haemorrhage (meaning 'flow of blood') is the medical term used to describe blood loss. Severe haemorrhage can lead to a condition conventionally termed 'shock'.

Shock is the result of any condition in which the ability of the blood to transport oxygen and nutrients to the tissues is suddenly reduced. Although blood loss is one major cause, there are a number of other causes, which are also discussed in this chapter.

One important emergency treatment for haemorrhage is transfusion of blood to replace the plasma and blood cells that have been lost. Transfusion can also be used in other conditions, such as in the treatment of two types of anaemia already described, thalassaemia and rhesus disease of the newborn. The common conditions in which transfusion of blood, or one of its component parts, is performed are explored in this chapter.

The conditions that can result from diseases of the spleen are described at the end of this chapter. Strictly speaking, the spleen is part of the lymphatic system, but it is included in this section because it plays such an important role in the physiology of the blood.

Acute blood loss

The sudden loss of a large volume of blood is a major trauma to the body. It most commonly occurs as a result of physical injury. Road traffic accidents and bleeding during surgery are the most significant causes of sudden blood loss in the UK.

There are also some common internal causes of haemorrhage. These include bleeding from gastrointestinal disease, such as peptic ulcer, and oesophageal varicose veins in liver disease. Occasionally, bleeding from a tumour in the bowel or the lung can be very severe. Another site from which a lot of blood can be lost is the uterus, following childbirth or miscarriage.

The body can usually withstand the sudden loss of less than 500 millilitres of blood. This corresponds to about one-eighth of the circulating volume. This is the amount of blood that is withdrawn from the vein of a blood donor in one session. Nevertheless, it is not uncommon for blood donors to feel dizzy or faint immediately after giving blood. This symptom arises because the body has not had time to adjust to the sudden reduction in volume of the blood.

When the blood volume is suddenly reduced as a result of haemorrhage, there is an immediate drop in blood pressure. This can be compared to suddenly releasing air from a bicycle tyre so that the tyre pressure drops. A sudden drop in blood pressure causes an immediate drop in the amount of oxygen and nutrients that can reach the tissues. The brain responds most rapidly to this change, as it requires an adequate level of oxygen and glucose to function well. The lack of oxygen and glucose in the brain is the cause of dizziness and fainting, and if the drop is very severe the person may lose consciousness.

There are 'sensors' in the circulation that can detect a sudden drop in blood pressure. The most important of these are situated in the aorta and the carotid vessels of the neck. These are part of a negative-feedback loop (see Chapter 1.1c), which ensures that the blood pressure is kept at a steady level. As soon as the blood pressure drops, the sensors trigger a series of bodily changes to ensure that the tissues regain a supply of oxygen and nutrients. It is not necessary to go into too much detail about the mechanism of the negative-feedback loop. However, it is helpful to understand that one of the results of a drop in blood pressure is that a range of hormones, including adrenaline, renin, and the body's natural steroid, cortisol, are released into the bloodstream. All these hormones have effects on the body that tend to increase the blood pressure. They also tend to increase the availability to the tissues of nutrients stored in the body. Adrenaline, renin and cortisol are all released from the region of the body in which the kidneys are located. Adrenaline and cortisol are made in the adrenal glands, and renin in the kidneys themselves.

These responses include an increase in the heart rate, constriction of the blood vessels, particularly in the superficial parts of the body (leading to coldness of the hands and feet), conservation of water by the kidneys, release of sugar into the blood from the liver, and the emotional response of panic or fear (see Q3.4d-1).

To summarise, after an initial drop in blood volume from haemorrhage, there are a number of bodily responses that have the effect of increasing the supply of blood and nutrients to the tissues, and in particular to the deep organs. From a patient's point of view, the experience of acute blood loss will bring about symptoms of dizziness and feeling faint. There will also be profound symptoms resulting from the bodily reaction to this blood loss. The patient will have a racing heart, and clammy and cold hands and feet. They will pass very little urine. The dizziness and faint feeling might be overcome by a sense of urgency, panic or fear.

If blood loss continues, these bodily reactions are not sufficient to protect the tissues from lack of oxygen and sugar. The patient will feel increasingly cold at their core. The heart rate might slow down again as the body 'gives up'. Faintness and confusion may increase, and gradually the patient will lose consciousness. Without urgent medical treatment, the patient in this state is very close to death.

Shock

'Shock' is the medical term used to describe the syndrome of these bodily responses to a sudden reduction in the supply of oxygen and nutrients to the tissues. However, sudden haemorrhage is only one cause of shock (see Q3.4d-2).

Shock can result from three other medically significant causes: acute heart failure, acute allergic reaction and severe infection.

Shock resulting from acute heart failure

In acute heart failure, the pumping action of the heart suddenly deteriorates. This may be due to cardiac arrest or another arrhythmia, weakening of the heart muscle following a heart attack, or compression of the heart through injury.

Shock resulting from acute allergic reaction (anaphylaxis)

Anaphylactic shock is the most severe form of allergic reaction. In cases of severe allergy there is a dramatic release of a number of chemicals of inflammation into the bloodstream. The function of these in health is to cause dilatation of the blood vessels and leakage of fluid into the tissues. However, in excessive quantities they cause a life-threatening reaction involving widespread swelling of the tissues, spasm of the bronchi and bronchioles (asthma), and a sudden drop in blood pressure.

Shock resulting from severe infection (endotoxic shock)

In very severe infection, toxins released by the infectious organism can cause a similar reaction of dilatation of all the blood vessels in the body. This is a life-threatening condition called 'endotoxic shock'.

Fainting

Profound emotion can also lead to a sudden drop in blood pressure, so much so as to cause fainting (see Chapter 3.2a). This reaction will rarely lead to a prolonged condition of shock in the medical sense of the term, because it is so readily reversed by the bodily reactions triggered by the sudden drop in blood pressure. However, technically speaking, for the brief period leading up to the faint, the body is in the state of shock. Although there are no life-threatening consequences, there is no doubt that the body in such a situation has had to respond in a sudden and profound way, and will need some time to recover and regain a state of balance. This temporary but unbalanced state is what is being described when we hear on the news that people involved in traumatic situations have been treated for 'shock'.

The treatment of shock

Treatment of shock should always involve treating the cause with measures including stemming blood loss, treating heart failure, and treating any infections with antibiotics.

Treatment of the temporary shock that results from emotional trauma involves allowing the person to rest, giving sweet warm drinks and emotional support. However, when the state of shock is very profound, this has to be treated as an urgent priority. Patients in severe shock are ideally managed in an intensive care unit, with close monitoring of the important body functions.

In situations in which fluid has been lost from the circulation, it can be replaced by rapid infusions of saline and blood. When it is the cardiovascular system and not the volume of blood that is the problem, a wide range of drugs, including adrenaline, are given to encourage the heart to beat faster and the blood vessels to constrict. The insertion of an intravenous cannula (tube), fed via the superficial veins of the neck deep into the right side of the heart (a central line), may be necessary so that fluid pressures can be assessed accurately.

Information Box 3.4d-I

Shock: comments from a Chinese medicine perspective

In Chinese medicine, an emotional or physical shock is believed to deplete the Kidneys, and in particular the Jing, which is a deep reserve of condensed Qi. In conventional medicine terms, the body responds to the state of shock by the release of powerful hormones, many of which either originate from or affect the kidneys. This response draws on stored nutrients in the body. Here the possible correspondence with the Chinese medicine view is clear.

In the case of haemorrhage, treatment with blood and fluids is an appropriate energetic remedy because it replaces the lost Blood and Yin. Treatment of other forms of shock with drugs that stimulate the kidneys and cardiovascular system, such as adrenaline, boost Kidney and Heart Yang. In doing so they draw on the body's deep reserves of Yin and Yang, and so are ultimately depleting. Although life-saving in the short term, these treatments are ultimately suppressive in nature.

Blood transfusion

In many situations the transfusion of whole blood or components of the blood is a life-saving treatment when the body requires replacement of these substances.

Ideally, blood donors are healthy individuals. In the UK, blood donors are volunteers, who are asked a series of 'screening' questions in order to exclude potential donors who may have come in contact with any of the infectious diseases that affect the blood, such as human immunodeficiency virus

(HIV) and hepatitis. In addition, a simple blood test is used to exclude people who are anaemic.

All donated blood is screened for infectious diseases, such as HIV, hepatitis and syphilis, and is treated to kill infectious agents. The blood is then typed according to the ABO and rhesus blood groups.

In very severe acute blood loss, whole blood is occasionally used as the replacement treatment. However, in most cases only one part of the blood is required by the patient. For these cases, the blood is separated into its component parts of plasma, white cells, platelets and red cells. The plasma proteins can be separated from the plasma so that people who are in need of clotting factors or antibodies might be given these factors only.

The risks of blood transfusion

Blood transfusion carries risks, and for this reason should not be performed unless considered absolutely necessary. These risks include the transmission of infection and the problems that can result from incompatibility with the blood of the recipient.

Despite screening and treatment for infections, there is always a risk that donated blood carries infectious agents. Recent history provides tragic examples of the problems caused by the transmission of infections such as HIV and hepatitis C and D via donated blood products. These were infections which, at the time of the transfusions, were not fully recognised. It has been estimated that before hepatitis C testing was introduced in 1991, up to 1% of all transfusions led to this form of hepatitis in the recipient. It is very possible that there are still some infections, not yet isolated, which might in the future be found in donated blood.

Although the risks of infection from transfusion of blood products are considered to be very low, they are of course increased in those people who require repeated transfusions. This is the reason why so many patients with haemophilia, who need regular transfusions of clotting factors, have developed hepatitis C and HIV in recent years (see Chapter 2.1c).

The other risk of transfusion comes from incompatibility. Ideally, before each transfusion, the blood of the donor and the recipient is 'cross-matched'. This is a laboratory test to rule out the possibility of an immune reaction that could lead to damage of either the donated or the recipient's blood cells. The test involves checking that antibodies to the red blood cells are not present. Again, although cross-matching very much reduces the risk of major immune reactions, it is not fail-safe.

Incompatibility reactions are more common in patients who receive repeated blood transfusions because they gradually build up immunity to all the foreign blood cells that their body encounters. This can become very problematic in conditions such as thalassaemia, in which repeated transfusions are necessary.

A mild reaction may simply involve a fever or rash, which settles down over a few hours. This is thought to result from immune reactions between the plasma proteins or white cells of the recipient and donor. Mild reactions are common. However, in rare cases, this reaction is very severe, leading to high fever and a form of anaphylactic shock. In this life-threatening situation the patient may need to be given intravenous adrenaline, antihistamines and corticosteroids to reverse the reaction.

Incompatibility of red cells is a very serious situation. The damaged red cells can clump to cause infarction and will release a lot of haemoglobin into the circulation. This can damage the kidneys, and the bilirubin that is formed leads to a severe form of jaundice.

The clinical uses of transfusion of blood products

Blood is most commonly used in the UK to replace losses that have occurred through haemorrhage from injury, disease or surgery. Unless blood loss is very severe, red cells are transfused, rather than whole blood, as this minimises the risks of incompatibility from the other parts of the blood. Fluid losses are replaced by intravenous saline solution.

As described in Chapter 3.4c, red cells are also used in certain types of anaemia, such as aplastic anaemia and thalassaemia, to increase the numbers of red cells in the circulating blood. These transfusions have to be repeated at regular intervals because the life of red cells in transfused blood is no more than 1–2 months.

Platelets may be used in severe cases of thrombocytopenia and bone marrow failure, to increase the clotting function of the blood.

Plasma is used to provide clotting factors in situations such as severe infection and trauma, when the body's own supply of clotting factors has been used up.

Individual clotting factors can be given to patients with haemophilia. Nowadays these can be treated to kill all viruses, and so do not carry the risks of the cell-containing blood products.

Antibodies can be obtained from the pooled plasma of many donors. These are most commonly used in the practice of vaccination to generate 'passive' immunity. This is only a temporary immunity because the antibodies have a life of about 3 months. Preparations of human antibodies are called 'immunoglobulins', and are most useful in vulnerable people who have had recent exposure to a dangerous disease such as rabies, when there is no time for the patient to develop their own immune response.

Information Box 3.4d-II

Transfusion: comments from a Chinese medicine perspective

In Chinese medicine, the transfusion of blood products would appear to be a form of Nourishing Blood and Yin. However, transfused blood can never perfectly match the requirements of the patient. The presence of foreign antigens and antibodies, as well as infectious agents in blood products, is a potential form of Xie Qi, which can have damaging effects on the body by leading to the Invasion of Pathogenic Factors and depletion of Vital Substances.

Conversely, the donation of blood will deplete the Blood, Yin and Qi of the donor. Although the lives of many people depend on blood donation, blood donors should be made aware of the way in which it can cause depletion. In fit individuals, the losses can be made up through attention to rest and diet. Blood donation may not be advisable in those who are already deficient in Blood and/or Qi.

The disorders of the spleen

In this concluding section of this chapter the ways in which the spleen is affected by disease are explored (see Q3.4d-3).

The spleen is composed of two different sorts of tissue, called the 'white pulp' and the 'red pulp' because of their physical appearance.

The role of the white pulp is as part of the immune system. This part of the spleen can be compared to a very large lymph node through which all blood flows. The spleen houses many lymphocytes, some of which mature as they rest within it. The spleen is important in the development of immunity to disease and the production of antibodies.

The primary role of the red pulp in health is to ensure the removal of ageing and misshapen red blood cells and platelets. This leads to the release of iron and bilirubin into the circulation. This role of the red pulp is also shared by the liver and bone marrow. The red pulp also has the capability of housing bone marrow tissue. This means that, in times of stress, extra blood cells can be made within the spleen. This capability is also shared by the liver.

Information Box 3.4d-III

The spleen: comments from a Chinese medicine perspective

In Chinese medicine, the roles of the spleen recognised by conventional medicine cannot be directly attributed to the Spleen Organ. In turn, the digestive function of the Spleen Organ is more properly attributed to the various functions of the conventional gastrointestinal system. However, the main role of the red pulp of the spleen can be seen to overlap with this function, in that it breaks down the ageing blood cells and enables the nutrients contained therein to be recycled for further use in the body.

Another function of the red pulp is that it literally 'holds blood'. Up to one-third of the platelets are stored within the spleen, from where they can be released when necessary. Here is a remarkable correspondence with the ancient Chinese view that one function of the healthy Spleen is to hold blood and so to prevent bleeding.

The role of the white pulp of the spleen in the immune system much more closely fits with the combined roles of Wei Qi and its foundation Kidney Jing. As discussed in Chapter 2.1d, these are the Substances that are seen in Chinese medicine to be important in protecting the body from invasion by Pathogenic Factors of external origin.

Rupture of the spleen

This is probably the most common condition to affect the spleen and is a consequence of modern life. This is because the trauma that is associated with a serious road traffic accident very commonly involves the spleen. It is a complication of seat belts that they can forcefully compress the abdomen in an accident that has occurred at high speed, and in this way the spleen can be damaged. However, the damage that can result from not wearing a seat belt is potentially far more severe than rupture of the spleen.

The spleen has a delicate lining and is very vulnerable to trauma. Once damaged, bleeding from the spleen can be profuse. It is a surgical emergency, often requiring a large transfusion of blood. Occasionally, the damage is so severe that repair is impossible, and the spleen is removed to stop the bleeding.

Loss of the spleen (asplenism)

The spleen is most commonly removed because of damage in traumatic accidents as described above. However, there are certain conditions in which the spleen is removed for medical reasons in a surgical operation known as a 'splenectomy'. These include those conditions in which there is a need to preserve red blood cells or platelets, which are usually removed by the spleen. Splenectomy may be performed for these reasons in conditions such as thalassaemia and thrombocytopenia.

Sometimes the spleen has to be removed because it has become too large. This can be a problem because a large spleen will cause excessive destruction of blood cells and can lead to anaemia and thrombocytopenia.

In the short term, the loss of the spleen leads to a build up of platelets because these can no longer be removed from the blood as rapidly, and this may lead problems with excessive blood clotting. However, in a few weeks this problem settles down as the liver and the bone marrow begin to take over this role of the red pulp of the spleen.

The major long-term problem with splenectomy is that there is a risk of the patient developing overwhelming infections. For a reason that is unclear, patients are particularly at risk of infections caused by the very common respiratory bacterium *Streptococcus pneumoniae*. For this reason, all patients are given a vaccination to protect against streptococcal infections. Some patients may be prescribed regular penicillin to reduce further the risk of infections.

Information Box 3.4d-IV

Loss of the spleen: comments from a Chinese medicine perspective

In Chinese medicine, loss of the spleen does not directly correspond with Spleen Deficiency, as digestive symptoms are not prominent. Much of the role of the red pulp is not lost, but it is taken over by the liver and bone marrow. The main problem that results from splenectomy is impaired immunity, and in particular to an infection that normally leads to Wind Heat progressing to Lung Heat. This suggests that loss of the Spleen must in some ways be regarded as equivalent to a form of Depletion of Wei Qi and possibly also of Kidney Jing.

Enlarged spleen (hypersplenism)

In health, the spleen is about the size of a large fist and sits at the back of the abdominal cavity, resting against the tenth to twelfth ribs on the left. It normally cannot be felt on examination of the abdomen.

In certain conditions the spleen can enlarge to an enormous size. Sometimes the spleen can be felt extending below the umbilicus in the front of the abdomen. This can occasionally result from infections, and tropical infections in particular. However, glandular fever is the most common cause of temporary enlargement of the spleen in the UK, and leads to the common symptom of pain under the ribs on the left-hand side. Occasionally, the enlargement of the spleen in glandular fever can be so rapid as to lead to rupture, although this complication is very rare.

> **Information Box 3.4d-V**
>
> **Enlargement of the spleen: comments from a Chinese medicine perspective**
>
> The condition of an enlarged spleen can lead to anaemia and bleeding due to excessive destruction of the red cells and platelets. This would be consistent with the symptoms associated with Deficiency of Blood and Yin, with Spleen Qi not holding Blood.

Another cause of a very enlarged spleen is cancer of the blood cells (leukaemia and lymphoma), which is described in the next chapter. In these cancers the spleen enlarges as it fills up with excessive cancerous white blood cells.

The main problem of an enlarged spleen is that it can cause excessive destruction of the red cells and platelets. If this becomes a severe problem, the spleen can be surgically removed (see Q3.4d-4).

The red flags of haemorrhage and shock

Red flags are those symptoms and signs that indicate that referral to a conventional doctor is to be considered. The red flags of the conditions discussed in this chapter are described in Table 3.4d-I. This table forms part of the summary on red flags given in Appendix III, which also gives advice on the degree of urgency of referral for each of the red flag conditions listed.

Table 3.4d-I Red Flags 19 – haemorrhage and shock

Red Flag	Description	Reasoning
19.1	**Continuing blood loss**: any situation in which significant bleeding is continuing for more than a few minutes without any signs of abating, except within the context of menstruation	An adequate volume of blood in the circulation is essential to maintain the blood pressure required to enable adequate perfusion of the organs and tissues of the body. If the blood pressure drops too low, the syndrome of shock develops, which is defined as 'a situation in which there is a failure of the circulatory system to maintain adequate perfusion of vital organs' If bleeding is continuing unabated, and this is of particular concern if the bleeding is from an internal location, then the patient needs to be referred for fluid replacement and medical or surgical intervention to prevent further blood loss Administer basic first aid to accessible bleeding sites whilst help arrives
19.2	**Features of severe blood loss leading to shock**: refer if blood has been lost and the following symptoms and signs have been present **for more than a few minutes**, or are **worsening**: **dizziness**, **fainting** and **confusion**; **rapid pulse** of more than 100 beats/minute; **blood pressure less than 90/60 mmHg**; **cold and clammy extremities**	If the symptoms of shock (see notes above) are developing, this is an emergency situation Administer basic first aid to bleeding sites. Ensure that the patient is lying down and is kept warm as you wait for help to arrive
19.3	**General symptoms of shock: dizziness**, **fainting** and **confusion**; **rapid pulse** of more than 100 beats/minute; **blood pressure less than 90/60 mmHg**; **cold and clammy extremities** Refer if these symptoms are **worsening** or **sustained** (more than a few seconds)	Shock can also result from an allergic reaction (anaphylactic shock), in the situation of overwhelming infection (endotoxic shock), in the situation of extreme dehydration (hypovolaemic shock), and failure of the heart to maintain an adequate circulation (cardiogenic shock resulting from damage to the heart muscle or heart valves, or from an arrhythmia) Sustained shock is always a situation in which treatment is required as an emergency, as the vulnerable organs of the brain, kidneys and heart are at risk of damage from inadequate levels of oxygen and nutrients A faint can produce a syndrome that is akin to shock, but the drop in blood pressure is always short lived and the person should start to recover within seconds. In the case of a faint the drop in blood pressure follows a sudden slowing of the heart rate, so a weak and slow pulse would be the norm in the few seconds following a faint, and this should return to a normal within 1–2 minutes. There is no need to refer in this situation
19.4	Additional symptoms of **anaphylactic shock: widespread inflammatory response – warm extremities**, **puffy skin**, **difficulty breathing**	In anaphylactic shock the drop in blood pressure is a result of an extreme allergic reaction. In this case the collapse may be preceded by a hives-like swelling of the skin and worsening asthma. This is an emergency situation as the symptoms can worsen rapidly to a state of respiratory and circulatory collapse

Self-test 3.4d

Acute blood loss, transfusion and disorders of the spleen

1. You are called out to see an elderly patient who has collapsed in your clinic waiting room. You find that she is slumped on her chair but is conscious. She says that she feels slightly sick and light-headed, but has no other symptoms. When you take her pulse you find that it is deep, weak and fine. The rhythm is regular but the rate is 100 beats/minute. Her hands are cold and clammy. As you talk to her she complains that the sensation of light-headedness is worsening. When you take her pulse again you find that the rate has increased to 110 beats/minute.
   (i) What medical condition do these symptoms suggest?
   (ii) What do you think are possible causes in this patient?
   (iii) What should be your course of action?
2. You are treating a 25-year-old student for mild eczema. He is generally fairly fit. Your Chinese medical diagnosis of his condition is Damp Heat with underlying Blood Deficiency. He tells you that this week he is going to give blood as he has been doing every 6 months for the past 3 years. How might you respond to this information?

Answers

1. (i) These symptoms suggest the medical condition of shock.
   (ii) Shock can result from the emotional disturbance that can lead to a faint (temporary), acute blood loss, acute heart failure, severe allergy (anaphylaxis) or very severe infection (endotoxic shock).

   In this patient the symptoms and signs are worsening. This is not characteristic of a simple faint. The most likely cause in this elderly person is acute heart failure, either as a result of a silent heart attack leading to a weakened heart muscle, or from the sudden onset of an arrhythmia.

   It is also possible that this patient has suddenly developed some internal bleeding. The most likely site for this is from the stomach or bowel. Bleeding in these sites may not become apparent for some time. Another possible site for severe and sudden internal bleeding is from a ruptured aortic aneurysm.

   NB: Do not get confused by the lack of symptoms. In some elderly people, even very severe internal disease may lead to vague symptoms only, such as feeling sick.

   (iii) You should telephone for an ambulance as a matter of urgency. While you are waiting, you should ensure your patient is kept warm and help her to lie down. You should not give her anything to eat or drink, as she may require emergency surgery if internal bleeding is the cause of the shock. As long as she consents to this, there is no reason why you should not give your patient emergency acupuncture treatment whilst you are waiting for the ambulance to arrive.
2. You may wish to advise this patient on the Chinese medical view of the energetics of blood donation. Choosing words and phrases to match your patient's outlook, you could explain that in Chinese medicine loss of the blood would be seen as a Depletion of some of the Vital Substances of the body. Although these may be recovered by proper attention to rest and diet, this may be more problematic in this particular patient as he is already deficient in Blood. It is also important that you inform your patient that if he donates blood in the UK, he may not be permitted to do so within 4 months of last receiving acupuncture treatment unless that treatment was offered by a qualified Healthcare Professional registered with a statutory body.

Chapter 3.4e Cancer of the blood cells

LEARNING POINTS

At the end of this chapter you will:
- be able to recognise the main features of leukaemia, lymphoma and myeloma
- understand the principles of treatment of the cancers of the blood cells
- be able to recognise the red flags of cancer of the blood cells.

Estimated time for chapter: 90 minutes.

Introduction

This chapter is concerned with the three main types of cancer of the white blood cells: leukaemia, lymphoma and myeloma. These are the focus of a single chapter because, as blood is a fluid tissue, cancer of the blood has characteristics that are different to the solid cancers described in Chapter 2.3a.

The cancers of the blood are relatively rare. Leukaemia and lymphoma are particularly well known because, although rare, they are two of the most common forms of cancer that affect children and young adults. These are also unusual forms of cancer in that often they can be cured by medical treatment, particularly in young people.

This chapter focuses on the clinical features and treatment of these three most common forms of cancer.

Leukaemia

'Leukaemia' is a term derived from the Greek words meaning 'white blood'. This description refers to the fact that the numbers of white blood cells in the circulating blood can be greatly increased in some forms of leukaemia. Leukaemia results from a cancerous mutation in a single immature white blood cell within the bone marrow. The cancerous change means that this single cell multiplies at an uncontrolled rate, just as occurs in solid cancers.

The cause of leukaemia

In most individual cases no cause can be found for the cancerous change. However, it is recognised that certain environmental factors increase the risk of leukaemia. There is clear evidence of a link between leukaemia and exposure to radioactive 'fallout' after an atomic explosion, such as occurred in the communities living close to Hiroshima. It is also clear that high doses or cumulative exposure to x-rays can increase the risk of developing leukaemia. Certain chemicals, including benzene, and drugs, including some used in cancer chemotherapy, are also known to increase the risk of leukaemia.

The tendency to leukaemia runs slightly in families, suggesting a genetic susceptibility. It is also more common in people with Down syndrome.

The types of leukaemia

There are many different types of leukaemia and these can be categorised according to the exact type of white blood cell that has mutated, the surface chemistry of the cancer cells and the form of their chromosomes. Each type of leukaemia can also be broadly categorised as either acute leukaemia or chronic leukaemia. This categorisation is made on the basis of the speed of development of the leukaemia. Acute leukaemia is the type that most commonly affects children and young adults.

Acute leukaemia

In acute leukaemia the cancerous white blood cells multiply extremely rapidly and cause symptoms because they take over the bone marrow space. This leads to the life-threatening syndrome of bone marrow failure, which was described in Chapter 3.4c (see Q3.4e-1).

Acute leukaemia can be diagnosed on the basis of a FBC and blood film, and a bone marrow investigation, in which the excessive numbers of white blood cells can be clearly measured and seen.

Without urgent treatment, the patient will inevitably succumb to severe infection or haemorrhage within days or weeks of diagnosis. Bone pain may be a prominent symptom.

The treatment of acute leukaemia should take place in a specialised environment in which the patient is kept at low risk of infection. Any infections that develop are treated with high-dose intravenous antibiotics. Anaemia and thrombocytopenia may require transfusions of red cells and platelets, respectively.

The cancer is treated with cycles of chemotherapy (including drugs such as vincristine, prednisolone, asparaginase and doxorubicin) over the course of 6–12 months. In cases in which it is assessed that there is a high risk of spread of cancer cells to the nervous system, the chemotherapy is given into the spinal fluid as well as intravenously. The treatment itself damages the already depleted cells of the bone marrow, and so the patient has to be intensively nursed during this period. In some types of acute leukaemia the cancer cells are rapidly destroyed by the treatment. If the patient can survive the risky period of treatment, they may be left with no measurable evidence of leukaemia. However, although there is no evidence of leukaemia, it is still possible that a few cancer cells remain in the body. This state is called 'remission'.

In the most common form of childhood leukaemia, up to 90% of children enter complete remission. However, in adults, and in other forms of acute leukaemia, the success rate is not so high. Without more intensive 'consolidation' treatment, after months to a few years the leukaemia reappears, this time in a form that is more resistant to treatment. Therefore, to prevent these relapses, further 'maintenance' chemotherapy may be given, or a bone marrow transplant may be performed.

Bone marrow transplant involves replacing the potentially cancer-containing bone marrow of the patient with a sample of healthy bone marrow. This can involve use of the patient's own bone marrow, which is withdrawn by a needle just after remission has been induced by chemotherapy. It can only be hoped that this sample does not contain lingering cancer cells. Alternatively, transplant involves the use of marrow from a donor, who ideally is a close relative of the patient.

The principle of bone marrow transplant is first to totally kill all remaining bone marrow after remission has been induced by high-dose chemotherapy (cyclophosphamide) and irradiation. This is a most risky time for the patient, as all the blood-forming stem cells have been removed and the patient becomes totally dependent for a time on transfused blood products. The healthy bone marrow sample is then injected into one of the patient's veins. The stem cells within the sample find their way into the patient's marrow spaces and start to multiply. If successful, the transplant will 'take' and new blood cells will start to be produced.

There is a risk that marrow from a donor will not 'take' because the white cells within it start to damage the patient's tissues, which they recognise as 'foreign' (so-called 'graft-versus-host' disease). This is more likely to occur if a non-relative's marrow is used. To prevent this, the patient has to stay on immunosuppressive medication for life (see Chapter 2.2c).

Up to one-third of patients who receive donated marrow die during the treatment. The risks are lower with the use of the patient's own marrow, but the risks of cancer recurrence are greater. In those who survive the treatment, bone marrow transplant can bring about cure of the leukaemia, but in every case a very careful risk–benefit analysis has to be made. For this reason, bone marrow transplants are generally performed in the forms of leukaemia that are less likely to respond to chemotherapy alone.

The long-term effects of cancer chemotherapy on children cannot be estimated fully because this form of treatment has only been used widely with success over the past three or four decades. There is no doubt that the physical depletion that results from the toxic drugs and corticosteroids given at such a vulnerable time in development is great, and problems in lung function, thyroid function, fertility and growth may become apparent. It is increasingly being recognised that the psychological impact of having a life-threatening disease for a period of 2 years or more in childhood is also very significant. In addition, the time scale and severity of treatment cause shock waves that affect all the close relatives of the sick child.

Chronic leukaemia

Chronic leukaemia is a disease of older people. In chronic leukaemia, the onset of the disease is much slower than in acute leukaemia. The underlying cause is the same, a multiplication of a cancerous white blood cell. Chronic leukaemia is also classified on the basis of cell type, and also the chromosomal status of the cells. The different manifestations include chronic myelocytic leukaemia (CML), chronic lymphocytic leukaemia

Information Box 3.4e-I

Acute leukaemia: comments from a Chinese medicine perspective

The stem cells in the bone marrow, viewed from the perspective of Chinese medicine, could be seen as one of the physical roots of Blood and Yin, as these are the source of the healthy blood cells. In this way they could be seen as corresponding to Kidney Jing. The stem cells are crowded out in acute leukaemia. Therefore, in Chinese medicine acute leukaemia could be interpreted as severe deficiency of Jing, Blood and Yin. The immune deficiency and bleeding suggest that there is additional deficiency of Spleen and Lung Qi.

The cause of these deficiencies is the rapidly dividing cancerous white cells. These can be likened to Phlegm. This is a comparison that accords with the appearance of the swollen lymph tissue which develops in some forms of leukaemia.

Chemotherapy would be seen as Clearing of Phlegm but depleting of Jing, Blood and Yin because it too destroys bone marrow tissue. This has to be suppressive in nature, because the root cause is not treated. Many individuals can survive this depletion, probably because they have deep reserves of Vital Substances, which can be built up once the Phlegm has been cleared. This might explain why children have the best chances of a cure from leukaemia.

Bone marrow transplant literally replaces the lost vital substances of Jing, Blood and Yin. However, as with blood transfusion, there is a high risk of the introduction of Pathogenic Xie Qi with the treatment.

(CLL), and a cluster of conditions of abnormal cellular development of the bone marrow called myelodysplastic syndromes.

Because of the slow onset, less acute symptoms such as enlarged lymph nodes or recurrent low fevers may be the first symptoms. Sometimes the diagnosis is made by chance because a FBC blood test is taken for another unrelated reason.

As the condition progresses, the multiplication of cancer cells tends to become more active and a transformation to acute leukaemia can develop. Treatment with chemotherapy (including chlorambucil, corticosteroids, alpha-interferon and imatinib), can slow the disease, but is not expected to be curative. However, a few patients can be cured with a combination of chemotherapy and a bone marrow transplant. Even if cure is not achieved, symptoms can be held at bay by intermittent drug treatment, and in some cases they may not necessarily lead to premature death.

Information Box 3.4e-II

Chronic leukaemia: comments from a Chinese medicine perspective

The Chinese medicine interpretation of chronic leukaemia is similar to that of acute leukaemia. The chances of long-term survival are lower, possibly because the reserves of Vital Substances are much lower in older people.

Lymphoma

Lymphoma is a tumour of the white blood cells that originates not in the bone marrow but in lymph tissue. The most common site for a lymphoma to develop is in a lymph node, but it can also occasionally emerge from within the lymphoid cells that line the respiratory tract or the gastrointestinal tract.

One type of lymphoma, called Hodgkin's disease, is particularly common in young adults. This tumour predominantly affects the lymph nodes of the neck and is potentially curable.

As well as an abnormal swelling of a lymph node, Hodgkin's disease can lead to symptoms such as fevers, itching and loss of appetite. Often the disease can be diagnosed early in its development because the swollen lymph nodes in the neck are very noticeable.

Other forms of lymphoma may have similar symptoms, although these can also affect deep lymph nodes or other sites such as the bowel, and so diagnosis may be delayed. In advanced lymphoma, a number of lymph nodes as well as the spleen and liver may be found to be enlarged by cancerous white blood cells. If untreated, lymphoma causes death for reasons similar to other solid tumours.

Early Hodgkin's disease is unusual in that it can be cured by radiotherapy to the affected nodes alone. Although this carries risks of long-term damage to the healthy tissues that have been irradiated, this treatment has a very high cure rate of over 95%.

Advanced Hodgkin's disease may also be cured by a combination of chemotherapy (usually the ABVD regimen of adriamycin, bleomycin, vinblastine and dacarbazine) and radiotherapy, although the success rate is lower. If Hodgkin's disease recurs after treatment, it is almost never curable.

Some of the other lymphomas can be cured by radiotherapy alone or by a combination of chemotherapy (including chlorambucil, alpha-interferon, rituximab, and the CHCP regimen of cyclophosphamide, hydroxydaunorubicin, vincristine and prednisolone together with rituximab) and radiotherapy. Most non-Hodgkin's lymphoma is less responsive to treatment, and the tumour eventually reappears in a form that cannot be cured.

Myeloma

Myeloma is a rare cancer of those white cells that produce antibodies. It predominantly affects elderly people. The cancerous cells cause three main problems which are characteristic of myeloma.

First, the myeloma cells multiply within bone tissue, and this causes weak areas of bone that are prone to fracture and which are a source of intense pain. Second, the myeloma cells release excessive amounts of protein into the bloodstream. This protein is similar in form to the antibody protein, immunoglobulin, but has no value in protection against infection. In high concentrations it tends to cause damage to the kidneys

Information Box 3.4e-III

Lymphoma: comments from a Chinese medicine perspective

In Chinese medicine, lymphoma, like most solid tumours, could be seen as Phlegm with Blood Stagnation against a background of Depletion of Yin and/or Yang.

and can lead to kidney failure. Finally, in advanced disease, the cancerous cells take over the bone marrow and cause bone marrow failure.

The progression of myeloma can be slowed down by chemotherapy. In elderly patients the chemotherapy used (usually melphalan or cyclophosphamide with prednisolone and thalidomide) has a much lower risk of bone marrow failure than that used in leukaemia. In younger people, a more aggressive combination of drugs may be used (such as the VAD regimen: vincristine, adriamycin and dexamethasone), and bone marrow transplant may be considered.

Eventually, the cancerous cells in myeloma progress to a form of acute leukaemia. Patients usually die either from bone marrow failure or from kidney failure. Even with treatment death occurs on average at 3–4 years after diagnosis (see Q3.4e-2).

The red flags of leukaemia and lymphoma

Red flags are those symptoms and signs that indicate that referral to a conventional doctor is to be considered. The red flags of the conditions discussed in this chapter are described in Table 3.4e-I. This table forms part of the summary on red flags given in Appendix III, which also gives advice on the degree of urgency of referral for each of the red flag conditions listed.

Information Box 3.4e-IV

Myeloma: comments from a Chinese medicine perspective

In Chinese medicine, the interpretation of myeloma could be similar to that of leukaemia, because the symptoms are comparable. The presence of bone pain suggests that Blood Stagnation contributes to the symptoms.

Table 3.4e-I Red Flags 20 – leukaemia and lymphoma

Red Flag	Description	Reasoning
20.1	**Features of bone marrow failure**: symptoms of progressive **anaemia** (see Red Flags Table A18 in Appendix III), recurrent progressive **infections**, progressive **easy bruising**, **purpura** and **bleeding**	The bone marrow contains the stem cells for the three major cellular components of the blood: the red cells, platelets and white blood cells. Bone marrow can fail to produce healthy blood cells if infiltrated by cancer, damaged by medication (including cancer chemotherapy) or radiation, and sometimes as a result of an autoimmune disease. Bone marrow failure is a life-threatening situation
20.2	**Multiple enlarged lymph nodes** (>1 cm in diameter) but painless, with no other obvious cause (i.e. known glandular fever infection)	Groups of lymph nodes can be found in the cervical region, in the armpits (axillary nodes) and in the inguinal creases (groin). In health, the lymph nodes are usually impalpable masses of soft tissue, but they can enlarge and become more palpable when the node is active in fighting an infection or if it is infiltrated by tumour cells. If a number of nodes are enlarged (to >1 cm in diameter) this may signify a generalised infectious disease such as glandular fever The other important cause of widespread lymph node enlargement (lymphadenopathy) is cancer, and in particular the cancers of the white blood cells: leukaemia and lymphoma If multiple enlarged lymph nodes are found it is best to refer for a diagnosis, and as a high priority if the patient is unwell
20.3	**A single markedly enlarged lymph node** (>2 cm in diameter) with no other obvious cause	Even in the situation of infection it is unusual for a lymph node to become grossly enlarged. Cancerous infiltration can lead to a firm, enlarged lymph node, which may be painless. This is particularly typical of lymphoma Unexplained fever, weight loss and itching are other symptoms which, together with lymph node enlargement, are suggestive of lymphoma

Self-test 3.4e

Cancer of the blood cells

1. A 58-year-old new patient of yours tells you that he has been given a diagnosis of chronic leukaemia. His story is that he went to the doctor because he had found swollen lymph nodes in his neck and armpits. A blood test was abnormal, and the doctor referred him to a haematologist for further tests, including a bone marrow examination. A diagnosis of chronic lymphocytic leukaemia (CLL) was made.

   The patient's doctor has told him that his form of leukaemia is slow growing and will need treatment only if he develops further symptoms. This patient has come for acupuncture because he hopes that alternative treatment can complement his conventional treatment and help him fight the cancer.

   (i) What do you think could be the long-term outlook for your patient?

   (ii) What sort of red flags might alert you to the fact that his disease might be progressing more rapidly?

   (iii) Should you have any concerns about using acupuncture on this patient?

Answers

1. (i) CLL, although incurable, may run a very slow course with the time scale of 9–10 years, after which the progression of the disease leads to bone marrow failure. This patient has not been offered any chemotherapy, which suggests that his disease poses no immediate threat and is slow growing.

   The patient can expect to be given intermittent courses of chemotherapy (by mouth) at the times when the progression of his disease has appeared to accelerate. He will remain under the close supervision of his haematologist, who will keep a check on the progression of disease through regular physical examination and blood tests.

   (ii) Features of disease progression include enlargement of the liver and spleen and then the development of bone marrow failure.

   The first sign of bone marrow failure is anaemia. You might first notice that the patient is experiencing the symptoms of anaemia. Recurrent infections and signs of excessive bruising and bleeding are strong signs that the bone marrow has been severely depleted and the CLL is at an advanced stage.

   (iii) In all the blood cancers, acupuncture will only potentially become problematic if the patient is in a state of bone marrow failure, when the reduction in white blood cells and platelets leads to a susceptibility to infections and bleeding. The risks for your patient at this early stage of disease are no different than they would be for any of your patients.

   However, it would be good practice to make formal contact with the patient's haematologist to check that he or she is happy for you to commence treatment. In the letter you could explain that you will be treating their patient, and that, as a member of a recognised professional body, you use sterile needle technique and shallow insertions. Explain that you are aware of the risks of treating in the case of bone marrow failure, but that you understand that there are no such risks at the present time.

Diseases of the nervous system

4.1

Chapter 4.1a The physiology of the nervous system

LEARNING POINTS

At the end of this chapter you will:

- understand the mechanisms by which nerve cells can enable communication between one part of the body and another
- understand how the parts of the nervous system are grouped into the central nervous system, the peripheral nervous system and the autonomic nervous system
- be able to describe the main functions of the different parts of the brain.

Estimated time for chapter: Part 1, 120 minutes; Part 2, 100 minutes.

Introduction to the nervous system

This chapter focuses on the physiology of the nervous system. Together with the endocrine system, the nervous system is one of the topics explored in this text which arguably has the most relevance to the understanding of the physical basis of holistic approaches to healing. This is because, together with the endocrine system, the nervous system is involved in the process of communication of one body part with another. Together, these systems form, from a medical perspective, part of the physical foundation of what makes the body an integrated whole. It is important to point out that some holistic practitioners, (exemplified by Myers (2001) who writes about muscle trains), also propose that the myofascial system (comprising the muscles and the body-wide interconnected web of connective tissue that links them with the periosteum of the bones) is another integrated body system that is a medium for the communication of 'energy' between disparate body parts.

The complexity of the nervous system is so great that it is very likely that it can never be fully understood by human minds. The number of brain cells alone approximates 10 billion, while the total number of connections made between these cells runs into the trillions. These connections are unique to each individual, not only as a consequence of a particular genetic make-up, but also because these connections continually form and reform in response to the personal experiences of that individual.

In the light of this complexity, it could be said that only the most basic features in this mysterious neural landscape have been understood and described by scientists. The subtleties that form the foundations for many aspects of human experience, such as the diverse emotions and spiritual experiences, have simply not yet been mapped. It is very possible that these experiences, and also the subtle phenomena that holistic therapists attribute to the movement of 'energy' described as Qi or Prana, could be explained scientifically if this unmapped part of the nervous system were explored using reductionist experimental methods. However, it may be that such knowledge will always be out of reach of the scientific experiment, being protected within the complexity of the structure of the individual human brain.

For this reason it may well be that the mechanism of the more subtle energetic approaches to healing will never be fully explained by science. For example, there is strong scientific evidence to support the role of acupuncture in the modulation of pain, but little or no evidence to explain the more subtle effects on the body's function, emotions, and even the destiny of an individual, as described in Chinese medicine theory. However, this does not mean that a physical mechanism for these subtle effects does not exist, but possibly that it is far too delicate and complex for current scientific experiment (and possibly for the human mind) to explain in physical terms.

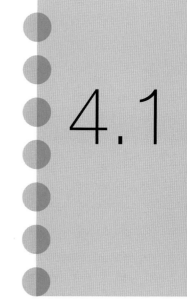

This chapter explores only the most basic of the principles of the physiology of the nervous system. Nevertheless, it might be helpful to consider that the structures described here are those parts of the body that house those aspects which many complementary therapists might recognise as essential foundations to health, such as the control of homeostasis, thoughts, emotional feelings and even the spirit.

As there is a great deal of material to study, the chapter is divided into two parts. If you are following this text as part of a study course, you are recommended to work through this chapter in two separate study sessions. Part I describes the nervous tissue, which is the basic building material for the nervous system. The three parts of the nervous system, the central nervous system, the peripheral nervous system and the autonomic nervous system, are then introduced. Finally, the central nervous system is explored in more detail. In Part II the peripheral nervous system and the autonomic nervous system are described in more detail.

Part I: The physiology of the nervous system

The nerve cells (neurons)

The foundation of the nervous system is the nerve cell, which is scientifically termed the 'neuron'. Nerve cells have the ability to relay messages between each other, and are specialised to perform this role.

The way in which this communication occurs can be compared to an old fashioned telephone exchange, which allows communication to take place between any two households that are connected to that exchange. In a telephone exchange the physical basis of the communication is electrical current, which is conducted from households through telephone wires to the exchange. The telephone acts as the receiver of information, as well as relaying the message from the household at the other end of the line. At the exchange the telephone message from one household can be specifically processed and directed to another household by means of a telephone operating system. The presence of the exchange dramatically reduces the need to have wires linking every home with all the others in the system. Each home needs to be connected only to the exchange, and similarly each body part needs to be connected only to the central nervous system in order to have a nerve-mediated influence on another body part.

In the nervous system some of the specialised nerve cells are able to receive information from the environment and translate it into an electrical message (akin to the telephone receiver). Nerve cells that receive external information and relay it to the nervous system are known as 'sensory nerve cells' (also known as 'effector nerve cells'). This term reflects the fact that these nerve cells 'sense' the environment.

Other cells are adapted to act like the telephone wires to the exchange, and relay the message via the spinal cord to other nerves cells or to the brain. The spinal cord and the brain can be seen as the telephone exchange, from which messages originating in the body are redirected to other parts of the nervous system. The nerve cells that link up different parts of the nervous system in this way are sometimes called 'connector nerve cells'.

Within the body's 'telephone exchange' the message is processed and leads to one or more response messages, which are relayed back out to the body. The nerve cells that relay messages back out to the body to bring about a change in the body's function are called 'effector nerve cells' or 'motor nerve cells'. In this text the term 'motor nerve cell' is used to describe these nerve cells. It may help to remember this term by reflecting that a motor in mechanical terms is a structure that converts energy into action. It is the same for motor nerve cells, because they allow the transformation of the energy of the electrical message that they are carrying into the action of a contraction of a single muscle cell fibre.

A simple example to illustrate this system is the bodily response to an unexpected pin prick. The message of pain is sensed and relayed by sensory nerve cells to the spinal cord. Messages returning via motor nerve cells from the spinal cord in response to this pain lead to action in the form of a rapid withdrawal of the body from the offending pin. This example describes the most basic form of reflex, which will be explained in more detail presently.

The physiology of the nerve cell

The membrane that surrounds each nerve cell is very sensitive to changes in its environment. External changes to which a nerve cell is sensitive are termed 'stimuli' (singular 'stimulus'). Sensory nerves, depending on their specific role, can respond to a diverse range of external stimuli, such as pressure, light, heat, cold and irritants. All other nerve cells respond to the stimulus of chemicals called 'neurotransmitters', which are released from the nerve cells that are near to them.

A stimulus will cause the membrane of a nerve cell to change so that an electrical impulse is transmitted to all parts of the cell membrane. The ability to convert an external stimulus to an electrical charge is called 'irritability'. The transmission of the electrical impulse to all parts of the cell is called 'conductivity'. It is these properties of irritability and conductivity that allow a stimulus at one part of the cell to be transmitted, in an electrical form, to all other parts of the cell.

All nerve cells are closely linked to other nerve cells by means of fine-branching extensions of the cell membrane called 'dendrites' (from the Greek meaning 'little trees').

Figure 4.1a-I illustrates a generalised nerve cell, and shows the long extension of the axon and the smaller tree-like extensions called dendrites. The branching dendrite-like structures at the bottom of the axons have endings called 'boutons', which are adapted to release tiny quantities of neurotransmitter chemicals from secretory vesicles inside the cell. The axon is an extension that can be very long, and for this reason it can also be termed a 'nerve fibre'. For example, the nerve cells that relay information from the feet have axons or nerve fibres that run from the spinal cord right down to the toes.

When a nerve cell receives a stimulus, the electrical impulse is conducted to the tips of all the dendrites and also down the length of the axon. Some axons are coated in a white substance called 'myelin'. This myelin sheath is simply represented in Figure 4.1a-I, but the structure of myelin is complex as it is actually a fine layer of fatty substance secreted between layers of a glial cell membrane wrapped many times around the nerve

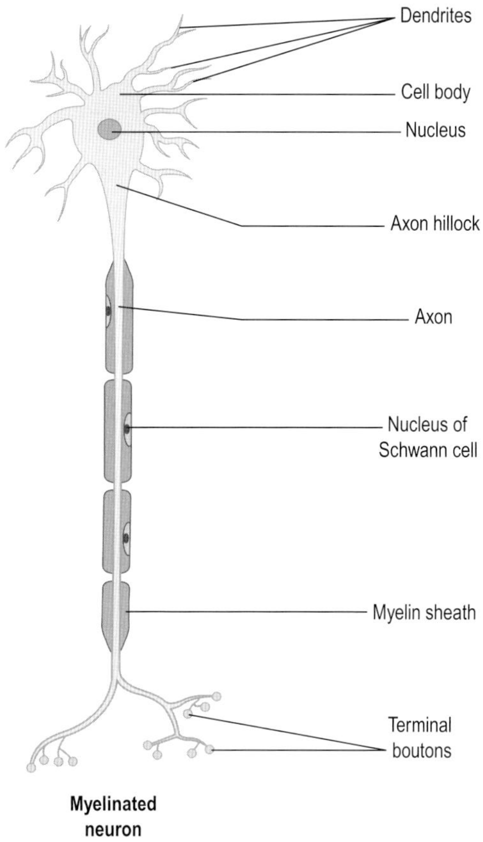

Figure 4.1a I • The structure of a typical neuron.

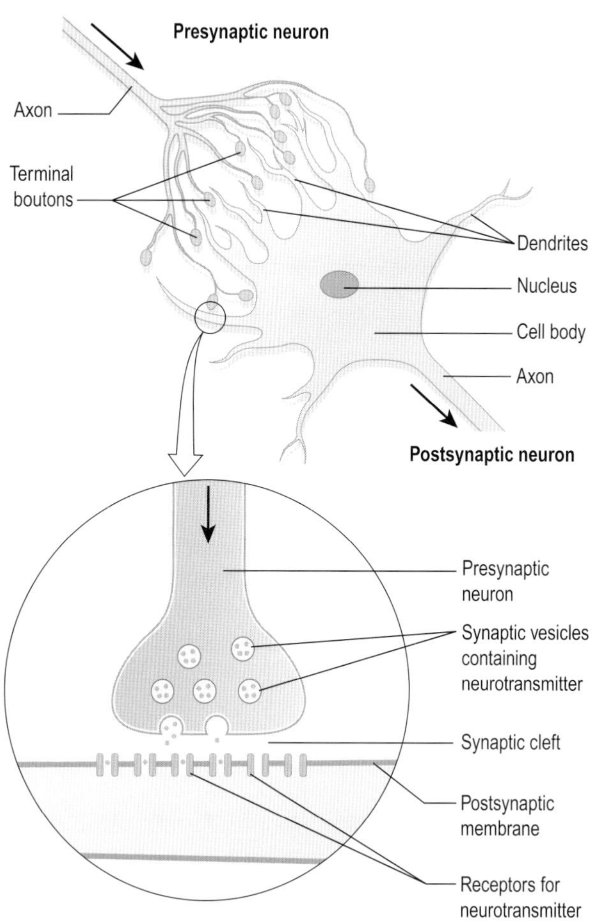

Figure 4.1a-II • A synapse.

fibre. The glial cell that forms myelin in this way is called the 'Schwann cell'. Myelin enables these cells to transmit an impulse more quickly than those cells that do not have this coating.

The tips of the dendrites make contact with other nerve cells. In the case of motor nerves, the tips of some of the axons make contact with muscles. The way in which dendrites or axons make contact with other nerve cells is shown in Figure 4.1a-II. In can be seen from the figures that the branching ends of the axons come very close to the dendrites of another nerve cell. However, they do not actually touch, but leave a tiny gap called a 'synapse' or "synaptic cleft".

When an electrical charge reaches the branching end of the axon it causes an internal change in the cell, which leads to a release of neurotransmitter from the branching tips of the axon at the terminal boutons. This chemical can diffuse across the synapse, and may act as the stimulus for the nerve cell on the other side of the gap. In some cases the neurotransmitter has the opposite effect and reduces the irritability of the nerve cell on the other side of the synapse. In this case, instead of acting as a stimulus, the neurotransmitter inhibits further stimuli for a brief period. This complex process involving both an electrical charge and a release of chemicals is the basis for communication between nerve cells, and also between a nerve cell and a muscle.

As stated earlier, the number of synapses in the body runs into trillions. Whenever a single cell is stimulated, impulses are transmitted via its axons to a number of other cells. Some of these impulses will lead to the stimulation of a series of cells in connection with the first cell. Of course, all these cells have their own connections with many other cells, and this can lead to a 'chain reaction' of impulses, which can spread through the nervous system. However, there will also be inhibition of other cells, which may in turn lead to another chain reaction of inhibition of other cells in the nervous system.

This series of chain reactions from a single stimulus is how an experience such as a single pin prick not only causes a withdrawal from the source of pain, but also leads to the felt experience of pain, an emotional response to the pain, an expressed cry of indignation, and the laying down of memory about the incident, among many other possible responses (see Q4.1a-1 and Q4.1a-2).

Nerve cells are highly active because they constantly manufacture neurotransmitter chemicals. The manufacture of substances within the cell requires basic nutrients and energy in the form of energy-charged adenosine triphosphate (ATP), and takes place within the endoplasmic reticulum and the Golgi body (see Chapter 1.1b). The neurotransmitters are exported to the outside environment by the process of exocytosis of vesicles, which is one of the methods of active transport described in Chapter 1.1b. This process also requires energy in the form of ATP.

Because of its intensive energy requirements, the nerve cell is absolutely reliant on a high level of oxygen and glucose to perform this function. A nerve cell that is even temporarily starved of these nutrients cannot function well, and is more likely to die than some other types of cell. Once a nerve cell has died it cannot be replaced, because nerve cells are one of the few types of cells in the body that do not divide. However, although nerve cells cannot be replaced, new connections between remaining cells can be made, as dendrites from nerve cells can grow out and make new contacts with other cells.

Sometimes the loss of nerve cells can be overcome by this mechanism of new growth, although full recovery may take some time. In other cases, the loss of nerve cells leaves a permanent deficit, as occurs in the case of many strokes.

Glial cells (neuroglia)

Glial cells (also known as 'neuroglia') are the connective-tissue cells of the nervous system. They form about one-third of all nervous tissue. These cells act as the scaffolding that holds the nerve cells in place. Unlike nerve cells, glial cells can replicate. For this reason almost all cancers of the nervous system are derived from the glial cells rather than from nerve cells.

A type of glial cell called the 'astrocyte' protects nervous tissue from toxins in the blood by forming a layer around the blood vessels that enter the nervous system. This is called the 'blood–brain barrier'. Some drugs cannot penetrate the blood–brain barrier, a property which has been utilised by drug manufacturers. For example, the newer types of beta blocker drugs are less likely to cause emotional and sleep disturbance because they have been designed not to be able to cross the blood–brain barrier. However, many other drugs, such as alcohol and nicotine, cross this barrier very easily.

Another type of glial cell, called the 'oligodendrocyte', is responsible for the manufacture of the myelin that enables rapid conduction of electrical impulses down the nerve cell axons.

The last type of glial cell, called the 'microglia', is derived from the leukocyte. It is similar to the macrophage in ordinary connective tissue, and can phagocytose (see Chapter 1.1c) unwanted cellular material.

The composition of nervous tissue

The nerve cells and the supporting glial cells are the main components of all parts of the nervous system, from the brain and spinal cord, right down to the thread-like branching nerves that penetrate all the body tissues. The structure and consistency of the different types of nervous tissue depend on the relative proportion of cell bodies and axons (nerve fibres).

The tissue that makes up the brain contains many cell bodies and is very soft in consistency, rather akin to a thick blancmange. This explains why it can be so easily damaged by violent shaking or a blow to the head, and why it requires the rigid casing of the skull for protection. The cell bodies are concentrated in particular areas within different parts of the brain and, when very closely packed, have a greyish colour. This is the origin of the term 'grey matter', which in common usage refers to the part of the brain that does the thinking. The nerve fibres or axons running from these cell bodies to different parts of the brain, or down to the spinal cord, tend to run together rather like all the telephone wires running from one group of houses to the exchange. These 'pathways' of thousands of nerve fibres are called 'tracts'. They have a white appearance because of the white myelin, and are described as the 'white matter'.

In the spinal cord, the tracts of nerve fibres are very prominent. Thousands of nerve fibres run up and down the length of the spinal cord, allowing communication between different parts of the body and the brain. These also appear as white matter when the spinal cord is dissected. However, in the core of the spinal cord are dense clusters of the nerve cell bodies of connector and motor neurons. On dissection these are seen as a central H-shaped area of grey matter. Figure 4.1a-III shows a diagram of a cross-section of the spinal cord, illustrating the appearance of the white and grey matter. Like the brain, the spinal cord is of a very soft consistency and is also vulnerable to injury.

Figure 4.1a-III also shows the two 'roots' of the nerve fibres that leave this part of the spinal cord. These meet to leave the vertebral column as a single spinal nerve containing thousands of nerve fibres. With the exception of the nerves that supply the head and the neck, all the bodily nerves originate from spinal nerves. In this case, the word 'nerve' means thousands of nerve fibres bundled together, rather than a single cell (correctly called 'nerve cell', "nerve fibre" or 'neuron').

All the nerves that run outside the spinal cord consist entirely of sensory and motor nerve fibres, and have originated from the anterior (containing motor fibres) and posterior (containing sensory fibres) spinal nerve roots (see Figure 4.1a-III). The cell bodies of the motor nerve fibres sit within the grey matter of the spinal cord. However, the cell bodies of the sensory nerve sit outside the spinal cord, mostly within the spinal root ganglion on the sensory nerve root. This is seen as a swelling in Figure 4.1a-III. The spinal root ganglion is, therefore, a little mass of grey matter. (NB: The sensory nerves of the autonomic nervous system have their cell bodies in ganglia situated further away from the spinal cord, as described later in this chapter.)

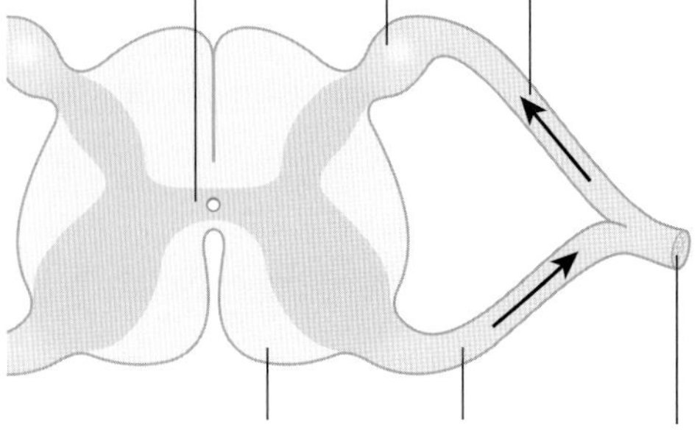

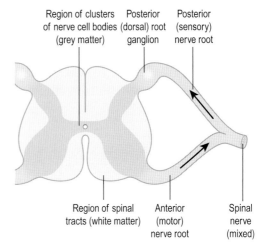

Figure 4.1a-III • A section of the spinal cord showing the nerve roots on one side.

The parts of the nervous system

The nervous system is conventionally described as being composed of three interrelated parts: the central nervous system (CNS), the peripheral nervous system (PNS) and the autonomic nervous system (ANS).

The CNS consists of the brain and the spinal cord. It is protected by a thick fibrous coat and sits within the brain and the vertebral column. The brain is further divided on an anatomical basis into the upper brain (cerebral hemispheres), hindbrain (cerebellum) and brainstem (the midbrain, the pons and medulla oblongata).

The largest part of the PNS consists of 31 pairs of spinal nerves, which emerge from the spinal cord to pass through the spaces between each vertebra and through the holes in the sacrum bone known as the 'sacral foramina'. These nerves contain sensory and motor nerve fibres, and divide to penetrate most of the body tissues. The motor nerve fibres of this part of the PNS are primarily concerned with the voluntary control of muscle action.

The PNS also embraces 12 pairs of cranial nerves, which originate not from the spinal cord but from the lower portions of the brain itself. These also contain sensory and motor nerve fibres. Although some of the motor nerve fibres in the cranial nerves are concerned with the voluntary control of muscular action (e.g. the nerve that supplies the masseter muscle, the muscle of chewing), many carry nerve impulses to control involuntary muscle action (e.g. the vagus nerve, which supplies the cardiac muscle).

Those nerves in the PNS which are involved in the involuntary control of body activity are conventionally considered as a separate system, the ANS. Strictly speaking, the ANS is a subdivision of the PNS.

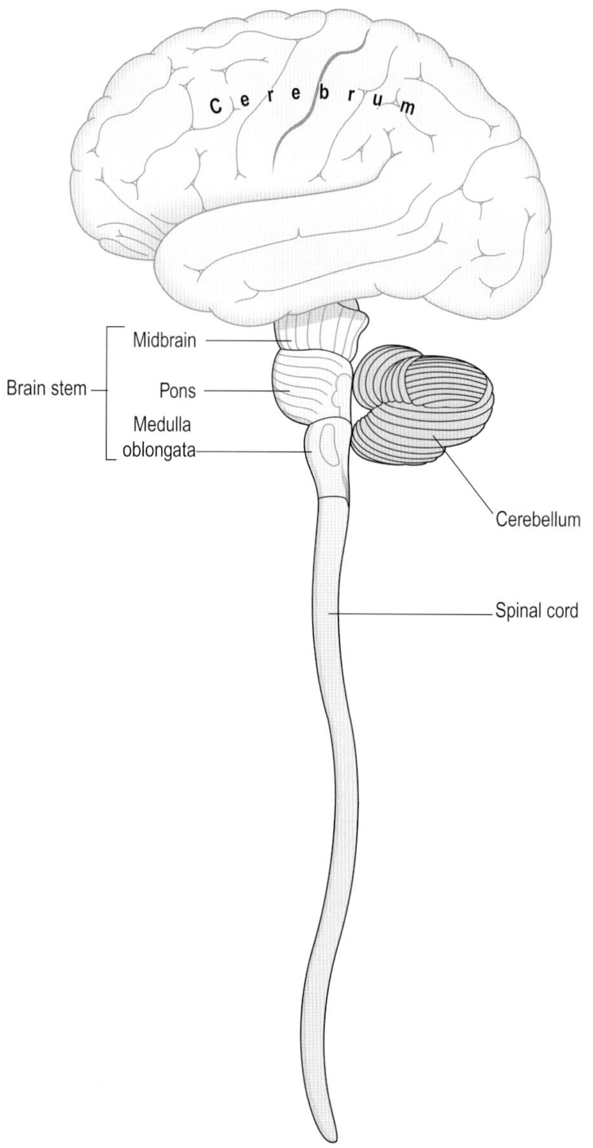

Figure 4.1a-IV • The parts of the central nervous system.

The central nervous system

The CNS consists of the brain and the spinal cord, and sits protected within spaces formed within the bony architecture of the brain and the vertebral column. Figure 4.1a-IV illustrates the structure of the main parts of the CNS. Note that this diagram is not drawn to scale; the spinal cord is, in reality, much longer than indicated in this drawing.

This delicate nervous tissue of brain and spinal cord is protected within the bony housing of the skull and vertebral canal by three layers of tissue, the dura mater, arachnoid mater and the pia mater, which collectively are called the 'meninges'.

The meninges

The meninges (Figure 4.1a-V) consist largely of fibrous tissue. The outermost layer, known as the 'dura mater' (dura) is composed of dense white fibrous tissue, the outer layer of which is adherent to the skull, where it forms the periosteum (see Chapter 4.2a) and the bony margins of the vertebral canal (central canal) right down to the coccyx. In certain regions in the skull the dura splits into two layers, and venous blood courses in the spaces between them in canals called 'sinuses'. An epidural anaesthetic is one that is injected carefully in the lumbar region of the spinal cord so that the anaesthetic drug collects outside the dura and so acts to numb the lower thoracic and lumbar spinal nerve roots as they course down to supply the abdomen and legs.

Beneath the layers of the dura is the subdural space. This contains fluid which separates the dura from the next layer, the arachnoid mater, which is also composed of fibrous tissue. The arachnoid mater loosely follows the internal contours of the dura mater. Veins also pass through the subdural space. These can become vulnerable to damage in old age as the substance of the brain shrinks, and there is more possibility of traction on these vessels if the skull is suddenly moved as can occur in a fall. This is the cause of subdural haemorrhage (see Chapter 4.1d).

Beneath the arachnoid mater is the subarachnoid space, which separates the arachnoid mater from the deepest meningeal layer, the pia mater. The delicate pia courses along the surface of the brain and the spinal cord, and in some areas there is quite a pronounced space between it and the arachnoid mater. This space is filled with a fluid known as

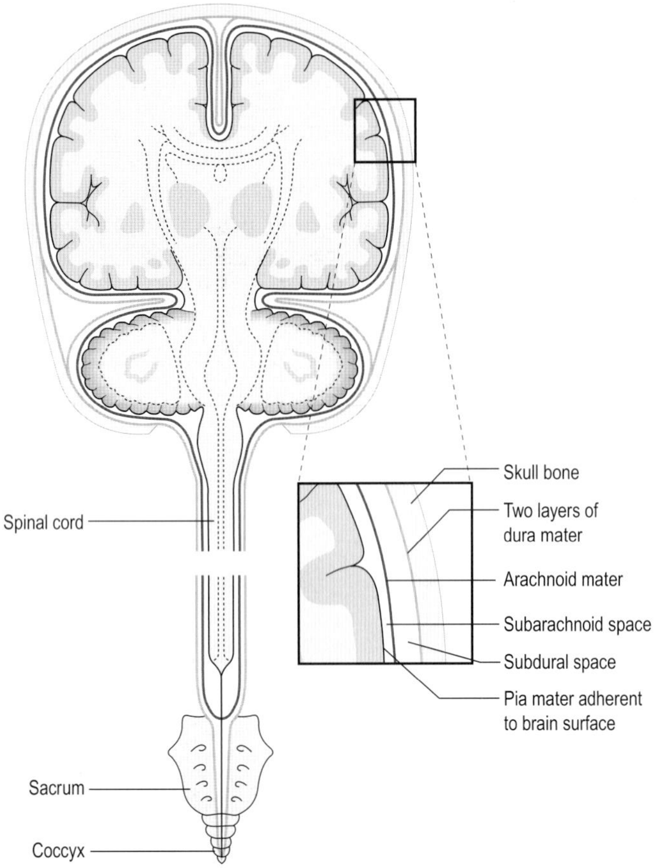

Figure 4.1a-V • The meninges covering the brain and the spinal cord.

'cerebrospinal fluid' (CSF). This space is in connection with the CSF, which bathes internal portions of the brain within the chambers known as 'ventricles'. It is in the subarachnoid space that the major arteries which course along the surface of the brain are located, and it is into this space that blood can leak should one of these arteries become damaged. This is the situation of subarachnoid haemorrhage (see Chapter 4.1d). A lumbar puncture is an investigation that involves inserting a needle into the region of the subarachnoid space as it widens out in the lower lumbar area below the termination of the spinal cord (see Figure 4.1-V) so that a sample of CSF can be obtained (see Q4.1a-3-Q4.1a-6).

Cranial therapists claim that they can detect the pulsations of the CSF within the meningeal membranes. These pulsations are proposed to be transmitted throughout the whole body via the myofascial system. Cranial therapy works to influence deep structures by allowing the release of the myofascial system, through very gentle manipulation techniques, and through such manipulation effect healing at physical, emotional and spiritual levels.

The cerebrum

The cerebrum is the upper part of the brain (see Figure 4.1-IV), and is divided into two cerebral hemispheres. These have a convoluted surface, giving this part of the brain a cauliflower-like appearance. Despite this visual comparison with a lowly vegetable, the cerebrum is the most complex part of the brain, and is the part that is most enlarged in human beings compared to other animals.

The cerebrum deals with the most complicated aspects of nervous activity. To use once again the example of the pin prick, although the reflex withdrawal from the pain need not involve the brain at all, the emotional experience of pain, the cry of indignation and the laying down of memory about the event all involve the nerve cells in the cerebral hemispheres. In keeping with this complexity, the cerebrum contains a lot of grey matter (nerve cell bodies) concentrated on its convoluted surface. This part of the cerebrum is called the 'cerebral cortex'. The functions of particular parts of the cerebral cortex have now been extensively mapped. For instance, the voluntary control of movement of all the body parts can be located onto precise segments of a single ridge of cortex, called the 'motor area', situated on the side of each cerebral hemisphere. The complexity of such representation is illustrated in Figure 4.1a-VI.

In order to comprehend the complicated effects of cerebral diseases it helps to understand that, if parts of the cerebrum are lost through injury or disease, the precise function of those parts is also lost. For example, a person who has a small stroke (see Chapter 4.1d) that damages a part of the motor area of the cortex only will suffer an inability to move the corresponding part of their body. In this situation, other functions such as sensation and speech will be unaffected. In contrast, a person who has a stroke that affects the visual

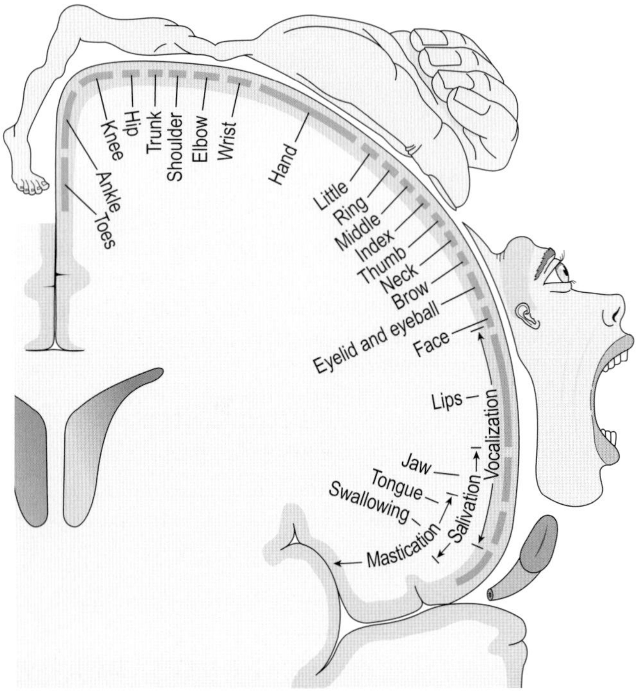

Figure 4.1a-VI • The mapping of the motor cortex to bodily function • This diagram illustrates how different strips of the motor cortex have been mapped to muscle function in the body. The distorted humanoid figure is called a 'homunculus' and is drawn to illustrate that some parts of the body (the hand, face and tongue) have disproportionate representation on the motor cortex, in keeping with the complexity of their muscle action.

cortex only will suffer from visual problems, while movement will be unimpaired.

Tracts of white matter (nerve fibres) descend through the brain from the cerebral cortices (plural of 'cortex'). These connect with other parts of the brain, and also with the spinal cord. The two halves of the upper brain are intimately connected with each other by a wide tract of nerve fibres called the 'corpus callosum'. The tracts of fibres that link the cortices with the rest of the body tend to cross over (decussate) within the brainstem, so that the left side of the brain controls the right side of the body, and vice versa. For this reason the left side of the brain is the dominant hemisphere in a right-handed person.

Deep within the cerebral hemispheres are islands of grey matter called 'nuclei'. These have essential control functions. The largest of these nuclei are the basal ganglia (important for the control of movement), the thalamus (important for the control of sensation) and the hypothalamus (important for the control of the hormones of the pituitary gland and for other aspects of homeostasis such as temperature control).

The main areas and functions of the cerebral cortex are illustrated in Figure 4.1a-VII. The cortices are each anatomically divided into four lobes named after the skull bone that overlies them. Functions can therefore be associated anatomically with lobes; for instance, vision is a function of the occipital lobe. The areas associated with speech production (frontal lobe) and processing of language (temporal lobe) are concentrated on the so-called 'dominant hemisphere' only, which is usually on the left-hand side in right-handed people and the right-hand side in left-handed people. In contrast, the areas responsible for spatial awareness (parietal lobe) tend to be more developed on the non-dominant side of the cerebrum (see Q4.1a-7 and Q4.1a-8).

The brainstem

The brainstem consists of the midbrain, the pons variolii (the pons) and the medulla oblongata (the medulla) (see Figure 4.1a-IV). These three sections of the brain contain large tracts of white matter which carry nerve fibres between the cerebrum and the spinal cord.

All three of these areas of the brain contain nuclei of nerve cell bodies which have the function of the control of the most basic aspects of maintaining life in a complicated organism. For this reason, the structure of these areas is not too dissimilar to the equivalent parts of the brain in other animals. For example, the control of breathing, heart rate and blood pressure is coordinated by specialised centres of nerve cells in the medulla. Because these functions are all essential for life, these specialised areas of the brainstem are called 'vital centres'. Other centres in this part of the brain control the reflex actions of coughing, vomiting and sneezing.

A specialised area in the brainstem called the 'reticular activating system' (RAS) is responsible for the control of how much sensory information gets through to the cerebral cortex. It is the RAS that controls our level of awareness of the environment, and which allows us to focus on one thing to the exclusion of all others in certain circumstances. It is believed that sleep, a time in which our conscious awareness is very much inhibited, is controlled in part by the RAS (see Q4.1a-9).

The cerebellum

The cerebellum, or hindbrain, sits at the back of the brainstem. A hand placed over the upper part of the back of the neck and supporting the base of the skull (while covering the area that includes acupoints Fengfu Du-16 and Fengchi GB-20) will have the palm overlying the cerebellum.

The cerebellum is another control centre of the brain. It is responsible for the smooth coordination of movement and balance. To perform this function it receives information from the muscles, ears and eyes about the position of the body.

It is believed that the cerebellum also holds memory about repeated actions, so that with practice these can be performed smoothly and without conscious effort. For example, it is

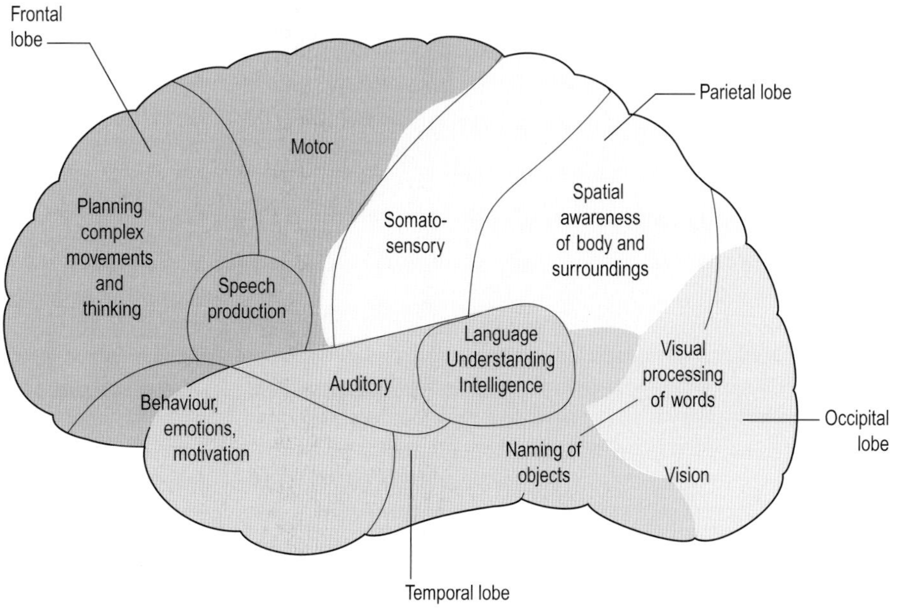

Figure 4.1a-VII • The lobes and functional regions of the cerebral cortex.

the cerebellum that allows a person who is driving to perform a complex task such as changing gear and signalling when decelerating towards a junction, even while focusing consciously on a conversation on the radio.

In a disease that damages the cerebellum only, the conscious mind and the vital centres are left intact. A person with such a condition will have no problem with thinking and the physical body will be in generally good health. However, balance will be poor, speech will be clumsy and the most simple tasks will have to be performed slowly and deliberately, with many errors of movement occurring as the task is undertaken.

The spinal cord

The spinal cord is the long extension of nervous tissue that leaves the brain at the base of the brainstem. It projects through the large hole at the base of the skull called the 'foramen magnum', and extends down as far as the first or second lumbar vertebrae. The spinal cord is protected as it runs in the vertebral canal (also known as 'spinal canal'), formed by the ring-shaped vertebrae that sit one on top of the other. The solid vertebral bodies lie in front of the spinal cord, and the spinous and transverse processes project out to the back and the side of the vertebral rings that embrace the cord along it length. A section of the thoracic spinal cord is illustrated in Figure 4.1a-VIII.

As shown in Figure 4.1a-IX, the 31 pairs of spinal nerves leave the cord at regular intervals. These spinal nerves project out of the meningeal membranes, which protect the cord and leave the vertebral column through spaces between the vertebrae. Figure 4.1a-X illustrates the base of the spinal cord as it looks on a vertical section of the vertebral column. This diagram shows how the cord only goes down as far as the first lumbar vertebra. The labels T1, T7, T12, L1, S1 and S3 point to the solid bodies of three thoracic vertebrae, one lumbar vertebra and two of the sacral vertebrae which are fused to form the sacrum bone. This diagram also shows the spinous processes projecting back from the vertebral canal. These processes are linked by a tough fibrous ligament, not shown in this diagram, which runs from the base of the skull to the sacrum. It is this ligament that is penetrated when a lumbar puncture is performed.

Figure 4.1a-IX shows the paired spinal nerves. In this diagram the nerves are cut off just at the point where they exit the vertebral canal between the vertebrae. This shows how the lower thoracic, lumbar and sacral nerves descend by increasing lengths through the vertebral canal before they actually leave the space between the vertebrae.

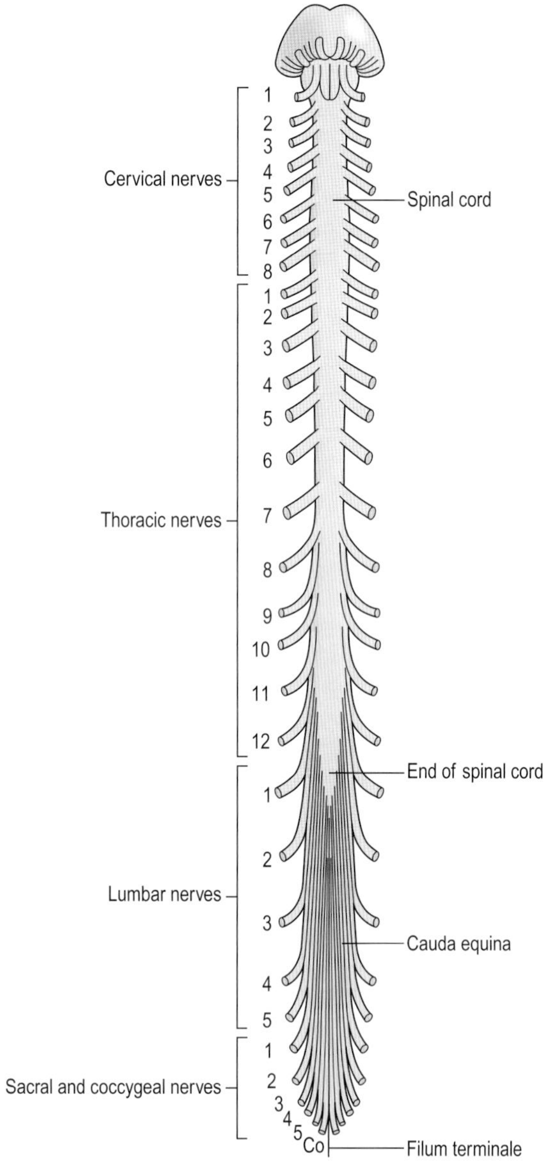

Figure 4.1a-IX • The spinal cord and spinal nerves.

The first to seventh cervical nerves leave above the corresponding cervical vertebra. However, the eighth cervical nerve leaves below the seventh cervical vertebra. The 12 thoracic and five lumbar spinal nerves all exit below the corresponding thoracic and lumbar vertebrae. The sacral and coccygeal nerves all leave through gaps in the fused sacrum and bones of the coccyx.

With this information it is possible to work out which spinal nerve emerges at a particular spinal level. For example, the level L2/L3, the level at which the acupoints Mingmen Du-4 or Shenshu Bl-23 are situated, is also the level of the emergence of the second lumbar spinal nerve from the vertebral column.

The spinal cord consists of tracts of white matter containing vertically ascending and descending nerve fibres, and a core of grey matter containing cell bodies. This core is approximately H-shaped when seen in horizontal section (see Figure 4.1a-VIII).

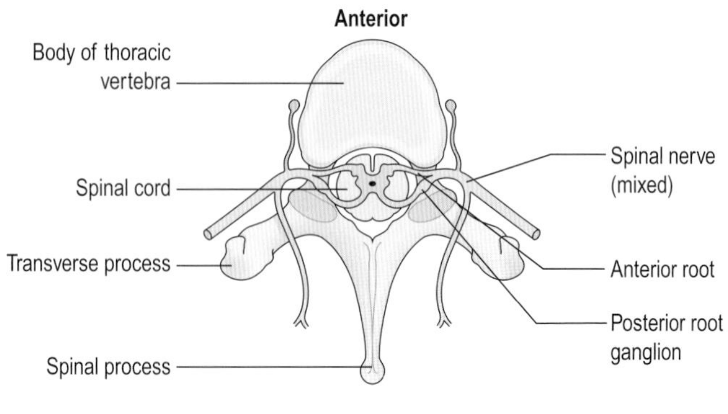

Figure 4.1a-VIII • Horizontal section through the vertebral column and spinal cord at the level of the thorax.

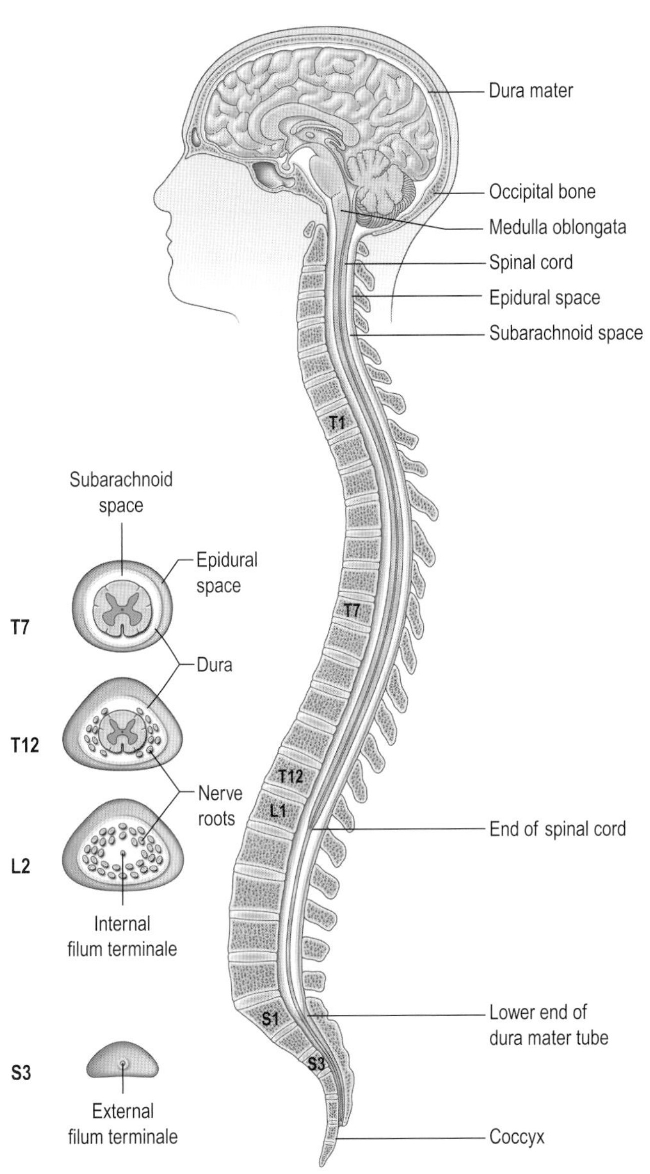

Figure 4.1a-X • Section of the distal end of the vertebral canal. This diagram also shows horizontal sections of the spinal column at four levels. These illustrate how the spinal cord terminates at the level of L1/L2 and distal to this only nerve roots travel in the spinal canal.

Some of the nerve fibres in the white matter of the spinal cord travel to and from the brain, whereas others simply link different levels in the spinal cord.

The spinal cord receives sensory information from most parts of the body below the head and the neck through sensory nerve cells that enter the cord through the sensory root of the spinal nerves. The muscle action within the body is controlled by information carried by motor nerve cells that leave the spinal cord at the motor root of the spinal nerves. (see Figures 4.1a-III and 4.1a-VIII).

The grey matter in the spinal cord can be considered as having a similar function to the nuclei of the brain. Some basic aspects of muscle movement are controlled by the clusters of nerve cells in the spinal cord alone. The protective reflex arc and spinal tone are two such aspects that function adequately without any input from the nerve fibres of the brain.

The protective reflex arc

The protective reflex of withdrawal from pain is one example of a movement that is controlled by the spinal cord alone. Once again the example of the response to a pin prick of the finger is a useful illustration. In this case, the pain of a pin prick leads to impulses in the sensory nerves that supply the finger. These travel up the arm to where the nerves enter the spinal cord at the thoracic level of T6/T7. Here the sensory nerve cells make connections with a number of motor nerve cells in the spinal cord by means of connector nerve cells. These motor nerve cells send impulses down to various muscles in the arm and shoulder to cause a withdrawal of the arm from the pain. In such a reflex, the brain is not involved. A diagrammatic representation of a simple reflex arc is given in Figure 4.1a-XI. In this case the diagram illustrates the "knee jerk" reflex which is an involuntary response to the stretch of the patellar tendon.

Spinal tone

The spinal cord is responsible for maintaining a constant level of contraction, or tone, in the body muscles. This is essential as a background upon which upright posture and smooth body movements can occur. The existence of this tone is clear in the situation when all connection between the limbs and the brain is lost, as can occur in an injury of the spinal cord. In this situation, the muscles do not just go limp and useless. Instead they manifest a sometimes intense level of this sustained contraction, a result of impulses from motor nerves originating in the spinal cord. In this situation this tone tends to cause the lower limbs to extend out straight, and the upper limbs to flex so that a bend is held at the elbow. This limb position is characteristic of patients who have suffered a spinal injury at a high level such as at the neck. In such patients the involuntary muscular contraction is often over forceful and over time the muscles become tight and contracted.

The reason why this excessive level of tone is not experienced in a healthy person is that nerve impulses originating from the brain are transmitted down the spinal cord to partially inhibit the spinal motor nerves, and to reduce the muscle tone to a level that enables upright posture and smooth movements.

Motor nerve cells that originate in the spinal cord are called 'lower motor neurons'. Motor nerve cells that originate in the brain and descend to control the function of lower motor nerves are called 'upper motor neurons'. This distinction is important to make, as it will help in understanding the underlying problems in the severe diseases that cause impaired muscular movement, such as multiple sclerosis, motor neuron disease and stroke.

In a simple reflex arc and the production of tone after a spinal injury it is the lower motor nerves only that are responsible for the muscle contraction. However, in most other movements the action of the lower motor nerve cells has been stimulated or inhibited by the impulses from upper motor nerves originating from the brain (see Q4.1a-10).

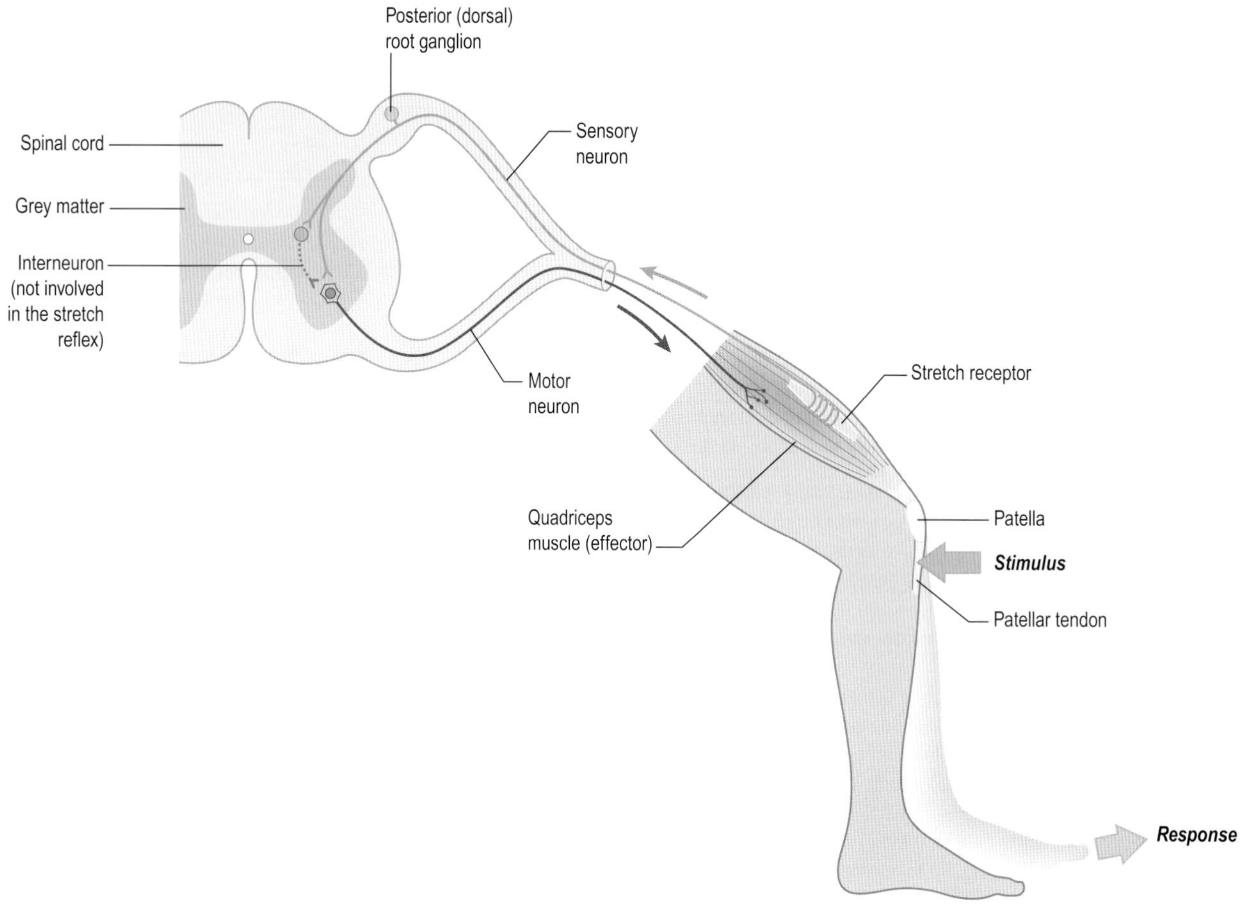

Figure 4.1a-XI • A simple reflex arc.

Part II: The physiology of the nervous system

The peripheral nervous system

The peripheral nervous system (PNS) consists of all the parts of the nervous system that exist outside the protective skeletal casing of the skull and the vertebral column. It comprises the 31 pairs of spinal nerves and the 12 pairs of cranial nerves. The autonomic nervous system (ANS) is the part of the PNS which is concerned with the involuntary control of the deep organs, blood vessels and glands, and thus it is essential for the maintenance of homeostasis.

The spinal nerves

The structure of the spinal cord was described at the end of Part I of this chapter. The 31 pairs of spinal nerves, which leave the cord at regular intervals (see Figure 4.1a-IX), divide to form the largest part of the PNS.

All the spinal nerves are mixed nerves in that they carry both motor and sensory nerve fibres to all the parts of the body that they supply. In the spinal nerves, the motor nerve fibres are largely responsible for the voluntary movement of the skeletal muscles (this includes reflex actions such as the withdrawal of parts of the body from painful stimuli). However, some of the motor fibres divide away from the spinal nerves close to their exit from the vertebral column to control the contraction of the smooth and cardiac muscle of the blood vessels, deep organs and glands. These functions are mainly not under the control of the will. These involuntary motor nerves are considered to be part of the ANS.

The first pair of spinal nerves (the first cervical nerves) passes out of the vertebral column between the skull and the first cervical vertebra. All the other cervical nerves, the thoracic nerves and first four lumbar nerves pass out between the vertebrae that make up the vertebral column. The fifth lumbar nerve exits between the fifth lumbar vertebra and the sacrum. The sacral nerves leave via holes (foramina) within the sacrum, and the coccygeal nerves leave at the level of the fusion of the bones of the sacrum and the coccyx. The names of the spinal nerves are usually abbreviated according to the associated spinal level. For example, the third cervical nerve is called C3, and the fifth lumbar nerve is called L5.

After its exit from the vertebral column, each spinal nerve divides many times to form all the nerves that together carry motor and sensory nerve fibres to most parts of the body below the head and the neck.

The cranial nerves

In addition to the spinal nerves, 12 pairs of nerves (the cranial nerves) leave the base of the brain to supply the tissues of the head and the neck. In addition, the tenth cranial nerves (the vagus nerves) each divide to form nerve branches, which extend deep into the thorax and abdomen to supply the deep organs within. The optic nerves, which supply the eye, and the auditory nerves, which supply the ear, are two other examples of cranial nerves.

The cranial nerves are named either by a name derived from a Latin root or by a number (abbreviated as the Roman numeral). For example, the optic nerve is also known as the second cranial nerve (II), and the vagus nerve is also known as the tenth cranial nerve (X).

Unlike the spinal nerves, not all the cranial nerves are mixed nerves. Three of the pairs of cranial nerves carry only sensory fibres (e.g. the optic nerve, which leads from the retina of the eye to the brain). Five pairs carry only motor nerve fibres (e.g. the oculomotor nerves, which supply some of the muscles that move the eye). The remaining four pairs of cranial nerves are mixed nerves. Like the spinal nerves, these four pairs of mixed cranial nerves also carry motor nerves, which are responsible for involuntary action of the muscles that control the functions of the deep organs and glands.

The cranial nerves pass out from the bony skull through holes in or between the cranial bones (e.g. through the hole at the back of the orbit, the cavity which cradles the eyeball).

In these paragraphs on the PNS, only those aspects of the cranial nerves that are responsible for sensation and the voluntary control of the skeletal muscles are considered. Those nerve fibres that are responsible for the involuntary control of smooth muscle and cardiac muscle in the blood vessels, deep organs and glands are generally considered as forming a distinct system, the ANS. This system is discussed in the last part of this chapter.

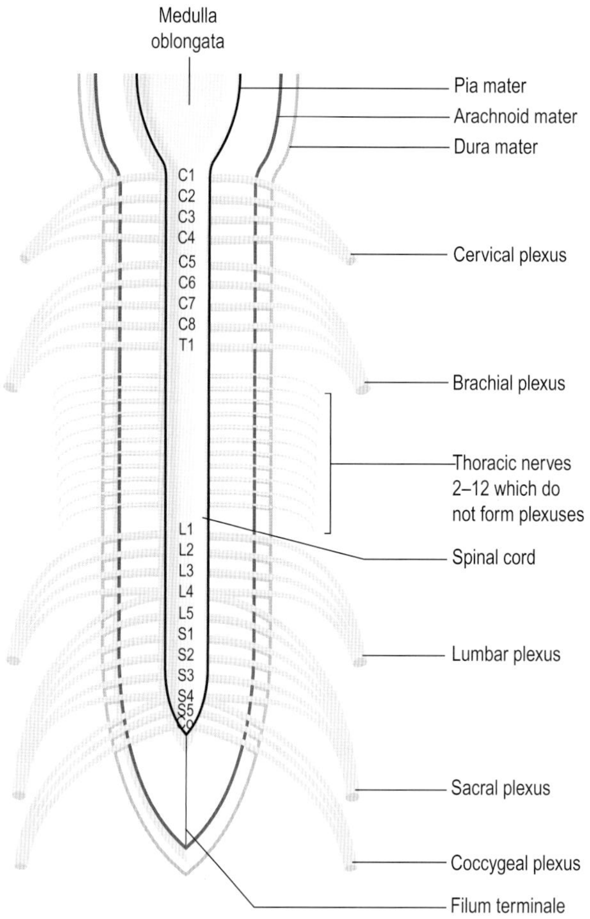

Figure 4.1a-XII • Diagrammatic representation of the level of the five major nerve plexuses.

The division of the spinal and cranial nerves

Each spinal and cranial nerve branches in a tree-like fashion to 'supply' a particular portion of the body. In the cervical, lumbar and sacral regions, the adjacent spinal nerves intermingle with each other close to the spinal cord before they separate out again into a number of nerve branches that then supply the tissues of the neck, arm, leg and genital areas. This intermingling forms a net-like web of nerves called a 'plexus'. Figure 4.1a-XII illustrates the location of the major nerve plexuses.

The major nerve branches that emerge from the plexuses are given descriptive names derived from Latin. For example, the radial nerve is the nerve in the arm that runs close to the radius bone, and the peroneal nerve describes the nerve in the leg that runs close to the peroneal muscles.

The intermingling of fibres in the plexuses is important to understand because the nerve branches that emerge from each plexus contain nerve fibres that originate from more than one spinal nerve. For example, the sciatic nerve, which emerges from the buttock to descend down the leg, carries fibres that originate from five spinal nerves (L4, L5, S1, S2 and S3). This may seem to be a rather esoteric point, but is very relevant to an understanding of the physical effect of acupuncture and other manipulative therapies.

Dermatomes

The parts of the body that are supplied by each spinal and cranial nerve are clearly understood. The areas of skin and tissue supplied by the sensory nerves of each spinal nerve have been mapped, and are much the same for each person. These areas are called 'dermatomes', and are illustrated in Figure 4.1a-XIII. Dermatomes represent those strips of skin and areas of the body that are supplied by the individual spinal and cranial nerves. Although the diagram suggests that there is a clear demarcation between dermatomes, in reality this is not the case, there being considerable overlap of the regions supplied by adjacent spinal nerves. Nevertheless, these diagrams can be very useful for health practitioners because they indicate which spinal nerve supplies the nerves to whatever body part is a source of symptoms or a focus for treatment. Some dermatomal diagrams also indicate which nerve branch (e.g. the radial nerve or the sciatic nerve) supplies a particular area. Figures 4.1a-XIV and 4.1a-XV show examples of such diagrams for the arm and the leg, respectively (see Q4.1a-11).

Although the aim of dermatomal diagrams is to illustrate the distribution of the sensory nerves, they can also give

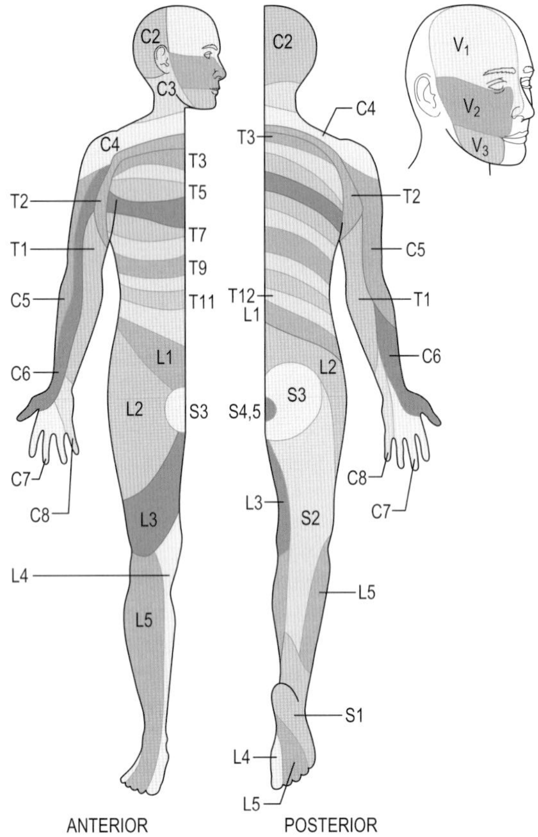

Figure 4.1a-XIII • Dermatomes of the spinal roots and the three divisions of the fifth (V) cranial nerve on the face (the trigeminal nerve).

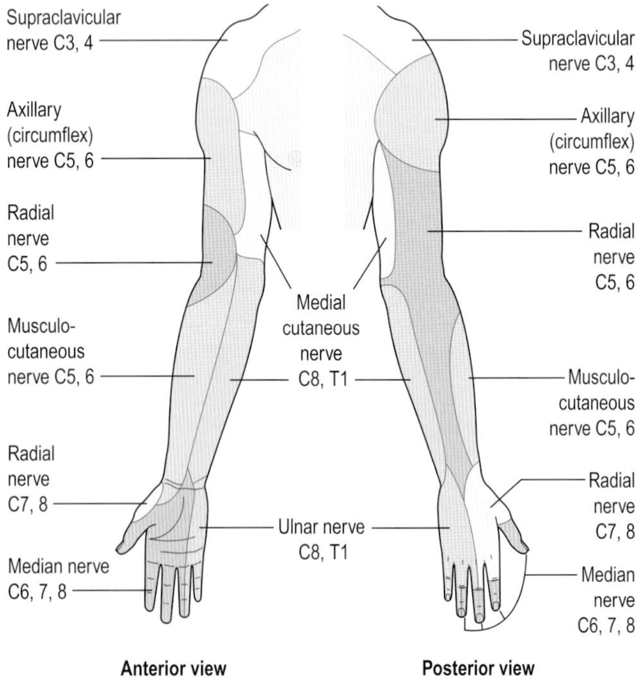

Figure 4.1a-XIV • Dermatomes of the nerves that supply the arms.

approximate information about the motor nerves that supply the muscles in a particular region. For example, the muscles that control plantar flexion of the wrist and gripping of the fingers are largely supplied by motor nerves that originate from the C6, C7, C8, T1 spinal nerves. Just as they direct the sensory nerve fibres from these spinal nerves away from the area, the ulnar and median nerves and their branches direct these motor nerve fibres to this part of the lower arm.

Referred pain

Referred pain is the term used to describe the situation in which pain originating in one part of the body is experienced elsewhere. In general, referred pain is felt either as a cutaneous or muscular sensation, when in fact the pathology is in a deeper part of the body. In sciatica, the problem usually lies either in the structure of the lumbar and sacral bones at the base of the back, where there can be bony or muscular impingement on the L5–S3 nerve roots, or in the proximal region of the sciatic nerve itself as it emerges from the sacral plexus and enters the buttock muscles. However, sciatic pain is experienced at the back of the leg and the foot. The pain is experienced in the leg and foot because the brain misinterprets the origin of the irritation as coming from the distal ends of the spinal nerve branches that terminate in the dermatome, rather than the correct site, which is far more proximally located.

Another cause of referred pain is the pain that originates from the deep organs. Compared to the skin and the skeletal muscles, the deeper body parts do not have a very full sensory nerve supply. For example, there is not a general awareness of how the spleen feels, or of the opening of our heart valves. If a deep organ is in distress, the pain from the organ and its surrounding tissues results in sensory messages that travel to the spinal cord through the spinal nerves which supply nerve fibres to that organ. However, the brain interprets these messages as coming from the nerves that supply its particular dermatome. The organs are connected by nerves often to a number of spinal levels, which means that deep organ pain is often vague and difficult for the patient to localise. In some cases, the dermatome overlies the position of the organ, but in others the pain is felt in a distant site. For example, gallbladder pain may be referred to the shoulder tip, the region of the C4 dermatome, because fibres from the C4 spinal nerve supply the diaphragmatic region as well as the shoulder (see Q4.1a-12).

The autonomic nervous system (ANS)

As mentioned earlier in this chapter, the motor nerve fibres of the spinal nerves and the mixed cranial nerves are involved in the involuntary control of the deep organs, blood vessels and glands. It is this aspect of the function of the nervous system that is called the 'autonomic nervous system' (ANS). The term 'autonomic' refers to the fact that the function of the ANS is largely outside the control of the conscious will.

The ANS controls the automatic functions of the body such as breathing, the pumping of the heart, the maintenance of blood pressure, sweating, salivation and the function of the digestive system. It not only keeps these functions going, but also enables them to be modified so that the total function

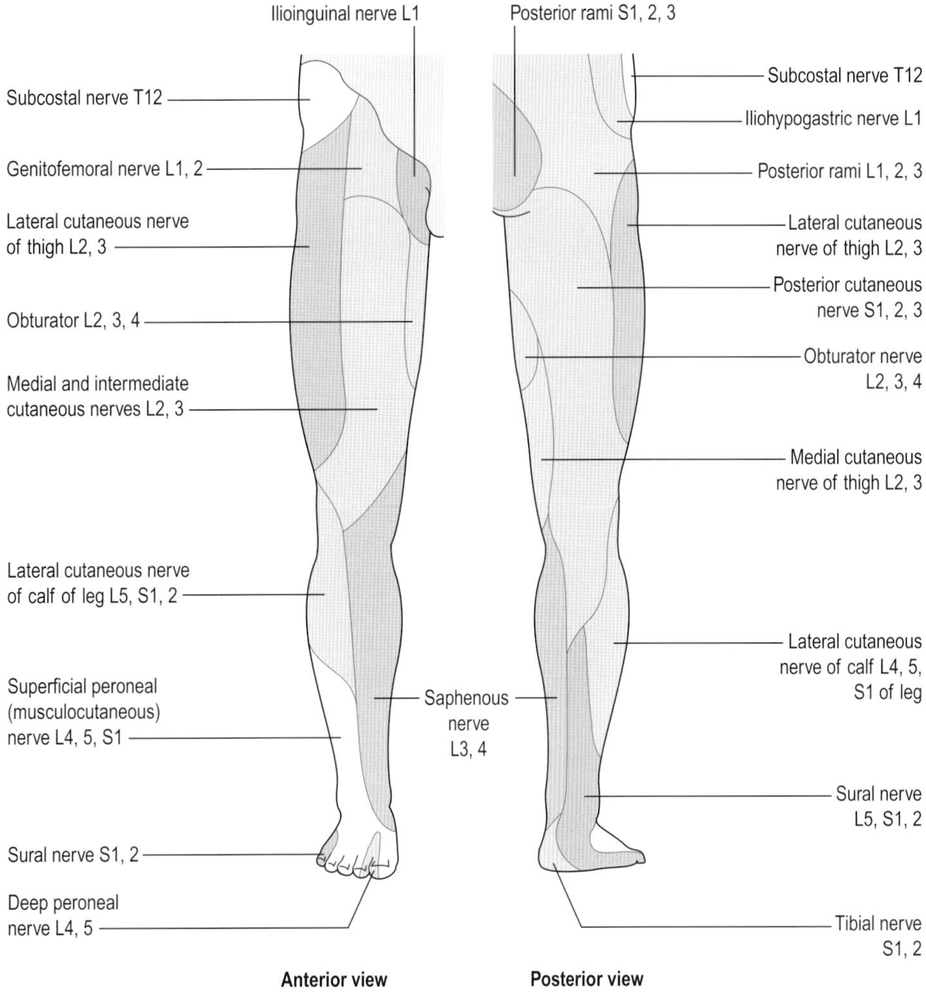

Figure 4.1a-XV • Dermatomes of the nerves that supply the legs.

Information Box 4.1a-I

The dermatomes: comments from a Chinese medicine perspective

The discussion about referred pain shows a recognition in conventional medicine terms that distant parts of the body are linked because they are associated with the same spinal levels. For example, there is a link in the nervous system between the heart and the front of the arm and the neck. In this example, the spinal levels of C3 through to T6 are linked, probably by connector nerve cells in the spinal cord.

In the examples of referred pain, the site of the pain from these deep organs can relate to the position of channels and points that have a close connection with the treatment of these conditions from the Chinese medicine viewpoint.

The referred pain in a heart attack is felt not only in the centre of the chest, but down the arm in the area of the Pericardium and Heart channels, and up the neck, through which the deep pathway of the Heart channel runs. The referred pain of cholecystitis is felt at the shoulder, over which the Gallbladder channel passes. The referred pain of the ovary is felt on the front and inner aspect of the thigh, over which pass the Stomach, Spleen and Liver channels. In all three conditions, points can be chosen from these channels to relieve the symptoms.

It is now scientifically accepted that acupuncture has a measurable analgesic effect mediated by impulses travelling up to the spinal cord by sensory nerves. Acupuncture stimulation appears to modulate nervous activity in the spinal cord at the level of the stimulated spinal nerve, which then results in inhibition of pain-carrying nerve fibres associated with the same spinal level. Impulses also travel up from the affected spinal cord level to the regions of the midbrain that deal in the general modulation of pain. This supports the observation that acupuncture can have both a local and general effect on the experience of pain. The neurotransmitters B endorphin and metenkephalin are recognised as two chemical mediators that are instrumental in these acupuncture effects.

The non-analgesic effects of acupuncture are less well explained scientifically. These include improvements in wound healing, nausea reduction, treatment of addiction, improved organ function, stimulation of the immune system and enhancement of mood. However, given the complex interconnections of the nervous and endocrine systems, it is feasible that acupuncture-mediated stimulation of nerves at a particular spinal level may have diverse ramifications both at a neural and the endocrine level.

of the body is responsive to its precise requirements at any one time. For example, the ability of the cardiovascular system to modify the pulse rate and blood pressure according to the needs of the body is mediated by the ANS.

In a healthy person, the ANS is always working to return the body to a state of homeostasis. Often it has to undo the imbalance in homeostasis that has been induced by the actions commanded by the conscious mind. For example, when a person decides to start running for a 'not-to-be-missed' bus, the ANS brings about a series of changes in the body to ensure that the cells receive a steady supply of oxygen and nutrients, and that the body does not get overheated. In this sort of situation, it is the ANS that temporarily 'shuts down' unnecessary functions, such as the production of urine and digestion, and speeds up the heart and respiratory rate, increases blood pressure and promotes sweating. The ANS even alters aspects of the mind, so that a state of daydreaming is replaced by one of focus and determination. After the bus has been caught and the pressure is off, the ANS continues to act to ensure that the body gradually returns to a balanced resting state.

The ANS is made up of two parts, which work in an opposing manner. The SNS tends to predominate in stressful situations, such as the previously mentioned situation of running for a bus. The parasympathetic nervous system (PSNS) predominates during rest, such as in the recovery period after running for the bus.

Information Box 4.1a-II

The sympathetic nervous system: comments from a Chinese medicine perspective

The sympathetic chain of ganglions is situated in the part of the back that runs from T1 to L3. This is the part that curves outwards between the natural inward curves formed by the neck and the small of the back. Although all of the back is considered as Yang in Chinese medicine, this section of the back is its most Yang aspect.

A noteworthy point is that the inner line of the Bladder channel, which is considered in Chinese medicine to have a profound influence on the function of the deep organs, runs on the surface of the skin overlying the position of the sympathetic ganglia. It is possible that needling points along this section of the bladder line may exert a profound influence on the organs by affecting the nerve impulses within the sympathetic ganglia. This nervous tissue is particularly concentrated in three main ganglia: one at the level of T12, one at the level of L1 and one at the level of L3. These would correspond in level to the position of the major points on the back affecting the Spleen, the Stomach and the Kidney (acupoints Pishu Bl-20, Weishu Bl-21 and Shenshu Bl-23), respectively.

The sympathetic nervous system

It might be said that the SNS acts to promote the more Yang aspects of the maintenance of homeostasis. It is most active when the mind has been alerted, or when the body has been injured, and prepares the body for quick responses, including meeting a challenge head on or the decision to escape (fight or flight).

The nerve cells of the SNS originate in the brainstem, and descend to connect with nerves in the spinal cord between T1 and L3. From these levels, fibres leave the spinal cord through the spinal nerves and intermingle with each other in a chain of nervous tissue that runs on either side of the spinal column at the back of the abdominal and thoracic cavities. There are a number of cell bodies, known as the 'sympathetic ganglia', within this chain of nervous tissue, and thus it can be compared to the grey matter of the brain and the spinal cord (the term 'ganglion', from the Greek meaning 'lump', is used in this case to refer to a cluster of nerve cell bodies). Figure 4.1a-XVI illustrates how nerve fibres leave the sympathetic ganglia to travel to all body parts, and indicates the wide range of tissues and organs that are influenced by the sympathetic nerves.

As mentioned above, the sympathetic part of the ANS is sometimes described as the part of the nervous system that prepares the body for fight or flight. It causes physical changes that allow the body to expend energy in a focused way, such as was described in the example of running for the bus. The various actions of the SNS are listed in Figure 4.1a-XVI, and it might become clear that all these changes, such as dilatation of the pupil, inhibition of mucus secretion, increased heart rate and reduced peristalsis, are appropriate ones for a body that is about to go into action.

The SNS also directly stimulates one endocrine gland, the adrenal medulla (the central part of the adrenal gland), which is situated just above the kidneys. This causes the release of the hormones adrenaline and noradrenaline into the bloodstream. These hormones help the body to deal with impending stress, and complement the function of the sympathetic nerves, as they have effects such as stimulation of the heart rate, increase of blood pressure, widening of the bronchioles and increased mental alertness.

The parasympathetic nervous system

In contrast to the sympathetic system, the parasympathetic nervous system (PSNS) might be described as promoting the maintenance of homeostasis. It is most active when the mind and body are at rest.

The parasympathetic nerves originate in the brainstem and the sacral part of the spinal cord. In particular, the vital centres in the brainstem, which deal with essential functions such as respiration and the heart rate, contain many parasympathetic nerve cells. These nerve cells have fibres that leave the cord either through the four pairs of mixed cranial nerves (the oculomotor, facial, glossopharyngeal and vagus nerves) or within the S2, S3 and S4 spinal nerves. The mixed cranial nerves have parasympathetic branches that extend to supply the deep organs and glands of the head, neck and abdomen down to the upper part of the large intestine. The parasympathetic fibres in the sacral spinal nerves supply the lower part of the large intestine, the bladder and the genital organs. Figure 4.1a-XVII illustrates the structure of the PSNS.

The PSNS promotes those aspects of bodily function that work to nourish and build up the body's reserves. It enables

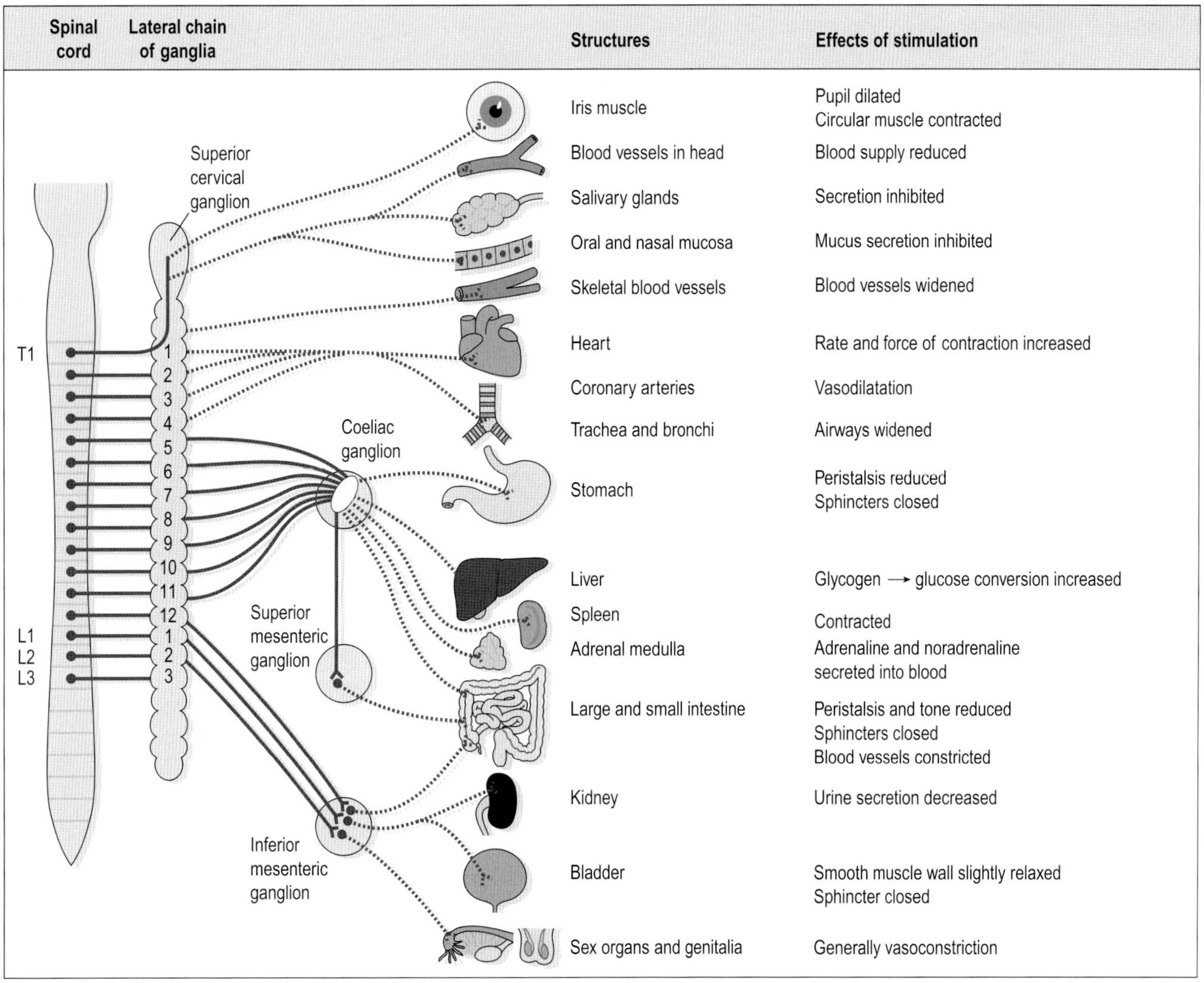

Figure 4.1a-XVI • The structure and influence of the sympathetic nervous system (SNS).

the body to make use of the resting periods to perform functions such as the digestion of nutrients and the clearance of wastes from the kidneys and the bowel. It is noteworthy that it is when the PSNS is active that sexual function is promoted. This suggests that sex is an activity that ideally takes place when the person is at rest, and has the purpose of nourishing and building up the individual as well as the creation of a new life. It is clear that excessive sympathetic nervous activity, such as would occur in a stressful period or even a situation of excitement, tends to counteract this parasympathetic action, and can lead to impotence.

Figure 4.1a-XVII shows how the various organs and glands are supplied by nerves that originate from the brainstem and the sacral spinal cord. The parasympathetic nerves increase secretions from the eye, the mouth and the digestive tract. Although not indicated in this diagram, the production of mucus of the respiratory tract is also increased. These secretions are all protective and nourishing to the organs that produce them. The heart and respiratory rate slows with parasympathetic stimulation, and digestion, defecation and urination are also promoted.

Information Box 4.1a-III

The parasympathetic nervous system: comments from a Chinese medicine perspective

In contrast to the SNS, the outflow of the parasympathetic nerves emerges from the regions of the spinal column in which there is an inward curve (the neck and the small of the back). These could be described as the more structurally Yin regions of the spine because of their inward curvature. The activity of the PSNS aids assimilation and storage of nutrients. It also increases bodily secretions, which are protective and nourishing to the organs that produce them. Such activities would be interpreted as Yin in Chinese medicine terms.

It is interesting to consider that much of the lifestyle advice of Chinese medicine focuses on activities that promote the action of the PSNS. Regular relaxed meals, regular times of sleep, gentle exercise and meditation will all have this effect. The hands-on therapies such as massage, shiatsu and reflexology will tend to stimulate the PSNS. The approach of craniosacral therapy, in particular, focuses on the two regions of the spine from which the parasympathetic nerves emerge.

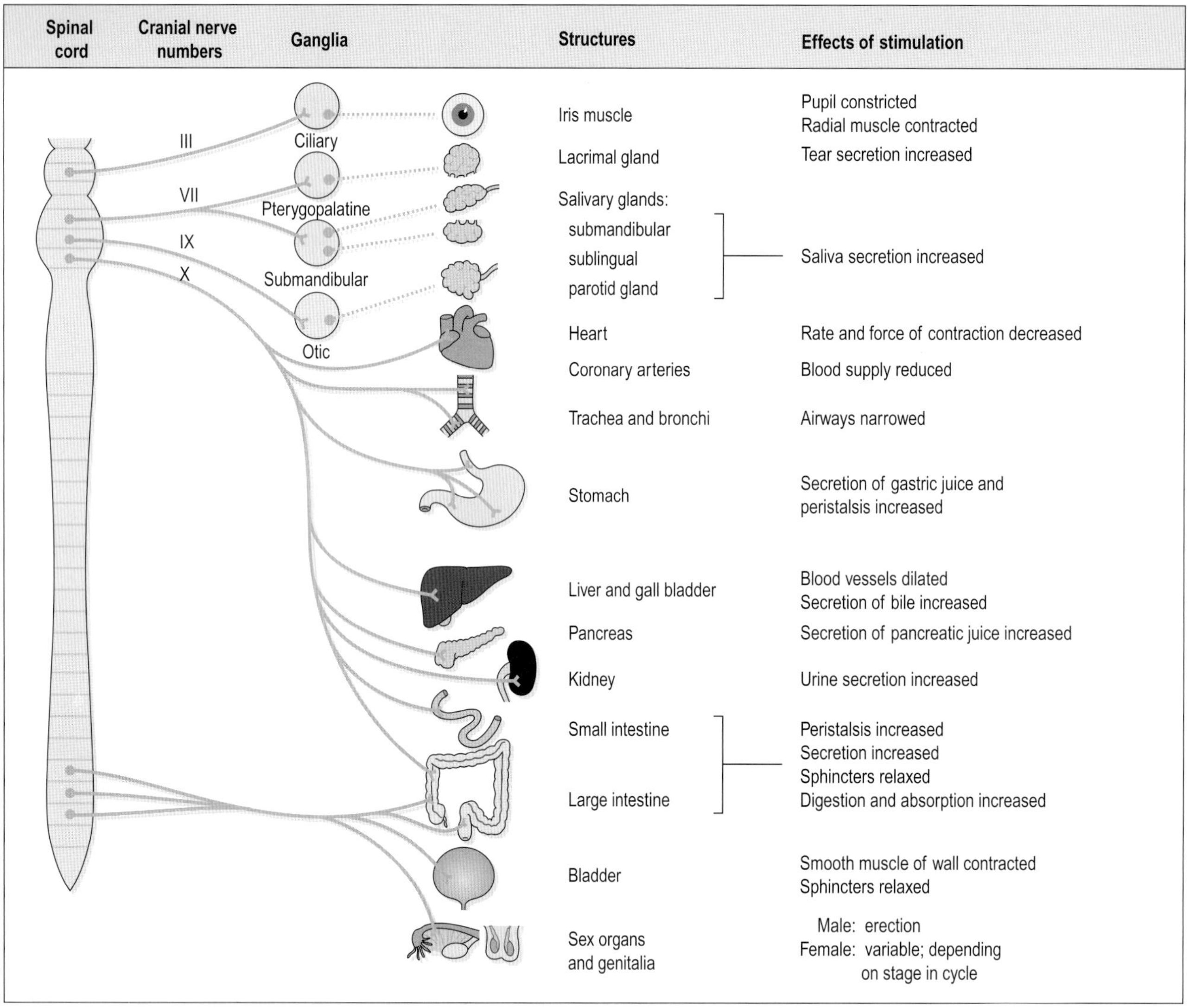

Figure 4.1a-XVII • The structure and influence of the parasympathetic nervous system (PSNS).

The balance between the sympathetic and parasympathetic systems

The PSNS can be seen as the aspect of the ANS that always tends to increase in function when the mind and body is at rest. When the mind and body are at rest, the centres of nerve cells in the brainstem and in the spinal cord automatically cause the PSNS to stimulate all the organs and glands of the body. When the mind is alerted or when the body has been injured, messages are relayed to inhibit the action of the parasympathetic centres in the brainstem, and the sympathetic nerve centres in the brainstem come into action instead.

It would make sense that the periods of stress that lead to sympathetic stimulation should be short-lived, so that a time of parasympathetic stimulation can allow the body to recover from the stress. It is part of human life to have to deal with stress, not least because the creative and competitive aspects of human nature often lead us to instigate situations of stress. This is not necessarily a bad thing, as long as there are adequate periods of recuperation between these stressful episodes.

It is not easy to assess what the ideal balance of parasympathetic and sympathetic stimulation should be, and this ideal may vary from individual to individual, depending on personality amongst other things. However, what seems to be clear is that many people in modern society do not have sufficient periods of parasympathetic activity to make up for the times during which their SNS is overactive.

Persistent stress, be it social, spiritual or physical, leads to excessive stimulation of the fight-or-flight response of the sympathetic nerves. Blood pressure and heart rate become persistently high, digestion worsens, the blood sugar levels rise, muscle tension is increased and the mind is unable to relax. This, of course, becomes a vicious circle, as a tense body and alerted mind further stimulate the sympathetic nerves. In such a situation, if the body and mind could be allowed to rest, the activation of the PSNS would help the organs to begin the self-healing process of the body. This is why rest is so important, as it allows the heart and blood vessels to relax, nutrients to be well absorbed, wastes to be fully cleared, and muscles and joints to be free of tension.

Information Box 4.1a-IV

The autonomic nervous system (ANS): comments from a Chinese medicine perspective

The healthy function of the ANS, with an ideal balance between the opposing aspects of the SNS and PSNS, is a fundamental requirement for the maintenance of health, both from a conventional and a complementary medical viewpoint. It would make sense that complementary therapies, including Chinese medicine, which focus heavily on allowing the body to regain balance, have their profound effects at the level of the ANS. In Chinese medicine, treatments that tonify Yin or treatments that are reducing would seem to promote parasympathetic aspects of function, while treatments that tonify Yang would appear to promote sympathetic aspects of function.

One could argue that, if the more profound aspects of the mechanism of acupuncture are to be communicated to a conventionally trained practitioner, they might best be explained in terms of the function of the ANS. For example, it might be suggested that the acupuncture needle, by stimulating sensory nerves, leads to impulses that arrive at the corresponding spinal level of the spinal cord. It can then be explained that this is scientifically recognised to be the mechanism by which acupuncture leads to the reduction of pain. However, it can also be suggested that these impulses in the spinal cord may also modulate the nervous activity of the ANS, particularly of those autonomic nerves that emerge from the spinal level of the dermatome which is needled. In this way the parasympathetic and sympathetic aspects of the functions of the blood vessels, deep organs and glands may be affected.

One could add that, in most treatments, it would seem that acupuncture, and the lifestyle advice which goes with it, enhances in particular the function of the parasympathetic aspect of the ANS. To support this suggestion, scientific studies of the action of electroacupuncture have demonstrated that electrostimulation leads to predictable modification of organ function normally controlled by the autonomic nervous system.

Self-test 4.1a

The physiology of the nervous system

1. What is the most basic response that a person might have if they accidentally pick up a very hot plate?
   How is this response mediated by the nervous system (i.e. describe which sorts of nerves and connections are involved)?
2. Describe in no more than two sentences the position and important functions of the following parts of the brain:
   (i) the cerebral cortex
   (ii) the cerebellum
   (iii) the brainstem
   (iv) the basal ganglia.
3. List three bodily changes that might be promoted by the PSNS.

Answers

1. The most basic response to a burn to the hand is to recoil by reflex from the source of the pain. This might cause the person to drop the hot plate. The mechanism of this basic reflex is that the pain stimulates the endings of sensory nerve cells in the hand. These nerves send impulses to the spinal cord (at the approximate level of C6–C8) via the sensory root of the spinal nerves. In the spinal cord the sensory nerve fibres synapse with connector nerve cells. The connector nerve cells in turn stimulate the motor nerve cells that supply the muscles of the arm and the hand. This causes the reflex withdrawal away from the pain.
   In addition, other impulses travel via connector neurons up to the brain, and these lead to the more complex responses to the situation such as the perception of pain and an angry response to the incident.
2. (i) The cerebral cortex is the outermost layer of the cerebral hemispheres, or upper brain. It consists of grey matter, and is responsible for the conscious perception of sensation, the voluntary control of movement, and higher functions such as thought, responsibility, emotions and the will.
   (ii) The cerebellum, or hindbrain, sits at the back of the brainstem and below the cerebral hemispheres. It is responsible for the unconscious coordination of movement and balance, and for the memory of complex physical tasks.
   (iii) The brainstem links the spinal cord with the cerebellum and the cerebral hemispheres, and so is an important area for the relay of nervous impulses. It is particularly responsible for the control of the involuntary but essential body functions, and is the origin of the autonomic nervous system.
   (iv) The basal ganglia are nuclei of grey matter deep within the cerebral hemispheres, and are responsible for the control of the smoothness of muscle movement.
3. You might have listed any three of the following functions of the PSNS:
   - constriction of the pupil
   - increased secretions from the eye and digestive and respiratory tracts
   - increased peristalsis of the digestive tract
   - increased storage of glucose and other nutrients by the liver
   - opening of the bowels
   - increased production of urine
   - slowing of the heart and respiratory rate, and narrowing of the bronchioles
   - improved sexual function.

Chapter 4.1b The investigation of the nervous system

LEARNING POINTS

At the end of this chapter you will:
- be able to recognise the main investigations used for neurological disease
- understand what a patient might experience when undergoing these investigations.

Estimated time for chapter: 60 minutes.

Introduction

The investigation of the nervous system is managed within the hospital speciality of neurology. Because most of these investigations are highly technical, in the UK most are arranged for a patient only after referral to a hospital specialist called a 'neurologist'. An investigation of the nervous system might involve:

- a thorough physical examination
- investigations to examine the structure of the nervous system (magnetic resonance imaging (MRI), computed tomography (CT) scan and angiography)
- examination of the cerebrospinal fluid (CSF) and biopsy
- investigation to examine the function of the brain and spinal cord (electroencephalography (EEG))
- investigations to examine the function of the peripheral nerves (electromyography (EMG) and nerve conduction studies)

These investigations are considered briefly in turn below.

Physical examination

The physical examination of the nervous system involves the stages listed in Table 4.1b-I. Most aspects of the nervous system cannot be examined directly. Instead, much of the examination of the nervous system involves looking for the physical signs that can result from damage to specific parts of the nervous system.

Table 4.1b-I The stages of physical examination of the nervous system

- **Examination of the general appearance**: this can reveal the characteristic features of neurological disease that affect the facial appearance, movements and posture, such as Parkinson's disease and stroke
- **Examination of the retina**: by means of an ophthalmoscope
- **Examination of the cranial nerves**: a systematic examination that tests functions of the body which are controlled by the cranial nerves. These include:
  - the sense of smell and taste
  - the acuity of vision and the extent of the visual fields
  - the eye movements and the reactions of the pupil to light
  - the sense of hearing
  - the sensation of the dermatomes of the face
  - the strength of the facial muscles and the muscles of the palate and the tongue
  - the strength of the muscles of the neck and shoulders
- **Examination of the spinal nerves**: a systematic examination that involves testing of the following functions of the spinal nerves:
  - the sensation of the skin across the various dermatomes
  - the strength of the muscle groups in the limbs
  - the stretch reflexes of the important muscle groups such as the triceps, quadriceps and gastrocnemius
- **Examination of the cerebellum**: testing the balance and coordination of skilled movements
- **Examination of the cerebral cortex**: this can include a wide range of specialised tests designed to expose specific defects in functions such as speech, memory and the ability to recognise objects by their shape

Examination of the general appearance

This can reveal the characteristic features of neurological disease that affect the facial appearance, movements and posture, such as Parkinson's disease and stroke.

Examination of the retina by means of ophthalmoscope

This is the one aspect of physical examination that involves direct visualisation of an aspect of the nervous system. The retina at the back of the eye consists of layers of specialised sensory nerve cells called 'rods' and 'cones'. All the nerve fibres of these converge at a place called the 'optic disc', which is located just off the centre of the retina. From here they run down the optic nerve to the brain (the diseases that affect the eye are discussed in more detail in Chapter 6.1d). The appearance of this layer of nervous tissue and the root of the optic nerve can be seen using an ophthalmoscope. In addition to the conditions that affect the eye itself, this examination can reveal changes which occur as a result of increased pressure within the brain.

Examination of the cranial nerves

This is a systematic examination that tests the functions of the body that are controlled by the cranial nerves. These include:

- the sense of smell and taste
- the acuity of vision and the extent of the visual fields
- the eye movements and the reactions of the pupil to light
- the sense of hearing
- the sensation of the dermatomes of the face
- the strength of the facial muscles and the muscles of the palate and the tongue
- the strength of the muscles of the neck and shoulders.

Examination of the spinal nerves

This is a systematic examination that involves testing of the following functions of the spinal nerves:

- The sensation of the skin across the various dermatomes: by testing for the ability to sense a pin prick, heavy pressure and light touch from cotton wool.
- The strength of the muscle groups in the limbs: motor nerves are tested by systematically checking the strength of the various muscle groups of the body.
- The stretch reflexes of the important muscle groups such as the triceps, quadriceps and gastrocnemius: a light hammer is used to test the 'stretch reflexes' of some of the major muscle groups, for example the 'knee jerk'. In the knee-jerk test, the hammer is used to apply a sudden stretch to the patellar tendon, which attaches the quadriceps group of muscles, through the patella, to the upper part of the tibia. In healthy people there is a spinal reflex that causes the suddenly stretched muscle to contract. In the knee-jerk reflex the stretch of the patellar tendon causes the lower leg to kick upwards involuntarily as the knee joint is extended (see Figure 4.1a-XI). In conditions in which the upper motor neurons that descend from the brain to the spinal cord are affected by disease these reflexes will be excessive as a result of reduced inhibition of spinal tone. The reflexes will therefore be increased in conditions such as stroke or multiple sclerosis. In conditions in which the lower motor neurons that leave the spinal cord to supply the muscles are diseased, the stretch reflexes will be absent. Motor neuron disease is an example of such a condition. Also, any condition that impairs the sensory nerves which supply the tendons will also cause the stretch reflexes to be absent. This can occur in severe diabetes for example.

Examination of the cerebellum

This involves testing the balance and coordination of skilled movements.

Examination of the cerebellar cortex

The examination of the cerebral cortex can include a wide range of specialised tests designed to expose specific defects in functions such as speech, memory and the ability to recognise objects by their shape.

Magnetic Resonance Imaging (MRI) and Computed Tomography (CT) scan

The structure of the brain and the spinal cord can be examined in detail by means of MRI. The patient lies on a bed that is moved into a cylindrical scanner. A very strong magnetic field is used to produce detailed images of 'slices' of the body. MRI produces high-resolution images of nervous tissue, and in this respect for many neurological diseases it is a superior investigation to CT scanning (Figures 4.1b-I and 4.1b-II).

MRI is not believed to carry the long-term risk that exposure to the X-radiation that is used to produce CT scans carries does. However, many patients find this painless procedure an ordeal

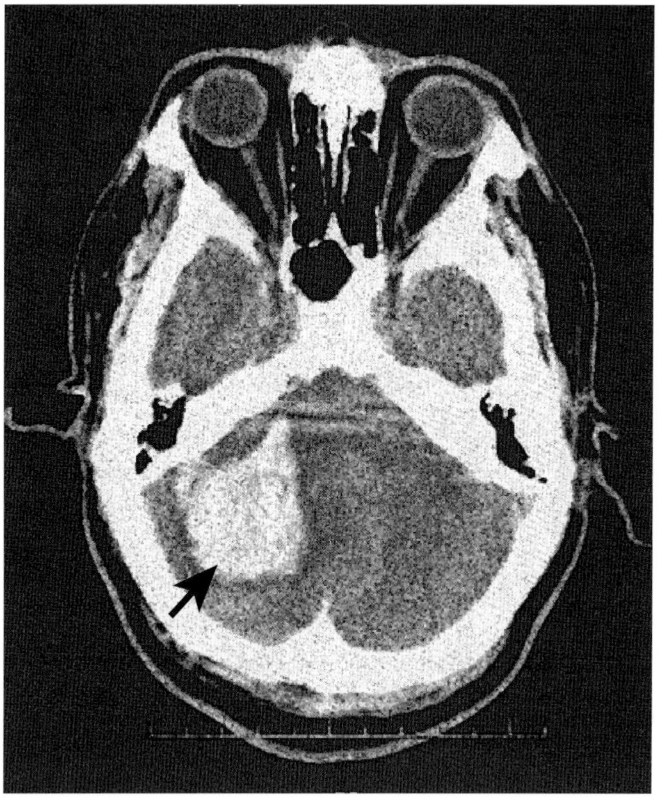

Figure 4.1b-I • CT scan of the brain showing an area of haemorrhage in the cerebellum (arrow) • A horizontal 'slice' taken at the level of the eyes. The eyeballs and optic nerves can be seen anteriorly, and the sphenoid bone of the skull is in the middle of the image.

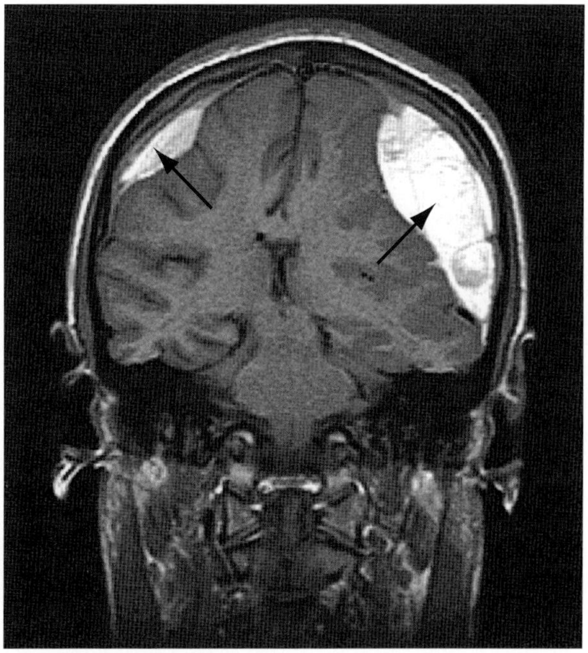

Figure 4.1b-II • MRI scan of the brain showing two areas of subdural haemorrhage (arrows) • A vertical 'slice' showing cervical vertebrae inferiorly. Note the very distinct contrast between the grey and white matter of the brain, a characteristic of a high-definition MRI image.

because it involves spending about 30 minutes keeping very still within the noisy enclosed space of the MRI scanner. Very small children and some adults cannot tolerate this, and may have to be given a general anaesthetic to undergo an MRI scan. The patient undergoing a CT scan has a very similar experience, as the external structure of the CT scanner is similar to that of the MRI scanner.

Before the development of CT and MRI scanners, plain X-ray images of the skull and spinal cord were very often used, although the information that these tests could give was never very specific. An invasive test called 'myelography', involving injection of a 'dye' into the subarachnoid space (the dye mixes with the CSF) was also commonly used to expose the structure of the spinal cord. However, this carried risks of inflammation of the meningeal membranes, and commonly had the side-effect of prolonged headaches. Myelography is no longer performed in most neurology departments, as it has been replaced by MRI.

Angiography

Angiography is described in detail in Chapter 3.2b on the cardiovascular system. The same technique is used in the investigation of diseases of the brain and spinal cord to produce images of the main blood vessels that lead to and supply the brain, although advances in MRI have led to this procedure being far less frequently performed.

Angiography can reveal the narrowing of the carotid and vertebral vessels in the neck. This narrowing can lead to emboli, and so is a risk for recurrent strokes. Angiography can also show up areas of the blood vessels that are dilated by aneurysms.

Despite being used as part of the prevention and treatment of stroke, angiography of these delicate vessels in itself carries a risk of stroke. Doppler (ultrasound) imaging is a useful non-invasive alternative investigation for the carotid and vertebral arteries of the neck.

Examination of the cerebrospinal fluid

A sample of cerebrospinal fluid (CSF) can be obtained by means of the technique known as 'lumbar puncture'. The unsedated patient is either seated or lying on their side in the fetal position. A needle is inserted into the L2/3 or L3/4 intervertebral space as far as the subarachnoid space, so that a few millilitres of CSF can be withdrawn.

Lumbar puncture is used most frequently to diagnose the infective organism in meningitis. It can also show characteristic changes in more rare conditions such as multiple sclerosis. The technique can also be used to treat certain diseases of the brain, as drugs can be injected directly into the CSF (e.g. for administering chemotherapy in the treatment of leukaemia).

The most common problem that occurs with lumbar puncture is that the patient can suffer from recurrent headaches as a result of the drop in the volume of the lubricating CSF. This complication affects up to one-third of patients. The patient is requested to keep lying down for 24 hours after the procedure in order to prevent this occurring.

The spinal cord terminates above the L2 level, and so there should be no risk of damage to the spinal cord from this test. Nevertheless, the needle can irritate or damage one of the lumbar spinal nerves that descend through the space, so leading to referred pain in the affected dermatomes, and possible numbness and weakness of associated muscles. This is a very rare complication.

It is in the diagnosis of meningitis that lumbar puncture carries the most risk. In severe meningitis, the inflammation of the brain can cause the CSF to be under great pressure. The sudden release of pressure that follows withdrawal of CSF can result in the brainstem being forced downwards against the base of the skull. This can be a fatal complication. Because of this real risk, if possible, all patients with meningitis should have a CT scan to look for signs of brain swelling before the lumbar puncture is performed.

Biopsy

In cases of suspected infection or cancer, a sample of tissue can be removed from the brain or other parts of the nervous system by means of a small probe. The biopsy is guided with the help of CT and MRI scans.

Electroencephalography (EEG)

The technique of EEG can be compared to electrocardiography (ECG) in that it detects electrical changes originating from a deep organ via electrodes placed on the skin. Both techniques are completely non-invasive. EEG exposes the electrical changes that are a reflection of the electrical activity of the brain, commonly called the 'brainwaves'.

The activity of the nerves in the brain leads to characteristic patterns of brainwaves, which vary according to the state of consciousness. The EEG of a person who is actively thinking is different to that of a person who is asleep. The brainwaves in sleep go through phases according to the depth of sleep, so that deep sleep can be differentiated from the dreaming state, in which there are spontaneous bodily movements and rapid eye movements (REM). Interestingly, the brainwaves that occur in a state of deep meditation (alpha waves) are very similar to those that occur in a stage of the healthy sleep cycle. It is known that the alpha brain rhythm is associated with a predominance of the parasympathetic part of the ANS.

In certain diseases, in particular during an epileptic seizure, the brainwaves look abnormal. The EEG is used most commonly to diagnose epilepsy. An EEG study may be combined with a video recording of the patient's behaviour, so that in the case of epilepsy a seizure can be captured on video and compared with the brainwaves that were occurring at the same time.

Electromyography (EMG)

This less commonly performed technique measures the electrical activity within a muscle. It involves the insertion of a very fine needle into a muscle. EMG can detect disorders of both the muscle and the motor nerves that supply the muscles.

Nerve conduction studies

This is another type of study that detects electrical changes, this time in the peripheral nerves. In nerve conduction studies one part of the nerve is stimulated with a small electrical impulse. The time for the impulse to be recorded further down the nerve is measured. This test can detect problems that affect the structure of the peripheral nerves (e.g. the damage caused by compression of the median nerve in carpal tunnel syndrome). A particular form of nerve conduction study assesses, by means of a surface electrode, the brain response to the stimulation of the eye or the ear. These 'cerebral evoked potentials' give information on the health of the neural pathways that link the sense organs with the cerebral cortex.

Self-test 4.1b

The investigation of the nervous system

1. You have referred a 50-year-old patient to his GP because you are concerned that the headaches he has been experiencing have been getting progressively worse. The GP has referred this man to a neurologist for further examination. When the patient asks the GP what he thinks the problem is, she explains that she believes the headaches are probably a form of migraine, but says that the referral is necessary in order to undertake tests to exclude a more serious diagnosis (such as cancer). What tests do you think this patient might have to undergo?

Answers

1. The patient will first undergo a thorough physical examination to look for any defects in function of the cranial nerves, the spinal nerves, the cerebellum and the cerebral cortex. His eyes will be examined using an ophthalmoscope to look for any evidence of swelling of the brain. Only if particular defects are found on this examination, or if the history is very uncharacteristic of one of the benign causes of headache, would this man have to undergo further tests.

   Of the possible further tests, MRI would be the most helpful, because if the findings are normal this will exclude all possible sinister causes of headaches. If a tumour is revealed by MRI, then further tests would be required to diagnose and stage the tumour. A biopsy of the tissue would be required, necessitating a minor MRI-guided operation.

Chapter 4.1c Disorders of the central nervous system: impairment of consciousness

LEARNING POINTS

At the end of this chapter you will:

- be able to recognise the main conditions that cause loss of consciousness
- be able to recognise the red flags of loss of consciousness
- understand the consequences of a raised intracranial pressure
- be able to recognise the red flags of raised intracranial pressure.

Estimated time for chapter: 60 minutes.

Introduction

Consciousness can be defined as a state of wakefulness in which there is awareness of self and surroundings. Consciousness results from the healthy functioning of certain parts of the brain. If these parts are damaged by disease, consciousness can be impaired. This can manifest as sleepiness or confusion, and can progress to stupor, when it is very difficult to rouse the patient to respond to external stimuli. A coma is a state of unrousable unconsciousness. If extreme, there are no responses at all, even to the most painful stimuli (see Q4.1c-1).

The cerebral cortices are responsible for the complex higher functions of the brain, including thinking, memory, conscience and will. If a small area of a cerebral cortex is damaged, a clearly defined disability may result. However, if the whole of the cerebral cortex is poorly functioning, such as might occur in advanced dementia or meningitis, then confusion followed by a lack of consciousness will develop.

The reticular activating system (RAS) in the brainstem is responsible for wakefulness. The RAS is responsible for switching off the consciousness in sleep, but can also be damaged in certain disease states. In particular, metabolic disturbances, such as hyperglycaemia in acute diabetes, uraemia in kidney failure or drug intoxication, can affect the functioning of the brainstem and lead to loss of consciousness. Similarly, raised pressure within the skull can cause compression of the brainstem against the base of the skull and lead to loss of consciousness.

Unconsciousness resulting from disease of the cerebral cortex

The cells of the brain, and the cerebral cortex in particular, are very sensitive to anything that disturbs the homeostasis of their immediate environment. Reduction in the levels of oxygen and glucose, or the presence of toxins or certain drugs can impair the function of brain cells much more rapidly than the cells of many other tissues of the body. Fever is another cause of impaired brain function, particularly if very high or if it rises rapidly. Physical trauma can also lead to a disturbance in the function of the cortex, which may only be temporary. Nevertheless, even if the damage is not long-lasting, a profound change in consciousness can occur for the period leading up to recovery.

This sensitivity to lack of oxygen and glucose, toxins, fever and trauma is very marked in young children and elderly people, which means that a state of confusion or drowsiness can result from what might appear to be a fairly minor bodily disturbance. For example, small children and old people can easily become poorly responsive or confused as a result of an infection or a high fever.

The effect of an oxygen or glucose imbalance

In general, even in severe disease, the bodily responses to a disturbance in homeostasis will ensure that an adequate supply of oxygen and glucose to the brain is maintained. The action of the sympathetic aspect of the ANS is very important in this respect. A simple faint can lead to loss of consciousness, but the SNS immediately responds to reverse the impaired blood flow to the brain, so that consciousness returns within a matter of seconds. The sympathetic nerves initiate an increase in the heart and respiratory rate, an increase in blood pressure, and a constriction of peripheral blood vessels so that more oxygenated blood is redirected to the brain and other essential organs. Glucose stores are released from the liver in response to sympathetic nervous activation.

Inadequate oxygen to the brain can result from insufficient atmospheric oxygen, such as might occur at high altitude. However, the most common cause is cardiac or respiratory failure, in which the heart and the lungs fail to ensure that sufficient oxygenated blood reaches the brain. For example, confusion and coma can be the result of very severe heart failure or chronic obstructive pulmonary disease (COPD). If these conditions cannot be treated, death will follow.

Insufficient blood glucose can result from the drug treatment of diabetes. This can lead to the progression of confusion, coma and death if not reversed.

The effect of drugs and toxins

The brain cells are also very sensitive to the build up of certain drugs and toxins. If these are present in excess, consciousness will be impaired, but the dysfunction is very often reversible. In fact, this sensitivity to drugs is utilised in conventional medicine when general anaesthetics are administered. Alcohol and sleeping tablets are other examples of widely used drugs that can also easily cause a reversible loss of consciousness.

In certain diseases a build up of toxins can occur. Kidney and liver failure are both conditions that can lead to confusion and coma for this reason. In both these conditions, without medical intervention the toxins will rapidly lead to death.

Other diseases alter the delicate balance of the chemical reactions that go on within all the cells of the body. These are known collectively as 'metabolic diseases' (metabolic imbalance is classed in Chapter 2.2a as one of the seven fundamental processes of disease). In some metabolic diseases the balance of acidity and salts in the blood becomes progressively disturbed. These disturbances can affect the function of the brain cells. Often, it is a disease of an endocrine organ that is the cause of this metabolic imbalance. It is for this reason that conditions such as pituitary disease, hypothyroidism and diabetes, if untreated, can lead to coma and death.

The effect of physical trauma

The brain is very vulnerable to physical trauma. A sudden blow to the head or a physical shaking can lead to a degree of swelling of the damaged brain tissue. This leads to a build up of pressure within the enclosed space of the skull. If this swelling is minor it may settle down within hours or days. In such cases the pressure causes a temporary dysfunction of the cortical brain cells and may even lead to a loss of consciousness. As the swelling settles down the patient may recover within a short time and regain normal function, although he or she will often have a period of memory loss relating to the time just before the injury and leading up to the period of recovery. This is the state which is described as 'concussion'.

In a more severe head injury the cells of the cortex and other parts of the brain may sustain permanent injury. If a patient with this sort of injury recovers from the coma, they will be left with a permanent loss of cortical function. If the damage is confined to one area of the cortex, the patient will suffer from a permanent deficit in the function that is controlled by that area of the brain. This is akin to the consequences of a stroke. These 'focal' problems of cortical function are described in Chapter 4.1d.

However, more commonly, a severe traumatic injury leads to loss of nerve cells throughout the cortex and other parts of the brain, so that the loss of function is much harder to define. In such cases there may be a change in aspects of the personality, memory loss and difficulties with perception and movement. This is the underlying problem that affects boxers who have become 'punch drunk'. In this case, it is repeated 'knock-outs' that have led to a cumulative and permanent loss of brain cells, a condition known as "dementia pugilistica".

If the cortical damage is very severe, consciousness may never be recovered. This leads to the condition known as 'persistent vegetative state' (PVS). In PVS the vital functions such as breathing and respiration, and the basic reflexes, such as coughing, remain intact, but the patient is unable to perceive anything about the environment and has lost awareness of self.

The other major consequence of head injury is that the pressure within the enclosed space of the cranium can increase to such an extent that the deeper parts of the brain such as the brainstem are also compressed. This can result purely from swelling of the brain, but may be compounded by internal bleeding.

Unconsciousness resulting from damage to the brainstem

The brainstem contains the RAS. If this part of the brain is damaged the patient will lose the state of wakefulness, and if the damage is severe will become unrousable. The most common causes of damage to the brainstem are stroke and raised intracranial pressure.

Brainstem stroke

The brainstem can be damaged by a stroke (see Chapter 4.1d), which causes a sudden reduction in oxygen supply to this vital part of the brain. Often these strokes are fatal because the vital centres of respiration and heart rate are damaged. Sometimes, it is consciousness only that is lost, and this can result in a permanent comatose state.

Suddenly raised intracranial pressure

A sudden increase in pressure in the intracranial space (the space within the enclosed skull) can cause severe damage to the brainstem. This is because the brainstem can be rapidly forced down against the opening of the foramen magnum and thus receive the brunt of the pressure. This situation carries a high risk of death, because the vital centres of the brainstem can be damaged.

The most common cause of this situation is the head injury that can result from high-speed road-traffic accidents. A combination of brain swelling and bleeding into the brain leads to a rapid rise in pressure within the cranium. In such cases there is a rapid loss of consciousness. A severe warning sign of brainstem damage is that the pupils become tightly constricted. Such a scenario is a neurosurgical emergency. The patient requires surgery immediately to drain any blood and fluid from the brain to relieve the pressure.

The other well-known cause of this sudden increase in pressure is severe bacterial meningitis (see Chapter 4.1e), in which an infection of the meninges leads to swelling and inflammation. As mentioned in Chapter 4.1b, in such a case the risk of damage can be increased by the procedure of lumbar puncture.

The role of the brainstem in death

Even if very severe damage is sustained to the cerebral cortex, such as in the case of PVS, life is maintained because the vital centres of the brainstem are intact. Although the causes of death are diverse, the final event that leads to death is always loss of function of the brainstem. It is this relatively small area of the brain which, figuratively speaking, holds the key to life and death.

However, in most deaths, the sequence of events is that the whole brain is affected either by lack of oxygen and glucose in the blood supply, or by a build up of toxins. This would be the case in death caused by heart attack, bronchopneumonia or liver failure, for example. This means that the cells of the cerebral cortex as well as those in the brainstem start to dysfunction. The person will drift or fall rapidly into unconsciousness, depending on the speed of events. Once the vital centres of the brainstem stop functioning, death will ensue within seconds to minutes, as the whole of the brain loses its already impaired blood supply.

Information Box 4.1c-I

Loss of consciousness: comments from a Chinese medicine perspective

In Chinese medicine, the state of consciousness reflects a healthy Shen. The Shen is the aspect of vital energy that is housed by the Heart Organ. When consciousness is impaired, the Shen is described as Obstructed in Chinese medicine. Obstruction of the Shen is said to occur following Obstruction to the Orifices of the Heart. Two of the most important Pathogenic Factors associated with this syndrome are Phlegm and Heat. The underlying mechanism of some of the causes of impaired consciousness described in the text can be attributed directly, from a Chinese medicine viewpoint, to Phlegm or Heat.

The obstruction to blood flow from atheroma, the underlying mechanism of many strokes, can be seen as a manifestation of Phlegm in the blood vessels. It is described in Chapter 5.1c how hypothyroidism is a condition that leads to accumulation of Phlegm. Any form of swelling of the brain will place pressure on the brainstem, and this will affect consciousness. This can result from metabolic diseases, head injury or from a tumour. Swelling of tissues may also be a manifestation of Damp or Phlegm.

High fever or infections such as meningitis represent Heat. Heat and Damp predominate in uncontrolled diabetes. Severe bleeding (reckless haemorrhage) is also seen as a manifestation of Heat. If this occurs into the brain, consciousness will be depressed.

Raised intracranial pressure

It has just been described how a sudden rise in intracranial pressure can cause severe damage to the brainstem and result in a loss of consciousness. However, there are a number of causes of a gradual rise in intracranial pressure which give rise to less dramatic symptoms.

There are three main reasons for a rise in intracranial pressure: swelling of the brain tissue, accumulation of CSF within the ventricles of the brain, and the development of a swelling or tumour within the brain. The term 'space-occupying lesion' is used to describe the latter cause. (The word 'lesion' in medical usage refers to any area of damage to the body that results from a disease process.)

In swelling of the brain tissue, the main symptom of raised intracranial pressure is impaired or lost consciousness, because the swelling develops rapidly as a result of inflammation. In contrast, the pressure that develops from accumulation of CSF and most space-occupying lesions (with the exception of the swelling that results from a haemorrhage) is gradual in onset, and impaired consciousness is not a prominent symptom until very late in the progression of the underlying condition.

Swelling of the brain from inflammation

As described earlier, inflammation can result from infections such as meningitis or encephalitis, or can be a response of the brain cells to toxins or drugs. In these sorts of cases the swelling of the brain tissue causes rapid changes in consciousness because it is primarily the cells of the cortex that are affected.

The inflammation of the brain that occurs following trauma can be much more severe, and can lead to compression of the brainstem. Again, in this case there is a rapid loss of consciousness.

Accumulation of cerebrospinal fluid

If the CSF cannot drain freely from the ventricles of the brain, the pressure of fluid within the ventricles will build up. The ventricles expand under this pressure and the surrounding brain tissue becomes compressed. This is called 'hydrocephalus' (from the Greek meaning 'water in the head'). Hydrocephalus can result from a congenital malformation of the structure of part of the brain, although the symptoms of this may not become apparent until adult life. In severe cases, the baby is born with an enlarged head, because the increased pressure has caused expansion between the not yet fused bones of the cranium.

Hydrocephalus can also develop in adult life. In most cases this is due to an obstruction in the flow of CSF by a brain tumour or from the scarring that follows an episode of meningitis or a brain haemorrhage. Hydrocephalus is occasionally found during may also be a the investigation of an elderly person with dementia. In these poorly understood cases, the pressure of the CSF is normal and the condition is called 'normal pressure hydrocephalus'.

Space-occupying lesions

A space-occupying lesion refers to any product of a disease process that takes up the limited space within the skull. This may be a brain tumour, an abscess or a collection of blood that has formed following a haemorrhage. All these conditions are described in more detail in the following chapters in this section. If the development of the space-occupying lesion is gradual, there will be a gradual increase in pressure within the skull.

The symptoms of a gradual rise in intracranial pressure

The three main symptoms of a gradual rise in intracranial pressure are headaches, vomiting and blurred vision. All these symptoms are progressive over a period of weeks to months. These symptoms should always be regarded as red flags of severe disease.

The headaches are characteristically worse in the morning because the pressure in the skull is increased after a night of lying down. The headache tends to wear off as the day goes on.

The vomiting is also worse in the morning, and need not be accompanied by nausea. This symptom is described as 'effortless vomiting'. The vomiting is probably a result of pressure on the vomiting centre in the brainstem.

The blurred vision occurs at a later stage, and is a result of pressure on the nerves that leave the brain to supply the retina of the eye. This produces a characteristic swollen appearance of the optic disc when the eye is examined using an ophthalmoscope.

The treatment of raised intracranial pressure

In all cases, whether the onset is rapid or gradual, treatment should be focused on reversal of the cause of raised pressure in the skull. This is undertaken as a matter of urgency.

In hydrocephalus, the CSF can be enabled to drain freely by means of the surgical insertion of a fine tube known as a 'shunt', which leads from the ventricles of the brain either into a large blood vessel or into the peritoneal cavity. This tube is passed from the brain through the deep tissues of the body and is left in place. It contains a tiny pump, which can be massaged through the skin to prevent it from becoming blocked. There is a risk of infection of this 'foreign body', so frequent courses of antibiotics may be necessary.

A space-occupying lesion has to be removed or drained by means of surgery. In the case of a brain tumour, after surgery, radiotherapy and steroids may be given to reduce further the size of the mass for as long as possible (see Chapter 4.1d) (see Q4.1c-2).

The red flags of loss of consciousness and raised intracranial pressure

Any patients with undiagnosed features of raised intracranial pressure will benefit from referral to a conventional doctor for assessment and/or treatment. Red flags are those symptoms and signs that will indicate that referral is to be considered. The red flags of raised intracranial pressure are described in Table 4.1c-I. This table forms part of the summary on red flags given in Appendix III, which also gives advice on the degree of urgency of referral for each of the red flag conditions listed.

Table 4.1c-I Red Flags 21 – raised intracranial pressure

Red Flag	Description	Reasoning
21.1	**Features of a rapid increase in intracranial pressure**: a rapid deterioration of consciousness leading to coma. Irregular breathing patterns and pinpoint pupils are a very serious sign	An increase in the pressure within the skull seriously threatens the integrity of the structure of the brain. If the pressure rapidly increases (usually as a result of a sudden intracranial haemorrhage or bleeding from a fractured skull) there can follow downwards pressure via the soft tissue of the brain onto the brainstem. The brainstem is the seat of the basic vital functions such as breathing and maintenance of consciousness. As the brainstem becomes compressed, the patient will lose consciousness and eventually will stop breathing. Constriction of the pupils is a result of compression of the nerve that leaves the brain at the level of the brainstem to supply the internal muscles of the eye. This is a grave warning sign of impending serious brain damage. Ensure that the patient is in a safe and warm place, and ideally in the recovery position (unless neck trauma is suspected), until help arrives
21.2	**Features of a slow increase in intracranial pressure**: progressive headaches and vomiting over the time scale of a few weeks to months. The headaches are worse in the morning and the vomiting may be effortless. Blurring of vision may be an additional symptom	Intracranial pressure will slowly increase if there is a gradual development of a "space-occupying lesion such as a brain tumour, abscess in the brain or accumulation of poorly draining cerebrospinal fluid. The pressure will be worse when the patient has been lying down, and so the symptoms are characteristically worse in the morning. Symptoms include blurring of vision, effortless vomiting (i.e. not much preceding nausea) and headache

Self-test 4.1c

Disorders of the central nervous system: impairment of consciousness

1. A new patient describes how he was involved in a car accident 5 years ago, after which he was in a coma for 3 days. Since that time he has suffered from a weakness of his right side, has poor memory and has frequent emotional outbursts. He is hoping that acupuncture can help him.
   What is the physical nature of the damage this man has sustained from his injury?
   In light of this, do you think that acupuncture might be of help in his situation?
2. A 40-year-old patient has been attending for the past month for treatment of headaches. These headaches started 3 months ago when the patient was involved in a stressful relationship break-up. The headaches have always occurred in the morning, but over the past 2 weeks have been progressively worse each day, despite your treatment. In the last week the patient has vomited with the headache, although he describes feeling much better after lunch-time.
   How would you respond to this scenario?

Answers

1. This patient appears to have sustained permanent loss of brain cells as a result of his injury. The one-sided weakness suggests some focal damage to the motor area of one cerebral hemisphere. The memory loss and emotional outbursts may be due to permanent loss of brain cells throughout the cerebral cortex.
   Nevertheless, even if all these symptoms reflect a loss of brain cells, which cannot be recovered, acupuncture, particularly involving scalp points, may well be of help as there is always potential for the brain to adapt and heal, although the improvement that can be expected may be limited depending on the degree of damage to the brain cells. Remember that, even though brain cells cannot be replaced, the connections between those remaining can be reformed. Memory loss and emotional outbursts may not necessarily reflect permanent cortical damage, as the shock of a traumatic accident and the development of a physical disability can lead to an emotional disturbance, which has its roots in depression rather than physical damage to the brain.
2. This patient is demonstrating the red flags of a gradual rise in intracranial pressure, with morning headaches and vomiting. The fact that the headaches are getting progressively worse is a serious sign. You should refer this patient for investigation to exclude hydrocephalus or a space-occupying lesion such as a brain tumour.

Chapter 4.1d Disorders of the central nervous system: haemorrhage, stroke and brain tumours

LEARNING POINTS

At the end of this chapter you will:

- be able to recognise the different conditions that can result from a haemorrhage within the skull
- be able to recognise the causes and possible outcomes of a stroke
- understand how a brain tumour might cause symptoms
- be able to recognise the red flags of these serious conditions.

Estimated time for chapter: 100 minutes.

Introduction

This chapter describes some serious conditions that affect the function of the brain, beginning with an exploration of the ways in which bleeding within the enclosed space of the skull (intracranial haemorrhage) can affect the brain. The chapter then examines the causes of stroke (one of these being brain haemorrhage) and the physical basis for the many different symptoms of stroke. Finally, the symptoms and treatment of brain tumours are described.

Intracranial haemorrhage

Haemorrhage within the skull has different consequences according to the site of bleeding. Conventionally, bleeding from within the skull is categorised according to its origin in relation to the three meningeal membranes. 'Extradural haemorrhage' refers to bleeding that occurs between the skull bones and the outer dural membrane of the skull. 'Subdural haemorrhage' describes bleeding that occurs between the dural membrane and the arachnoid mater. 'Subarachnoid haemorrhage' refers to bleeding that occurs in the space between the arachnoid and the pia mater; this is the space through which the CSF circulates. 'Intracerebral haemorrhage' refers to bleeding that occurs within the brain tissue itself.

Extradural haemorrhage

This occurs most commonly as a complication of a head injury in which the skull is fractured. The bleeding comes from the damaged blood vessels that normally run up the inside of the skull. Initially, the person who has had the injury may be conscious, but as the blood begins to accumulate along one side of the brain, the brain and brainstem gradually become compressed. Within a matter of minutes to hours the person will develop weakness of one side of the body, confusion and, eventually, coma. Without emergency surgery to drain the blood, the pupils will become constricted and death will follow due to compression of the vital centres of the brainstem.

Emergency surgery involves drilling a hole through the skull bones to drain the blood and surgical attention to any major bleeding blood vessels. In some cases this essential treatment can permit full recovery.

Subdural haemorrhage

A subdural haemorrhage occurs more commonly in the elderly. It is the result of bleeding from the veins that run between the dural and arachnoid membranes. In elderly people the supportive tissues around these veins become weak, so that the veins are liable to break more easily. This can occur as a result of a fairly minor fall or knock to the head. Subdural haemorrhage is more likely if the person is a heavy drinker.

In contrast to extradural haemorrhage, the bleeding is usually much more slow. A mass of clotted blood, called a 'haematoma', develops over the course of days to weeks. This gradually increases the intracranial pressure. The symptoms are of gradually developing drowsiness, confusion and headaches. Because the symptoms are often vague, the condition may not be diagnosed for some time.

The treatment is surgical drainage of the clotted blood, but it may be too late to reverse some of the damage to the brain that has occurred as a result of the bleed.

Subarachnoid haemorrhage

In subarachnoid haemorrhage the bleeding is from the arteries that pass through the subarachnoid space to enter the base of the brain. The bleeding is rapid, and thus symptoms develop quickly. In 80% of cases there is an underlying problem in the structure of these arteries, which has commonly been there from birth. The most common form of structural problem is the berry aneurysm (see Chapter 3.2c), which is a small rounded dilatation of the artery.

The leaking blood mixes with the CSF in the subarachnoid space, and therefore can circulate around the brain and spinal cord. The blood increases the pressure within this space and also stimulates an inflammatory response. The sudden increase in pressure causes an intense headache, which can be described as feeling like a hit to the back of the head. For this reason this type of headache is termed 'thunderclap headache'. The patient is in intense pain and needs to lie still. Vomiting is common. If the bleed is very large, the patient can rapidly become unconscious. In this case the patient will die if this serious bleed is not treated urgently.

The inflammation of the membranes is technically called 'meningitis', even though there is no infectious cause. This will disturb the function of the brain cells so that, following less severe bleeds, the patient may become drowsy or comatose over the period of a few days after the bleed.

All patients with a sudden onset of a very severe headache which appears out of the blue and which does not abate within a couple of hours should be assessed medically as a matter of urgency. The possibility of a bleed will be assessed by means of a CT scan, which can confirm the presence of bleeding. If the scan is inconclusive, a lumbar puncture may be performed to look for evidence of blood in the CSF. If bleeding is confirmed, then MRI-guided angiography may be used to locate the source of the bleeding. In up to 50% of cases of thunderclap headache these tests show no abnormalities, the patient recovers and the diagnosis remains uncertain.

The development of a subarachnoid haemorrhage is a very severe condition. Over half of all patients die before reaching hospital. Up to one-fifth of the remainder will die in hospital because the bleeding cannot be prevented or because the damage to the brain is already very severe. The immediate treatment is bed rest and management of any hypertension. Intravenous steroids and the calcium-channel blocker nimodipine may be prescribed to reduce brain swelling and prevent spasm of the cerebral blood vessels. Surgical treatments attempt to stop the bleeding from the artery by means of application of a metal clip. Increasingly, angiographic treatments are employed, including the insertion of platinum coils into the damaged blood vessels.

Of the 50% of patients who survive a subarachnoid haemorrhage, some will be left with a permanent disability resulting from brain damage, and some will develop hydrocephalus because of the scarring that has resulted from the inflammation. However, others will make a full physical recovery from this life-threatening condition.

Intracerebral haemorrhage

In intracerebral haemorrhage the bleeding occurs deep in the substance of the brain from one of the intracerebral arteries. This is usually a result of weakening of the arteries by atheroma, and may be precipitated by a rise in blood pressure, which puts strain on the already weakened arteries.

The blood spreads into the surrounding brain tissue and causes damage to the brain cells. It also has effects on more distant parts of the brain due to increased pressure. The result is that a specific aspect of the function of the brain is immediately lost, and very often this is accompanied by a severe headache. Intracerebral haemorrhage is one of the important and life-threatening causes of the condition called 'stroke', which is discussed below.

Information Box 4.1d-I

Intracranial haemorrhage: comments from a Chinese medicine perspective

The rapid bleeding and loss of consciousness associated with extradural and subarachnoid haemorrhage suggest that the Chinese medicine diagnosis could be Extreme Heat causing Obstruction of the Orifices of the Heart. The intense pain that can accompany these conditions reflects Stagnation of Qi and Blood.

In subdural and intracerebral haemorrhage, pain can be a less prominent feature, and the bleeding is more contained. In subdural haemorrhage, the blood congeals to form a mass of clot. In intracranial haemorrhage the underlying cause is usually atheroma in the cerebral arteries. This suggests that Phlegm is possibly an additional Pathogenic Factor in both these conditions.

Stroke

'Stroke' is the term used to describe a condition in which there is a sudden loss of function of part of the brain. The other commonly used medical term to describe a stroke is 'cerebrovascular accident' (CVA).

There are a number of causes of stroke, but cardiac emboli, hypertension and atheroma are the most important underlying conditions. The symptoms of the stroke depend on exactly which part of the brain has been damaged.

Stroke most frequently results from infarction of part of the brain (cerebral infarction). Common causes of a cerebral infarction are the formation of a blood clot which blocks an artery within the brain, and blockage by an embolus (usually a blood clot originating either in the chambers of the heart or from a distorted carotid artery) which has lodged within the artery in the brain. About one-third of strokes result from an intracranial haemorrhage. Although these are usually a result of atheroma in the blood vessels and hypertension, haemorrhage can also occur as a result of trauma.

Rarely, infarction occurs because of inflammation of the arteries of the brain (arteritis). Syphilis used to be one of the most common cause of arteritis of the arteries of the brain, but nowadays most cases are due to autoimmune disease (most commonly systemic lupus eryhtematosus (SLE) and temporal arteritis).

A rapidly growing tumour can also mimic a stroke, as it can lead to a sudden loss in brain function. Tumours are another cause of intracerebral haemorrhage, and so can also cause stroke in this way (see Q4.1d-1).

The conditions that lead to increased clotting (such as pregnancy) and problems with heart valves and heart rhythm (especially atrial fibrillation) are important causes of thrombosis and embolism.

Transient ischaemic attack (TIA)

A TIA is the consequence of a small embolus that lodges only temporarily within a branch of an artery in the brain. As the embolus usually consists of a tiny blood clot, this may simply break up with time. The temporary blockage of the circulation to the part of the brain causes a loss of function of that part, but only for a period of seconds to a few hours. Because the blockage is temporary, the brain cells can recover, and the person regains completely normal function after the event. If the blockage stays in place for longer than a few hours, the risk of permanent damage to the brain cells increases and full recovery from the event becomes less likely.

Blood clot emboli can arise for a number of reasons. The most common cause is from atheroma in the blood vessels of the neck that lead up to the brain. The carotid arteries (in the region of acupoint Renying St-9) are a common site for atheroma. Twisting and compression of the atheromatous vessels of the neck during neck movements may promote the development of emboli relatively easily.

The heart can also be a source of emboli (see Chapters 3.2f and 3.2g). The conditions of atrial fibrillation, damaged or replaced heart valves and endocarditis can all lead to the formation of emboli which can travel through the circulation to the brain.

Occasionally, emboli will develop in circumstances in which the blood is more prone to clot. For example, rarely, TIAs can occur in women who are pregnant, or those on the combined oral contraceptive pill. They are also more likely in smokers or those with a serious underlying disease such as cancer.

The symptoms of a TIA are indistinguishable from those of a small stroke, the only difference being that they are temporary. Symptoms such as blindness, inability to speak clearly, memory loss and one-sided limb weakness may develop only to recover again within minutes to hours.

A TIA is a serious occurrence because it is a warning of an impending stroke. Statistics show that within 5 years nearly half of all people who have suffered a TIA will have had a stroke, and a quarter will have died either from heart disease or stroke.

The patient with a TIA is investigated by means of an echocardiogram for underlying causes such as atrial fibrillation and damaged heart valves. A Doppler/ultrasound scan of the vessels of the neck can reveal the presence of atheroma and assess its extent. Angiography can be used to complement this investigation of the arteries of the neck. A CT scan or MRI may be performed to check that there has been no permanent brain damage.

The symptoms of TIA and stroke

The symptoms of stroke depend on which area of the brain has been damaged and how much damage has been caused. In a TIA or a small stroke, the symptoms generally reflect the fact that the damage is limited to a fairly small part of the brain. On the other hand, a stroke that results from a large haemorrhage or infarction of a major artery may lead to profound disability, coma or instantaneous death.

Nevertheless, there are some relatively small parts of the brain that have important functions, and if these are damaged by a stroke the patient may be left severely disabled. Problems such as loss of speech, blindness, one-sided weakness of a limbs, loss of memory and loss of balance may all result from damage to a relatively small area of the brain. In a TIA these problems are temporary, but in an established stroke these symptoms will persist to a greater or lesser extent.

In contrast, sometimes an established stroke may result in very few persisting symptoms. For example, sometimes a CT or MRI scan performed for another reason, reveals the signs of a past stroke, even though the patient has no history of any symptoms.

A large stroke can cause the loss of a number of functions of the brain. One common form of large stroke is one which affects a deep portion of one part of the cerebrum. This is called a 'cerebral stroke'. A cerebral stroke may result in loss of sensation and movement on the whole of one side of the body. If there is total paralysis of one side of the body this is called 'hemiplegia', while if there is some muscle strength remaining, then the term 'hemiparesis' is used. In hemiplegia and hemiparesis the weakness of the muscles results from damage to the upper motor neurons, which run down the spinal cord. The lower motor neurons, which lead from the spinal cord to the muscles themselves, are left intact. This means that the spinal reflexes that work to provide tone to these muscles are not impaired. Therefore, in hemiplegia and hemiparesis the limbs are not floppy, and instead there is increased muscle tone. The leg tends to assume an extended posture, and the arm becomes flexed at the shoulder and the elbow. The tendon reflexes, if tested using a tendon hammer, are increased. The sensitivity of this reflex is so great that the whole limb can go into an involuntary twitching movement called 'spasm' at unpredictable times. This can be both painful and embarrassing for the patient.

In addition, comprehension and production of speech may be lost. Loss of speech is termed 'aphasia', whereas partial impairment of speech is called 'dysphasia'. When the ability to articulate speech has been lost, difficulty in swallowing may also be present. This is a severe symptom as it can cause choking on food and drink.

A stroke to the posterior part of the cerebrum will damage the visual higher centres, so that difficulty in comprehending visual images or total blindness may result.

Strokes that affect the anterior part of the cerebrum may have less clearly defined physical effects, but can bring about a change in personality. Apathy, inappropriate social behaviour and impairment of intellectual function may be the result of such a stroke.

A stroke that damages the cerebellum will lead to clumsy movements, awkward speech and inability to maintain a steady balance.

A stroke that damages the brainstem often causes extremely severe symptoms because it can damage the vital centres in the brainstem. A brainstem stroke often leads rapidly to coma and death. A smaller brainstem stroke may leave the vital centres intact, but may damage the reticular activating system (RAS) or other centres which deal with bodily reflexes and balance. Therefore, various symptoms such as drowsiness, vomiting, hiccuping and dizziness can result from a less severe brainstem stroke.

One rare form of brainstem stroke causes serious damage to the fibres that link the brain through the spinal cord to the outside world. This stroke will leave the patient conscious, and with intact sight and hearing, but bodily sensation and the ability to move the body is lost. The patient is left totally paralysed but aware. The only possible form of communication is through blinking of the eyes. The medical term for this condition is 'locked-in syndrome'.

In some people, particularly those with hypertension, a number of small strokes occur in succession. These lead to a cumulative loss of function of the brain, which may superficially appear to result in a gradual decline in the intellectual and physical ability of the patient. In fact the decline occurs in a number of small steps. Over the course of time, memory and intellect deteriorate, and the patient becomes clumsy. The pattern is very like Alzheimer's disease, but can be distinguished by means of CT scan or MRI. This condition is called 'multi-infarct dementia', and is the second most common cause of dementia after Alzheimer's disease. It is also recognised that a stroke may trigger an Alzheimer-like dementia process.

Treatment of TIA and stroke

The treatment of TIA is to deal with the underlying cause and thus prevent the occurrence of a stroke in the future. In all cases patients should be prescribed either regular low-dose aspirin or warfarin (see Chapter 2.2d) to reduce the risk of the formation of emboli. Clopidogrel and dipyridamole are two platelet-inhibiting medications that might be used as alternatives. If heart emboli are confirmed, then evidence suggests that warfarin is the most effective anticoagulant to prevent stroke, but otherwise low-dose aspirin is the drug of choice because of its low risk of side-effects. These relatively simple therapies have been shown to be life-saving. Atrial fibrillation and endocarditis are treated medically. Smokers are urged to give up, and the oral contraceptive pill and hormone replacement therapy should be stopped.

Some patients will respond very well to a surgical operation to remove the atheroma from the vessels of the neck. This operation carries a significant risk (3%) of death, and so is only undertaken in those cases in which the potential benefit appears to be high on the basis of general health and angiographic assessment.

There is sadly very little that can be done to reverse the damage to the brain cells that has occurred as a result of a stroke. For this reason, many patients with TIAs or a mild stroke might not even be sent into hospital, although all should be referred to a specialist to rule out underlying preventable causes.

Most patients who have suffered from a stroke will undergo MRI or a CT scan to determine whether or not the cause is infarction (by thrombosis, embolism, arteritis or compression) or haemorrhage. Tests are performed for underlying conditions, such as atheroma of the neck vessels, hyperlipidaemia, hypertension, atrial fibrillation or autoimmune disease, which then can be treated. In the case of infarction, the patient will be prescribed a regular dose of aspirin, dipyridamol, clopidogrel or warfarin to prevent further clotting of the blood. This, of course, would not be appropriate treatment in the case of intracerebral haemorrhage. If the patient can be seen in a specialist unit within 3 hours of onset of the stroke, 'clot-busting' treatment may be considered for cerebral infarction. The drug tPA (tissue plasminogen activator) may be prescribed under close medical supervision.

Recovery from a stroke is known to be maximised if the patient is referred to a specialist stroke unit. Unfortunately, in the UK there are not enough stroke units to admit every patient who has suffered a stroke. In general, young patients who have suffered a severe stroke are the most likely to receive the specialised care offered by a stroke unit.

The aim of the treatment of stroke is rehabilitation, which is a process that enables the patient to regain as many of the activities of daily living (such as washing, dressing, self-feeding) as possible. Rehabilitation is not the same as recovery. It involves accepting that a disability is present, and then finding new ways to deal with life's challenges while living with that disability.

One of the principles of rehabilitation is to enable the patient to relearn certain activities so that different parts of the brain can be encouraged to take up the role of those parts that have been permanently lost. In this process, new connections will form between the remaining brain cells, and remarkable recovery can be achieved for up to a year after a stroke, and even after this time the patient may continue to make physical improvements.

Skilled physiotherapy is a fundamental aspect of stroke rehabilitation. The patient is encouraged to start using their muscles as soon as possible after the stroke and to relearn basic activities such as how to balance and walk. The physiotherapist will teach the patient with a hemiparesis how to prevent the limb muscles from becoming tight and contracted.

Speech therapy may be required in cases of aphasia and dysphasia. Speech therapists are also skilled in dealing with difficulties in swallowing.

Occupational therapists work with the patient to help them relearn the more complex activities that are important for a dignified and independent life, such as dressing and washing, making a cup of tea and using the telephone. An occupational therapist might recommend that specialised physical aids such as stair-lifts, raised toilet seats and modified kitchen appliances are installed in the patient's home.

A hospital social worker may counsel the patient about the possibility of returning to work and eligibility for various state benefits.

Stroke care is one of the many examples in the care of complicated physical illness in which a 'multidisciplinary approach' is ideal. Hospital doctors, the GP, the therapists described above, and the social worker may communicate with each other to coordinate the aspects of care for an individual patient.

The long-term outcome in stroke

The majority of patients who die directly as a result of a stroke will do so within the month following the stroke. Haemorrhagic strokes and large brainstem strokes tend to have the worst outcome. Patients with a large cerebral infarction, particularly one that affects swallowing, also do not generally do very well. This is because the problem of choking on food and drink, combined with impaired free body movement, carries a high risk of the patient of developing bronchopneumonia.

Many people who have had a stroke will go on to have a second or third stroke. In the majority of cases, because atheroma is an underlying problem, there is also a high risk of death from a heart attack.

Overall, of those who survive a stroke, about one-third will regain independent activities, and about one-third will require long-term institutionalised care.

Brain tumours

Tumours within the tissue of the brain are common. Approximately 10% of all forms of primary cancer arise from the brain. Secondary brain tumours arising from cancers elsewhere in the body, in particular from the lung, the breast, the stomach, melanoma and the prostate, are also common, constituting 30% of all brain tumours.

Primary brain tumours almost always arise from the neuroglial cells, which form the connective tissue of the nervous system. These tumours tend not to metastasise outside the nervous system, and instead cause damage by spreading within the tissue of the brain.

The symptoms of a brain tumour develop for two main reasons. The first is that the growth causes local damage to the surrounding tissue of the brain. According to the position of the tumour, the symptoms will be similar to those of a stroke affecting the corresponding part of the brain. The main difference is that with a tumour the symptoms are usually progressive rather than sudden in onset. For example, a brain tumour in one cerebral hemisphere may lead to a gradually worsening numbness and weakness of the opposite side of the body, a hemiparesis. Eventually, total paralysis, a hemiplegia, may develop. All this might occur over the course of days to weeks. In contrast, a stroke in the same part of the brain will lead to a sudden development of a hemiplegia. Sometimes the damage caused by a tumour is a trigger for an epileptic seizure. For this reason any person who has suffered with an epileptic seizure for the first time in their life should be investigated by means of a CT scan or MRI to exclude a brain tumour.

The second problem that can be caused by a tumour is a gradual rise in intracranial pressure, as discussed in the previous chapter (see Q4.1d-2).

The different types of brain tumours

Approximately 70% of primary brain tumours are malignant, the most common being astrocytomas and oligodendrogliomas. These strange names refer to the glial cell of origin of the tumour. Despite being malignant, some of these tumours are slow growing and develop gradually over the course of many years. Others are highly malignant and will cause death within months.

Information Box 4.1d-II

Stroke: comments from a Chinese medicine perspective

In Chinese medicine, the syndrome that corresponds to most forms of acute stroke is described as Wind Stroke. This term reflects the rapid onset of changing symptoms that occurs in a stroke.

In Chinese medicine, Wind Stroke is seen to occur due to a combination of factors. Wind causes the sudden onset of profound symptoms, and is understood to arise from underlying Liver Yin deficiency. Symptoms of mental confusion, numbness and slurred speech are described in terms of Phlegm or Phlegm Fire,and stiffness and pain in the limbs in terms of Blood Stagnation. Deficiency of Qi and Blood in the Channels predispose to the invasion of Wind and Phlegm and the development of Blood Stasis in the limbs and face.

In many cases, depletion of the Kidneys is an important underlying factor. Kidney Yin deficiency can lead to Liver Yin deficiency, and then to Liver Yang Rising and Liver Wind. Deficiency of Jing will deplete the Marrow, and this will fail to nourish the Blood. Blood Deficiency and Stasis is the result.

These Chinese medicine interpretations correspond to the modern medical understanding of stroke. In cerebral infarction stroke occurs because of insufficient blood supply to a part of the brain. The Chinese medicine interpretation of this would be Blood Deficiency and Blood Stasis. Very often, atheroma is an underlying problem. Atheroma may be understood in terms of a combination of Phlegm and Stagnation, as it is a substantial obstruction which impedes smooth flow of blood.

The bleeding from an intracerebral haemorrhage is very often associated with atheroma and hypertension. As profuse bleeding represents Heat, the Chinese medicine interpretation of this could be a combination of Wind and Phlegm Fire.

In stroke the substance of the brain itself is damaged. This would be interpreted as Jing (Essence) deficiency. Another possibility is that the tissue of the brain may be a physical location for the mysterious Orifices of the Heart and an aspect of the physical housing for the Shen. This can explain why a stroke can lead to symptoms such as mental confusion, loss of memory, intellect and personality change, all of which are properties of Obstructed Shen.

The remaining one-third of brain tumours are relatively benign. These can often be removed surgically, but may have caused irreparable damage to a part of the brain before they are diagnosed. The meningioma arises from the arachnoid membrane and can grow slowly to a large size. This growth will gradually damage a part of the cortex of the cerebral hemispheres by direct pressure. Also, if not diagnosed early, the tumour can lead to a rise in intracranial pressure.

The neurofibroma is a tumour that can arise anywhere in the body from a peripheral nerve. It can develop within the skull from the root of a cranial nerve. The most common form of this tumour arises from the auditory nerve (VIII), which arises close to the cerebellum and passes through a hole in the side of the skull to the ear. This tumour is also known as an acoustic neuroma. The symptoms include one-sided deafness and dizziness (vertigo). Eventually, pressure on the cerebellum can cause unsteadiness and clumsy gait (ataxia).

Pituitary tumours

Strictly speaking, pituitary tumours do not arise from nervous tissue, as they originate from the endocrine cells of the pituitary gland. Nevertheless, they develop at the site of the pituitary gland, which lies at the base of the brain within the skull, at the level of the eyes.

A pituitary tumour can grow so that pressure is exerted on the optic nerves, which lead from the eyes to the back of the brain, and so it can cause visual disturbances. It can also lead to symptoms of a gradual rise in intracranial pressure.

The most important symptoms of these tumours result from damage to the pituitary gland or from the production of excessive quantities of a single hormone, or both these problems. These aspects of pituitary tumours are discussed in more detail in Chapter 5.1e.

Treatment of brain tumours

Many patients with brain tumours and features of pressure effects initially will be given a high dose of a corticosteroid medication called dexamethasone. This has the effect of reducing swelling of the brain tissue and can cause a dramatic reduction in symptoms, irrespective of whether the tumour is malignant or benign.

If possible, the tumour is removed either completely or in part by surgery. This will be curative in operable benign tumours but, as mentioned previously, the patient may be left with a permanent disability due to localised brain damage.

Many patients will require long-term anti-epileptic medication to prevent the seizures that can result from the damage caused by the tumour.

In the case of malignant tumours, chemotherapy and radiotherapy to the brain may also be prescribed. These therapies can slow the progression of the tumour, but are rarely curative. In most patients with malignant tumours the growth will gradually spread again. Only half of patients with a malignant primary brain tumour will still be alive 5 years after the date of diagnosis (see Q4.1d-3).

> **Information Box 4.1d-III**
>
> **Brain tumours: comments from a Chinese medicine perspective**
>
> As with all forms of cancer, in Chinese medicine the substantial nature of a brain tumour would be interpreted in terms of Phlegm and Blood Stagnation. The fact that the site of the tumour is in the brain suggests that Kidney or Essence Deficiency is the most significant underlying problem that has preceded the development of the Pathogenic Factors.

The red flags of intracranial haemorrhage, stroke and brain tumours

Any patients with undiagnosed features of intracranial haemorrhage, stroke or brain tumours will benefit from referral to a conventional doctor for assessment and/or treatment. Red flags are those symptoms and signs that indicate that referral is to be considered. The red flags of these conditions are described in Table 4.1d-I. This table forms part of the summary on red flags given in Appendix III, which also gives advice on the degree of urgency of referral for each of the red flag conditions listed.

Chapter 4.1e Disorders of the central nervous system: headache and infections

LEARNING POINTS

At the end of this chapter you will:
- be able to recognise the main conditions that cause the symptom of headache
- be able to recognise the red flags of headaches
- understand the ways in which infectious disease can affect the central nervous system.
- Estimated time for chapter: 100 minutes.

Introduction

This chapter focuses on those conditions that cause the symptom of headache. Headache is a very common symptom, familiar to most people. In most cases, headaches have no underlying measurable physical basis. These headaches are usually ascribed a diagnosis of either tension headache or migraine. However, some headaches are much more sinister, for example, the early morning headaches of raised intracranial pressure and the thunderclap headaches of a subarachnoid haemorrhage introduced in Chapters 4.1c and 4.1d.

Table 4.1d-I Red Flags 22 – brain haemorrhage, stroke and brain tumour

Red Flag	Description	Reasoning
22.1	**Progressive decline in mental and social functioning**: increasing difficulty in intellectual function, memory, concentration and use of language	Gradual loss of mental function can result from a range of slowly developing brain disorders, including dementia, recurrent small strokes, extradural haemorrhage and slow-growing brain tumour Remember that, in the elderly in particular, depression can manifest in this way, and the symptoms may resolve with antidepressant medication.
22.2	**A temporary loss of brain function** (usually less than 2 hours long), such as loss of consciousness, loss of vision, unsteadiness, confusion, loss of memory, loss of sensation or limb weakness	A temporary loss of brain function is most commonly seen as part of the syndrome of migraine, in which case it usually is part of a pattern with which the patient is familiar. In migraine, the blood flow to a portion of the brain is temporarily reduced as a result of spasm of an artery. A simple migraine does not merit referral The most common cause of temporary loss of consciousness is a simple faint. This benign syndrome does not merit referral. It is characterised by low blood pressure and a slow but regular pulse, and is triggered by prolonged standing, stuffy conditions and/or emotional arousal. A person who has fainted should start to recover almost immediately after the collapse If these sorts of symptoms occur for the first time, and are not obviously due to a faint, then it is important to exclude the more serious syndrome of transient ischaemic attack (TIA) in which a branch of a cerebral artery has been blocked by the temporary lodging of a small blood clot. A TIA is a warning sign of the more permanent damage that results from stroke, and the patient needs referral for diagnosis and treatment
22.3	**A persisting loss of brain function**, such as loss of consciousness, loss of vision, unsteadiness, confusion, loss of memory, loss of sensation or muscle weakness	Any development of symptoms that suggest a persisting loss in brain function merits referral to exclude stroke or a rapidly growing brain tumour. Some of these symptoms can also result from disease of the spinal cord (e.g. multiple sclerosis) or of a peripheral nerve (e.g. Bell's palsy)
22.4	**A loss of brain function that is progressive** over the course of days to weeks: this is more suggestive of a brain tumour than a stroke	See Red Flag 22.3; progressive symptoms of loss of brain function are more suggestive of brain tumour than stroke
22.5	**Features of a slow increase in intracranial pressure**: progressive headaches and vomiting over the time scale of a few weeks to months. The headaches are worse in the morning and the vomiting may be effortless. Blurring of vision may be an additional symptom	Intracranial pressure will slowly increase if there is a gradual development of a "space-occupying lesion such as a brain tumour, abscess in the brain, extradural haemorrhage or accumulation of poorly draining cerebrospinal fluid. The pressure will be worse when the patient has been lying down, and so the symptoms are characteristically worse in the morning. These include blurring of vision, effortless vomiting (i.e. not much preceding nausea) and headache
22.6	**Features of a rapid increase in intracranial pressure**: a rapid deterioration of consciousness leading to coma. Irregular breathing patterns and pinpoint pupils are a very serious sign	An increase in the pressure within the skull seriously threatens the integrity of the structure of the brain. If the pressure increases rapidly (usually as a result of a sudden intracranial haemorrhage or bleeding from a fractured skull), there can follow downwards pressure via the soft tissue of the brain onto the brainstem. The brainstem is the seat of the basic vital functions such as breathing and maintenance of consciousness. As the brainstem is compressed the patient can lose consciousness and eventually will stop breathing. Constriction of the pupils is a result of compression of the nerve that leaves the brain at the level of the brainstem to supply the internal muscles of the eye. This is a grave warning sign of serious brain damage

Self-test 4.1d

Disorders of the central nervous system: haemorrhage, stroke and brain tumours

1. The wife of a 40-year-old patient of yours telephones to see if you can come for an emergency home visit. Her husband has been suffering from a very severe headache for the past 3 hours. It came on suddenly and he has taken to his bed, which is not at all like him. He has vomited with the pain. How might you respond to this request?
2. A new patient, a 65-year-old retired teacher, describes to you that over the past 3 weeks she has suffered from three episodes, each lasting only a few minutes, during which she feels very dizzy and sick. The room feels as if it is spinning and she has to lie down. After a short period of time she feels 'right as rain' and can get on with her daily activities.
   (i) What do you think might be the cause of these episodes?
   (ii) How might you advise this patient?
3. You have been treating a 50-year-old patient for some months for mild headaches that had developed during the past year. He now describes that one side of his face has become numb. He otherwise feels well. Would you refer this patient for a medical opinion?

Answers

1. The sudden onset of a severe headache that is not usual for a patient should be taken seriously, as it may indicate the onset of a subarachnoid haemorrhage. You should advise the patient's wife to call the on-call doctor or paramedics straight away so that the patient can be assessed medically.
2. (i) There is a possibility that these three episodes could represent transient ischaemic attacks (affecting the brainstem).
   (ii) It would be advisable to ensure that your patient visits her GP so that these episodes can be investigated and preventive treatment considered.
3. The development of a patch of numbness on the face in the context of a recent history of headaches could represent the progression of symptoms from a brain tumour. Although there may be a more benign explanation for this persisting neurological deficit, it would be best to refer this patient to their GP for investigations to exclude this important possible diagnosis.

Because recurrent headache is a problem very commonly presented to complementary therapists, the important distinction between benign symptoms and those that should be referred for further investigation is emphasised in this chapter.

The chapter concludes with an overview of the different ways in which infection can affect the brain. Three of the most common forms of brain infection are meningitis, encephalitis and brain abscess. All of these have headache as a primary symptom, so it makes sense to include them in this chapter.

The mechanism of headache

Contrary to popular understanding, the pain of a headache does not result from the brain tissue itself. The brain is supplied by hardly any pain nerve fibres. Headache in fact results either from sensations that originate from tissues outside the skull (e.g. the blood vessels and muscles of the neck and scalp) or from the tissues that surround the brain within the skull (e.g. the meninges and the blood vessels that supply the inner aspect of the skull bones).

The exact source of the pain in most benign headaches is poorly understood, although tenderness in the muscles of the scalp and neck frequently accompany benign headaches. It is conventionally recognised that the tenderness can be localised by the patient to very precise areas, and these are recognised as muscle trigger points by body therapists and as the equivalent of Ah Shi points in Chinese medicine. It is also well recognised that treatment of trigger points either by massage, manipulation or needling can relieve headache.

Benign headaches

In benign headaches there is no measurable physical basis for the symptoms. Because of this, the symptoms that result from a benign headache, even if very severe and debilitating, are not a source of serious concern to conventional practitioners (see Q4.1e-1).

Conditions that give rise to symptoms but which have no measurable physical basis are called 'functional syndromes'. Benign headaches, such as migraine, are an example of functional syndromes. It is important to recognise that, although the physical basis is not measurable, it does not mean that there is no physical basis. Instead, the term 'functional' implies that, whatever the mechanism of the underlying cause, it is too subtle to be assessed by currently available medical investigations and is unlikely to progress to a serious condition.

Tension headaches

Tension or stress headaches are the most common form of benign headache. The most common symptoms of tension headache include a feeling of tightness around the head, a pressure behind one or both eyes, and throbbing or bursting sensations. Usually these symptoms come on gradually, at any time of the day, and will ease off gradually. Sometimes a tension headache can last for days on end.

Many people recognise that certain situations will trigger their symptoms. Very often emotional stress is an underlying factor. In other people more physical causes such as muscle tension around the neck and shoulders, eye strain, sinusitis and toothache precede the development of the headache. Some people can attribute their headaches to certain foods or drinks, such as chocolate, coffee, oranges or alcohol. Headaches of a similar nature are a common symptom accompanying an infection such as a common cold or influenza. Tension headaches are also common premenstrually, in pregnancy and after childbirth.

In the absence of more worrying features, the most common practice is to reassure the patient, who may be concerned about a more serious underlying cause, and to recommend a painkiller. Aspirin and paracetamol are most frequently recommended, although increasingly many people use more potent preparations, including non-steroidal anti-inflammatory drugs (NSAIDs), such as ibuprofen, or morphine-related drugs, such as codeine. It is not uncommon for some people with recurrent tension headaches to self-medicate with the maximum dose of these drugs for days on end.

Many people find that regular massage of areas of chronic tension (trigger points) in the muscles of the neck and the upper shoulders can prevent tension headaches from developing.

The reassuring feature of a tension headache is that the symptoms are not progressive over the course of a period of weeks to months. In most cases the headaches have a familiar pattern of symptoms, and although they may get worse and more frequent during times of stress, they will settle down again when the pressure is off.

Information Box 4.1e-I

Tension headache: comments from a Chinese medicine perspective

In Chinese medicine, the syndrome of pain that is conventionally termed 'tension headache' can be attributed to a range of syndromes according to the precise nature and location of the symptoms. External Full conditions that can cause headache include invasion of Wind Cold, Wind Heat and Wind Damp. Internal Full conditions include Liver Qi Stagnation, Liver Yang Rising, Liver Fire Blazing, Stomach Fire and Blood Stagnation. Internal Empty conditions include Blood Deficiency, Qi Deficiency and Kidney Deficiency. In all these conditions the underlying syndrome leads to a Stagnation of Qi and Blood in the scalp or the neck, and this is the manifestation that leads to the pain.

All painkillers act by moving Qi and Blood. With the possible exception of aspirin in a case of Wind Cold invasion, none of them addresses the root cause of the imbalance. Aspirin may release the exterior in an invasion of Wind Cold and so may be an appropriate energetic remedy. All the other preparations are suppressive in nature.

In some types of headache, in addition to the effects of suppressed symptoms, the drug-induced disease caused by the medication may also worsen the root imbalance. For example, aspirin can cause Stomach Heat, and so may worsen the underlying problem in a Stomach Heat headache, even though it can improve the symptoms temporarily. Paracetamol and the morphine-related drugs are toxic to the liver, and so may worsen the underlying imbalance in headaches caused by Liver Qi Stagnation and Liver Yang rising.

Migraine

In contrast to the possible muscular origin of tension headache, the pain of migraine is believed to originate from the blood vessels that supply the brain within the skull. The vessels are thought to constrict and then expand during a migraine attack, and this leads to the symptom of a throbbing headache. The one-sided nature of the syndrome is attributed to the fact that this problem only affects the vessels on one side of the brain.

Migraine is distinguished from tension headache on the basis of some characteristic features. In contrast to tension headache, many people report that a migraine attack might come on at a time when stress has been relieved, such as the weekend after a busy working week. Very often a dietary trigger can be found. Chocolate, coffee, cheese, monosodium glutamate and red wine are among the most common dietary triggers for migraine. The experience of migraine often changes at puberty, during pregnancy or during the menopause. Some people get better and some people get worse after these times of major hormonal change.

The classic syndrome of migraine involves a period of a few minutes to hours of some warning symptoms called an 'aura', although most (90%) patients with migraine do not experience an aura. It is believed that the aura results from constriction of the blood vessels that supply a defined part of the brain. For this reason, the symptoms of an aura can be very like a stroke or TIA.

The most common form of aura that migraine patients experience involves visual disturbances, often including flashing lights or some loss of vision. Some experience a characteristic mood change, dizziness or a strange smell, and others experience a temporary weakness of one half of the body (hemiparesis) or inability to speak (aphasia).

The migraine headache itself is characteristically one sided, often located behind or above one eye. In a severe case the patient may feel nauseous and may have diarrhoea or vomiting. Many people need to lie down in a darkened room. The headache usually lasts for a few hours. When it wears off some people report that they experience a period of a day or so of exhaustion, and some describe a lightened mood, sometimes described as euphoria.

Some migraines are not so severe, and so in many cases it is difficult to distinguish them from tension headaches.

The treatment of migraine involves treatment to relieve the acute attack and treatment aimed at prevention of future attacks. Migraine will settle down without any treatment, but many people find that the pain and nausea is so debilitating that they seek medication. If migraine is relatively infrequent, painkillers are generally prescribed, although commonly much stronger preparations are required to have any effect on the pain of a bad migraine. Tablets that contain a combination of paracetamol and a morphine-related drug such as codeine (Co-codamol) are commonly prescribed. Recently high dose aspirin (900 mg) has been found to be particularly effective for the treatment of migraine. Antinausea medication such as metaclopramide (Maxolon) may also be prescribed for an acute migraine attack.

The triptan drugs such as rizatriptan or sumatriptan are prescribed to treat very severe symptoms. These are available in a tablet and injection form, and it is advised that they are taken as early as possible to abort a migraine attack. These drugs give marked relief in over one-third of patients, and so are commonly prescribed. The triptans reverse the dilatation of the blood vessels in the brain, but can have side-effects resulting from constriction of other blood vessels in the body. For example, angina is a known side-effect. For this reason, triptans should not be given to people with heart disease or uncontrolled hypertension.

To prevent further attacks it is helpful if the patient can determine whether there are any avoidable triggers for the migraine. Keeping a headache diary can be useful in clarifying a link with dietary or other lifestyle factors. The offending trigger can then be avoided if possible.

All women with focal (classic) migraine should use alternative forms of contraception to the oral contraceptive pill, as the risk of stroke is increased in women with migraine who take the pill.

There are a range of drug preparations that can be taken regularly to avoid migraine (i.e. for prophylaxis). These tend to be considered if attacks occur more than twice a month. Pizotifen is a commonly prescribed preparation. This has the side-effect of drowsiness and weight gain, but will often reduce the frequency of attacks. Beta blockers can also reduce the frequency of migraine. Propranolol is one of the most commonly prescribed beta blockers. Antidepressants such as amitriptyline can also help reduce frequency of attacks. If these fail, sometimes the antiepileptic medications valproate, gabapentin or topiramate may be effective for prophylaxis

Information Box 4.1e-II

Migraine: comments from a Chinese medicine perspective

In Chinese medicine, the intensity and one-sided frontal position of the typical migraine suggests that the pain is a manifestation of a mixed or full condition. Liver Yang Rising, Liver Fire Blazing and Stomach Heat might all give rise to the symptoms of migraine. A dislike of bright light suggests an imbalance of the Liver. Nausea, vomiting and diarrhoea can be attributed to Stagnant Liver Qi invading the Stomach and Spleen.

The fact that migraine is recurrent suggests that there is a longstanding tendency to imbalance of the Liver Organ. Pent-up emotions are likely to be a common underlying cause of Stagnation of Liver Qi. The underlying pathology of dilatation of blood vessels suggests that Heat is present, either as a result or as a cause of the Stagnation.

The simple painkillers tend to move Blood and Qi. The triptans cause constriction of blood vessels, and so could be described in terms of Clearing Heat, but at the expense of causing more Stagnation (constriction of blood vessels) of Blood and Qi. These preparations are all suppressive in nature.

The drugs used to prevent migraine all have in common the tendency to promote Damp or Phlegm or Yang Deficiency, a fact evidenced by the side-effects of treatment such as weight gain, coldness, drowsiness and sluggishness. These treatments are all suppressive in nature.

Cluster headache

Cluster headache is a debilitating form of headache characterised by recurring bouts of intense pain centred over one eye. The bout of pain lasts for up to several hours and can be so severe as to cause vomiting. The affected eye may become bloodshot and the eyelid may droop. The attacks often occur at night, and can recur over a period of about 4–8 weeks. Sometimes there can be a long remission of months to years before the next series of attacks.

The frequency of attacks peaks between the ages of 20 and 55 years, after which they generally become less severe and less frequent. They are more common in men.

The headaches do not appear to be related to migraine. Inhalation of 100% oxygen may be prescribed during an acute attack, and drugs as diverse as calcium-channel blockers, lithium and steroids have been prescribed in attempts at prophylaxis.

Information Box 4.1e-III

Cluster headache: comments from a Chinese medicine perspective

In Chinese medicine, the intense pain of a cluster headache represents severe Blood Stagnation in the region of the Gallbladder channel. In the light of the intensity of the attacks, the underlying syndrome would appear to be either Liver Yang Rising or Liver Fire Blazing.

Less benign causes of headache

Conditions such as intracranial haemorrhage and the causes of raised intracranial pressure have been described in earlier chapters as very serious causes of headache. The two remaining important serious causes are temporal arteritis, an inflammatory condition which affects older people, and the various infections that can affect the brain and the meninges.

Temporal (giant cell or cranial) arteritis

Temporal arteritis is an inflammatory condition of possible autoimmune origin, which almost always affects people over 50 years of age. Men are affected more commonly than women. The underlying problem is an inflammation of the blood vessels (vasculitis) of the brain and scalp. In about one-quarter of cases the patient also suffers from the condition of polymyalgia rheumatica.

Inflammation of the blood vessels that supply the temples (temporal arteries) is a common feature of the condition. This leads to a severe one-sided headache (in the region of acupoint Taiyang M-HN-9), and exquisite tenderness in this region across which the inflamed artery runs. Commonly, tenderness may radiate back over the scalp to the base of the skull on the same side. The artery can be thickened and distorted in shape. There can also be pain in the face, jaw and mouth, particularly on chewing.

The headache and facial pain of temporal arteritis are red flags of a very serious complication of the condition. This is a result of inflammation of the retinal artery, which can lead to sudden and irreversible blindness in one eye.

Temporal arteritis should be referred as a matter of urgency. A blood test generally shows a very high erythrocyte sedimentation rate (ESR) and C-reactive protein (CRP) (see Chapter 3.4b), which is highly suggestive of the diagnosis. Treatment is urgent administration of high-dose corticosteroids (60 mg/day). In most cases this will lead to the reversal of the symptoms, and markedly reduces the risk of developing permanent visual impairment. Rapid withdrawal of this medication may result in recurrence of the symptoms, and the patient may have to remain on very gradually reducing doses of steroids for a period of months to years, while activity of the condition is assessed by means of serial ESR tests.

The diagnosis of arteritis is usually confirmed by means of a biopsy of the temporal artery, although this test is often only performed after treatment has been established.

Information Box 4.1e-IV

Temporal arteritis: comments from a Chinese medicine perspective

In Chinese medicine, the pain of temporal arteritis corresponds to Blood Stagnation in the region of the Gallbladder and Stomach channels. The late age of onset and underlying inflammation suggest that Yin Deficiency (in particular of Liver Yin) and Heat are underlying factors. As with other autoimmune diseases, Damp and Phlegm are likely to be present. The evidence for this is in the thickened and distorted blood vessels.

The sudden onset of blindness is very similar to that which might occur in a small stroke, and therefore might represent a stirring up of Phlegm by Wind. This Obstructs the Orifices of the Heart (as the Heart, together with the Liver, is the Organ responsible for clear vision) and may lead to a sudden loss of vision.

Infections of the brain

The brain is affected by infectious agents in three ways: meningitis (inflammation of the meninges), encephalitis (inflammation of the substance of the brain, and brain abscess (a localised collection of pus within the brain). Headache is a symptom that is common to all of these serious types of infection.

Meningitis

Meningitis literally means inflammation of the meninges, and can have a variety of causes. Upper respiratory tract organisms are the most common cause of meningitis.

Most often the condition of meningitis gives rise to severe symptoms that develop over the course of a few hours. This is known as 'acute meningitis', and is most commonly the result of bacterial or viral infection. A more slowly developing form of meningitis is also recognised. This is termed 'chronic meningitis'.

The bacterial causes of acute meningitis can lead to the most severe infections because they tend to cause more pus formation and therefore more damage to the lining of the brain. One of the most common bacterial causes is meningococcus (*Neisseria meningitidis*). This organism leads to an infection called 'meningococcal meningitis'. Two of the other important bacterial causes of meningitis are pneumococcus (*Streptococcus pneumoniae*) and *Haemophilus influenzae*.

Common viral causes of acute inflammation of the meninges include mumps and *measles*. In general, viral meningitis is less severe than bacterial infection, and is commonly followed by full recovery. In rare cases, infection with the human immunodeficiency virus (HIV) can cause a form of meningitis.

Chronic meningitis is a condition that results from a slowly developing infection. This can be a result of tuberculosis infection, or can occur as a form of opportunistic infection in conditions that lead to impairment of the immune system. In acquired immunodeficiency syndrome (AIDS), for example, fungal and tuberculous infection can lead to vague symptoms that develop over the course of a few weeks.

Acute meningitis is characterised by a triad of symptoms which, if found together, should always be taken seriously. These are severe headache, neck stiffness and fever. Nausea and vomiting are also commonly present. The headache is characteristically intense. The patient prefers to lie still in a darkened room, sometimes lying with the neck arched backwards. This extended head position is particularly noticeable in young children.

Neck stiffness refers to the resistance that is felt by an examiner trying to move the patient's head freely at the neck. In meningitis there is muscle spasm in the upper back and neck, and free movement is involuntarily resisted.

Fever is usually, but not always, high. In uncomplicated meningitis the patient remains fully conscious. In practice, if any patient has a severe headache, nausea and fever, it is wise to refer them to their GP or medical emergency department for an urgent medical opinion.

Another very serious sign, which is unique to meningococcal meningitis, is the development of a bruising rash. This rash, which may be confined to only one part of the body, is a result of inflammation of the blood vessels following infection of the blood (septicaemia). The blood vessels leak blood into the tissue, so that the marks of the rash look deep red or purplish in colour and (unlike most rashes) they do not fade (blanch) when pressure is applied to them. If a person with the symptoms of meningitis develops this rash, they should be referred to hospital as a matter of urgency.

Without treatment the infection of acute bacterial meningitis can spread into the brain tissue, and the resulting tissue swelling can cause severe pressure on the brain. This will cause the patient to fall into a coma. Death may follow as the vital centres of the brain become irreversibly damaged.

An episode of viral meningitis will generally settle down over the course of a few days, although the patient may experience persistent headaches for a prolonged period following the infection.

The treatment for acute bacterial meningitis is primarily by means of intravenous antibiotics. In an urgent case benzylpenicillin or an equivalent antibiotic will be given before any tests are performed because the condition can deteriorate very rapidly. If in hospital, the patient might also be given intravenous steroids to reduce swelling of the brain tissue.

In a less unwell patient, tests to confirm the diagnosis should first be performed before antibiotic treatment is given.

These tests include blood samples to culture for bacteria. Many patients are then given a CT scan, which may show the accumulation of pus within the subarachnoid space. If there is no warning sign of increased intracranial pressure from the CT scan, a lumbar puncture (see Chapter 4.1b) is performed to obtain a sample of cerebrospinal fluid. The fluid obtained will show increased leukocytes and many bacteria in a bacterial infection. It is very helpful to confirm the type of bacteria so that appropriate antibiotic treatment can be chosen.

Even with rapid and appropriate treatment, 15% of patients with bacterial meningitis will die. A proportion of those who recover will have some persisting damage, most commonly deafness due to damage to the nerve that leads from the base of the brain to the ear. Many more will suffer from a prolonged syndrome of weakness and recurrent headaches.

In a case of meningococcal meningitis, the close contacts of the patient will also be offered antibiotic treatment in the form of a very short course of rifampicin or ciprofloxacin, as it is known that close contacts are more likely than the average person to be 'carrying' the meningococcus as part of the 'healthy' bacteria that reside in their respiratory tract. However, studies of healthy people show that many people (up to 25% is some groups of young people) do carry this bacterium harmlessly. It remains a mystery why only a tiny proportion of those who carry the meningococcus will actually develop meningitis.

Vaccines are available to prevent two forms of bacterial meningitis. The HiB and meningitis C vaccines are offered to all babies as part of the UK routine immunisation schedule at 2, 3 and 4 months of age.

The symptoms of chronic meningitis are much slower to develop. Vague recurrent headaches, low fevers, exhaustion and nausea are typical symptoms, which can be present for weeks before a diagnosis is made. Treatment of chronic meningitis is by means of appropriate antibiotic therapy.

Information Box 4.1e-V

Acute meningitis: comments from a Chinese medicine perspective

In Chinese medicine, the symptoms of acute meningitis would closely approximate to an extreme Wind Heat invasion. The headache is due to Stagnation of Blood and Qi in the head as a result of Wind. The high fever is a manifestation of extreme Heat. In bacterial meningitis, the development of pus is an indication that Phlegm is also present. Wind and Phlegm can combine to obstruct the Orifices of the Heart and this can manifest as impaired consciousness.

In conventional medicine terms, antibiotic treatment acts by clearing the pathogens, and this could be described symptomatically in Chinese medicine as Clearing of Wind Heat and Phlegm. The drawn-out period of recovery in some people with meningitis may be a reflection of residual Pathogenic Factors.

The fact that bacterial meningitis is often caused by a bacterium commonly found in the respiratory tract suggests that an underlying susceptibility, possibly in the form of Wei Qi deficiency or Yin deficiency, plays a part in the development of meningitis.

Encephalitis

Encephalitis is a condition in which the substance of the brain is inflamed. This is a deeper condition than meningitis. In most cases, encephalitis is caused by viruses, although bacteria and fungi are common causes in people who are immunocompromised (e.g. those with AIDS).

Some brain infections lead not to inflammation but degeneration, and result in a syndrome of dementia similar to Alzheimer's disease. Prion disease, such as Creutzfeldt–Jakob disease (CJD) and new-variant CJD (attributed to bovine spongiform encephalitis (BSE) infection), are two examples. Degeneration of the brain is also a late manifestation of syphilis and HIV infection.

In the UK, the most common viruses to cause encephalitis include mumps, measles and herpes simplex, the virus which causes cold sores. Sometimes the infection, such as viral meningitis, is relatively mild. The patient develops headache and fever, but will recover within a few days.

In more severe infections, headaches and fever are followed by drowsiness, confusion and mood changes. Herpes simplex is the most common cause of severe encephalitis in the UK. If untreated, features of localised brain damage, including epileptic fits (see Chapter 4.1f) and loss of consciousness, might develop. Permanent brain damage or death can be the result of severe infections.

Rabies is a well-known form of encephalitis which is transmitted through the bite of an infected animal. Without urgent treatment the encephalitis caused by rabies is always fatal.

Encephalitis is diagnosed by means of CT scans, and MRI and EEG recordings. Herpes simplex infection can be treated with an intravenous antiviral drug called aciclovir although the impact of this drug on the infection and on long-term recovery is not as great as with antibiotics and bacterial meningitis.

Vaccines are available to protect against encephalitis caused by mumps and measles, although these are very rare complications of these previously common infections. These vaccines are offered to all children in the UK as part of the measles–mumps–rubella (MMR) vaccine. Rabies vaccine is available to protect travellers to areas in which rabies is endemic.

Information Box 4.1e-VI

Encephalitis: comments from a Chinese medicine perspective

In Chinese medicine, the symptoms of encephalitis, like meningitis, suggest an Invasion of Wind Heat. Drowsiness and loss of consciousness are a result of obstruction of the Orifices of the Heart.

Encephalitis is a rare infection, but is caused by common viruses. This suggests that, as with meningitis, there is a pre-existing susceptibility in the patient. Deficiency of Wei Qi or of Yin are likely to be present in someone who develops viral encephalitis.

Myalgic encephalomyelitis (chronic fatigue syndrome)

Myalgic encephalitis (ME) is one of the many terms used for an increasingly described syndrome of chronic tiredness and aching muscles. The currently medically preferred term for this syndrome is 'chronic fatigue syndrome'. The name 'myalgic encephalitis' literally means 'inflammation of the brain and spinal cord (encephalomyelitis) with aching muscles (myalgia)'. Although it can affect all groups of people, it has been reported to be common in young people, especially women, from high-achieving backgrounds, and students who have a tendency to overwork. A history of trauma such as whiplash may also be present.

The symptoms that can be experienced in ME include fatigue (by definition affecting more than 50% of the day and lasting over 6 months), poor concentration and memory, swollen and tender lymph nodes, mood changes, unrefreshing sleep, and muscle and joint aches. The nature of the fatigue is characteristic in that muscles become progressively more fatigued with recurrent use. The condition can be extremely debilitating, but is not life-threatening.

Despite its medical name, ME is considered by the medical profession to be a functional syndrome. This means that there are no easily measurable physical changes consistently found in patients who complain of the symptoms characteristic of the syndrome. This is why many doctors believe that 'chronic fatigue syndrome' is a better term to describe the condition.

Scientific studies have shown that the blood supply to parts of the brain is reduced in patients who have the symptoms of ME, which does indicate that there is some physical basis to the condition. Also, there is evidence that there is abnormal mitochondrial function in some patients, which points to problems in the cellular production of energy in the form of ATP. This is supported by research evidence that treatment with the drug NADP, a precursor of ATP, showed some promising results in symptom reduction in chronic fatigue syndrome.

However, because of the lack of simple tests to diagnose the condition, ME is often diagnosed after a long period of excluding other conditions. Although some cases follow a viral infection, such as influenza or glandular fever, this is not a consistent finding, which means that an infective cause is generally not medically recognised. In some cases, the symptoms develop slowly over the course of a few months. In these cases it is often impossible to pinpoint a particular infection that might have been the trigger for the symptoms

In the UK, most patients who seek help from an NHS doctor will, at best, be offered psychological therapies, including counselling and antidepressant medication, together with graded exercise programmes. It is generally believed that it is important to help the patient see their symptoms as possibly having a psychological component, and it appears that patients who are resistant to accepting this possibility have a worse prognosis.

Information Box 4.1e-VII

Myalgic encephalitis (chronic fatigue syndrome): comments from a Chinese medicine perspective

In Chinese medicine, the symptoms of myalgic encephalitis, or chronic fatigue syndrome, correspond to one or more of Residual Pathogenic Factor, Latent Heat or the Lesser Yang pattern according to the Six Stages theory. Damp and Heat are the predominant Pathogenic Factors in these conditions. There is often an underlying deficiency syndrome, such as Qi Deficiency, or Deficiency of Kidney Yin and Yang.

Brain abscess

A brain abscess results from a localised area of pus-producing infection within the brain. The area of pus expands to produce a mass, which compresses adjacent parts of the brain, and so the symptoms of a gradual rise in intracranial pressure can develop (see Chapter 4.1c).

The source of infection is usually an area of the body that is close to the brain, commonly the middle ear and the sinuses. However, an abscess can develop through spread of infectious organisms in the blood from a more distant source, such as from pneumonia or endocarditis. Although tuberculosis is a rare cause of a brain abscess in the UK, tuberculous brain abscess is relatively common worldwide.

The symptoms of a brain abscess can be very similar to those of a brain tumour (see Chapter 4.1d), and similarly there can be a long delay before the correct diagnosis is made. The symptoms may persist in a vague form for weeks before the patient becomes very unwell. Common symptoms include vague headache, low fevers, and the progressive signs of brain damage, such as hemiparesis or epileptic fits.

The brain abscess is diagnosed and clearly localised by means of CT scan or MRI. Some abscesses will respond to antibiotic treatment alone, but in many cases a surgical operation is required to drain the pus. However, despite treatment, up to one-quarter of people with a brain abscess will die from the damage caused by the infection (see Q4.1e-2).

The red flags of headache

Some patients with headache will benefit from referral to a conventional doctor for assessment and/or treatment. Red flags are those symptoms and signs that will indicate that referral is to be considered. The red flags of headache are described in Table 4.1e-I. This table forms part of the summary on red flags given in Appendix III, which also gives advice on the degree of urgency of referral for each of the red flag conditions listed.

Table 4.1e-I Red Flags 23 – headache

Red Flag	Description	Reasoning
23.1	**Features of a slow increase in intracranial pressure**: progressive headaches and vomiting over the time scale of a few weeks to months. The headaches are worse in the morning and the vomiting may be effortless. Blurring of vision may be an additional symptom	Intracranial pressure will slowly increase if there is a gradual development of a space-occupying lesion, such as a brain tumour, abscess in the brain, extradural haemorrhage or accumulation of poorly draining cerebrospinal fluid. The pressure will be worse when the patient has been lying down, and so the symptoms are characteristically worse in the morning. These include blurring of vision (especially after coughing or leaning forward), effortless vomiting (i.e. not much preceding nausea) and headache
23.2	**A sudden very severe headache that comes on out of the blue:** the patient needs to lie down and may vomit. There may be neck stiffness (reluctance to move the head) and dislike of bright light	The sudden very severe headache (like a hit to the back of the head) is a cardinal symptom of the potentially devastating subarachnoid haemorrhage. This is a bleed from an area of weakness in one of the arterial branches that course round the base of the brain (the circle of Willis). Subarachnoid haemorrhage may result from an inherited malformation and so may develop out of the blue in a seemingly fit person
23.3	**A severe headache that develops over the course of a few hours to days with fever**, together with either **vomiting** or **neck stiffness**. Suggests acute meningitis or encephalitis	Meningitis and encephalitis are infections (of the meninges and brain tissue respectively) that can be caused by a wide range of infectious organisms. Although headache and fever are common co-symptoms in benign infections such as tonsillitis, the triad of headache, vomiting and fever is more suggestive of brain infections, and needs to be treated with caution. Additional symptoms such as reluctance to move the head, arching the back of the neck and dislike of bright lights may also be present, and if so are sinister signs. There may be a purpuric rash (see Red Flag 23.4), but the absence of a rash does not rule out the diagnosis
23.4	**A severe headache that develops over the course of a few hours to days with fever and with a bruising and non-blanching rash**. Suggests **meningococcal meningitis**	See Red Flag 23.3. In the form of meningitis caused by the meningococcus there can be a serious form of pus-producing infection of the meninges, a risk of septicaemia (and endotoxic shock; see Red Flag Table A19 in Appendix III) and the development of an irregularly distributed purpuric (like a shower of small bruises) rash. This is an emergency situation
23.5	**A severe one-sided headache over the temple occurring for the first time in an elderly person**	One-sided headaches are common and usually benign, but an unusual, severe, persistent, one-sided headache in an elderly person should be taken seriously as it could reflect the inflammatory condition of temporal arteritis In this condition, which is a form of vasculitis, the arteries supplying the head can become inflamed and thickened, and this carries the risk of obstruction by blood clot. There is a significant risk of thrombosis of a cerebral (brain) artery or retinal artery in temporal arteritis, and this is minimised by treatment with corticosteroid medication Temporal arteritis is more likely to develop in people who have also been diagnosed with polymyalgia rheumatica (see Red Flag Table A28 in Appendix III)
23.6	**A long history of worsening (progressive) headaches**, with generalised symptoms such as fever, loss of appetite and exhaustion	Recurrent headaches are common and are usually benign. They are often categorised by doctors as either migraine or tension headaches Consider referral if there is a progression in severity of the headaches or if there are other symptoms not usually associated with benign headache, such as fever, loss of appetite, weight loss or other neurological symptoms Benign headaches should respond significantly to your treatment, so also consider referral of recurrent headaches if there is no improvement within 1–2 months

Self-test 4.1e

Disorders of the central nervous system: headache and infections

1. A long-standing patient of yours, Harry, who is 75 years old, has been suffering from his worst migraine ever for the past 24 hours. In some ways the pain is similar to his usual pattern of migraines, in that it is focused to the side of one eye and that the area is very tender to the touch, but the pain is much worse than usual. He has also noticed that the side of his face and jaw is aching, which is not usual for his migraines. He is concerned because he thought he had 'grown out' of his migraines, as the last one was 2 years ago and was relatively mild.
   (i) What are your thoughts about the possible causes of Harry's pain?
   (ii) Would you refer Harry for a medical opinion?
2. John is 45 years old. He has had a flu-like illness for the past 2 days, but over the last 6 hours has developed a severe headache. He needs to lie in bed and keep his head very still. His wife is concerned because his temperature has stayed over 40°C for the past 24 hours, despite taking the full recommended dose of paracetamol. John has not vomited, and he does not have a rash.
   (i) What are the possible causes of John's headache?
   (ii) Would you refer John for a medical opinion?

Answers

1. (i) It is possible that Harry is suffering from another migraine. The other possibility is that he may have developed temporal arteritis. His age, the severity of the pain, and the facial pain are consistent with this diagnosis.
   (ii) Because of the risk of loss of sight in one eye, it would be wise to refer Harry to his GP for an urgent medical opinion.
2. (i) It is possible that John is suffering from the flu, as severe headache is a common result of high fevers. Nevertheless, unless you feel confident that you can assess and exclude neck stiffness, you are not in a position to exclude a possible diagnosis of meningitis.
   (ii) Unless you feel very confident that the headache is not sinister, and that you can keep in touch with the family, it would be wise for you to recommend that the GP is called out to assess John's physical state. You should definitely refer if there is no improvement within 2 hours of acupuncture treatment.

Chapter 4.1f Disorders of the central nervous system: dementia, epilepsy and other disorders

LEARNING POINTS

At the end of this chapter you will:

- be able to name the main features of the remaining important diseases of the brain
- understand the principles of treatment of a few of the most common diseases
- be able to recognise the red flags of these diseases.

Estimated time for chapter: 100 minutes.

Introduction

This chapter completes the overview of disorders that affect the functioning of the brain. The information covered will fill all the important remaining gaps concerning the conditions that affect the CNS, and for this reason this chapter introduces a range of very diverse conditions.

The conditions to be explored in this chapter are:

- Dementia:
  - Alzheimer's disease
  - multi-infarct dementia
  - infectious causes of dementia.
- Epilepsy.
- Disorders of movement:
  - Parkinson's disease
  - Huntingdon's disease
  - benign tremor
  - tics and spasms.
- Multiple sclerosis.
- Motor neuron disease.
- Cerebral palsy.

Dementia

'Dementia' is a general term applied to the range of conditions that lead to a widespread and permanent impairment of the function of the cortex of the brain, as well as certain subcortical areas. In most cases this impairment is progressive, so that the patient will suffer a gradual loss of the higher functions for which the cortex of the brain is responsible. This means that memory, thinking, comprehension, calculation, orientation, language and judgement are all gradually impaired.

Despite these losses, consciousness remains relatively intact, so that the person with dementia can remain fully alert until very advanced stages of the condition. Psychiatric problems are well recognised in patients with dementia, particularly in the early stages of a progressive dementia. Depression, paranoia, agitation and aggression are particularly common.

As the damage to the cortex progresses, the person with dementia gradually becomes less able to perform basic activities of daily life, such as washing and dressing. Incontinence can develop and movements become more clumsy. Life expectancy is shortened, as in this state the person becomes more immobile and prone to infections. Bronchopneumonia is a common terminal event in patients with advanced dementia.

Dementia can be described as pre-senile and senile. This arbitrary classification is used to describe dementia that occurs before and after the age of 70 years, respectively. There is no clinical distinction between these two classes of dementia.

As the condition of dementia progresses, the impact on the carer, often an elderly spouse, becomes very great. The incidence of depression in the carers of people with dementia is known to be high. This is now recognised to be an important problem, so that the ideal approach to the care of a person with dementia should also embrace the needs of the carers of that person. In many cases, as with a severe stroke, a multidisciplinary team of health professionals coordinates the care of a person with dementia.

> **Information Box 4.1f-I**
>
> **Dementia: comments from a Chinese medicine perspective**
>
> In Chinese medicine, dementia corresponds in part to Jing Deficiency, reflected by the fact that the substance of the brain is lost in the progression of the condition. Phlegm would also appear to be prominent in the condition. The difficulties in functions such as thinking, concentration, memory, which in health are the manifestation of a balanced Shen, are often associated with Phlegm obstructing the orifices of the Heart.

Alzheimer's disease

Alzheimer's disease is the most common form of progressive dementia. It becomes more common in older age groups but can develop in people as young as 40 years old. The tendency to develop Alzheimer's disease can run in families, and there is very commonly a strong family history of the condition if the disease develops at a very early age. Alzheimer's disease is also particularly common in people who have Down syndrome, in whom features of this dementia can also appear at an early age.

In Alzheimer's disease there is a characteristic degeneration of the cells of the cortex. Plaques of a thick substance called 'amyloid' develop in the tissue of the brain. There is also a reduction in the quantities of a range of neurotransmitters, including acetyl choline, a fact that has been focused on in the development of drug treatments for the disease.

Ideally, a patient with suspected Alzheimer's disease needs to be investigated carefully in order to exclude treatable causes of cognitive impairment such as hypothyroidism, pernicious anaemia and subdural haematoma. This would involve tests of mental ability, blood tests and a CT scan or MRI.

There is now good evidence that the cholinesterase inhibitors such as donepezil, rivastigmine and galantamine cause moderate improvement of memory and motivation at all stages of the disease process, and the drug memantine seems to be of benefit in more advanced stages. It is always worth treating hypertension in people with Alzheimer's disease, as high blood pressure is linked with worsening disease. Gingko biloba, fish oils, statins and vitamin E are recommended by some authorities as improving brain function, but clinical evidence is not yet conclusive for the benefit of any of these treatments.

Even with drug treatment, the condition is always slowly progressive. Most patients will have died within 10 years of the first diagnosis.

Multi-infarct dementia

This second most common form of dementia was explained in Chapter 4.1d as one of the syndromes that can result from recurrent strokes. The underlying physical problem in multi-infarct dementia is usually atheroma or hypertension, or a combination of both.

> **Information Box 4.1f-II**
>
> **Alzheimer's disease, multi-infarct dementia and prion disease: comments from a Chinese medicine perspective**
>
> In Chinese medicine, the development of amyloid plaques could be interpreted as Accumulation of Phlegm. The general degeneration of the cortex could also reflect Jing Deficiency.
>
> The underlying energetic problem of multi-infarct dementia is likely to be a combination of Phlegm and Blood Stagnation, as these are the Pathogenic Factors that correspond to the development of atheroma. The infarcts that result lead to loss of brain tissue, and this corresponds to Jing deficiency.
>
> In prion disease, the irreversible change of brain proteins into masses of prion proteins might be suggestive of the Accumulation of Phlegm. The rapid development of symptoms and the irregular writhing and twitching movements that can occur in these disorders suggest that Liver Wind is an additional important pathogenic factor.

Infectious causes of dementia

Various infections can cause a gradual degeneration of the brain tissue and thus lead to a dementia.

The prion diseases Creutzfeldt–Jakob disease (CJD) and new variant CJD are both recognised to lead to a form of rapidly developing dementia due to a characteristic degeneration of the brain tissue. This degeneration has been likened to a sponge, in that multiple tiny areas of brain tissue are lost throughout the brain. The degeneration is not wholly confined to the brain cortex, which means that disorders of movement are also prominent in these conditions.

Although CJD can develop out of the blue for no understood reason, it is also known to be contracted if a patient is exposed to the nervous tissue of an infected person. Until fairly recently, the surgical use of corneal grafts and injections of hormones, such as growth hormone derived from human brain tissue, were two mechanisms whereby CJD was transmitted from one person to another, symptoms appearing often after a delay of about 5 years. New variant CJD is believed, but not proven, to originate from the ingestion of nervous tissue in the meat from cattle infected with the bovine spongiform encephalopathy (BSE) prion.

The venereal disease syphilis can lead to a form of inflammation and degeneration of the nervous system, which can then progress to the symptoms of a dementia. This is increasingly a very rare condition, because syphilis can be completely cured in its early stages by means of early antibiotic treatment. Before such treatment was available, the syphilis organism could lie dormant for many years after an initial infection, and then reappear in a form that could cause damage to the nerves, spinal cord and brain. This form of syphilis was termed 'general paralysis of the insane', because the dementia was combined with impairment of movement and sensation.

HIV is also well known to cause a form of dementia in advanced stages of infection. The development of this dementia is rapid, and is very often the cause of death in people with AIDS.

Epilepsy

'Epilepsy' is a term used to describe a range of conditions in which the common event is that a large number of nerve cells in the brain discharge simultaneously. A single episode of simultaneous discharge of nerve cells leads to what is termed an epileptic 'fit' or 'seizure'. Epilepsy is only diagnosed if there is tendency to experience recurrent seizures. This affects about one person in 200 of the general population.

An epileptic seizure occurs when the discharge of one set of nerve cells in the brain is not limited adequately. This means that a chain reaction takes place, in which all the adjacent nerve cells discharge and then cause the discharge of their neighbouring cells. This chain reaction is sometimes so great that a wave of electrical discharge spreads across the surface of the brain. In other cases the area of discharge is limited to one part of the brain.

This loss of limitation of the nerve cell impulses can occur in any person under certain conditions. For example, extreme lack of oxygen, low blood sugar, very high temperatures or certain chemicals can induce fits in many people. However, in some people fits occur much more readily. It is known that this tendency to epilepsy runs in families.

Alcohol abuse is a well known cause of fits. These particularly occur either during a drinking 'binge' or on withdrawal of alcohol. Usually the fits will cease if the alcohol problem is dealt with.

Fits are more likely to occur if there is an area of brain damage, even if this area is so small that it does not cause any other problems for the patient. For this reason, epilepsy is a well-known complication of birth trauma (causing brain damage to the baby), brain tumours and abscesses, brain surgery, strokes and head injury. However, in most cases, the reason for the development of epilepsy is unknown, in that there is no identifiable area of brain damage.

The characteristics of an epileptic seizure depend on the site of origin of the discharging brain cells and on how far this discharge spreads across the brain. In current medical practice, epilepsy is classified according to the type of seizure. If a seizure represents a widespread discharge of nerves across the brain, it is known as a 'generalised seizure', whereas if it is confined to a defined area of the brain it is called a 'partial seizure'. In a generalised seizure consciousness is always impaired or lost.

In established epilepsy, some people will experience a 'prodrome' of a couple of days leading up to a fit, in which there is a subtle change of personality, mood or energy levels. Also, many patients often recognise a warning sensation in the few seconds to minutes prior to seizure, similar to the warning sensation experienced by some migraine sufferers. This warning is also called an 'aura'. In epilepsy, the common types of aura include a characteristic mood, a recurrent memory or a strange smell.

Some sufferers of epilepsy recognise that there are particular triggers for attacks. These include tiredness, emotional upset, high fevers and exposure to rapidly flashing lights.

Generalised seizures: grand mal (tonic–clonic) seizures

In a grand mal seizure the discharge of the brain cells affects the motor cortex so that the muscles of the body are stimulated to contract simultaneously. This causes the body to go rigid, and the patient often lets out a cry before falling to the ground. This state of muscular contraction, which lasts for 10–30 seconds, is called the 'tonic phase'. The muscles then go into repeated and rhythmic cycles of contraction and relaxation, so that the patient lies in an unconscious state while the body undergoes coarse shaking movements. At this stage the patient may froth at the mouth, and can go blue in the face as breathing is impaired. This is called the 'clonic phase', and usually lasts for a few seconds to a few minutes. During this phase the bladder or the bowel may empty involuntarily.

After the grand mal (or tonic–clonic) seizure the patient can remain in an unconscious or drowsy state for up to several hours. In severe cases, the clonic state does not settle down. This is called 'status epilepticus', and is a medical emergency if it last for more than a few minutes. This is because in status epilepticus there is an increasing risk with time that the brain becomes starved of oxygen and permanently damaged.

The onset of grand mal epilepsy most commonly occurs either between 3 and 7 years of age or in the teenage years. In these cases there is usually no obvious underlying cause. If this form of epilepsy occurs after the age of 25 years, a distinct area of brain damage, such as a brain tumour or brain abscess, is more likely to be the underlying cause.

Generalised seizures: petit mal (absence) seizures

In petit mal epilepsy the seizure is not associated with any disorder of movement. Instead, the patient suffers a brief (few seconds) loss of awareness known as an 'absence'. To an onlooker, the person suddenly becomes vacant, may even stop in mid-speech or activity, and can go pale. When the seizure is over the person may carry on the activity they were performing as if nothing has happened.

Petit mal epilepsy is most common in young children, who may grow out of it as they enter their teens. Rarely, some children with absence attacks may go on to develop grand mal epilepsy. The condition is sometimes confused with dreaminess, and so may not be diagnosed for some time. This can become a real problem in the education of the child. It is now known that a child with petit mal epilepsy misses out on a lot more learning than would be represented by the time of the absence attacks alone, and can develop learning difficulties without appropriate teaching support.

Partial seizures

In partial seizures only a small portion of the brain is affected by the discharge of brain cells. The resulting seizure can be compared in some ways to a transient ischaemic attack, in which there is also a temporary loss of function of a small area of the brain. In some cases there is also impairment of consciousness.

A motor partial seizure involves the motor cortex on one side of the brain, so that the patient will experience a rhythmic jerking of all or part of one half of the body. In many cases, the development of this type of epilepsy signifies a progressive but localised condition of the brain such as a tumour.

A temporal partial seizure involves the cortex of the temporal lobe of one side of the brain. This can have very diverse symptoms, including the experience of a strange mood or smell, a period of loss of memory, a changed personality state and visual hallucinations. For this reason, temporal lobe epilepsy can easily be misdiagnosed as a psychiatric or personality disorder. These temporal lobe seizures are also known as 'complex partial seizures'.

Diagnosis of epilepsy

The first aspect of diagnosis is to confirm that a fit has actually occurred. This is not always as straightforward as might be expected, as a number of other conditions, including fainting, transient ischaemic attacks and psychiatric disorders, can mimic epileptic fits.

The electroencephalogram (EEG) is used to assess the 'brainwaves' or the electrical activity of the brain. An EEG recording taken during a fit is almost always abnormal. Therefore, the ideal is to obtain an EEG reading when a fit actually occurs. This is not always possible if fits are infrequent.

In some people, the EEG is abnormal in between fits. This is highly suggestive of epilepsy, although this is not always the case. For this reason, a patient with possible epilepsy may be exposed to certain triggers, such as rapidly flashing lights, during the EEG recording, to see if any abnormalities of brain activity are induced.

A CT scan or MRI is always performed to look for any structural abnormalities of the brain. This is of particular importance in adult-onset epilepsy, in which an underlying disease such as cancer or stroke might explain the development of the seizures.

Treatment of epilepsy

An isolated fit is never diagnosed as epilepsy, and so medication would not be offered unless the seizures became recurrent. Nevertheless, an isolated seizure does have considerable impact on the life of an adult patient. In the UK, for example, according to the Driver and Vehicle Licensing Agency (DVLA) legislation, anyone who has had an epileptic fit or unexplained loss of consciousness is not allowed to drive for the following 12 months. Heavy goods vehicle (HGV) drivers who have suffered a seizure will lose their HGV licence for the next 10 years.

Patients who are prone to recurrent seizures are advised to avoid activities that may put their own lives or those of other people at risk should they happen to have a seizure. For example, activities such as climbing, swimming alone, and the use of heavy machinery are discouraged. Driving is permitted in people with controlled epilepsy, as long as there have been no seizures in the daytime for at least one year. Fits that occur during sleep are much more common and are not considered to be a reason to avoid driving, as long as they have occurred only in sleep for over 3 years.

The treatment of status epilepticus includes first-aid measures to ensure that the patient can breathe freely. The patient should be encouraged to lie on their side in the 'recovery position' and restrictive clothing should be loosened. If the seizure has been ongoing for more than 3 minutes, the medical treatment is a tranquilliser such as lorazepam or diazepam, which is inserted by means of a rectal tablet (suppository) or by intravenous injection. In the very unusual case of this having no effect, the situation becomes an emergency. The patient in resistant status epilepticus may require ventilation in an intensive care unit.

Prevention of recurrent seizures involves prescription of one or more drugs. Different types of seizures tend to respond to different groups of drugs. All these drugs are given the general name of 'anticonvulsants' or 'antiepileptics' (see *British National Formulary*, Section 4.8). Anticonvulsant medication acts by preventing the spread of electrical discharge in the brain, which seems to encourage the inhibitory aspect of the nervous system (see Chapter 4.1a under The Physiology of the Nerve Cell).

All the anticonvulsant drugs have significant side-effects. The ideal treatment involves only one of these preparations, because it is recognised that side-effects are more troublesome, and the likelihood of toxicity increases, if they are used in combination. It sometimes takes a number of years to establish which medication is the most suitable for a particular patient in terms of effectiveness and minimisation of side-effects. This is a particularly difficult process in adults who drive, because driving is not permitted in a patient with epilepsy for a year after any change in medication, because of the risk of recurrence of fits.

The drugs most commonly used in generalised epilepsy include carbemazepine, lamotrigine, sodium valproate, topiramate and vigabatrin. Phenytoin used to be widely prescribed, but is less used now as newer agents with better side-effect profiles and a lower risk of toxicity have been introduced.

All these medications are introduced initially as the sole drug at a low dose, and gradually increased in dose until the frequency of seizures is brought under control. Sometimes perfect control can never be achieved. Some preparations require the patient to have regular blood tests to ensure that the levels of the drug in the blood are within a safe threshold.

All these drugs in excessive doses lead to a condition of drowsiness, confusion, stumbling speech and staggering gait. Even in safe doses, most patients experience a degree of drowsiness or clumsiness when on medication.

In addition, each drug has characteristic side-effects that can have a significant impact on the quality of life. These include rashes, weight gain, swollen gums, dizziness, blurred vision and excessive body hair (depending on the particular drug). The three commonly prescribed preparations, carbamazepine, sodium valproate, and phenytoin, are all potentially harmful to the developing fetus, so pregnancy should be avoided.

Withdrawal from anticonvulsant medication should be very slow and controlled because of the high risk of recurrence of seizures. For this reason, drug withdrawal should never be undertaken outside of medical supervision. All patients who withdraw from medication are obliged to abstain from driving for the period of the withdrawal and for 6 months afterwards.

All patients with epilepsy in the UK should be under the supervision of a hospital neurologist. Some may also have access to a specialist epilepsy nurse, who will be experienced in carefully guiding and supporting patients through the complex medical and social issues that arise from having epilepsy.

Information Box 4.1f-III

Epilepsy: comments from a Chinese medicine perspective

In Chinese medicine, the sudden loss of consciousness and spasm of muscles of a grand mal seizure are usually described as a manifestation of Liver Wind stirring upwards and causing Phlegm to obstruct the Orifices of the Heart. A petit mal seizure, although less dramatic, has similar characteristics in terms of sudden onset and loss of awareness. These also imply that Wind and Phlegm are important Pathogenic Factors.

In partial motor seizures, the most prominent feature is the sudden onset of twitching muscles. This is indicative of Wind in Chinese medicine. In partial temporal lobe epilepsy, the various rather vague perceptual symptoms would also appear to result from Phlegm impeding the functions of the Shen. Sudden onsets of conditions are themselves often indicative of Wind.

The underlying syndromes in a person with epilepsy are likely to be those that predispose to the development of Liver Wind and Phlegm. These include Deficiency of Liver and Kidney Yin and Spleen and Stomach Deficiency. In the many cases in which the onset is in childhood, this is highly suggestive that Jing Deficiency is an additional factor.

All anticonvulsant medication is suppressive in nature, as evidenced by the fact that seizures often return with greater severity on withdrawal of medication. The side-effects of drowsiness and clumsiness, with dizziness, confusion and loss of balance, if drugs are taken in excessive dose, all suggest that these drugs are Phlegm Forming. The drugs appear to act by damping down the Stirring up of the Wind (their physical action is to increase the action of the inhibitory nerves of the brain), but do not address the main root cause of the problem, which of course is the accumulation of Phlegm.

The various additional side-effects are due to drug-induced disease. Swollen gums indicate Heat and Phlegm in the Stomach, and rashes indicate Heat in the Blood. Most of the drugs are toxic to some degree to the liver, and side-effects that indicate Stagnation of Liver Qi are also common, including depression and increased risk of suicide.

Parkinson's disease and other disorders of movement

There are a number of disorders of movement that result from disease of the brain. The most important movement disorder by far, in terms of the number of people affected and severity of disease, is Parkinson's disease, also known as 'paralysis agitans', a Latin term which succinctly describes the distressing nature of the disability that develops in this condition.

Parkinson's disease

Parkinson's disease is a progressive disorder affecting one in 200 of the UK population over the age of 65 years. It is the result of degeneration of a part of the brain called the 'basal ganglia'. These clusters (nuclei) of nerve cells, situated deep within the cerebral hemispheres, play a part in the smooth control of muscle action.

In most cases the cause of the condition is unknown, although in some there is a family history. Occasionally, Parkinson's disease can develop following a head injury. It is a well-known complication of the frequent knock-outs experienced by boxers.

An important cause of a syndrome called 'parkinsonism', which is very like Parkinson's disease, is the prescription of some of the major tranquilliser drugs used to treat serious mental illness such as schizophrenia and bipolar disorder. This syndrome occurs because these drugs work by lowering the levels of a neurotransmitter in the brain called dopamine. The levels of dopamine are known to be disturbed in major mental illnesses. However, dopamine is also important for the correct function of the basal ganglia. A person on high doses of this sort of medication is very likely to develop the symptoms of Parkinson's disease within a few days of the onset of treatment. This is a significant cause of discomfort and also stigmatisation. Parkinsonism is largely reversible on withdrawal of treatment.

In Parkinson's disease, degeneration of a specific part of the basal ganglia, and loss of dopamine-producing cells, leads to a characteristic syndrome of stiffness of muscles, difficulty initiating movements and tremor.

The first symptom frequently is of gradual onset of stiffness of muscles initially affecting the limbs, but later involving facial and body muscles. Often the onset of this stiffness is asymmetrical, so that one side of the body is more severely affected than the other.

In addition to this stiffness, a difficulty in initiating movement develops. Actions such as standing from sitting or getting out of bed become difficult. The rapid responsiveness of the facial muscles is lost so that a person with Parkinson's disease can look permanently blank and emotionless. This, of course can affect social interactions.

A coarse tremor (with a rate of 4–6 beats/second) develops in the hands and limbs, and progresses over a period of years to affect the whole body. This tremor is improved during the performance of an action such as picking something up, and is worse at rest. Strong emotion can also cause worsening of the tremor.

Gradually, the posture is affected, so that the person develops a stoop, and has a characteristic shuffling gait. Balance is impaired, and falls are common. These can have serious consequences in elderly people. Sleep may be impaired, and bowel and bladder function problematic. Depression is a common and serious problem. In late stages of the disease speech becomes difficult to comprehend, and difficulty swallowing and dribbling of saliva are common.

Usually the disease progresses slowly over the course of 10–15 years. Death usually occurs from bronchopneumonia, a result of immobility and the inability to clear secretions from the throat.

The UK National Institute of Health and Clinical Excellence (NICE) recommends that anyone with suspected Parkinson's disease should be referred at the point of diagnosis to a specialist team comprising a neurologist, physiotherapist and specialist nurse, because of the complex mix of medical and social needs affecting anyone with this diagnosis.

Exercises to maintain mobility and balance are recommended from the outset. For example, tai chi is recognised to help strengthen the postural muscles and prevent falls and may be recommended. Medication is deferred until symptoms are very significant, as it does not prevent progression and the beneficial effects of the drugs wear off with time.

Parkinson's disease is most commonly treated with two main types of drug. One mimics the action of dopamine (the so-called dopaminergic drugs). Increasingly, newer agents such as ropinirole may be introduced as the first treatment, but the most established dopaminergics are forms of L-dopa, a chemical precursor of dopamine. The common preparations of this drug are called cocareldopa and cobeneldopa.

The effects of each dose of the dopaminergic type drugs are to reverse the symptoms of Parkinson's disease, but this effect wears off with increasing rapidity as time progresses. This means that eventually the patient may have to take a number of doses throughout the day.

L-dopa preparations can have severe long-term effects on the nervous system (after about 5 years), which is the reason why treatment is delayed for as long as possible. Immediate side-effects include nausea, confusion and hallucinations. Long-term effects include uncontrollable muscle movements. Another problem with long-term treatment is that the periods of relief from symptoms can be interspersed with periods of 2–4 hours of a greatly reduced ability to move (on–off syndrome), which are very unpleasant for the patient. One extra drug, entacapone, which slows the breakdown of the dopa-related drugs by the body, may be prescribed together with dopa-related to prevent on–off syndrome.

Another type of drug, selegiline, may be introduced at an earlier stage in the disease. This drug increases the action of the dopamine that is produced in the brain. It may also be used together with L-dopa preparations, because it seems to overcome, at least for a few years, the rapid end-of-dose deterioration of these drugs. The short-term side-effects of selegiline are similar to those of the L-dopa drugs, in that they include nausea, and psychiatric disturbances.

Experimental studies involving the insertion of cells removed from the brains of aborted human fetuses into the brains of people with Parkinson's disease have received a lot of media attention in recent years. There have been mixed reports about the benefits of such an approach, which still remains within the realm of research rather than clinical practice.

Information Box 4.1f-IV

Parkinson's disease: comments from a Chinese medicine perspective

In Chinese medicine, a root cause of tremor is considered to be insufficient Blood and fluids to nourish the channels and sinews. This can result from longstanding Qi and Blood Deficiency. The channels and sinews are then vulnerable to Wind. Liver Wind is the most likely description in Chinese medicine for the manifestation of tremor in Parkinson's disease.

Liver Wind may develop as a consequence of Liver and Kidney Yin Deficiency, as it does in the development of Wind Stroke. Liver Yang Rising can also lead to the generation of Liver Wind, so that long-term suppressed emotion may also be causative in Parkinson's disease. Phlegm Heat or Phlegm Fire can be important in some cases, because Phlegm Heat obstructs and dries the channels and sinews.

The drug treatments for Parkinson's disease therefore act by subduing Wind and clearing Phlegm. They do not attend to the root cause of the problem, and so are suppressive in nature. Nausea and psychiatric disturbances suggest that these drugs may themselves be Phlegm forming. The development of chronic disorders of movement after prolonged drug treatment suggests the reappearance of Wind in a different manifestation.

Drugs used in major mental illness that are also a cause of the syndrome of parkinsonism have a number of features that suggest that they are both Heating and Phlegm forming. Other side-effects of these drugs indicate that they lead to the generation of Wind (the complex energetics of these powerful drugs is discussed in more detail in Section 6.2).

Huntingdon's disease (HD)

Huntingdon's disease is another degenerative disorder of the deep nuclei in the brain known as the basal ganglia (see Chapter 4.1a). In this condition, different parts of the basal ganglia are affected than in Parkinson's disease, and the result is a progressive disorder of movement called 'chorea' (from the Greek word meaning 'dance'). Chorea consists of jerky and fidgety extra movements of the limbs and the body, which can progress from one body part to another. Other parts of the brain also degenerate in this condition, leading to a form of dementia.

Huntingdon's disease tends to affect people in middle life. It is almost always inherited from one parent, who passes the gene for the disease to the children. There is a 50% chance of a child developing the condition if one parent carries that gene (it is an autosomal-dominant condition; see Chapter 5.4c).

Because the disease usually develops after childbearing years, it is not usually known that there is a risk of the children having the disease until a few years after they are born, when one parent develops the condition. A genetic test is available that can offer the children of a person with Huntingdon's disease the opportunity of knowing whether or not they too carry the gene.

The progression of Huntingdon's disease is such that death occurs within 10–20 years of diagnosis. There is no satisfactory treatment for the condition. Tetrabenazine may help mitigate the chorea in some patients, but this drug can cause depression, which limits its usefulness.

Information Box 4.1f-V

Huntingdon's disease: comments from a Chinese medicine perspective

In Chinese medicine, the dementia of Huntingdon's disease most clearly corresponds to Jing Deficiency. The chorea is the result of Liver Wind, which in this case can possibly to be attributed to Kidney and Liver Yin Deficiency.

Benign (essential) tremor

Benign essential tremor is a condition in which there is a fine tremor of the limbs, often including the head and the body. This tremor is similar in quality to the tremor that may be experienced by most people in an extreme state of anxiety. The difference with benign tremor is that, although it is worsened by a nervous mood, it is present all the time. The tremor is not as coarse as the tremor of Parkinson's disease, and so the two conditions are easily distinguished by an experienced doctor. In some cases the tremor has been present since youth, and in these cases it is often an inherited condition (also autosomal dominant). In other cases the tremor develops as a consequence of ageing. Although the tremor may be progressive, it rarely hinders daily activities in a significant way.

Occasionally, beta blockers (propranolol) are given to ease the tremor. This is because they block the action of adrenaline, one of the natural contributors to a benign tremor. Interestingly, alcohol in small doses can also reduce the shaking movements of this condition.

Information Box 4.1f-VI

Benign essential tremor: comments from a Chinese medicine perspective

In Chinese medicine, a benign tremor would normally be diagnosed as a manifestation of Liver Wind. Qi and Blood Deficiency or Kidney and Liver Yin Deficiency may be underlying conditions.

From a conventional medical perspective, the release of adrenaline leads to this physical manifestation of fear. In Chinese medicine, the tremor that results from adrenaline could be described in terms of Empty Heat and Wind, which can result from Kidney Yin that is deficient in relation to Kidney Yang. By blocking the action of adrenaline, beta blockers, which also have side-effects of slowed heart rate and feelings of cold and depression, might be seen as suppressing Kidney Yang.

Tics and spasms

There are a few diverse conditions in which repetitive unwanted movements (tics) occur. The most common form of tic is benign and appears in early childhood. The child can pass through a phase of performing habitual movements such as blinking or screwing up the face. These often settle down as the child grows up. More pronounced tics can last throughout life or can develop in adult life. Other conditions can involve unpredictable limb movements, in which the muscles can go into painful spasms (also known as 'dystonias').

Information Box 4.1f-VII

Tics and spasms: comments from a Chinese medicine perspective

Most unwanted movements are seen in Chinese medicine to correspond to Liver Wind. If spasm of muscles (interpreted as tendons and sinews in Chinese medicine) is also prominent, this suggests an additional imbalance within the Liver, such as Liver Qi Stagnation or Liver Blood deficiency.

Multiple sclerosis

Multiple sclerosis (MS) is a common degenerative disease of unknown cause that affects the nerve cells of both the brain and the spinal cord, but not the peripheral nerves. The condition can first appear at any time in teenage and adult life. Most commonly, MS affects young women. It is also more common in people who have spent their childhood in countries a long way from the equator (such as northern Europe, Canada and the northern USA). This suggests that there is some sort of environmental trigger that affects a growing child in a cold climate, but no trigger has yet been isolated. Some studies of large populations suggest that a diet high in animal fats might be contributory in increasing the risk of MS, but this link has not been proven.

The underlying problem in MS is that small patches, called 'plaques', develop within the CNS in which the myelin coating of the nerve fibres has degenerated. It is now recognised that an abnormal immune response is responsible for this damage to the myelin, and axon death follows the loss of the myelin. This means that the ability of the nerves to transmit 'messages' through the affected areas is lost. The plaques can develop in a wide range of sites, and thus can cause a wide range of neurological problems, hence the other name for MS, 'disseminated sclerosis'.

The pattern of the condition is that it commonly starts with a period in which there is a sudden and rapid deterioration of the function of an aspect of the nervous system, sometimes triggered by stress, heat or exercise. Frequent first symptoms include the sudden onset of blurred vision, or numbness and weakness of one or both limbs, or slurred speech. This sudden deterioration is termed a 'relapse'.

In the majority of cases, a relapse is followed after a few weeks by a period in which the symptoms may get partially and sometimes completely better. This improvement is called a 'remission'. However, in most people with MS the period of remission is followed by a further relapse, this time leaving the nervous system in a more damaged state than before. Thus, with a cycle of relapses and remissions, most people with MS become progressively more disabled over the course of 10–30 years. In approximately 30% of cases, the remissions are less prominent, and the pattern is instead one of a progressive decline. In a very few cases, the decline between relapses is not so rapidly progressive, and permanent severe disability never develops.

The disabilities that can affect a person with advanced MS depend on the site of the CNS in which the plaques are most prominent. Common problems include weakness and numbness of the limbs due to damage to the nerves that travel down the spinal cord to supply the limbs. Upper motor neurons are affected (see the section Spinal Tone at the end of Part I of Chapter 4.1a), leading to increased tone of the affected limbs, and the limbs can easily go into painful spasms. This condition can progress so that the patient becomes wheelchair bound.

Damage to the sensory nerves of the bladder and the bowel can result in incontinence. Damage to the cerebellum can cause difficulty in balance and clumsiness. Speech becomes difficult to understand. Damage in the cortex of the brain can affect personality and intellect. This means that a form of dementia may complicate long-term MS. Even in the early stages of the disease, mood can be affected. In particular, a state of euphoria is well known in people with MS. However, violent mood swings, depression and irritability are also common.

MS may be diagnosed by means of an MRI, which reveals the plaques as small patches throughout the CNS. A lumbar puncture may be performed and characteristic antibodies may be found in the cerebrospinal fluid. There is increasing interest in using assays for antibodies to myelin proteins, as these are raised in people with MS, and early studies suggest they might have a predictive role in that high levels are correlated with increased chances of rapid relapse.

A person who is suffering from an acute relapse is usually offered treatment of high doses of intravenous corticosteroids (methylprednisolone). Although this treatment seems to reduce the initial extent of the disability experienced during the relapse, there is no evidence that it affects the long-term outcome of the condition. The side-effects of these treatments, in particular weight gain and muscle weakness, can in some cases hinder the person's ability to recover from the damage caused by the relapse.

There is a small range of new drugs available that seem to have a modest effect on the relapse rate in primary progressive MS. Interferon-beta, glatiramer and the immunosuppressant azathioprine all seem to reduce the relapse rate, but have a less marked effect on reducing long-term disability. The interferons have side-effects including flu-like symptoms and depression, which may make them very difficult for some people to tolerate as long-term treatments.

Natalizumab is a very new drug which carries significant risks of side-effects, but seems to lead to an impressive reduction in relapse rate (reduced by two-thirds). It is currently reserved for use only in those patients whose relapses are continuing despite treatment with interferon-beta.

Patients may find that linoleic acid supplements and regular vitamin B_{12} injections help with chronic tiredness.

The main aspect of treatment in advanced MS is multidisciplinary support of the patient and their family. In this way it is comparable to the treatment of the disability caused by stroke. Physiotherapy is essential to prevent tightening of the muscles of the limbs. Drugs may be prescribed to help mitigate discomfort from spasms and nerve pain. These include the antiepileptic drugs carbamazepine and gabapentin, and the antidepressant amitriptyline. Occupational therapists can advise on methods by which the progressive disabilities can be overcome with the use of physical aids. Advice from a social worker may be needed to discuss plans for future employment and to help acquire appropriate state benefits. The MS Society can be a valued source of support for people in the UK with MS.

Information Box 4.1f-VIII

Multiple sclerosis: comments from a Chinese medicine perspective

In Chinese medicine, multiple sclerosis (MS) is a type of atrophy syndrome (Wei Syndrome). It is considered to be a manifestation of a combination of Damp obstructing the channels (causing heaviness, numbness and tingling) and Deficiency of Kidney and Liver Yin (causing dizziness, problems with vision, difficulty in urination and weakness of the muscles). Muscle spasms are due to the generation of Liver Wind. A sudden shock leading to depletion of Spleen and Heart Qi is also considered to be an additional factor in some cases. The observations that MS is more prevalent in a cold climate and in populations that have a diet high in animal fats are consistent with the Chinese medicine interpretation that Damp is an important factor in the development of MS.

The action of steroid medication might be described in terms of clearing Damp from the channels. However, its side-effects demonstrate that it is in the long-term Damp/Phlegm forming and depleting of Yin. It therefore seems to be having a suppressive action in the treatment of MS.

(For more detail about the Chinese medicine interpretation of MS and Wei Syndrome, see: Maciocia 1994, Chapters 28 and 29).

Motor neuron disease

Motor neuron disease (MND), as its name implies, is a degenerative condition that affects the motor neurons within the brain and spinal cord. It may help for you now to turn back to the section entitled Spinal Tone at the end of Part I of Chapter 4.1a to remind yourself of the distinction between upper and lower motor neurons.

MND is much rarer than multiple sclerosis. It tends to affect men in middle life more often than women, and is of unknown cause. The loss of the motor neurons in MND is progressive, and leads to death usually within 3 years of diagnosis. Rarely, some patients survive for as long as 10 years.

There are two main forms of MND. The first, amyotrophic lateral sclerosis (ALS) (also known as Lou Gehrig's disease) includes a subcategory called 'progressive bulbar palsy' (PBP). ALS results from degeneration of motor nerve cells in the motor cortex and the spinal cord, and manifests as progressive weakness, first of the limbs and then of the muscles of speech, mastication and swallowing. In PBP only the upper and lower motor neurons that govern swallowing, speech and chewing are affected. The progression of this form of MND is usually rapid over the course of about 3 years, and death tends to result from pneumonia resulting from poor swallowing mechanisms and aspiration of fluid into the lungs. PBP tends to run an even shorter course. In about one-third of patients a form of dementia also becomes apparent.

The other form of MND is called 'progressive muscular atrophy' (PMA) and this form tends to affect lower motor neurons in the spinal cord. The patient will present with progressive weakness. PMA tends to run a longer course than ALS and is not associated with dementia.

The first symptom to appear depends on which motor nerves are affected first. In the most common form of MND the lower motor neurons that lead to the muscles of the limbs are affected first. This leads to weakness and wasting of the muscles. Eventually, the limbs become flaccid and lifeless. As the nerve cells supplying the muscles die, this causes a fine twitch to be seen on the surface of the muscles, which appears like a constant rippling motion under the surface of the skin. There is no pain or loss of sensation in MND.

In less common forms of MND the upper motor neurons are affected first. If this occurs within the spinal cord, the result is a gradual paralysis of the muscles of the limbs and body, but without the wasting. The tone of the paralysed muscles is increased, as commonly occurs in multiple sclerosis. Spasm and tightening of the muscles occurs, and this can be very painful.

If the upper motor neurons of the brainstem are affected, this affects the action of the cranial nerves. The patient loses the ability to speak freely, and swallowing becomes difficult. This is the most serious aspect of MND, because impaired swallowing will eventually lead to choking on excess saliva, development of bronchopneumonia and death.

The only drug that is licensed for the treatment of MND is riluzole, which is reported to increase life expectancy in ALS by 3 months only. Riluzole counteracts the action of the excitatory neurotransmitter glutamate, which is believed to have a causative role in MND, although for reasons which are as yet unclear. Riluzole is only licensed in the UK for used in ALS, and not for PMA.

Information Box 4.1f-IX

Motor neuron disease: comments from a Chinese medicine perspective

In Chinese medicine, motor neuron disease is another atrophy syndrome. The underlying causes could include invasion of Damp in the channels, on top of a range of possible conditions of depletion, including Stomach and Spleen Qi Deficiency, Heart and Spleen Qi Deficiency, and Kidney and Liver Yin Deficiency. The rippling of the muscles that follows lower motor nerve degeneration in MND reflects Wind in the channels.

Cerebral palsy

'Cerebral palsy' is a broad term used to describe a non-progressive defect within the CNS that occurs either before birth or in early childhood.

The most usual cause of cerebral palsy is that the baby in the womb is starved of oxygen for a short time. This can occur either before or during labour. Another well-known cause is the bursting of blood vessels in the brain of the baby during a traumatic labour. Immature clotting mechanisms mean that even a small injury might lead to a significant bleed and damage to the brain. After birth, the fits that can occur in high fever, or other causes of coma, can leave the baby with an area of permanent brain damage.

Cerebral palsy is much less common than it used to be. Some of this decline can be attributed to improved antenatal care and the specialist care of high-risk pregnancies. Two oral doses of vitamin K, which is essential in the production of four of the 12 clotting factors in the liver, are offered to all newborn babies in the UK to improve immature clotting mechanisms and help prevent intracranial bleeding.

In many cases, cerebral palsy is not diagnosed for some months to years after birth. This is because some of the disabilities that result from the area of brain damage are not apparent in the immature nervous system of an infant. The most common situation is that the baby is found not to be attaining the usual milestones of development (child development is explored in more detail in Section 5.4) and is then referred for a neurological examination.

In some cases, the disability is confined to the physical realm. In these cases there may be problems such as a hemiplegia (see Stroke, Chapter 4.1d), paralysis of both legs (diplegia), muscle spasms or difficulties with production of clear speech. Because of the increased tone of the affected limb muscles and problems with spasms, the (now outdated) term 'spastic' used to be applied to children with these sorts of disabilities.

However, many children with cerebral palsy have, in addition to physical problems, learning difficulties, which can vary from being mild to very severe. Epilepsy is also very common in children with cerebral palsy.

It is recognised that early diagnosis is important so that the child can receive appropriate treatment, such as physiotherapy, and the family can be offered support in caring for the child (see Q4.1f-1).

Information Box 4.1f-X

Cerebral palsy: comments from a Chinese medicine perspective

In Chinese medicine, the loss of the functioning of an aspect of the brain will nearly always correspond to Jing (Essence) Deficiency. Other syndromes depend on the exact nature of the disability. Phlegm is an important additional factor, particularly in cases in which there is epilepsy or in which intellect has been impaired.

The red flags of dementia, epilepsy and the other disorders of the central nervous system

Some patients with dementia, epilepsy and the other disorders of the CNS will benefit from referral to a conventional doctor for assessment and/or treatment. Red flags are those symptoms and signs that will indicate that referral is to be considered. The red flags of these conditions are described in Table 4.1f-I. This table forms part of the summary on red flags given in Appendix III, which also gives advice on the degree of urgency of referral for each of the red flag conditions listed.

Self-test 4.1f

Disorders of the central nervous system: dementia, epilepsy and other disorders

1. You have a 65-year-old patient, Mary, who is a widow. You have been treating her since she suffered a couple of small strokes 2 years ago. You have noticed that she has become distinctly more vague over the past 6 months. She has confused the times of the last two appointments and is concerned that her memory is going. She lives on her own, and rarely visits her GP.
   (i) What are possible reasons for Mary's symptoms?
   (ii) How would you manage this situation?
2. A new patient who is 35 years old tells you with embarrassment that over the past 3 months he has woken a couple of times to find that he has wet the bed. When this has happened he says that he feels even more groggy than usual in the morning. He has tried cutting down on drinks in the evening, but this does not help. What is the possible serious explanation for this symptom?
3. Jane has made an emergency appointment because she has woken to find that her vision is blurred in both eyes, so much so that she cannot read the print in a newspaper. She also feels a bit dizzy and unsteady and has a deep aching feeling behind both eyes. How would you deal with this situation?

Answers

1. (i) You have noticed a change in Mary over the past 6 months, and she has noticed that her memory is worsening. This could be purely the result of a form of depression. However, you cannot exclude the early onset of a form of dementia. Multi-infarct dementia is a possibility in view of the fact that Mary has suffered some small strokes in the past.
   (ii) As Mary lives on her own, and is not in regular touch with her GP, it would be wise to encourage her to make an appointment with the GP to talk about the problem, so that the practice team are aware that this is happening to her. It would be helpful for you to write to or telephone the GP to express your concerns about the progressive nature of the condition, as Mary may not be able to describe the situation with clarity herself.
2. This man might have been suffering from nocturnal epileptic fits. In view of the relatively late age of onset, this form of epilepsy might have an underlying structural cause, such as a small stroke or a tumour. For these reasons you should refer this man to his GP.
3. Jane is experiencing significant visual loss. The fact that both eyes are affected and that she is also feeling dizzy and unsteady tells you that the underlying problem is located in more than one site in the central nervous system.
   The suddenness of the development of these symptoms is highly suggestive of multiple sclerosis (MS). This is not a medical emergency, and so It is appropriate to give Jane an acupuncture treatment, as she has requested, but you must make sure that she arranges to visit the GP that day. Because of the dizziness and visual disturbance it is imperative she must not drive.
   The purpose of the referral is to ensure that Jane receives a firm diagnosis as soon as possible, and is offered the option of steroid treatment if the diagnosis of MS is confirmed. You could offer to treat her on a very frequent basis, and reassure her that you would be willing to talk with her about the pros and cons of any medication she might be offered by the neurologist.

Table 4.1f-I Red Flags 24 – dementia, epilepsy and other disorders of the central nervous system

Red Flag	Description	Reasoning
24.1	**Progressive decline in mental and social functioning**: increasing difficulty in intellectual function, memory, concentration and use of language	Gradual loss of mental function could result from a range of slowly developing brain disorders, including dementia, recurrent small strokes, extradural haemorrhage and a slow growing brain tumour Remember that, in the elderly in particular, depression can manifest in this way, and the symptoms may resolve with antidepressant medication
24.2	**Recent onset of confusion** (i.e. evidence of an acute organic mental health disorder) such as confusion, agitation, visual hallucinations and loss of ability to care for self	Organic mental health disorders are, by definition, those that have a medically recognised physical cause, such as drug intoxication, brain damage or dementia. They are characterised by confusion or clouding of consciousness, and loss of insight. Visual hallucinations may be apparent, as in the case of delirium tremens (alcohol withdrawal) Referral has to be considered if you recognise that the patient or other people are at serious risk of harm if you do not disclose the patient's condition. As it may be very difficult for you to assess this risk fully, it is advised that unless you are absolutely sure of the patient's safety you should refer him or her to professionals who are experienced in the treatment of mental health disorders Referral in such a situation may result in the serious outcome of the patient being detained against their will in hospital under a section of the Mental Health Act. As this may be a situation in which you may need to breach patient confidentiality, you may wish to seek advice from your professional body about how to proceed

Table 4.1f-I Red Flags 24 – dementia, epilepsy and other disorders of the central nervous system—Cont'd

Red Flag	Description	Reasoning
24.3	**A temporary loss of brain function** (usually lasting less than 2 hours). Features may include: loss of consciousness, loss of vision, unsteadiness, confusion, loss of memory, loss of sensation, limb weakness	A temporary loss of brain function is most commonly seen as part of the syndrome of migraine, in which case it usually is part of a pattern with which the patient is familiar. In migraine, the blood flow to a portion of the brain is temporarily reduced as a result of spasm of an artery. A simple migraine does not merit referral The most common cause of loss of consciousness is a simple faint. This benign syndrome does not merit referral. It is characterised by low blood pressure and a slow but regular pulse, and is triggered by prolonged standing, stuffy conditions and/or emotional arousal. A person who has fainted should start to recover almost immediately after the collapse If these symptoms occur for the first time it is important to exclude the more serious syndrome of transient ischaemic attack (TIA), in which a branch of a cerebral artery has been blocked by the temporary lodging of a small blood clot. A TIA is a warning sign of the more permanent damage that results from stroke, and the patient needs referral for diagnosis and treatment
24.4	**A persisting loss of brain function** (lasting more than 2 hours). Features may include: loss of vision, unsteadiness, confusion, loss of memory, loss of sensation and muscle weakness	Any development of symptoms that suggest a persisting loss in brain function merits referral to exclude stroke or a rapidly growing brain tumour. Some of these symptoms can also result from disease of the spinal cord (e.g. multiple sclerosis) or of a peripheral nerve (e.g. Bell's palsy)
24.5	**A first ever epileptic seizure** Generalised tonic–clonic seizure: convulsions, loss of consciousness, bitten tongue, emptying of bladder and/or bowels. This is an emergency if the fit does not settle down within 2 minutes Generalised absence or complex partial seizures: defined periods of vagueness or loss of awareness or mood or personality changes Focal simple seizures: episodes of coarse twitching of one part of the body	Anyone who may have experienced a first epileptic seizure needs to be referred for diagnosis and advice about driving and personal safety The only symptom a patient might experience of nocturnal seizures might be a sensation of grogginess in the morning and a wet bed. In such a case the patient will have no memory of the episode of urination. The patient must be strongly urged not to drive until they have received medical advice Absence and complex partial seizures may also be difficult to recognise; but are important to refer if suspected, as there is real risk of harm if an episode occurs when performing a risky activity such as climbing or driving A first epileptic seizure may rarely result from a brain tumour If a tonic–clonic seizure is ongoing, and particularly if it lasts for more than 1 minute, it could develop into an emergency situation and help needs to be summoned with urgency. It is important to ensure that the fitting patient is in the recovery position while you are waiting for help to arrive
24.6	**Fit in a child**: refer any child who has suffered from a suspected blank episode (absence) or seizure	Epilepsy most commonly first presents in childhood, and is more common in children who have experienced febrile convulsions. Early diagnosis is important so that early management can help prevent deleterious effects on education and social development
24.7	**Progressive coarse tremor appearing in middle to late life**	A fine symmetrical tremor that is worse with anxiety and overarousal is common and benign, particularly in the elderly In contrast, Parkinson's disease presents with a progressive tremor that is far more coarse and which characteristically causes the movement of repeated opposition of thumb and fingers (the so-called 'pill-rolling tremor'). Combined with this there will be increased stiffness of the muscles (the arms will be felt to resist passive movement). Parkinson's disease commonly affects one side more than another in its early stages Commonly, treatment is delayed for as long as is reasonable in Parkinson's disease, so there is no need for high-priority referral, but referral is advised so that the patient can benefit from the support of a specialist team of health professionals

Chapter 4.1g Disorders of the spinal cord and peripheral nerves

LEARNING POINTS

- At the end of this chapter you will:
- be able to name the main features of the important diseases of the spinal cord and the peripheral nerves
- understand the principles of treatment of these diseases
- be able to recognise the red flags of these diseases.

Estimated time for chapter: 120 minutes.

Introduction

This final chapter is concerned with the neurological disorders that have their origin outside the brain, either within the spinal cord or the peripheral nerves. The conditions to be explored in this chapter are:

- Disorders of the spinal cord:
  - spinal cord compression
  - spina bifida
  - poliomyelitis.
- Disorders of the spinal nerve roots:
  - lumbar spondylosis
  - sciatica
  - cervical spondylosis.
- Disorders which affect the nerve plexuses:
  - cervical rib
  - malignant infiltration.
- Disorders of the peripheral nerves:
  - Guillain-Barré syndrome
  - polyneuropathy
  - mononeuropathy
  - carpal tunnel syndrome
  - meralgia paraesthetica
  - Bell's palsy
  - trigeminal neuralgia
  - multiple mononeuropathy
  - leprosy
  - herpes zoster (shingles).
- Disorders of the neuromuscular junction:
  - myasthenia gravis.

Disorders of the spinal cord

It might be helpful to turn back to Chapter 4.1a to revise the structure of the spinal cord and how the peripheral nerves arise from it. (This information can be found from the section entitled The Spinal Cord up to the end of Part I, and information on the spinal nerves from the beginning of Part II up to the end of the section entitled Referred Pain.)

Spinal cord compression

The nervous tissue of the spinal cord is very delicate and is vulnerable to permanent damage by compression. Sudden spinal cord compression can result from traumatic injury to the spine in which a fracture or dislocation of one or more vertebrae can cause narrowing of the spinal canal. A more gradual onset of compression can result from a tumour or an abscess developing within the spinal canal. Occasionally, an intervertebral disc can prolapse (slip) and compress the posterior aspect of a part of the cord. This rare form of prolapse most commonly affects the sacral levels of the cord. Arthritic changes of the vertebrae can also lead to a deformity of the spinal cord that is so great as to cause compression. This most commonly affects the lower cervical and sacral cord.

The various symptoms of cord compression are the result of the combined damage to the sensitive meninges that surround the cord, damage to the spinal nerves emerging from the cord at the level of the compression, and damage to the nerve cells and nerve fibres situated in the spinal cord at that level. The way in which these symptoms manifest of course depends on the level of the compression. For example, a sudden compression at the level of T5 from a fracture dislocation between the T5 and T6 vertebrae will lead to pain in the region of the compression (from damage to the bones and meninges) and pain in the dermatome of skin supplied by the T5 spinal nerves. In this case the area of skin is a band that encircles the chest approximately at the level of the nipple. The pain will be worse on coughing or straining because these actions further increase the pressure within the spinal canal.

The most significant symptoms of compression result from the damage done within the cord itself. This can result in damage to the nerve fibres that travel through the cord at that level. The function of these fibres is to connect all parts of the body supplied by spinal nerves originating at positions lower than that level with the brain.

If the compression is very severe or the cord is actually severed, all connection between those parts of the body supplied by the more distal spinal nerves and the brain is lost. The result is total paralysis of all voluntary muscles in these parts of the body, and total numbness of these parts of the body. For example, in the case of a serious compression at the level of T5, the patient will become paralysed from the lower chest down and will be numb from the chest down. Voluntary control of the bladder and bowels is lost. Total paralysis of the lower limbs is termed 'paraplegia' (if partial it is termed 'paraparesis'). However, the spinal reflexes responsible for the maintenance of tone in the lower limbs and for the involuntary control of the bladder and bowel are not affected. The tone of the muscles in the legs can be excessive, because the control that is normally exerted on these reflexes by the brain is lost. This means that muscle spasms can occur. This is the reason for the term 'spastic paraplegia'.

In the case of an injury at the level of the cervical vertebrae (colloquially termed a 'broken neck'), the connection is lost between the brain and the spinal nerves that supply the arms. This means that all four limbs become paralysed, a condition termed 'tetraplegia' (also known as quadriplegia).

In a cervical cord compression the muscles that supply the chest wall are also paralysed, and this severely impairs the action of inspiration. An injury above the level of C3–4 has the added serious consequence of causing paralysis to the diaphragm, so that unassisted breathing is not possible at all.

In the acute compression of the cord that occurs from traumatic injury, the condition is a surgical emergency. Without very prompt attention, permanent damage to the cord will occur. Even with very careful support, it is rare for a person who suddenly has developed these sorts of symptoms to recover fully from the injury.

A more slowly developing cause of compression will, of course, cause a more gradual progression of these sorts of symptoms. For example, the typical scenario that follows from the growth of a tumour within the spinal cord is that pain develops in the dermatome supplied by the spinal root, and there is a gradual and patchy onset of numbness and weakness in the parts of the body supplied by spinal nerves distal to the tumour.

Patients with suspected acute or gradual cord compression are diagnosed by means of an MRI. In many cases of progressive cord damage, urgent removal of the cause of the problem (known as 'spinal decompression') can arrest the symptoms and may be followed by recovery of some of the lost function. Intravenous steroids may be given in the acute situation to reduce swelling of the cord, and anticoagulants to prevent blood clotting from reduced muscle movement. Tumours may be treated by one or more of surgery, chemotherapy and radiotherapy.

However, following a traumatic compression to the spinal cord, many patients will have to learn to live with a serious and permanent disability. Any patient who develops paraplegia or tetraplegia requires skilled and prolonged nursing care. The ideal is for the patient to be nursed within a specialised spinal unit that puts an emphasis on rehabilitation. The aim of rehabilitation is to enable the patient to return to an active role in society.

Special attention has to be given to the function of the bladder and bowel. In the initial stages after injury the bladder may not void at all. A urethral catheter is intermittently inserted to enable complete drainage of the bladder. This has the potential complication of increasing the risk of infections of the bladder. These bladder infections have a tendency to spread to involve the kidneys in a patient who is immobile. If they occur, they are treated promptly with antibiotics. Some people manage to start to learn to void without use of a catheter at all as the bladder is under reflex spinal control. Others, even without this reflex, can learn to self-catheterise. Elderly people are more likely to have to depend on an indwelling catheter.

Similarly, initially the patient will be faecally incontinent. However, with time the bowel starts to empty regularly, and a form of continence can be achieved, although a pattern may take some weeks to establish following the injury.

The problem of permanently contracted muscles has to be avoided. This means that the patient requires intensive physiotherapy to the limbs to enable the muscles to be stretched regularly. Drugs such as baclofen and dantrolene that inhibit spasms are given frequently to prevent contractures. These can have side-effects such as severe nausea, confusion and other mental disturbances, which can markedly affect the quality of life of the patient. The paralysed patient has to be turned regularly in bed, or moved in position within a wheelchair, to prevent pressure sores developing. A chronic pressure sore is a serious problem in paraplegia, as once established it is very difficult to heal. The chronic infection from a pressure sore can have a very debilitating effect.

With time, many patients regain mobility with the help of specially adapted lightweight wheelchairs. Although all will continue to require regular support from a multidisciplinary team of carers, many will be able to return to an active life in their own homes.

The patient with a spinal cord injury remains at risk of recurrent infections of the chest and the kidneys. These complications can lead to an early death, either from respiratory failure or from chronic kidney failure.

Other causes of damage to the spinal cord

Some other rare conditions can cause localised damage to the cord, leading to a condition similar to cord compression. For example, vitamin B_{12} deficiency (pernicious anaemia) involves spinal cord damage as well as a form of dementia. Also, occasionally the damage caused by the plaques of multiple sclerosis can be localised to one part of the cord, and might produce similar symptoms, although in both these conditions the pain is not so prominent. Inflammation of the cord can occur as a result of radiotherapy or some rare infections. This too will produce similar symptoms.

Information Box 4.1g-I

Spinal cord injury: comments from a Chinese medicine perspective

In Chinese medicine, the symptoms that arise from severe damage in spinal cord injury correspond to deficiency of Jing. It is another example of an atrophy syndrome (see Chapter 4.1f). Numbness and weakness correspond to Damp obstructing the channels together with Deficiency of Yin (Kidney and Liver). Spasticity is a manifestation of Liver Wind in the muscles. Lack of control of the urethra and the anus would also fit with severe Kidney Deficiency.

Spina bifida

Spinal bifida is a congenital structural abnormality of the spinal cord in the lumbosacral region. In severe cases, the posterior part of the cord is undeveloped, and the residual part of the cord opens out onto the skin, where it is covered by a membrane-bound sac called a 'meningocoele'. This requires immediate surgery at birth to protect the cord from rupture of the sac and subsequent infection. Surgery cannot amend the damage caused by the lack of the nerves in this part of the cord. In severe spina bifida, the child might have a spastic paraplegia, numbness of the lower limbs, and incontinence of the bladder and bowel. In some cases, these problems can be associated with other abnormalities such as hydrocephalus.

In less severe cases the abnormality is not apparent at birth, and only becomes apparent as the child fails to reach the expected milestones of development, such as sitting, crawling and walking. This situation of undiagnosed spina bifida is becoming increasingly rare because the condition can be detected from the prenatal ultrasound scan which most pregnant women in the UK undergo. This means that appropriate care for the child can be offered at a very early stage.

It is now known that adequate dietary levels of certain vitamins early in pregnancy are important in the prevention of spina bifida. In particular, there is very strong evidence that a regular dose of folic acid, taken in the first weeks of pregnancy (ideally from preconception to at least 20 weeks) reduces the risk of this abnormality. It is also for this reason that foods such as bread and breakfast cereals are often fortified with this vitamin.

Information Box 4.1g-II

Spina bifida: comments from a Chinese medicine perspective

In Chinese medicine spina bifida might be described as Deficiency of Jing and Yin together with accumulation of Damp in the channels. In this case the cause of the Jing Deficiency is congenital rather than severe trauma, but otherwise the energetic interpretation of the syndrome is comparable to that of a spinal cord injury.

The strong link that exists between spina bifida and deficiency of folic acid in pregnancy suggests that folic acid plays a role in nourishing the Jing of the fetus.

Poliomyelitis (polio)

Poliomyelitis is a viral infection that has a propensity for the nervous system. The virus is excreted in the faeces, and so is passed on through contact with faeces. In most cases of polio infection (95%) there are very few symptoms. The remaining 5% of people who contract the infection suffer from a flu-like illness with muscle aches. However, less than one in five of these will go on to develop the severe condition of paralytic poliomyelitis. In these cases the virus has invaded some of the lower motor nerve cells in the spinal cord that lead to all the voluntary muscles. The result is a paralysis of the affected muscle groups. The paralysis leads to a flaccid limb, without tone, and in this way is different to the paralysis caused by spinal cord compression. There is no loss of sensation in polio.

In paralytic polio the patient experiences a flare up of symptoms about 4–5 days following recovery from the flu-like illness, a headache (due to a form of meningitis) and the development of weakness of some of the muscles. The muscle weakness is not necessarily symmetrical.

Polio tends to affect children less severely than adults. Whereas a child characteristically might develop weakness in one or both lower limbs, an adult might develop a tetraplegia or difficulty swallowing due to damage to the lower motor nerve cells originating in the cervical cord and the brainstem.

The incidence of polio worldwide has dropped markedly since the introduction of vaccination. It is the aim of the World Health Organization to coordinate the vaccination campaign so that polio, like smallpox, becomes totally eradicated. The initial aim of the programme was total eradication by the year 2000. This looked tantalisingly close, as in 1994 the Americas were declared polio free, and in 2000 the Western Pacific followed. In 2002 Europe was declared polio free, but in six countries, including Afghanistan, India and Nigeria, the disease remained endemic. Since that time there has been a resurgence of cases in many countries in Africa, not helped by political unrest in many of these countries and the disruption that such unrest causes to the success of health programmes.

In the UK almost all of the very few new cases of polio were diagnosed either in people who had contracted the condition overseas or who had developed polio as a result of a very rare complication of the live vaccine (now totally replaced by inactivated vaccine). Nevertheless, in some developing countries polio is still an endemic disease. In these countries, people who have the lifelong disabilities that have resulted from a childhood polio infection (usually a single wasted and useless limb) are a common sight.

Disorders of the spinal nerve roots

The spinal nerves (nerve roots) that emerge from the spinal cord can be selectively damaged in some conditions. These conditions will lead to a characteristic syndrome of one-sided pain, sensory loss and weakness, depending on the site of the damage.

Lumbar spondylosis and sciatica

'Sciatica' is the term used to describe a pain that has its origin in the lumbar and sacral spinal nerves. This pain is referred down one or both legs, along the distribution of the sciatic nerve. The symptoms include pain and/or tingling that radiates down the buttock and the back of one leg to the foot. There may be patchy numbness of the skin in the region affected by the pain, and weakness of some of the muscles of the lower leg. The pain is typically provoked by movements that affect the lower back, particularly bending forward. Sciatica is often, but not always, associated with low back pain.

Sciatica results from damage to one or more of the lumbar or sacral spinal nerves that emerge from the very base of the spinal cord. The spinal cord actually terminates at the level of L1/L2 vertebrae. The lower lumbar and sacral spinal nerves leave the base of the cord at this level, and then travel downwards within the spinal canal to their points of exit at the sacral and lumbar intervertebral spaces.

The lumbar and sacral spinal nerves can be damaged by anything that compresses them, either as they descend through the spinal canal, or as they emerge through the intervertebral spaces in the lower lumbar or sacral regions of the back. The

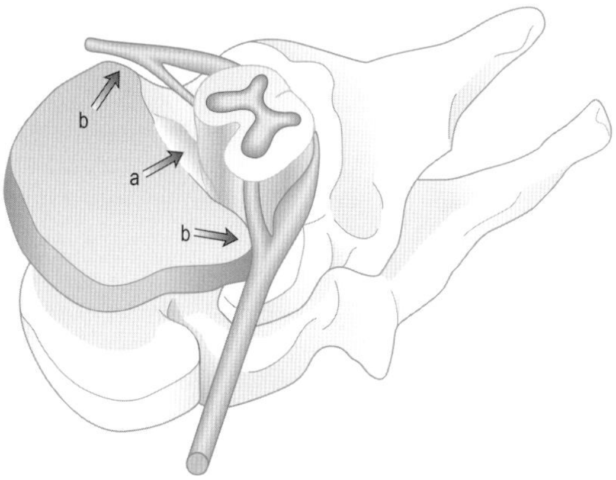

Figure 4.1g-I • Central (a) and lateral (b) disc protrusion • Diagram showing compression of cord and spinal nerve roots, respectively.

most common cause of compression of the spinal nerves is the protrusion (prolapse) of an intervertebral disc, either between the L5/S1 vertebrae or between the S1/S2 vertebrae. (for more detail about intervertebral disc prolapse see Chapter 4.2e). Prolapsed discs will tend to compress the L5 and S1 nerve roots.

Figure 4.1g-I illustrates how a prolapsed disc can compress the spinal nerve roots. This diagram shows how the bulging of the posterior part of an intervertebral disc can affect either the spinal nerves (b) or the cord itself (a), depending on the site of the bulge. Bulging that is slightly to one side (b) is by far the more common situation.

The other common cause of compression of the spinal nerves is osteoarthritis of the vertebrae (see Chapter 4.2f). The arthritic changes to the vertebral bones can lead to narrowing of the intervertebral spaces as well as of the spinal canal itself.

The term 'spondylosis' is used to describe the degenerative processes that lead to both disc prolapse and arthritic deformity of the vertebrae. Therefore, 'lumbar spondylosis' is the medical term applied to these degenerative causes of sciatica and low back pain.

Sciatica may also occur simply as a result of tension in the muscles and ligaments that support the vertebrae. Tension causes the vertebrae to be squeezed close together and cramps the spaces through which the spinal nerves should exit. This form of sciatica is typically less severe and tends to appear and disappear according to factors such as overwork, tiredness, mood and the weather.

Rarely, a tumour of the spinal canal, or one that is situated close to the lumbosacral spinal column, may cause sciatica. In this case, the sciatica is slowly progressive. Progressive sciatic pain should, therefore, be taken as a red flag of serious disease.

The arthritic changes of lumbar spondylosis may be seen on an X-ray image of the spine, although there is a poor correlation between the changes seen on the X-ray image and the severity of symptoms. The most informative investigation is MRI, which will usually show the site of the compression of the spinal nerve, and whether or not a disc prolapse is present.

The treatment of sciatica and low back pain is described in more detail in Chapter 4.2e.

Information Box 4.1g-III

Sciatica: comments from a Chinese medicine perspective

In Chinese medicine, the pain and numbness of sciatica is ascribed to Damp Cold (or, more rarely, Damp Heat) in the Gallbladder and Bladder channels. An underlying Deficiency of the Kidneys is very often the reason why sciatica has developed.

Cervical spondylosis

The same process of degeneration of the intervertebral discs and the vertebral bones also commonly occurs in the cervical spine. In this case the C7 spinal nerves are most frequently affected. This leads to pain and tingling that radiates down one arm to the hand, numbness of the skin of the arm and weakness of the muscles of the forearm and the hand.

The treatment of cervical spondylosis is discussed in Chapter 4.2e.

Information Box 4.1g-IV

Cervical spondylosis: comments from a Chinese medicine perspective

In Chinese medicine, the symptoms of cervical spondylosis would also be ascribed to Damp Cold or Damp Heat leading to Qi and Blood Stagnation, this time in the channels of the arm. Again, because the degeneration of the spine is the underlying cause, a Kidney Deficiency is likely to be present. Contributory neck and shoulder muscular tension would correspond to Qi Stagnation.

Disorders of the nerve plexuses

The nerve plexuses are the networks of nerves formed by the intermingling of the spinal nerves that supply the arms and the legs. If these are affected by disease a complex pattern of symptoms can develop because a number of peripheral nerves will be damaged.

The two brachial plexuses involve the C5 to T1 spinal nerves, and are situated deep in the upper chest at the level of the clavicle. The nerves that supply the shoulder, the arm and the upper chest emerge from the brachial plexus.

The two lumbosacral plexuses involve the L4 to the coccygeal nerves and are situated deep in the lower abdomen and pelvis close to the lumbar spine and sacrum. The nerves that supply the buttocks, leg and genitals emerge from this plexus.

Cervical rib

The brachial plexus can be affected by a rare condition in which there is an additional rudimentary rib attached to the C7 vertebra, the so-called 'cervical rib'. This can stretch the lower nerve roots of the brachial plexus and cause pain and numbness on the underside of the arm and the ulnar border of the forearm and hand. This extra rib can also compress the major artery that supplies blood to the arm and hand. If one-sided, this can lead to a very weak pulse on that side. Usually, a cervical rib causes no symptoms, but if they do occur the condition can be treated surgically.

Information Box 4.1g-V

Cervical rib: comments from a Chinese medicine perspective

In Chinese medicine, the symptoms of a cervical rib correspond to a Stagnation of Qi and Blood in the Heart and Small Intestine channels of the affected arm. Although the pulse may be very abnormal on the affected side, this perhaps should be taken as a feature of the condition rather than as a reflection of the whole energetic balance of the body.

Malignant infiltration of a nerve plexus

The more serious condition that can affect the nerve plexuses is infiltration by a tumour. The most common cancer-related plexus problem results from *lung cancer* that invades the brachial plexus having spread from the upper portion of a lung. This causes pain down the arm of the same side and wasting of the muscles of that arm. The pain of cancerous infiltration of the nerves can be very severe.

Information Box 4.1g-VI

Malignant infiltration of a nerve plexus: comments from a Chinese medicine perspective

In Chinese medicine, the pain of malignant infiltration corresponds to Blood Stagnation in the affected channels, and is a manifestation of the underlying cancerous process.

Disorders of the peripheral nerves

The peripheral nerves comprise the cranial nerves and the spinal nerves, and include all the nerves that emerge from the nerve plexuses. These nerves branch to supply all the muscles of the body with motor or autonomic nerve endings. They also carry sensory nerve fibres from all superficial parts of the body. Therefore, a condition that damages a peripheral nerve will have two effects: it will cause weakness and wasting of the muscles supplied by that nerve, and also will cause a loss of sensation of the part of the body supplied by that nerve. Sometimes the affected nerve gives rise to pain or tingling rather than numbness. The pain from a damaged nerve is called 'neuralgia', and is characteristically severe.

A condition that affects a number of peripheral nerves is called a 'polyneuropathy', and one that affects a single nerve is called a 'mononeuropathy'. A polyneuropathy typically affects long nerves most severely. This means that the nerves which supply the hands, the legs and the feet are most damaged. The patient with this form of polyneuropathy develops what is called 'glove and stocking' numbness, because of the area of skin affected, and weakness of the muscles of the hands and the legs. Balance can be impaired, because the sensation of the bones of the feet and ankles is also lost.

In both types of neuropathy, if prolonged, the numbness can result in recurrent injury to the affected area, because the protective mechanism of pain has been lost.

Information Box 4.1g-VII

Neuropathy: comments from a Chinese medicine perspective

In Chinese medicine, the numbness of neuropathy would usually correspond to Damp and/or Blood Deficiency, and the weakness to Deficiency of Liver and Kidney Yin. This is another form of atrophy syndrome. Injuries that result from the numbness reflect Stagnation of Blood and Qi.

Guillain-Barré syndrome (postinfective polyneuropathy)

This syndrome tends to follow 1–3 weeks after an infectious illness. It is thought to be the result of autoimmune damage to the peripheral nerves which has been triggered by the infectious process. The patient initially develops a glove-and-stocking numbness, and weakness of the hands and legs. In many patients there is a slow but sure recovery of the nerves over the following few weeks. However, in some cases (about 20%) the polyneuropathy is rapidly progressive so that shorter nerves become affected. This includes the respiratory and facial muscles. This deterioration can occur rapidly, over the course of a few days, and can lead to a medical emergency as the patient may require assisted ventilation to support the failing respiratory muscles.

A preparation of antibodies, called 'gamma-globulin', appears to slow the progress and severity of the condition. This is given to patients with severe Guillain-Barré syndrome.

In severe cases recovery may require several months, during which time the patient is almost totally paralysed. In these cases recovery is often not complete, so that some residual numbness and weakness of muscles remains. The mortality associated with the severe form of this condition is 10%.

Information Box 4.1g-VIII

Guillain-Barré Syndrome: comments from a Chinese medicine perspective

In Chinese medicine, Guillain-Barré syndrome with peripheral numbness and weakness, like all forms of polyneuropathy, corresponds to Damp in the channels, with Liver and Kidney Yin Deficiency. In this case the origin of the Damp is possibly a Residual Pathogenic Factor following an infectious disease. Full Heat from an infection may have contributed to weakening of the Yin.

Polyneuropathy in chronic illness

There are a number of chronic conditions in which polyneuropathy can develop. The most common of these is diabetes mellitus, in which, because wound healing is poor, numbness can be a source of serious medical complications. Small wounds to the numb skin of the feet, in particular, can easily develop into chronic ulcers, and eventually the foot may require amputation.

Numbness of the hands and feet can also develop in severe kidney disease and advanced cancer.

Certain vitamin deficiencies, if prolonged, can lead to a polyneuropathy because the vitamins are essential for the maintenance of healthy nerves. In particular, deficiencies of thiamine (vitamin B_1), pyridoxine (vitamin B_6) and vitamin B_{12} may lead to nerve damage.

Polyneuropathy caused by toxins

A number of drugs and toxins can damage the peripheral nerves. Alcohol is the most important of these in the UK in terms of number of people affected. With high alcohol intake over a length of time, loss of sensation of the feet and legs and muscle weakness can develop, and lead to a vulnerability to injury and an impairment of balance. This problem with balance is over and above that caused by the direct effects of alcohol itself. The nerve damage often persists even after abstention from alcohol.

Some of the drugs that cause polyneuropathy include phenytoin (an anti-epileptic drug), gold (an antirheumatoid medication), and vincristine and cisplatin (chemotherapeutic drugs).

Mononeuropathy from nerve entrapment

A single peripheral nerve can be damaged by excessive pressure as it passes through the tissues. Some nerves are more vulnerable to this problem than others because they travel through areas that are more exposed to damage, or because they pass through a very tight anatomical space. The loss of function that results from damage to a single nerve is sometimes termed a 'palsy'. For example, a 'median nerve palsy' is the cause of the carpal tunnel syndrome.

Carpal tunnel syndrome is an entrapment neuropathy that results from the compression of the median nerve as it passes over the wrist bones (in the region of acupoint Daling PC-7) to supply the muscles of the thumb and skin of the radial side of the hand. The cause is usually an accumulation of fluid within the limited space of the soft tissue of the wrist (known as the 'carpal tunnel') through which the nerve passes. Carpal tunnel syndrome can occur out of the blue, but it is often associated with more generalised conditions, in particular pregnancy, hypothyroidism and obesity.

The symptoms include numbness and tingling of the radial side of the hand and weakness of grip. There may be pain and aching in the hand and forearm, which is particularly bad at night, and is helped by dropping the arm out of bed.

Treatment includes taking the pressure off the nerve by splinting the wrist in an extended position. Corticosteroid injections may be given. If the pain and weakness is persistent, a surgical operation is performed on the wrist to reduce the pressure in the carpal tunnel.

Meralgia paraesthetica is an entrapment neuropathy of the lateral cutaneous nerve of the thigh. This is a sensory nerve that supplies the outer aspect of the skin of the thigh. The entrapment occurs as the nerve passes through the femoral canal (in the region of acupoint Qichong St-30). This causes numbness, tingling and pain on the outer aspect of the thigh.

Meralgia paraesthetica is fairly common in pregnancy and can also be a problem in obesity. This is because in both these conditions there is additional pressure on the femoral canal. If the condition develops during pregnancy it usually settles after delivery.

Information Box 4.1g-IX

Carpal tunnel syndrome and meralgia paraesthetica: comments from a Chinese medicine perspective

In Chinese medicine, the numbness and weakness of carpal tunnel syndrome corresponds to Damp and/or Blood deficiency. The Pericardium and Lung channels are particularly affected.

The numbness of meralgia paraesthetica corresponds to Damp and/or Blood deficiency. The Stomach channel is affected.

Bell's palsy and facial weakness

Bell's palsy is the result of inflammation of the facial nerve (the seventh cranial nerve), which supplies the muscles of the face. The facial nerve carries very few sensory fibres, which means that numbness is not a symptom. It is believed that the inflammation is due to a viral infection of the facial nerve, which causes swelling of the nerve as it passes through the bone of the skull close to the ear.

The symptoms are of a sudden onset of weakness of one side of the face, sometimes following a brief episode of earache on the affected side. The corner of the mouth droops and the eyelid may be unable to close completely. In serious cases this problem, if prolonged, can lead to ulceration of the eye and damage to the cornea. The patient may also notice an altered taste on one side of the tongue.

In most people improvement begins spontaneously after 2 weeks and complete recovery can be expected, although recovery can be slow and incomplete in a minority of cases. Corticosteroids are often given by mouth for a week or so early in the course of the condition to reduce the swelling and damage to the nerve. A minor operation may have to be performed to encourage the eyelid to close and thus prevent ulceration of the cornea of the eye.

A more serious cause of damage to the facial nerve is pressure on the nerve from a brain tumour. For this reason, if a person with Bell's palsy does not start to recover at all within 2 weeks they may be referred for further neurological investigations including MRI.

Weakness of the facial muscles can occur in other conditions. The most common cause is a one-sided stroke, although this will usually be accompanied by symptoms of weakness in other parts of the body. In a stroke, the eyelids and the forehead muscles are not affected.

Myasthenia gravis is a condition that causes a more symmetrical facial weakness; it is described in more detail at the end of this chapter.

Information Box 4.1g-X

Facial weakness: comments from a Chinese medicine perspective

In Chinese medicine, the symptom of facial weakness is considered to be caused by Wind Invasion of the channels of the face. Bell's palsy is attributed to external Wind, whereas facial weakness occurring in a stroke is due to internally generated Wind.

Trigeminal neuralgia

Trigeminal neuralgia (TGN) is a condition in which the nerve that carries the sensory nerve fibres that supply the skin and soft tissues of the face becomes excessively sensitive. This nerve is the fifth cranial nerve, also known as the 'trigeminal nerve'. The pain of trigeminal neuralgia is experienced as a severe stabbing or electric-shock-like sensation that radiates down the face from the area in front of the ear. The condition predominantly affects elderly people.

Light touch, shaving, washing and exposure to a cool breeze can trigger an attack of this pain, which then can occur repeatedly over the course of a period of hours. There may be gaps of weeks to months between attacks.

Although the majority of cases have no precipitating cause, in a significant minority (14%) the nerve has been irritated by a structural change such as a tumour or aneurysm. For this reason many cases will be investigated by means of MRI.

The most effective painkillers for the intense pain of TGN are the antiepileptic medications carbamazepine, phenytoin, lamotrigine and gabapentin, all of which have an inhibitory effect on the nervous system. In very severe recurrent cases, the nerve may be deadened by injection with alcohol. This will leave the patient with a permanently numb face. Alternatively, in some cases the blood supply of the nerve root can be decompressed by delicate microsurgery, with good results.

Information Box 4.1g-XI

Trigeminal neuralgia: comments from a Chinese medicine perspective

In Chinese medicine, the symptoms of trigeminal neuralgia also correspond to Wind or Wind Cold Invasion. The intense pain indicates a Blood Stagnation, which results from the Wind Invasion. The fact that this is a disease of the elderly suggests that an underlying Deficiency of Blood or Qi is likely to be present also.

Multiple mononeuropathy

Multiple mononeuropathy is a condition in which a number of peripheral nerves are damaged, but not usually in the symmetrical way in which a polyneuropathy first presents. In the UK, it is most commonly a result of the damage to the circulation to the nerves which occurs in diabetes. The patient with this condition will have repeated episodes in which the function of single nerves is lost. This occurs suddenly as the arterioles that supply the nerves undergo thrombosis.

For example, a sudden onset of numbness and weakness affecting the ulnar side of the hand (ulnar nerve palsy) might be followed by an inability to raise the foot and numbness on the border of the shin (common peroneal nerve palsy), and so on.

Other causes of multiple mononeuropathy include advanced cancer, and HIV infection. Leprosy, which is described below, is the most important cause worldwide.

Information Box 4.1g-XII

Multiple mononeuropathy: comments from a Chinese medicine perspective

As with the other mononeuropathies, the numbness and weakness correspond to Damp and/or Blood Deficiency. The progressive nature of the problem indicates an underlying Deficiency of Yin.

Leprosy

Leprosy is an infection that occurs in tropical and warm temperate regions. It primarily affects the peripheral nervous system, but can spread via the nerves to affect the soft tissues. The infectious agent, *Mycobacterium leprae*, is from the same family as the organism that causes tuberculosis. It is uncertain exactly how the organism is transmitted from one person to another. It is possible that organisms are transmitted by nasal secretions, as it is known that millions of organisms may be expelled from the nose each day by an infected individual. Whether these then infect skin or the respiratory tract of a contact is, as yet, unknown. After the initial infection there can be a delay of a few months to a few years before symptoms appear.

The manifestation of the leprosy infection depends very much on the state of the immune system of the individual. In those with good immunity, the infection is localised to one part of the body and is not contagious. This is known as 'paucibacillary leprosy' or 'tuberculoid leprosy'. In this form of leprosy, a single peripheral nerve becomes damaged and thickened. The skin supplied by this nerve becomes numb and loses some of its pigment. The pale patch that results can have slightly thickened edges. As with other mononeuropathies, the muscles supplied by the nerve become weak and wasted.

In people with poor immunity, the number of nerves affected increases, and the damage done by the organism to the skin supplied by those nerves is greater. This is called 'lepromatous leprosy' or 'multibacillary leprosy'. In severe cases there is a multiple mononeuropathy, with weakness or paralysis of a number of muscle groups, numerous numb patches of skin, and gross thickening of areas of the skin, particularly on the face. In severe lepromatous leprosy, the face can become very deformed by the thickened skin. The inflammation affects deeper tissues also. The cartilage of the nose erodes and the testes atrophy. The prolonged numbness of the limbs leads to loss of fingers and toes as a result of chronic injury not prevented by the usual withdrawal response to pain.

It is no wonder that leprosy used to be such a dreaded disease, and that in many countries 'lepers' were exiled from their own communities. Despite this fear, the condition is not very contagious, with only one in 100 of people who have been in close contact with a person with advanced leprosy going on to develop the disease.

Lepromatous leprosy can be treated by long-term antibiotic therapy. Because the bacterium is slow growing, and able to 'hide' within the nervous system, a daily dose of the antibiotic dapsone and low-dose clofazimine is recommended to be taken for a minimum of 2 years. In addition, additional antibiotics (rifampicin and high-dose clofazimine) are given once a month. This regimen is a difficult one to stick to for anyone, and more so for people who live in poverty in rural areas. Ideally, treatment is administered from a specialist centre. In tuberculoid leprosy, 6 months of treatment is the maximum that would be prescribed to eradicate the infection.

In established leprosy, the damage already done to the nerves, soft tissues and the skin cannot be reversed by drug treatment. Physiotherapy and surgery are also important aspects of the treatment of the deformities caused by this infection.

> **Information Box 4.1g-XIII**
>
> **Leprosy: comments from a Chinese medicine perspective**
>
> In leprosy, in addition to Damp (numbness) and Blood Deficiency (pale skin patches), the thickening of the skin suggests that Phlegm is an important additional Pathogenic Factor. The fact that an impaired immunity predisposes people to severe leprosy suggests that there is an underlying severe Deficiency Syndrome. Kidney Yin Deficiency is the most likely.

Varicella zoster (shingles)

'Varicella zoster' is the name given to the chickenpox virus. The condition of shingles is a late consequence of a chickenpox infection, and usually occurs decades after an initial childhood infection. It is common, affecting up to 20% of people in the UK in their lifetime.

It seems that, following some cases of chickenpox, the virus is not fully cleared from the body, but instead 'hides' within the sensory nerve cell bodies that sit next to the spinal nerves close to the spinal cord. It is believed that during the episode of chickenpox the virus travels up to this site via the sensory nerve fibres that supply the areas of infected skin. In this way an episode of shingles involves the recurrence of a skin infection by the virus, but this time localised to the dermatome supplied by a single spinal nerve.

The virus spreads from its hiding place close to the spinal cord via the nerve ending of the spinal nerve so that the skin of the dermatome first becomes painful for a day or so, and only then develops crusting and weeping spots akin to the original chickenpox. Shingles is contagious at this stage, although the condition that would be transmitted would be chickenpox rather than shingles. The appearance is of a strip of red crusting skin localised to one half of the body only.

Shingles develops at a time when the natural immunity is low, either as a result of ageing, or because of stress or another ongoing illness. In frail people, the skin infection can be very severe and painful. In particular, shingles that affects one of the facial dermatomes can be very debilitating, particularly if it is close to the eye. A shingles infection that affects the nerve that supplies the cornea of the eye (the ophthalmic division of the fifth (trigeminal) cranial nerve) can be so severe as to threaten the sight.

Recovery of the crusting rash occurs over a matter of days. However, in up to one in 10 people the area of skin which was affected is left in a very sensitive and painful state. This pain can be intense, prolonged and draining, and does not respond to conventional painkillers. It can last for a period of months to years. In some people, treatment with anti-epileptic or antidepressant medication (e.g. carbamazepine, gabapentin, lamotrigine or amitriptyline) can be of help.

The acute infection of shingles can be treated with the antiviral drug aciclovir given in tablet form. Some studies demonstrate that if this drug is given to people with shingles in its very early stages, the prolonged pain that follows the infection can be reduced in severity.

> **Information Box 4.1g-XIV**
>
> **Shingles: comments from a Chinese medicine perspective**
>
> In Chinese medicine, the rash of shingles corresponds to an invasion of the channels by Wind Damp and/or Wind Heat. If very painful, it is suggestive of Heat.

Disorders of the neuromuscular junction

'Neuromuscular junction' is the term given to the specialised synapse at which the branches (dendrites) at the very end of a motor nerve make contact with a muscle fibre. The dendrites of the stimulated nerve release a neurotransmitter into the space of the synapse. Receptors on the muscle fibre respond to these molecules by causing a muscle contraction. The most important disorder of the neuromuscular junction is myasthenia gravis.

Myasthenia gravis

'Myasthenia gravis' is a term which literally means 'severe weakness of muscles'. It is an organ-specific autoimmune disease of unknown cause, but tends to affect women twice as often as men. Commonly, young adults are affected.

In myasthenia gravis, antibodies are found that target the receptors for the acetylcholine neurotransmitter in the neuromuscular junction. This means that the 'message' of the stimulated motor nerve cannot get through effectively to the muscle to bring about a contraction. In addition, in 70% of young patients the thymus gland, a small lump of lymphoid tissue deep in the chest, is found to be enlarged. In a small proportion of these people a tumour, called a 'thymoma', is found within the thymus.

The characteristic symptom of myasthenia is that muscles are weak, and that the weakness increases after repeated action of a particular muscle. This is known as 'fatigability'. The facial muscles and the muscles that cause flex of the shoulders and hips are most affected. This means that double vision, drooping eyelids, difficulty swallowing and chewing, and difficulty standing from sitting may all occur. In severe cases, the action of breathing may be impaired. However, there is one form of myasthenia in which the eye and eyelid muscles only are affected.

Because the first symptoms are often vague, the patient who complains of periods of weakness and fatigue may not be correctly diagnosed for some time. In most cases there is a gradual, but slow, progression of symptoms. In severe cases respiratory failure may develop.

Diagnosis may be confirmed by testing for antibodies to the acetylcholine receptor. A CT scan should be performed to exclude tumour of the thymus in the chest.

Myasthenia gravis is treated with drugs that prevent the normal removal of the neurotransmitter at the neuromuscular junction. Pyridostigmine is the most widely used drug. The side-effects of diarrhoea, abdominal pain and excessive salivation are partly a result of the effect this drug has on parts of the body that are not affected by the myasthenia. These drugs do not alter the course of the disease.

In severe cases corticosteroids and other immunosuppressants, such as azathioprine or methotrexate, can also reduce the symptoms by inhibiting the immune damage to the neuromuscular junction.

In people with a large thymus gland or a thymoma, a surgical operation is performed to remove the gland. This operation can also lead to some relief from symptoms in up to half of patients (see Q4.1g-1).

The red flags of diseases of the spinal cord and peripheral nerves

Some patients with diseases of the spinal cord and peripheral nerves will benefit from referral to a conventional doctor for assessment and/or treatment. Red flags are those symptoms and signs that will indicate that referral is to be considered. The red flags of these conditions are described in Table 4.1g-I. This table forms part of the summary on red flags given in Appendix III, which also gives advice on the degree of urgency of referral for each of the red flag conditions listed.

Table 4.1g-I Red Flags 25 – diseases of the spinal cord and peripheral nerves

Red Flag	Description	Reasoning
25.1	**Any sudden or gradual onset of objectively quantifiable muscular weakness** (e.g. weak grip, difficulty in standing from sitting) For Bell's palsy (facial muscular weakness) – see Red Flag 25.2	It is important to distinguish true muscle weakness from a perception of muscle weakness (a common complaint, particularly in people who are depressed). In true muscle weakness there is real limitation in performing simple day-to-day activities such as brushing teeth and walking Asking the patient to move muscles against resistance is a simple way of gauging the strength of their muscles, and is particularly effective in demonstrating if the weakness is not symmetrical (e.g. a one-sided weakness of grip would be very clearly felt on resisted movements of the hands and arms) Muscle weakness may result from conditions of the brain, spinal cord, peripheral nerves, the neuromuscular junction, as well as the muscles themselves. As so many of these conditions are potentially serious, it is wise to refer anyone with muscle weakness for a medical diagnosis The rare condition of Guillain-Barré syndrome can lead to a rapidly progressive weakness of the limbs. This would be accompanied by numbness of the hands and feet (a peripheral neuropathy). If the person is unable to walk, refer urgently, as the condition rarely can progress to affect the respiratory muscles

Table 4.1g-I Red Flags 25 – diseases of the spinal cord and peripheral nerves—Cont'd

Red Flag	Description	Reasoning
25.2	**Bell's Palsy** (facial weakness)	Bell's palsy is usually the result of a viral infection affecting the facial nerve, in which case the onset is dramatic, with facial paralysis developing over the course of 1–2 days. The person may be unable to move their mouth or lift their eyebrows, and importantly not be able to close the eye on the affected side. In rare cases, the palsy may be the result of more serious underlying conditions, such as tumour, multiple sclerosis or Lyme disease Bell's palsy requires high-priority referral, as early treatment with antiviral and corticosteroid medication may improve the chances of full resolution of symptoms. Also, the health of the cornea of the eye needs to be assessed regularly in the early stages (it can become damaged if the eyelid cannot close fully)
25.3	**Any sudden or gradual onset of unexplained measurable numbness or pins and needles** (either generalised or localised)	Numbness can arise from problems in the brain, spinal cord and the peripheral nerves. All of these have potentially serious underlying causes, so if the cause is unclear the patient should be referred for a medical diagnosis Vague numbness is a subjective complaint which is commonly described, but when tested the person can actually distinguish between different types of touch on the 'numb' area. Measurable numbness here refers to the finding that there is an inability to feel or distinguish between the pain of a pin prick and the touch of a piece of cotton wool The most common cause of measurable numbness, however, is compression of the nerve roots in either the neck or the sacral region as a result of osteoarthritis of the spine and sacrum and increased muscle spasm (e.g. in piriformis syndrome). These are benign causes of numbness and are distinguished by having a one-sided distribution on either the side of an arm and hand or down the back of the leg (this is sciatica). In this case, if your diagnosis is correct, treatment (with acupuncture and massage and specific muscle-stretching exercises) should relieve the numbness as the muscle tension resolves. Refer if there is no improvement in 1 week
25.4	**Cauda equina syndrome: numbness of buttocks and perineum** (saddle anaesthesia) with bilateral numbness or sciatica in the legs. Difficulties in urination or defecation are serious symptoms	The cauda equina (horse's tail) is the bunch of nerves that descend from the bottom of the spinal cord from the level of L1–2 downwards. These nerve roots supply sensation and motor impulses to the perineum, buttocks, groin and legs. Cauda equina syndrome suggests the compression of a number of these roots (usually from a central prolapsed disc, but possibly from tumour or other spinal growth). This is a serious situation, as prolonged compression to the perineal supply can lead to permanent problems with urination, defecation and sexual function. Refer as a high priority
25.5	**The features of early shingles**: intense one-sided pain, with overlying rash of crops of fluid-filled reddened and crusting blisters The pain and rash correspond in location to a neurological dermatome The pain may precede the rash by 1–2 days	Shingles is an outbreak of the chickenpox virus (varicella zoster) that has lain dormant within a spinal nerve root since an earlier episode of chickenpox. It tends to reactivate when the person is run down, exposed to intense sunlight and in the elderly Warn the patient that the condition is contagious, and advise that immediate treatment with the antiviral drug aciclovir has been proven to reduce the severity of prolonged pain after recovery of the rash (in this way you are allowing the patient the opportunity of making an informed decision about choosing conventional treatment)
25.6	**Trigeminal neuralgia** (and other forms of one-sided facial pain). Lancinating pain on one side of the face, which radiates out from a focal point in response to defined triggers. May be associated with twitching (tic doloreux)	Trigeminal neuralgia is excruciating facial pain, often triggered by light touch or wind, which radiates from a defined point in a predictable distribution on one side of the face. The common (and 'benign') form may be the result of pressure on the trigeminal nerve within the skull by a blood vessel, but rarely is the result of something more serious, such as a brain tumour or multiple sclerosis. For this reason, a person with unexplained facial pain should be referred for full investigation. Microsurgical treatments have recently been found to have success in intractable cases. Acupuncture is recognised by doctors to be a reasonable pain-relief option for this debilitating condition

Self-test 4.1g

Disorders of the spinal cord and peripheral nerves

1. A new patient or yours suffered a spinal injury after a rock-climbing accident 4 years ago. Over the telephone, while arranging the appointment, he explains that his injury is at the L1 spinal level and that he is now wheelchair bound. What other physical problems would you expect that this patient might experience in everyday life?
2. Sarah is a 30-year-old mother of two. Although she is a regular patient, you haven't seen her for the past fortnight because she has been recovering from a severe bout of flu. Now she mentions that, although she feels better, she has a strange sensation of numbness in her hands and feet, which started 2 days ago. She also feels that she has become clumsy, and drops things very easily.
   (i) What is a possible diagnosis?
   (ii) Would you consider referral?
3. Gerald is 78 years old and thinks he might have shingles. For the past 2 days he has noticed a painful red rash on one side of his chest, and he is feeling a little under the weather. When you examine him, you discover red crusting and weeping spots running in a strip around the left side of Gerald's chest just below the nipple.
   (i) How would you manage this situation?
   (ii) Would your management be any different if the shingles was on Gerald's face?

Answers

1. A spinal injury at the level of L1 will leave a patient numb from the L1 level downwards (just below the umbilicus). There will be a spastic paraplegia, and the patient might be troubled by muscle spasms and contractures. He will require a catheter to permit good drainage of the bladder and will be prone to bladder infections.
2. (i) The numbness that Sarah describes is characteristic of a polyneuropathy. In view of the recent history of infection, postinfectious polyneuropathy (Guillain-Barré syndrome) is a possible diagnosis. Multiple sclerosis is another possible diagnosis, although it would be unusual for the numbness and weakness to be confined to the hands and the feet.
   (ii) You should refer Sarah to get a formal medical diagnosis, particularly in view of the fact that Guillain-Barré syndrome can be rapidly progressive in some cases.
3. (i) Gerald should be informed that his shingles is infectious and he should avoid contact with people who have not already had chickenpox. There is a risk that Gerald will suffer from severe pain following the shingles, particularly in view of his age. Although prompt treatment to clear Wind, Heat and Damp may well reduce the risk of this, it would be good practice to inform Gerald that the medical advice would be to take aciclovir to reduce the risk of long-term pain (although this is a suppressive approach). He then has the option of choosing to take this medication in addition to acupuncture.
   (ii) Facial shingles is often a more severe condition, and there is a risk of eye involvement, which can threaten sight in the long term. You should refer Gerald straightaway so that the extent of the problem can be diagnosed formally. In this case, he will almost certainly be offered a 5–7 day course of aciclovir.

The musculoskeletal system

4.2

Chapter 4.2a The physiology of the musculoskeletal system

LEARNING POINTS

At the end of this chapter you will be able to:

- describe the structure and function of the different types of bones
- describe the different types of joints and their functions
- describe how the skeletal muscles act to maintain posture and allow movement.

Estimated time for chapter: 120 minutes.

Introduction

The musculoskeletal system consists of the bony skeleton, the joints and the muscles. Its functions are to support the soft tissues of the body, to protect the deep organs and to enable the movements of the body. In addition, as described in Stage 3, the bones contain the marrow spaces in which most of the maturation of the blood cells takes place.

This chapter considers in turn the physiology of the bony skeleton, the joints and the muscles. It is assumed that the reader has a basic knowledge of the shape, position and names of the bones, joints and muscles.

The physiology of the bony skeleton

All bone consists of a combination of a hard, non-living substance containing salts of calcium and phosphorus together with a vast number of living bone cells. The non-living part of bone is structured upon a scaffolding of numerous connective-tissue fibres. It is this complex material that persists after death when the rest of the body has decayed. Nevertheless, in life, this seemingly fixed aspect of bone is constantly in a state of change, as the bone cells are always active in reshaping this hard material according to the needs of the body.

There are two main types of bone tissue. Compact bone is a dense, but very strong material present in all bones at their margins. Cancellous bone is more spongy and filled with red marrow, and is particularly rich in the shafts of the long bones and the ribs, the centre of the vertebral bodies and the core of the pelvic bones. In both types of bone a rich network of vessels supplies the bone cells, the osteocytes, with blood and lymph fluid.

The bony skeleton is made up of four different types of bones, categorised according to their shape: the long bones (e.g. the femur and the humerus), the irregular bones (e.g. the vertebrae and the carpal bones), the flat bones (e.g. the sternum and the skull) and the sesamoid bones (e.g. the patella and the pisiform bone). In terms of physiology, the important distinction to be made is between the long bones and the three other types of bone (irregular, flat and sesamoid) (see Q4.2a-1).

Long bones

The long bones (Figure 4.2a-I) in the body are the radius, ulna and humerus of the arm and the femur, tibia and fibula of the leg. They are characterised by a shaft and two widened ends known as 'epiphyses'. The shaft is composed of dense, strong compact bone, with a central hollow that is filled with fatty yellow bone marrow. The epiphyses are the site of bone growth in the child, and are largely composed of soft, spongy cancellous bone containing bloody red marrow, all bounded by a rim of strong compact bone. The epiphyses are covered with hyaline cartilage in the regions where they make joints with other bones; elsewhere the long bones are bounded by a fibrous coat called the 'periosteum'. Underneath the periosteum lie clusters of osteblasts and osteoclasts, the bone-forming cells that are responsible for bone remodelling and

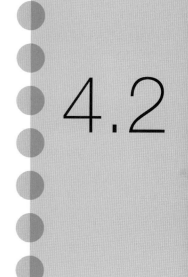

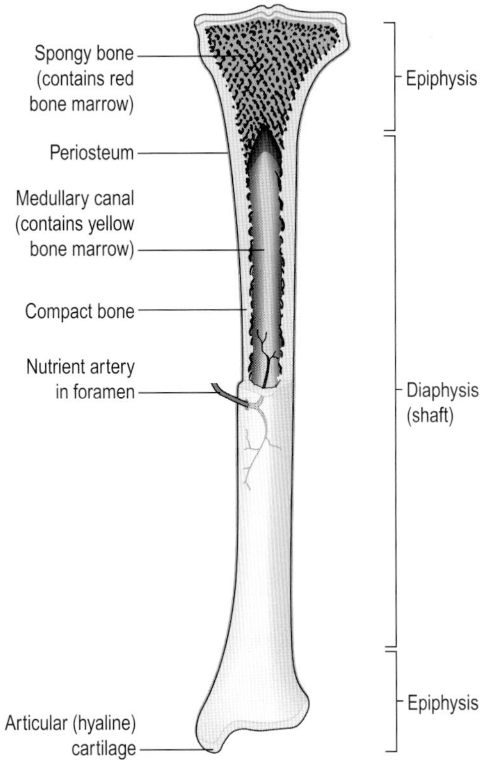

Figure 4.2a-I • The structure of a long bone (partially sectioned).

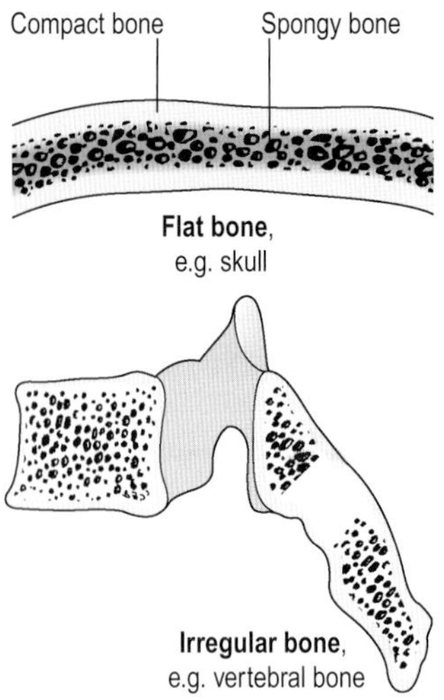

Figure 4.2a-II • The structure of flat and irregular bones (sectioned).

production. These cells are stimulated to form and reshape new bone when the periosteum or underlying bone becomes damaged. The design of the long bones confers strength, which is necessary for their main functions of locomotion, posture and manipulation.

Short, irregular, flat and sesamoid bones

The short bones are less strong than the long bones because they are composed largely of spongy, cancellous, red, marrow-containing bone, and are bounded by a relatively thin protective rim of compact bone. This structure (Figure 4.2a-II) supports their functions of intricate movements (in the back, hands and feet), protection (skull bones, pelvis and ribs) and bone marrow production (see Q4.2a-2).

The blood-forming marrow

It is the red marrow that is the site of the development of the blood cells. This marrow is abundant in the vertebrae and the flat bones of the skull, ribs, sternum and pelvis.

The growth of bone in childhood and adolescence

An understanding of how bones grow is relevant to the pathology of a number of the diseases of bone. In the fetus there is initially no hard bony material. Instead, at the future site of the long and irregular bones, soft cartilage, a form of connective tissue, appears. At the site of the flat bones a soft-tissue membrane develops. Gradually, as birth approaches, osteoblast cells within these areas of soft tissue secrete the hard substance that will form the non-living part of bone. This process of transformation of soft tissue into hard bone is called 'ossification'. When bone has ossified, some of the osteoblasts mature into the bone cells situated deep within bone, where they are known as 'osteocytes'.

This means that in the newborn only a small part of each of the bones is mature hard bone. For example, at the time of birth, only the centres of the skull bones have ossified. The edges of these flat bones are still thick membrane, which allows for some flexibility of movement between the skull bones (very important during childbirth). This soft membrane is most prominent in the diamond-shaped 'soft-spot' (the fontanelle) which can be felt on the top of the head of most babies under 1 year of age.

The bones do not fully ossify until early adulthood. Until then, there are still some areas of cartilage or membrane that are actively forming new bone and allowing for growth. Because of this, the approximate age of a child can be estimated from an X-ray image of the bones, which shows the state of progression of ossification of the bones. Puberty is a time during which the surge of sex hormones causes an initial spurt of growth of long bones followed by ossification of the growth centres in the long bones (see Chapter 5.2a). This is why growth slows considerably once puberty has been reached.

The continued growth of bones

After early adulthood the bones do not change significantly in size. Nevertheless, the osteoblasts remain active in secreting new bone. This laying down of new bone is counterbalanced by the activity of another type of bone cell called the 'osteoclast'. The osteoclasts act continually to digest old bone and to return the calcium, phosphorus and other nutrients within the bone back to the circulation for reuse. This process, known as ‘remodelling’, allows bones to become stronger in areas in which there is perpetual physical stress (e.g. the upper part of the femur in someone who is physically active) and allows for the repair of bones in the case of fracture.

The rate of remodelling of bone is influenced by various hormones of the endocrine system. The thyroid hormones, growth hormone from the pituitary gland and insulin from the pancreas stimulate the correct development and ossification of the bones. In puberty, testosterone and oestrogen stimulate the growth spurt, and also the changes that differentiate the male and the female adult skeletons. Oestrogen also helps to maintain the calcium content of bones in premenopausal women. In addition, two hormones secreted from the region of the thyroid gland, calcitonin and parathyroid hormone, are essential in the control of the balance of the activity of the osteoblasts and the osteoclasts.

Vitamin D is an essential factor in the maintenance of the non-living (calcified) part of bone. In vitamin D deficiency the bones become softened. This leads to bowing of the bones during childhood (rickets) and pain and weakness in adulthood (osteomalacia). These conditions are discussed in more detail in Chapter 4.2d.

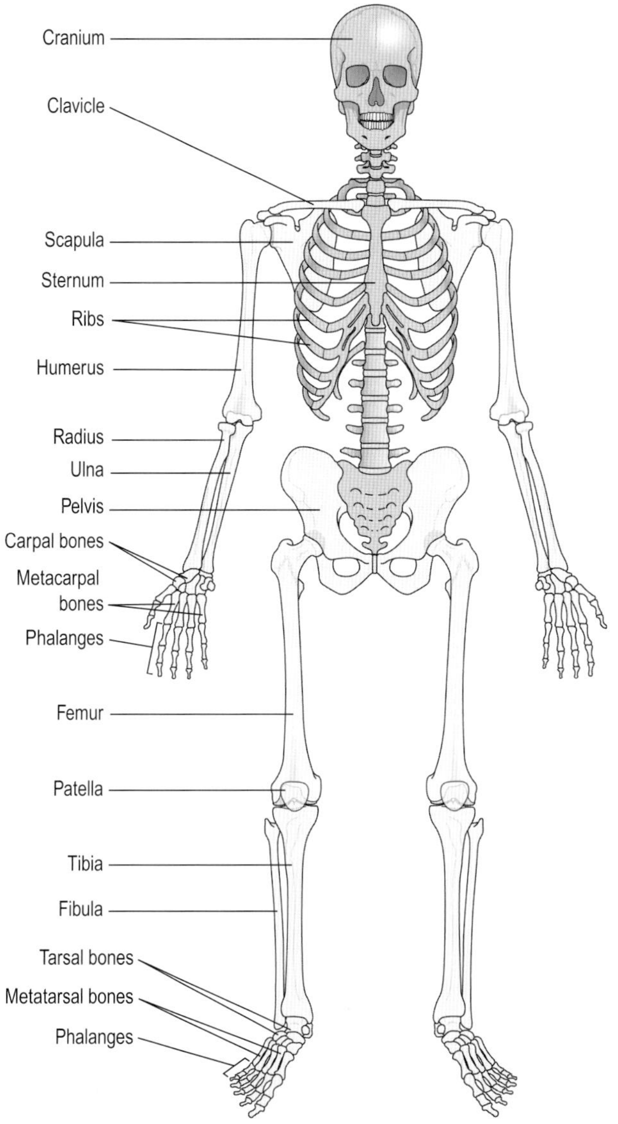

Figure 4.2a-III • The skeleton: anterior view (the bones of the axial skeleton are shaded).

The structure of the skeleton

The skeleton can be considered as consisting of two parts: the axial skeleton and the appendicular skeleton. The axial skeleton (shaded bones in Figure 4.2a-III) forms the central bony core of the body, and consists of the skull, vertebral bones, sacrum, coccyx, ribs and sternum. All these bones are either flat or irregular, and so each is composed of a core of red-marrow-containing cancellous bone surrounded by a thin rim of compact bone. The skull and the vertebral column support and protect the fragile structure of the brain and spinal cord. The ribs and sternum likewise support and protect the lungs and the heart in the thorax, and the organs of the upper abdomen, including the liver, kidneys, pancreas and the spleen.

The appendicular skeleton (unshaded bones in Figure 4.2a-III) is so called because it consists of the appendages to the axial skeleton. These are the shoulder girdle (clavicles and shoulder blades), the upper limbs, the pelvic girdle (the hip bones) and the lower limbs. The bones of the shoulder girdle and the pelvic girdle are flat bones. The bones of the limbs are either long bones or irregular bones.

The healing of bones

Healthy bones are strong and slightly flexible. In health, bones will only break if exposed to significant trauma. Fractures of healthy bone can be classified as simple, compound or greenstick. If a fracture occurs because the bone is weakened in some way by an underlying disease process, it is described as a ‘pathological fracture’.

A simple fracture describes when the ends of the bone do not protrude through the skin, whereas a compound fracture involves a break to the skin by the sharp end of the fractured bone. A greenstick fracture occurs in the flexible bones of young children. In this fracture, the break is incomplete, as the bone is far less brittle than the fully ossified adult bone. This means that the bone bends like a green stick, rather than snapping into two.

The healing of broken bones can be compared to the healing of wounds in that it is the formation of a blood clot in the space between the broken ends that initiates the healing process. Figure 4.2a-IV illustrates the stages in the healing of the broken shaft of a long bone. The blood clot stimulates the inward movement of phagocytes and osteoblasts. The phagocytes remove unwanted debris, while the osteoblasts lay down an initially chaotic mass of new bone called ‘callus’. The callus is gradually remodelled by osteoclasts into new, ordered compact bone. In adults this process takes weeks to months, but it is significantly quicker in children (see Q4.2a-3 and Q4.2a-4).

Information Box 4.2a-I

The bones: comments from a Chinese medicine perspective

In Chinese medicine, the bones and bone marrow have a relationship with two of the extraordinary Yang organs: the Bones and the Marrow.

The Marrow corresponds to the substance that nourishes and forms nervous tissue and the bone marrow, and which is produced by Kidney Essence. Therefore, if the Kidneys are deficient, the bone marrow will be weak.

The Bones correspond directly to the physiological bones. They are nourished by Kidney Essence and Marrow, and will also become weak if the Kidneys are deficient.

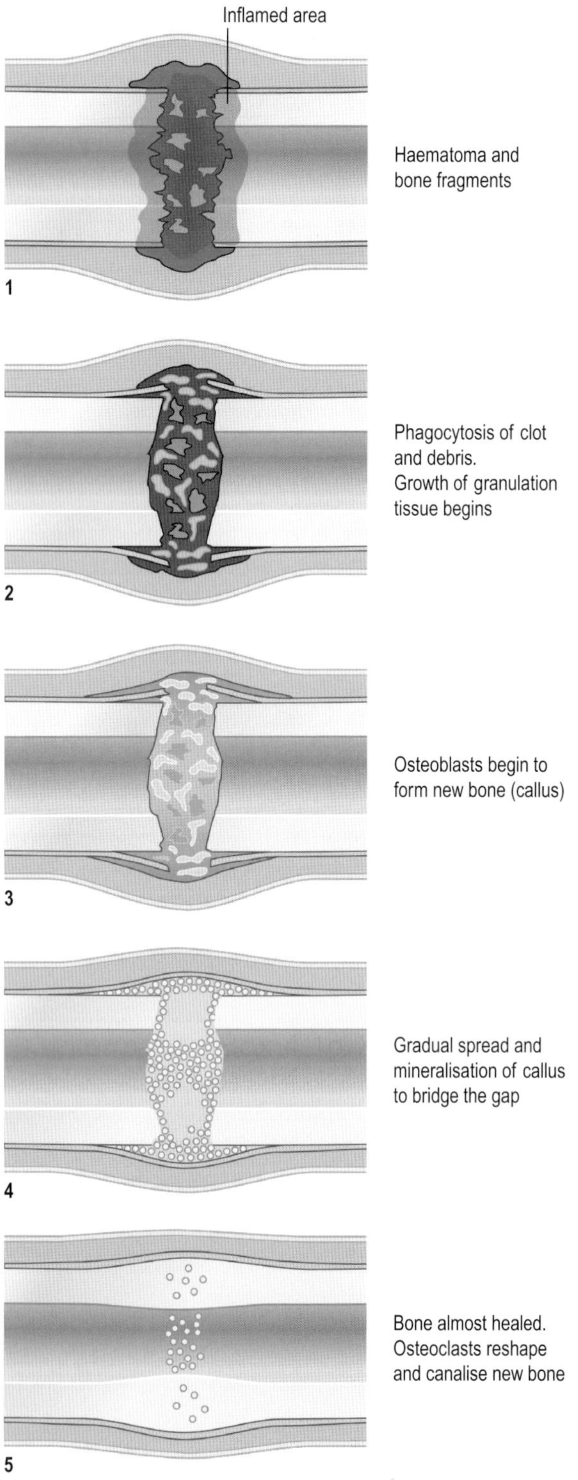
Inflamed area
Haematoma and bone fragments
1
Phagocytosis of clot and debris.
Growth of granulation tissue begins
2
Osteoblasts begin to form new bone (callus)
3
Gradual spread and mineralisation of callus to bridge the gap
4
Bone almost healed.
Osteoclasts reshape and canalise new bone
5

Figure 4.2a-IV • The stages in bone healing.

The physiology of the joints

The joints are the sites in the body at which two or more bones come together. They are essential for allowing free, but controlled, movement of the body (see Q4.2a-5).

There are three categories of joint in the body: the fixed or fibrous joints (e.g. the sutures of the skull), the slightly movable or cartilaginous joints (e.g. symphysis pubis and intervertebral joints) and the movable or synovial joints (e.g. the elbow, knee and ankle).

Fibrous joints involve two edges of bone that are linked by tough strands of fibrous connective tissue. The suture lines of the skull are an example of fibrous joints (Figure 4.2a-V). The movement at a fibrous joint is limited.

Cartilaginous joints offer the potential for more movement because the bones in these joints are linked by a pad of fibrocartilage, which has more spring and bulk than the fibrous strands of a fibrous joint. In the pubis symphysis and in between the vertebral bodies this fibrocartilage pad has a shock-absorbing function (Figure 4.2a-VI).

Synovial joints offer the most movement and have the most complex structure (Figure 4.2a-VII). The internal surface of the bones in synovial joints is lined with glassy smooth hyaline articular cartilage, and the rest of the joint space is bound by a fibrous joint capsule (the capsular ligament). The internal surface of the joint is lined with a fluid-secreting synovial membrane. The term 'synovial' has its root in the Greek word 'ovum' meaning egg. This is because the lubricating fluid contained within these joints has been likened in consistency to the white of an egg. The whole joint is given stability by means of fibrous bands (the ligaments) that link the bones and also by the muscle insertions (the tendons), which cross the joint to insert close to its margins.

Some of the synovial joints have unique additional features, for example the knee joint illustrated in Figure 4.2a-VII contains thickened C-shaped cartilage pads, which sit on the tibial plateau, and two cruciate (crossing) ligaments, which run through the joint space to provide anterior to posterior stability.

Close to the large joints such as the knee, hip and shoulder are fluid-filled sacs lined with synovial membrane called 'bursae' (singular 'bursa'). The purpose of a bursa is to prevent friction between the layers of tissue overlying the joint.

There are a wide range of structures of synovial joints, although all have the same basic features listed above. Diverse examples include the ball-and-socket joint of the hip, the hinge mechanism of the elbow, the pivot provided by the atlantoaxial

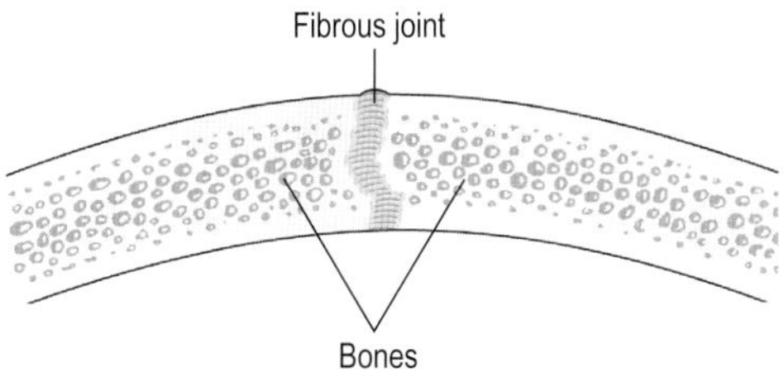

Figure 4.2a-V • An example of a fibrous joint: a suture line of the skull.

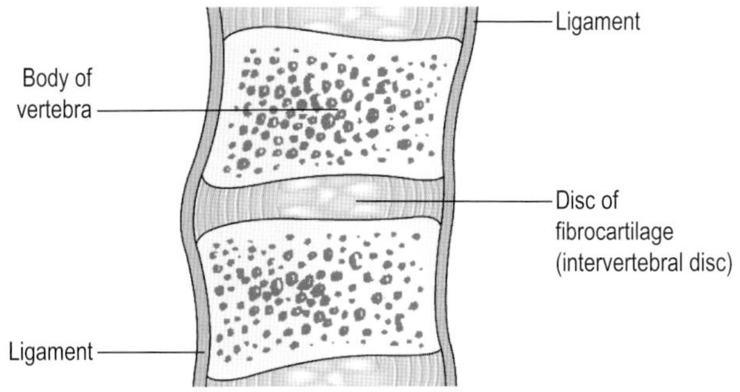

Figure 4.2a-VI • An example of a cartilaginous joint: the intervertebral joint.

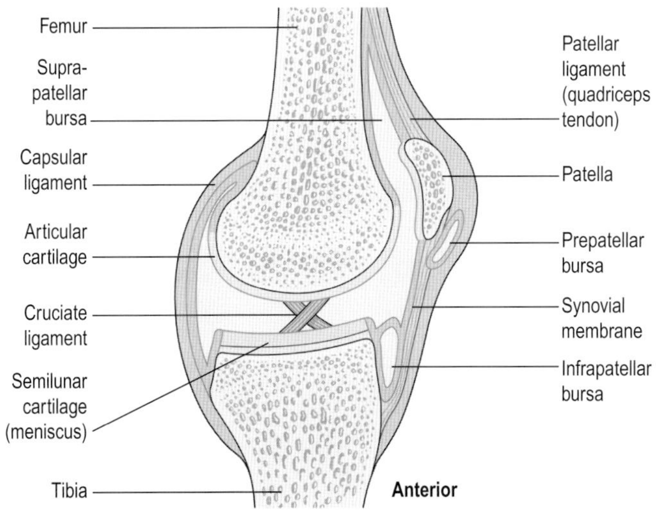

Figure 4.2a-VII • An example of a synovial joint: section of the knee joint viewed from the front.

Information Box 4.2a-II

The joints: comments from a Chinese medicine perspective

The physiological joints are made up of bone, ligaments and synovial fluid, further supported by muscles. In this way their health is dependent on Kidney Essence, Liver Qi and Blood, and Gallbladder Qi, all of which are said to have direct correspondences with these aspects.

The fluid that lubricates the joints in Chinese medicine is called Ye, and is under the control of the Spleen and the Kidneys.

joint (between the C1 and C2 vertebrae) and the complementary saddle shapes of many of the small bones of the hands and feet (see Q4.2a-6-Q4.2a-8).

The physiology of the skeletal muscles

The muscles that are responsible for the movement of the bony joints are all largely composed of skeletal muscle fibres (cells). The muscle fibres run parallel to one another within each muscle, and are bound together by fibrous connective tissue. The muscle fibres converge at two or more fibrous structures, called 'tendons', at the extremities of the muscle. Tendons usually insert into a part of the bony skeleton, but in some muscles they attach to the connective tissue of the skin (e.g. in the muscles of facial expression). The fibrous tissue of muscles (including the tendons) is glistening white and contains blood vessels and fat cells. This is the tissue that gives a raw steak its streaky appearance (see Q4.2a-9).

The muscle fibres contract in unison in response to motor nerve impulses (see Chapter 4.1a). Each muscle fibre receives electrical impulses from a nerve fibre via a specialised synapse called the 'motor end plate'. At this synapse, the electrical impulse travelling down the nerve fibre leads to the release of a neurotransmitter chemical. This chemical stimulates the changes within the muscle fibre that culminate in a temporary contraction. The contraction is sustained only for as long as the nerve continues to stimulate the motor end plate.

Muscles act because they are attached to at least two separate parts of the body, and because they can contract. When a muscle contracts, it draws the two or more parts of the body to which it is attached closer together, and this leads to movement.

Most skeletal muscles never attain a state of full relaxation. There is always a low level of nervous stimulation to the muscles, which gives them a firmness known as 'tone'. This background level of tone is essential for correct posture. It is generated as a result of reflex nervous activity at the level of the spinal cord, and is modified further by nervous impulses originating from higher control centres in the brain (see Chapter 4.1a). If the nerve supply to a muscle is cut off, the muscle becomes completely flaccid, and loses the springy quality that is the normal state in good health.

Muscles act in a variety of ways, of which the biceps brachii, the buccinator and the pelvic floor muscles are good examples. These three muscles have the diverse effects of limb movement, facial expression and support of soft tissues respectively. The biceps (brachii) muscle of the upper arm is an example of a muscle that acts over a synovial joint (the elbow). The biceps has two tendon insertions on the scapula at its proximal end and a single distal insertion into the radius. The flat buccinator muscle of the cheek is an example of a muscle that inserts only into the connective tissue of skin to allow for the movements of the mouth. The muscles of the pelvic floor insert into bone (they are slung between the ischium of the pelvis and the sacrum and coccyx), but do not cause movement at a joint. Instead, by contracting they give support to the tissues of the pelvic floor and are important for maintaining continence of faeces and urine.

Information Box 4.2a-III

The muscles: comments from a Chinese medicine perspective

The muscles are made up of flesh, tendons and sinews. Their health is dependent on healthy Spleen, Liver and Gallbladder Qi.

Spleen Qi is more responsible for the springy fleshy quality resulting from healthy muscle tone, whereas Liver and Gallbladder Qi are responsible for the power of contraction and the movement that results.

The knots and excessive tone often felt in overtense muscles are usually a reflection of Liver Qi (and Blood) Stagnation. This, in turn, is more likely to occur in muscles that are weak as a result of Spleen Qi Deficiency.

Information Box 4.2a-IV

The musculoskeletal system: comments from a Chinese medicine perspective

In summary, a healthy musculoskeletal system is dependent on the health of the Kidney, Liver, Gallbladder and Spleen Organs. Kidney Essence is of particular importance to the bones. Healthy Blood and Yin are important for lubricating and nourishing the muscles and joints, as well as for preventing Stagnation of Qi. Hence, muscle and joint pains, stiffness or inflamed tendons can result if Blood and Yin, in particular of the Liver, are deficient.

Self-test 4.2a

The physiology of the musculoskeletal system

1. Why do you think it is that long bones are mostly made of compact bone, whereas the other types of bone are mostly composed of cancellous bone?
2. How is synovial fluid made? What is its purpose?
3. Why is it that our muscles can never be fully relaxed?

Answers

1. The long bones need to be strong because they have to withstand recurrent stress from lifting and weight bearing. Compact bone is a tissue that provides strength in the direction required. Strength is less important in the other bones. In the other bones (irregular, flat and sesamoid), cancellous bone minimises the weight of the bone and provides a site for the manufacture of the blood cells.
2. Synovial fluid is made by the cells of the synovial lining that covers the ends of the bones and the lining of the capsular ligament on the inside of the joint space. The fluid provides lubrication for the joint, contains immune cells, and also allows the passage of nutrients to the cartilage that covers the bony ends within the joint.
3. The muscles of the body are never in a state of full relaxation, even in sleep, because there is always a 'background' level of nervous stimulation of the muscles, which gives each muscle its tone. Without tone the muscles would become flaccid.

Chapter 4.2b The investigation of the musculoskeletal system

LEARNING POINTS

At the end of this chapter you will:

- be able to recognise the main investigations used for diseases of the musculoskeletal system
- understand what a patient might experience when undergoing these investigations.

Estimated time for chapter: 30 minutes.

Introduction

Diseases of the bones, joints and muscles are investigated within two distinct conventional specialities. Diseases that are likely to require medical treatment with drugs are referred to a physician known as a rheumatologist, while those conditions that are likely to require surgery are referred to an orthopaedic surgeon.

An investigation of the musculoskeletal system might involve:

- a thorough physical examination
- investigations to examine the structure of the bones, muscles and joints (X-ray imaging, ultrasound imaging, magnetic resonance imaging (MRI) and bone scans)
- examination of the blood to look for disturbances in the hormones and chemicals that reflect bone disorders and autoimmune diseases
- examination of the synovial fluid of a joint
- arthroscopy, the endoscopic examination of the interior of a joint.

These investigations are considered briefly in turn below.

Physical examination

The physical examination is a very important aspect of the examination of the musculoskeletal system. A skilled examiner can identify the site and nature of a wide range of musculoskeletal problems without the need for further investigations. For each joint and muscle group there is a range of specific physical tests that can be performed to examine for particular disorders. For example, the FABER (flexion, abduction and external rotation) test is used to examine for a painful disorder of the hip joint.

The physical examination of the musculoskeletal system involves the stages listed in Table 4.2b-I.

X-ray imaging

X-ray imaging is the most common investigation performed for musculoskeletal disease. This is because it is relatively cheap, quick to perform, and often produces an excellent picture of the bony structure of the body. The disadvantage of X-ray imaging is that it exposes the patient to radiation, although this

Table 4.2b-I The stages in the physical examination of the musculoskeletal system

- *Examination of the gait, posture and general appearance*: this can reveal the characteristic features of musculoskeletal disease, such as a characteristic limp, areas of one-sided muscle wasting or postural deformity due to arthritis
- *Examination of the muscle groups*: looking specifically for areas of wasting or fine twitching, feeling for knots or swellings, and assessing the strength of the muscle groups
- *Examination of the bones*: looking specifically for areas of deformity or shortening, feeling for deformity, swellings or areas of tenderness, and percussion of the bones to examine for deep tenderness
- *Examination of the joints*: looking specifically for redness, swelling and deformity, feeling for heat and tenderness, and passively moving a joint to assess range of movement and the strength of the muscles that cause movement of the joint (active movement). In the case of a localised joint problem, the joint is examined using a range of specific tests

is considered to be of minimal risk if X-ray imaging is only required on rare occasions during the lifetime of a patient.

However, X-ray images cannot reveal much information about muscle problems, and will only reveal changes of arthritis at a late stage in the condition, when the bony surfaces of the joint have become eroded. For this reason, the general medical view is that X-ray images are not helpful in the diagnosis of most cases of low back pain, which are usually the result of muscle strain, prolapsed disc or early arthritis, none of which are revealed on an X-ray image.

Ultrasound scan

This can be a useful and non-invasive test for the examination of a joint and the soft tissues that surround it. It is of particular value in the examination of the shoulder.

Magnetic resonance imaging (MRI)

MRI provides very high-quality information about joints and muscles, and reveals the structure of the low back in detail. However, it is expensive and can be uncomfortable for the patient to experience.

Bone scans

Bone scans involve the injection of a radioactive substance into the bloodstream. This substance is concentrated in areas of bone in which there is active growth, which are then revealed by scanning the body for radioactivity. This is useful for revealing areas where there may be a fracture or the site of bone cancer.

A DXA scan is a specialised form of X-ray imaging used to investigate the condition of osteoporosis. This form of bone scan does not necessitate injection of a radioactive substance. Instead, it uses a low-dose of X-rays to assess the degree of osteoporosis. The DXA scan is most usually performed in menopausal women and other people at risk of osteoporosis to assess need for medical treatment for this condition.

Blood tests

There are numerous blood tests that can give some information about certain diseases of the musculoskeletal system. A serum sample can give information about the levels of the mineral salts of calcium and phosphorus in the blood, as well as whether or not levels of hormones such as parathyroid hormone and calcitonin are within the normal range.

The erythrocyte sedimentation rate (ESR) and C reactive protein (CRP) tests can indicate whether an inflammatory process is going on. There is a range of autoantibodies that can be assayed from a serum sample if an autoimmune disease is suspected. In the case of a chronic autoimmune disease, such as rheumatoid arthritis, a full blood count (FBC) may reveal anaemia of chronic disease.

Examination of the synovial fluid of a joint

Synovial fluid may be withdrawn from a joint by means of a needle and syringe for examination in the case of arthritis. If the joint is very swollen with fluid, this simple procedure may also give the patient relief from discomfort. In some cases, after withdrawal of the fluid, a corticosteroid drug may be injected directly into the joint through the same needle.

The fluid may reveal the microorganisms and pus characteristic of infection, and so can be a guide for appropriate antibiotic treatment. In the case of arthritis due to simple inflammation (e.g. autoimmune disease or osteoarthritis) the fluid will be clear. In gout the fluid will contain the microscopic crystals that are the cause of the pain.

There is a small risk of introducing infection into the joint with this procedure.

Arthroscopy

Arthroscopy is a procedure that enables the examination of the interior of a joint, usually the knee. It involves the insertion of a fine endoscope into the joint space via a small incision in the skin overlying the joint. A general anaesthetic is usually given. In this way, the integrity of the joint cartilage and any other structures, such as ligaments within the joint, can be examined. In some cases, surgery to the damaged structures within the joint (e.g. a tear in the cartilage within the knee) may be carried out at the same time.

Even if no surgery is carried out, many people report that chronic knee pain is relieved (usually temporarily) following arthroscopy.

Self-test 4.2b

The investigation of the musculoskeletal system

1. A 35-year-old female patient is referred to a rheumatologist because she has developed a painful condition of the joints in which a number of the joints (wrists, elbows, hips and knees) are swollen and warm. One knee in particular is very swollen with fluid. The patient is unwell and slightly feverish, and the joints feel very stiff in the mornings. The GP suspects rheumatoid arthritis. What investigations do you think this patient might have to undergo?
2. Faith is 55 years old. She has pain in the centre of her back. The GP suspects osteoporosis and is considering prescribing treatment to help prevent fractures. What investigations do you think the GP might perform?

Answers

1. The patient will be given a thorough physical examination in which the swollen joints are assessed and any joint deformities noted.

   Blood tests will be ordered to examine for autoantibodies and anaemia in particular. A serum sample may also reveal some features suggestive of gout, which can also rarely give rise to a painful arthritis such as in this case.

   X-ray images of the joints will be requested, although these may be normal at an early stage of an inflammatory arthritis. Nevertheless, they will be useful as a baseline against which to compare any future X-ray images should the condition progress. Other imaging tests are not likely to be helpful in this case.

   Fluid may be withdrawn from the swollen knee joint to exclude the presence of infection or crystals, and to provide the patient with some relief from discomfort.

   An arthroscopy would be unnecessary in this case.
2. Faith may undergo X-ray imaging of the painful part of her back. This might reveal the 'thinning' of the bones, which is characteristic of osteoporosis, and might also show if any of the vertebrae have become compressed as a result of the condition.

   Blood tests might be performed to check that the mineral salts and hormones are within the normal range, which they should be in simple osteoporosis.

   The other imaging test that can be useful is the DXA scan, which uses low-dose X-rays to assess the degree of osteoporosis in different parts of the body. This too can be used as a baseline against which progression of the condition and response to treatment can be assessed.

   Examination of joint fluid and arthroscopy are not relevant to this case.

Chapter 4.2c The treatment of musculoskeletal pain

LEARNING POINTS

At the end of this chapter you will:

- be able to describe the mode of action of the simple analgesics, the non-steroidal anti-inflammatory drugs and the opioid analgesics
- understand the principles of treatment with analgesics
- be able to describe how muscle relaxants and corticosteroid preparations may be used to relieve musculoskeletal pain
- be able to describe the use of non-drug methods of pain relief in conventional medicine.

Estimated time for chapter: 60 minutes.

Introduction

This chapter explores the way in which conventional medicine manages the problem of pain due to musculoskeletal disease. The approach to musculoskeletal pain can be broadly categorised into disease modification and symptom relief.

Disease modification involves the use of medication which actually alters the progression of the underlying disease. Because the disease has been slowed or halted, symptoms abate. The disease-modifying treatments are described in the next three chapters on diseases of the musculoskeletal system because they vary according to the disease being treated.

Symptom relief involves the use of medication or other therapies to block the sensation of pain. It does not attempt to alter the underlying disease process. Almost by definition, symptom relief is suppressive in nature. The most common form of symptom relief in musculoskeletal pain is the use of painkillers. The medical term for a painkiller medication is an 'analgesic'.

Analgesics in musculoskeletal disease

Musculoskeletal disease is the most common reason for the prescription of analgesics. Analgesics are also used for a wide range of other conditions, including headache, menstrual pain and the pain of cancer. The analgesics used can be broadly categorised into simple analgesics, non-steroidal anti-inflammatory drugs (NSAIDs) and opioid (morphine-like) analgesics. These might be prescribed on their own or in combination with each other. There are, in fact, many analgesic preparations that contain a combination of two drugs that are believed to complement each other in their mode of action (e.g. co-codamol and co-dydramol, which combine paracetamol with codeine and dihydrocodeine, respectively). Other compound analgesics incorporate non-analgesic drugs such as caffeine or decongestant medication.

A vast range of analgesics is available for direct sale to the public. Many of these are compound preparations. These are listed at the end of Section 4.71 of the *British National Formulary*.

Simple analgesics

The simple analgesics are aspirin and paracetamol. Aspirin is anti-inflammatory in action, which means that it inhibits the chemical communication between the leukocytes that maintain the process of inflammation. Therefore, aspirin acts to reduce the heat (fever), redness, pain and swelling that are characteristic of inflammation. Paracetamol has a poorly understood mechanism of action. It is believed not to be anti-inflammatory. However, its effect is similar to that of aspirin in that it can reduce pain and fever.

Aspirin also reduces the tendency of platelets to stick together. This is why it is of value in the prevention of thrombosis and embolism. For this effect, a very low dose (75 mg) is required daily. The analgesic dose is much higher (up to 600 mg four times a day).

Aspirin tends to irritate the lining of the digestive tract, although in most cases this effect is mild and painless. However, in some people this can result in severe inflammation, with bleeding into the stomach (gastritis). Other side-effects include asthma and rashes. In children under the age of 12 years there is a very small risk of a severe form of inflammation of the liver called Reye's syndrome.

Paracetamol has few side-effects in low doses, but in overdose it is highly toxic to the liver.

Simple analgesics are recommended for mild pain. Aspirin should not be given to children, and ideally should not be taken at analgesic doses for a long-standing (chronic) condition because of the risk of stomach irritation.

Information Box 4.2c-I

Simple analgesics: comments from a Chinese medicine perspective

In Chinese medicine, the reduction in pain from the simple analgesics corresponds to Movement of Stagnation and Clearance of Heat. In pain relief the action is suppressive in nature, as it clears the symptom locally without necessarily addressing the underlying cause.

Aspirin is believed to be generally Warming and Dispersing in nature. In some cases it may enable the clearing of Wind Cold by causing sweating and the Release of the Exterior. The Warm nature is evidenced by the side-effect of Heat in the Stomach. Asthma and rashes suggest that, in some people, aspirin may also depress Lung Qi and permit Wind Heat Invasion.

In high doses, the liver toxicity described in conventional medicine strongly suggests that paracetamol stagnates and damages the Liver Qi from a Chinese medicine viewpoint.

Non-steroidal anti-inflammatory drugs (NSAIDs)

The NSAIDs are a family of drugs that have an anti-inflammatory effect similar to that of aspirin. Like aspirin they can reduce pain, fever, redness and swelling, and they also have side-effects which include gastric irritation, asthma and rashes.

Commonly prescribed NSAIDs include ibuprofen and diclofenac.

NSAIDs generally have a more powerful effect than aspirin, and are particularly useful in any pain that has inflammation as its root cause. Therefore they are useful in the inflammatory conditions of the musculoskeletal system such as arthritis, tendon and ligament injuries, and most bony pain, including fractures. NSAIDs at maximum dose can be safely used in combination with paracetamol or with opioid analgesics to increase the effect of pain relief.

The side-effect of gastric irritation is less marked than for aspirin. Nevertheless, it is recommended that NSAIDs are taken with food. However, NSAIDs can also be toxic to the kidneys in susceptible people, particularly if taken at a high dose for a prolonged period. For this reason they should be used with caution in the elderly or in combination with other medication that may affect the kidney function.

The cyclo-oxygenase-2 NSAIDs (etoricoxib and celecoxib), which are selective inhibitors, were developed to minimise the risk of upper gastrointestinal bleeding, and short-term data suggest that they do indeed carry a low risk of bleeding events in clinical practice. However, there does seem to be an association between these cox-2 inhibitors and adverse thrombotic cardiac events, and so their use is reserved only for those situations when older generation NSAIDs cannot be used and risk of cardiovascular disease is low.

For reasons that are unclear, the response in terms of pain relief of an individual to different NSAIDs is unpredictable. For this reason a number of these drugs may be tried in succession before the best effect is found.

Information Box 4.2c-II

Non-steroidal anti-inflammatory drugs: comments from a Chinese medicine perspective

In Chinese medicine, the energetic action of NSAIDs is similar to that of aspirin. In the long term, the warming nature of these drugs may deplete Blood and Yin, primarily of the Liver and Kidney.

Opioid analgesics

This range of painkillers is so called because their action is similar to that of the naturally occurring drug opium. They all appear to mimic the effect of the body's natural painkillers, the endorphins, and act within the spinal cord and the brain to reduce the sensation of pain.

The opioid analgesics provide strong pain relief, although they do not reduce inflammation directly. They are generally only used in musculoskeletal conditions when pain is very severe (e.g. after acute trauma such as a fracture). They may safely be used in combination with aspirin, paracetamol or the NSAIDs. The opioid analgesics include codeine, morphine, buprenorphine, diamorphine (heroin), dihydrocodeine, pethidine and tramadol.

The opioids are highly addictive, and also induce bodily tolerance to the effects of the drug. This means that, with recurrent use, increasing doses may be required to maintain a steady level of pain relief. They may induce a sense of euphoria or well-being.

The most common adverse side-effect is nausea and vomiting. This means that an anti-sickness medication may have to be prescribed at the same time. Constipation is also a common side-effect. With very high doses the depth of breathing may be inhibited, and the patient may fall into a stupor. In overdose, death may result from respiratory failure.

Information Box 4.2c-III

The opioids: comments from a Chinese medicine perspective

In Chinese medicine, the pain-relieving effect of the opioids seems to correspond to the Movement of Stagnation. This effect is suppressive in nature. The side-effects of euphoria and stupor may reflect the effect of Heat (at the Blood Level) on the Heart Organ. Constipation is also a result of Heat, in this case in the Small and Large Intestine. Suppression of respiration may reflect a depression of Lung and Kidney Qi. Nausea and vomiting might be seen as a manifestation of rebellion of Stomach Qi.

Other drugs used for symptom relief in musculoskeletal disease

The two other classes of drugs that are used for symptom relief in musculoskeletal disease are the muscle relaxants and the corticosteroids.

Muscle relaxants

An important drug used to relax tense muscles in musculoskeletal conditions is diazepam. This drug is most commonly prescribed for its effect in calming anxiety in minor mental illness (see Section 6.2).

In certain painful conditions of the joints and muscles, in particular low back pain, reflex muscle spasm can worsen the underlying pain and may slow healing by making the whole area surrounding the injury rigid. In cases such as these, diazepam may be prescribed for a short period (ideally a few days at the most) to relieve the pain and tension caused by the muscle spasm.

The side-effects of diazepam include drowsiness and unsteadiness of gait, but these are not usually problematic in short-term use for an acute musculoskeletal problem. Diazepam is also highly addictive, but again this should not be a problem when used in the short term.

Information Box 4.2c-IV

Diazepam: comments from a Chinese medicine perspective

From a Chinese medicine perspective, the calming and slowing effect of diazepam could correlate with a Cooling effect, and thus a depression of Yang, in particular of the Heart. Side-effects of drowsiness and unsteadiness indicate that in excess it might be seen as Phlegm Forming.

Corticosteroids

Corticosteroids may be used for their disease-modifying properties in the forms of arthritis that result from autoimmune disease (e.g. rheumatoid arthritis). In this case they are given regularly by mouth to calm the underlying inflammatory process.

Corticosteroids may also be administered by injection to reduce local inflammation in a wide range of musculoskeletal conditions. The injection can be directed into a joint in cases of arthritis, or around a tendon in cases of tendonitis (e.g. tennis elbow). The injection may bring about a rapid relief in the symptoms of inflammation, and can be relatively long acting (days to weeks).

The side-effects are mostly a consequence of the locally high concentration of steroid in the tissues. They include wasting of the tissues below the skin (fat atrophy) and, in rare cases, weakening of the connective tissue of the tendons themselves. Occasionally, tendons may rupture as a result. The anti-inflammatory properties of steroids may promote the development of infection (unchecked by the immune system), which can have disastrous effects within a joint.

Information Box 4.2c-V

Corticosteroid injections: comments from a Chinese medicine perspective

The effects of corticosteroid injections might be interpreted as Clearing of Heat by Moving of Stagnation. These effects are suppressive. Other side-effects (e.g. irritation of the stomach lining) suggest that corticosteroids are actually Heating in nature. Fat atrophy and wasting of tendons could be a manifestation of depletion of Yin and Qi of the tissues.

Non-drug methods of pain relief in musculoskeletal disease

Many patients with chronic musculoskeletal disease are referred to an orthopaedic physiotherapist who may use one or more of the following approaches to relieve pain. Unfortunately, because of the time-consuming nature of many of these therapies, they are not always available free of charge within the UK National Health Service (NHS).

Advice and training on posture and physical exercises

This is very commonly offered, as it is considered a therapy that can help patients to help themselves. Usually, a few appointments are offered to teach the patient some basic exercises to help strengthen muscles or stretch out tense areas. It is probably true that if all patients could stick to an allotted exercise regimen much discomfort from muscular and arthritic problems would be relieved. Unfortunately, many people are not able to generate the commitment required for a regular exercise and posture routine, particularly if little long-term follow-up of their progress is arranged.

Manipulation and massage

Some physiotherapists are skilled in the manipulation of joints and massage of tense muscles. These therapies can relieve muscle spasm, but may need to be repeated to be of long-term benefit. Heat and ice packs may also be used to relieve pain and swelling.

Information Box 4.2c-VI

Exercises, massage and manipulation: comments from a Chinese medicine perspective

The Chinese medicine interpretation of attention to appropriate exercise and correction of posture is that it helps to move Stagnant Qi and benefits the Kidneys. This is an energetically appropriate treatment, as long as it is not too strenuous.

Massage and manipulation would be seen as moving Stagnant Qi and Blood. If an underlying imbalance is not attended to, this form of therapy can be suppressive in nature, dissipating a symptom without addressing the underlying cause.

Ultrasound, TENS and local acupuncture

These three approaches are used by physiotherapists to relieve the pain in localised musculoskeletal problems. Ultrasound therapy involves focusing ultrasound waves so that they are concentrated at the site of the injury. TENS (transcutaneous electrical nerve stimulation) involves the passage of a low-voltage electrical current across the affected area of the body via electrode pads fixed to the skin. The acupuncture offered in the NHS often involves the use of local and tender (Ah-shi) points.

The mechanism of all three approaches is not clearly understood in conventional terms, although there is a belief that all have a similar action in stimulating suppressive neurotransmitters (including endorphins) within the spinal cord and the brain.

Information Box 4.2c-IX

Ultrasound, TENS and local acupuncture: comments from a Chinese medicine perspective

In Chinese medicine, all three of these treatments will move Blood and Qi Stagnation and may enable the Clearance of Pathogenic Factors. However, if the underlying imbalance is not attended to, all three may be suppressive in action.

Anaesthetic and surgical approaches to pain relief

In some cases of severe intractable pain, specialised procedures can be performed to reduce the sensation of pain. These involve the deadening or destroying of nerves or nerves roots within the peripheral nervous system. These procedures are carried out by anaesthetists or surgeons. It is extremely rare for these procedures to be necessary in musculoskeletal pain, although they may be used in cases of severe chronic low back pain.

Self-test 4.2c

The treatment of musculoskeletal pain

1. A 60-year-old patient is taking three 200 mg tablets of ibuprofen a day for a constant pain in both hips. This pain has been diagnosed as early osteoarthritis. Because she gets slight indigestion if she takes any more tablets than this, her GP recommends that she also takes up to 4000 mg/day of paracetamol to relieve her pain. She finds she often needs to take all these tablets. Do you think that this approach to symptom relief is a reasonable one in conventional terms?
2. A 27-year-old gardener has suffered a sudden onset of back pain while digging. He is in so much pain that he is unable to drive himself home, and finds that his only relief is to lie flat on the floor. The GP examines him on a home visit and finds excessive muscle spasm in the lumbar area. Flexion of the hip joint induces pain on the left-hand side which radiates into the buttock and down the back of the leg (sciatica).
   (i) What medication do you think the GP might prescribe?
   (ii) Assuming that the condition is much better 5 days later, but is still very tense and painful, what other additional treatment approaches might the GP consider?

Answers

1. The GP has prescribed reasonably in conventional medicine terms. Ibuprofen is the best choice for arthritis, as long as the patient can tolerate its side-effects. In the short term, maximum-dose paracetamol is considered relatively safe, and may complement the action of the ibuprofen.
   Nevertheless, both these treatments are suppressive, and in the long term may be causing increasing energetic imbalance. This issue is not really accepted in conventional medicine, although serious adverse effects such as gastritis and kidney damage are, of course, recognised as rare complications of this treatment.
2. (i) If the pain is very severe the GP might consider giving a single dose of an opiate mediation by injection, but this would be unusual. The most usual approach would be to offer a regular dose of a NSAID, with the option of a combined paracetamol and opiate preparation (e.g. co-codamol). In addition, diazepam might be prescribed for a few days to relax the muscle spasm. Current advice is for the patient to continue to move the back gently as soon as possible (mobilisation rather than bed rest; see Chapter 4.2f).
   (ii) If the patient is improving but pain and spasm are persisting, the GP might consider referral to a physiotherapist so that the patient can be taught some back and postural exercises. The physiotherapist might also choose to offer additional therapies such as massage, TENS and acupuncture, according to his or her interest, training and the time available. If the problem persists the GP might decide to refer the patient to an orthopaedic surgeon for further investigation of the back pain (see Chapter 4.2e).

Chapter 4.2d The diseases of the bones

LEARNING POINTS

At the end of this chapter you will:

- be able to name the main features of the most important diseases of the bones
- understand the principles of treatment of a few of the most common diseases
- be able to recognise the red flags of the diseases of the bones.

Estimated time for chapter: 120 minutes.

Introduction

This chapter is concerned with the important diseases that affect the bones. The diseases of the bone marrow have already been summarised in Chapter 3.4e. The conditions studied in this chapter are:

- Generalised disorders of the formation of bone (see Q4.2d-1):
  - osteoporosis
  - Paget's disease.
- Rickets and osteomalacia (vitamin D deficiency).
- Inherited or childhood bone disorders:
  - achondroplasia
  - brittle bone disease.
- Infection of the bones:
  - osteomyelitis.
- Tumours of the bone:
  - benign tumours
  - malignant osteosarcoma.
- Metastatic disease of the bone:
  - myeloma.

Generalised disorders of the formation of bone

Osteoporosis

'Osteoporosis' is a term used to describe a condition in which the actual amount of bony material within the bones is decreased, meaning that there are more spaces within the bone tissue. This has the effect of weakening the bones, and the bones look pale on an X-ray image. In laymen's terms, the bones in osteoporosis are 'thin'. In conventional medical terminology the term 'low bone density' means the same thing.

The solidity or density of bone normally rapidly increases as a response to the hormone surge of puberty. At this time the bones in a healthy adolescent become more heavy and resistant to fracture. From the age of about 40 years onwards there is a progressive natural decline in this density of bone. This decline is called 'bone loss'. In men the bone loss continues gradually into old age. In some women the rate of bone loss increases very rapidly at the menopause, when the natural levels of oestrogen suddenly drop, and bone density can suddenly become significantly reduced over a relatively short period of a few years.

Certain factors reduce the rate of bone loss. These include a healthy vitamin- and calcium-rich diet and a moderate level of physical activity from childhood. Weight-bearing physical activity (e.g. walking and running rather than swimming) is known to be particularly important in the maintenance of good bone density.

Factors that increase the rate of bone loss include a poor diet, physical inactivity, reduced levels of oestrogen in women (including early menopause), smoking and chronic diseases. The amenorrhoea that affects some women athletes and women with anorexia will lead to thinned bones if prolonged. It follows that excessive physical activity may not necessarily be so beneficial to the bones in women. Numerous pregnancies and prolonged periods of breastfeeding will also deplete calcium reserves in the bone. It is now known that it is very significant if any of these factors are present in adolescence, as the bones will then never achieve the optimum starting point of bone density after the growth spurt. This is of concern in westernised countries today in which adolescents tend to live an increasingly sedentary existence and eat a highly processed diet. In addition, particularly in girls, eating disorders are increasingly prevalent in younger age groups.

Osteoporosis is of enormous health concern in developed countries, in which there is an increasing proportion of the population who are elderly. Osteoporotic hip fractures will affect 15% of all women and 5% of men from the age of 60 years. A hip fracture can have disastrous consequences in an elderly person. A high percentage of people who suffer from these fractures either die as a direct result of the injury or complications of the fracture, or suffer from long-term disability.

The symptoms of osteoporosis can be broadly categorised according to the age and sex of the patient, although there is much overlap between the categories.

In some postmenopausal women a very rapid decline in cancellous bone mass causes the vertebrae in the cervical and thoracic spine to thin very quickly. These spongy bones are then at risk of collapsing under the weight of the head and upper body. This form of 'crush fracture' can be very painful and will lead to progressive bowing forward of the upper back. In extreme cases, a so-called 'dowager's hump' results. In addition, there is particular thinning of the distal end of the radius, which means that a fall onto the outstretched hand may lead to a fracture of the wrist (Colles' fracture).

In more elderly people (over the age of 70 years) the strength of the compact bone of the long bones is more gradually reduced, and it is at this stage that hip fracture becomes more common. The vertebrae of the spine also soften and compress down, but because the bone loss is less abrupt, sudden painful crush fractures are less common.

The ideal approach to the management of osteoporosis is prevention. Ideally, this begins in adolescence with a calcium-rich diet and regular moderate weight-bearing exercise. Women, in particular, should also be encouraged to keep up a calcium-rich diet, particularly when breastfeeding. All people should keep up a steady level of activity throughout adult life in order to minimise the rate of bone loss.

Osteoporosis can be graded in severity by means of a DXA scan, in which bone density of the lumbar spine and hip are assessed. The results are expressed in the form of a 'T score', in which a negative value suggests lower than predicted bone density for a young healthy adult. A T score below –1 would lead a doctor to consider preventive medical treatment.

Hormone replacement therapy (HRT) used to be a widely prescribed preventive treatment for osteoporosis in perimenopausal and postmenopausal women. However, recent clinical research following large groups of women on HRT has prompted the UK Committee on the Safety of Medicines (CSM) to advise that HRT is no longer recommended as a principal ("first-line) treatment. This guidance has come in the light of an established link between HRT and an increased risk of breast cancer, ovarian cancer and endometrial cancer. The clinical studies also demonstrated that HRT has a less protective effect against the development of coronary heart disease than was previously believed.

The bisphosphonates form a class of drugs that is increasingly used in established early osteoporosis. These drugs prevent the action of the osteoclasts in breaking down bone, and do seem to slow bone loss, and reduce the fracture rate. Alendronate and clodronate are two types of bisphosphonate in common use. Nausea and oesophagitis are unwelcome common side-effects. These drugs may be prescribed together with calcium and vitamin D.

Calcium and vitamin D in a low-dose preparation may be prescribed together as a preventive treatment in elderly people. This treatment, which is less well supported by evidence of benefit than the biphosphonates, should be unnecessary if dietary intake is adequate, but a poor diet and poor absorption may work together in old age to reduce intake of calcium.

A late preventive measure is to prevent the occurrence of falls in the elderly. Exercise programmes can improve muscle strength and improve balance, and therefore may prevent falls. Regular Tai Chi classes are one of the active measures that have been shown in experimental studies to reduce the incidence of falls in elderly people.

Paget's disease

Paget's disease is a disease of the ageing bones that affects up to 10% of adults by the age of 90 years. In this condition the process of bone remodelling is imbalanced, with both excessive absorption of old bone (by osteoclasts) and excessive formation of new bone (by osteoblasts) taking place.

The affected areas of bone may become enlarged and irregular, but the bones are actually structurally weak and more prone to fracture. An increased blood supply causes the affected bone to feel warmer than other parts of the body. Most patients with Paget's disease have no symptoms, although some bony deformities may be apparent such as bowed shin bones (Figure 4.2d-I) or an enlarged and irregular skull. The most common symptom, which still affects only a minority of patients, is aching in the affected bone. In some people a joint may become arthritic if the bony deformity affects the internal architecture of the joint. Fractures and bone cancer are very rare complication of Paget's disease.

Bisphosphonates (usually alendronate) may be given to treat the symptoms of Paget's disease, because of their effect on the osteoclasts. Surgery is occasionally necessary to correct a severe deformity.

Information Box 4.2d-II

Paget's disease: comments from a Chinese medicine perspective

In Chinese medicine, the irregular enlargement of the bones and increased blood supply might be seen as corresponding to an accumulation of Phlegm with Heat. The weakening of the affected bones suggests an underlying deficiency of Kidney Yin and Essence. The increased risk of cancer is consistent with the development of Phlegm against a background of Yin Deficiency.

As discussed earlier, bisphosphonates nourish Kidney Yin and Essence, but are suppressive in nature.

Information Box 4.2d-I

Osteoporosis: comments from a Chinese medicine perspective

In Chinese medicine, the thinning of bones in osteoporosis corresponds to deficiency of Kidney Jing. The gradual decline in bone density corresponds to the idea in Chinese medicine that Essence gradually declines from its maximum flourishing state in early adulthood. Attention to a healthy diet and moderate exercise will allow for a measured and natural decline of Kidney Yin and Jing, whereas under- or overexercising and undereating will deplete Kidney Yin and Jing. Pregnancy and breastfeeding are draining of Blood and Yin.

The hormone oestrogen is nourishing to the Spleen and to Yin, as evidenced by its beneficial effect on fleshiness and fertility. Hormone replacement therapy (HRT) likewise Boosts Yin, but this may be at the expense of drawing on reserves of Kidney Yin and Jing. The common side-effects of HRT include headaches, fluid retention and weight gain. There is also an increased risk of breast, ovarian and womb cancer. This suggests that there is additional Stagnation of Liver Qi and accumulation of Phlegm and Damp. These symptoms could be a form of drug-induced disease, as HRT is not identical to natural oestrogen. As HRT actually 'suppresses' the natural progression to the menopause, these symptoms may even be a form of expression of suppressed imbalance.

By slowing bone loss, bisphosphonates directly Boost the Kidneys and Jing, but are depleting to Spleen Qi and Stomach Yin, as evidenced by the very common side-effects of nausea and oesophageal ulceration. They are suppressive in nature. Vitamin D and calcium nourish the bones, and therefore are nourishing to the Kidneys and Jing. In normal dietary quantities this treatment is curative in nature.

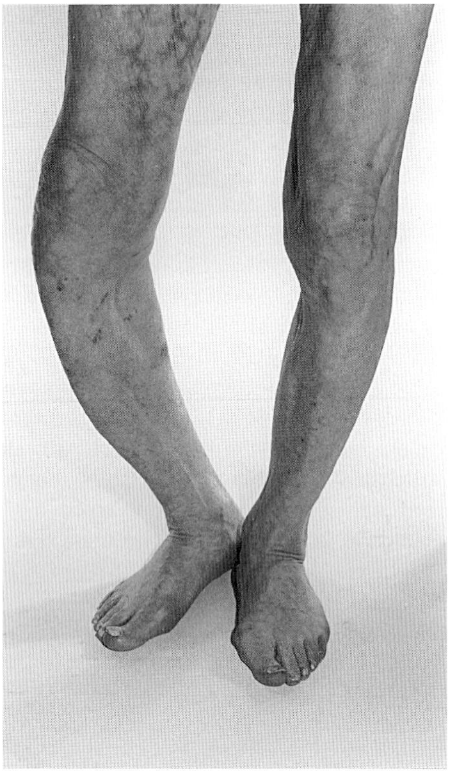

Figure 4.2d-I • Bowing of the legs in Paget's disease.

Rickets and osteomalacia (vitamin D deficiency)

The main source of vitamin D for humans is through manufacture of the vitamin in skin which is exposed to sunlight. In most people the diet is only a secondary source of vitamin D. This fat-soluble vitamin is found in animal fats, eggs and fish oils.

However sourced, vitamin D depends on healthy kidneys to be converted to a useful form in the body. When converted by the kidneys to the active form, vitamin D enables the hardening of new bone by promoting the absorption of calcium from the blood. In its absence, any new bone formed is too soft.

Rickets is the result of vitamin D deficiency in infancy and childhood, whereas osteomalacia is the result of vitamin D deficiency in adulthood. In westernised countries, a very common cause of both these conditions is the lifestyle of Asian immigrant girls and women. A combination of lack of exposure to sunlight and a vegetarian or vegan diet can lead to vitamin D deficiency. Chronic kidney disease is the other important cause of osteomalacia, because the diseased kidneys can no longer activate the vitamin D to a form that is useful to the body.

Rickets is rare in developed countries. When established, there is a characteristic widening of the wrist joints, grooving of the ribs at the level of the diaphragm, and a bowing outwards of the shin bones. The muscles are weak because these too depend on vitamin D for an adequate supply of calcium.

In adulthood, osteomalacia causes vague aches in the bones and muscle weakness, which may lead to a 'waddling' gait in advanced cases. Small areas of bone fracture can develop.

Simple attention to diet and exposure to sunlight can reverse cases of osteomalacia and prevent rickets. Medical treatment usually also includes vitamin D tablets taken by mouth.

> **Information Box 4.2d-III**
>
> **Rickets and osteomalacia: comments from a Chinese medicine perspective**
>
> In Chinese medicine, the symptoms of both rickets and osteomalacia correspond to Jing Deficiency. Vitamin D nourishes the Kidneys and Jing.

Inherited or childhood bone disorders

Achondroplasia (dwarfism)

Achondroplasia is an autosomal-dominant inherited genetic condition in which there is defective formation of bone and cartilage. This causes the long bones to fail to lengthen fully during childhood. An adult with achondroplasia has a trunk of normal length, but very short and broad legs and arms. The skull is enlarged in size and the face appears small, with a depressed nasal ridge. Because of the way this condition is inherited, there is a 50% chance of the children of a person with achondroplasia also developing the disorder.

> **Information Box 4.2d-IV**
>
> **Achondroplasia: comments from a Chinese medicine perspective**
>
> In Chinese medicine, the underlying problem of maturation of bone in achondroplasia suggests Jing Deficiency.

Brittle bone disease (osteogenesis imperfecta)

The term 'brittle bone disease' is used to describe a group of inherited conditions in which there is a defect in the structure of collagen, the connective tissue that supports bone. This means that the bones are unusually brittle.

In very severe types of this condition, the newborn baby develops multiple fractures and bony deformities. Early death is almost inevitable. In less severe forms, the child may be more prone to recurrent fractures, but may grow up to lead a relatively normal adult life as the bones strengthen in puberty. In one of the most common forms of brittle bone disease (osteogenesis imperfecta tarda) a cluster of other features is also often present, including deafness (otosclerosis), heart-valve disorders, weak teeth and a blue discoloration to the whites of the eyes. This form of brittle bone disease is autosomal-dominantly inherited, which means that the gene defect will be passed down to 50% of the children of someone with the condition.

> **Information Box 4.2d-V**
>
> **Brittle bone disease: comments from a Chinese medicine perspective**
>
> In Chinese medicine, brittle bone disease corresponds to Jing Deficiency.

Infections of the bone

Osteomyelitis

'Osteomyelitis' is the term used to describe an infection that has developed within bone tissue. It can develop as a result of direct contamination of bone, as might occur following a compound fracture, or from a traumatic penetration of the flesh, such as a gunshot wound. Alternatively, bacteria from an infected site (such as a boil) elsewhere in the body can lodge in the bone from the bloodstream.

People who have a depleted immune system from malnutrition or another chronic illness are more prone to osteomyelitis. Also, those with sickle cell anaemia may be particularly prone to developing infection in the areas of infarcted bone that can result from the condition.

Another cause of osteomyelitis is tuberculosis.The bones are a favoured site for infection in which the tuberculosis bacterium can thrive. A common location for tuberculous osteomyelitis is in the vertebrae. In this case, it can lead to collapse of the vertebrae.

Osteomyelitis is very difficult to treat because the bone tissue is relatively poorly supplied with blood and immune cells. It is common for an acute infection to become chronic. In some cases an abscess containing pus develops within the bone. This may start discharging through a sinus out onto the skin or towards other body parts (see Chapter 2.2b).

Treatment might involve a long course of high-dose antibiotics, in some cases initially given intravenously to maximise the concentration of drug in the bloodstream. In persistent cases the area of infected bone may need to be surgically excised. Some cases of chronic osteomyelitis will never heal fully.

> **Information Box 4.2d-VI**
>
> **Osteomyelitis: comments from a Chinese medicine perspective**
>
> In Chinese medicine, the infection of osteomyelitis might be seen as corresponding to Heat or Damp Heat against a background of Kidney or Jing Deficiency.

Tumours of the bone

Benign tumours

Occasionally, a smooth, rounded, hard lump of dense bone and cartilage tissue can start to project from the surface of a bone. This benign bony growth, known as an 'osteochondroma', is particularly common in the facial bones. In addition, chondromas, benign bony lumps derived from cartilage, can develop, usually from the ends of the bones of the fingers and toes. Both these forms of benign growth are usually painless, and once developed may change either very slowly or not at all. They are only removed for cosmetic reasons.

Occasionally, an area of dense bone develops deep within the bone tissue. This benign condition, known as 'osteoid osteoma', can lead to a sensation of deep throbbing pain because of the increased pressure within the bone. It is a recognised cause of intense bone pain in young adults. In this case, a surgical operation might be performed to remove the internal growth of dense bone tissue.

> **Information Box 4.2d-VII**
>
> **Benign bone tumours: comments from a Chinese medicine perspective**
>
> The dense tissue of benign tumours of the bone is likely to be described as a manifestation of Phlegm. Pain would suggest additional Blood Stagnation.

Malignant osteosarcoma

Osteosarcoma is a rare primary cancer of bone tissue. It most commonly affects children and young adults, with boys being more commonly affected than girls. However, it can also affect elderly people, and sometimes occurs as a very rare complication of Paget's disease.

This malignant tumour commonly develops close to the end of a long bone, especially the femur, in young people. The symptoms include deep pain, a limp and fever.

Often a plain X-ray image is sufficient to confirm a diagnosis of malignancy, but a biopsy of the bone is performed to grade the tumour.

Treatment is by means of immediate amputation, as the tumour is very aggressive and needs to be removed to avoid

> **Information Box 4.2d-VIII**
>
> **Osteosarcoma: comments from a Chinese medicine perspective**
>
> The fact that osteosarcoma is usually a young person's disease suggests that there is an underlying inherited weakness, possibly of Jing. The tumour itself is often regarded, like most tumours, as a manifestation of Phlegm and Blood Stagnation.

rapid progression. This treatment, together with intensive chemotherapy (doxorubicin and cisplatin), has improved a previously very poor average length of survival, and total cure is now achieved in approximately 50% of cases.

Metastatic disease of the bone

Secondary bone cancer is by far the most common form of bone cancer. Cancers that are particularly likely to metastasise to bone include cancers of the lung, breast, prostate thyroid and kidney.

The most common symptom of secondary bone cancer is pain, which can be very intense and boring in quality. The bone may be particularly tender to percussion, which is a feature of deep bone pathology. In some cases the first symptom is an unexpected (pathological) fracture. The fracture is the result of the underlying weakness of the cancerous bone. As secondary cancer indicates that the condition is in an advanced stage, the patient may also experience symptoms of exhaustion, fevers, weight loss and appetite loss.

In addition to the solid cancers, myeloma is the cancer of the white blood cells that particularly affects the bone (see Chapter 3.4e). Myeloma tends to cause multiple small erosions in the bone. When myeloma is in an advanced stage, the weakening caused by these erosions can be similar in effect to that of severe osteoporosis. The patient becomes prone to fractures, particularly of the marrow-containing ribs and vertebrae.

Treatment of secondary bone cancer is almost never curative, because the disease is at such an advanced stage. Nevertheless, chemotherapy may be given to slow the progression of the disease and reduce its severe symptoms. Pain can be reduced by means of analgesics; NSAIDs can be particularly effective in bone pain. Localised radiotherapy to an affected bone might also temporarily reduce pain significantly (see Q4.2d-2).

Information Box 4.2d-IX

Secondary bone cancer: comments from a Chinese medicine perspective

In Chinese medicine, the pain of secondary bone cancer indicates Blood Stagnation against a background of severe Kidney Deficiency.

The red flags of diseases of the bone

Some patients with bone diseases will benefit from referral to a conventional doctor for assessment and/or treatment. Red flags are those symptoms and signs that will indicate that referral is to be considered. The red flags of the diseases of bone are described in Table 4.2d-I. This table forms part of the summary on red flags given in Appendix III, which also gives advice on the degree of urgency of referral for each of the red flag conditions listed.

Self-test 4.2d

The diseases of the bones

1. Harry is 75 years old. He mentions to you that he suffers from 'rheumatics'. When you question him further, he tells you that he has aching in his bones, particularly along his shin bones. He also says that he has started suffering from headaches, although these are not very severe. When you examine Harry, the areas that ache do not seem to be tender. However, you notice that his tibial bones seem slightly bowed outwards and irregular in shape.
   (i) What is the most likely diagnosis?
   (ii) Would you refer in this case?
2. Marjorie reached the menopause when she was 48 years old. She is now 55 years old and is suffering from some aching pain in the centre of her back. Her GP has told her that this is a sign of osteoporosis, and is recommending that Marjorie takes alendronate, one of the bisphosphonate drugs, to strengthen her bones. Marjorie would prefer to take hormone replacement therapy (HRT), as she has heard this is good for the bones, and wants to hear your opinion about this medication. How might you deal with this situation?

Answers

1. (i) The most likely diagnosis is Paget's disease. This is a fairly common cause of aching in the affected areas of bones in elderly people, and it particularly affects the lower legs and the skull bones.
   (ii) If Harry is referred and the diagnosis is confirmed (on the basis of an X-ray image), he would be offered simple painkillers or bisphosphonates if the pain is unremitting. As these treatments are not curative, Harry could choose to defer accepting treatment until he had seen how the symptoms respond to your treatment.
2. You might first of all choose to examine Marjorie's back. The pain of osteoporosis of the vertebrae is characteristically located in the midline, and the spines of the affected vertebrae may be tender on deep pressure or percussion. Ideally, the severity of the osteoporosis would be assessed by means of a DXA scan. The result of this could guide current management and provide a baseline against which the results of future scans can be compared. Marjorie could request that her GP arranges this for her if this has not been done already.

   Assuming that you agree that this is the diagnosis, you could present Marjorie with the pros and cons of HRT. You can explain that the evidence suggests that HRT certainly does delay the sudden loss of bone that occurs in some women at the time of the menopause, and this is reflected by a reduction in the risk of fracture. However, the side-effects include headaches, weight gain and mood changes. Recent clinical studies show that HRT carries a slightly increased risk of cancer of the breast, ovary and womb, and for this reason it is no longer considered the first choice of treatment for the prevention of osteoporosis. Alendronate does not carry such risks, but does lead to unpleasant digestive symptoms in some people (nausea and oesophagitis). It is currently considered to be the first treatment of choice for osteoporosis.

   From an alternative point of view, HRT can be seen as suppressive of the natural process of entering the menopause, and may also introduce some unwanted energetic effects. Alendronate would appear to boost Kidney Qi, but also by a suppressive mechanism, and also is Heating and Depleting of Stomach and Spleen Qi. If the DXA scan shows that the osteoporosis not too far advanced, a more holistic approach would embrace a diet rich in calcium-containing foods and regular gentle exercise to strengthen the bones. Acupuncture and/or herbal treatment might be offered to strengthen Kidney Qi, Yin and Essence.

Table 4.2d-I Red Flags 26 – diseases of the bones

Red Flag	Description	Reasoning
26.1	**Bone pain**: bone pain originating from bone is characteristically fixed and deep. It may either have an aching or boring quality Tenderness on palpation and on percussion (weighty tapping with the fingertip of the skin overlying the bone) indicates a structural abnormality such as a fracture Boring back pain at night suggests that the origin is from bones rather than muscles. This symptom might suggest bone cancer	It is worth referring any severe or persistent pain that you believe to be originating from bone, as this more often than not results from an infective, cancerous or degenerative condition of the bone Possible causes of bone pain include traumatic bruising or fracture, osteomyelitis (bone infection), tumour, Paget's disease, osteoporosis and osteomalacia The collapse of vertebrae in osteoporosis can lead to a sudden onset of vertebral pain and radiated pain round to the front of the body along the line of the affected spinal nerve. Although not usually serious in itself, an osteoporotic collapse needs to be referred for treatment of severe pain, consideration of medical management of the osteoporosis, and exclusion of weakening of bones by cancer deposits, as this can mimic osteoporosis

Chapter 4.2e Localised diseases of the joints, ligaments and muscles

LEARNING POINTS

At the end of this chapter you will be able to:
- describe the different disease processes that affect individual joints, ligaments and muscles
- recognise the ways in which these processes lead to the various musculoskeletal conditions specific to the different anatomical regions of the body
- recognise the red flags of the localised disorders of the joints, ligaments and muscles.

Estimated time for chapter: 120 minutes.

Introduction

In this and the next chapter the diseases of the joints, ligaments and muscles are studied together, because symptoms arising from these three different structures often overlap, and under certain conditions may co-exist. This chapter focuses on conditions that are localised to a single part of the body only, while the following chapter explores those diseases that tend to affect a number of muscles and joints in the whole body (generalised or systemic diseases).

The conditions considered in this chapter are:

Localised disease processes affecting the joints, ligaments and muscles

- Joint disorders:
  - arthritis
  - damage to internal structures of the joints
  - joint cysts.
- Bursal disorders:
  - bursitis.
- Ligament disorders:
  - sprains
  - hypermobility.
- Muscle disorders:
  - myofascial nodules
  - cramp
  - muscle tears
  - haematomas.
- Tendon disorders:
  - strains
  - tendon rupture
  - tendonitis
  - enthesopathy
  - repetitive strain disorder
  - tendon swellings.
- Fascial disorders:
  - fasciitis
  - contracture.

The following specific disorders of the musculoskeletal system are all manifestations of one or more of the disease processes listed above. These disease processes are described in detail in this chapter. Table 4.2e-I clarifies which disease processes are relevant for each of these specific disorders and so the underlying pathology of each can be more clearly understood.

Specific disorders of the various anatomical regions

- The neck:
  - muscle pain
  - spondylosis
  - whiplash.
- The shoulders:
  - frozen shoulder
  - subacromial bursitis.
- The elbow:
  - epicondylitis
  - bursitis.
- The hand and wrist:
  - tenosynovitis
  - ganglion
  - Dupuytren's contracture
  - trigger finger.
- The lower back:
  - muscular lower back pain

  - spondylolisthesis
  - spondylosis
  - disc prolapse
  - spinal stenosis.
- The hip:
  - osteoarthritis
  - bursitis
  - femoral neck fracture.
- The knee:
  - medial and lateral ligament strain
  - patellar bursitis
  - chondromalacia patellae
  - meniscal and cruciate ligament tears
  - Baker's cyst.
- The lower leg, foot and heel:
  - hallux valgus and bunion
  - plantar fasciitis
  - Achilles tendonitis
  - tear of Achilles tendon
  - calcaneal bursitis
  - shin splints.

Localised joint disorders

Arthritis

The main pathological processes that affect the internal structure of the joints are inflammation and degeneration. The term 'arthritis', literally meaning 'inflammation of the joints', is confusingly often used to describe both these processes.

Arthritis can be caused by a wide range of different factors. It may affect a single joint, or may occur as part of a generalised or systemic disease in which a number of joints are affected. In systemic arthritis the joints are often affected in a symmetrical fashion.

In inflammatory arthritis, the affected joints tend to be hot and painful. In synovial joints, the inflammation affects the synovial membrane lining the interior of the joint. The inflammation can then lead to excessive fluid production from the membrane and, if prolonged, damage to the cartilage of the joint. The inflamed joint is, therefore, swollen and may become deformed as the internal structure becomes destroyed.

Inflammatory arthritis of a single joint can result from infection within the joint, a condition known as 'septic arthritis'. This infection can originate from another site in the body, or can arise as a result of a penetrating injury into the joint. Joint infection is very serious because, like osteomyelitis, the infectious agents are relatively protected from the immune system and thus the infection can progress rapidly. The production of pus can result in permanent inflammatory damage to the interior of a joint.

In septic arthritis, the patient is very unwell with a red, tense and very painful joint and a high fever. However, these symptoms may be less marked in people with chronic illness, such as diabetes or rheumatoid arthritis, or in the elderly. The treatment is hospitalisation and urgent administration of antibiotics, ideally by intravenous injection for the first week. Up to 12 weeks of antibiotic treatment may be given to ensure eradication of the bacterium.

Some infectious diseases can lead to a generalised form of arthritis (see Chapter 4.2f).

Crystal arthritis is a form of non-infectious inflammatory arthritis that can appear very like septic arthritis. It is caused by the formation of small crystals within the joint fluid which are highly irritating and thus cause inflammation. Gout is the most common form of crystal arthritis (see Chapter 4.2f).

Bleeding is another cause of inflammation in a joint. This usually occurs as a result of an injury, but may occur spontaneously in a person who suffers from a clotting disorder such as haemophilia. The technical term for blood in a joint space is 'haemarthrosis'. The blood cells within the joint break down and are highly irritating to the synovial membrane. They then induce severe inflammation. Like infection, a haemarthrosis can also result in permanent damage to the structure of the joint. This is one mechanism for the severe disability that can develop in people with haemophilia.

Other non-infectious systemic conditions can affect the joints, leading to a generalised inflammatory arthritis. The underlying cause of inflammation may be a deposition of autoantibodies within the joint, as occurs in rheumatoid arthritis and systemic lupus erythematosus (SLE). In other conditions the direct cause may be unclear (e.g. in ankylosing spondylitis and inflammatory bowel disease). If the inflammation occurring in these conditions is prolonged, the joints may become permanently deformed (for more detail on generalised arthritis see Chapter 4.2f).

The joints can also become damaged as a result of a process that is largely degenerative, and which leads to thinning or destruction of the protective cartilage that covers the ends of the bones within the joint. This process, known as 'osteoarthritis', is loosely described as 'wear and tear' by many doctors to their patients. Osteoarthritis is more likely to occur in joints that have become damaged through injury or overuse, or in those that are held slightly out of alignment due to chronic muscle tension. Conversely, wear and tear may occur because of excessive laxity of the ligaments (hypermobility), so that the joint is repeatedly taken through a much wider range of movements than those for which it is designed. A rather confusing layman's term for hypermobility is 'double jointedness'.

Generalised osteoarthritis usually occurs as a part of the ageing process and tends to affect the joints in a symmetrical fashion (see also Chapter 4.2f).

Damage to the internal structures of the joints

As described in Chapter 4.2a, some of the synovial joints contain additional structures. The joint between the femur and the tibia at the knee is a good example of such a joint. First, it contains two C-shaped pads of cartilage, which act as cushions for the condyles of the femur upon the table of the tibia. Secondly, two thick ligaments (cruciate ligaments) cross within the joint to prevent the joint from dislocating in an anterior or posterior direction. An injury to the knee, particularly if the joint is twisted, can cause a tear in the cartilage or a rupture of one of the two ligaments. The pain and disability resulting from damage to these structures might be intensified by the swelling caused by bleeding into the joint, a "traumatic haemarthrosis".

Torn cartilage may prevent full mobility of the joint. A sign of this is that the joint may lock in a flexed position. Particles of broken cartilage can also impair the mobility of the joint and be a cause of pain and inflammation. A torn ligament will reduce the support to the knee joint and cause it to be prone to further injury. In both situations, if not well healed, the risk of future osteoarthritis of the knee is increased. Injuries of the internal structure of the knee can be clearly visualised by means of MRI. Injuries to either the cartilage or the cruciate ligaments usually require surgical repair if severe. This may be performed by means of the arthroscope.

Information Box 4.2e-I

Arthritis and damage to the internal structures of the joints: comments from a Chinese medicine perspective

.In Chinese medicine, the pain of arthritis is usually described as a form of Painful Obstruction Syndrome and is a manifestation of Blood and Qi Stagnation. In most cases there is also evidence of a Pathogenic Factor (Bi Syndrome). Inflammatory arthritis always involves Heat, but Wind and Damp may also be present. Degenerative arthritis may simply reflect underlying Deficiency, particularly of the Kidneys, but very often Damp or Cold has also lodged in the affected joints to give symptoms of stiffness and deep pain.

The pain from an injury to the internal structures of the joint may well reflect Blood and Qi Stagnation. If adequate healing fails to occur, chronic Qi and Blood Deficiency of the joint can develop, and Pathogenic Factors such as Damp and Cold may invade.

Joint cysts and ganglions

These are fluid filled cysts that appear close to the margin of a synovial joint. The cyst is an out-pouching of the synovial membrane, and is filled with synovial fluid. Cysts generally appear as part of a degenerative process. The most common site for a joint cyst is at the edge of the wrist joint, where it appears as a smooth, firm, slightly compressible lump (ganglion). Joint cysts at the back of the knee (Baker's cysts) may also be degenerative, but can develop as part of a generalised inflammatory disorder such as rheumatoid arthritis. Joint cysts are usually painless, but may ache or lead to restriction of movement of the affected joint.

Occasionally, the cyst can burst and release fluid into the surrounding tissues. This may lead to resolution of the problem, although commonly the cyst will reform. Rupture of a large cyst such as a Baker's cyst can cause marked inflammation. In the case of a Baker's cyst the inflammation can mimic that of a deep vein thrombosis because the released fluid tracks down the muscles of the calf to cause a tender and swollen calf muscle.

The most effective form of treatment of these cysts is surgical removal. Fluid can be drawn out of the cysts by syringe for relief of discomfort, but fluid tends to reaccumulate in a short space of time.

Information Box 4.2e-II

Ganglia: comments from a Chinese medicine perspective

In Chinese medicine, the development of a joint cyst would possibly be described as accumulation of Phlegm caused by Stagnation of Body Fluids.

Bursal disorders

Bursitis

A bursa is a space lined with synovial membrane and filled with fluid. Its function is to reduce friction to the tissues surrounding a joint. A bursa can become inflamed, particularly if the tissues surrounding the joint are under excessive pressure or misuse. This condition is known as 'bursitis' and is characterised by the bursa swelling up with excess fluid, and becoming hot, red and painful. Student's elbow (the olecranon bursa), housemaid's knee (suprapatellar bursa) and clergyman's knee (prepatellar bursa) are three examples of bursitis from pressure and overuse.

Bursitis is usually treated by means of rest of the overused tissues and NSAIDs. In persistent cases, a corticosteroid injection might be used to reduce the inflammation.

Information Box 4.2e-III

Bursitis: comments from a Chinese medicine perspective

In Chinese medicine, an attack of bursitis might be described as local Blood and Qi Stagnation with Heat.

Ligament disorders

Sprains

The ligaments are the tough fibrous structures made of fibrocartilage which bind bone to bone around the joints. Some ligaments fuse into the joint capsules (also known as the 'capsular ligament'), while others are external to the joint. In some cases the ligaments are found within the synovial joint cavity (e.g. the cruciate ligaments).

In the case of an injury that puts a stretching tension on a ligament, some or all of the fibres in a ligament may become torn, and bleeding can occur in the ligament tissue. A common example of this is the injury that might occur when someone 'turns on their ankle', so that the ligament which links the external malleolus of the fibula to the talus of the foot (in the region of acupoint Qiuxu GB-40) is suddenly stretched. This sort of injury is called a 'sprain'.

In a mild injury only a few fibres of the ligament are torn. The person may feel momentary discomfort, but the problem then subsides. In a more severe tear there may be marked swelling and bruising from the damaged ligament, and the injury may take weeks to heal. A severe tear, even when healed, may leave the joint vulnerable to a recurrence of the injury, as the repaired ligament is never quite as strong as before. This problem of persistent weakness is due to the fact that ligaments do not heal as efficiently as other tissues such as skin or muscle.

The conventional way of treating an acute ligament strain involves rest of the affected area, application of ice to reduce swelling, use of a compression bandage such as Tubigrip, and elevation of the affected part to reduce swelling (RICE). This treatment reduces the amount of bleeding into the ligament, but will slow healing if prolonged. RICE can be maintained for the first 24 hours after the injury. Thereafter, gentle heat applied to the injury will be more beneficial. Some severe ligament tears may require physiotherapy, a plaster splint or surgery to allow optimum healing.

Information Box 4.2e-IV

Acute sprain: comments from a Chinese medicine perspective

In Chinese medicine an acute sprain might correspond to acute Blood and Qi Stagnation. Chronic weakness of a previously sprained ligament corresponds to local Qi Deficiency, and the area may become vulnerable to invasion by Pathogenic Factors (especially Damp and Cold).

Hypermobility

'Hypermobility' is a term used to describe excessive joint laxity. Some people are born with this tendency. If severe it may represent a rare inherited deficiency of connective tissue. Hypermobility may also be acquired through long-term strenuous stretching exercise, such as gymnastics, particularly if performed during childhood. Although the joints of most adults are far too inflexible, a hypermobile joint is not necessarily a good thing. This is because the increased range of movement puts excessive strain on the internal structures of the joint and may lead to the development of osteoarthritis in later life.

Information Box 4.2e-V

Hypermobility: comments from a Chinese medicine perspective

In Chinese medicine, the range of movement associated with hypermobility might point to an instability of the joint corresponding to a Deficiency in Liver Blood and Qi.

Muscle disorders

Myofascial nodules (trigger points)

Myofascila nodules are lumps, commonly called 'knots', which can be felt within the body of tense muscle. They are often very tender. Myofascial nodules form as a result of a localised area of tensely contracted muscle fibres. If a nodule has only recently developed, deep massage of the area of the knot may cause it to relax and disappear. More long-standing nodules may become fixed as structural changes take place in the tensed area of muscle.

These nodules are commonly found in the muscles of the back of the neck, upper back and shoulders, lower back and overlying the sacrum. In particular, the trapezius muscle is commonly affected. The nodules can develop in any skeletal muscle as a result of excessive tension held in the muscle body. They are often the underlying cause of musculoskeletal pain when there is no other structural damage to be found. Muscle tension may have a postural or an emotional root, and is very commonly a combination of the two. It can also develop as a result of a local painful musculoskeletal problem. For example, pain from disease of the intervertebral joints in the lower back can lead to tension (spasm) of the lumbar muscles. This initially protective reflex can result in the development of painful myofascial nodules in the lumbar muscles and, if the joint problem persists, may become chronic in nature.

The pain from myofascial nodules can cause tension to spread to other local muscle groups, so that a whole anatomical region, in particular the shoulder and back of the neck, can become stiff and knotted. Often, pain is referred to other parts of the body. For example, headache is a very common consequence of muscle tension in the shoulders and upper neck. The patient will tend to want to rub or hold the affected area, and the pain can be greatly helped by a prolonged stretch of the affected muscle, application of warmth or massage. Acupuncture is medically recognised to be an effective treatment for tender myofascial nodules (also known as 'trigger point acupuncture').

Information Box 4.2e-VI

Myofascial nodules: comments from a Chinese medicine perspective

In Chinese medicine, myofascial nodules correspond to areas of Qi and Blood Stagnation. Sometimes they are at the site of known acupuncture points, and can be viewed as a form of Ah-shi point. This has implications for how the nodules are treated. They point to disharmony in the Organ that dominates the area in which the nodule has developed. Very commonly, this disharmony is within one of the Yang Officials, in particular the Gallbladder, Small Intestine, Triple Burner or Bladder. Referred pain is commonly felt along the pathway of the associated channel.

Treatment directed at the trigger points alone, such as massage, cupping and acupuncture, can be very helpful in relieving symptoms, but may not deal with the deep root of the problem (usually a form of Deficiency). If this is the case, the patient will need to return again and again for treatment, and the practitioner needs to consider additional methods of treatment to focus directly on the root problem.

Muscle cramp

Cramp is a sudden painful contraction of a large muscle group. The mechanism of cramp is poorly understood, but is commonly explained as a result of build-up of waste products in a muscle. This theory fits with the observation that cramp commonly occurs in overexercised muscle in which the requirements of the metabolism of the muscle may exceed the blood supply. Cramps in the legs (particularly in the calf and feet) become increasingly common in old age. In this case, they must be distinguished from the cramping pain that can result from arteriosclerosis of the arteries of the legs.

An acute cramp may be relieved by forcibly stretching the muscle. Chronic night-time cramps may be relieved in some people by the medication quinine sulphate taken on a regular basis.

> **Information Box 4.2e-VII**
>
> **Acute cramp: comments from a Chinese medicine perspective**
>
> In Chinese medicine, an acute cramp would correspond to Blood and Qi Stagnation. It tends to develop against a background of Deficiency of Liver Blood and Yin.

Torn muscle and muscle haematoma

Just as a ligament can be torn during an acute injury, so can the fibres of a muscle. Muscle fibres can tear when unexpected strain is placed on a muscle group, especially if those muscles are contracted. This is a common injury to affect the hamstring muscles (at the back of the upper leg) and the abdominal muscles, both in the context of strenuous exercise. The term 'strain' is used to describe a torn muscle or tendon.

An area of torn muscle will become inflamed as a result of cell damage and bleeding, and if the tear is severe the affected area may become tender and warm. Rarely, a large bleed into the body of the muscle may lead to the formation of a tender, hot lump called a 'haematoma'. This is a common occurrence in people who have a disorder of clotting such as haemophilia.

Usually, muscle tears heal well because muscle fibres have a very good blood supply. Like ligament sprains, if severe, the tear is treated with RICE (see ligament sprains, above) for the first 24 hours. This treatment helps to prevent excessive bleeding into the area. A haematoma may impair healing as the mass of clotted blood can be a continuing trigger for inflammation, and scarring and contracture of the muscle can develop. For this reason, a large-muscle haematoma may have to be drained surgically to permit full healing. Muscle contractures are a serious consequence of muscle bleeds in haemophilia.

> **Information Box 4.2e-VIII**
>
> **Muscle tears: comments from a Chinese medicine perspective**
>
> In Chinese medicine, a muscle tear corresponds to Blood and Qi Stagnation. A haematoma reflects Blood Stagnation and may also be a reflection of additional Heat. Scarring of a poorly healed muscle reflects local Blood and Qi Deficiency, with persistent Qi Stagnation.

Tendon disorders

Tendon strains and rupture

As the tendon is the site at which the muscle inserts into bone, tendon strains also result from acute trauma or misuse of muscles. The strain can occur at the very point at which the tendon inserts into the bone, or at any position along a tendon up to its insertion into the muscle belly. In very severe cases the tendon can be totally ruptured. A common example of this is the rupture of the Achilles tendon, which can occur following a forceful landing on the feet when the gastrocnemius muscle is contracted.

Tendons do not heal as well as muscle tissue, as their structure and blood supply is more like that of ligaments. Treatment of a severe tendon strain involves RICE (see ligament sprains, above), followed by prolonged immobilisation of the area. If there has been a rupture, reparative surgery may be necessary. If the injury is less severe, gentle use of the affected tendon may actually aid healing.

> **Information Box 4.2e-IX**
>
> **Tendon strains: comments from a Chinese medicine perspective**
>
> A tendon strain corresponds to Blood and Qi Stagnation. If healing is poor, this is due to long-term local depletion of Blood and Qi.
>
> Although sprains and strains commonly affect young healthy people, they are more likely to occur within the context of an underlying state of Blood and Qi Deficiency or Stagnation. For example, a Liver Blood deficient person who turns their ankle would be seen as more likely to sustain an injury to the ankle ligaments than someone who is in good health.

Tendonitis and tenosynovitis

'Tendonitis' is a term used to describe a condition in which tendons become inflamed. Some tendons, for example the extensor tendons of the hand, travel within fluid-filled sheaths, which protect and lubricate the tendons. If these tendons become inflamed, the term 'tenosynovitis' more correctly describes the condition.

The most common cause of tendonitis is repetitive misuse of the muscles attached to the inflamed tendon. For example, repetitive use of clippers or scissors may lead to tenosynovitis of the extensor tendons of the hand, and repetitive twisting actions of the wrist may lead to tendonitis of the tendon of the extensor carpi radialis as it inserts into the lateral epicondyle of the elbow (known as 'lateral epicondylitis' or 'tennis elbow').

Tendonitis presents with inflammation of the area affected, and pain on performing the movement that has caused the problem. In tenosynovitis, the tendon sheaths may be swollen with fluid, and crackling sensations (crepitus) may be felt over the affected area if the tendons are moved.

Conventional treatment is with NSAIDs and advice to rest the affected part. Many cases will settle down over 2–3 days, but in some cases they can become chronic. In such cases, a corticosteroid injection may be offered.

Information Box 4.2e-X

Tendonitis and tenosynovitis: comments from a Chinese medicine perspective

In Chinese medicine, tendonitis and tenosynovitis represent severe Blood and Qi Stagnation. They often occur against a background of local or general Blood and Qi Deficiency (possibly caused by the overuse of the area). Liver Blood Deficiency is a common underlying deficiency.

Enthesopathy

'Enthesopathy' is the medical term used to describe inflammation of the area at which a tendon or ligament inserts into the bone in the region of a joint. Strictly speaking, tennis elbow is an example of an enthesopathy. Enthesopathy may also occur as a result of a more generalised inflammatory condition such as rheumatoid arthritis or ankylosing spondylitis (see Chapter 4.2f).

Repetitive strain injury

Repetitive strain injury (RSI) is a term used to describe a painful condition that affects the muscle groups which have to perform repetitive movements, often in the context of a stressful work situation. More recently, the terms 'work-related upper-limb injury' and 'chronic upper-limb pain syndrome' have been introduced to describe the same condition. RSI is a well-recognised problem for people engaged in work that demands repetitive movements, for example typing or the playing of a musical instrument. It is also recognised that there are often underlying emotional or stress-related problems. The cause of the pain can be one or both of small-muscle and tendon strains or chronic tendonitis.

Initial treatment may involve rest, which often means time off work. Ideally, the sources of stress in the working environment should be tackled. Advice about posture and personal stress management might be given. The Alexander technique can be of particular benefit. It is not uncommon for patients to be prescribed counselling, beta blockers or antidepressants to deal with the underlying emotional issues.

Information Box 4.2e-XI

Repetitive strain injury: comments from a Chinese medicine perspective

In Chinese medicine, the pain of repetitive strain injury represents Blood and Qi Stagnation, but there is likely to be an underlying condition of Deficiency, in particular of Liver Blood Deficiency and Spleen Qi Deficiency.

Tendon swellings (trigger finger)

Trigger finger is a condition in which a swelling develops on a flexor tendon of a finger just at the point at which it enters the tendon sheath. This is usually a painless condition, but can cause a problem in free movement of the finger. The affected finger tends to lock in a fully flexed position, and will only open with a degree of force, and with a clicking sensation.

De Quervain's syndrome is pain and swelling over the region of the styloid process of the radius (in the region of acupoint Yangxi LI-5) because of thickening of the tendons of abductor pollicis longus and extensor pollicis brevis. The pain is worst when lifting something like a teapot.

For these conditions patient may be offered a corticosteroid injection, which can reduce the swelling on the tendon. Severe cases may be offered surgery.

Fascial disorders

The 'fascia' is the term used to describe the fibrous connective tissue that surrounds the muscles and tendons and holds them in place. In some parts of the body the fibres of the fascia coalesce to form thick sheets of tissue, which have both a protective and structural role. For example, the palmar and plantar fasciae are sheets of connective tissue that lie within the palm of the hand and sole of the foot, respectively. These overlie and protect the flexor tendons of the hands and feet.

Fasciitis

Fasciitis is a condition in which there is inflammation of the fascial tissue. The most common site for this to occur is in the sole of the foot (plantar fasciitis). Plantar fasciitis can occur as a result of excessive walking, but may also develop as part of a more generalised inflammatory disorder such as ankylosing spondylitis (see Chapter 4.2f).

Fasciitis can be very painful. It is treated with rest of the affected area, NSAIDs and, occasionally, corticosteroid injections.

Dupuytren's contracture

This is a disorder in which bands of the palmar fascia become thickened and contracted. If severe, over the course of months to years the contraction can pull the fingers, particularly the fourth and fifth fingers, into a permanent state of flexion. Most commonly, this disorder affects middle-aged men and has no obvious cause. In some cases there may be an associated liver disorder or alcohol problem.

Information Box 4.2e-XII

Dupuytren's contracture: comments from a Chinese medicine perspective

In Chinese medicine, Dupuytren's contracture would represent Liver Blood Deficiency and Liver Qi Stagnation. Because of the affected area, there may also be an imbalance in the Heart or Pericardium Officials.

Carpal tunnel syndrome

The carpal tunnel is a space running through the wrist that is bounded by a band of thick fascia (the flexor retinaculum), which helps to hold the small bones in place. Figure 4.2e-I illustrates the structure and location of the flexor retinaculum. Inflammation of the soft tissue within this space can cause compression of the median nerve. This leads to the symptoms that comprise carpal tunnel syndrome. This condition, an entrapment neuropathy, is described in Chapter 4.1g.

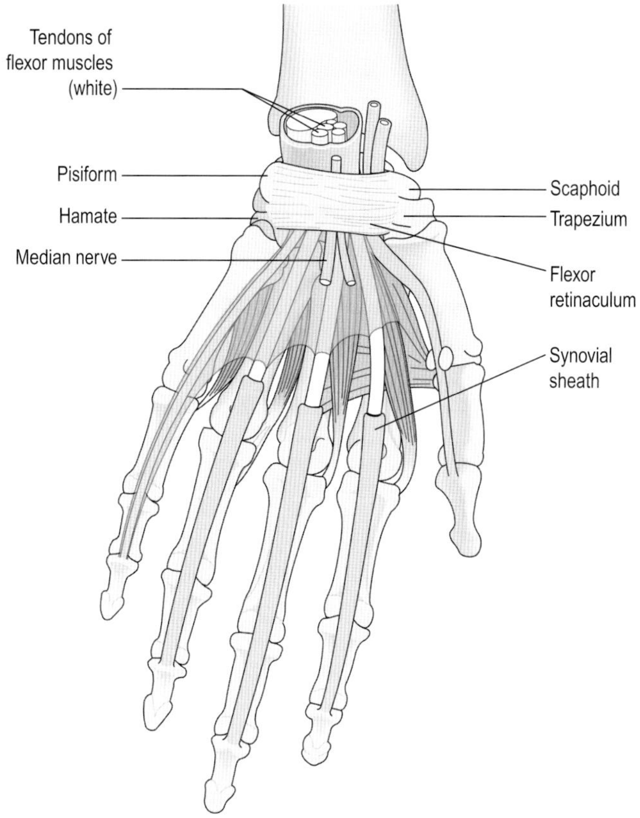

Figure 4.2e-I • The carpal tunnel and synovial sheaths in the wrist and hand.

Specific localised problems according to anatomical region

Specific localised musculoskeletal problems were listed at the beginning of this chapter. All these conditions result from one or more of the types of muscle and ligament disorder described above. The nature of the pathology of each of these conditions is listed in Table 4.2e-I. It can be seen from this table that the pathology of most of these conditions has already been described and so by using the Table 4.2e-I as a guide, the underlying disease process for each of these conditions can be understood.

The exception to this rule relates to those conditions that are the most common cause of pain in the neck and the lower back. A summary of these conditions now follows.

Chronic neck and back pain

In many cases, chronic neck and back pain begins simply as a result of long-standing tension in the supporting muscles of the neck and back. The muscles in such a case will feel tense and have knotted areas containing myofascial nodules that are particularly tender. It is at this stage that alternative treatments such as massage, osteopathy and acupuncture can be most effective, and may be curative.

Spondylosis

If muscle tension is held for a long time, fibrous changes develop within the muscles, with the result that they lose their ability to fall into a fully relaxed state. Moreover, some of the myofascial nodules can become permanent fibrous structures. The continual tension placed on the fibrous joints of the vertebral column is likely to speed up the degenerative process of osteoarthritis which, as has been previously discussed, is a natural tendency of ageing joints. However, held tension is not the whole story. Some people are more likely to develop osteoarthritis than others simply because of an inherited tendency to the condition.

Osteoarthritis of the fibrous intervertebral joints leads to deformity of the vertebral bodies, and pain and stiffness of the facet joints, which in health permit free movement of one vertebra upon another. The most characteristic deformity is the development of bony outgrowths, called 'osteophytes', which project horizontally outwards from the bodies of

Table 4.2e-I The pathology of the common localised musculoskeletal disorders: the underlying pathology of each of these conditions is described in detail in the body of the text of Chapter 4.2e

Anatomical region	Name of condition	Underlying pathology
Neck	Muscle pain Spondylosis Whiplash	Muscle strain and myofascial nodules Degenerative arthritis and nerve compression Complex ligament sprains, and muscle and tendon strains
Shoulders	Frozen shoulder Subacromial bursitis	Tendonitis or inflammation of the fibrous ligaments of the joint capsule Bursitis
Elbow	Medial and lateral epicondylitis	Tendonitis
Hand and wrist	Tenosynovitis Ganglion Dupuytren's contracture Trigger finger	Tenosynovitis Joint cyst Fascial contracture Tendon swelling
Lower back	Muscle pain Spondylolisthesis and spondylosis Disc prolapse Spinal stenosis	Muscle strain and myofascial nodules Degenerative arthritis and nerve or spinal cord compression Degenerative arthritis of a fibrous joint Degenerative arthritis and nerve compression
Hip	Osteoarthritis Trochanteric bursitis	Degenerative arthritis Bursitis
Knee	Osteoarthritis Medial and lateral ligament strain Patellar bursitis (housemaid's and clergyman's knee) Chondromalacia patellae Meniscal and cruciate tears Baker's cyst	Osteoarthritis Chronic sprain Bursitis Degenerative arthritis Degeneration of the structures inside a joint Joint cyst
Lower leg, foot and heel	Hallux valgus and bunion Plantar fasciitis Calcaneal bursitis Achilles tendonitis Achilles tendon tear Shin splints (pain in the front of the calf from overuse – common in joggers)	Degenerative arthritis and bursitis Fasciitis Bursitis Tendonitis Strain Fasciitis of the tibialis anterior muscle fascia

the vertebrae. Together, these bony changes are called 'spondylosis'. Spondylosis develops most prominently in the cervical and lumbar spine, but can appear at any intervertebral joint. Cervical and lumbar spondylosis are described in Chapter 4.1g.

The osteophytes in spondylosis may place pressure on local tissues, including nerve fibres, and be an additional cause of pain. Therefore, the symptoms of spondylosis might include chronic pain, stiffness and reduction of free movement. There may also be referred pain in the distribution of an affected nerve root (lumbar and upper sacral spondylosis is one possible cause of sciatica).

It makes sense that spondylosis can be prevented by attention to minimising held muscle tension earlier in life. Regular gentle stretching exercise, focus on good posture and relaxation will help to minimise the tendency to the formation of spondylosis and will also reduce its symptoms.

Intervertebral disc prolapse

The increased pressure on the fibrous pad (disc) that separates the individual vertebrae may cause a protrusion of its soft core (known as a 'herniation' or 'prolapse'), so that a bulge projects, usually posterolaterally, out of the joint.

Intervertebral disc prolapse may lead to pressure on one of the posterior nerve roots of the spinal cord and, if this is the case, will cause symptoms of pain, numbness and weakness affecting the distribution of the nerves in the nerve root. There may be additional back pain, as the injury may trigger increased muscle spasm in the surrounding area. Sometimes the prolapse can occur gradually as a response to chronic muscle tension, but often will develop suddenly because of an acute increase in pressure within the disc. Common causes of acute herniation of a disc are digging and lifting of heavy weights. In a weak back, a small turn or a cough may be enough to cause an acute prolapse.

Disc prolapse can affect young people, in whom the cause is excessive tension of the muscles of the lower back. In some cases, there is also a degree of inherited structural deformity of the vertebrae or their ligaments. In later life, disc prolapse is also associated with the changes of spondylosis, in which case a degree of degeneration of the intervertebral disc may have predisposed to the condition.

In both spondylosis and disc prolapse there are underlying structural changes that are often irreversible. Nevertheless, exercises and lifestyle changes focusing on the reduction of muscle tension may well be of benefit in reducing symptoms, but are unlikely to cure the problem completely.

In conventional medical practice the pain of spondylosis and disc prolapse is notoriously difficult to investigate and treat. The symptoms of both can be indistinguishable from the pain and nerve compression caused by simple muscle tension or muscle strains. The bony changes of spondylosis can be seen on an x-ray image, but are very commonly not associated with pain, so that such images are usually unhelpful. The investigation of choice is MRI, because this can differentiate between bone, muscle and nerve root, and can often show the precise physical cause of the pain. MRI is uncomfortable for the patient and expensive to the health service, so its use is usually reserved for severe intractable cases of low back and neck pain.

Treatment initially involves pain relief, usually with a combination of paracetamol and a NSAID. In an acute situation, opiate analgesics and muscle relaxants may be needed in the short term to relieve pain and reduce spasm of the supporting muscles. In persistent or severe cases, the patient may be offered advice and treatment from a physiotherapist. In some cases, surgery may be required to decompress the soft tissue around compressed nerve roots, remove the bulging part of a prolapsed disc, or to stabilise the intervertebral joints.

Information Box 4.2e-XIII

Low back and neck pain: comments from a Chinese medicine perspective

In Chinese medicine, low back and neck pain usually correspond to a combination of Damp and Cold Invasion, Blood and Qi Stagnation and underlying Deficiency, usually of the Kidney/Bladder and Liver/Gallbladder Officials.

The red flags of localised disorders of the diseases of the joints, ligaments and muscles

Some patients with localised disorders of the joints, ligaments and muscles will benefit from referral to a conventional doctor for assessment and/or treatment. Red flags are those symptoms and signs that will indicate that referral is to be considered. The red flags of the localised disorders of the joints, ligaments and muscles are described in the Table 4.2e-II. This table forms part of the summary on red flags given in Appendix III, which also gives advice on the degree of urgency of referral for each of the red flag conditions listed.

Self-test 4.2e

Localised disorders of the joints, ligaments and muscles

1. Jim is an enthusiastic footballer who is dismayed to discover that he has developed a knee problem. This resulted from what felt like a minor injury during a tackle, but now, 3 hours after the match, his knee is tense, swollen, hot and painful, and also can become fixed from time to time in a flexed position, which feels very alarming.
   (i) What is a possible diagnosis(es)?
   (ii) In addition to the complementary therapy that you practise, what simple treatment might you recommend?
   (iii) Would you refer Jim to see a doctor?
2. Harriet is a keen university rower, but her performance has been hindered by the development of pain at the back of her hands and thumbs when she rows. Over the past 2 days this pain has become excruciating. When you examine her you find that the backs of her hands are puffy, warm and tender to touch. She is reluctant to move her fingers. Any extension of her fingers or thumb makes the pain worse. She feels slightly sick and unwell with the pain.
   (i) What is the most likely diagnosis?
   (ii) Would you refer Harriet to a doctor?

Answers

1. (i) Jim has suffered a traumatic injury to his knee. The fact that the joint has swollen suggests that there has been some damage to the internal structures of the knee. The fluid could be the result of inflammation or blood infiltration. Therefore there is a possibility that Jim has developed a haemarthrosis. The locking of the knee in a flexed position is a sign of a tear in the cartilage (meniscus) of the knee, and is probably the cause of the bleeding.
   (ii) You might suggest that Jim follows the principles of RICE (rest, ice, compression and elevation) treatment to minimise bleeding, although this is less effective for bleeding deep within a joint.
   (iii) Jim should see a doctor that day. It may be that a severe haemarthrosis requires draining to minimise the risk of permanent joint damage. If the injury is considered severe, he may be offered immediate arthroscopic treatment of the torn meniscal cartilage.
2. (i) This sounds like an acute case of tenosynovitis, induced by overuse of the extensor tendons of the fingers whilst rowing.
   (ii) Despite the apparent severity of Harriet's symptoms (all a result of acute inflammation) they should respond to rest and complementary medical approaches. You might suggest that she finds a way of splinting the hands in one position for a couple of days to enable total rest of the tendon sheaths. If you were to refer her, the doctor would prescribe NSAID painkillers and might offer a corticosteroid injection if the problem does not settle.

Table 4.2e-II Red Flags 27 –localised disorders of the joints, ligaments and muscles

Red Flag	Description	Reasoning
27.1	**Features of traumatic injury to a muscle or joint** (which may require surgical treatment or immobilization): sudden onset of pain or swelling in a joint (possible haemarthrosis), sudden severe pain and swelling around a joint with reluctance to move (sprain or strain or possible fracture), sudden onset of tender swelling in a muscle (possible haematoma), locking of the knee joint (meniscal cartilage tear)	If there are any of these features of traumatic injury to a muscle or joint, and if you are not familiar with sports injuries, it is wise to refer for appropriate immediate assessment (including x-ray imaging) and orthopaedic management The rest/ice/compression/elevation (RICE) formula should be considered if there is significant inflammation (redness and swelling). Rest means ensuring that the injured region is immobilised, and this needs to be effected by means of recognised first-aid approaches (e.g. splints, bandages and slings)
27.2	**Features of intervertebral disc prolapse and severe nerve root irritation**: sudden onset of low back pain so severe that walking is impossible; severe sciatica, difficulty urinating or defecating	In most cases disc prolapse is not an emergency condition, and may do very well with appropriate acupuncture, cupping and massage techniques. Even with sciatic pain you can expect that your treatment might bring relief without need for referral In most cases the referred pain and weakness indicates compression of one or more of the L3, L4, L5 or S1 nerve roots, and the symptoms are usually one sided. Expect at least partial relief of these symptoms within a few days of treatment However, medical treatment (anti-inflammatory and muscle relaxant medication) can be very useful if the pain is very severe and there is a lot of muscle spasm that is not responding to your treatment Difficulty in urination or defecation or sacral numbness are rare but serious signs that indicate compression of the delicate lower sacral roots. If these symptoms are apparent, refer for assessment as a high priority (see Red Flag 29.3, below)
27.3	**Cauda equina syndrome: numbness of the buttocks and perineum** (saddle anaesthesia) with bilateral numbness or sciatica in legs. Difficulties in urination or defecation are serious symptoms	The cauda equina (horse's tail) is the bunch of nerves that descends from the bottom of the spinal cord from the level of L1–2 downwards. These nerve roots supply sensation and motor impulses to the perineum, buttocks, groin and legs. Cauda equina syndrome suggests the compression of a number of these roots (usually from a central prolapsed disc, but possibly from tumour or other spinal growth). This is a serious situation, as prolonged compression to the perineal supply can lead to permanent problems with urination, defecation and sexual function. Refer as a high priority
27.4	**Features of septic or crystal arthritis:** a single hot swollen and very tender joint. Patient is unwell. Not usually associated with injury, but may occasionally be caused by a penetrating injury of the joint space	A hot, swollen joint is a sign of possible joint infection. This presents a grave risk to the health of the joint and needs to be referred so that infection can be excluded However, the most common cause of a single hot and swollen joint is gout (crystal arthritis), which can respond well to acupuncture alone. If this is the case the doctor may wish to prescribe anti-inflammatory medication, but after diagnosis has been confirmed it is worth using needles in the first instance and reserving medication if there is no benefit within 3–7 days
27.5	**Unexplained intense persistent shoulder pain** unrelated to shoulder movement (for more than 2 weeks)	Shoulder pain that seems to be unrelated to shoulder movement might be referred from a tumour at the apex of the lung (Pancoast tumour). A frozen shoulder is the most common (and benign) cause of shoulder pain, and is characterised by an inability to use the affected joint. Refer any case in which the pain does not fit this picture

Chapter 4.2f Generalised diseases of the joints, ligaments and muscles

LEARNING POINTS

At the end of this chapter you will:

- be able to name the main features of the most important generalised diseases of the joints and muscles
- understand the principles of treatment of a few of the most common diseases
- be able to recognise the red flags of the generalised disorders of the joints, ligaments and muscles.

Estimated time for chapter: 120 minutes.

Introduction

Chapter 4.2e focused on those conditions of the joints, ligaments and muscles that are localised to a single part of the body only. This chapter explores those diseases that tend to affect a number of muscles and joints in the whole body (generalised or systemic diseases).

The conditions considered in this chapter are (see Q4.2f-1):

- Arthritis:
  - osteoarthritis
  - rheumatoid arthritis
- Other forms of inflammatory arthritis:
  - arthritis in autoimmune disease
  - ankylosing spondylitis
  - psoriatic arthritis
  - gout
  - arthritis due to infection.
- Disorders of the muscles and ligaments:
  - fibromyalgia
  - polymyalgia rheumatica
  - muscular dystrophy.

Arthritis

The different types of arthritis are summarised in Chapter 4.2e. In this chapter, those generalised conditions that manifest in these diverse forms of arthritis will be summarised.

Osteoarthritis

As described in Chapter 4.2e, osteoarthritis (OA) is a progressive degenerative disorder of the synovial joints. It is the commonest joint disorder, affects women three times more than men, and usually is symmetrical.

Figure 4.2f-I illustrates the parts of the body that tend to affected by OA. It can be seen that the hips, knees, ankles and small joints of the fingers (metacarpophalangeal and interphalangeal joints) are most commonly affected.

The underlying process of disease in OA is focal degeneration of the hyaline cartilage that lines the ends of the bones inside a synovial joint. By a mechanism which is poorly understood, in some cases the bone around the joint also degenerates and becomes deformed in shape. The edges of the bony joint become 'lipped' with spiky protuberances of bones called 'osteophytes' (literally meaning 'bony leaves'). Figure 4.2f-II illustrates the cartilage thinning and osteophyte formation in early OA of the knee joint.

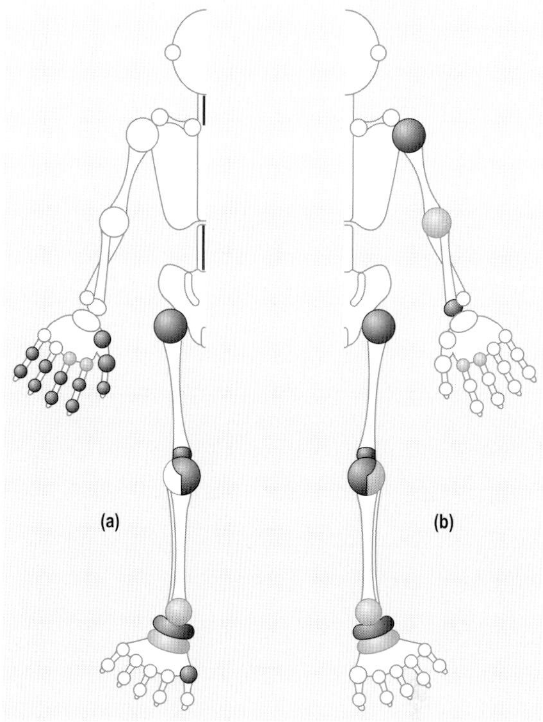

Figure 4.2f-I • Typical distribution of the joints affected in generalised osteoarthritis.

The development of OA is so common in old age that it can almost be seen as part of the normal ageing process. Most people over 60 years old will have features of OA on x-ray images, even if they have no symptoms.

The tendency to develop a severe disabling form of OA runs in families. In addition, any joint that has been subjected to stress or trauma in earlier life is more likely to develop OA with the progression of time. Strenuous exercise is not good for the joints, particularly in women. It is known that women who are involved in weight-bearing exercise (running, aerobics,

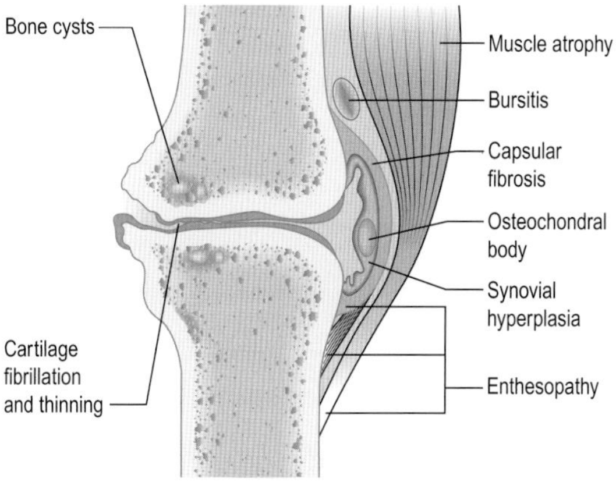

Figure 4.2f-II • Diagram of the knee showing early osteoarthritis.

squash, tennis, etc.) are 2–3 times more likely to develop OA of the hip and the knee. Also, joints that are not held in correct alignment due to anatomical deformity, hypermobility of ligaments or chronic muscle tension are more prone to developing OA. Another factor that may make the development OA worse is a diet low in antioxidants such as vitamin C.

The development of severe symptoms of OA may be prevented by attention to the following factors:

- avoidance of repetitive stressful use of the joints earlier in life (such as might occur in competitive sports and certain occupations)
- loss of weight (symptoms are much worse in obese people)
- adoption of exercise routines that relax and strengthen the muscles around the joints so that the joints are held in the correct anatomical alignment (gentle swimming, Tai Chi and gentle yoga can all be very helpful in relieving the chronic pain of OA)
- maintenance of a diet rich in antioxidants, including vitamin C.

Joints affected by OA can ache, and tend to feel stiff in the morning, although gentle mobilisation will improve this stiffness. Heat often helps the pain. A severely affected large joint may accumulate excess synovial fluid, and can appear puffy.

In many people, particularly women, the first features of OA may be a painless deformity of the small joints of the hand. This commonly starts to occur in late middle age, often around the time of the menopause in women. The distal interphalangeal joints and the first metacarpophalangeal joints are particularly affected. Irregular swellings protrude from the edges of the bone at these joints, so that the ends of the fingers develop a characteristic deformity (known as Heberden's nodes) (Figure 4.2f-III). In some people this process, known as nodular OA, will cause achy pain and inflammation of the joints of the hand. In most painful cases the pain and the swelling will settle down over the course of a few years, although the deformity of the joints will persist, and may progress.

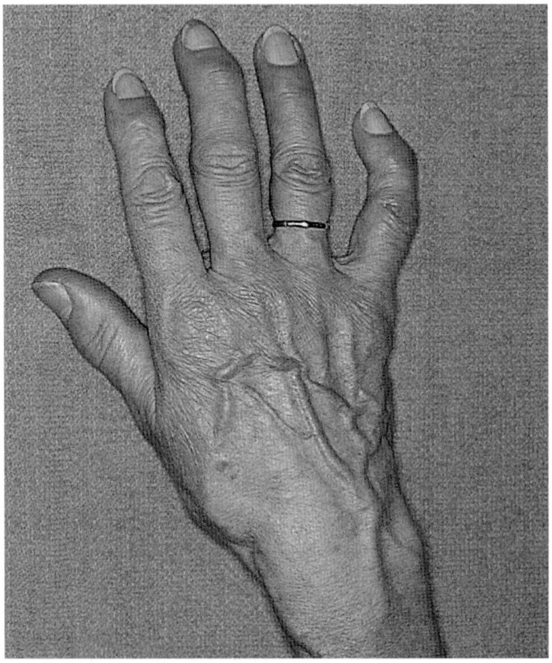

Figure 4.2f-III • Nodal osteoarthritis • Heberden's nodes of the distal interphalangeal joints and marked deformity of the middle finger proximal interphalangeal joint.

Less commonly in nodular OA, the minor changes in the hands are accompanied by aching and stiffness of the large joints, which in some cases progresses steadily to a disabling condition. The hips and/or the knees are the most commonly affected joints. Hip pain tends to be felt deep in the low buttock (often in the region of acupoint Huantiao GB-30) and radiates into the groin. Weight-bearing exercise is uncomfortable. The knee pain of OA is felt deep in the joint and may be associated with crunching noises (crepitus) as the joint is moved. In both types of OA the muscles that support the joint may become very thin and wasted. This appears to be a reflex response to the pain in a joint, although it is not helpful for the patient. The weakened muscles cannot support the joint as well, and may contribute to worsening of the symptoms.

Degeneration of the joints can also affect the intervertebral joints, in particular of the cervical spine and the lumbar spine. These changes may or may not co-exist with symptoms of OA elsewhere in the body. These are the changes known as 'cervical spondylosis' and 'lumbar spondylosis' which were discussed in the previous chapter.

OA can lead to marked deformity, such as significant bony swelling around the joints of the hands and the knee, but may give rise to very few symptoms. In these cases there is no need for treatment. If symptoms develop, the patient could first be advised about lifestyle changes, such as attention to a healthy diet and weight loss, and be given a simple exercise routine to strengthen the affected joints. Most conventional practitioners would be happy for their patients to seek complementary approaches, such as acupuncture, for the symptoms of early OA, although these are not usually provided by the UK National Health Service.

Analgesics form the mainstay of the treatment approaches for OA, ideally starting with paracetamol before NSAID medication is commenced. Corticosteroids may be injected into affected joints, but it is recognised that this procedure should not be performed repeatedly. Glucosamine is a supplement also recognised to be of benefit in mild to moderate OA when prescribed on a once daily basis, although the mechanism of action of this naturally occurring mucopolysaccharide is currently unknown.

In very severe OA of the large joints, joint-replacement surgery can transform the pain and disability caused by the condition. In both hip- and knee-replacement surgery the worn-out ends of the bones forming the joint are removed and replaced by plastic or metal replacement parts or 'prostheses'. These do not provoke an immune response because they are not of antigenic material, and many patients recover remarkably quickly from the operation. In about 1% of operations a serious complication such as infection or loosening of the joint prosthesis develops. Often the patient then requires a repeat operation, but the chances of full recovery are diminished. Thrombosis of the leg veins is also a possible complication, although all patients are now protected from this by means of antithrombosis medication during the period of the operation and hospital stay.

> **Information Box 4.2f-I**
>
> **Osteoarthritis: comments from a Chinese medicine perspective**
>
> In Chinese medicine, the presenting features of osteoarthritis (OA) would be described as Bi Syndrome. The aching and stiffness is characteristic of Cold (Painful) and Damp (Fixed) Bi, whereas the deformities that develop in the late stages of the condition reflect Phlegm (Bony) Bi. There is always an underlying Deficiency of the Kidneys, and particularly so in OA of the knee. OA of the hip suggests that there is an additional imbalance of the Gallbladder and Liver Organs.
>
> The analgesics used in OA are suppressive in nature. Joint replacement does not affect the underlying imbalance, but strengthening the integrity and mobility of the joints would appear to be a local form of nourishing Kidney and Liver Qi and Yin. For this reason, glucosamine might be described as a Kidney Yin tonic.

A replacement joint is said to last about 10 years before it may need further replacement, but many joints appear to survive longer than this.

Rheumatoid arthritis

Rheumatoid arthritis (RA) is a symmetrical inflammatory and deforming arthritis. It is the result of an autoimmune process. The underlying problem in RA is that the body develops autoantibodies which are targeted at the synovial membrane that overlies the cartilage within synovial joints. Other tissues may well be affected by autoimmune damage. This means that RA is an example of a multisystem autoimmune disease.

The synovial lining of the joints in RA becomes very inflamed and thickened. It spreads within the joint space as a boggy tissue called 'pannus' and deprives the cartilage in the joint of nutrients. Pannus also causes thinning and destruction of the bone adjacent to the joint. As the disease progresses, the joint becomes more deformed.

RA is common, affecting 1–3% of the population, but is far less common than OA. It generally starts at an earlier age than OA (from 30–50 years of age) and affects women more commonly than men, particularly in younger age groups. There is a tendency for it to run in families, but less markedly so than for OA. RA is more common in damp and cold climates. RA can affect children. Childhood arthritis has slightly different features to adult RA and is discussed in more detail in Section 5.4.

The first symptoms are pain and stiffness of the joints associated with a sense of illness and fever. Stiffness is characteristically worse in the morning and, unlike the stiffness of OA, which improves within a few minutes with movement, may persist for more than an hour after waking. The joints most commonly affected are the small joints of the hands and feet, and the wrists, elbow, knees and ankles. The affected joints are usually warm, tender and slightly swollen. In some people the condition begins with brief episodes of inflammation of a single joint, which may only last for 1–2 days, and then eventually develops into a more generalised form of arthritis.

Up to 25% of cases of RA can be expected to recover completely after the initial flare-up. In some cases the acute condition lasts only a matter of months before it settles down again without leaving any permanent damage, and in other cases, despite a course of a few years, the condition settles down leaving only minimal damage. However, the usual pattern is that the initial condition persists, flaring up from time to time, and over the course of a few years leads to progressive damage to the joints and other parts of the body. In these cases, the initially swollen joints become permanently deformed by the development of pannus within the joint.

In very severe cases the following problems may develop:

- In the hands and feet the fingers and toes tend to point in the ulnar direction, and to assume permanent misshapen positions (Figure 4.2f-IV).
- The muscles around the shoulder may waste and the tendons may rupture, leading to an inability to perform basic activities of daily living such as washing and dressing.
- The knees may become very swollen and deformed, although the hips are only rarely affected.
- RA in the neck can be of very serious consequence because parts of the bony vertebrae may become weakened or destroyed. The vertebrae may slip slightly against one another and place excessive pressure of the spinal cord. This may lead to spinal cord compression (see Chapter 4.1g), which requires emergency surgery.

The other parts of the body that can become affected in RA are shown in Figure 4.2f-V. Other aspects of musculoskeletal damage include muscle wasting around affected joints, for the same reason as it occurs in OA. The tendons can become inflamed (tendonitis), which means that they can become swollen, painful and may rupture. Also, the synovial membrane inside a bursa may become inflamed, leading to a tense, swollen, hot lump within the soft tissue close to a joint (bursitis). Another cause of lumps in the soft tissue is the formation of nodules. These lumps are unique to RA. They tend to form close to the elbow and other parts of the body exposed to recurrent pressure. Nodules are the result of a focus of autoimmune damage within the soft tissue.

The autoimmune process of RA can also lead to progressive scarring of the lung tissue, damage to single nerves (mononeuropathy) and polyneuropathy (see Chapter 4.1g), inflammation of the white of the eye (scleritis), dry eyes, kidney

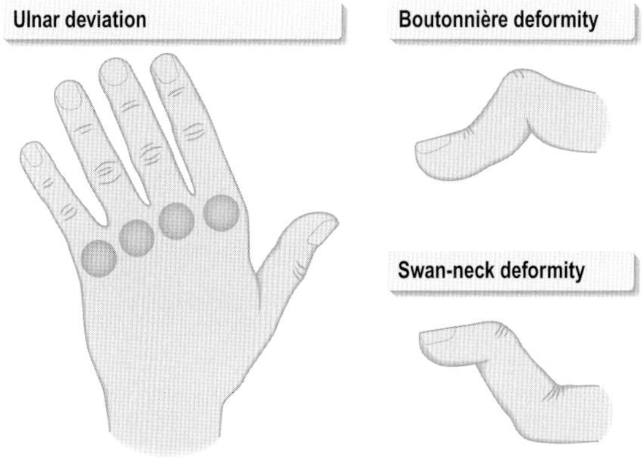

Figure 4.2f-IV • Characteristic hand deformities in rheumatoid arthritis.

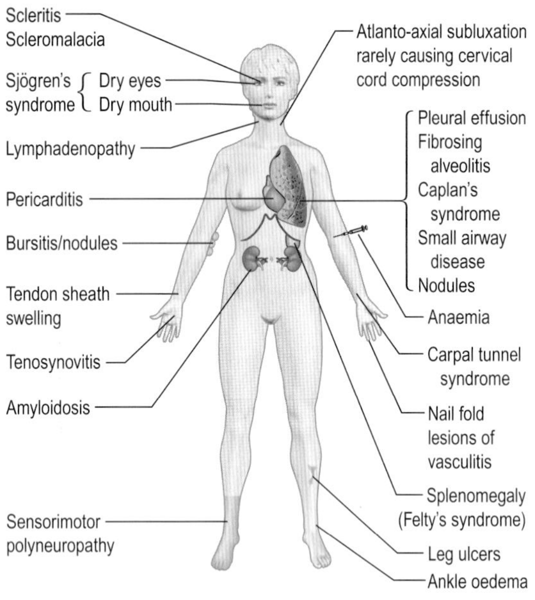

Figure 4.2f-V • Systemic complications of rheumatoid arthritis.

damage and inflammation of the small blood vessels of the skin (vasculitis). In addition to these problems, anaemia of chronic disease and depletion of immune cells may also occur.

RA is diagnosed on the basis of the characteristic clinical features, X-ray images of the joints and by means of blood tests. In RA a FBC will often reveal anaemia of chronic disease, and the ESR and CRP are raised, indicating an inflammatory process (see Chapter 3.4b). In about 70% of cases a particular antibody, called 'rheumatoid factor', is present in the serum. These so-called seropositive cases of RA are more likely to progress to severe multisystem forms of the disease. It follows that in 30% of cases this specific antibody is not detectable, and in these instances the diagnosis is made mainly on the basis of the joint changes found on examination.

Treatment involves both symptom control, usually by means of NSAID medication, and a disease-modifying approach. Disease-modifying antirheumatoid drugs (DMARDs) are prescribed because they tend to inhibit the destructive inflammatory process. Some of the DMARDs are immunosuppressants used in other conditions such as cancer control. The DMARDs include leflunomide, sulfasalazine, methotrexate, gold (auranofin), penicillamine and hydroxychloroquine. Sulfasalazine is one of the most commonly prescribed DMARDs. It is also used in other forms of arthritis, such as ankylosing spondylitis and psoriatic arthritis. This is the same drug that is used to treat and prevent relapses of ulcerative colitis. All DMARDs have a number of potentially serious side-effects. These include damage to the blood cells, liver damage, kidney damage, visual damage and severe skin rashes, depending on the individual drug.

The current medical opinion is that DMARDs may be prescribed early after the diagnosis of RA (especially if seropositive for rheumatoid factor) despite their potential side-effects, because they will reduce the risk of long-term damage to the interior of the joint by inflammation. Because the patient requires monitoring for adverse effects and response to treatment, all patients with RA are best managed by a hospital specialist. Usually only one drug is prescribed at a time, and is initially given for a few weeks to months to see how well the patient responds. Poor response or the development of side-effects will necessitate a change to another DMARD.

Corticosteroids are powerful disease-modifying drugs, but are used only in very severe intractable cases of RA because of the problems with long-term side-effects (see Chapter 2.2c). Corticosteroids are also given in RA by injection into inflamed joints or around inflamed tendons. In cases in which there is multisystem involvement, with the threat of damage to major organs such as the kidney, corticosteroids used to be the only option available to prevent disease progression. However, a new range of immune-system-modifying drugs are now increasingly being prescribed instead of oral steroids in severe cases of RA that is unresponsive to DMARDs. These counteract the action of a mediator of the immune response called 'tumour necrosis factor' (TNF), which is recognised to be overactive in RA. These drugs include infliximab and adalimumab (anti-TNF antibodies) and etanercept (a TNF receptor blocker).

Physiotherapy is an important aspect of the treatment of RA. In acute flare-ups, the damage to the joints can be minimised by splinting the joints in a fixed position. In between flare-ups, graded exercises and hydrotherapy can aid mobility and muscle strength.

Surgery may be performed for a range of reasons in severe RA. The excess pannus in an inflamed joint can be removed surgically to minimise deformity early in the condition. Surgical alteration of the shape of some of the bones close to the joints may relieve pressure points that have developed as a result of joint deformity. With advanced technology, the large joints of the body can now all be replaced with plastic and metal prostheses. In the case of impending cervical cord compression, a surgical approach may be necessary to stabilise the cervical vertebrae.

Information Box 4.2f-II

Rheumatoid arthritis: comments from a Chinese medicine perspective

In Chinese medicine, the initial presentation of rheumatoid arthritis (RA) with hot and stiff joints corresponds to Hot and Damp (fixed) Bi. In some cases, Cold and Damp Bi may have been the first presentation, but the Cold rapidly turns to Heat. The progression of the condition to the development of permanent deformity is an indication of the accumulation of Phlegm (Bony Bi). Rheumatoid nodules also correspond to Phlegm. The wasting of muscles and tendons, the weakening of the bones and the damage to other systems of the body indicate a severe underlying Deficiency of Spleen Qi, Liver Yin and Kidney Yin and Yang.

The NSAIDs are warming and initially Clear Heat by Moving Stagnation. The DMARDs and corticosteroids also have Warming properties. The long-term problem with these drugs is that they appear to deplete Blood and Yin, as evidenced by blood disorders and heat symptoms. All the drugs used to treat RA are suppressive in nature.

Arthritis in other autoimmune diseases

A few of the other multisystem autoimmune diseases involve the musculoskeletal system, and this is the reason for their alternative collective name of 'rheumatic autoimmune disease'.

The most common of these conditions which affects the joints rather than the muscles is systemic lupus erythematosus (SLE). SLE is a condition in which autoantibodies cause damage to the kidneys, skin and hair follicles, the lining of the lungs and the heart as well as the joints. It tends to affect women significantly more than men. The diagnosis can be confirmed by the presence of antinuclear antibodies (present in 95% of cases) and anti-double-stranded DNA antibodies (present in 60% of cases). The affected patient suffers from symptoms in episodes known as 'relapses'. These can then subside ('remit'), leaving disease-free intervals. Important symptoms include tiredness and fever, a facial rash, and muscle and joint aches. A serious relapse can involve symptoms of damage to deep organs, including the heart, lungs, kidneys and brain, and if signs of organ damage are apparent, immunosuppressant drugs including hydroxychloroquine, cyclophosphamide and high-dose corticosteroids, may be prescribed. Low-dose steroids or azathioprine may be used as maintenance treatment to prevent relapses occurring in vulnerable patients in remission. More recently, the antibody drug Rituximab, which targets the overactive B lymphocytes in SLE, has shown some promising benefits.

The other rheumatic autoimmune diseases include systemic sclerosis and dermatomyositis.

Ankylosing spondylitis

Ankylosing spondylitis is an inflammatory arthritis that primarily affects the vertebrae and sacroiliac joints. It tends to cluster in families, and its effects are more serious in men than women.

The cause of the inflammation is unknown, although it is known that almost all people who develop ankylosing spondylitis are more likely to have a certain type of genetic make-up (known as HLA B27), which is found in 8% of the population. It is believed that this genetic constitution gives susceptibility to developing the condition. There is as yet no evidence of any autoimmune damage in ankylosing spondylitis.

The condition usually first presents with episodes of pain in the sacroiliac joints in early adulthood. The pain can radiate into the buttocks, and as with most forms of arthritis the pain and stiffness are worse in the morning. At an early stage of the disease the patient may also be prone to other inflammatory musculoskeletal conditions, such as inflammation of the joints between the ribs over the front of the chest (costochondritis) or within the soft tissue of the heel (plantar fasciitis). Inflammation of the interior of the eye (uveitis) is also relatively common in people with ankylosing spondylitis. In some people the large joints, in particular the hip, are affected.

In severe cases, the mobility of the sacroiliac joints and the intervertebral joints gradually becomes greatly reduced as bony osteophytes grow out and cause the bones to fuse across the joints (the term 'ankylosing' refers to this phenomenon). In severe cases, the ribs cannot expand freely as their joints are also affected, and breathing becomes laboured. The thoracic part of the chest and the neck can become very bowed, so much so that the person may be unable to look straight ahead.

This severe degree of rigidity can be prevented, at least in part, if the condition is diagnosed early and the patient encouraged to perform regular back exercises. NSAIDs and sulfasalazine may be prescribed for their symptom-relieving properties, as pain relief will enable exercises to be performed more freely. The new anti-TNF drugs infliximab, adalimumab and etanercept, which are known to be of benefit in advanced RA, are licensed for use in ankylosing spondylitis, although long-term benefit is yet to be proven.

Although the majority of patients with ankylosing spondylitis live normal lives, nearly a fifth become moderately to severely disabled by the condition.

> **Information Box 4.2f-III**
>
> **Ankylosing spondylitis: comments from a Chinese medicine perspective**
>
> In Chinese medicine, the symptoms of ankylosing spondylitis (AS) of stiffness, rigidity and pain in the sacroiliac joints and hips suggests a diagnosis of Qi Stagnation in the Liver and Gallbladder Channels against a background of a Kidney Deficiency.
>
> The symptomatic treatments, NSAIDs and sulfasalazine, are both Warming in nature and can move Stagnation, although in the long run will be depleting to Yin and Blood. A gentle exercise programme is an energetically appropriate approach, as it will enable the Movement of Stagnation without being depleting.

Psoriatic arthritis

Psoriasis is a fairly common inflammatory scaling disorder of the skin (see Chapter 6.1c). Up to 8% of people with psoriasis will develop one of a number of forms of arthritis. In some cases the arthritis appears before the skin disorder. It can be triggered by exposure to damp and cold climates.

The arthritis is typically symmetrical and inflammatory in nature. The most common form involves the finger joints only, and in this case deformities and pitting of the nails are common. In other forms the arthritis can be much more widely distributed and can be very similar to RA. In addition, it is not uncommon for tendonitis and bursitis to occur. It is a characteristic of psoriatic arthritis that, as well as the synovial membrane becoming inflamed, the bone adjacent to the joint can become eroded. In less than 5% of cases this bony erosion is so severe that the integrity of joints is seriously compromised (Figure 4.2f-VI).

In most cases NSAIDs are all that is needed to provide symptom relief. In more serious cases, sulfasalazine or other immunosuppressants may be prescribed to control the progression of the disease.

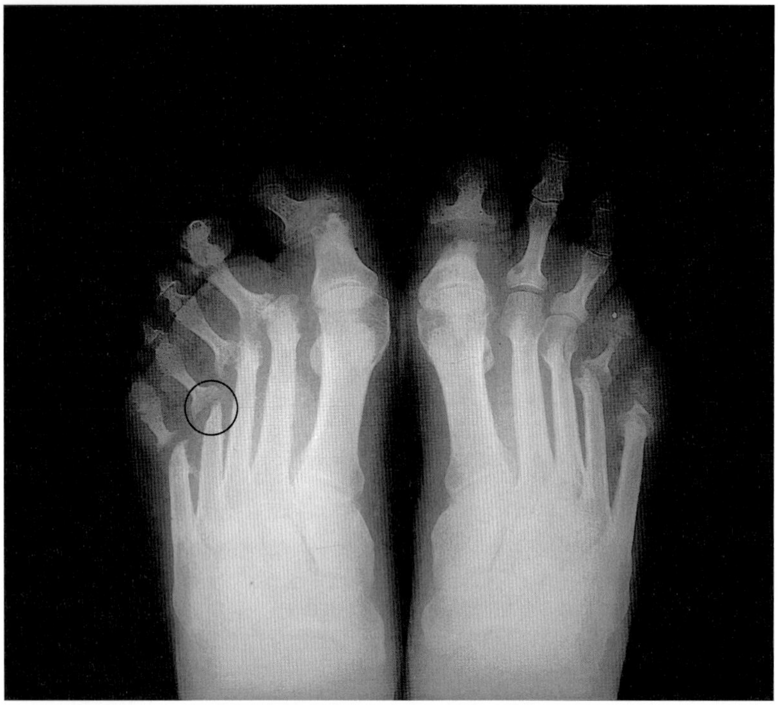

Figure 4.2f-VI • X-ray image of feet in psoriatic arthritis, showing deformities of the toes • The circled area shows a total loss of bone on the head of the fourth metatarsal and a hollowing of the proximal end of the fourth proximal phalanx.

> **Information Box 4.2f-IV**
>
> **Psoriatic arthritis: comments from a Chinese medicine perspective**
>
> In Chinese medicine, the diagnosis of psoriatic arthritis is similar to that of rheumatoid arthritis, in that it would correspond to a form of Damp and Hot Bi against a background of Deficiency. In some cases this may be precipitated by an initial invasion of Damp Cold. In psoriasis the scaling, inflamed skin would be attributed to Heat (and sometimes Damp) upon an underlying Deficiency of Blood and Yin.

Gout

Gout is an inflammatory arthritis that results from the formation of crystals of uric acid (also known as 'urate') within the synovial fluid. Uric acid is a by-product of the normal metabolic processes of the body. It is produced in excess if there is a high amount of cholesterol, beer, offal, fish and shellfish in the diet, or if there is a high turnover of cells in the body, such as might occur in cancer. Uric acid is usually excreted by the kidneys so that its levels do not rise too high. However, excretion from the kidneys may be impaired in certain situations, including following excessive exercise, in starvation and following excessive alcohol intake. Certain drugs, including thiazide diuretics and aspirin, can also impair the excretion of uric acid.

If the concentration of uric acid in the blood becomes too high, which might occur as a combination of excessive production of uric acid and impaired excretion, crystals of uric acid can come out of solution within the synovial fluid. The crystals are engulfed by leukocytes, but this then causes these cells to rupture and release inflammatory chemicals into the joint. This triggers the process of inflammation.

Commonly, the arthritis of gout is confined to a single joint, often the first metatarsophalangeal joint (at the base of the big toe). However, large joints, such as the knee or ankle, might also be affected. The affected joint becomes acutely inflamed and swollen, and is intensely painful. The attack may be precipitated by a 'binge' of drinking and eating to excess or by a period of dehydration. Not uncommonly, a prescription of diuretics can provoke an attack. Men are affected more often than women, and attacks are more likely in older people. Less commonly, the arthritis can be more generalised, and affects a number of joints. This form of gout is more prevalent in elderly people.

If the uric acid level is very high, the crystals may form not only in the joint but also in the soft tissues. This leads to large, slightly inflamed, white deposits called 'tophi'. Tophi might appear in various sites, including the tissues surrounding joints and the ear lobes. In these cases there is a possibility that crystals may also be deposited within the delicate tissue of the kidney. This is a serious situation that requires prompt medical treatment.

Gout is diagnosed by examination of joint fluid for crystals (not always performed) and by a serum blood test for uric acid levels, which will show high–normal to high levels.

An acute attack of gout is treated by encouraging a high fluid intake, and prescription of NSAIDs to calm down the inflammation and relieve the intense pain.

If attacks are frequent and do not respond to dietary advice and alcohol reduction, allopurinol is prescribed to be taken on a regular basis. This drug reduces the production of uric acid in the body. A severe but very rare side-effect is depletion of blood cell production in the marrow. More commonly, skin rashes may occur.

Information Box 4.2f-V

Acute gout: comments from a Chinese medicine perspective

In Chinese medicine, the intense pain of acute gout would correspond to Heat and Damp Bi. Tophi would be described as a manifestation of Phlegm. Foods that precipitate attacks tend to be Damp Heat forming, as is alcohol. The most likely site for an attack is the big toe, and this position might suggest an underlying Liver or Spleen disharmony. An underlying Deficiency of Kidney Yin may also be present.

Arthritis in infectious disease

A temporary generalised arthritis is a very common occurrence either during or following a number of viral infections. For example, the childhood infection of rubella often causes joint aches, particularly in adults who contract the infection. Chickenpox, glandular fever and mumps are other common causes. In some cases the aching of the joints can persist for a few days to weeks after the infection has settled down.

Some bacterial infections may also affect the joints. The most common of these in the UK is the sexually transmitted disease of gonorrhoea. The infection by the *Gonococcus* bacterium spreads from the genital tract, and leads to a fever and a prolonged period of joint aches and swelling. Gonococcal arthritis is most common in women and homosexual men. It responds to antibiotic treatment.

Information Box 4.2f-VI

Arthritis associated with acute infections: comments from a Chinese medicine perspective

In Chinese medicine, acute arthritis associated with infection might often correspond to Wind and Heat Bi following an invasion of Wind Heat.

In some susceptible patients an inflammatory arthritis (not unlike early RA or ankylosing spondylitis) develops as a delayed reaction to infection by some of the gastrointestinal or sexually transmitted organisms (including *Salmonella*, *Shigella* and *Chlamydia*). In most cases this arthritis will settle down within weeks, but in some a progressive condition develops. In severe cases, attacks of uveitis might occur, and episodes of tendonitis and plantar fasciitis can develop (as can occur in ankylosing spondylitis). This 'reactive arthritis' is treated with NSAIDs. If the arthritis is progressive, DMARDs and corticosteroids, as used in RA or ankylosing spondylitis, may be prescribed. The new anti-TNF drugs infliximab, adalimumab and etanercept may have a role in severe, unremitting cases.

Rheumatic fever is a rare complication of infection with the *Streptococcus* bacterium (most commonly in the form of tonsillitis). It is much more common in the Middle and Far East, eastern Europe and South America. It mostly tends to affect children and adolescents. In this condition the bacterial infection triggers a delayed autoimmune response, which primarily affects the joints but can also affect the heart, skin and nervous system.

Information Box 4.2f-VII

Reactive arthritis: comments from a Chinese medicine perspective

The Chinese medicine interpretation of reactive arthritis would be similar to that for rheumatoid arthritis or ankylosing spondylitis. In reactive arthritis, it is likely that the initial infection has led to the accumulation of the Pathogenic Factors of Damp and Heat.

Rheumatic fever follows on from a streptococcal infection with a sudden onset of high fever, joint pains and malaise. The joints are red, swollen and exquisitely tender, and the pain and swelling 'flits' from one joint to another. In some cases there are irregularities of the heart rhythm and heart murmurs due to inflammation of the pericardium and heart valves. There may also be a pink skin rash, which spreads across the skin. A very severe late complication is Sydenham's chorea (also known as St Vitus' dance), which is a disorder of movement and speech resulting from damage to the nerve centres deep in the brain.

Treatment of rheumatic fever includes bed rest and antibiotics to eradicate the streptococcal infection. The joint pains respond to high-dose aspirin. Corticosteroids may be given to limit damage to the heart.

In most cases the symptoms subside within 3 weeks, but in some patients symptoms persist for much longer and the arthritis can become long-standing.

About one-tenth of those who experience inflammation of the heart and valves in the acute infection will go on to develop progressive valve damage in late adulthood (see Chapter 3.2g).

Information Box 4.2f-VIII

Rheumatoid arthritis: comments from a Chinese medicine perspective

In Chinese medicine, an attack of rheumatoid arthritis might be diagnosed as Wind Heat Invasion with Wind (Moving) and Heat Bi. The development of cardiac complications suggests that the Heat in this condition can be very full and can damage Heart Yin.

Generalised disorders of the muscles and ligaments

Fibromyalgia (fibrositis)

'Fibromyalgia' is a term used by some conventional practitioners to describe a condition in which the muscles, particularly of the back and shoulders, are tense and very tender.

The tenderness is often focused in certain defined areas called 'trigger points'. Often a 'knot' or area of very tense muscle is located at a trigger point. Fibromyalgia is recognised to be more common in women and to be associated with emotional disharmony of one sort or another.

A patient with the symptoms of fibromyalgia may also suffer from the symptoms of other functional conditions such as - irritable bowel syndrome (IBS), myalgic encephalomyelitis (ME), premenstrual syndrome (PMS) or recurrent headaches.

NSAIDs may be given to relieve the pain, and counselling or antidepressants may be considered to treat the emotional foundation of the condition. It is recognised that the trigger points may be relieved by corticosteroid injections, deep massage or acupuncture.

> **Information Box 4.2f-IX**
>
> **Fibromyalgia: comments from a Chinese medicine perspective**
>
> In Chinese medicine, fibromyalgia represents Liver Qi and Blood Stagnation. There may be an underlying Deficiency of Spleen Qi and/or Liver Blood.

Polymyalgia rheumatica

Polymyalgia rheumatica (PMR) is an inflammatory condition of the arteries which leads to severe pain and stiffness in the large muscle groups of the shoulders and hips. Like another inflammatory disorder of the arteries, temporal arteritis (see Chapter 4.1e), it is a condition that primarily affects elderly people. Women are affected more commonly than men.

The patient is often unwell, with fever, exhaustion and depression. There may be an overlap with the symptoms of temporal arteritis. If a one-sided headache develops it should be treated very seriously as a warning sign of an impending loss of vision or stroke.

In terms of blood-test abnormalities, PMR is associated with a raised ESR, mild anaemia and a raised alkaline phosphatase level on testing of liver function.

Treatment is initially with a moderate dose of corticosteroids (10–15 mg/ daily), which always leads to a dramatic reduction in symptoms and an improvement in well-being. Most people need to be on this medication for at least a year, and for about a quarter of these this treatment has to be life-long in order to keep symptoms at bay.

As long-term steroid treatment can cause osteoporosis, patients being treated for PMR will also often be prescribed 'bone-protecting' drugs such as a bisphosphonates, calcium and vitamin D.

> **Information Box 4.2f-X**
>
> **Polymyalgia rheumatica and arteritis: comments from a Chinese medicine perspective**
>
> In Chinese medicine, the symptoms of arteritis might suggest Heat and Stagnation in the blood vessels. As this is a condition of elderly people, there is a possibility that the Heat may have been generated as a result of chronic deficiency of Kidney Yin. The intense aching and stiffness of polymyalgia is also a reflection of severe Qi Stagnation, and its distribution often relates to the Gallbladder and Bladder channels.
>
> Corticosteroids are Warming in nature and Clear Stagnation by Moving Qi. In the long term they will further deplete Kidney Yin and Jing.

Muscular dystrophy

The muscular dystrophies are a group of inherited disorders that result in a progressive degeneration of skeletal muscle. In some forms the cardiac muscle is also affected.

Duchenne muscular dystrophy is the most common form, affecting 1 in 4000 male infants. The genetic defect leads to an absence of a protein essential for the maturation of skeletal muscle. The muscular dystrophy becomes obvious in early childhood, when the child loses the ability to run with ease or to stand up from the floor without support. By the age of 10 years the muscles of the limbs are very wasted, and the child becomes severely disabled. Death is inevitable between the ages of 15 and 25 years, and usually results from respiratory infections.

There are less severe forms of muscular dystrophy. Of the two next most common forms, one results in a severe but not life-threatening disability by early adulthood, and the other causes a relative muscle weakness, particularly of the upper body, but life expectancy is normal.

For all forms of muscular dystrophy, the only treatment is supportive, including physiotherapy to prevent muscle contractures. Genetic counselling with respect to future pregnancies may be offered to parents and siblings.

> **Information Box 4.2f-XI**
>
> **Muscular dystrophy: comments from a Chinese medicine perspective**
>
> In Chinese medicine, the symptoms of muscular dystrophy would indicate Jing Deficiency. Weak and wasted muscles are an indication of additional Deficiency of Spleen and Liver Qi.

The red flags of generalised disorders of the joints, ligaments and muscles

Some patients with the generalised disorders of the joints, ligaments and muscles will benefit from referral to a conventional doctor for assessment and/or treatment. Red flags are those symptoms and signs that indicate that referral is to be considered. The red flags of the generalised disorders of the joints, ligament and muscles are described in Table 4.2f-I. This table forms part of the summary on red flags given in Appendix III, which also gives advice on the degree of urgency of referral for each of the red flag conditions listed.

Table 4.2f-I Red Flags 28 – generalised diseases of the joints, ligaments and muscles

Red Flag	Description	Reasoning
28.1	**Features of a degenerative arthritis which may benefit from joint replacement**: severe disability from long-standing pain and stiffness in the hips, knees or shoulders	Many complementary therapies can provide very helpful supportive treatment in advanced osteoarthritis of the hip, knee or shoulder. Referral needs to be considered if the condition is deteriorating to a point where activities of daily living are becoming compromised. Refer relatively early, as the patient may need to be put on a waiting list, meaning that surgical treatment may only come after a delay of some weeks to months
28.2	**Any features of an inflammatory arthritis**: symmetrical pain, stiffness and swelling of the joints or symmetrical stiffness and pain in the sacroiliac joint. May be associated with a fever or sense of malaise	All episodes of inflammatory arthritis (distinguished from osteoarthritis by fairly rapid onset over days to weeks rather than months to years, joint swelling, fever and general malaise) are best investigated by a conventional practitioner so that autoimmune disease or other serious underlying disease can be excluded. Some forms of inflammatory arthritis are erosive, and powerful medical approaches need to be considered to prevent progression and permanent joint damage
28.3	**Features of polymyalgia rheumatica**: prolonged pain and stiffness and weakness of the muscles of the hips and shoulders associated with malaise and depression. Refer urgently if there is a sudden onset of a severe one-sided temporal headache or visual disturbances	Polymyalgia rheumatica is an inflammatory condition of the muscles of the shoulders and hips that predominantly afflicts people over the age of 50 years. Because it is inflammatory in nature there may be associated malaise, but the main symptoms are pain and weakness of the shoulder and hip muscles. Difficulty in standing from a sitting position is a classic sign of weakness in the hip muscles There is an increased risk of the serious condition of temporal arteritis, and referral would enable the patient to make a decision about whether to take the medical treatment of corticosteroids (see Red Flag Table A23 in Appendix III)

Self-test 4.2f

The generalised diseases of the joints, ligaments and muscles

1. Stephen is 25 years old. He has noticed some uncomfortable back pain for some time now, especially in his lower back. His back feels particularly bad in the morning, and gets better as the day goes on. There is no history of sudden injury or exertion to explain the pain. When you examine his back you find tenderness that symmetrically overlies the sacroiliac joints. Stephen's posture is slightly hunched.
   (i) What inflammatory condition could this be?
   (ii) Would you refer Stephen for conventional investigation?
2. Gladys is 75 years old. Recently she has been feeling very tired and a bit out of sorts. She has been feeling achy for a few weeks now, especially in the shoulders. It is a real effort now even to lift her arms to brush her hair or wash. She also finds it quite an effort to stand when she has been sitting in an armchair. What is the serious conventional diagnosis that these symptoms suggest?

Answers

1. (i) This may be early ankylosing spondylitis. It is otherwise very unusual for a young man to suffer from symmetrical sacroiliac pain without a history of injury. The other possibility is a reactive arthritis following an infection or inflammatory bowel disease.
   (ii) You would be wise to refer Stephen to his GP so that he can be correctly diagnosed and, if ankylosing spondylitis is confirmed, advised about a programme of preventive exercises.
2. This is a classic history of polymyalgia rheumatica. If Gladys is referred to her GP and the diagnosis confirmed, she will be prescribed a high-dose steroid medication. You need to discuss this possibility with her. If she would like to defer referral and see how your treatment helps, you need to warn her of the warning sign of a severe one-sided temporal headache. She needs to be told that if she develops this, she should make an urgent appointment with her GP to exclude temporal arteritis.

The urinary system

4.3

Chapter 4.3a The physiology of the urinary system

LEARNING POINTS

At the end of this chapter you will be able to:

- explain the basic structure of the kidneys and the urinary tract
- describe the principles of how the blood that flows through the kidneys is filtered to produce urine
- describe the roles of the kidney in the excretion of wastes, the homeostasis of the concentration of the blood, the manufacture of red blood cells and the control of blood pressure.

Estimated time for chapter: 120 minutes.

Introduction

The urinary system consists of the kidneys, the ureters, the bladder and the urethra. The urinary system may also be called the 'renal system', although strictly speaking 'renal' (from the Latin term for kidney) is a term that refers to the kidneys alone. The Greek term for kidney is 'nephron', and hence the study of the kidneys is called 'nephrology'.

The component parts of the urinary system are illustrated in Figure 4.3a-I. It can be seen how the kidneys are situated in the upper part of the back of the abdomen. They rest protected against the ribs between the levels of T11 and L3. The influential acupoints on the back of the Kidney Organ (Shenshu Bl-23) lie directly over the lower parts of the kidneys. The ureters run from the medial aspect of each kidney, down the posterior border of the abdominal cavity, to open into the bladder. The bladder sits protected within the pelvis. Note from the diagram how small the bladder is. Even when uncomfortably full the bladder rarely rises very much higher than the level of the pubic symphysis (the region of acupoint Qugu Rn-2). The urethra (similarly spelled to the more proximal ureter, but a different anatomical structure) is the tube that links the bladder to the external world. It is very short in women, but longer in men because of its passage through the penis.

The major function of the kidneys is to maintain homeostasis of the composition of the blood by excreting wastes and controlling the concentrations of the various mineral salts within the blood. It does this by the formation and excretion of urine, which is a solution of wastes and salts. Other important functions include the control of the blood pressure, control of the development of the red blood cells by the secretion of the hormone erythropoietin, and production of active vitamin D.

The function of the ureters is to allow the free drainage of the urine into the bladder. The bladder is a reservoir that contains this steady flow of urine from the kidneys until there is an appropriate time for its expulsion. This happens through the process of urination (also known as 'micturition'), in which the bladder contracts and the urine passes through the urethra and out of the body.

The physiology of the kidneys

The position and structure of the kidneys

The kidneys sit at the back of the upper abdominal cavity embedded in fat. The adrenal glands sit on the top of each kidney, but do not have a direct link with the role of the urinary system. However, both the adrenal glands and the kidneys have functions that would be understood in Chinese medicine as being related to the Kidney Organ. The kidneys sit very close to a number of other deep organs, including the spleen, pancreas, liver, duodenum and the large intestine.

The tissue of the kidney consists of thousands of tiny tubes called 'nephrons'. Each of these tubes has its origin in the outer parts of the substance of the kidney (the renal cortex). The nephrons converge to open out into wider tubes called 'collecting tubules', which drain into a space in the core of the kidney called the 'renal pelvis'. The renal pelvis drains

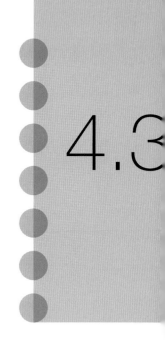

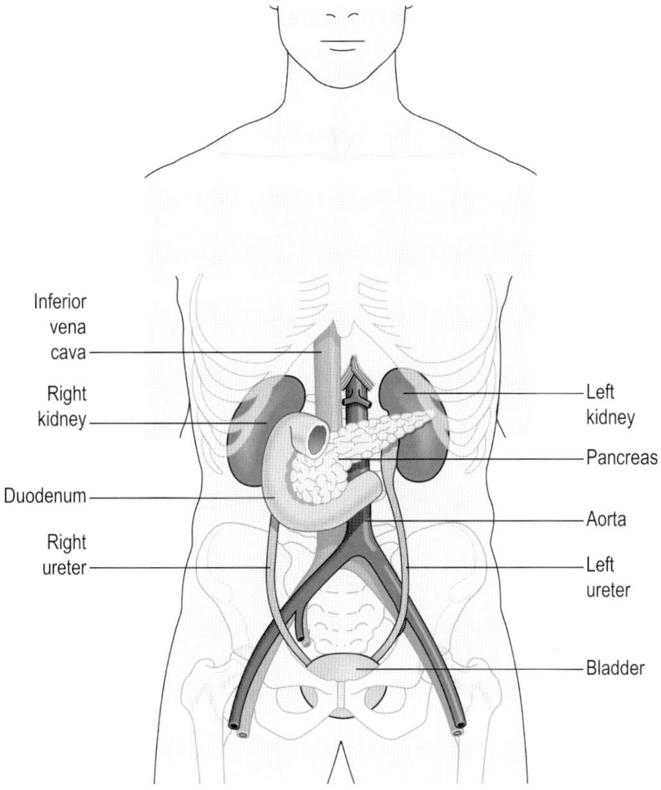

Figure 4.3a-I • The component parts of the urinary system (excluding the urethra) and related abdominal structures.

downwards into the ureter. The collecting tubules are situated in the deeper tissue of the kidney, which is known as the 'renal medulla'. Figures 4.3a-II and 4.3a-III illustrate the external and internal structure of the kidneys in some detail. Figure 4.3a-II shows the position and size of the adrenal glands, and Figure 4.3a-III indicates the location of the renal cortex, medulla, pelvis and ureter.

These diagrams clarify how the kidneys receive their blood supply from a large branch of the aorta called the 'renal artery'.

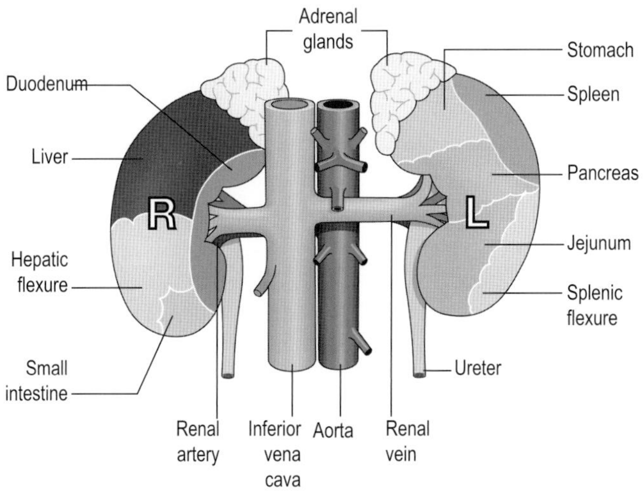

Figure 4.3a-II • Anterior view of the kidneys.

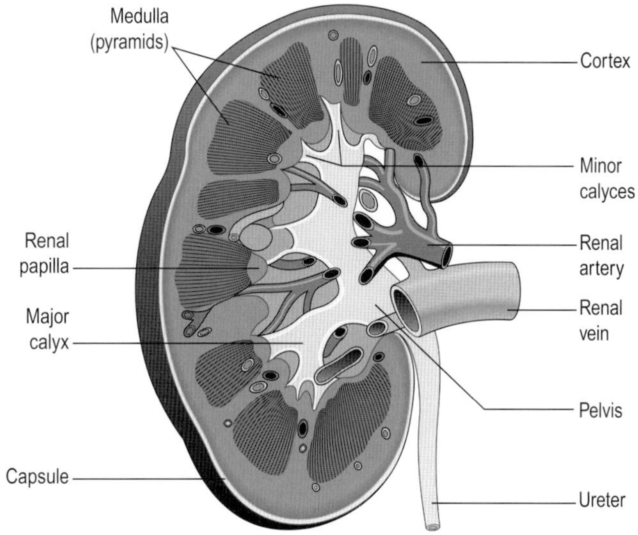

Figure 4.3a-III • Longitudinal section of the right kidney.

This artery branches within the substance of the kidney to provide each nephron with its own arteriole. The blood supply to the kidney is very rich. About one quarter of all the blood that has left the heart is directed from the aorta through the kidneys. This is very important because it ensures that the blood undergoes a continual and efficient process of being cleansed and returned to a state of balance.

The formation of urine in the kidneys

Figure 4.3a-IV shows how the blood that reaches the nephron first enters a cluster of capillaries called the 'glomerulus'. Here, because of a sudden restriction of easy flow, fluid containing salts, wastes and water is forced out of the glomerulus. From here this fluid passes into the cup-like origin of the nephron. However, substances such as plasma proteins and blood cells are too large to be squeezed out, and so these remain within the blood vessel. This process of draining water and small molecules from the blood into the nephron is called 'simple filtration'.

This fluid then drains down through the tube of the glomerulus towards the collecting tubule. However, it does not yet have the composition of urine. During its passage through the nephron some of the fluid and the salts are reabsorbed back into the bloodstream. The diagram indicates how the arteriole travels on to supply the rest of the nephron with a blood supply for this purpose. Substances can also be secreted from the blood in the arteriole into more distal parts of the nephron.

These two processes of reabsorption and secretion not only make the original fluid that has been drained out of the glomerulus much more concentrated (it is nearly 200 times as concentrated as plasma fluid), but they also allow for a subtle control of its composition according to the body's requirements. For instance, if the person is dehydrated, more water than normal is reabsorbed, and if the person is depleted in salts, more salts are reabsorbed.

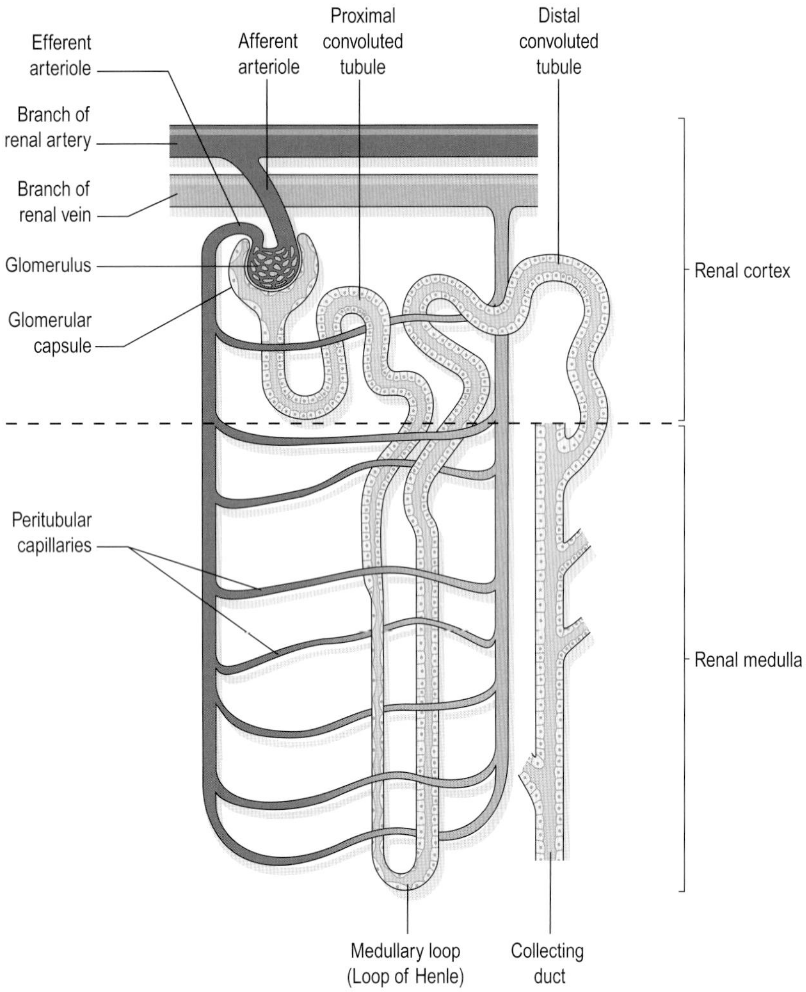

Figure 4.3a-IV • A nephron and the associated blood vessels.

The reabsorption and secretion of the fluid in the nephron are under the control of a number of hormones, including parathyroid hormone (which regulates calcium and phosphate levels), antidiuretic hormone (ADH) (which regulates the concentration of the blood) and aldosterone from the adrenal glands (which regulates the amount of sodium and potassium in the blood).

The fluid that leaves the nephron to enter the collecting tubule, and thence the renal pelvis, has the composition of urine. This yellow-coloured fluid consists mostly (96%) of water, with a further 2% being urea (the waste product of protein metabolism) and the remaining 2% comprising a range of other salts including sodium, potassium and uric acid. In a healthy adult, approximately 1–1.5 litres of urine are passed a day, although this can vary from as little as 500 millilitres to as high as 3 litres, depending on the balance of fluid intake and other fluid losses.

Diuretic drugs that act on the kidney tend to inhibit the amount of water that is reabsorbed, and so increase the volume of urine entering the renal pelvis. Some diuretic drugs may also affect the reabsorption of salts. This is why some diuretics can lead to sodium or potassium depletion, and others may cause a build up of uric acid (predisposing to an attack of gout) (see Q4.3a-1 and Q4.3a-2).

The kidneys and the formation of the red blood cells

Erythropoietin (EPO) is a hormone that is made within the kidneys in response to low levels of oxygen in the bloodstream. It is an essential factor in the production of red blood cells from the bone marrow. When blood oxygen levels drop, the secretion of EPO is stimulated, and this in turn increases the production of red blood cells from the bone marrow. These blood cells are then available to carry more oxygen, and thereby to increase the level of oxygen in the blood.

The kidneys and the control of blood pressure

Healthy kidneys are essential for the control of blood pressure, and disease of the kidneys is one of the causes of hypertension. In addition, the kidneys act in a situation of shock (low blood pressure) to conserve fluid, and so to prevent its loss into the urine. There are at least two important hormone systems that cause the kidney to excrete more fluid when the blood pressure is high and to conserve fluid when the blood pressure drops.

The hormones involved in the kidneys' control of blood pressure include aldosterone, renin, angiotensin I and II, and atrial natruriectic factor (ANP). The drugs known as the ACE inhibitors and the angiotensin II receptor blockers, which are used in the treatment of hypertension and heart failure, act by blocking the formation of one of these hormones (angiotensin II).

The kidneys and vitamin D metabolism

Although vitamin D is mostly manufactured as a response to the action of sunlight on the skin, it requires conversion within the kidneys to become active in the body. For this reason, kidney disease can be a cause of the disease of weakening of the bones known as 'osteomalacia'.

The physiology of the ureters

The ureters receive a steady flow of urine from the renal pelvis at a rate of 20–100 millilitres/hour. These structures run down the back of the abdominal cavity and enter the bladder where it sits within the pelvis. The flow of urine is aided by waves of muscular contractions that are generated by the smooth muscle fibres within the ureter walls.

The urine that enters the bladder passes through a narrowing, akin to a valve, as it enters the bladder. This important structure prevents the return of urine back into the ureter (known as 'reflux') from the bladder. The urine enters the bladder in little spurts, which occur every 10 seconds or so.

The physiology of the bladder

The bladder is a hollow, pear-shaped organ, the function of which is to act as a reservoir for urine. Figures 4.3a-V and 4.3a-VI show a vertical section through the pelvis of a woman and a man, respectively. These diagrams illustrate the position of the bladder within the pelvis. Note how in the woman the bladder sits just in front of the cervix and womb. In the man the prostate gland sits at the neck of the bladder, surrounding the first part of the urethra.

The bladder is lined by a form of epithelium called 'transitional epithelium' which has the ability to stretch. Within the wall of the bladder are sheets of smooth muscle, which together are called the 'detrusor muscle'. When the detrusor muscle contracts, it forces urine out through the urethra.

In a healthy adult the desire to urinate arises when the bladder contains more than 300 millilitres of urine. At this stage, the stretch of the bladder muscle stimulates nerve impulses so that the bladder contracts spontaneously (this is a spinal reflex). Indeed, this is what occurs both in the newborn and in someone who has had a spinal injury. However, in the healthy adult, although the sensation of a desire to urinate occurs at this stage, the brain exerts an inhibitory control on this reflex until an appropriate time arises for it to occur. This voluntary control of bladder function is usually learned during the third year of life.

The physiology of the urethra

The urethra is the canal that leaves the neck of the bladder and links it to the exterior. In women, the urethra is about 4 centimetres long, and it opens to the exterior just in front of the vaginal orifice. In men, the urethra first passes through the tissue of the prostate gland and then travels through the length of the penis to the orifice at the tip of the glans penis. Ducts open out into the first part of the male urethra through which the seminal fluid and semen are passed during ejaculation.

In both women and men the urethra passes through the region of the body called the 'perineum' which forms the floor of the pelvis. In doing so, it passes through the pelvic

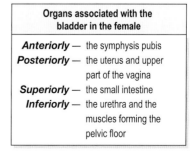

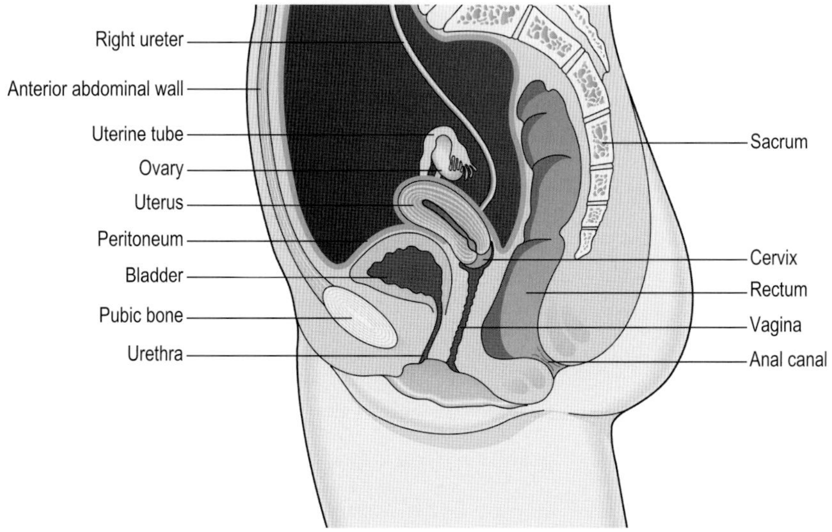

Organs associated with the bladder in the female	
Anteriorly —	the symphysis pubis
Posteriorly —	the uterus and upper part of the vagina
Superiorly —	the small intestine
Inferiorly —	the urethra and the muscles forming the pelvic floor

Figures 4.3a-V • The pelvic organs associated with the bladder in the female.

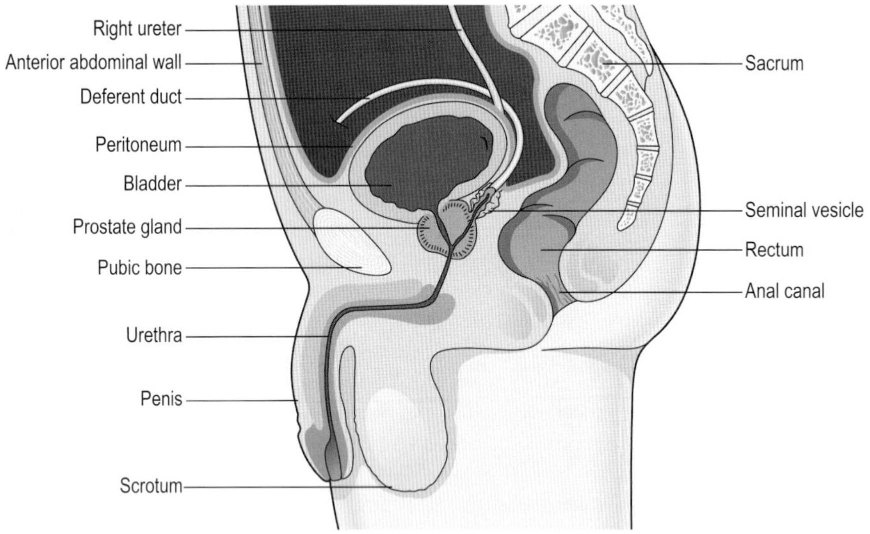

Organs associated with the bladder in the male
Anteriorly — the symphysis pubis
Posteriorly — the rectum and seminal vesicles
Superiorly — the small intestine
Inferiorly — the urethra and prostate gland

Figures 4.3a-VI • The pelvic organs associated with the bladder in the male.

floor muscles, which are slung between the pubic bone and the base of the sacrum and coccyx.

At the origin of the urethra is a smooth muscle ring called the 'internal urethral sphincter'. This sphincter is generally maintained in a state of contraction, thus holding the urine within the bladder. In addition to the internal sphincter, the muscles of the pelvic floor provide an additional 'external urethral sphincter' as a result of their generally high level of tone. Together, these factors exert a closing pressure on the urethra, which is released when the person intends to urinate.

Self-test 4.3a

The physiology of the urinary system

1. The urine in the bladder is usually sterile (i.e. free from infectious agents). If bacteria enter the bladder and multiply, this sort of infection is called cystitis.
   (i) Why do you think cystitis is more common in women than in men?
   (ii) Why do you think cystitis is common, but kidney infections rare?
2. In severe chronic kidney disease the tissue of the kidney, including the nephrons, has become permanently damaged. How do you think this might affect:
   (i) the levels of waste products in the blood, such as urea
   (ii) the health of the bones
   (iii) the health of the blood cells
   (iv) the blood pressure?

Answers

1. (i) Cystitis is more common in women for anatomical reasons. The length of the female urethra is considerably less than that of men, and thus the barrier to developing infection is reduced. Cystitis is even more common in postmenopausal women. This is because the female hormone oestrogen maintains the health of the lining cells of the vagina and the urethra. The levels of oestrogen drop after the menopause, and this leads to dryness of the vagina and weakening of the lining of the urethra.
   (ii) Although cystitis is common, it rarely spreads up the ureters to involve the kidney because of the structure of the junction between the ureters and the bladder, which prevents backflow of urine into the ureters from the bladder.
   In pregnancy, the effect of the hormone progesterone causes the muscular wall of the ureter to relax more than usual, and this can permit some backflow of urine up the ureters. Therefore, because there is a significant risk of progression to a kidney infection, in pregnancy cystitis is treated at an early stage with antibiotics.
2. (i) The levels of waste products such as urea will rise in progressive chronic renal disease. This is the basis of one of the serum blood tests for kidney function, which uses the level of urea and other waste products as a measure of the health of the kidneys.
   (ii) The bones are affected in chronic renal disease partly as a result of the lack of active vitamin D. This means that calcium is not absorbed from the diet and osteomalacia develops.
   (iii) The blood cells are affected in chronic renal disease because there is a lack of erythropoietin. This hormone is an essential factor in the manufacture of red blood cells within the bone marrow. Therefore, in chronic renal disease a severe form of "anaemia of chronic disease" develops.
   (iv) Healthy kidneys are essential for the control of blood pressure because, in health, there are at least two important hormone systems that cause the kidney to excrete more fluid when the blood pressure is high and to conserve fluid when the blood pressure drops. In some forms of chronic renal failure the blood pressure can start to rise as these systems are disrupted. This can cause further worsening of the kidney disease, as the delicate structure of the kidneys can be damaged in the state of chronic hypertension.

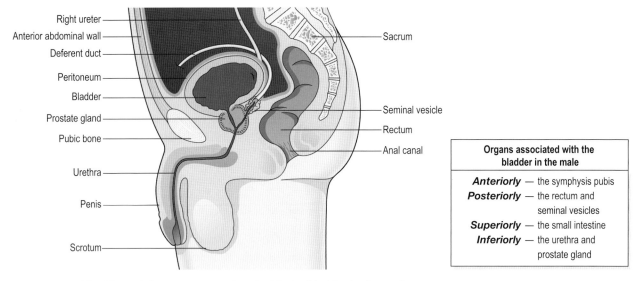

Information Box 4.3a-I

The urinary system: comments from a Chinese medicine perspective

According to traditional Chinese medicine, the functions of the Kidneys and Bladder are considered to be as follows:

- The Kidneys:
  - store Essence (Jing) and control birth, growth, reproduction and development
  - produce Marrow, fill up the brain and control bones
  - govern water
  - control the reception of Qi
  - open into the ears
  - manifest in the hair
  - control the lower two orifices
  - house the Will.
- The Bladder:
  - removes water by the power of Qi transformation.

However, according to Chinese Medicine, it is not only the Kidneys and Bladder that play a part in fluid balance and the excretion of waste. The Lungs, Spleen, Small Intestine and Triple Burner also have specific functions, which are described by Maciocia (1989) as follows:

The Lungs control dispersing and descending: The Lungs have the function of spreading the body fluids around the body in the form of a 'fine mist'. If impaired, fluid may accumulate in the form of oedema (often of the face).

The Lungs regulate the water passages: The Lungs also direct fluids down to the Kidneys and Bladder. If this function is impaired there may be urinary retention.

The Spleen governs transformation and transportation: One aspect of this is the transformation, separation and movement of fluids. In Chinese medicine the dirty part of the fluids ingested gets sent to the Small Intestine. If this function is impaired Phlegm or Damp will accumulate, sometimes in the form of oedema.

The Small Intestine controls receiving and transforming and separates Fluids. The Small Intestine first receives food and drink from the Stomach. The Clean part is sent to the Spleen, and the Dirty part to the Large Intestine (solid) and to the Bladder (fluid). This function of separation is powered by Kidney Yang.

The Triple Burner. The Simple Questions states: 'The Triple Burner is the organ in charge of irrigation and it controls the water passages'. It is the Lower Burner aspect of the Triple Burner which is directly related to the excretion of fluids. This is the aspect which directs the separation of the food essences into a dirty and clean part, and which facilitates the excretion of the dirty fluid as urine. In this way the Lower Burner is a summary of the function of the Spleen and Small Intestine.

So here it becomes clear that the Chinese medicine interpretation of the function of the urinary system is not that straightforward. First, most of the functions of the Kidney Organ do not relate directly to functions of the urinary system (e.g. storage of Essence, production of Marrow (with the exception of the effect of erythropoietin on red blood cell production), reception of Qi, opening into the ears, manifesting in the hair and housing Will power). Secondly, the actual function of the urinary system, which is to permit the continual cleansing of the blood of wastes and the removal of excess fluid into the urine, would seem to be controlled in Chinese medicine by a number of Organs (i.e. the Kidney, the Bladder, the Stomach and Spleen, the Small Intestine and the Triple Burner).

It is important to bear this in mind when considering specific diseases of the urinary system, and attempting to draw conclusions about a Chinese medicine interpretation. It is important to remember that an imbalance may be described as involving one or more of these six Chinese medicine organs.

Chapter 4.3b The investigation of the urinary system

LEARNING POINTS

At the end of this chapter you will:

- be able to recognise the main investigations used for diseases of the urinary system and male reproductive organs
- understand what a patient might experience when undergoing these investigations.

Estimated time for chapter: 60 minutes.

Introduction

Diseases of the urinary system are investigated within three distinct conventional specialties. Medical conditions that affect the kidney are treated by a renal physician within the speciality of renal medicine or nephrology. Conditions that affect the ureters, bladder and urethra, and also those conditions of the kidney that may require surgery, are treated by a surgeon called a 'urologist' within the speciality of urology. Conditions that affect the male reproductive organs are also commonly treated by a urologist. However, those conditions that result from sexually transmitted diseases are treated by a genitourinary physician within the speciality of genitourinary medicine or sexual medicine.

The investigation of the urinary system involves:

- a thorough physical examination
- examination of the urine
- examination of the blood to assay waste products and salts in the serum, autoantibodies and other markers of specific diseases, and also to look for anaemia
- imaging tests to examine the structure of the urinary system, including ultrasound scan, CT scan and plain X-ray images
- imaging tests to examine the function of the urinary system, including intravenous urography (IVU), cystourethrography and radioactive isotope scans
- examination of the inside of the bladder (cystoscopy)
- biopsy of the kidneys
- urodynamic studies.

These are each considered briefly in turn below.

Physical examination

The physical examination of the urinary system involves the stages listed in Table 4.3b-I.

Examination of the urine

The most common urine tests require a 'midstream' sample of urine (MSU). This means that the specimen is taken only after a flow of urine from the urethra has been established. The sample ideally should be free from contamination by the bacteria of the skin, although this is not always possible to ensure, particularly when collecting urine from small children. Any sterile container is suitable for a urine specimen.

Healthy urine is pale yellow and clear. The first urine passed in the morning is usually the most concentrated, and can have a deep amber colour. Visual assessment of urine may reveal a pink discoloration suggestive of blood, or cloudiness suggestive of infection. Both these findings are abnormal, but commonly result from benign causes. For example, a large amount of beetroot in the recent diet as well as some drugs can cause the urine to become pink.

The simplest quantitative test of urine involves 'dipping the urine' with a plastic strip that holds tiny indicator cards. These cards change colour according to the concentration of a range of factors within the urine. Use of the plastic dipsticks, commonly termed 'stix' or 'multistix', can give an instantaneous indication of the amount of sugar, blood, protein and white blood cells in the urine, to name just a few of the factors that can be detected. This test is not as reliable as a laboratory test, but is very commonly used in general practice to check for blood in the urine (haematuria), to give an indication of undiagnosed or poorly controlled diabetes, and to give added weight to a provisional diagnosis of urine infection.

Urine may be sent to a laboratory for microscopic examination. This may reveal the presence of microorganisms and excessive white blood cells in the case of infection. It will also confirm the presence of red blood cells in the urine. In the diseases (classed as glomerulonephritis) that affect the structure of the tubules of the kidney, unusual tube-shaped 'casts' of protein may be seen in the urine.

The urine can also be analysed for the substances that are dissolved within it. In addition to the usual body wastes, drugs and hormones can also be found in the urine. Therefore, a urine test can detect the presence of illicit drugs or increased levels of hormones. The protein in the urine should be at a very low level, but in severe kidney disease it may be present in vast quantities. Both the total protein and the albumin (the most common protein in the plasma) levels may be assessed from a urine sample. A 24-hour collection of urine may be used to quantify accurately the protein loss in kidney disease, and can also be used to assess the rate at which blood is filtered by the kidneys (glomerular filtration rate).

Table 4.3b-I The stages in the physical examination of the urinary system

- *Examination of the general appearance* for the pallor of anaemia and the 'smoky yellow' tinge of uraemia (this develops in chronic renal failure)
- *Assessment of the blood pressure*
- *Examination of the ankles* for evidence of oedema
- *Examination of the abdomen* for abnormal enlargement of the kidneys or a distended bladder (the kidneys and bladder are usually not palpable in the abdominal examination, so if they can be felt, this is a sign of distension or enlargement)
- *Examination of the male genitalia and prostate gland*: the prostate gland is examined by means of the insertion of a gloved finger through the anus into the rectum.
- *Examination of the female genitalia*: internal vaginal examination can identify uterine prolapse and posterior prolapse of the bladder wall, both causes of urinary incontinence.

Examination of the blood

A serum sample of blood can be analysed to reveal the disturbances in blood chemicals that result from kidney failure. In particular, the by-products of protein metabolism (urea and creatinine) may be increased in quantity. In severe kidney disease there may also be disturbances of the concentration of the basic mineral salts, such as sodium, calcium and potassium, in the blood. The level of creatinine may be inserted into a mathematical formula that incorporates the age, ethnicity and sex of the patient to generate an estimate of the amount of fluid filtered by the kidneys in a fixed amount of time. This is the estimated glomerular filtration rate (eGFR), which is a useful indication of the progression of chronic kidney disease, a condition that becomes increasingly prevalent with ageing.

Other factors that indicate a specific cause of kidney disease may also be assayed (e.g. autoantibodies in systemic lupus erythematosus (SLE)). In disease of the prostate gland, a particular protein called prostate-specific antigen (PSA) is assayed, as this is more likely to be raised if cancer is present.

A full blood count (FBC) may reveal the anaemia of chronic disease that can accompany chronic kidney disease.

Imaging tests to examine the structure of the urinary system

Ultrasound, magnetic resonance imaging (MRI) and computed tomography (CT) scans are used to visualise the shape of the kidneys, ureters and bladder. The images obtained may be used to examine gross defects, such as the presence of cancer or obstruction to the outflow of urine from the bladder, but cannot reveal the more subtle changes that occur in most diseases of the urinary system. An ultrasound scan obtained by means of a probe passed into the anus may also be used to examine the prostate gland.

A plain X-ray image, although it cannot show any detail about the soft tissues, may be used to reveal the presence of kidney stones, also known as 'calculi'. Figure 4.3b-I shows the X-ray images of the passage over time of a calculus down the left ureter.

A catheter (a plastic tube) may be passed into the bladder via the urethra to inject a 'dye' which is opaque to X-rays into the bladder. This test, known as 'cystography' or 'urography', can show up defects in the structure of the bladder.

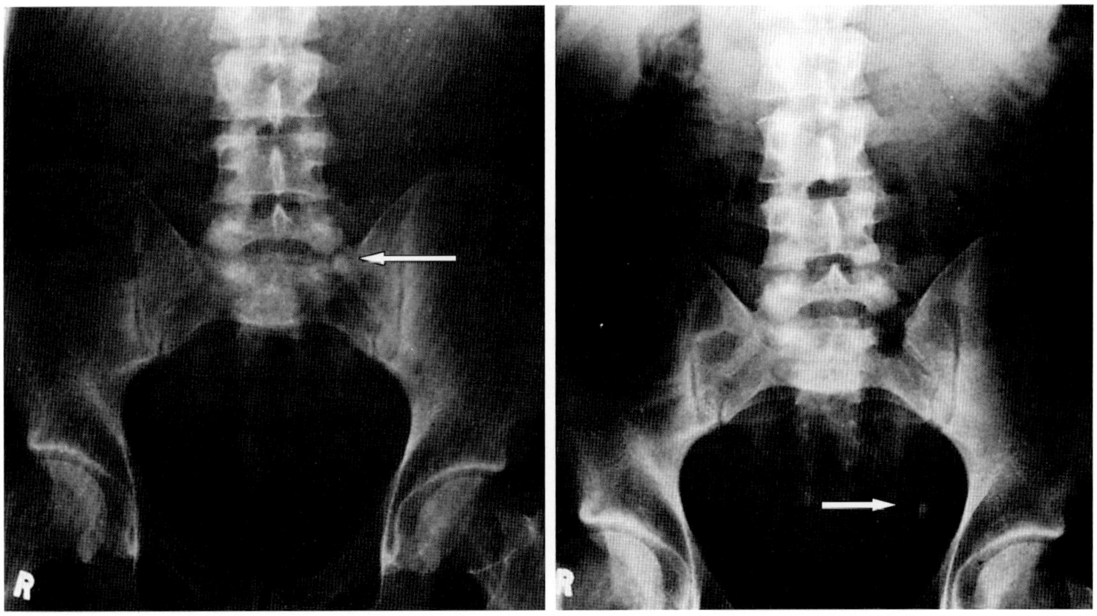

Figure 4.3b-I • X-ray images of calculi at different levels of the left ureter.

Imaging tests to examine the function of the urinary system

Until recently, the most common of the imaging tests of function would involve the intravenous injection of a solution that contained iodine. This solution, when concentrated, shows up on X-ray images. After injection, serial X-ray images can be taken of the abdomen. The whole procedure, known as an 'intravenous urogram' (IVU) or 'excretion urogram', reveals the passage of the 'dye' through the urinary system, from when it is first concentrated from the blood by the kidneys and then drained into the bladder. This test can reveal abnormalities in the structure of the kidneys and ureters, as well as in their function of filtering the blood. An excretion urogram is shown in Figure 4.3b-II. An increasingly popular and more accurate form of the IVU is the CT urogram in which the CT scanner is used to locate the obstruction in the urinary system instead of a series of X-ray films.

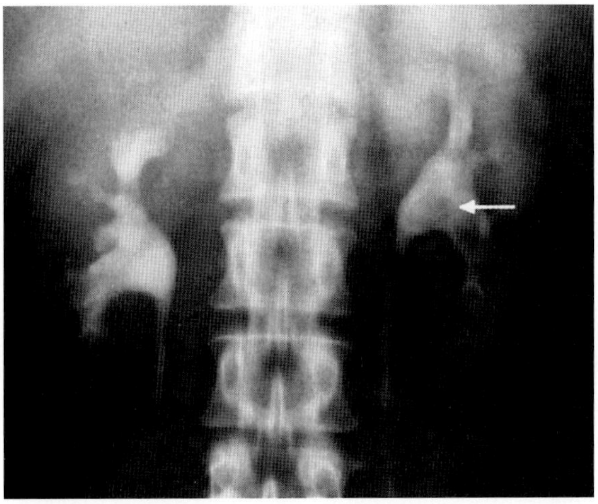

Figure 4.3b-II • Excretion urogram showing a pale patch of contrast in the calyx of the left kidney • The pale patch represents a large calculus (kidney stone).

The function of the bladder may be visualised by requesting the patient to urinate after 'dye' has been inserted into the bladder for cystography. An X-ray image taken during contraction of the bladder will reveal any abnormalities in the way in which it empties. This test is known as 'micturating cystourethrography' (MCU).

A radioactive chemical (containing a radioactive isotope) known as DMSA can be used to assess the filtration function of the kidneys more accurately than the IVU. As in the IVU, DMSA is injected intravenously, and is filtered and concentrated in the kidney. The amount of radioactivity that builds up in the kidneys over the next few hours is then assessed by means of a gamma scanner. The radioactivity dies off very quickly, and so this test is not considered to be harmful to the patient.

Cystoscopy

In cystoscopy, a fibre-optic telescope is inserted into the urethra so that the inside of the bladder can be seen directly. The patient is usually heavily sedated, or has a general anaesthetic. Biopsies of the bladder can also be taken by means of the cystoscope.

Renal biopsy

Under guidance from an ultrasound scan, a needle may be directed through the skin into the kidney to remove a small sample of tissue for examination. This procedure carries a small but significant risk of bleeding into or around the kidney.

Self-test 4.3b

The investigation of the urinary system

1. One of your patients goes to the local hospital department of renal medicine every 6 months because she has an abnormality of her kidneys which may lead to progressive kidney failure. This pattern of attendance would be normal in the routine hospital follow-up of a chronic disease. What investigations do you think she might have to undergo as part of her hospital appointment?
2. Gerald is in his mid-70s, and is experiencing increasing difficulty in passing urine. He is referred to a urologist for investigation of possible disease of the prostate gland. What investigations do you think Gerald might have to undergo? (As you think about your answer, bear in mind that severe obstruction to the flow of urine, such as can result from enlargement of the prostate gland, may eventually lead to kidney damage due to back-pressure.)

Answers

1. This patient will be given a brief physical examination which focuses on the assessment of blood pressure, a visual assessment of skin colour and an abdominal examination.

   A serum blood sample will be taken to measure the levels of urea and creatinine, to estimate the glomerular flitration rate (eGFR) and to make a full blood count for anaemia. Other tests for specific diseases such as systemic lupus erythematosus will be done if relevant to the case.

   The patient may be requested to bring in a 24-hour collection of urine, or alternatively will be asked to provide a midstream urine (MSU) sample for analysis for protein and other chemicals. Depending on the nature of the underlying disease, the structure of the kidneys may be assessed by means of an ultrasound scan, and the function by means of a radioisotope scan (although this is not usual in the routine follow-up of an already diagnosed chronic disease).
2. Gerald will be given a brief physical examination which focuses in particular on the abdomen and the prostate gland. The suprapubic area will be palpated to exclude an enlarged distended bladder.

   Blood tests for kidney function (urea and creatinine) and prostate-specific antigen (PSA) will be performed. A full blood count may also be done to exclude the anaemia that can accompany severe disease such as prostate cancer.

   An ultrasound scan of the bladder and prostate may be performed. If impaired renal function is suspected, an intravenous urogram may be booked to exclude dilatation of the ureters and damage to the kidneys due to back-pressure of urine from the bladder.

Urodynamic studies

Urodynamics is the study of the pressure of the urine in the bladder and the flow of the stream of the urine from the urethra. Specialised tests to measure the pressure within the bladder and the flow rate are used mostly to investigate the underlying problem in cases of incontinence or obstructed flow of urine. They may be used in combination with MCU.

Chapter 4.3c Diseases of the kidneys

LEARNING POINTS

At the end of this chapter you will be able to:
- describe the different disease processes that can affect the kidney
- describe the difference between acute renal failure and chronic kidney disease
- name some of the main features of acute renal failure and chronic kidney disease.

Estimated time for chapter: Part I, 100 minutes; Part II, 60 minutes.

Introduction

The conditions studied in this chapter are (see Q4.3c-1):
- Part I – disease processes that affect the kidney:
  - glomerulonephritis – nephritic syndrome and nephrotic syndrome
  - acute and chronic pyelonephritis
  - kidney and ureteric stones
  - polycystic kidney disease
  - interstitial nephritis
  - haemolytic uraemic syndrome
  - hypertension and the kidneys
  - diabetes and the kidneys
  - cancer of the kidney.
- Part II – serious consequences of disease of the kidney:
  - acute renal failure
  - chronic kidney disease.

All the common diseases of the kidney described in this chapter may be so severe as to lead to either sudden (acute) or gradual (chronic) failure of the kidney to perform its necessary functions.

Part I: Disease processes that affect the kidney

Glomerulonephritis

'Glomerulonephritis' is a term used to describe a broad range of conditions that affect the structure of the cup-like origin of the tubules in the kidney and the cluster of blood vessels within this cup known as the 'glomerulus'. In glomerulonephritis the filtering process is impaired. This has the consequence that red blood cells and protein may leak out of the blood into the urine, and also that excess salts, wastes and water may be retained in the circulation.

In medical textbooks, the condition of glomerulonephritis is categorised according to the precise pathological changes occurring in the glomerulus, and these categories are assigned descriptive terms such as 'minimal change', 'membranous glomerulonephritis' and 'mesangiocapillary glomerulonephritis'. This categorisation, which is based on the results of kidney biopsy and is important for predicting prognosis, does not relate directly to the condition that may have caused the disease process. For this reason it is not described further in this chapter.

The causes of glomerulonephritis

Glomerulonephritis can be caused by a variety of underlying disease processes, but also commonly develops without any recognised cause. In many cases the problem results from the deposition of autoantibodies within the glomerulus. Autoantibodies stimulate the immune response, and the inflammation that results leads to glomerular damage. Autoantibodies may develop as a delayed response to infection, as part of an established autoimmune disease such as systemic lupus erythematosus (SLE), or as a reaction to certain drugs. They may also account for many of the cases of glomerulonephritis of unknown cause.

The *Streptococcus* bacterium, which is a common cause of sore throat and tonsillitis, used to be a very common cause of antibody-related glomerulonephritis. Post-streptococcal glomerulonephritis tends to lead to a characteristic cluster of symptoms known as 'nephritic syndrome' or 'acute nephritis' (see below). 'Bright's disease' is an old-fashioned name for nephritic syndrome. This term used to be almost synonymous with 'post-streptococcal kidney disease' (see Q4.3c-2).

Other infectious agents that may cause the development of damaging autoantibodies include viruses, such as measles and hepatitis, bacteria, such as *Salmonella*, and parasites, such as malaria.

Glomerulonephritis may also be part of the disease process of a multisystem autoimmune disease. SLE is the most common specific autoimmune disease known to cause glomerulonephritis. In SLE, chronic kidney disease resulting from severe persistent cases of glomerulonephritis is the most common cause of death.

Some drugs may also trigger the development of damaging autoantibodies. The drug which most commonly has this effect is penicillamine, which is prescribed as a disease-modifying treatment in rheumatoid arthritis.

The consequences of glomerular damage

The effects of glomerulonephritis can be broadly divided into four categories, although in practice, for any individual patient, it may be difficult to assign them to a category. The categories are:

- haematuria (blood in the urine)
- proteinuria (protein in the urine)
- nephritic syndrome (blood and protein in the urine, with high blood pressure and oedema)
- nephrotic syndrome (excessive protein in the urine leading to severe oedema).

Haematuria and proteinuria in glomerulonephritis

Some forms of glomerulonephritis cause sufficient damage to the glomerulus to bring about a leakage of red blood cells, protein or both. This leakage may not be sufficiently severe to be visible to the patient, and instead may be picked up on routine urine testing. Greater numbers of red blood cells might cause the urine to appear pink or smoky coloured, and excess protein might cause the urine to appear frothy. There may be no other symptoms.

Nevertheless, despite the mildness of the symptoms, the finding of even small amounts of blood or protein in the urine in the absence of urinary infection can be a warning sign of a progressive disease of the kidney. Chronic kidney disease can be the long-term consequence of glomerulonephritis which may be signalled by haematuria or proteinuria. For this reason, all patients who are found to have unexplained haematuria or proteinuria above a certain level will be referred to a renal physician for further investigations.

Some forms of glomerulonephritis that cause haematuria or proteinuria may respond to treatment with immunosuppressant drugs, including corticosteroids. Other immunosuppressant medications that may be prescribed at the same time include azathioprine, cyclophosphamide and chlorambucil. All these drugs can have a wide range of toxic effects.

Nephritic syndrome (acute nephritis or Bright's disease)

'Nephritic syndrome' is a term used to describe a glomerulonephritis that causes severe symptoms to appear rapidly. In nephritic syndrome the patient, commonly a child, becomes unwell with fever, vomiting and pain in the back. There may be a history of a streptococcal infection within the past 2–4 weeks, although streptococcal infection is not always the cause. The face becomes puffy with oedema and the blood pressure is raised. The urine may be pink or smoky coloured with red blood cells. In severe cases the production of urine becomes severely reduced as the filtration function of the kidney is extremely impaired. The patient is then at risk of death from acute kidney failure or malignant hypertension.

Information Box 4.3c-I

Glomerulonephritis: comments from a Chinese medicine perspective

In Chinese medicine, the underlying pathological process of damage to the structure of the kidney in glomerulonephritis suggests that Internal Heat (which may have had External origins if following an infection) is causing Kidney Yin depletion. Blood in the urine can be a result of transmission of Heart Fire via the Small Intestine or Damp Heat in the Bladder. Protein in the urine may be interpreted as the draining of Essence from the Kidneys.

The predominant energetic effect of immunosuppressant drugs such as azathioprine and cyclophosphamide is that of Heating and may cause severe damage to Blood and Yin.

A patient with nephritic syndrome requires close medical observation. In most childhood cases there is full recovery from the condition after 4–7 days, although a minority of cases take a more chronic course. In contrast to the forms of glomerulonephritis that cause haematuria and proteinuria alone, most of these chronic cases of nephritic syndrome do not respond to immunosuppressant drugs. In post-streptococcal nephritis a course of penicillin is given to ensure eradication of the *Streptococcus*.

In the acute cases, as the tissue of the kidneys recovers, the toxins and excess salts that have built up in the body are cleared by means of profuse urination. However, in rare cases, the patient may die during the acute illness from acute renal failure and from damage caused to the brain by a rapidly rising blood pressure. Convulsions may develop in these severe cases. This consequence can be prevented with the help of emergency dialysis, which takes over the function of the failing kidney (see later in this chapter).

In the more chronic cases, and more commonly in adults, there may be persisting damage to the kidneys. This damage can progress to chronic kidney failure over the course of months to years.

Nephrotic syndrome

Other forms of glomerulonephritis cause the 'filter' of the kidney to leak large amounts of protein. This protein is lost into the urine, which becomes frothy as a result. The main plasma protein to be lost is albumin, but other proteins, including immunoglobulin (the protein that forms the plasma antibodies), are lost as well. When excessive amounts of protein are lost into the urine, a condition known as 'nephrotic syndrome' results. As albumin is the most abundant plasma protein, this is found in high concentrations in the urine.

Other causes of nephrotic syndrome include the kidney damage that develops in some cases of diabetes, rare drug reactions and allergic reactions.

> **Information Box 4.3c-II**
>
> **Nephritic syndrome: comments from a Chinese medicine perspective**
>
> In Chinese medicine, some of the symptoms of nephritic syndrome would appear to result from Full Heat. This may originate from a Wind Heat invasion in the case of post-streptococcal disease. Heat in the Heart is transmitted via the Small Intestine to the Bladder, causing scanty urination and haematuria. Heat obstructing the Orifices of the Heart may lead to the confusion and coma that result from acute renal failure.
>
> Hypertension in nephritic syndrome can lead to convulsions. In Chinese medicine terms these are most likely to result from Heat causing damage to Kidney Yin. Liver Yin is then not nourished, and this leads to Hyperactivity of Liver Yang, which rises and stirs up Liver Wind.
>
> A sudden development of facial oedema is characteristic of invasion of Wind Water. Proteinuria is a manifestation of Essence draining from the Kidneys.

It is important for the plasma to be maintained at a certain concentration to give it sufficient osmotic pressure to remain in the circulation. The protein albumin plays a very important role in giving the plasma this adequate level of concentration. If albumin is lost, the plasma becomes too dilute, and the plasma fluid tends to move by osmosis into the more concentrated tissue fluid. Excessive fluid collecting in the tissues is called 'oedema'. In nephrotic syndrome, the severity of the proteinuria results in severe oedema. The patient develops very swollen ankles and legs, and eventually fluid collects in a wide range of body regions, including the abdomen, within the lungs, the facial tissues and the male genitalia.

In nephrotic syndrome, the changes in the constitution of the plasma mean that clotting becomes a problem, and there is a slightly increased risk of venous thrombosis. Loss of antibodies means that the patient with nephrotic syndrome is more prone to infection. Hyperlipidaemia can also develop.

The patient with nephrotic syndrome is treated by means of diuretic medication to encourage loss of the excess tissue fluid, and restriction of salt in the diet. ACE inhibitor medication is prescribed, as this tends to reduce proteinuria, partly by reducing blood pressure. Anticoagulant medication may be given by injection to prevent blood clots. Statins may be prescribed to reduce the hyperlipidaemia. Some cases will respond to corticosteroid medication or to other immunosuppressant drugs; this is particularly true in many of the cases that start in childhood.

> **Information Box 4.3c-III**
>
> **Nephrotic syndrome: comments from a Chinese medicine perspective**
>
> In Chinese medicine, the excessive oedema and proteinuria of nephrotic syndrome is usually associated with a chronic deficiency of the Lungs, Spleen and Kidneys. The accumulation of oedema corresponds to Damp or Damp Heat.
>
> Proteinuria is seen as the draining of Essence from the Kidneys. The Deficiency of Original Qi of the Kidneys which results gives rise to Stagnation of Blood, as Original Qi is necessary to enable smooth movement of Blood in the vessels. This is reflected in the increased risk of thrombosis in nephrotic syndrome.

In children, the underlying glomerulonephritis will very often (in 95% of cases) disappear after a few weeks of treatment with corticosteroids. In many of these cases the remission is permanent, and the kidneys return to a healthy state. In most adults, and the remaining childhood cases, a more chronic course develops, in which the proteinuria has to be controlled by ongoing immunosuppressant medication. In some cases the damage to the kidney progresses and chronic kidney disease results.

Acute and chronic pyelonephritis

'Pyelonephritis' is a term that describes the inflammation which results from infection in the kidney. In most cases this infection has spread from the bladder. Acute and chronic pyelonephritis are two distinct syndromes with different manifestations.

Acute pyelonephritis

Acute pyelonephritis is usually the result of a spread of a bacterial infection in the bladder. It is an uncommon consequence of a bladder infection, and usually indicates underlying chronic disease or depletion in the patient. The exception to this is in pregnancy, when apparently healthy women can develop a kidney infection. This vulnerability in pregnancy to kidney infection is believed to be the result of the effect of the hormone progesterone which causes excessive relaxation of the 'valve' at the site of the insertion of the ureters into the bladder.

The diseases that may predispose to acute pyelonephritis include diabetes and those that result in damage to the structure of the urinary tract. Therefore, the presence of kidney stones and inherited abnormalities of the structure of the kidneys are risk factors for kidney infections. In addition, anything that obstructs the easy flow of urine from the bladder will increase the risk of bladder infections and kidney infections. Prostate disease in men is the most common cause of obstruction to the flow of urine (see Chapter 4.3d).

Information Box 4.3c-IV

Acute pyelonephritis: comments from a Chinese medicine perspective

In Chinese medicine the symptoms of acute pyelonephritis correspond to Damp Heat in the Bladder. There is usually an underlying deficiency of Kidney Yin, which predisposes to the development of Damp Heat.

Information Box 4.3c-V

Reflux nephropathy: comments from a Chinese medicine perspective

In Chinese medicine, reflux nephropathy represents Kidney Yin Deficiency against a background of Jing Deficiency. These deficiencies predispose to Damp Heat in the Bladder, which can further worsen the underlying Yin Deficiency.

The symptoms of acute pyelonephritis include high fever, malaise and loin pain. The urine is often cloudy, and may contain many white and red blood cells and bacteria. In most patients the attack will settle with a course of appropriate antibiotics. However, in rare cases, some areas of the kidney may be scarred and be left with a permanently reduced function. In those who are susceptible, recurrent attacks may cause progressive kidney damage. For this reason, antibiotic treatment is considered to be essential in the treatment of kidney infections.

Chronic pyelonephritis (reflux nephropathy)

'Chronic pyelonephritis' and 'reflux nephropathy' are synonymous terms used to describe a long-standing condition of the kidneys that results from repeated kidney infections. It is now believed that in all cases the damage to the kidneys actually began in childhood as a result of an anatomical abnormality of the ureters. This abnormality is a weakness of the valve that normally prevents reflux of urine from the bladder into the ureters. The vesico-ureteric reflux (VUR) which results allows the passage of any bacteria in the bladder up the ureters towards the kidneys. In many cases, VUR affects only one of the two ureters.

This problem can begin in infancy, and in particular in baby girls, in whom the passage of bacteria into the bladder is a fairly common event. In a healthy bladder, this transient infection is cleared, usually with few symptoms. However, in the case of a baby with VUR, bacteria may start to colonise in the kidneys. This might be the cause of a feverish illness, but alternatively can lead to a more slowly developing but progressive scarring of the affected kidney. This underlying infection may remain undetected for years. A chronic infection of the kidney can then become the source of repeated bladder infections.

It is now considered good medical practice to refer all children who suffer from recurrent bladder infections for investigation of the urinary tract to exclude VUR. Sadly, in many cases of VUR, many years elapse before the underlying cause is diagnosed, by which time permanent scarring of the kidney may have developed.

If VUR is diagnosed before damage to the kidney has developed, the renal function of the child is closely monitored and urine infections are rapidly treated. It is no longer considered helpful to operate to correct VUR, but in some cases it may be considered appropriate to remove a very damaged kidney if only one side has been affected, as this would otherwise remain as a persistent source of recurrent infections.

The condition that results from long-term scarring of the kidneys due to VUR is termed 'chronic pyelonephritis' or 'reflux nephropathy'. The affected patient may suffer form long-term ill-health and recurrent urinary infections. The damage to the kidney, if severe, is progressive and can lead to hypertension and, eventually, chronic kidney disease in adulthood.

Kidney and ureteric stones (calculi)

Kidney stones

Kidney stones are the result of crystals forming in concentrated urine from substances that usually remain dissolved in the urine. The most common form of stone is made of calcium oxalate, but calcium phosphate and uric acid are also common constituents. Some individuals have a tendency to form these crystals more than others, often for reasons that are unclear. However, there are some known risk factors for the development of kidney stones.

A state of dehydration, which can occur in hot, dry climates or hot working environments, will lead to the production of very concentrated urine. Kidney stones are, therefore, more common in hot countries, and in particular in the Middle East.

High levels of chemicals such as calcium salts, oxalic acid and uric acid in the urine can also lead to stone formation. Calcium appears in excess in the urine in people who have too much calcium or vitamin D in their diet. This also occurs in those who have a disorder of the metabolism of their bones which causes too much calcium to be released from the bones into the bloodstream. This can develop in advanced bone cancer, in people who have to undergo prolonged bed rest, and in cases in which the parathyroid glands are overactive. Oxalate can appear in excess in the urine from an excessive dietary intake of spinach, rhubarb and tea. Excessive uric acid is found in the urine if there is a high dietary intake of cholesterol, beer, offal, fish and shellfish. It also occurs in conditions in which there is a high turnover of cells in the body, such as in cancer. There can also be an inherited tendency to the excessive production of oxalic and uric acid in the urine.

A crystal is more likely to develop in concentrated urine if there is a particle within the urine or an irregularity in the urinary tract around which it can form. Therefore, the sludge that can develop in the urine in urinary infections can encourage stone formation. Recurrent infections can lead to the formation of very large irregular stones.

Kidney stones cause damage in a variety of ways. They can lodge in the form of tiny crystals within the substance of the kidney and there act as a focus for inflammation. The damage that can result from stones can also be a focus for acute pyelonephritis. Alternatively, larger stones can obstruct the outflow of urine from the kidney. This might result in increased pressure and dilatation within a large section of a kidney, and eventually loss of function of that portion of the kidney. A stone that dislodges from the kidney and impacts within a ureter can cause excruciating colicky pain as the ureter contracts in a wave-like pattern around the obstruction.

Ureteric stones

Very often kidney stones that leave the kidney cause no symptoms and are passed painlessly in the urine out of the urethra. The most common symptom is pain as the stone travels down the ureter towards the bladder. In many people this pain is transient, and the pain subsides once the stone has left the ureter. However, in those in whom the stone impacts in the ureter, the pain can be very intense. The pain of a ureteric stone tends to peak every few minutes and radiates from the loin (kidney area) round to the suprapubic area. In men the pain can radiate into the testicle on the affected side. In some cases the stone can damage the lining of the ureter and can cause a small amount of blood to enter the urine.

A ureteric stone may totally obstruct the flow of urine from the kidney on the affected side. In this case, as well as being very painful, it is a threat to the health of thc kidney, as obstructed urine places pressure on the kidney tissue.

A ureteric stone can be diagnosed on the basis of the history alone, but is confirmed by means of a plain X-ray image and, if this is not clear, a CT scan. An ultrasound scan will reveal whether or not the impacted stone is causing any back-pressure within the kidney.

If the pain is very intense, the patient is given intramuscular non-steroidal anti-inflammatory drugs (NSAIDs) or opiate pain relief. This may actually allow movement of the stone, as analgesic drugs can cause the ureters to relax, as well as relieving pain. However, stones larger than 1 centimetre in diameter usually require surgical removal.

The development of the endoscope has meant that kidney and ureteric stones are less of a problem to remove than they used to be. 'Keyhole' surgery, which relies on an endoscopic technique, is usually possible for renal stones (percutaneous nephrolithotomy). This means that the patient is left with only a tiny scar. Alternatively, ultrasound shock waves (lithotripsy) can be directed towards the impacted stone, which may then break up so that the fragments pass into the bladder. In intractable cases, an operation is required that leaves the patient with a diagonal scar in the loin (kidney) region.

The best treatment for kidney and ureteric stones is prevention. Those who are at increased risk of developing stones are advised to maintain a high fluid intake. In 'stone formers', dietary sources of calcium, oxalic and uric acids should be kept to a minimum.

> **Information Box 4.3c-VI**
>
> **Kidney stones: comments from a Chinese medicine perspective**
>
> In Chinese medicine, the formation of stones is equated with Phlegm. Damp Heat on a background of Kidney Yin Deficiency is likely to be a precursor to this. The pain of ureteric stones results from Blood Stagnation. Analgesic drugs move Stagnation in the short term.

Miscellaneous disorders of the kidney

Polycystic kidney disease

Autosomal-dominant polycystic kidney disease (ADPCKD) is a relatively common inherited disorder of the kidneys in which the kidneys develop large fluid-filled cysts during adult life. It affects 1 in 1000 people. The cysts gradually destroy the substance of the kidney so that chronic kidney disease develops in middle to late adult life. The first symptoms are usually haematuria or loin pain (i.e. pain in the kidney area) as a cyst ruptures. Occasionally, severe hypertension or the development of chronic kidney disease is the first sign of the disease. People with ADPCKD are also more prone to developing liver cysts, mitral valve problems and subarachnoid haemorrhages.

There is no treatment for ADPCKD except for the symptoms of pain, hypertension and chronic kidney disease as they develop (see later in this chapter). Patients may be screened by means of cranial arteriography for the berry aneurysms that can predispose to subarachnoid haemorrhage.

There is a genetic test for ADPCKD so that people from affected families can be screened for the disease, and so that those who are planning a family can receive genetic counselling.

> **Information Box 4.3c-VII**
>
> **Polycystic kidney disease: comments from a Chinese medicine perspective**
>
> In Chinese medicine, the symptoms of polycystic kidney disease are a manifestation of deficiency of Kidney Jing and Yin.

Interstitial nephritis

Like glomerulonephritis, interstitial nephritis (also termed 'tubulointerstitial nephritis') is a form of inflammation of the tissue of the kidney. In this case, the inflammation is not of the glomerulus, but of the tissue that surrounds the tubules.

The most common cause of this inflammation is the infection of acute pyelonephritis, but there are important non-infectious causes which are more likely to lead to permanent kidney damage. The most important non-infectious cause in developed countries is the recurrent use of analgesic tablets. The most troublesome drug from this point of view used to be a paracetamol-like drug called phenacetin, although this is not now prescribed by doctors in the UK. Paracetamol is far less likely to have this effect on the kidneys. However, the NSAIDs may also, on rare occasions, cause this condition if taken on a repeated basis over the course of 3 years or more. A prescription of this length is not uncommon in many people with chronic musculoskeletal disease.

Analgesic-related interstitial nephritis can result in a long-term scarring of the kidney tissue, which can develop into chronic kidney disease. For this reason, anyone who is taking

NSAID-related analgesics on a long-term basis should have regular blood tests to check that the function of the kidneys is not being affected.

Progressive interstitial nephritis can also result from some chronic diseases, most importantly diabetes and sickle cell disease.

> **Information Box 4.3c-VIII**
>
> **Interstitial nephritis: comments from a Chinese medicine perspective**
>
> In Chinese medicine, the symptoms of interstitial nephritis suggest a progressive depletion of Kidney Yin. The damaging effect analgesic drugs could be attributed to their Heating properties.

Haemolytic uraemic syndrome

Haemolytic uraemic syndrome (HUS) is a condition in which the primary problem is the formation of fibrin and the breakdown of the red blood cells within the small blood vessels of the circulation (haemolysis). In HUS this serious complication usually follows an infection, particularly of the gastrointestinal or respiratory tracts. A specific strain of the bacterium *Escherichia coli* (known as O157) has recently been associated with HUS. It is believed that in HUS the infectious agent somehow causes damage to the lining of the blood vessels, which then triggers the clotting cascade and damage to the red blood cells.

This damage affects the renal arterioles in particular, with the result that the glomeruli become damaged. The affected patient, commonly a child, develops haematuria and high blood pressure, and kidney function starts to deteriorate. In some cases this deterioration is so rapid that it leads to acute renal failure. However, in most cases, with adequate medical supervision, there can be full recovery from the condition. An outbreak of *E. coli* O157 food poisoning in Scotland in 1996 was complicated by the development of HUS in a number of patients. The mortality in this outbreak demonstrated that the complications of HUS were more likely to be fatal in the elderly.

> **Information Box 4.3c-IX**
>
> **Haemolytic uraemic syndrome: comments from a Chinese medicine perspective**
>
> In Chinese medicine, the interpretation of haemolytic uraemic syndrome would be similar to that of acute nephritic syndrome, in that an invasion of Wind Damp Heat is the initiating factor. Haematuria corresponds to Heat transmitted from the Small Intestine, or to Damp Heat in the Urine. The Full Heat causes damage to Kidney Yin, which in those who are depleted already, such as the elderly, can have life-threatening consequences.

Hypertension and the kidneys

Hypertension can in itself lead to damage to the kidneys. One of the effects of hypertension is that it causes narrowing and rigidity of the blood vessels by the process of arteriosclerosis. This results in a reduced blood supply to the kidney and also in structural damage to the glomeruli. The reduced delivery of oxygen to the kidneys triggers a hormonal response which is intended to improve the blood supply to the kidneys in the situation of shock. This response involves hormones called 'renin' and 'angiotensin', which both act to increase the blood pressure. What would be an appropriate response in the case of shock is actually an inappropriate response in the case of arteriosclerosis, as a vicious cycle of increasing hypertension is set up. The ACE inhibitors and angiotensin II receptor antagonists are classes of antihypertensive medication that act to prevent the action of angiotensin, and so directly break this negative cycle of events.

The damage to the glomeruli also reduces the function of the kidneys, so that in some people with sustained hypertension permanent renal impairment can develop.

Kidney disease can itself be a cause of hypertension, because it too can lead to the inappropriate production of renin and angiotensin. Kidney disease also leads to the retention of salt and water in the circulation, which also tends to increase the blood pressure. These factors can cause a vicious circle of escalating hypertension, as the hypertension in kidney disease further reduces the blood supply to the already damaged kidneys.

For this reason, many patients with diverse forms of kidney disease will develop hypertension. In acute kidney disease, such as the nephritic syndrome and HUS, the rise in blood pressure can be very rapid, whereas in chronic kidney disease a more gradual rise is usual. Patients with one-sided kidney disease can also develop hypertension in later life. This is an important reason why some people will have a diseased kidney removed (e.g. in one-sided reflux nephropathy).

The treatment of hypertension resulting from kidney disease involves strict attention to a reduction of salt in the diet, and the use of diuretics and ACE inhibitors.

> **Information Box 4.3c-X**
>
> **Hypertension and the kidney: comments from a Chinese medicine perspective**
>
> In Chinese medicine, the hypertension that results from underlying kidney disease might result from Deficiency of either Kidney Yin or Yang, or both. Kidney Yin Deficiency is seen to predispose to the development of Liver Fire, and Yang Deficiency to the accumulation of Phlegm Damp. In severe kidney disease, it is likely that a combination of these two syndromes contributes to the development of the hypertension.

Diabetes and the kidneys

The kidneys can be damaged in a variety of ways in diabetes mellitus. Diabetes is a condition in which a persistently raised level of blood sugar leads to damage of the small and medium-sized blood vessels. This damage affects the renal arteriole and the glomerulus.

In up to one-third of patients who have been diagnosed with type 1 (juvenile onset) diabetes, serious damage to the kidneys will become apparent in later life. The glomerular damage leads to progressive proteinuria, which if unchecked can lead to nephrotic syndrome. The reduction in the blood flow resulting from the narrowed renal arteriole can cause hypertension, which in turn can further worsen the glomerular damage. On top of these two causes of kidney damage, the diabetic patient is also prone to urinary infections because of excessive amounts of glucose in the urine. These infections can lead to acute pyelonephritis in the already damaged kidney. Chronic kidney disease is a common end result of diabetic kidney disease.

The rate of progression of diabetic kidney disease can be prevented by meticulous control of the blood sugar. Patients should receive regular screening for traces of protein in the urine and blood tests for abnormalities of kidney function such as a decline in the eGFR. It is considered very important that hypertension is controlled to a level of less than 130/80 mmHg, ideally by ACE inhibitors, and that any urine infections are treated rapidly by means of appropriate antibiotics.

Cancer of the kidney

The most common tumour of the kidney is the renal cell carcinoma. This affects men approximately twice as often as women, and has an average age of onset of 55 years.

The presenting symptoms are usually haematuria or loin pain, although diagnosis may not occur until after more generalised symptoms of cancer such as fever and weight loss have developed. In localised renal cell carcinoma, the treatment involves removal of the affected kidney. In some patients this surgery can be curative. Surgery may also be performed if the cancer has already spread to lymph nodes and other organs (in particular the other kidney, liver, bone and lungs). In about one-fifth of patients with metastatic disease, chemotherapy with alpha-interferon and interleukin-2 can give a very good response rate in the short term. However, the long-term outlook is poor for those with metastases, with only 5% still alive after 5 years from diagnosis, compared with 45% for those who present without metastases.

The kidney is also the site for one of the most common tumours of infancy known as a 'nephroblastoma' (Wilms' tumour). Common first symptoms of this tumour are haematuria and abdominal swelling. It has a much better prognosis than renal cell carcinoma, in that most children are cured of this tumour by a combination of surgery, radiotherapy and chemotherapy.

> **Information Box 4.3c-XI**
>
> **Cancer and the kidney: comments from a Chinese medicine perspective**
>
> In Chinese medicine, a tumour of the kidney may represent Phlegm and/or Blood Stagnation. A deficiency of Kidney Yin and/or Yang is likely to be an underlying factor. In Wilms' tumour Jing Deficiency is contributory.

Part II: Serious consequences of disease of the kidney

The most serious consequence of kidney disease is that the kidney totally fails to perform its functions of filtering the blood and forming concentrated urine. If these functions are lost, fluid, salts and waste products build up in the blood to cause severe illness. 'Acute renal failure' describes an abrupt failure of the kidney function occurring over the course of hours to weeks. 'Chronic kidney disease' (formerly known as 'chronic renal failure') is a term used to describe a gradual loss of kidney function, which can develop over the course of weeks to years. Patients who are developing chronic kidney disease may experience a sudden rapid deterioration of renal function, in which case the term 'acute on chronic renal failure' may be applied.

Acute renal failure

The causes of acute renal failure

Acute renal failure (ARF) can have a variety of causes. A potentially reversible cause is an insufficient blood supply to the kidneys. This means that the kidneys are simply unable to perform their filtration function adequately because they are not receiving sufficient fluid to do so. This can occur as a result of sudden blood or fluid loss. Therefore, haemorrhage from serious trauma, fluid loss from burns, and dehydration from severe diarrhoea and vomiting can all lead to acute renal failure in this way. The impaired blood supply that can result from a heart attack or heart failure can also cause ARF for the same reason. However, in these cases, as long as the situation of impaired blood supply does not continue for too long, the ARF can be reversed if the blood supply can be restored to normal.

ARF can also result from damage to the tissues of the kidney. Most commonly, this form of ARF is due to a condition known as 'acute tubular necrosis', in which the cells of the tubules die for a variety of reasons. The most common reason for this to occur is a prolonged reduction of blood supply to the kidneys for the reasons listed above. The cells die simply because of lack of oxygen and basic nutrients. Toxic reactions to drugs are also a common cause of this form of ARF. Diuretics, NSAIDs and ACE inhibitors are well known for causing this severe reaction in very rare cases.

The kidney tissue can also be damaged by haemoglobin circulating free in the blood. This reason for ARF most commonly develops following a serious traumatic accident, during which damage to blood vessels and tissues leads to the release of haemoglobin from the blood cells. In this case the damage caused to the kidneys by the haemoglobin is often compounded by a sudden loss of blood supply to the kidneys.

ARF can also develop in pregnancy. The most common cause is the complex cycle of events that develops starting with pre-eclampsia. In this condition of late pregnancy, the initial signs of raised blood pressure and loss of protein in the urine can be overtaken by a serious condition called 'eclampsia', in which the blood pressure rises to life-threatening levels and the tubular cells of the kidney die from the resulting poor blood supply. Patients with eclampsia can die from a combination of malignant hypertension and ARF. Another cause of ARF during pregnancy is the sudden blood loss that can occur either from a tear of the placenta (abruptio placentae) or from the womb after the delivery of the baby.

The symptoms of acute renal failure

ARF initially leads to the formation of very small quantities of urine. The levels of toxins such as urea and creatinine start to rise rapidly in the blood as the kidneys are unable to clear them. This condition, known as 'acute uraemia', will lead to nausea, drowsiness, fits and eventually coma, depending on the rate of accumulation of the toxins. The patient may develop symptoms from overload of fluid in the circulation, including breathlessness due to pulmonary oedema. The situation of uraemia resulting from ARF is a medical emergency. Ideally, patients with ARF should be nursed in an intensive-care setting.

The treatment of acute renal failure

The treatment depends very much on an accurate diagnosis of the underlying cause of the ARF. In the situation in which a temporary impairment of blood supply to the kidney is suspected, the prime aim of treatment is to restore the blood supply to the kidney. This may mean giving a blood transfusion in the case of severe haemorrhage, or a fluid infusion in the case of dehydration. In the case of heart attack or heart failure, drugs may be given to improve the pumping action of the heart. If there has been no damage to the tubular cells of the kidney, these treatment approaches may be sufficient to reverse the ARF.

If the ARF is due to damage to the tubular cells, the cause of the damage needs to be removed. Shock or dehydration needs to be treated, but with great care, as fluid overload is a potential problem with ARF. Toxic drugs are withdrawn in the case of drug-related tubular necrosis. In the case of eclampsia, delivery of the baby by caesarean section can halt the negative cycle of events.

Assuming that the cause of the ARF can be removed, the patient with tubular damage then requires intensive care to support them over the period of the next 7–21 days, which is the time required for the damaged tubular cells to recover. Early specialist care in this situation is vital, as the patient will require very careful monitoring of the circulatory and urinary systems, and may require emergency dialysis (see later in this chapter) to clear excess fluid, salts and toxins from the blood.

Up to 50% of people who suffer from acute tubular necrosis will die from the acute illness. Many who survive will regain normal function of the kidneys. However, a proportion will be left with permanent damage, which may lead to a state of chronic renal failure.

> **Information Box 4.3c-XII**
>
> **Acute renal failure: comments from a Chinese medicine perspective**
>
> In Chinese medicine, acute renal failure may correspond to Depletion of Kidney Yin and Yang with sudden accumulation of Heat and Damp. Fits and coma correspond to the Stirring up of Liver Wind (following severe Kidney Yin Deficiency) and to Heat obstructing the Orifices of the Heart.

Chronic kidney disease

The symptoms of chronic kidney disease

'Chronic kidney disease' (chronic renal failure) is a term used to describe a state of gradually deteriorating kidney function. In chronic kidney disease, the ability of the kidneys to filter the blood and concentrate the urine is lost over a period of weeks to years. Over this time the levels of urea and creatinine in the blood rise slowly, causing the patient to feel unwell and the skin to itch.

This state of 'chronic uraemia' is only life threatening when the levels of urea and creatinine reach very high levels. Features of fluid retention, with oedema, may develop, and the blood pressure tends to rise. Loss of the hormone erythropoietin leads to a severe form of anaemia. Loss of the ability to activate vitamin D contributes to a form of osteomalacia. Impotence is also a known consequence of chronic kidney disease.

The causes of chronic kidney disease

Chronic kidney disease can develop as a result of a wide range of disease processes. These include diabetes, hypertension, glomerulonephritis (all forms), infection (in particular infection leading to reflux nephropathy following vesicoureteric reflux), interstitial nephritis, damage by kidney stones, and congenital abnormalities (including polycystic kidney disease). In addition, any of the causes of acute renal failure may lead to permanent kidney damage if not successfully treated. Diabetes accounts for half of all cases of symptomatic chronic kidney disease and hypertension for a further quarter, most of which develop in the eighth decade of life (see Q4.3c-3).

One other important cause of chronic kidney disease is obstruction to the outflow of urine. The underlying causes of this problem are discussed in Chapter 4.3d, as it primarily relates to the bladder and the prostate gland. As urine outflow obstruction is usually gradual in onset, the damage caused by back-pressure on the kidneys is also gradual, but can be so severe as to lead to chronic kidney disease. A sudden obstruction to the ureter from a large ureteric stone can cause a sudden onset of acute renal failure in someone who has only one kidney.

The treatment of chronic kidney disease

In the early stages of chronic kidney disease the patient may remain without symptoms and the condition is only apparent through recognition of abnormal blood test results such as a low eGFR or a high creatinine level. In symptomatic cases the symptoms can be controlled by means of salt, potassium, phosphate and protein restriction, and meticulous attention to blood pressure control. A genetically engineered form of erythropoietin is now available so that the severe anaemia of chronic disease can be prevented. Activated vitamin D can be given in the form of a drug, although this has to be monitored with care, as there is a risk of developing excessive levels of calcium in the blood. All this treatment should be provided and monitored by a team of specialist physicians based within a hospital renal unit.

The ideal treatment for chronic kidney disease is prevention of progression, and so accurate treatment of the cause and meticulous attention to blood pressure and blood sugar levels (in diabetes) is crucial. Once the inevitable progression appears to be apparent, the best treatment is considered to be kidney transplantation at an early stage in the disease, before the health of the body has been too affected by the long-term state of uraemia. If a suitable kidney for transplantation is not immediately available, the patient will eventually require regular dialysis to take over the detoxifying and fluid-balancing functions of the failing kidneys.

Dialysis

'Dialysis' is a general term that is used to describe any method by which the blood is filtered artificially. In haemodialysis, the blood of the patient is redirected through a machine designed to filter the blood of toxins and to remove excess fluids and salts. The flow of blood through the machine must be rapid for the dialysis to work adequately. To enable this to happen, a surgical operation is performed whereby the blood in an artery (usually the brachial artery at the elbow) is directed into a local vein. This operation, known as 'creating a fistula', leads to the formation of a pulsatile and tense blood vessel that lies close to the surface of the skin. A fistula (Figure 4.3c-I) permits repeated ready access to a good blood supply for the purposes of haemodialysis.

At the time of haemodialysis, a large-bore needle is inserted into the fistula so that blood can be passed through the dialysis machine. This blood is returned to the body through another needle inserted into a distal portion of the fistula. The whole process takes about 4–5 hours and needs to be repeated two or three times a week. If the frequency of dialysis is too low, the patient will develop signs of chronic uraemia, including tiredness, itching and poor sleep.

Haemodialysis is an efficient method of dialysis, but carries some problems for the patient. First, it is disruptive to normal life to have to attend the haemodialysis unit on a very frequent basis; and, secondly, some people feel quite unwell from the rapid changes in blood composition that result from haemodialysis.

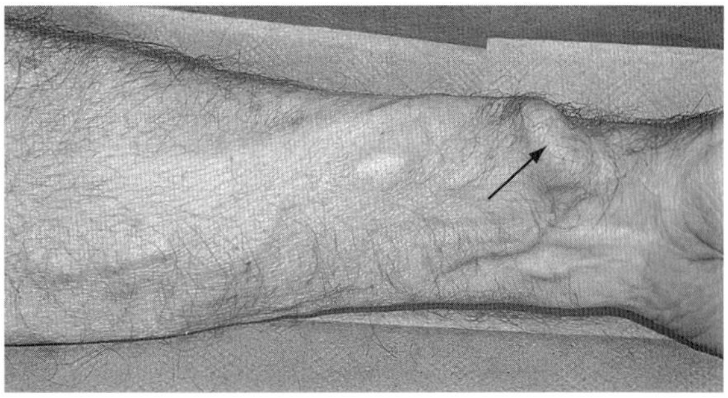

Figure 4.3c-I • An arteriovenous fistula in the right forearm.

Peritoneal dialysis (chronic ambulatory peritoneal dialysis (CAPD)) is a form of dialysis that does not require the blood to be circulated through a machine. Instead, it relies on the peritoneal space (the space inside the abdomen that surrounds the abdominal organs) to be the site of dialysis. For peritoneal dialysis to take place, a soft plastic tube (catheter) has to be inserted by a surgical procedure so that it rests permanently with its tip in the peritoneal space. The location of the CAPD catheter is shown in Figure 4.3c-II.

Peritoneal dialysis can be performed by the patient at home. In peritoneal dialysis 1.5–3 litres of sterile dialysis fluid are drained into the peritoneal space through the plastic tube and kept within the space for 20–30 minutes. The peritoneal lining acts as the kidney, and toxins and excess salts and fluid can move out of the blood in the abdominal tissues by diffusion into the dialysis fluid. After about half an hour the fluid is drained back out of the abdominal space through the tube by the patient and discarded. This all has to be performed with a strict attention to sterile procedure, as infection in the peritoneal space can lead to severe illness.

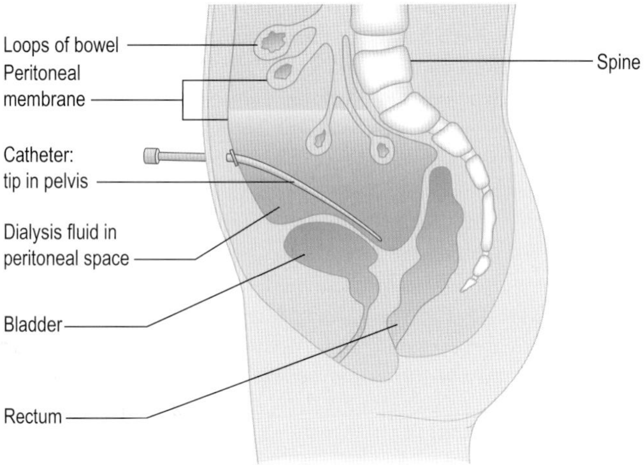

Figure 4.3c-II • The position of the catheter used for chronic ambulatory peritoneal dialysis (CAPD).

Some patients can continue for years being fully reliant on one of the forms of dialysis to perform the function of their failed kidneys. However, the problem remains that the life of a dialysis patient is dominated by the technicalities of the dialysis, and also with dealing with its complications.

Moreover, dialysis can never fully reverse the state of chronic uraemia, so that the patient will always be less well than someone with normal kidney function. A successful kidney transplant offers much more day-to-day freedom and well-being than dialysis, but unfortunately is not possible for all people with chronic kidney disease.

Kidney transplantation

The success of transplantation depends on the availability of a donor kidney that is as accurately 'matched' to the tissues of the recipient as possible. The ideal is for a patient to receive a kidney from a twin, in which case there is no risk of rejection of the donated organ by the immune system. Kidneys from any other source will carry antigens on the kidney tissue that are recognised as foreign by the recipient's body.

It is understood that the kidneys from some donors carry more foreign antigens than others. The process of tissue typing involves comparing the antigens on a donor kidney with those of the potential recipient. Only if a fairly close match (it will never be perfect) is achieved will the transplantation operation go ahead. Once the kidney has been transplanted, the recipient will have to remain on life-long immunosuppressant medication to prevent rejection of the donated organ.

Donor kidneys most often come from young people who have suffered an accidental death. The ideal situation is that the kidney is removed from a patient who has suffered brain-stem death, but whose vital functions have been maintained by means of a life-support machine. In this situation the donated kidney is likely to be very healthy.

In the UK, the removal of the organ always requires the consent of the patient's family if the donor is under 16 years old, and usually also requires evidence that the patient also wished for their organs to be donated after death. After tissue typing, the pattern of antigens in the donor kidney is compared with those of all the patients on the national waiting list for transplantation. A combination of close match and urgency of need are the criteria by which a suitable recipient is chosen. The transplantation operation is then organised as a matter of urgency. However, because of the low availability of organs, many patients remain on the waiting list for years.

In rare cases, the organ may be removed from a living close relative who wishes to donate one of their kidneys. The donor, whether alive or dead, is always screened thoroughly for evidence of infectious disease and cancer, but the risks of transmitted disease from the donor organ can never be ruled out totally.

The operation itself carries risks, particularly if the patient is in a fairly advanced state of chronic kidney disease. In particular, the blood supply to the new organ may be lost because of thrombosis. In some patients, the new organ becomes damaged by the inflammation resulting from rejection by the immune system. These 'rejection episodes' are particularly common in the first few months after transplantation. Most are reversible by treating with increased doses of immunosuppressant medication, but some lead to death of the new organ.

A combination of immunosuppressant drugs is used in transplant patients. These most commonly include corticosteroids, and the drugs azathioprine, ciclosporin and tacrolimus. The latter two drugs, like many of the early antibiotics, are derivatives of naturally occurring fungi.

All these drugs can have serious side-effects. Azathioprine may cause bone marrow failure, ciclosporin can cause kidney damage, and tacrolimus can damage the kidneys and the nerves. All these drugs will also depress the healthy response to infection, so that the transplant patient is more at risk of developing opportunistic infections.

However, despite the risk of side-effects and infections, many patients who have had a successful transplant are able to tolerate these drugs and continue to live a normal life.

Information Box 4.3c-XIII

Chronic renal failure: comments from a Chinese medicine perspective

In Chinese medicine, the features of chronic renal failure correspond to severe depletion of Kidney Yin and Yang. This is always associated with depletion of Lung and Spleen Yang. Fluid retention and hypertension might represent accumulation of Phlegm and Damp. Anaemia corresponds to Blood Deficiency, and osteomalacia to Jing Deficiency. The itch, drowsiness and coma that develop in advanced uraemia may be consequences of Heat and Phlegm, which eventually obstruct the Orifices of the Heart.

The action of dialysis probably permits some clearance of accumulated Pathogenic Factors, including Heat and Damp, and acts by supporting the Kidney Yin and Yang.

Transplantation might be considered to Nourish Kidney Yin and Yang, although at the cost of the introduction of Pathogenic Factors in the form of foreign antigens (Wind Heat and Wind Damp most commonly). Immunosuppressant medication is suppressive in nature, but is necessary to prevent the negative effect of these Pathogens.

The red flags of the diseases of the kidneys

Some patients with diseases of the kidneys will benefit from referral to a conventional doctor for assessment and/or treatment. Red flags are those symptoms and signs that indicate that referral is to be considered. The red flags of the diseases of the kidneys are described in Table 4.3c-I. This table forms part of the summary on red flags given in Appendix III, which also gives advice on the degree of urgency of referral for each of the red flag conditions listed.

Table 4.3c-I Red Flags 29 – diseases of the kidneys

Red Flag	Description	Reasoning
29.1	**Blood in the urine: refer all cases in men**; refer in women except in the case of acute urinary infection	The most common and benign cause of blood in the urine is bladder infection (cystitis) in women. If the symptoms are suggestive of this diagnosis (burning on urination, low abdominal pain, cloudy or blood-stained urine) there is no need to refer straight away. Treat with complementary medicine, recommend a high fluid intake and only refer if the symptoms are not settling within 3 days However, blood in the urine is not normal in men, who should be protected from infection by their relatively long urethras. Refer all cases of blood in the urine in men, and in women if there are either no other symptoms (blood may be coming from a kidney or from a tumour) or if there is pain in the loin (suggesting a spread of infection to the kidneys or kidney stones)
29.2	**Unexplained oedema** (excess tissue fluid, manifesting primarily as ankle swelling extending to more than 2 cm above the malleoli)	'Oedema' means excess tissue fluid and tends to manifest in the lower regions of the body, first appearing as ankle swelling. Mild ankle swelling can develop as a result of inactivity and overheating, but should never extend to more than a couple of centimetres above the malleoli. If the oedema is severe it may affect the lower part of the calf, and can also accumulate in the scrotum, buttocks and lower abdominal tissue If the oedema is due to excess tissue fluid it will tend to 'pit', meaning that sustained pressure will leave an indentation in the skin Oedema can have a range of causes, and most of these, including kidney disease and chronic heart failure (see Red Flags 15, Table 3.2f-I), are potentially serious. If the patient is accumulating significant oedema (more than mild ankle swelling), they should be referred for investigation of the cause
29.3	**Acute loin pain**: often comes in waves; patient may vomit and collapse	This is characteristic of an obstructed kidney stone. The pain may radiate round to the suprapubic region, particularly if the stone moves some way down the ureter. Encourage drinking of fluids
29.4	**Persistent loin pain** (i.e. pain in the flanks either side of the spine between the levels of T11 and L3)	Persistent achy pain (for longer than 1 week) in one or both loins might be an indication of kidney disease. It would be wise to refer if there is no obvious muscular explanation. Refer as a high priority if there are coexisting symptoms of urinary or generalised infection (fever and cloudy urine)
29.5	**Features of acute pyelonephritis**: fever, malaise, loin pain and cloudy urine suggest an infection of the kidneys	While bladder infections are usually self-limiting, particularly in women, features that indicate the infection has ascended the ureters to affect the kidney imply a more serious situation. Acute pyelonephritis carries a risk of permanent scarring of the kidneys and merits medical attention (treatment with antibiotics)
29.6	**Features of vesico-ureteric reflux disease (VUR) in a child**: any history of recurrent episodes or a current episode of cloudy urine or burning on urination should be taken seriously in a prepubescent child	Urine infections are common in young children but need to be taken seriously, particularly if there is a history of recurrent infections. The small child is more vulnerable to VUR, which means that when the bladder contracts some urine is flushed back towards the kidneys. In the case of infection of the bladder, VUR can lead to infectious organisms causing damage to the delicate structure of the kidney. Sometimes this damage occurs with very few symptoms, but if cumulative and undetected can lead to serious kidney problems and high blood pressure in later life For this reason it is wise to refer all prepubescent children with a history of symptoms of urinary infections, to exclude the possibility of VUR

Self-test 4.3c

The diseases of the kidneys

1. Sarah is 12 years old. She suddenly comes down with a fever, and complains of nausea and low backache. Her mother notices that her face and ankles seem puffy.
   (i) What kidney disease might account for these symptoms?
   (ii) What might be unusual about Sarah's urine?
   (iii) What other illness might she have experienced in the past few days to weeks?
   (iv) Would you refer Sarah for a conventional opinion?
2. Jim is a 55-year-old insulin-dependent diabetic. He describes an episode of pain that he suffered the previous day which started in the mid-back on the left-hand side and then moved round to the front of his abdomen before fading away. He describes the pain as having peaks, which felt like a knife twisting in his flesh, and which made him sweat. In all, the episode lasted about half an hour.
   (i) What do you think might have been the cause of Jim's pain?
   (ii) Is there any reason why Jim as a diabetic might have been more susceptible to this condition?
   (iii) Would you refer Jim to his doctor concerning this episode?
3. Janice, aged 35 years, knows that she has polycystic kidney disease. Her father died of the condition 10 years ago (when he was in his 60s). Janice recently had a genetic test to show that she too carries the gene. An ultrasound scan of her kidneys performed after confirmation of the diagnosis has shown that she has some cysts developing in both kidneys, but she was told that she may not experience any symptoms for some years yet.

   There is little that can be done for polycystic kidney disease except to treat the symptoms as they arise. Do you think that having the genetic test, so that an early diagnosis can been confirmed, might have been of any help to Janice? If so, why? Can you think of any negative consequences of receiving a diagnosis so early?

Answers

1. (i) Sarah's symptoms are consistent with an onset of acute nephritic syndrome.
   (ii) The urine could be pink or smoky coloured from the presence of red blood cells.
   (iii) Sarah might have a recent history of a streptococcal infection, such as a sore throat, tonsillitis or scarlet fever. This would fit with a diagnosis of post-streptococcal nephritis.
   (iv) You should refer Sarah as a matter of urgency, as acute nephritis can have life-threatening consequences because of rapidly rising blood pressure.
2. (i) The symptoms of this episode are highly suggestive of the passage of a left-sided kidney stone through the ureter into the bladder.
   (ii) Diabetics are more prone to urinary infections, which can encourage the formation of urinary stones.
   (iii) As Jim is diabetic, in this case it would be good practice to encourage him to report the episode to his GP. The development of the stone may be a signal that he is suffering from recurrent urinary infections. As these can be a factor in the development of kidney disease in diabetes, it may be appropriate for Jim to have further tests of his renal function at this stage.
3. An early diagnosis can help some people prepare themselves for the development of a chronic disease. Janice may choose to change her lifestyle and improve her health as much as possible so that she is as fit as she can be at the time when the function of her kidneys starts to decline. It is particularly important for her blood pressure to be maintained at a low level, and so early diagnosis should prompt her to ensure her blood pressure is monitored on a regular basis.

   Although polycystic kidney disease leads to inevitable renal failure, Janice's later life might be transformed if she has a renal transplant. This is likely to be most successful if performed early in the development of renal failure, so by having an early diagnosis, Janice is in a good position for being placed on the transplant waiting list at the best possible time for her.

   Another important consequence of having an early diagnosis is that Janice can be given counselling concerning the risk of conceiving a child with the polycystic kidney disease gene. The disadvantage of an early diagnosis is that some people may respond negatively, and may not be able to cope emotionally with the prospect of impending chronic disease.

   An unfortunate disadvantage of early diagnosis of a chronic illness like polycystic kidney disease is that the patient may have to pay very high premiums if he or she has to take out a life or health insurance policy.

Chapter 4.3d Diseases of the ureters, bladder and the urethra

LEARNING POINTS

At the end of this chapter you will be able to:
- name the most common causes of urinary tract obstruction
- describe how urinary tract obstruction can affect the function of the urinary system
- describe the different disease processes that affect the ureters, bladder and urethra.

Estimated time for chapter: 90 minutes.

Introduction

In this chapter the diseases of the ureters, bladder and the urethra are considered together because they share the function of collecting urine as it drains from the kidney.

The conditions studied in this chapter are:
- Urinary tract obstruction:
  - hydronephrosis
  - prostatic enlargement.
- Lower urinary tract infection:
  - cystitis
  - prostatitis
  - urethritis.

- Incontinence:
  - stress incontinence
  - urge incontinence
  - overflow incontinence
  - neurological incontinence.
- Tumours of the lower urinary tract:
  - cancer of the bladder
  - prostate cancer.

Urinary tract obstruction

The outflow of urine from the urinary tract can be blocked at any level in its passage from the pelvis of the kidney down to the distal urethra, and this can impact on the function of the kidneys. For example, kidney stones can impact in the ureter to cause acute one-sided urinary obstruction. In contrast, the condition of chronic kidney disease can develop from gradual obstruction of the lower urinary tract (e.g. in prostate disease).

There are numerous possible causes of obstruction to the outflow of urine from one or both kidneys. Internal obstruction to the urine flow in the ureters may result from stones, blood clots or urinary tumours. External compression of the ureters may be the result of intra-abdominal cancer or the enlargement of the womb that occurs in pregnancy.

Obstruction of the ureters is usually one-sided, and will affect the function of the kidney on that side. In most cases of one-sided ureteric obstruction, the filtering function of the kidneys is not jeopardised because the other kidney is able to perform this role alone. However, if the other kidney is diseased or missing, ureteric obstruction will lead to acute renal failure if not adequately treated.

Obstruction of the flow through the bladder and the urethra will always affect both kidneys, as the pressure of the accumulating urine builds up within both ureters. Causes include large bladder tumours, impaired muscle contraction of the bladder (due to a neurological disorder that affects the nerve supply to the bladder) and enlargement of the prostate gland in men. Tightening (stricture) of the urethra can develop as a consequence of infection or damage, and this too may be sufficient to cause partial or complete obstruction.

Hydronephrosis

Prolonged urinary obstruction leads to a condition of one or both kidneys called 'hydronephrosis'. In hydronephrosis the affected kidney becomes dilated with the accumulating urine, and the ureter becomes distended down to the point of the obstruction. If the obstruction occurs suddenly, the build up of pressure in this system is acute and can lead to a rapid loss of function of the affected kidney(s). The more usual case is that the obstruction is partial or gradual, in which case the function of the affected kidney(s) is progressively reduced, but not lost totally.

Hydronephrosis can be seen by means of an abdominal ultrasound scan, but the best test to confirm its presence is the IVU, because this can also reveal loss of function of the affected kidney(s).

Symptoms of urinary obstruction

The symptoms of gradual obstruction may be minimal in the early stages, although, if affecting both kidneys, will lead to the symptoms of chronic kidney disease if persisting for some time (see Chapter 4.3c). If one-sided obstruction is gradual, there may actually be no symptoms. This is not necessarily a good thing, because the obstruction may have led to total loss of function of the kidney before the diagnosis is made.

In some cases the distension of the kidneys, particularly if rapid in development, will cause loin pain. The pain is worsened by drinking a large volume of fluid. Sudden obstruction of the ureters by a stone or blood clot will lead to the characteristic pain of ureteric colic.

If an obstruction affects both sides of the urinary system, the patient will notice a sluggishness of urine flow, or no urine flow at all if the obstruction is sudden and total. In sudden obstruction of the urethra, the bladder becomes very distended over the course of a few hours. This condition, known as 'acute retention of urine', can be extremely uncomfortable. In severe retention, the top of the distended bladder can be felt as high as the level of the umbilicus (it normally never rises above the level of the pubic bone).

Gradual obstruction of the urinary tract leads to stagnation of urine flow, and this can predispose to the development of infection, particularly if the bladder is affected. Cystitis and acute pyelonephritis may therefore also complicate the condition of urinary obstruction.

Prostatic enlargement

In men, the prostate gland sits at the base of the bladder, where it encircles the first section of the urethra. Enlargement of the prostate gland, known as 'benign hyperplasia', is a very common feature of ageing in men, and commonly becomes apparent after the sixth decade of life. In some men this enlargement causes narrowing of the urethral passageway through the prostate so that the free flow of urine is restricted.

A less common cause of prostate enlargement is prostate cancer. Often, in cases of prostate cancer, benign hyperplasia coexists. The diagnosis of prostate cancer should be considered in all men who have symptoms of an enlarged prostate.

A first symptom of prostatic enlargement is that the urine flow becomes less powerful than it used to be. There may be difficulty starting the flow (leading to a need to wait for a few seconds to start to urinate) and also some dribbling at the end of urination. As the condition progresses, these symptoms worsen. The man might have to get up more than once a night to pass urine, and each time he may need to stand for some minutes while waiting for a small dribble to appear. In severe prostatic obstruction the quality of life can be markedly diminished.

The muscle wall of the bladder is affected by having to deal with the increased pressure of urine within it. In mild cases, the muscle wall thickens so that the bladder can still perform its function of emptying all the urine within it. However, in severe prostatic disease the muscle eventually weakens so that the bladder cannot fully expel all the urine. There is then an increased risk of infection due to stagnation of urine in the bladder. The increased pressure is transmitted to the ureters, which dilate, leading to hydronephrosis.

Patients with symptoms should be investigated to exclude the possibility of prostate cancer and also of damage to other parts of the urinary system. In all but the mildest cases, further tests should be carried out to check that the kidney function and emptying of the bladder is normal. At the least, this would require an ultrasound scan of the bladder while voiding urine, and a serum blood test for kidney function.

Those with distressing symptoms and all those with features of impairment of bladder and/or kidney function should be offered treatment. Some patients will respond very well to drugs such as tamsulosin, doxazosin and finasteride (see the case of Ian described in the questions in Chapter 1.2a), although many people cannot tolerate these drugs because of side-effects of dizziness and tiredness (tamsulosin and doxazosin) and impotence (finasteride).

Treatment of severe prostatic enlargement involves surgery. The most common operation performed makes use of an endoscopic tool inserted via the urethra to cut a wider channel through the prostate. Operations of this type, known as 'transurethral resection of the prostate' (TURP) or the less invasive 'transurethral incision of the prostate' (TUIP), carry a risk of haemorrhage into the urethra. To minimise this risk, the patient is left with an indwelling plastic catheter in the urethra for a few days after the operation. This keeps the enlarged channel through the urethra open and compresses any bleeding points. The bladder is continually flushed with saline through this tube for the first couple of days to prevent the accumulation of clots in the bladder or the urethra.

Nevertheless, with TURP blood loss is common, and patients who have had this operation frequently require a blood transfusion, or at least iron tablets, after the operation. In most cases the operation will reduce symptoms and improve quality of life, as well as relieve the pressure on the kidneys. Impotence and infertility (due to ejaculation of semen into the bladder) are common side-effects following TURP, but are less problematic after TUIP.

Information Box 4.3d-I

Urinary obstruction: comments from a Chinese medicine perspective

In Chinese medicine, urinary obstruction in general would correspond to Deficiency of Kidney Yang, the motive force of the Kidneys. There may also be Deficiency of Spleen Yang. Ming-Men Deficiency is a specific syndrome of old age and chronic illness, in which weakness of the Ming Men (which then fails to warm the Spleen and Kidney Yang) causes lack of strength when urinating.

Retention of urine is usually thought to correspond with Damp or Damp Heat in the Middle Jiao, against a background of Spleen and Kidney Yang Deficiency.

Kidney failure following on from obstruction is an indication of Kidney Yin Deficiency, which often coexists with Kidney Yang Deficiency. Infections represent Damp in the Bladder. An enlarged prostate may be said to represent the accumulation of Phlegm.

Infections of the lower urinary tract

Cystitis (bladder infections)

The infections of the lower urinary tract originate from bacteria, which most usually have entered the urethra through its external orifice. Very commonly, bacteria from the patient's own 'healthy' bowel bacteria are the cause. The most common organisms recognised to cause bladder infections (cystitis) include *Escherichia coli*, and *Proteus* and *Enterococcus* species.

Bacteria are more likely to enter the urethra in women, because of the short female urethra, and in young children (especially girls) who wear nappies. Postmenopausal women are even more prone to infections because of the change in the urethral lining that occurs after the menopause. The physical stress on the female urethra from sexual intercourse can precipitate a first attack of cystitis (formerly termed 'honeymoon cystitis'). The insertion of a plastic catheter into the bladder is also a known risk factor for cystitis.

It is also believed that changes to the 'healthy' bacteria of the vagina can increase the risk of cystitis in susceptible woman. Tight clothing, overwashing, or the use of perfumed soaps or talcum powders may all have this effect.

Once bacteria have entered the bladder, they have to multiply and cause damage to lead to a case of cystitis. In most people, the flow of urine in a healthy bladder can prevent this, and simply washes the bacteria out of the bladder again. Cystitis is, therefore, more common in those who have obstruction to the flow of urine and those who drink very little fluid. It is also more common in children with vesico-ureteric reflux and people with diabetes.

Cystitis is more common in pregnancy because of combined hormonal and pressure effects on the urinary system. These reduce the smooth, free flow of urine through the ureters and bladder of a pregnant woman.

Cystitis is usually a mild condition that clears to leave no persisting damage to the urinary system. It is usually only of serious consequence to those who already have underlying disease of the urinary system. In these cases the infection may become recurrent and can cause worsening of the underlying condition.

Cystitis can also predispose to the development of kidney stones in those who are susceptible to forming them.

The symptoms of cystitis include painful and difficult urination and low abdominal pain. The urine may be smelly, cloudy or blood stained, but can appear clear, even in established infection. In severe cases the patient can feel very unwell, with fever and malaise. These general symptoms are more usual if the infection spreads up the ureters to involve the kidneys (acute pyelonephritis), in which case loin pain is often experienced. In young children, the symptoms are less specific. A child with cystitis may simply appear unwell with fever and irritability.

In most cases a simple bout of cystitis will clear of its own accord. The symptoms and speed of clearance can be helped by drinking plenty of fluids. Drinking cranberry juice is sometimes recommended by conventional doctors. Most doctors in the UK will readily prescribe an antibiotic because the response to this treatment is very rapid. Often this treatment is given 'blind' in the form of a broad-spectrum antibiotic that is likely to target the most common organisms. In most cases a short course of 1–3 days may be sufficient to clear the infection from the urinary system, so side-effects are minimised.

A case of cystitis in someone who has an underlying problem of the urinary system, or in someone with diabetes, is treated more intensively. A sample of urine is taken to ensure that it is clear what type of organism has caused the infection. In this case antibiotics are strongly advocated, and the course may last 5–7 days. The antibiotics are chosen to target the particular organism identified from the urine culture. In the case of people who suffer from recurrent infections, long-term antibiotic treatment might be recommended in an attempt to clear the urinary system of any bacteria that may be being harboured in an area of damaged tissue.

Some people experience the distressing symptoms of cystitis but all the tests of the urine come back as normal. In some of these cases the patient may be shown to have a physical cause such as a sexually transmitted infection of the urethra, or inflammation of the urethra following sexual intercourse. In other cases, 'stress' may be a prominent feature, and the symptoms may be classed as a functional disease (irritable bladder) akin to irritable bowel syndrome.

> **Information Box 4.3d-II**
>
> **Cystitis: comments from a Chinese medicine perspective**
>
> In Chinese medicine, urinary infections of the bladder often represent Damp Heat or Damp Cold in the Bladder. There is likely to be an underlying Spleen or Kidney Deficiency.

Prostatitis

On rare occasions, a bacterial infection can spread from the urethra to affect the prostate gland, which then becomes inflamed and swollen. The symptoms of prostatitis include pain in the perineum and the testicles, and occasionally a discharge from the urethra. Prostatitis may be a complication of a sexually transmitted disease, but may simply complicate a urinary infection.

Prostatitis is difficult to treat, as the infection is deep seated. A 4–6 week course of antibiotics may be prescribed.

> **Information Box 4.3d-III**
>
> **Prostatitis: comments from a Chinese medicine perspective**
>
> In Chinese medicine, prostatitis represents Damp Heat in the Lower Jiao and/or Liver and Gallbladder.

Urethritis

Inflammation of the urethra is almost always a complication of a sexually transmitted infection such as gonorrhoea or *Chlamydia*.

Incontinence

Incontinence is defined as a condition in which there is an involuntary flow of urine from the bladder through the urethra. A small degree of incontinence is an extremely common, but underreported, symptom, particularly in women after they have had children. Incontinence is often a cause of great distress, but may be kept secret because of embarrassment.

Stress incontinence

Stress incontinence is an involuntary leakage of urine that occurs when a relatively full bladder experiences an additional external pressure. The leakage is due to weakness of the external urethral sphincter, which consists of the muscle of the pelvic floor (the perineal muscles). This muscle group can become weakened by childbirth and also by losing tone through ageing. The atrophy of the urethra that can occur when the levels of oestrogen decline can lead to the worsening of stress incontinence after the menopause. In some female patients stress incontinence coexists with a degree of prolapse of the womb, another long-term muscular problem associated with childbirth.

In stress incontinence, the patient, who is almost always a woman, will lose an amount of urine upon laughing, coughing or sneezing. In mild cases, the leakage can be contained by a thin sanitary towel, but in more severe cases a much larger volume of urine can be lost.

Urge incontinence

Urge incontinence also affects women much more frequently than men. In this condition, the bladder muscle becomes unstable and may suddenly contract with little or no warning. There may be a sudden and intense urge to urinate, which cannot be suppressed for more than a few seconds, meaning that the patient has to rush to find a toilet. Flooding is an unfortunate consequence of urge incontinence.

Frequently, stress and urge incontinence coexist. Sometimes an increase in pressure within the abdomen can trigger not only a small stress incontinence leakage, but also a full contraction due to bladder instability.

Overflow incontinence

Overflow incontinence is a problem that results from obstruction to the outflow of urine from the bladder. The overflow occurs when the bladder is already quite distended with urine, and the pressure within is high. This form of incontinence is usually in the form of slight dribbling. It is most commonly caused by prostatic enlargement.

Treatment of stress, urge and overflow incontinence

Treatment of these forms of incontinence depends on an accurate diagnosis of the cause. Urodynamic studies are used to assess the changes in pressure within the bladder and the flow rate of urine as it empties. These can help distinguish between urge and stress incontinence in particular.

Mild urge and stress incontinence can both respond very well to simple lifestyle advice. A trained incontinence adviser is invaluable in enabling patients to follow this advice correctly. Stress incontinence may be improved dramatically by means of regular perineal exercises that build up the strength of the pelvic floor muscles. The same exercises can be used by younger women after childbirth to prevent the development of stress incontinence. Urge incontinence can be helped by bladder training, which involves concentrating on a programme of regular and complete emptying of the bladder.

Medication may be prescribed to help prevent incontinence. Duloxetine is an antidepressant which is also licensed for the treatment of stress incontinence. Drugs such as oxybutynin calm down an overreactive bladder muscle and so may be of help in urge incontinence.

There is a wide range of incontinence pads and aids available which may help cope with a mild problem. In men a condom (sheath) can be used to drain leaked urine down a plastic tube into a bag discreetly attached to the thigh.

For more severe stress incontinence, surgical repair of the weak supporting muscles of the bladder may be recommended. The results of this operation are now recognised to not always be very satisfactory to the patient, so it is performed less frequently than it used to be. The repair operation may be performed at the same time as a hysterectomy to correct the problem of a prolapsed womb.

Neurological incontinence

In neurological incontinence the control of the bladder is lost because of damage to the nerves that supply the bladder. This might be the result of disease of the brain or spinal cord (e.g. stroke, multiple sclerosis or spinal injury) or can be the result of a disorder that causes damage to the peripheral nerves (e.g. diabetes).

In this condition, because the incontinence is often total, the treatment that offers the patient the most freedom in daily life is an indwelling plastic catheter. This plastic tube allows drainage of the urine from the bladder into a plastic bag, which can be emptied at intervals. The main disadvantage of indwelling catheters is that they are frequently the cause of recurrent urinary infections. In some cases patients can be taught to "intermittently self catheterise" which means that the catheter is used only for voiding the bladder at intervals (usually four times a day) and so does not needs to be indwelling.

Tumours of the lower urinary tract

The most important tumours to affect the urinary tract are those of the bladder and of the prostate. The rare forms of cancer that affect the ureters and urethra are similar in type to the cancer that more commonly develops in the bladder.

Information Box 4.3d-IV

Incontinence: comments from a Chinese medicine perspective

In Chinese medicine, incontinence corresponds to either Lung Qi Deficiency, a Deficiency of the Kidneys, or both. The Kidney Deficiency can be of Yin or Yang. Kidney Qi not Firm describes a syndrome of nocturnal incontinence. It is an aspect of Kidney Yang Deficiency.

Cancer of the bladder (transitional cell carcinoma)

Malignant tumours of the bladder affect men four times more often than women. They are associated with cigarette smoking and also exposure to certain drugs and environmental toxins. Bladder cancer has been linked to industrial exposure in the rubber and chemical industries. The tropical infection schistosomiasis is an important worldwide cause of bladder cancer. In schistosomiasis, the cancer results from the chronic inflammation of the bladder caused by the disease.

The first symptom of bladder cancer is usually blood in the urine. Alternatively, the first symptoms may mimic a bout of cystitis, including pain on urination and abdominal pain. In the case of cancer these symptoms will not respond fully to antibiotic therapy.

The diagnosis may be suggested by an ultrasound scan, but is confirmed by means of a cystoscopy during which a biopsy of the tumour can be obtained. If the tumour is localised it may be successfully treated by burning (diathermy) with an electrical probe inserted via the cystoscope. The patient is then instructed to return for a 'check cystoscopy' at regular intervals to look for and treat any recurrences of the tumour. Four out of five patients who have a localised bladder tumour will still be alive 5 years after the first diagnosis, and a proportion of these will be cured.

A more advanced tumour may be treated with a variety of approaches, including infusion of chemotherapy into the bladder, radiotherapy and surgical removal of the bladder. There is very little chance of cure of bladder cancer if the cancer has spread to other tissues at the time of diagnosis.

Information Box 4.3d-V

Bladder cancer: comments from a Chinese medicine perspective

In Chinese medicine, bladder cancer corresponds to Phlegm and/or Blood Stagnation. There is likely to be an underlying Deficiency of Kidney Yin and/or Yang.

Prostate cancer

Prostate cancer is a very common development in the ageing prostate gland. In many cases the cancer is slow growing and causes few symptoms. It is estimated that 80% of men have islands of cancer cells within their prostate gland by the age of 80 years, but only in a minority of these will the cancer cells be any threat to their health. More malignant prostate tumours grow to a size that causes urinary obstruction. The cancer spreads very commonly to bone, so that bone pain may be also a first symptom.

A malignant prostate may feel hard and irregular on rectal examination, but this is not a reliable sign. An ultrasound scan of the prostate may reveal a characteristic irregular swelling of the gland, and can give a good estimate of the size of the tumour for the purposes of staging.

A blood test for a chemical called prostate-specific antigen (PSA) is more likely to show a raised PSA level if cancer is present, but the results of this test can be confusing, which has brought its value as a cancer screening test into doubt. Prostate cancer can only really be confirmed by means of tissue biopsy. The tissue sample may be obtained by means of a transrectal ultrasound (TRUS) guided approach or at the time of a TURP for prostatic enlargement. X-ray imaging or a bone scan may be performed to exclude or assess the presence of bony metastases. This is important for the staging of the tumour. Localised prostate cancer is assigned a Gleason Score, which rates the invasiveness of the tumour on a scale from 2 to 10. This score is based on the microscopic appearance of the biopsy. A Gleason Score of 6 or less indicates that the cancer is not likely to spread beyond the prostate gland.

Treatment of symptomatic disease confined to the prostate involves removal of the prostate gland or radiotherapy. Removal of the prostate gland carries the risks of incontinence and impotence (erectile dysfunction). In localised prostate cancer, the radiotherapy can take the form of the insertion of radioactive pellets into the prostate gland, which then act over the course of time. This treatment is known as 'brachytherapy'. If the disease has spread outside the prostate gland, radiotherapy can again be beneficial. Radiotherapy carries no risk of incontinence, but does carry a significant risk of erectile dysfunction.

Drugs may be used to hinder the further spread of prostate cancer that has already spread beyond the prostate gland. It is known that the cancer regresses if the effects of testosterone can be eliminated. A radical solution to this used to be removal of the testes, but currently most men prefer to take tablets (cyproterone) or have an injection (e.g. goserilin) which act to suppress the action of testosterone in the body. These approaches carry the side-effects of loss of libido and hot flushes.

The prognosis in most cases of metastatic prostate disease is not very good. The majority of patients are not alive 5 years after diagnosis, although it must be remembered that many patients are elderly at diagnosis, so in some of these cases death may have been as a result of other causes.

Information Box 4.3d-VI

Prostate cancer: comments from a Chinese medicine perspective

In Chinese medicine, prostate cancer corresponds to Phlegm and/or Blood Stagnation against a background of severe Deficiency, in particular of Kidney Yin and Yang.

The red flags of the diseases of the ureters, bladder and urethra

Some patients with diseases of the ureters, bladder and urethra will benefit from referral to a conventional doctor for assessment and/or treatment. Red flags are those symptoms and signs that indicate that referral is to be considered. The red flags of the diseases of the kidneys are described in Table 4.3d-I. This table forms part of the summary on red flags given in Appendix III, which also gives advice on the degree of urgency of referral for each of the red flag conditions listed.

Self-test 4.3d

The diseases of the ureters, bladder and the urethra

1. A 60-year-old patient admits with embarrassment that, whenever she gets up from sitting or coughs, she leaks a small amount of urine. She says that this symptom has become progressively worse over the past few years, and now she often has to change her underwear despite wearing a sanitary towel all the time.
   (i) What sort of incontinence is this?
   (ii) For what reasons might you consider a referral to a conventional practitioner?
2. David is a 70-year-old long-standing patient of yours. You find out one day that he has been having trouble urinating for the past few months. He regularly gets up to urinate at least twice a night, and has a very weak stream of urine. David says that he knows that it is due to his age, and that the problem does not trouble him. When you suggest that he should go for a check up, he is reluctant to trouble his GP with the problem. Would you persist in encouraging him to visit his GP? If so, why?

Answers

1. (i) This is a typical description of fairly severe stress incontinence.
   (ii) You might consider a referral so that the diagnosis can be confirmed, and so that your patient may have access to specialist advice about management of stress incontinence. There is a possibility that her quality of life might be improved by repair surgery, so she may also benefit from a surgical opinion.
2. The chances are that David has benign enlargement of his prostate gland and this is causing obstruction to the flow of the urine from his bladder. However, there is also a possibility that he has prostate cancer. For this reason you should ask him if he has any recently developed pain in any part of his bones, which may suggest metastatic disease.

   David describes fairly severe symptoms because the flow of his urine is very weak. This means that there may be incomplete emptying of his bladder, and a possibility of increased pressure in the ureters and kidneys.

   It is advisable that David sees his doctor for some simple tests to rule out the possibility of prostate cancer and to check that his kidneys are not being affected by the obstruction.

   However, he is well, and there may be no underlying serious problem. A middle way would be to treat his Kidney energy for a month or so and suggest referral if there is no improvement, and certainly if there any worsening, of symptoms by then.

Table 4.3d-I Red Flags 30 – diseases of the ureters, bladder and urethra

Red Flag	Description	Reasoning
30.1	**Acute loin pain**: often comes in waves; patient may vomit and collapse	This is characteristic of an obstructed kidney stone. The pain may radiate round to the suprapubic region, particularly if the stone moves some way down the ureter. Encourage drinking of fluids
30.2	**Blood in the urine (haematuria) or sperm (haemospermia): refer all cases in men**; refer in women except in the case of acute urinary infection	The most common and benign cause of blood in the urine is bladder infection (cystitis) in women. If the symptoms are suggestive of this diagnosis (burning on urination, low abdominal pain, cloudy or blood-stained urine), there is no need to refer straight away. Treat with complementary medicine, recommend a high fluid intake and refer only if symptoms are not settling within 3 days However, blood in the urine is not normal in men, who should be protected from infection by their relatively long urethras. Refer all cases of blood in the urine in men, and in women if there are either no other symptoms (blood may be coming from kidney or from tumour) or if there is pain in the loin (suggesting spread of infection to kidneys) Haemospermia is alarming to the patient but is usually benign, as it can result from slight trauma to the genitals. Nevertheless, refer to exclude a serious cause
30.3	**Features of recurrent or persistent urinary tract infection**: episodes of symptoms including some or all of cloudy urine, burning on urination, abdominal discomfort, blood in urine and fever, especially if occurring in men	Urinary tract infections are generally self-limiting and should clear up within 5 days. Refer anyone who has persistent symptoms in order to exclude an underlying disorder of the urinary system. Recurrent or persistent infections are particularly uncommon in men and are more likely to signify an underlying disorder of the urinary tract than they are in women
30.4	**Features of a urinary tract infection in someone in one of the following vulnerable groups**: pre-existing disorder of the urinary system, diabetes, pregnancy, prepubescent child	Refer someone who develops symptoms of a urinary tract infection straightaway for treatment if there is an underlying vulnerability such as known disease of the urinary system (e.g. kidney disease, kidney stones, bladder cancer and enlarged prostate gland) diabetes or pregnancy In both pregnancy and diabetes, there is a far higher risk of the infection ascending the ureters and damaging the kidneys. Urinary infections may also increase the risk of early labour or miscarriage
30.5	**Features of moderate prostatic obstruction**: enlargement of the prostate gland leads to symptoms such as increasing difficulty urinating, need to get up at night to urinate (nocturia)	Benign prostatic enlargement is common and the symptoms can respond to acupuncture treatment. However, the same symptoms can be caused by a prostatic tumour, and so it is wise to refer for further investigations, including physical (rectal) examination, kidney function tests and a blood test for prostate specific antigen (PSA)
30.6	**Features of acute pyelonephritis**: fever, malaise, loin pain and cloudy urine suggest an infection of the kidneys	While bladder infections are usually self-limiting, particularly in women, if there are features suggesting that the infection has ascended the ureters to affect the kidney, the situation is more serious. Acute pyelonephritis carries a risk of permanent scarring of the kidneys, and merits medical attention (treatment with antibiotics)
30.7	**Features of vesico-ureteric reflux disease (VUR) in a child**: any history of recurrent episodes or a current episode of cloudy urine or burning on urination should be taken seriously in a prepubescent child	Urine infections are common in young children but need to be taken seriously, particularly if there is a history of recurrent infections. The small child is more vulnerable to VUR, which means that when the bladder contracts some urine is flushed back towards the kidneys. In the case of infection of the bladder, VUR can lead to infectious organisms causing damage to the delicate structure of the kidney. Sometimes this damage occurs with very few symptoms, but if cumulative and undetected can lead to serious kidney problems and high blood pressure in later life For this reason it is wise to refer all prepubescent children with a history of symptoms of urinary infections to exclude the possibility of VUR
30.8	**Bedwetting in a child**: if persisting over the age of 5 years	Consider referral if the child is over 5 years old, so that physical causes can be excluded and parents can have access to expert advice
30.9	**Incontinence**: if unexplained or causing distress	A mild degree of stress incontinence (leakage of a small amount of urine when coughing or laughing) is common and benign in women, particularly after childbirth and the menopause. However, uncontrollable losses of large amounts of urine are not normal, and nor is bedwetting when asleep. In these cases investigations are merited to look for treatable causes such as a prolapsed uterus, prostatic obstruction and nocturnal seizures. Also refer so that the patient can have access to guidance and support from a specialist incontinence nurse

Diseases of the endocrine system

5.1

Chapter 5.1a The physiology of the endocrine system

LEARNING POINTS

At the end of this chapter you will:

- be able to describe the role of a hormone
- be able to describe the anatomical positions of the organs of the endocrine system
- understand the importance of the negative feedback loop in the function of the endocrine system
- be able to describe the function of those endocrine organs that are affected by the important endocrine diseases.

Estimated time for chapter: 120 minutes.

Introduction

The idea has already been introduced that the nervous and endocrine systems together can be considered as the foundation of that which makes the body an integrated whole. This is because they are both concerned with communication between one body part and another.

In the nervous system, the communication between one nerve and another takes place at a junction called the 'synapse'. At the synapse, the release of a tiny amount of a chemical known as a 'neurotransmitter' enables a change that has taken place in one nerve cell to be transmitted to other nerve cells. In the endocrine system, the communication is also based on the release of chemicals. These chemicals, released by specialised endocrine cells, are known as 'hormones'. Endocrine cells may be grouped together in organs known as 'endocrine glands', but also can be found loosely distributed within many of the organs and tissues of the body (see Q.5.1a-1).

In contrast to neurotransmitters, hormones can stimulate changes in bodily cells only after travelling to local tissues via the tissue fluid, or to distant sites through the bloodstream. However, once hormones reach their target cells, the way in which they lead to internal changes within those cells is remarkably similar to the effect of neurotransmitters on target nerve cells. Both hormones and neurotransmitters connect with protein 'receptors' on the target cell membrane. Through this connection, these chemicals lead to a change in the internal physiology of the cell. As increasing numbers of these chemicals are discovered by scientists and their functions described, it is becoming clear that many of those which act as hormones in the body can also be found within the nervous system, where they function as neurotransmitters.

Through communication by means of hormones, the endocrine system encourages the state of homeostasis to be maintained within the body. In order to fulfil this role, the endocrine system has always to be responsive to changes in the internal and external environments of the body (see Q5.1a-2).

Cholecystokinin (CCK) (originating from cells in the duodenum), adrenaline (from the adrenal medulla), erythropoietin (EPO) (from the substance of the kidney) and testosterone (from the testes) are examples of hormones that have their impact on the digestive, cardiovascular, blood and reproductive systems, respectively. CCK and EPO are examples of hormones that are not released from specific endocrine organs. CCK is released from endocrine cells scattered within the wall of the duodenum, and EPO is released from endocrine cells within the tissue of the kidney. In contrast, adrenaline and testosterone are examples of hormones that originate from specialised endocrine organs, namely the adrenal glands and the testes, respectively.

The organs of the endocrine system

Figure 5.1a-I illustrates the anatomical location of the organs of the endocrine system. This chapter focuses on the most basic physiology of those endocrine organs that are affected in the important endocrine diseases. These are:

- the pituitary and the hypothalamus
- the thyroid gland

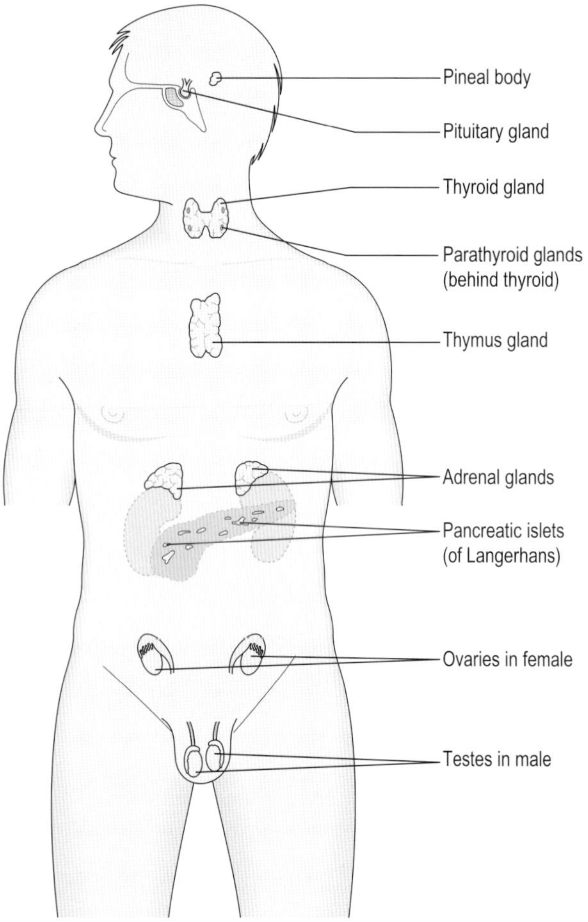

Figure 5.1a-I • The anatomical location of the organs of the endocrine system.

- the adrenal glands
- the endocrine part of the pancreas (pancreatic islets).

The role of the parathyroid glands in calcium homeostasis is described in Chapters 4.2a and 4.3a. The function of the ovaries and testes will be explored in Chapter 5.2a. The pineal gland and thymus gland will be not discussed further in this text.

The negative feedback loop

The negative feedback loop is the basic mechanism that underlies an important aspect of the action of these hormones. The negative feedback loop requires a detector to recognise a move away from balance, a control centre that recognises when the move has been so great that something has to be done about it, and an effector to bring about a change in the body to reverse the imbalance. A thermostat is a mechanical example of the negative feedback loop in action. The detector in this case is a thermometer. The control centre is the mechanism that is set to recognise when the temperature falls outside a desired range. The negative feedback loop is based on maximum desired temperature. When the temperature becomes too high, the effector, in this case the heating element, is switched off until the time when the temperature drops within the desired range once again.

Table 5.1a-I The release of cholecystokinin (CCK): an example of the negative feedback loop in the regulation of hormones
The endocrine cells of the duodenum are specialised to 'detect' increased levels of fat within the duodenum. They do this by means of specialised proteins on their cell membranes which, when they come into contact with fat, lead to internal changes within the cells. In this case the internal change is the onset of the manufacture of cholecystokinin (CCK). The control aspect is that it is only when the amount of fat is at a certain level that these cells are stimulated to release CCK into the bloodstream. CCK is the effector that travels within the bloodstream to lead to an appropriate release of bile from the gallbladder, which in turn helps to digest the fats. The release of CCK only ceases when all the fat has been digested and has left the duodenum. Incidentally, CCK also acts at the exocrine pancreas to stimulate the release of fat-digesting enzymes (amongst others) into the duodenum. This is another example of a negative feedback loop in action.

These rather abstract concepts, which were introduced in Chapter 1.1c, can now be placed in more concrete terms. Endocrine cells play the role of both detector and control centre, while the release of hormone corresponds to the effector of the negative feedback loop. As a thermostat is designed to keep ambient temperature constant, the endocrine negative feedback loops work to keep bodily variables such as blood sugar or blood calcium at a steady level. This chapter offers many more examples of this negative feedback loop in action (for example see Table 5.1a-I), as each of the important endocrine organs is described in turn.

The pituitary and the hypothalamus

The pituitary gland is a pea-sized organ that projects downwards from an area at the base of the brain called the 'hypothalamus'. The site of the pituitary is deep within the head, approximately at the level of the bridge of the nose (Figure 5.1a-II). The extra acupoint Yintang, which is considered in Chinese medicine to have a profound influence over mental functions, overlies the region of the pituitary and hypothalamus.

A 'stalk' projects downwards from the hypothalamus through which nerve fibres pass into the pituitary. A delicate network of blood vessels connects the two areas through this stalk. These blood vessels carry hormones from the hypothalamus to the pituitary.

An alternative term for the pituitary gland is the 'hypophysis'. The term 'adenohypophysis' refers to the anterior portion of the pituitary, which contains endocrine cells. The adenohypophysis is the source of six different hormones. The term 'neurohypophysis' refers to the posterior portion of the pituitary gland. This part receives nerve fibres from the hypothalamus, and is the source of two additional hormones, which are secreted directly into the bloodstream from the endings of these nerves.

Together, the hypothalamus and the pituitary perform a vital control function in the endocrine system. The hormones secreted by the hypothalamus and the pituitary affect the function of other endocrine organs, including the thyroid gland, the adrenal gland and the sex organs.

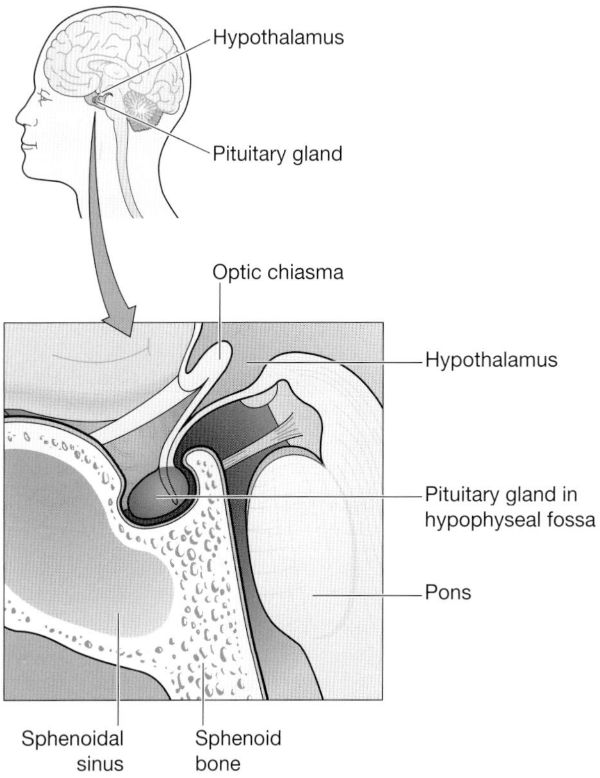

Figure 5.1a-II • The position of the pituitary gland and its associated structures.

The hormones of the hypothalamus are either secreted into the general bloodstream by the nerve endings of the neurohypophysis, or carried within the blood vessels of the pituitary stalk to act on the adenohypophysis. In contrast, all the hormones released by the pituitary gland travel within the bloodstream to have effects on distant endocrine organs as well as other parts of the body.

There are at least 13 hormones that are released by the hypothalamus and the pituitary gland. All of these are commonly described by conventional practitioners by their initials rather than their full medical names, and include growth hormone (GH), thyroid stimulating hormone (TSH), adrenocorticotrophic hormone (ACTH) from the pituitary and growth-hormone-releasing hormone (GHRH), corticotrophin-releasing hormone (CRH) and gonadotrophin-releasing hormone (GnRH) from the hypothalamus.

It is helpful to understand that the hormones of the hypothalamus are the mechanism by which the hormones of the pituitary are controlled. For example, the release of growth hormone (GH) from the pituitary gland can be increased and decreased by two different hormones (GHRH and GHIH) from the hypothalamus. This is one example of the close connection between the nervous system (hypothalamus) and the endocrine system (pituitary gland).

The hypothalamus lies deep within the substance of the brain, and thus can be influenced by complex internal factors, including the stage of psychological development and the emotions. This might explain why such factors can have profound effects on hormone-controlled events such as childhood growth, timing of puberty and breastmilk production.

Table 5.1a-II The hormones released from the anterior pituitary gland (adenohypophysis) and their functions

Hormone	Function
Growth hormone (GH)	Stimulates growth in many tissues
Thyroid-stimulating hormone (TSH)	Stimulates the production of thyroid hormones
Adrenocorticotrophic hormone (ACTH)	Stimulates the production of cortisol from the adrenal gland
Prolactin (PRL)	Stimulates breastmilk production
Follicle-stimulating hormone (FSH)	Stimulates the development of the ovarian follicle (the first half of the menstrual cycle)
Luteinising hormone (LH)	Stimulates ovulation and the maturation of the ruptured follicle (corpus luteum)

Table 5.1a-II lists the six hormones that are produced by the adenohypophysis.

The hormones oxytocin and antidiuretic hormone (ADH) are released from the neurohypophysis, but have their origins within nerve cells within the hypothalamus.

Growth hormone

Growth hormone is a hormone that stimulates the continued growth of the skeleton, muscles and soft tissues, including the major organs. This growth is not only essential during childhood, but is also important for the maintained health and liveliness of these tissues throughout adult life. Growth hormone affects the metabolism of the body, meaning that it alters the rate at which the complex chemical processes of the bodily tissues take place. Under the influence of growth hormone, the rate of protein and collagen synthesis increases, and the amount of sugar in the blood tends to rise to meet the body's increased requirements for energy.

Information Box 5.1a-I

Growth hormone: comments from a Chinese medicine perspective

A Chinese medicine energetic interpretation of this hormone has to be complex, as growth hormone affects the functioning of diverse tissues at a fundamental level.

Its role in continued growth suggests that its control is an aspect of Kidney Essence. Its role in the appropriate use of nutrients to build up the physical substance of the body suggests that it also plays a role in the transformation of Qi. Its control, therefore, can also be seen as an aspect of Original Qi and, in particular, Spleen Qi. Original Qi is, of course, closely related to Kidney Essence.

In excess, growth hormone leads to thickening of soft tissues and broadening of the bones (see Chapter 5.1e). This might be interpreted as accumulation of Damp and Phlegm. This again suggests that appropriate secretion of growth hormone is an aspect of the healthy function of the Spleen Organ.

Oxytocin

Oxytocin is important for contraction of the uterine muscle during labour and for the expression of breastmilk during suckling.

ADH, TSH, ACTH, FSH, LH and prolactin

The role of ADH was mentioned in Chapter 4.3a. This hormone is released in response to an increased concentration of the salts in the blood. It reduces the amount of water that is lost through the urine, and is important in the control of the homeostasis of the concentration of the blood. TSH and ACTH relate to the healthy function of the thyroid and adrenal glands, respectively. PRL, FSH and LH are all important in the physiology of the reproductive system. The function of these five pituitary hormones is described in more detail in Chapter 5.2a.

The thyroid gland

Figure 5.1a-III illustrates the thyroid gland, which is a bow-shaped organ situated just below the level of the laryngeal prominence (Adam's apple) in the neck. The bow shape is a result of the gland being formed by two lobes separated by a narrow bridge of tissue called the 'isthmus'. In health, the thyroid gland can be felt as a small region of vague softness below the voice box. This can be felt to rise and descend during swallowing.

The thyroid gland contains endocrine cells, which secrete two hormones, thyroxine (also known as T4) and tri-iodothyronine (T3). The thyroid gland draws upon iodine from the diet to manufacture sufficient quantities of these hormones. Iodine is found in seawater, and also in plant and animal products that originate from areas close to the sea. For this reason, iodine deficiency may occur in regions of the world that are distant from the sea, especially landlocked countries. However, in many developed countries, such as the UK, table salt contains additional iodine, meaning that iodine deficiency is rarely a problem.

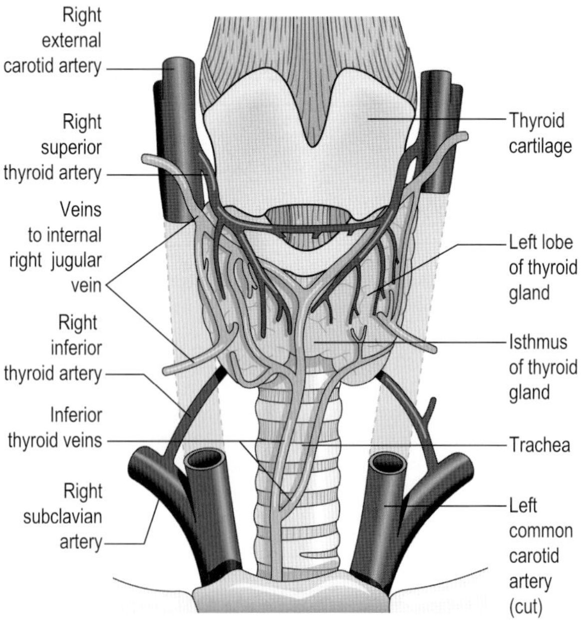

Figure 5.1a-III • The thyroid gland and its associated structures.

The thyroid hormones T4 and T3 are both released in response to TSH (thyroid-stimulating hormone) from the pituitary. The release of TSH is primarily controlled by the release of TRH (thyroid-releasing hormone) from the hypothalamus. This is the mechanism whereby the activity of the brain affects thyroid function.

Like growth hormone, the thyroid hormones play an important role in physical growth and the rate at which the cells of the body convert nutrients into energy (the metabolic rate). They are also important in the healthy development of the growing nervous system, the appropriate function of the cardiovascular system and the smooth functioning of the gastrointestinal system. If in excess, the thyroid hormones can cause an increased use of bodily nutrients, leading to the production of heat, weight loss, feelings of nervousness, a rapid heart rate and increased peristalsis in the bowel.

The negative feedback loop of control of the thyroid hormones is affected by factors such as exercise, stress, low blood glucose and malnutrition. All these factors increase the release of TSH from the hypothalamus, and thus increase the release of T4 and T3. Conversely, raised levels of thyroid hormones in the bloodstream will inhibit the release of TRH from the hypothalamus and TSH from the pituitary gland (see Q5.1a-3).

Information Box 5.1a-II

Thyroid hormone: comments from a Chinese medicine perspective

The Chinese medicine energetic interpretation of the thyroid hormones is complex. The thyroid hormones are important for growth and the appropriate use of nutrients at a cellular level. Both these aspects of their role suggest that their control reflects an aspect of Kidney Essence and Original Qi.

The consequence of an excessive secretion of thyroid hormones is the generation of a state similar to the general pattern described as Yin Deficiency (feelings of heat, anxiety and rapid heart rate). Insufficient secretion of thyroid hormones leads to a state that includes feelings of cold, lassitude, weight gain and slow heart rate (see Chapter 5.1c), which together can be compared to the pattern of Yang Deficiency. Thus these patterns suggest that the appropriate control of the thyroid hormones reflects an aspect of the fundamental balance of Yin and Yang.

As the seat of Yin and Yang lies within the Kidney Organ, here is another example of how the function of the thyroid gland might be closely related to the Kidney Organ in Chinese medicine. This fits with the fact that the deep pathway of the Kidney Organ passes through the throat and ends at the root of the tongue. Interestingly, the root of the tongue is the origin of the tissue of the developing thyroid gland in the embryo.

Calcitonin

Calcitonin is another hormone secreted by the thyroid gland. Together with the parathyroid hormone (PTH), it plays a role in calcium homeostasis. PTH is secreted by the cells of the four tiny parathyroid glands situated deep within the tissue of the thyroid gland.

Information Box 5.1a-III

Parathyroid hormone and calcitonin: comments from a Chinese medicine perspective

In Chinese medicine terms, the role of both these additional hormones secreted by the thyroid gland can also be linked to the Kidney Organ, in that they are fundamental to the health of the bony skeleton.

The adrenal glands

The adrenal glands are situated on top of the kidneys, deep in the back of the abdomen, approximately at the level of the lumbar vertebrae L1 and L2. Each gland contains two distinct areas of endocrine tissue. The outer part of each gland is called the 'cortex', and this is the source of three types of steroid hormones, known as glucocorticoids, mineralocorticoids and androgens. The androgens secreted by the adrenal cortex are male sex hormones, but have a minimal effect in comparison to the effect of those secreted by the sex organs. The inner part of the adrenal gland is called the 'medulla'. The adrenal medulla is the source of two hormones, adrenaline and noradrenaline, which play an important role in the sympathetic nervous system.

Glucocorticoids

The glucocorticoids include cortisol and corticosterone, and are essential for life. Their release is stimulated via the pituitary (by ACTH). Glucocorticoids are released in times of stress, and also their levels peak early in the morning in preparation for the time of waking up. They affect the way in which glucose is handled in the body, and increase the retention of salt and water in the body.

These hormones have the effect of preparing the body for sustained physical activity such as occurs on waking. They both enable the storage of glucose, and also increase its availability by breaking down other substances such as protein. By retaining salt and water, they increase the blood pressure, which is an appropriate response, if controlled.

Excessive stress will lead to excessive secretion of these hormones, and this can contribute to raised blood sugar (diabetes), muscle wasting and hypertension. Corticosteroids are synthetic forms of these hormones.

Mineralocorticoids

Aldosterone is the main mineralocorticoid hormone. It is secreted in response to a fall in sodium, and enables more sodium and water to be retained by the kidneys. It is also secreted in response to a reduced flow of blood in the kidneys (which stimulates the release of renin).

Aldosterone secretion, by increasing sodium and water retention, has the effect of raising the blood pressure. In the situation of prolonged stress, excessive secretion of this hormone will also contribute to hypertension.

Noradrenaline and adrenaline

Noradrenaline and adrenaline are released in response to activation of the sympathetic nervous system. Noradrenaline leads to increased constriction of blood vessels and so tends to raise the blood pressure. Adrenaline prepares the body in diverse ways to prepare for 'flight or fight'. In a situation of prolonged stress, both these hormones will contribute to the development of hypertension. In addition, adrenaline will lead to a sensation of anxiety, increased breathing rate and, eventually, weight loss (see Q5.1a-4).

Summary

In summary, the hormones of the adrenal gland function to enable the body to cope appropriately with the demands of physical and emotional stress. However, if stress is prolonged, this response can be harmful, as it can contribute to the development of hypertension, weight loss and diabetes.

Information Box 5.1a-IV

The hormones of the adrenal gland: comments from a Chinese medicine perspective

Again, from a Chinese medicine point of view, the energetics of these hormones are complex. In health, they all help the body to deal appropriately with physical and emotional demands, by ensuring adequate supplies of glucose to all the tissues and an adequate level of blood pressure. This can be equated to the role of Original Qi and Kidney Yang, which are both aspects of the function of the Kidney Organ.

In conditions of prolonged stress, the hormones are secreted in excess. The problems of excessive blood sugar and hypertension suggest an imbalance of Spleen Qi and hyperactivity of Kidney Yang. Features of Accumulation of Damp and Phlegm may be observed in glucocorticoid and mineralocorticoid excess (see Chapter 5.1e). See Chapter 2.2c for a more detailed Chinese medicine interpretation of the diverse effects of excessive synthetic corticosteroids.

The pancreas

The pancreas plays an important exocrine role in the production of several digestive enzymes, which are released into the duodenum to break down the nutrients in food leaving the stomach. Studded within the exocrine tissue of the pancreas are little islands (islets) of endocrine cells, which secrete a range of hormones. These hormones are important for controlling the way in which the body utilises glucose after it has been absorbed into the bloodstream. In a way this can also be seen as an aspect of the digestive function.

The two most well-recognised hormones secreted by the islets are insulin and glucagon. These two hormones act in complementary ways to ensure that the cells of the body have access to a continuous supply of glucose, whatever the external conditions may be. This means that, whether the prevailing condition is one of feast or famine, the body tissues can be adequately nourished, at least in the short term.

Insulin

Insulin is secreted in response to a rise in blood sugar, and acts to reduce the blood sugar levels so that they do not exceed a healthy level for the tissues of the body. It does this by:

- stimulating the conversion of excess blood glucose to glycogen, which can then be stored in the liver and muscles
- preventing protein and fat from being converted into sugar (thus counteracting one action of thyroxine)
- enabling the cells to take up glucose from the bloodstream (in the absence of insulin, cells are simply unable to utilise the glucose, however much there may be in the bloodstream; a state compared to 'starvation in the midst of plenty').

Glucagon

Glucagon is released in response to decreased levels of glucose in the bloodstream and acts to increase the blood sugar levels. It does this by:

- stimulating the conversion of glycogen stored in the liver into glucose
- stimulating the production of glucose from the breakdown of fats and proteins.

Information Box 5.1a-V

Insulin and glucagon: comments from a Chinese medicine perspective

The Chinese medicine interpretation of the endocrine aspect of the pancreas might be that it is also associated with the Spleen (Spleen/Pancreas) Organ. By ensuring an adequate level of glucose in the bloodstream, it continues the role of the digestive tract in providing nutrition for the cells of the body.

Summary

This concludes the introduction to the organs of the endocrine system. Perhaps more so than for any other system, the delicate nature of the function of this system can only really become apparent after studying what happens when the system becomes out of balance.

Self-test 5.1a

The physiology of the endocrine system

1. Describe (i) the similarities and (ii) the differences between a hormone and a neurotransmitter.
2. List:
   (i) three hormones released in the region of the thyroid gland
   (ii) three hormones released from the adrenal gland
   (iii) two hormones released from the pancreas.
3. Describe one important difference between the role of the hypothalamus and the role of the pituitary.

Answers

1. (i) Hormones and neurotransmitters are both chemicals whose role is to enable communication between one body part and another. Both are manufactured within specialised cells and are released (by the process of exocytosis) from those cells in response to defined changes that have occurred in those cells.

   Both hormones and neurotransmitters act to communicate with other cells by connecting with 'receptor' proteins in the membranes of those cells. This connection stimulates an internal change within the cell, and thus a change in one cell has been communicated to another.

   (ii) Hormones are released by specialised endocrine cells, which may either be loosely distributed within the tissue of another organ or grouped together as part of the tissue of an endocrine organ. Neurotransmitters are released by the specialised endings of the dendrites of nerve cells.

   Hormones are released into the tissue fluid surrounding the endocrine cells, and often travel long distances via the bloodstream to reach their target sites. Neurotransmitters travel a very short distance within the synaptic cleft before they reach their target site, on the membrane of a dendrite of another nerve cell.
2. (i) Thyroxine (T4), tri-iodothyronine (T3) and calcitonin are all released from the tissue of the thyroid gland. Parathyroid hormone (PTH) is released from the parathyroid glands, which are situated at the back of the thyroid gland.

   (ii) The glucocorticoids, cortisol and corticosterone, the mineralocorticoid, aldosterone, and androgens are released by the adrenal cortex. Noradrenaline and adrenaline are released by the adrenal medulla.

   (iii) Insulin, glucagon and various other digestive hormones, including somatostatin, are released from the endocrine pancreas.
3. To answer this question well you need first to make a distinction between the anterior pituitary (adenohypophysis) and the posterior pituitary (neurohypophysis). The neurohypophysis can be considered as a physical extension of the nerve cells of the hypothalamus. The two hormones released from the neurohypophysis are released in direct response to nervous messages reaching the hypothalamus. In this way they are similar in action to the hormone-releasing nerve cells of the hypothalamus itself.

   In contrast, the adenohypophysis contains hormone-secreting endocrine cells. The hormones of the pituitary are released in response to hormones that have been first released from the hypothalamus, and so can be seen as in the control of the hypothalamus. This is the important difference between the pituitary and the hypothalamus.

Chapter 5.1b The investigation of the endocrine system

LEARNING POINTS

At the end of this chapter you will:
- be able to recognise the main investigations used for endocrine disease
- understand what a patient might experience when undergoing these investigations.

Estimated time for chapter: 40 minutes.

Introduction

The investigation of the endocrine system is usually carried out within the hospital speciality of endocrinology. A patient with a suspected endocrine disease may be referred either to an endocrinologist or to a general physician with expertise in endocrinology.

The investigation of the endocrine system includes:
- a thorough physical examination
- blood tests to assess the levels of hormones in the blood
- urine tests to assess the levels of hormones excreted in the urine
- more complex blood and urine tests to assess the response of hormones to various stimuli (stimulation and suppression tests)
- imaging tests (in particular computed tomography (CT) scan and magnetic resonance imaging (MRI)) to visualise the structure of the endocrine organs.

Physical examination

With the exception of the thyroid gland and the testicles, most of the endocrine organs cannot be examined directly as part of the physical examination. However, much information can be gained by looking for the effects on the body that can result from endocrine disease.

The physical examination of the endocrine system involves the stages listed in Table 5.1b-I.

Table 5.1b-I The stages in the physical examination of the endocrine system

- *Examination of the general appearance*: this can reveal the characteristic features of many of the endocrine diseases, which can lead to marked changes in physical appearance. These include weight loss or weight gain, reduced or excessive body hair, changes to the texture of the skin and loss of muscle bulk. It is often possible for an experienced physician to be fairly sure of a diagnosis from a patient's physical appearance alone
- *Careful examination of all the other systems of the body*: as the endocrine diseases commonly result in changes in diverse body systems, a careful systematic approach to examination can reveal many characteristic changes, such as the increased pulse rate found in hyperthyroidism, or the changes of the retina that can develop in diabetes mellitus

Blood and urine tests

Simple blood tests can be used to assess the levels of the hormones in the blood. In some cases, the results alone may indicate whether or not endocrine disease should be suspected. For example, in suspected thyroid disease the most common first tests to be performed are serum tests to assess the levels of TSH, T4 and T3. Levels of these hormones that fall outside the normal range would be suggestive of thyroid disease. Such tests are easy for the doctor to perform, and not too inconvenient for the patient.

However, in other cases, because the level of the hormone varies dramatically throughout the day, and also according to individual need at the time, a single blood test cannot offer such conclusive results.

Sometimes a patient might be requested to collect all their urine over the course of 24 hours so that levels of hormone can be assessed from the urine. This has the advantage of overcoming the problem of varying levels throughout the day, but is well known for not being a very accurate method of assessment. Moreover, many patients find this an inconvenient and embarrassing test to perform.

Blood and urine tests may also be used to assess the effects on the body of the hormone in question. The most commonly performed test of this type is the assessment of the glucose (sugar) levels in the blood and the urine in cases of suspected diabetes mellitus. A raised blood glucose level is an indication of a lack of insulin, which is the underlying problem in diabetes mellitus. In both cases, a helpful result can be obtained by applying a drop of blood on a test card, or by dipping a test 'stick' into the urine.

The most accurate and clinically relevant form of assessing the blood glucose level is to take a specimen when the patient has been fasting for some hours. The least accurate means is to look for glucose in the urine. The latter may be performed to provide a very general overview of the problem, but the gold standard, the fasting blood sugar test, is obviously more inconvenient for the patient.

Stimulation and suppression tests

Stimulation and suppression tests are more complex forms of blood and urine tests. They usually involve assessing the hormonal response that takes place over a few hours following a certain 'stimulus' given to the body. For this reason, the patient may need to spend a day or more in hospital for such tests to be performed. The 'stimulus' is chosen to be something that would normally significantly increase (stimulation test) or decrease (suppression test) the level of the hormone in question.

In general, the stimulation test is used to investigate a disease resulting from insufficient hormone, and a suppression test is used to investigate a disease resulting from excessive secretion of a hormone. For example, suspected diabetes might be confirmed by using the glucose tolerance test. In this test, a patient who has been fasting from the previous night is given a glucose drink at a set time in the morning. Blood tests are taken at defined time intervals, including one just before the set time of the drink. The blood glucose can then be seen to rise and fall from the fasting period to a few hours after the drink. In health, the blood glucose never exceeds a predictable normal level, but in mild diabetes it may be seen to rise to above a healthy level, even though the level might then drop to within a healthy range after some time. Such an abnormality might not be picked up by a simple blood sugar test. The glucose tolerance test is an indirect form of a stimulation test. The glucose drink should, in health, lead to a release of insulin. The release of insulin in turn should prevent the rise in blood sugar from going too high. The fact that this fails to happen is an indication of insufficient release of insulin.

Another example is the test for a person with suspected disease of the adrenal cortex (Addison's disease). In this case the patient is given an injection of a synthetic form of the pituitary hormone ACTH. In health, this hormone stimulates the release of cortisol and corticosterone from the adrenal cortex. In a patient with Addison's disease, timed blood tests reveal a much lower rise in cortisol in the blood than would be expected. This is another example of a stimulation test that can reveal insufficient production of a hormone.

Stimulation and suppression tests are based on the complexities of endocrine physiology, a clear understanding of which is a challenge even for qualified doctors. From the perspective of a complementary medical practitioner, the important fact to appreciate about the investigation of endocrine disease is that a patient with suspected endocrine disease may be required to spend some time in hospital undergoing such tests.

Imaging tests

Very commonly, endocrine disease results from structural damage to an endocrine gland. In such cases the use of complex soft tissue imaging tests, such as the CT scan and MRI, can be helpful in defining the extent of the damage and whether or not the problem is operable.

For example, the pituitary gland can be clearly revealed by means of MRI. Figure 5.1b-I shows the sort of image that may be obtained. This image represents the upward growth of a pituitary tumour. Such growth can have marked endocrine consequences (as well as being very likely to impair vision by upwards pressure on the crossing of the optic nerve tracts) and also in the causation of headaches.

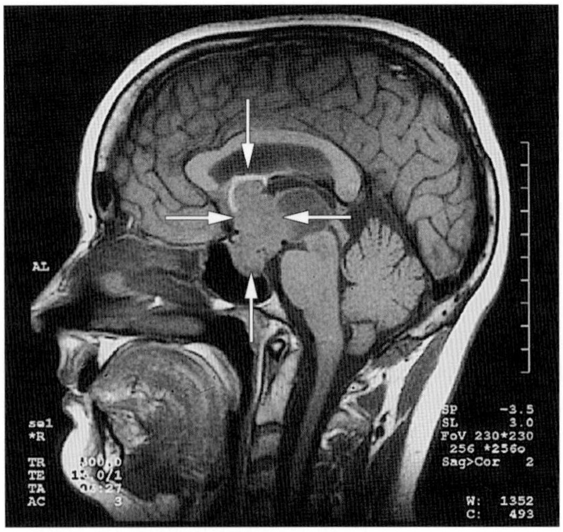

Figure 5.1b-I • MRI scan indicating a large pituitary tumour (extensive growth indicated by arrows).

Self-test 5.1b

The investigation of the endocrine system

1. Janet is a middle-aged patient of yours who has been treated for hypertension for 3 years. Now her doctor is concerned that the root of her problem might be the result of excessive levels of growth hormone from her pituitary gland. This fits with that facts that Janet's facial features have become more coarse over this time period and her shoe size has increased. The most likely cause of this syndrome is a tumour (usually benign) of the endocrine cells of the pituitary gland (see Chapter 5.1e).

   Janet has been referred to a hospital specialist for some tests. What sort of tests do you think she might have to undergo? You are not expected to predict the exact nature of the tests, but just the types of investigations used in endocrine disease which may be suggested.

Answers

1. Janet first will be given a thorough physical examination. She may be asked to bring photographs of herself in recent years, which may indicate a change in facial appearance. The specialist might observe that Janet's hands and feet are broad for her build. As excessive growth hormone can affect the cardiovascular system in particular, this system will be examined with care. An enlarged pituitary gland can affect the vision, so the eyes and vision will also be examined in detail.

   She will be given blood tests to assess the levels of growth hormone in her blood. She may also have to spend at least a few hours in hospital to undergo a suppression test (in this a case a glucose tolerance test, as glucose should have the effect of suppressing normal levels of growth hormone).

   As the concern is that there may be a tumour of the pituitary gland causing release of the excessive growth hormone, Janet may require more extensive hospital tests, possibly necessitating a stay as an inpatient. She will almost certainly undergo MRI of her head to visualise the pituitary gland. In addition, she may have to have further blood tests to check that the levels of the other pituitary hormones have not also been affected by the tumour.

Chapter 5.1c Diseases of the thyroid gland

LEARNING POINTS

At the end of this chapter you will be able to:

- recognise the features of the most important conditions that can affect the thyroid gland
- describe the clinical features of the syndromes of hypothyroidism and hyperthyroidism
- recognise the Red Flags of diseases of the thyroid gland.

Estimated time for chapter: 100 minutes.

Introduction

The conditions explored in this chapter are:

- Enlargement of the thyroid gland – the causes of goitre:
  - simple goitre
  - other causes of diffuse goitre
  - multinodular goitre
  - thyroid nodules and thyroid cancer.
- Hypothyroidism:
  - autoimmune hypothyroidism
  - iodine deficiency
  - congenital hypothyroidism
  - damage to the thyroid gland
  - pituitary disease.
- Hyperthyroidism (thyrotoxicosis):
  - Graves' disease
  - toxic nodular disease and thyroid cancer
  - acute thyroiditis
  - pituitary disease.

Enlargement of the thyroid gland: the causes of goitre

An enlarged thyroid gland is called a 'goitre'. Large goitres are visible as a fullness of the neck, whereas smaller goitres can only be felt on examination. A goitre is considered to be present if it can be felt as a swelling that moves up and down with swallowing. This swelling is more than the vague softness that is usually felt in the region of the thyroid gland. Most goitres are small, and may not be noticed by the patient.

A goitre can become so large as to cause symptoms. The most common symptom is of visible swelling and the cosmetic problems that accompany this. Only in rare cases are there other symptoms. These include discomfort in the neck, difficulty swallowing and restricted breathing.

A goitre does not necessarily mean that there is a problem with the production of the thyroid hormones. The various causes of goitre are described below.

> **Information Box 5.1c-I**
>
> **Goitre: comments from a Chinese medicine perspective**
>
> In Chinese medicine, the development of a goitre suggests the presence of Phlegm. The position of the goitre corresponds to the pathways of the Stomach and Large Intestine Channels, and so might also suggest imbalance in one or both of these Organs. If additional symptoms, such as discomfort or difficulty in swallowing, are present, this suggests additional Qi Stagnation.

Simple goitre

A simple goitre is a diffuse enlargement of the thyroid gland of unknown cause. It is not associated with any disturbance of the thyroid hormones. However, a simple goitre is most commonly seen in young women, either during puberty or during pregnancy, which implies that its development may be triggered by hormonal changes.

In most cases the simple goitre is small in size, and can regress if it appears during a time of hormonal change such as pregnancy. However, in some cases, surgery may be performed because of cosmetic unsightliness or, more rarely, because of pressure symptoms. The surgery leaves the patient with a horizontal scar that lies just above the level of the sternal notch (the region of acupoint Tiantu Rn-22).

Diffuse goitre

A diffuse swelling of the thyroid gland can develop for other reasons. Three fairly common autoimmune processes (atrophic thyroiditis, Hashimoto's thyroiditis and Graves' disease) are well recognised to cause a diffuse enlargement of the thyroid. All three of these conditions may also be associated with the syndromes of hypothyroidism and hyperthyroidism. In all these conditions, antithyroid antibodies lead to immune damage to the gland, which can result in tissue swelling. As with the simple goitre, autoimmune diffuse goitre is more common in women than in men.

More rare causes of a diffusely enlarged goitre in the UK include viral inflammation and iodine deficiency. In some developing countries, iodine deficiency is a common problem, and can lead to the development of a massive goitre (endemic goitre).

Multinodular goitre

A multinodular goitre is, as its name suggests, a thyroid gland that is enlarged due to the development of numerous benign nodules of thyroid tissue. This may, but not always, have the consequence of the production of excessive thyroid hormones, leading to the state of hyperthyroidism. This form of goitre is considered to be the result of a degenerative process of ageing.

Multinodular goitre is more common in elderly women, and may also be associated with local symptoms due to pressure effects from the irregularly enlarged gland.

Treatment for multinodular goitre is by means of surgery if there are symptoms due to pressure. Surgical removal of the thyroid is also performed if hyperthyroidism is present.

Thyroid nodules and thyroid cancer

Occasionally, a goitre develops as a result of a single enlarged area within a normal gland, known as a 'solitary nodule'. This is often caused by the same degenerative process that causes a multinodular goitre, but on rare occasions may also be a manifestation of tumour of the thyroid gland, and for this reason it requires careful investigation.

A tumour of the thyroid gland most commonly arises from the cells that produce the thyroid hormones. However, excessive production of these hormones is only a rare consequence of these tumours. This form of thyroid cancer is categorised as either a papillary, follicular or anaplastic carcinoma, according to the findings on examination of a biopsied tissue. Other more rare causes of a tumour within the thyroid gland include cancer of the calcitonin-producing cells (medullary carcinoma) and lymphoma.

Papillary and follicular carcinomas are by far the most common type of thyroid cancer. They are more common in young people and in women. They are often diagnosed before they spread from the thyroid gland, and are treated by total removal of the thyroid gland (thyroidectomy). A radioactive form of iodine is then given. This is concentrated by any remaining thyroid tissue, and is intended to kill off any remaining cancer cells. The majority of people who have this treatment at an early stage will have no recurrence, particularly if the diagnosis is made early in the disease. This treatment does however render the patient dependent on lifelong thyroid hormone replacement.

Papillary and follicular thyroid carcinoma, if not treated early, tend to spread to the lungs and bones. Anaplastic carcinoma is a disease of elderly people, and is a much more aggressive tumour. It spreads rapidly to local tissues and is usually fatal.

Information Box 5.1c-II

Thyroid cancer: comments from a Chinese medicine perspective

In Chinese medicine, carcinoma of the thyroid gland is also a manifestation of Phlegm, although pain in a rapidly enlarging nodule would indicate additional Blood Stagnation. As with all cancers, an underlying severe deficiency of Yin and Yang is likely to be present.

Hypothyroidism

'Hypothyroidism' is the term applied to the syndrome that results from inadequate production of the thyroid hormones. Another term that is commonly used to describe hypothyroidism is 'underactive thyroid'. Figure 5.1c-I lists some of the most common symptoms and signs that characterise this condition (see Q5.1c-1).

Many of the features of hypothyroidism result from the slowing down of the energy-producing processes of the cells. In health, these processes are dependent on the stimulus of thyroxine to allow the body to transform nutrition into energy. This is vital for continued activity, growth and maintenance of body temperature.

In early stages of the condition the patient will first experience symptoms of tiredness, sensitivity to cold and depression. It is only as the condition progresses that the more obvious features begin to appear. Therefore, the syndrome can be present for months or even years before a diagnosis is made. In elderly people, the diagnosis can be missed until very severe features such as confusion, dementia or hypothermia develop. In its most severe form, hypothyroidism can result in loss of consciousness, a condition termed 'myxoedema coma'. This is a medical emergency.

In most cases the diagnosis becomes clear following a blood test for TSH and T4. In established hypothyroidism due to thyroid disease, the T4 level is below the normal range, and the TSH is raised. The raised TSH level is the result of the response of the hypothalamus and the pituitary gland to the persistently low levels of thyroid hormones. In more borderline cases, the T4 levels are normal but the TSH is raised. This suggests that the failing thyroid gland is responding to the increased TSH and is managing to produce sufficient thyroid hormones. Patients with this sort of result may be treated conservatively (watching and waiting) or may be treated with thyroxine tablets if they have symptoms (see below).

Symptoms

- Tiredness
- Loss of appetite
- Weight gain
- Cold intolerance
- Depression
- Poor libido
- Joint and muscle aches
- Constipation
- Heavy periods
- Psychosis
- Confusion

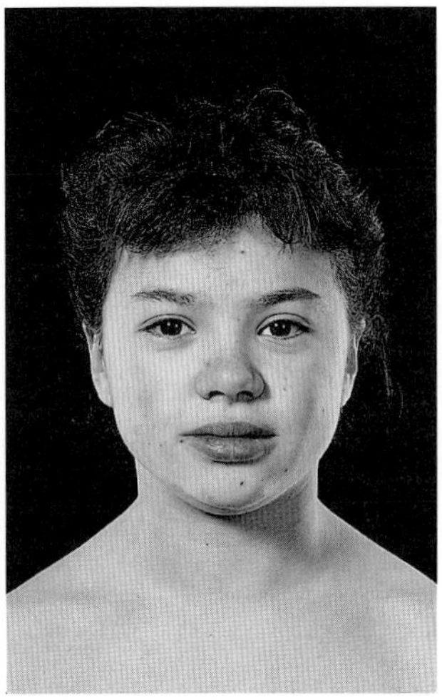

A history from a relative is often revealing
Symptoms of other autoimmune disease may be present

Signs

- Mental slowness
- Dementia
- Dry thin hair and skin
- Puffy eyes
- Obesity
- Hypertension
- Hypothermia
- Bradycardia
- Cold peripheries
- Oedema
- Deep voice
- Goitre
- Anaemia

Figure 5.1c-I • The symptoms and signs of hypothyroidism.

Treatment of most cases of hypothyroidism is with synthetic thyroxine (T4) in tablet form. This drug has the same structure as the natural hormone, but of course cannot currently be given in a dose that is tailored to the precise hour-to-hour needs of the body. The severe symptoms of hypothyroidism will abate over the course of a few months of adequate therapy, although swings in energy and mood may persist. Treatment is generally continued for life. The dose of the thyroxine is altered according to the results of regular blood tests for TSH and T4, and also the patient's symptoms.

Information Box 5.1c-III

Hypothyroidism: comments from a Chinese medicine perspective

In Chinese medicine, the syndrome of hypothyroidism primarily corresponds to depletion of Kidney Yang. In addition, Damp and Phlegm accumulation is apparent, and probably results from Deficiency of Spleen Yang. Interestingly, a yellow colouring (the cause, in part, of the characteristic 'peaches and cream' complexion) is well known in hypothyroidism.

Appropriate thyroxine replacement can be interpreted as being nourishing to Spleen and Kidney Yang. However, depending on the cause of hypothyroidism, it can be considered as either suppressive or curative. In cases in which there is some residual function of the thyroid gland, the treatment may be considered suppressive in that it does not target the root cause, and has the effect of inhibiting the natural response of the pituitary gland in producing TSH, which in turn stimulates the thyroid gland. However, in cases in which the gland has totally ceased to function, the treatment transforms the energetic imbalance and is undoubtedly curative in nature.

Autoimmune causes of hypothyroidism

The most common cause of hypothyroidism is a progressive autoimmune process which tends to run in families, and which affects women more than men. The antibodies are specific for thyroid cells, and lead to wasting of the thyroid tissue and accumulation of immune cells in the gland. In the most frequent form of autoimmune hypothyroidism, this process is often not associated with a goitre. A more rare form of autoimmune disease, known as Hashimoto's thyroiditis, is more likely to result in a firm, rubbery goitre. Treatment with thyroxine tablets will reverse the effects of this autoimmune destruction of the thyroid, but will have no effect on the root cause, for which there is no accepted treatment.

Information Box 5.1c-IV

Autoimmune hypothyroidism: comments from a Chinese medicine perspective

In Chinese medicine, the symptoms of autoimmune hypothyroidism correspond to Kidney and Spleen Yang Deficiency, leading to accumulation of Damp and Phlegm. This is consistent with all forms of hypothyroidism. The autoimmune process also suggests an underlying Jing Deficiency (see Chapter 2.1d).

Iodine deficiency

In areas in which dietary iodine is insufficient, endemic goitre may be common. In endemic goitre, the thyroid gland is basically healthy, but cannot make thyroid hormones because of insufficient iodine. The pituitary responds to low levels of thyroid hormones by producing high levels of TSH. The TSH stimulates the thyroid tissue excessively, and this causes the goitre. In some cases there may be mild hypothyroidism, but in many cases the excess stimulation is sufficient to cause the thyroid to manufacture sufficient thyroxine for the body's needs. Treatment of iodine deficiency is with dietary iodine replacement.

Information Box 5.1c-V

Iodine replacement: comments from a Chinese medicine perspective

In Chinese medicine, iodine replacement can be seen as nourishing to Spleen and Kidney Yang.

Congenital hypothyroidism

Congenital hypothyroidism is a condition in which the newborn baby is unable to produce thyroid hormones, most commonly because of an undeveloped thyroid gland. Because thyroid hormones are essential for healthy growth and development of the nervous system, if untreated this condition inevitably leads to poor health, permanent learning difficulties and short stature. The term 'cretin' was previously used to describe children who suffered the long-term effects of untreated hypothyroidism. As the problem affects 1 in 4000 births, cretinism used to be one of the most important causes of mental retardation.

In developed countries, severe problems from this condition have become extremely rare since the introduction of screening for hypothyroidism within the first few days of birth. A drop of blood is obtained from a prick to the baby's heel, and is placed on a card. It is then analysed for TSH and T4. If hypothyroidism is detected, the child is treated with daily thyroxine for life. This treatment reverses the problem before permanent developmental damage can occur.

Information Box 5.1c-VI

Congenital hypothyroidism: comments from a Chinese medicine perspective

In Chinese medicine, congenital hypothyroidism would be regarded as a manifestation of Jing Deficiency. By preventing this problem, thyroxine can be seen as nourishing Jing, as well as nourishing Kidney and Spleen Yang. In this context the treatment is curative in nature.

Damage to the thyroid gland

Physical damage to the thyroid gland can lead to reduced production of the thyroid hormones. Surgical thyroidectomy and medical (radioactive iodine) treatment of the thyroid gland for cancer or hyperthyroidism are both known to result in hypothyroidism. Lifelong thyroxine replacement may be necessary after such treatments. Other drugs are known to reduce the production of thyroid hormones. One of the most commonly prescribed is lithium, which is prescribed by psychiatrists for bipolar disorder. For this reason, people taking lithium are recommended to undergo regular blood tests for the thyroid hormones.

Pituitary disease

A very rare form of hypothyroidism springs from damage to the pituitary gland rather than the thyroid gland. In this case, the problem is the result of inadequate production of TSH. The most common cause of damage to the pituitary gland is a benign tumour. Pituitary hypothyroidism is also treated by means of synthetic thyroxine given as tablets.

Hyperthyroidism (Thyrotoxicosis)

Hyperthyroidism is a syndrome that results from excessive levels of thyroid hormones. It is also known as 'overactive thyroid' or 'thyrotoxicosis'. It is a more common condition than hypothyroidism, and tends to affect younger people. It is more common in women than men. Figure 5.1c-II lists some of the most common symptoms and signs that characterise this condition (see Q5.1c-2).

Most of these symptoms result from the effects of the increased thyroid hormones on the chemical processes of the cells. Increased amounts of the energy from food are diverted away from storage and tissue growth and into heat-producing processes. The patient therefore feels the characteristic restlessness, heat intolerance and raging appetite, despite an increased intake of food. The unmistakable changes that can affect the eyes (Figure 5.1c-III) only occur in the form of

Symptoms
- Weight loss
- Increased appetite
- Restlessness
- Muscle weakness
- Tremor
- Palpitations
- Thirst
- Diarrhoea
- Scanty periods
- Loss of libido
- Sweating

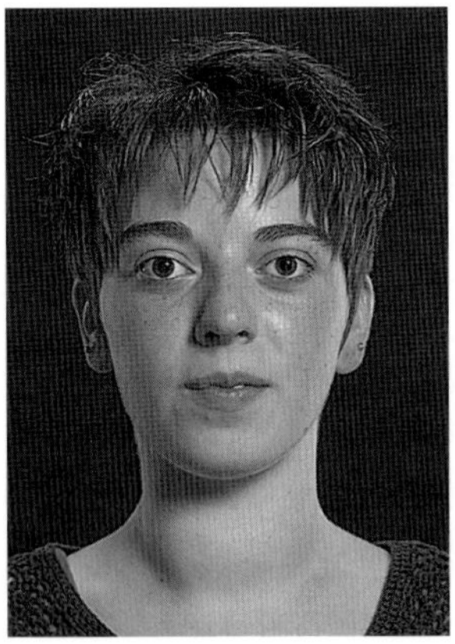

Signs
- Tremor
- Restlessness
- Sweating
- Irritability
- Tachycardia
- Warm peripheries
- Exophthalmos
- Goitre

Figure 5.1c-II • The symptoms and signs of hyperthyroidism.

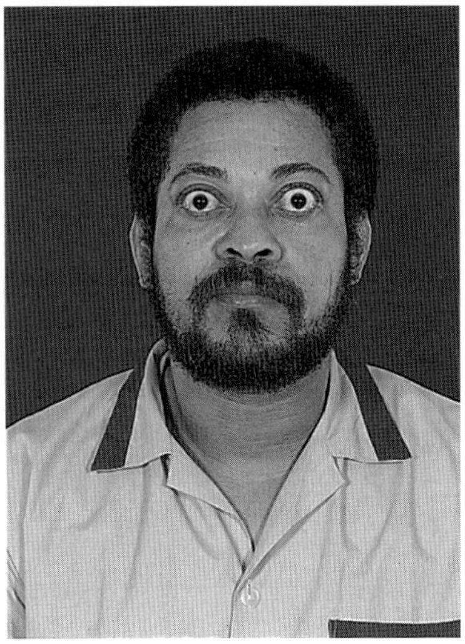

Figure 5.1c-III • Exophthalmos in Graves' disease.

hyperthyroidism called Graves' disease (see below). These result not from excessive thyroid hormones, but from the effect of the autoantibodies which are the cause of Graves' disease.

In early stages of hyperthyroidism the patient may complain only of anxiety or sleeplessness, and it is only in a more progressed stage of the condition that more obvious features such as weight loss and eye changes become apparent. In very severe cases the changes to the cardiovascular system can become life-threatening, as the overstimulated heart fails to cope with the work it has to perform. This can result in the development of atrial fibrillation or heart failure. In some cases the patient can become increasingly restless and irritable, and this can tip over into a full-blown psychosis, with delusions and the development of personality change.

Information Box 5.1c-VII

Hyperthyroidism: comments from a Chinese medicine perspective

In Chinese medicine, many of the features of hyperthyroidism correspond to the clinical picture of Yin Deficiency. Kidney Yin Deficiency is likely to be the root deficiency, although the features indicate that Deficiency of Heart and Liver Yin are also part of the picture. Raging appetite, psychosis and bloodshot eyes all suggest Full Heat, as these symptoms correspond to Stomach Fire, Phlegm Fire Obstructing the Orifices of the Heart, and Liver Fire.

Gascoigne (2001) comments that the Chinese view is that hyperthyroidism is a consequence of frustrated emotions, which lead first to Stagnation and then to Full Heat. It is the Full Heat that then damages the Yin of diverse organs, and which also encourages the accumulation of Phlegm in the form of a goitre.

Graves' disease

Graves' disease is by far the most common cause of hyperthyroidism. It is the result of the development of autoantibodies to thyroid cells. However, in contrast to autoimmune hypothyroidism, these antibodies tend to act rather like TSH, and initially stimulate rather than damage the thyroid cells. This has the result of causing excessive production of thyroid hormones.

Other autoantibodies that develop in Graves' disease also cause damage to the soft tissue of the eyes. This can have very severe consequences. Swelling of the soft tissue behind the eyes causes the eyes to bulge forward (see Figure 5.1c-III). This can sometimes be so severe that the eyelids are unable to close properly. Compression of the optic nerve behind the eye can threaten sight.

A diagnosis of advanced Graves' disease is often clinically obvious. However, in all cases a diagnosis of hyperthyroidism is confirmed by a blood test for TSH and T3, wherein the T3 levels are raised and TSH levels are very low. In addition, a blood test for the characteristic antibodies can confirm a diagnosis of Graves' disease.

There are three options for the treatment of Graves' disease. The most often first used treatment is the drug carbimazole. This works within 2–3 weeks to inhibit the production of the thyroid hormones, but the patient has to continue treatment for some months after this initial response. Beta blockers, such as propranolol, may also be given in the early stages to control symptoms such as anxiety, restlessness and palpitations. In about half of all patients this treatment is effective in restoring the thyroid activity to normal in the long term, but the remaining half of patients given carbimazole relapse within 2 years of treatment. These have then to turn to another treatment option.

Carbimazole has a rare serious side-effect in that in 1 in 1000 people it can suppress the activity of the bone marrow and lead to a life-threatening reduction in white blood cells. Other common side-effects include nausea, rashes and itching.

An alternative treatment option to carbimazole therapy is surgery to the thyroid gland. In this case some of the thyroid gland is removed (subtotal thyroidectomy) in the hope that this will restore normal function. The operation carries risks of damage to the nerve that supplies the vocal cords (in 1%) and also damage to the parathyroid glands, leading to problems in calcium balance (in 1%). More importantly, in up to 10% of people the operation is followed by hypothyroidism, requiring lifelong thyroxine replacement. In over 3% hyperthyroidism recurs after the operation.

An increasingly popular treatment option is the use of radioactive iodine therapy. This relies on a drug containing an iodine isotope which, when taken by mouth, is concentrated by the body in the thyroid tissue. The radioactivity causes progressive damage to the thyroid cells over the course of the next few months and can reverse the hyperthyroidism. Some people experience worsening of their symptoms before they get better with this treatment. Early concerns about increased risk of cancer do not appear to be founded. Because of these concerns, this therapy used to be reserved for the elderly, but now is increasingly being offered to younger people.

The most important complication of radioactive iodine therapy is progressive development of hypothyroidism. Because of this problem, patients are required to have regular blood tests to monitor thyroid hormone levels after both subtotal thyroidectomy and radioiodine treatment.

Information Box 5.1c-VIII

Treatment of hyperthyroidism: comments from a Chinese medicine perspective

In Chinese medicine, carbimazole, by inhibiting the production of the thyroid hormones, seems to prevent the development of Heat. Rashes and the very serious side-effect of bone marrow suppression may be evidence of suppression of this Heat to different and possibly deeper energetic levels of the body.

Radioactive iodine and surgery act in a different way because they actually lead to loss of thyroid tissue. They must also result in the Clearance of Heat in that they reduce the symptoms of hyperthyroidism. The fact that both these therapies have a high long-term incidence of hypothyroidism implies that they are ultimately Depleting of Qi, and in particular of Kidney Yang.

Toxic nodular disease and thyroid cancer

A multinodular goitre or a single nodule (see earlier in this chapter under Goitre) in the thyroid gland can occasionally produce excessive thyroid hormones, in which case the conditions are termed 'toxic multinodular goitre' and 'solitary toxic nodule', respectively. The clinical picture is similar to that of Graves' disease, but without the eye changes. These forms of hyperthyroidism rarely respond to carbimazole, and so are treated with either surgery or radioactive iodine.

Acute thyroiditis

Acute inflammation of the thyroid gland may follow a viral infection or, rarely, develop in a mother after delivery of a baby. The thyroid gland becomes slightly swollen and tender. There may be features of hypo- or hyperthyroidism, but these are usually self-limiting.

Pituitary disease

A TSH-secreting tumour of the pituitary gland is an extremely rare cause of hyperthyroidism. This, of course, is treated by surgery to the pituitary gland rather than by treatment of the thyroid gland.

The red flags of the diseases of the thyroid gland

Some patients with diseases of the thyroid gland will benefit from referral to a conventional doctor for assessment and/or treatment. Red flags are those symptoms and signs that indicate that referral is to be considered. The red flags of the diseases of the thyroid are described in Table 5.1c-I. This table forms part of the summary on red flags given in Appendix III, which also gives advice on the degree of urgency of referral for each of the red flag conditions listed.

Table 5.1c-I Red Flags 31 – diseases of the thyroid gland

Red Flag	Description	Reasoning
31.1	**Goitre**: refer only if symptoms of hyperthyroidism or hypothyroidism are present (see below), or if the goitre is tender, irregular or noticeably enlarging	A goitre is an enlarged thyroid gland. It can be felt and seen in the lower half of the neck, where it tends to fill the hollow that lies over the trachea and above the manubrium. A small symmetrical goitre is a not uncommon finding in women, particularly in puberty and pregnancy, and if no symptoms are associated, need not be a cause for referral in itself
31.2	**Features of hypothyroidism** (these tend to be progressive over the course of a few months) Symptoms: tiredness, depression, weight gain, heavy periods, constipation and cold intolerance Signs: dry puffy skin, dry and thin hair, slow pulse	The symptoms of hypothyroidism (underactive thyroid) overlap with those of depression, and a simple blood test can differentiate between the two syndromes. If prolonged, the state of hypothyroidism can have significant deleterious metabolic consequences, and medical replacement therapy is advised if the condition is not responding to complementary medical treatment
31.3	**Features of hyperthyroidism (**these tend to be progressive over the course of a few months) Symptoms: irritability, anxiety, sleeplessness, increased appetite, loose stools, weight loss, scanty periods and heat intolerance Signs: sweaty skin, tremor of the hands, staring eyes and rapid pulse	The symptoms of hyperthyroidism (overactive thyroid) overlap with those of an anxiety disorder, and a simple blood test can differentiate between the two syndromes. If prolonged, hyperthyroidism can have a significant impact on the cardiovascular system, and medical treatment is advised if the condition is not responding to complementary medical treatment High-priority referral may be indicated if the patient is very agitated, or if cardiac symptoms (chest pain, palpitations or breathlessness) are present

Self-test 5.1c

Diseases of the thyroid gland

1. You notice on examination of Jane, a 15-year-old new patient, that she has a smoothly enlarged thyroid gland which is visible as well as palpable. This gland rises and falls as you ask Jane to swallow. Jane has come for treatment of painful periods, although when you question her you have picked up some features of Spleen Qi Deficiency, including sweet cravings, a tendency to worry and weight gain.

   On examination her pulse is of normal rate and slightly slippery, and her tongue is normal in colour but has a thickish white coat and is swollen. How would you manage this situation?
2. Richard is a 35-year-old university lecturer. You have been treating him for anxiety, which has responded in part to your treatment but which has not ever left him so that he feels like he did 5 years ago. He says he used to be quite easy going, but now is jumpy and sleeps poorly. He feels very stressed about the demands of his work, and sweats easily when worried. He has lost weight through worry, although he thinks he is eating well.

In the morning before lectures, he often has to open his bowels a few times. His stools are loose.

On examination his eyes look normal, but his pulse is rapid at 94 beats/minute, and his hands are warm and sweaty. There is a fullness on examination of his neck, but you cannot be confident that it is a goitre. Thus Richard has some features of hyperthyroidism. Would you consider a referral?

Answers

1. The diagnosis is likely to be simple goitre. This is not associated with hypothyroidism or hyperthyroidism. There is no need in this situation to think about immediate referral. However, the fact that Jane has a goitre is of course of significance to your treatment, as it signifies accumulation of Phlegm. This is not inconsistent with your observation that Jane has an imbalance of Spleen Qi with evidence of accumulation of Damp.

   Nevertheless, you should be alert to the possible development of the features of hyperthyroidism or hypothyroidism, and consider referral if these should appear, or if the goitre should increase in size.

   There is no simple answer to whether or not you should discuss your finding with Jane, as she may well be oblivious of the fact that she has a goitre. It could be argued that in most cases it would be best to mention the goitre, as it may have been an unspoken source of anxiety which could then be discussed openly. You can encourage Jane that in many cases the goitre which appears during puberty will decrease in size.
2. Richard's symptoms could all be explained in terms of a purely emotional disorder, particularly if his work or personal situation has changed in the last 5 years. However, he does have warm hands, a high pulse rate and a possible goitre. These signs might tip the balance in terms of a more physical diagnosis. In this situation, particularly as your treatment is not wholly successful, it is advisable to refer to exclude a physical cause of Richard's symptoms.

Chapter 5.1d Diabetes mellitus

LEARNING POINTS

At the end of this chapter you will:

- understand the pathology of the two types of diabetes mellitus
- be able to describe how inadequate control of blood glucose can lead to disease
- be able to recognise the Red Flags of diabetes mellitus.

Estimated time for chapter: 120 minutes.

Introduction

'Diabetes mellitus' is the medical term used to refer to the syndrome that results from excessive levels of glucose (sugar) in the blood. In diabetes mellitus, raised blood glucose, conventionally termed 'hyperglycaemia', is the result of failure of the body either to produce adequate amounts of insulin or to respond to insulin properly (insulin resistance), or both.

The term 'diabetes mellitus' is derived from the Greek meaning 'excessive flow of urine (diabetes) which is very sweet (mellitus)'. The term is often shortened to the single word 'diabetes', although this does not clearly distinguish it from a much more rare condition known as 'diabetes insipidus'. In diabetes insipidus there is excessive flow of very dilute urine (hence the adjective 'insipidus'), which is the result of inadequate production of the pituitary hormone ADH.

The pancreatic hormone insulin plays two very important roles in the control of blood glucose. First, it ensures that the level of blood glucose never rises above a level that is healthy for the body. Secondly, it enables the cells of the body to take up glucose from the bloodstream. Without insulin, the cells cannot use the glucose circulating in the bloodstream, and will die rapidly unless the situation is reversed. For this reason, lack of insulin has been compared to the situation of 'starvation in the midst of plenty'.

The effects of diabetes are threatening to health in two broad ways. First, in acute diabetes an extreme lack of insulin leads to excessively high levels of blood glucose. This leads in a short space of time to the severe problems of dehydration and ketoacidotic coma. Secondly, in chronic diabetes, uncontrolled high levels of blood glucose have deleterious consequences on the various systems of the body.

The two types of diabetes

Diabetes can be broadly classified into two types, which are nowadays known as type 1 and type 2 diabetes. These were formerly called 'juvenile-onset' and 'late-onset' diabetes because, in general, type 1 diabetes affects young people and type 2 diabetes affects older people. However, this is by no means always the case, and so these terms have been largely abandoned in medical texts. Nevertheless, they still persist in common language, presumably because they are more descriptive.

Type 1 diabetes (insulin-dependent diabetes)

Type 1 diabetes is a result of the total failure of the insulin-producing cells of the pancreas to produce insulin. Once developed, it is irreversible, and without insulin replacement treatment it would lead to death within days. Type 1 diabetes is also termed 'insulin-dependent diabetes mellitus' (IDDM) because of the patient's absolute need for insulin replacement (see Q5.1d-1).

Type 1 diabetes used to be called 'juvenile-onset diabetes' because it primarily develops in children and young adults. The most common time of onset is between the ages of 10 and 13 years. For an unknown reason, the incidence has very much increased in recent years, particularly in children.

It is understood that type 1 diabetes develops because of autoimmune damage to the insulin-producing cells of the pancreas. Islet cell antibodies become apparent in the circulation years before clinical features of type 1 diabetes appear. The tendency for this to happen does run in families, but the actual trigger for the condition is not understood. The rapidly rising incidence suggests an environmental cause. Viral infection in early childhood is conventionally considered to be a possible trigger.

Clinical features of type 1 diabetes

In the early stages of type 1 diabetes there is still some residual production of insulin, so the symptoms appear gradually. However the severity of the symptoms means that this form of diabetes is usually diagnosed within days to a few weeks of onset. The first features include a general feeling of malaise, weight loss, thirst and increased urination.

All these symptoms are a result of the lack of insulin. Malaise and weight loss are due to the inability of the cells of the body to utilise the glucose they need, and thirst and increased urination are the consequence of increased levels of glucose in the blood. The glucose reaches such a high concentration in the blood that it starts entering the urine from the kidneys. The high level of glucose in the urine then encourages extra water to enter the urine from the bloodstream by the process of osmosis. The result is that large amounts of sugar-containing urine are produced, and the patient has to drink excessively to make up for this fluid loss.

If the condition is not treated as an emergency, eventually the levels of blood sugar become extremely high, and the patient becomes increasingly dehydrated. More importantly, the cells are deprived of glucose, and the body tries to derive energy by breaking down body fat and protein. Eventually, coma develops, as a combined result of dehydration, the build up of waste products from the breakdown of fat and protein, and the increased acidity of the blood that follows from this.

In the severe stages of acute diabetes, the patient becomes on the edge of a diabetic coma. In this situation, the patient becomes confused, dehydrated, the breathing is laboured and the breath has a characteristic slightly sweet smell. In this state, nausea, vomiting and severe abdominal pain are common.

Treatment of acute type 1 diabetes

Treatment is always a matter of emergency. If a coma has developed, the patient should be nursed in intensive care, as extremely careful control of the body chemistry is required. The main requirements are to replace fluids and to administer insulin, both of which are done in the initial stages by means of an intravenous drip.

If there are no complications, with this treatment the patient may be stable enough within a few days to eat and drink, and to no longer require an intravenous drip. From then on the patient will require regular injections of insulin, in doses tailored to meet individual day-to-day requirements. Most hospitals now have specialist diabetes nurses, whose role is to facilitate the newly diagnosed diabetic person's return to normal life. The initial meetings with this nurse specialist ideally should take place during this first hospital stay.

Type 2 diabetes (non-insulin-dependent diabetes)

Type 2 diabetes (non-insulin-dependent diabetes mellitus (NIDDM)) develops because of a combination of factors that affect the body's utilisation of glucose. The first is that the pancreas starts to fail to produce adequate amounts of insulin. This lack of insulin is not total, and in most cases at least half the insulin-producing cells remain functioning. The second factor is that the body tissues become less sensitive to the insulin that is secreted, a condition termed 'insulin resistance'. This latter factor is much more of a problem if the patient is overweight.

Type 2 diabetes is very common in older people. The age of onset is usually between 50 and 70 years of age, although on rare occasions it can develop in young people, particularly if obesity is present. In the UK, over 10% of people over the age of 70 years have this form of diabetes. It is very much more likely to develop if a close relative has been diagnosed with type 2 diabetes. It is also common in certain ethnic groups, in particular in those with South Asian, African or Caribbean ancestry.

Although the tendency to develop type 2 diabetes is strongly inherited, it is very much a disease of affluent populations. Obesity is present in 80% of patients with type 2 diabetes. A poor diet, with a high content of fatty and sugary foods, and low levels of exercise also contribute to the development of type 2 diabetes.

A syndrome similar to type 2 diabetes can also be triggered by certain drugs (most commonly thiazide diuretics and corticosteroid drugs) and during pregnancy. In these cases the clinical features may subside on withdrawal of the drugs or on delivery of the baby. However, in people who develop this form of temporary diabetes, it is known that there may be a tendency to develop type 2 diabetes at a later stage life.

Clinical features of type 2 diabetes

The onset of Type 2 diabetes may be much more insidious than in Type 1 diabetes. In some cases the patient may live for years with a raised level of blood glucose and be unaware of the fact. Sometimes, the diagnosis is only made after the patient has suffered a severe complication of prolonged hyperglycaemia such as a heart attack.

Most cases are diagnosed because of a combination of vague symptoms such as tiredness, frequent urination and thirst. Because of the vagueness of the symptoms, the patient may often have not felt right for some time before going to ask advice about the problem. This is in contrast with the onset of Type 1 diabetes.

The diagnosis of diabetes may also be made following routine 'stix' testing of the urine of patients who have visited a hospital doctor or a general practice for an unrelated reason. This is a practice which is very much encouraged, as it is known that early diagnosis may result in lifestyle changes and treatment choices which can prevent severe complications later on in the disease.

Treatment of acute type 2 diabetes

Only rarely do patients with Type 2 diabetes require hospital admission to control their diabetes after first diagnosis. However, in some cases, the blood glucose level can rise so high that the patient can become severely dehydrated. This can become a medical emergency, and particularly in elderly people.

Usually, the newly diagnosed patient with Type 2 diabetes is not acutely unwell. In this case they may first be encouraged to control their diabetes with lifestyle changes alone. In some people, a combination of attention to diet, cutting out alcohol, losing weight and increasing gentle exercise can be sufficient to control the problem entirely.

Diabetes and the kidneys

In chronic diabetes hyperglycaemia causes progressive damage to the blood vessels of the kidneys and so leads to the gradual development of chronic kidney disease and specific conditions such as nephrotic syndrome. The increased incidence of cystitis and pyelonephritis contributes to the kidney damage in diabetes. Kidney damage is the leading cause of premature death in insulin dependent diabetic people. Moreover, diabetes is the cause of 50% of cases of significant chronic kidney disease.

Diabetes and the eyes

Diabetes can lead to progressive damage to the small blood vessels of the retina. This can lead to permanent impairment of vision and, in some cases, blindness.

Diabetes and the nervous system

Damage to the small blood vessels that supply the nerves can lead to death of the peripheral nerves. This can lead to a progressive loss of sensation and muscle strength in the characteristic 'glove and stocking' distribution of a polyneuropathy. Alternatively, single nerves may suddenly die, leading to the features of a mononeuropathy. In this case the diabetic person might develop symptoms such as weakness of a muscle group in a limb or double vision.

The autonomic nerves can also be affected, leading to problems such as diarrhoea, erectile dysfunction, dizziness on standing and difficulty in passing urine.

Diabetes and the skin

The skin becomes vulnerable to damage in diabetes for three reasons. Poor circulation to large and small blood vessels impairs the nourishment of the skin. Infections of the skin are more likely and, for these two reasons, wounds are less likely to heal. This means that small injuries can become enormous problems for a diabetic person. A small wound might develop rapidly into an ulcer if not treated with adequate care. The third reason is that loss of sensation, in particular to the feet, means that small injuries are more likely, and are not protected because the patient is unable to feel pain.

Long-term management of diabetes

There are two central aims in the long-term management of diabetes:

- prevention of the recurrence of the acute state of hyperglycaemia and dehydration
- prevention of the long-term complications of diabetes, which result from chronically raised levels of blood glucose.

The long-term management of diabetes is discussed under the following subheadings:

- lifestyle factors
- medical control of hyperglycaemia
- screening for complications.

It is recognised that the adequate control of diabetes requires consistent attention to all three of these areas to achieve the best outcome for the patient. Education of the patient and their family is a necessary prerequisite to achieving the aims of long-term management. Ongoing support and education is, therefore, a core part of the management of diabetes.

Lifestyle factors

In both types of diabetes, careful attention to certain lifestyle factors is fundamental to achieving long-term control of the condition.

Diet is crucial in the management of both type 1 and type 2 diabetes. For both, a diet that minimises sudden peaks in blood glucose and which is low in unhealthy lipids is strongly advocated. Such a diet would be high in complex carbohydrates, such as sweet potatoes, pasta and brown rice (ideally comprising over one half of the total diet). Ideally, foods that have a low glycaemic index should be chosen over those that lead to a very rapid delivery of sugar to the bloodstream. Refined sugar (cakes, sweets and biscuits) should be kept to as low a level as possible, and alcohol should be cut out or kept to a minimum. Plenty of vegetables and fruit are advised (the sugars in fruits are less rapidly absorbed than refined sugars). Fats need to form much less than one-third of the diet, and unhealthy saturated fats and trans-fatty acids should be minimised. Protein should come in a low-fat form, such as lean meats, fish, pulses and eggs, and also should comprise no more than one-third of the diet.

Such a diet is no different from a typical 'healthy eating' diet which would be advocated for anyone by a conventional medical practitioner. This means that the diabetic person should not feel set apart by having to attend to this sort of dietary advice. However, in practice, because of cultural values about food, many people find this sort of advice very difficult to follow with ease.

Moderate exercise is also strongly advised, because physical fitness contributes to a smooth control of blood glucose. Moreover, physical exercise is known to improve blood lipid levels.

Smoking is a particular problem in diabetes because it also is very damaging to the circulation. People with diabetes will be counselled about stopping smoking.

Medical control of hyperglycaemia

In type 1 diabetes, because the insulin-producing cells of the pancreas have totally and permanently failed, insulin replacement is an essential aspect of the control of hyperglycaemia. In people with type 2 diabetes, although lifestyle changes may be sufficient to achieve adequate control, additional medical treatment will be required for most. Oral antidiabetic tablets, exenatide injections and insulin are the options for the medical treatment of type 2 diabetes.

Oral antidiabetic drugs

The oral antidiabetic drugs are medications that act either to increase the release of insulin from the remaining cells in the pancreas, or to increase the body's sensitivity to insulin. There are three classes of antidiabetic drugs that are most commonly prescribed and which are specifically recommended in current treatment guidelines. These are the sulphonylureas (which include tolbutamide and gliclazide), the biguanides (which include metformin) and the glitazones (which include pioglitazone and rosiglitazone).

Metformin is currently considered the first-line treatment for type 2 diabetes. Its advantages are that it carries no risk of hypoglycaemia and does not induce weight gain. Disadvantages are that a lot of people develop digestive side-effects. Sulphonylureas are the second-line choice, and are generally better tolerated than metformin. However, one unfortunate side-effect is that they promote weight gain, and they may cause the blood sugar to drop too low (hypoglycaemia).

If a single antidiabetic drug is not sufficient to achieve control in type 2 diabetes, two types of drug may be used in combination. If this approach also fails, insulin will be prescribed. The glitazones are new antidiabetic drugs that are generally reserved for cases in which metformin, sulphonylureas and insulin fail to suit the patient. They carry a known risk of inducing heart failure, which means the patients for whom they are prescribed need to be monitored carefully.

Insulin

Insulin is used in all cases of type 1 diabetes, and in cases of type 2 diabetes in which adequate control cannot be achieved by diet and tablets alone. It has to be given by injection. Insulin syringes have very fine needles, so that the pain of injection is less than that felt with a blood test or immunisation. The insulin can also be administered from a pen-shaped device, which holds a cartridge of insulin. The patient can then inject varying doses from the 'pen'. Diabetic people are taught to inject themselves into a pinch of the skin over the upper arm, buttock, thigh or the abdomen, and to vary the site of injection to avoid cumulative damage to the skin and soft tissues.

Insulin is either made from an extract of pig pancreas, or by a process that involves genetically engineered bacteria. Whereas pig insulin is similar to, but slightly different in structure from, human insulin, genetically engineered insulin ('human' insulin) is identical in structure to natural human insulin. Insulin is produced in three forms: short-, intermediate- and long-acting insulins. As their names suggest, these different preparations act over varying time scales in the body after injection.

Increasingly, diabetic people are taught to vary their doses of insulin according to their diet, level of exercise and the results of blood tests. They do this by using combinations of short- and intermediate-acting insulins given throughout the day. Most people require between two and four separate injections a day.

The ideal aim is to keep the level of blood glucose within a certain range. It is now accepted, at least for type 1 diabetes, that the more that this ideal can be attained, the lower the risk of the long-term complications. However, this is a taxing and complex process, and requires consistent attention to daily variations in diet and blood test results. Because of this, some people are much more able than others to control their diet and judge what doses of insulin they require, and so achieve better control of blood glucose. Some people may find the demands of a varying daily dose of insulin too difficult to deal with, and so will be prescribed a regular daily regimen of injections. The disadvantage of this is that blood sugar control is bound to be less than perfect, but this may be the only option for some people.

Some forms of diabetes are much more difficult to control than others, even with meticulous attention to diet and insulin dosage. If severe, these forms of diabetes are termed 'brittle', and unfortunately are bound to result in higher rates of long-term complications (see Q5.1d-2 and Q5.1d-3).

Monitoring of blood glucose

Although an ideal situation might be that the diabetic person is able to respond to minute-to-minute changes in blood glucose with an appropriate dose of insulin, this is not practical for daily life. Instead, the patient has to respond to as many blood test results as are acceptable. Nowadays, blood glucose levels can be fairly accurately assessed at home by means of a 'stix' test. This involves placing a drop of blood on a test strip, which is then inserted into a hand-held machine. This can be performed up to three times a day, and can inform what the next dose of insulin should be. Alternatively, a nurse can perform this test if the patient is unable to do it themselves, although this of course will not be possible on a frequent basis.

Urine 'stix' tests are easier for the patient to perform, but are less accurate. They are useful in that they can indicate that the blood sugar has been very high over the preceding few hours. They may induce a false sense of good control, even when this is not the case, as the blood glucose has to be very high in some people before glucose appears in the urine.

An additional blood test called HbA1c is performed in outpatient clinics. This test gives an indication of the general level of control over the past few weeks. This can be helpful in indicating whether or not a patient needs special support in regaining good long-term control of blood glucose.

Screening for complications

Screening for the complications of diabetes is a third essential aspect of treatment. This can be performed largely within general practice, although it is usual for most diabetics to attend a specialist hospital clinic at least annually. At the diabetes check-up appointment, the GP or hospital specialist should perform a physical examination to look for complications such as raised blood pressure, skin damage and numbness, and damage to the retina. Raised blood pressure is treated very attentively with drugs, as it is recognised that uncontrolled blood pressure can hasten kidney damage as well as increase cardiovascular complications. Any wounds to the skin should be given expert nursing care to promote healing. A urine test will be performed to look for protein and glucose and a blood test to check for HbA1c levels, high cholesterol and adequate kidney function. Many patients also attend an eye clinic at least annually so that the retina can be examined by means of a slit lamp. Laser treatment can be administered at the same appointment, and this can prevent progression of eye disease.

A multidisciplinary approach to diabetes management

The management of diabetes requires input from a range of medical disciplines. Because of this, ideally, a team of specialists including the GP, endocrinologist, diabetes specialist nurse and eye specialist should liaise to ensure a consistent approach.

Hypoglycaemia

'Hypoglycaemia' is a term used to describe a fall in the blood glucose level to below the normal range. Mild hypoglycaemia leads to a bodily response that results in feelings of panic or agitation, dizziness and sweating. The pupils are dilated. These features are largely a result of the reflex release of the hormone adrenaline from the adrenal gland. Hypoglycaemia, when very severe, leads to glucose starvation of the brain cells, which, in a short space of time leads to confusion and loss of consciousness. Death will follow if the blood glucose levels are not restored rapidly.

Hypoglycaemia and diabetes

Severe hypoglycaemia most commonly results from an inappropriately high dose of antidiabetic medication. Both the sulphonylurea class of antidiabetic drugs and insulin can induce a state of hypoglycaemia that is so severe as to be life-threatening. A common scenario is that a diabetic person whose disease is controlled on a regular dose of tablets or insulin either misses a meal or undertakes more exercise than is usual for them. In the initial stages, the person will feel agitation, sweating, a racing heartbeat and dizziness. It is important that people with diabetes become familiar with this pattern of symptoms, which are commonly described as a 'hypo'. If nothing is done to remedy this stage, the person can become so confused that they are no longer able to help themselves. This is a dangerous situation, as the person can then begin to lose consciousness.

Treatment for a hypo in diabetes is to restore the blood glucose level back to normal. In the early stages of the condition, eating some sweet food may be sufficient to bring this about. Most diabetic people on medical treatment will carry biscuits or glucose tablets on their person for dealing with a developing hypo as soon as possible. A glucose drink is also a very rapidly absorbed source of glucose. An alternative treatment is to inject a synthetic form of the hormone glucagon. This has the same effect as eating glucose in that it enables the release of glucose from glycogen stores in the liver. The advantage of glucagon is that it can be given quickly when the person is confused or comatose.

One problem that develops in advanced diabetes is the inability to recognise the early warning signs of a hypo. It is very important that friends and family are primed to recognise the confusion, irritability and clumsiness that can result, and are educated about encouraging sweet food intake and on how to administer glucagon.

Once hypoglycaemic coma is established, treatment must be given in hospital as a matter of urgency. Glucose is injected into a vein and glucagon is given at the same time. As long as brain damage has not occurred, the patient should make a rapid recovery back to full consciousness.

Other causes of hypoglycaemia

Severe hypoglycaemia can result from much more rare medical conditions. The most important of these is a tumour of the endocrine cells of the pancreas called an insulinoma.

The term hypoglycaemia is frequently used to describe a state which is experienced by seemingly healthy people, who become pale, weak and sweaty if meals are overdue. This condition is much more common in women than in men. A rapid intake of sweet or starchy food will reverse these symptoms. This syndrome is not conventionally recognised to be a result of *true* hypoglycaemia because studies of people experiencing these symptoms showed a very poor correlation of symptoms with low blood glucose levels. A psychosomatic cause is usually ascribed to cases in which these symptoms are common, but are non-progressive.

Secondary diabetes

Diabetes may also develop for other reasons, in which case it is called 'secondary' diabetes. These causes include other pancreatic diseases (e.g. chronic pancreatitis) and other endocrine diseases that affect the body's utilisation of glucose (e.g. Cushing's disease). In these cases the main treatment is of the underlying disease. However, if there has been permanent damage to the pancreas, the patient is treated in the same way as a patient with primary type 1 or type 2 diabetes.

Information Box 5.1d-I

Diabetes: comments from a Chinese medicine perspective

In Chinese medicine, diabetes used to be referred to as the thirsting and wasting disease (Xiao Ke). There are three components to the untreated condition, which are each related to one of the three Jiao. Excessive drinking is related to Upper Jiao wasting and is attributed to Lung Yin Deficiency with Heat. Excessive eating is related to wasting of the Middle Jiao, and this in turn is attributed to Stomach Yin Deficiency with Dryness and Heat. Excessive urination is related to Lower Jiao wasting, and this is attributed to exhaustion of Kidney Yin and Kidney Jing. Untreated acute diabetes can, therefore, be summarised in terms of Yin Deficiency with accumulation of Heat or Fire.

However, the diverse complications of long-term hyperglycaemia suggest that the energetic interpretation of long-term diabetes is more complicated. The vascular complications of stroke, heart attack and poor circulation are suggestive of Qi Deficiency with Qi and Blood Stagnation and accumulation of Damp or Phlegm. The Stagnation and Phlegm are possibly both long-term consequences of Heat. Numbness may relate to Blood Deficiency, Damp or Phlegm. Poor healing with a tendency to infections might relate to Blood and Qi Deficiency with Damp or Damp Heat.

In long-term diabetes, therefore, there is a state of overall deficiency together with accumulation of certain pathogenic factors. In particular, there are features of Yin Deficiency, Qi Deficiency and Blood Deficiency, together with accumulation of Heat, Stagnation, Damp and Phlegm. Dietary sugar is energetically Damp and Heat forming. It might be concluded from this that hyperglycaemia is a condition of Damp Heat.

Treatment with diet and exercise alone serves to nourish deficiency, reduce dietary sources of Damp and Heat, and clear Stagnation. Antidiabetic drugs and insulin, by reducing blood glucose levels and enabling the cells to utilise glucose, might be interpreted as both Clearing Heat and Nourishing Yin. Because antidiabetic medication can never be administered in precisely appropriate doses, it can have side-effects of hypoglycaemia and weight gain. This might be interpreted as Spleen Qi Deficiency with accumulation of Damp.

The Red Flags of Diabetes

Some patients with diabetes will benefit from referral to a conventional doctor for assessment and/or treatment. Red flags are those symptoms and signs that indicate that referral is to be considered. The red flags of diabetes are described in Table 5.1d-I. This table forms part of the summary on red flags given in Appendix III, which also gives advice on the degree of urgency of referral for each of the red flag conditions listed.

Table 5.1d-I Red Flags 32 – diabetes mellitus

Red Flag	Description	Reasoning
32.1	**Confusion/coma with dehydration (hyperglycaemia)**	These are serious symptoms of uncontrolled diabetes (when the level of glucose in the blood becomes too high) and are urgent red flags in their own right. If the patient is losing consciousness, ensure they are kept in a safe place in the recovery position until help arrives
32.2	**Hypoglycaemia** (due to the effects of insulin or antidiabetic medication in excess of bodily requirements): agitation, aggression, sweating, dilated pupils, confusion and coma	Confusion/coma can also be the consequence of a hypoglycaemic attack (a result of an excessive reaction to insulin or antidiabetic medication). This can be helped by urgent administration of glucose in a readily absorbable form (e.g. a glucose drink). If in doubt about the cause of the confusion in a diabetic, it is always appropriate to give glucose, as it is safe to do this whatever the cause. If the patient is losing consciousness, ensure they are kept in a safe place in the recovery position until help arrives
32.3	**Type I diabetes or poorly controlled type II diabetes**: short history of thirst, weight loss and excessive urination, which is rapidly progressive in severity	Thirst and excessive urination are due to the osmotic effect of glucose in the urine. Weight loss occurs because the tissues are unable to utilise the glucose in the situation where there is a lack of insulin. The patient is at high risk of coma because of rising levels of lactic acid. Refer as a high priority, and urgently if there are any signs of clouding of consciousness
32.4	**Type 2 diabetes**: general feeling of unwellness, with thirst and increased need to urinate large amounts of urine, which develops over the course of weeks to months	In type 2 diabetes the onset is more gradual and the situation is less urgent than in type 1 diabetes. Sustained levels of hyperglycaemia put the patient at increased risk of heart disease, kidney disease, vascular disease and chronic infections
32.5	**Increased tendency to infections** such as cystitis, boils and oral thrush (candidiasis)	An increased tendency to purulent, urinary and skin infections may indicate underlying type 2 diabetes
32.6	**Poor wound healing**, especially in the feet and legs	An increased tendency to poor wound healing may indicate underlying type 2 diabetes

Self-test 5.1d

Diabetes mellitus

1. You are called out of a consultation to the waiting room to see an elderly patient who is an insulin-dependent diabetic. She has slumped in her chair and is semi-conscious, with rambling speech. She is slightly sweaty, her pulse is rapid and thready, and her pupils appear slightly dilated.
   (i) What are three possible diagnoses?
   (ii) How would you manage this situation?
2. Janice is a 55-year-old housewife. She is overweight and is being treated for high blood pressure. She has come to see you because she feels tired all the time. When you question her, she tells you of features that suggest Yin Deficiency: dry mouth, thirst in the evenings and feelings of heat. She says that, recently, she has had to get up two times a night to go to the toilet. She attributes this to the fact that she is troubled with recurrent thrush, a problem that has only developed since she went through the menopause at the age of 50 years.

Would you refer Janice at this stage? If so, why?

Answers

1. (i) This diabetic patient is showing features that are highly suggestive of acute hypoglycaemia. However, she might have suffered from any of the other causes of acute confusion or loss of consciousness. In the case of a diabetic person, a heart attack or stroke are also strong possibilities.
   (ii) As with all cases like this, you should call for medical help as a matter of urgency. Calling for an ambulance would be appropriate. You should ensure that the patient is kept warm and comfortable. As she is semi-conscious, it is worth trying to encourage her to eat some sugar or take some highly sweetened drink. This will be of profound benefit in hypoglycaemia, and will do no harm if the cause is another condition.
2. Janice is showing features that could be attributed to the onset of type 2 diabetes. However, her symptoms could also be more functional in nature, and may not be explained by a defined medical complaint. Nevertheless, it would do no harm for her to see her doctor to exclude a diagnosis of diabetes, as this can be done very simply with a blood test. It would be wise to recommend that she makes an appointment to do this. If a diagnosis of type 2 diabetes is made, your treatment may be of great benefit in prompting her to make appropriate lifestyle changes and contribute to normalising her blood sugar levels.

Chapter 5.1e Diseases of the adrenal gland and the pituitary gland

LEARNING POINTS

At the end of this chapter you will be able to:
- describe the features of the common diseases of the adrenal gland
- describe the features of the common diseases of the pituitary gland
- recognise the Red Flags of these diseases.

Estimated time for chapter: 90 minutes.

Introduction

In comparison with the diseases of the thyroid gland and diabetes mellitus, the other endocrine diseases are rare. However, they can have long-term debilitating and sometimes life-threatening consequences, and for this reason merit further study.

The diseases studied in this chapter are:

- Diseases of the adrenal gland:
  - Cushing's syndrome
  - Addison's disease
  - Conn's syndrome
  - phaeochromocytoma.
- Diseases of the pituitary gland:
  - pituitary tumour and hypopituitarism
  - acromegaly and gigantism
  - short stature
  - Cushing's disease
  - diabetes insipidus.
- Other endocrine effects from tumours.

Diseases of the adrenal gland

Cushing's syndrome

'Cushing's syndrome' is the term used to describe the symptoms and signs that result from a long-term excess of glucocorticoid hormones (such as cortisol and corticosterone) in the body. Cushing's syndrome can also develop as a result of the long-term prescription of corticosteroid medication. This medication-induced form of Cushing's syndrome is, in fact, by far the most common form.

Disease of the adrenal gland can also be a cause of Cushing's syndrome. In this case, the excess glucocorticoid results from the growth of a benign or malignant tumour of the endocrine cells of the adrenal cortex. Figure 5.1e-I lists some of the most common symptoms and signs that characterise this condition.

Cushing's syndrome, if untreated, is a dangerous condition. Uncontrolled hypertension and increased blood glucose levels increase the risk of coronary heart disease. Premature death can occur from heart attack, heart failure or infection.

Addison's disease

Addison's disease most commonly results from an autoimmune loss of the endocrine cells of the adrenal cortex. The most significant consequence of this is that the adrenal gland gradually loses the ability to secrete sufficient cortisol and corticosterone. There is also loss of the ability to secrete aldosterone and the adrenal sex steroids. In common with many of the autoimmune diseases, Addison's disease primarily affects women of middle age and older. However, there are other, more rare causes. The next most common cause is secondary cancer

Symptoms

Abdominal weight gain, depression, scanty periods, thin skin, easy bruising, acne, facial hair, muscular weakness, poor growth in children

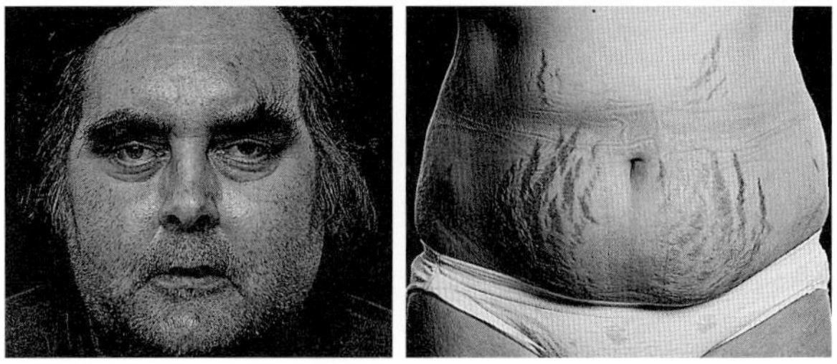

Signs

Moon face (fat deposition around face), acne, hirsutism, central obesity, thin skin, with stretch marks, bruising, hypertension, osteoporosis, proximal muscle wasting

Figure 5.1e-I • The symptoms and signs of Cushing's syndrome.

(metastases) developing in both adrenal glands. In certain cancers there is a marked tendency for secondary cancer to develop in the adrenal glands, and thus to destroy the healthy endocrine tissue. Figure 5.1e-II lists some of the most common symptoms and signs which characterise Addison's disease.

Addison's disease can be fatal within weeks to months if untreated. A severe complication of the undiagnosed condition is the Addisonian crisis. This is a consequence of an exposure to a stressor such as a severe infection or an accident. Because the body is unable to manufacture the steroid hormones that are required to cope with situations of stress, a person with Addison's disease can collapse with abdominal pain, vomiting and shock in such situations. This situation is treated as a medical emergency.

Information Box 5.1e-I

Cushing's syndrome: comments from a Chinese medicine perspective

In Chinese medicine, Cushing's syndrome would appear to embrace Kidney and Jing Deficiency (weak bones, vulnerability to infection), Spleen Deficiency (a tendency to bruising and stretch marks, weak muscles) and accumulation of Damp/Phlegm (weight gain, hypertension, extreme mood disturbances). There are also features of Full Heat (acne, raised blood sugar, tendency to gastritis and stomach ulcers).

Long-term treatment of Addison's disease is with daily doses of synthetic corticosteroid medication (cortisol or prednisolone) and a synthetic form of a hormone similar to aldosterone (fludrocortisone). This treatment has to be continued for life.

Information Box 5.1e-II

Addison's disease: comments from a Chinese medicine perspective

In Chinese medicine, the features of Addison's disease largely correspond to Kidney and Spleen Yang Deficiency. The dark pigmentation is consistent with a problem affecting the Kidney Organ.

Conn's syndrome

Conn's syndrome is a condition that usually results from an aldosterone-secreting tumour of the adrenal cortex. Aldosterone is responsible for maintaining salt and water balance and blood pressure. Excess secretion of aldosterone initially leads to high blood pressure. If this situation is untreated, the disturbance to the salts in the blood (low potassium) can become so severe as to be life-threatening. Conn's syndrome is an important cause of unexplained hypertension in young people.

Symptoms

A short history of:
weight loss, weakness, fever, scanty periods, depression, nausea, vomiting, fainting and abdominal pain

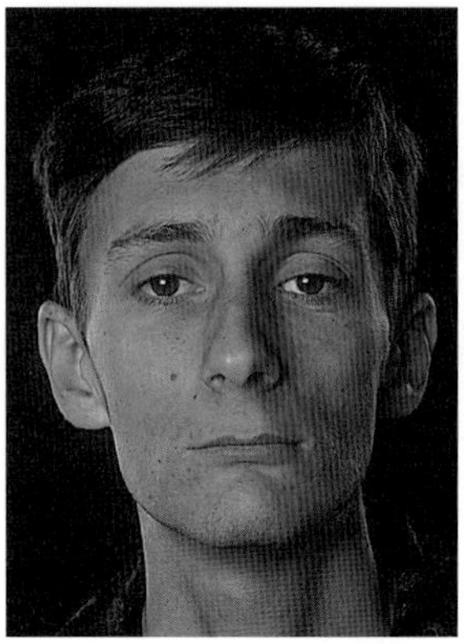

Signs

Pigmentation around new scars and on creases of palm, postural drop in blood pressure, wasting, dehydration, loss of body hair

Figure 5.1e-II • The symptoms and signs of Addison's disease.

Treatment is by means of surgical removal of the tumour. If this is not possible, a particular form of diuretic (spironolactone) can be used to counteract the effects of the excessive aldosterone.

Phaeochromocytoma

A phaeochromocytoma is a very rare tumour that secretes the catecholamine hormones adrenaline and noradrenaline in excess. The tumour usually develops from the endocrine cells of the adrenal medulla. However, in 10% of cases the tumour develops at another site in the sympathetic nervous system (usually alongside the spinal column). A patient with such a tumour may experience symptoms due to excessive release of the catecholamines. These commonly include panic attacks, palpitations, tremor and hypertension.

On diagnosis, the patient initially may require drug treatment to counteract the effects of the catecholamines (including beta blocker medication). Only once the drugs have been given for long enough for the patient to regain a stable state can an operation be performed to remove the tumour.

Diseases of the pituitary

Pituitary tumour and hypopituitarism

Pituitary tumours are the most common cause of pituitary disease. They may cause problems simply as a result of their growth into local tissue. Also, as occurs with some adrenal endocrine tumours, diverse syndromes can result from excessive hormone secretion from a pituitary tumour. However, tiny tumours of the pituitary, known as microadenomas, are very common incidental findings on MRI of the brain, and may never develop to lead to any symptoms.

The pituitary gland is cradled in a small cavity in the base of the skull just behind the sinus spaces at the side of the nose. The stalk of the pituitary lies very close to a crossing of the two optic nerves which carry nerve fibres from the back of the eye to the occipital lobe at the back of the brain.

A tumour of the pituitary can cause increased pressure within this bony cavity, and so can only easily expand upwards towards the stalk. This means that, as it grows, a pituitary tumour may readily cause loss of function of some or all of the remaining gland. This leads to a state known as 'hypopituitarism'. In hypopituitarism, there is impaired or absent secretion of the pituitary hormones. GH and LH are commonly affected first, but with progression of the tumour, FSH, ACTH and TSH will also be affected. Paradoxically, PRL (prolactin) may be secreted in excess in such cases.

Symptoms of hypopituitarism include loss of libido, impotence and menstrual disturbances due to loss of the control of such functions by LH and FSH. Excessive prolactin may lead to inappropriate secretion of milk from the nipples (in men and women) and infertility. Lack of GH, ACTH and TSH will all contribute to a condition of tiredness, slowness of thought and action (secondary hypothyroidism), and low blood pressure (secondary Addison's disease).

A pituitary tumour can also spread to damage other structures in the region. Headaches (due to local invasion of bone and meninges) and impairment of vision (due to damage to the optic nerves) can be the first symptoms indicating local spread of the tumour. Double vision can also develop as a result of damage to the cranial nerves which supply the muscles of the eye.

Some pituitary tumours may also secrete a particular pituitary hormone in excess. The most common hormones that are secreted include PRL (prolactin), GH (growth hormone) and ACTH. Prolactin-secreting tumours may lead to inappropriate milk production and infertility. The syndromes of excessive GH secretion (acromegaly and gigantism) and ACTH secretion (Cushing's disease) are described below.

Pituitary tumours are diagnosed by MRI. The patient has also to undergo detailed testing for visual defects. These tests can provide an additional indication of the extent of local spread of the tumour. Specific stimulation and suppression blood tests may be performed while the patient is in hospital in order to test for syndromes of hormone insufficiency or excess.

The tumour can be excised surgically, most often by a route that crosses the nasal (sphenoidal) sinus space through the nose. If the tumour is very large it is accessed via the frontal bone in the forehead.

Radiotherapy can be focused on the pituitary area in those cases that are partially or totally inoperable.

Medication (using a drug called bromocriptine or octreotide) can cause tumour shrinkage in some cases (in particular in those that secrete prolactin). Bromocriptine or cabergoline may be prescribed also simply to reduce the symptoms of hyperprolactinaemia.

In the case of hypopituitarism, the impaired secretion of pituitary hormones is treated by means of lifelong replacement with synthetic steroids, thyroxine and sex hormones.

Acromegaly and gigantism

Acromegaly and gigantism are the two possible consequences of excessive secretion of GH (growth hormone). These conditions almost always result from a GH-secreting pituitary tumour.

Acromegaly (literally meaning 'big extremities') is the syndrome that results when the problem occurs in adulthood. GH in excess will promote bone and soft tissue growth. It will also tend to increase the blood glucose level, and so is a rare cause of secondary diabetes. It can cause enlargement of the heart and a change in the dimensions of the large blood vessels, which together may have the outcome of heart failure and hypertension. It is also recognised that additional cancers are more likely to develop, presumably a consequence of the general growth-promoting properties of the hormone. Figure 5.1e-III lists some of the most common symptoms and signs that characterise acromegaly.

In the extremely rare situation of a GH-secreting tumour occurring in childhood, the condition of gigantism will occur. In this situation, because the bony epiphyses have yet to fuse, the excess hormone promotes growth of the long bones as well

Symptoms

Change in facial appearance, enlarged hands, feet and hat size, headaches, poor vision, excessive sweating, tiredness, scanty periods, deep voice

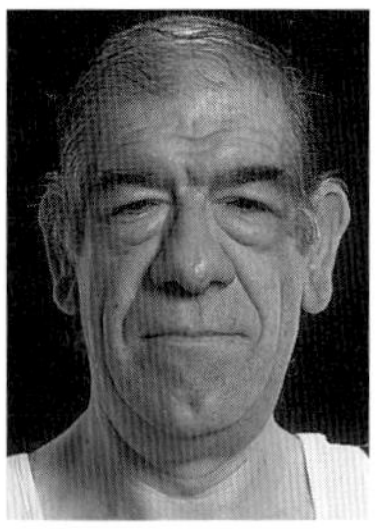

Signs

Coarse facial features, and thick greasy skin
Lower jaw projects further than upper jaw, gaps between teeth, spade like hands and feet, hypertension, oedema, weakness of muscles, glucose in the urine

Figure 5.1e-III • The symptoms and signs of acromegaly.

as the other tissues. This condition was the underlying problem for many of the record-breaking 'tallest men and women of the world' in the 20th century. Sadly, if untreated, gigantism leads to early death, usually from heart failure.

The treatment for acromegaly and gigantism is by means of treatment of the pituitary tumour (see above).

Short stature

A lack of GH is a rare but important cause of poor growth in childhood. The more common causes of poor growth are explored in detail in Section 5.4.

Cushing's disease

Cushing's disease is the result of excessive secretion of ACTH by a pituitary tumour. This was the cause of the syndrome that was initially reported by Cushing, and so this is why it is described as his disease.

The clinical features of Cushing's disease are very similar to those of the causes of Cushing's syndrome (see above). However, there are three other important features in Cushing's disease:

- pigmentation of the skin (due to the effect of ACTH on the melanin-producing cells of the skin)
- low levels of potassium in the blood (due to the effect of ACTH on the release of aldosterone)
- general features of a pituitary tumour with hypopituitarism may also be present.

Diabetes insipidus

Diabetes insipidus is a condition that develops as a result of lack of ADH (antidiuretic hormone). The consequence of this lack is that there is excessive production of very dilute urine (up to 10–15 litres in an adult), together with a compensatory increase in thirst. If very severe, the patient cannot keep up with the fluid requirements, and dehydration can result.

One of the most common causes of diabetes insipidus is surgery for a pituitary tumour, although in most cases this is only a temporary problem. Pituitary tumours themselves only rarely cause diabetes insipidus, because the ADH is actually produced in the hypothalamus, and even if the posterior pituitary is damaged, its production and release is not affected. Other more rare causes of reduced production of ADH include radiotherapy to the pituitary area and head injury.

Inherited diabetes insipidus may be the consequence of a defect in the hypothalamus, or of an abnormal response of the kidney to a normal level of ADH.

The treatment of diabetes insipidus is, ideally, of the underlying cause. Otherwise, a synthetic form of ADH, called DDVAP, can be given by nasal spray or injection once or twice daily.

Other endocrine effects from tumours

Apart from the tumours of endocrine tissue, other tumours can occasionally be a cause of a syndrome of excessive hormone production. This phenomenon is often the consequence of the secretion of hormone-like proteins from certain tumours that have become poorly differentiated (anaplastic).

The most common examples include the secretion of parathyroid-hormone-like protein from lung and breast cancers (particularly after there has been secondary spread), ADH-like protein from lung cancer, and ACTH from lung, thyroid and carcinoid tumours. Because these effects occur usually when the tumour is at quite an advanced stage, the treatment of the syndromes that result from the excessive hormones is usually palliative.

The red flags of the other endocrine diseases

Some patients with the less common endocrine diseases will benefit from referral to a conventional doctor for assessment and/or treatment. Red flags are those symptoms and signs that indicate that referral is to be considered. The red flags of the less common endocrine diseases are described in Table 5.1e-I. This table forms part of the summary on red flags given in Appendix III, which also gives advice on the degree of urgency of referral for each of the red flag conditions listed.

Table 5.1e-I Red Flags 33 –other endocrine disease

Red Flag	Description	Reasoning
33.1	**Features of Cushing's syndrome**: weight gain, weakness and wasting of limb muscles, stretch marks and bruises. Mood changes, hypertension, red cheeks, acne	Cushing's syndrome is due to chronically raised levels of corticosteroids and may result from medical treatment or from excessive bodily production. It carries serious health consequences in terms of increasing the risk of high blood pressure and diabetes and osteoporosis. Refer if the cause is unknown
33.2	**Features of Addison's disease**: increased pigmentation of skin, weight loss, muscle wasting, tiredness, loss of libido, low blood pressure, diarrhoea and vomiting, confusion, collapse with dehydration	Addison's disease is due to a lack of bodily corticosteroid, and the symptoms may develop gradually or may result in sudden collapse. The syndrome can also result from a sudden withdrawal from high doses of prescribed corticosteroid In both cases the situation is a medical emergency
33.3	**Features of the growth of a pituitary tumour**: progressive headaches, visual disturbance and double vision	The pituitary gland is situated at the base of the brain in the region of the crossing of the optic nerves and the passage of the cranial nerve which supplies the eye muscle. A tumour of the pituitary gland may cause early visual disturbance and double vision
33.4	**Features of hypopituitarism**: loss of libido, infertility, menstrual disturbances, tiredness, low blood pressure, inappropriate lactation	The pituitary is the source of the endocrine hormones that regulate growth, metabolism and the reproductive system. Damage to the pituitary gland can result in a complicated pattern of endocrine disturbance
33.5	**Features of hyperprolactinaemia**: inappropriate secretion of milk and infertility	Prolactin may be secreted in excess in all forms of pituitary disease, and so is a red flag for pituitary tumour
33.6	**Features of acromegaly (growth hormone excess)**: change in facial appearance (coarsening of features), increased size of hands and feet, enlarging tongue, deepening voice, joint pains and, if advanced, hypertension and breathlessness	Acromegaly commonly results from a pituitary tumour, and so symptoms of pituitary tumour growth (see Red Flags Table A22 in Appendix III) may also be present

Self-test 5.1e

Diseases of the adrenal gland and the pituitary

For the following case descriptions name:
(i) the most likely endocrine syndrome, and
(ii) the most likely cause of the syndrome.

1. John, aged 50 years, has been suffering from headaches and 'woolly vision' for some time now. Recently, he finds he sometimes has double vision, which is worrying him. He is feeling generally tired and out of sorts.
2. Ian, aged 57 years, is very alarmed to discover that a small amount of milky fluid has been coming out of both nipples for the past few days. He admits to you that he has not been interested in sex for some months now, and is convinced that the two things are related.
3. Anne, aged 44 years, has had a weight problem for a few years, but recently her weight has really soared, despite her trying to diet all the time. She is not sure if the blood pressure tablets she is getting from her doctor are making it worse. Also, her skin has changed: her face always feels flushed and is a bit spotty, and she gets bruises really easily. Because of all this she is feeling really down and not herself at all.
4. Ellen, aged 55 years, has lost a bit of weight recently. Together with this, she is feeling tired all the time and gets dizzy when she stands up suddenly. She is right off her food and gets occasional indigestion pain, which is not like her at all. Everyone tells her that she is looking unwell, and she thinks this is because her face is somehow darker and more unwell looking. She is really worried that she might have cancer, but cannot bring herself to make an appointment with her GP.

Answers

1. (i) John has features suggestive of a pituitary tumour, although there is nothing described to suggest a syndrome of excessive hormone secretion.
   (ii) The cause of this syndrome is enlargement of the tumour. This has caused damage to the remaining pituitary tissue, optic nerves and the nerves that supply the eye muscles.
2. (i) Ian has features suggestive of excessive secretion of the pituitary hormone prolactin.
   (ii) The cause of this syndrome may either be a tumour of prolactin-secreting cells in the pituitary, paradoxical secretion of prolactin as a consequence of a growing pituitary tumour, or (much less likely) secretion of a prolactin-like protein from a tumour elsewhere in the body.
3. (i) Anne has features of excessive production of the glucocorticoid hormones (also known as Cushing's syndrome).
   (ii) The disease that most commonly causes Cushing's syndrome is Cushing's disease, in which a pituitary tumour secretes excessive ACTH. However, the skin pigmentation that is a feature of Cushing's disease has not been described. An alternative cause is a hormone-secreting tumour of the adrenal cortex.
4. (i) Ellen has features of a lack of glucocorticoid hormones (also known as Addison's disease).
   (ii) The cause of this syndrome is most likely to be autoimmune destruction of the endocrine tissue of the adrenal cortex.

Diseases of the reproductive system

5.2

Chapter 5.2a The physiology of the reproductive system

LEARNING POINTS

At the end of this chapter you will:

- be able to describe the role of the reproductive system
- be able to describe the structure of the reproductive system in males and females
- be able to describe the role of the hormones FSH, LH, testosterone, oestrogen and progesterone in the reproductive system
- understand the physiology of sexual intercourse.

Estimated time for chapter: 120 minutes.

Introduction

The function of the reproductive system in both sexes is to ensure the reproduction of the human species. To do this, first, the reproductive system of each sex has to be able to produce healthy sex cells (gametes). These are the ova (singular ovum) from the female, and the spermatozoa (sperm) from the male. A second function of the reproductive system of each sex is to enable the meeting of these gametes (fertilisation) during the act of sexual intercourse.

The gametes originate from specialised cells called 'germ cells', which are formed within the ovaries in females and the testes in males. The gametes are the result of the particular form of cell division known as 'meiosis' (see Q5.2a-1).

After fertilisation, it is the role of the female reproductive system to provide a suitable environment for the implantation and nourishment of the fertilised egg (zygote). This role continues for the 40 weeks of pregnancy, as the zygote divides and enlarges through the stages of embryo and fetus in the womb. The female reproductive tract then has to ensure the safe expulsion of the fetus during labour. Finally, it has to undergo all the changes of the postnatal period, which allow the woman to return, as much as possible, to her pre-pregnant state.

Section 5.2 focuses on the male reproductive system and the non-pregnant female reproductive system. The study of the male reproductive system is conventionally termed 'andrology', and the study of the non-pregnant female reproductive system is termed 'gynaecology' (derived from the Greek words for man and woman, respectively). Section 5.3 is dedicated to the conditions of pregnancy, labour and the postnatal period. The study of these conditions is conventionally referred to as 'obstetrics'. The present chapter considers the physiology of the male and the female reproductive system in turn, and concludes with a brief discussion about the physiology of sexual intercourse.

The physiology of the male reproductive system

The male reproductive system consists of the testes, the epididymis, the urethra, the penis and associated glands, including the prostate gland. Figure 5.2a-I illustrates the anatomy of this system and Figure 5.2a-II shows the structure of the testis and scrotum in more detail.

The testes are the paired male sex glands, or gonads, and sit suspended from the perineum within the sacs formed by the scrotum. The two main products of the testes are spermatozoa (originating from the germinal, or germ, cells of the seminiferous tubules) and the male sex hormone testosterone (originating from the interstitial cells of Leydig).

The pituitary gland produces the two hormones follicle-stimulating hormone (FSH) and luteinising hormone (LH), which play an important role in the function of the testes. FSH stimulates the production of spermatozoa from the germ cells. LH stimulates the production of testosterone from the testes. The levels of both these hormones surge at puberty (see Q5.2a-2).

A mature sperm cell has a head, a body and a motile tail, which propels the sperm cell forwards by means of a whip-like motion. The formation of sperm is most efficient if it can take place at about 3°C below body temperature, which is aided by

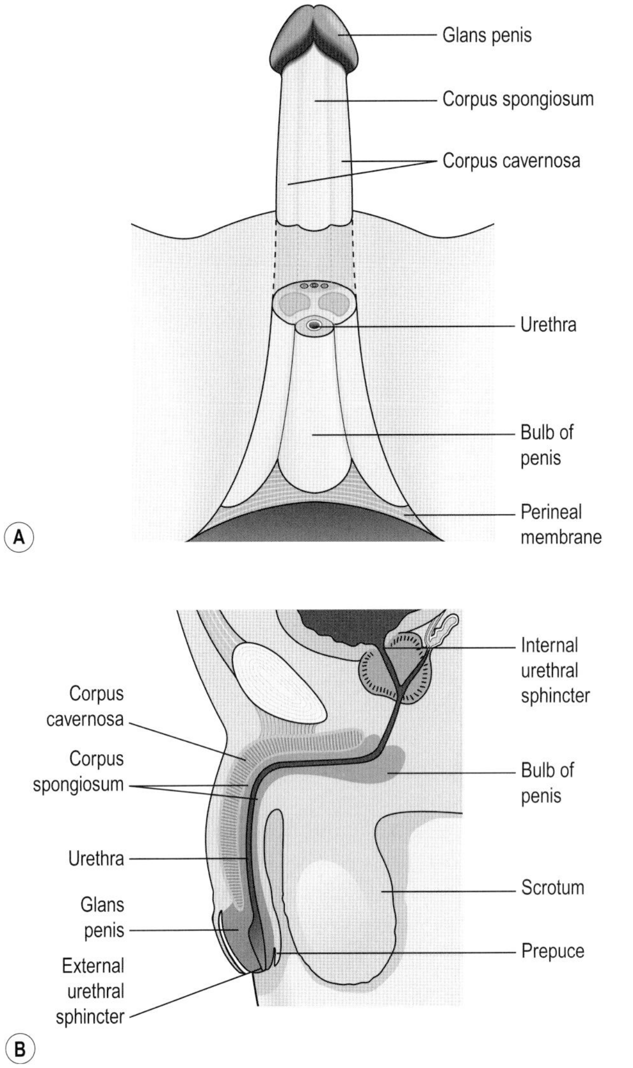

Figure 5.2a-I • The anatomy of the male reproductive system.

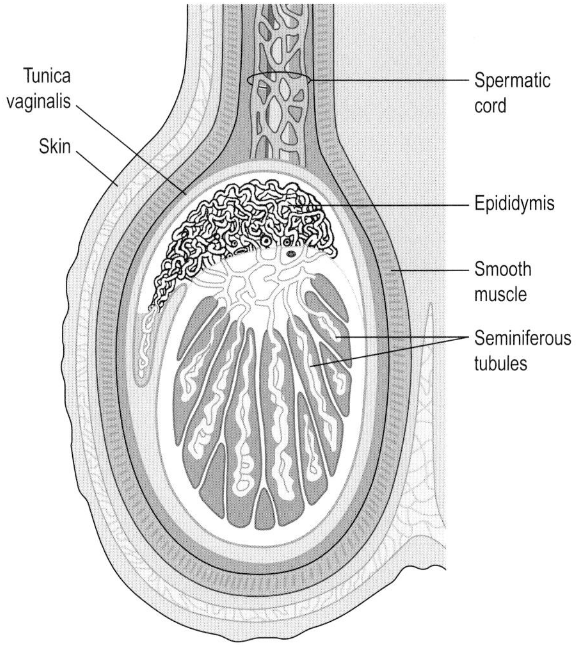

Figure 5.2a-II • The anatomy of the testis and the scrotum.

the fact that the testes sit in the scrotum. Spermatozoa are secreted from the germinal cells of the testis into the epididymis. The epididymis is a complex of very fine tubules, which store and direct spermatozoa towards the vas deferens. Testosterone is secreted from the cells of Leydig directly into the bloodstream. Thus the testis is, strictly speaking, both an exocrine and an endocrine gland.

The spermatic cords emerge from a gap in the musculature above the inguinal ligament and provide the testes with a blood and nerve supply. They also contain the vas deferens. The purpose of the vas deferens is to carry the spermatozoa away from the testes and the epididymis, and then to branch towards the urethra, from which the spermatozoa can be ejaculated. It is this tube that is severed and tied off in the procedure of vasectomy (see Q5.2a-3).

The prostate gland and seminal vesicles are exocrine glands that produce nutrient-rich lubricating fluid to maximise the survival of the spermatozoa and also to promote comfortable sexual intercourse. The seminal vesicles open out into the distal portion of the two vas deferens, and the prostate gland is situated at the base of the bladder at the point at which the vas deferens ducts enter the urethra. The prostate hugs the most proximal region of the urethra, which is why it is described as the 'prostatic urethra'. The fluids produced by these glands mix with the spermatozoa in the urethra during ejaculation to form semen (see Q5.2a-4-Q5.2a-6).

The onset of puberty in the boy

The pituitary gland responds to hormonal changes in the maturing hypothalamus to trigger the changes of puberty in both boys and girls. In both, puberty is preceded by a surge of growth hormone from the pituitary gland, and this becomes manifest as a prepubertal growth spurt. Then, in both, the pituitary starts to produce increasing quantities of LH. In boys, this stimulates the interstitial cells of the testes to produce testosterone, and it is testosterone that influences the tissues of the body to change and allows the secondary sexual characteristics to emerge. These include:

- enlargement of the testicles, penis and scrotum
- pubic hair growth in the groin and axilla
- increased facial and body hair, and thickening of the skin
- enlargement of the vocal cords and breaking of the voice
- increased muscle mass and bone density.

The female reproductive system

The female reproductive system lies at a deeper level in the body than in the male (Figures 5.2a-III and 5.2a-IV). The ovaries sit deep in the basin formed by the pelvis, and lie either side of the womb (uterus). The ovaries lie so that they are close to the openings of two tubes (the fallopian tubes) that extend sideways from the uterus. The uterus is a pear-sized organ sitting just behind and above the bladder, protected in

Information Box 5.2.a-I

The male reproductive system: comments from a Chinese medicine perspective

In Chinese medicine, the male reproductive system is dominated by the Kidney and Liver Organs. Healthy Qi and Kidney Essence (Jing) are key substances essential for male reproductive health.

The Kidney and Liver Channels pass across the anatomical location of the male genitalia. In both sexes, sexual maturation and fertility is underpinned by Jing, which is recognised to flow in 8-year cycles in men. Healthy Qi enables a healthy sexual response.

The Kidney Organ is said to control the two lower orifices. This is reflected in the fact that impotence and inappropriate seminal emissions are features of deficiency of both Kidney Yang (including Kidney Qi not firm) and Kidney Yin. In contrast, the Liver Organ appears to have more bearing on the external genitalia. Damp Heat in the Liver can manifest as soreness or itchiness of the scrotum, whereas Cold in the Liver Channel can give rise to deep pain in the scrotum.

front by the bridge formed by the pubic bone. The neck of the uterus (the cervix) opens into the bodily space called the 'vagina'. The entrance of the vagina, the vulva, is surrounded by the fleshy lips of the labia minora and labia majora in the perineum.

The vagina

The vagina is a tube-like space with tough muscular walls. It is approximately 8 centimetres long. The interior of the vagina is kept moist by secretions which originate from tiny glands in the cervix. The lining of the vagina is colonised by 'healthy' bacteria called *Lactobacillus acidophilus*. These secrete an acid called 'lactic acid', and so keep the interior of the vagina slightly acidic. Lactobacilli are the same type of bacteria that are used to turn milk into live yoghurt. The acidic environment created by the *Lactobacillus* helps keep the growth of less desirable bacteria and yeasts at bay.

In young girls, the opening of the vagina is partially closed by means of a thin sheet of tissue called the 'hymen'. A small opening in the hymen permits the escape of menstrual blood at the onset of puberty. The hymen is always stretched during first intercourse. Tearing of the hymen with a small amount of bleeding can happen at first intercourse, or may occur earlier in an active teenager. The finding of a torn hymen in a pre-pubescent child is not normal, and is an indicator of possible sexual abuse.

The uterus

The uterus is a hollow organ with three narrow openings formed by the cervix and the two fallopian tubes. The wall of the uterus is composed of a thick layer of smooth muscle called the 'myometrium'. The lining of the uterus is called 'endometrium'. This is composed of columnar epithelium and contains a large number of mucus-secreting glands. The thickness of this layer varies throughout the monthly menstrual cycle.

The endometrium extends to the lower third of the narrow entrance to the cervix, which is known as the 'cervical canal'. Below this there is a transition to squamous epithelium, which lines the vagina.

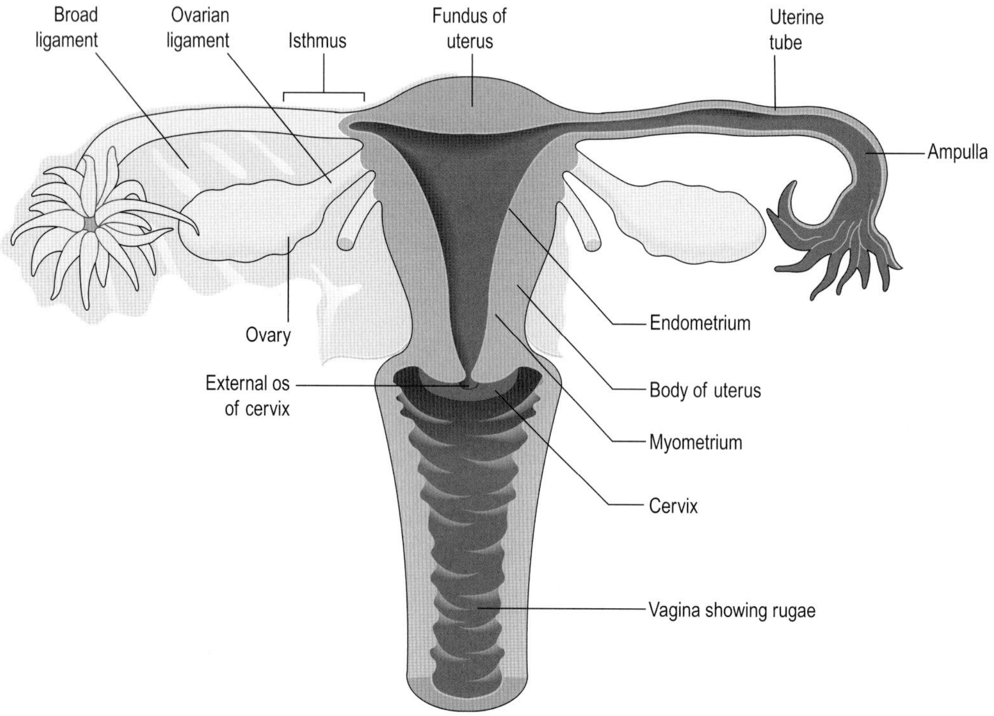

Figure 5.2a-III • The uterus and ovaries in the pelvis (anterior view).

Figure 5.2a-IV • The female reproductive system in the pelvis (lateral view).

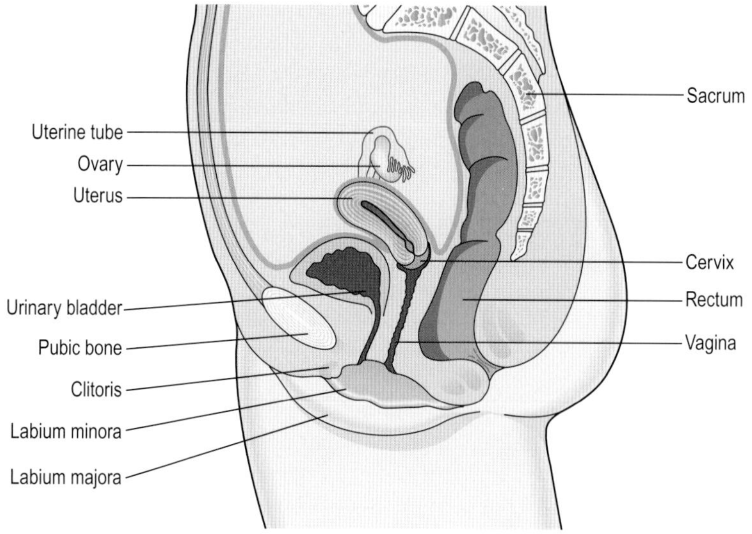

The fallopian tubes

The fallopian tubes receive the ovum (egg cell) from the ovary and aid in the transport of the ovum towards the space within the body of the uterus. To do this, the fallopian tubes have frond-like projections at their distal ends. These fronds and also the interior of the fallopian tube are lined with ciliated epithelial cells. When the ovum is released, ciliary movement wafts the ovum into and through the tube. The fallopian tube is the usual location for the fertilisation of the ovum and the spermatozoon. The fertilised zygote is then transported into the endometrium in preparation for implantation by means of the ciliary movement of the lining of the fallopian tubes (see Q5.2a-7).

The ovary

The ovary is the female sex gland, or gonad. The ovary originates from exactly the same embryonic tissue as the testis. During development of the male fetus, this embryonic tissue, originally positioned in the abdomen, develops into the testis and migrates into the scrotum under the influence of male sex hormones. In the female fetus, in the absence of these male hormones, the tissue remains where it is and develops into the ovary.

The ovary is the site for the maturation of the ova, and this takes place during the course of the first half of the menstrual cycle, during which usually only a single ovarian follicle enlarges. Ovarian follicles each consist of a single ovum and are lined by ovarian cells. By the time the female baby is born, her ovaries contain all the ova, each within its own ovarian follicle, that will be released during her childbearing years.

During the first half of the menstrual cycle, a single ovarian follicle begins the process of maturation (Figure 5.2a-V). This means that, over the course of approximately 14 days, the follicle enlarges and develops a fluid-filled cavity. This so called Graafian follicle then merges with the outer part of the ovary and ruptures to release the single ovum into the

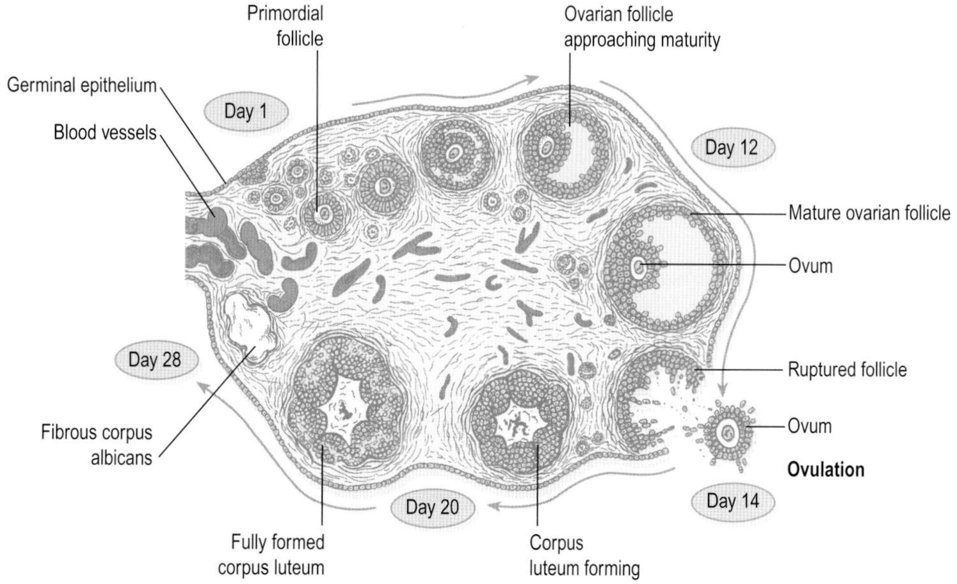

Figure 5.2a-V • Section of the ovary showing the development of one follicle over the course of one month.

space surrounding the ovary. This process of rupture and release is what is termed 'ovulation'. The whole process is stimulated firstly by FSH from the pituitary gland, and this explains its name. FSH is the same hormone that in men stimulates the development of spermatozoa from germinal cells.

During the first 14 days of the menstrual cycle, the multiplying follicle cells secrete the female sex hormone oestrogen, under the influence of FSH. The rising oestrogen levels have a suppressive (negative feedback) effect on the secretion of FSH. As The FSH levels start to drop, the pituitary then releases a surge of a second hormone, LH. It is this hormone that stimulates ovulation. After ovulation, the remaining follicle develops into a body known as the 'corpus luteum' (the origin of the term 'luteinising hormone'). The corpus luteum no longer produces oestrogen, and instead releases the other female sex hormone, progesterone.

The corpus luteum matures and then degenerates over the course of the next 14 days. As the corpus luteum degenerates, it ceases to produce progesterone. However, if fertilisation occurs, this degeneration does not happen, and instead the corpus luteum continues to develop. This occurs because, as the zygote multiplies and grows, it secretes the hormone human chorionic gonadotrophin (HCG) which stimulates the corpus luteum and prevents its degeneration. Thus, in early pregnancy the progesterone levels continue to rise.

To summarise; after puberty, the ovarian follicle is the source of a cyclical release of the female sex hormones. Oestrogen is released in the first half of the menstrual cycle, and progesterone in the second half of the menstrual cycle. This cycle is controlled by the cyclical release of the pituitary hormones FSH and LH (see Q5.2a-8).

The onset of puberty in the girl

As is the case for boys, in girls the onset of puberty is also stimulated by a rise in the production of FSH and LH. This usually occurs between the ages of 10 and 14 years.

Two to three years prior to this surge in FSH and LH in both boys and girls there is an increase in the release of GH from the pituitary gland. The release of GH stimulates the growth spurt that occurs in children just before puberty. In girls, the rise in FSH and LH stimulates the production of increasing amounts of oestrogen from the follicle cells of the ovaries. Initially, these pituitary hormones are not present in sufficient quantities to stimulate ovulation. However, the oestrogen produced affects diverse body tissues to bring about the early changes of puberty, including breast development and the growth of pubic hair. As puberty approaches, the levels of FSH and LH increase until ovulation is stimulated.

At approximately the same time as the onset of ovulation, menstruation begins. The onset of menstruation is termed the 'menarche'. It is recognised that ovulation may occur for a few cycles before the first menstrual bleed. This means that there is a possibility of pregnancy even before menstruation has started.

The onset of puberty in both girls and boys in westernised cultures is occurring at an increasingly early age. The average age of onset of menstruation is nearly 3 years earlier now than it was a century ago. This suggests that it is not purely biological 'programming' that stimulates the dramatic increase in the release of FSH and LH that initiates puberty. It is now believed that both nutritional and psychological factors also play a part in this hormonal change. These are believed to influence the physiology of the pituitary via the production of specific hormones from the hypothalamus.

A child who is less well nourished is more likely to experience a delayed onset of puberty. Conversely, a child who achieves a degree of psychological maturity, particularly with regard to understanding or experience of sexual matters, appears to experience an earlier onset of puberty. Both these factors tend to promote the earlier onset of puberty in girls who grow up in 'modern' cultures.

Menstruation

The changes that take place in the ovary after the onset of ovulation have a cycle of approximately 28 days, although any interval between 22 and 35 days is considered conventionally to be within the normal range. These changes are mirrored by cyclical changes in the uterus and vagina as well as many other tissues in the body. These changes are the result of the rise of oestrogen in the first half of the cycle and in progesterone in the second half of the cycle.

Oestrogen can be considered as a hormone that stimulates fleshiness. In the first half of the cycle, it continues to promote the healthy development of the breasts and pubic hair. It also stimulates and maintains the changes to the skin, body fat and bony skeleton (in particular the hips and pelvis) which are characteristic of the female body. In the uterus, it stimulates a thickening of the endometrium, with the development of deep mucus-forming glands and a rich supply of blood vessels. About 3 days before ovulation a thick sticky mucus is secreted from the cervix. This mucus encourages the passage of spermatozoa at the time when the woman is likely to be most fertile. This phase of the menstrual cycle is termed the 'proliferative phase', a term which refers to the changes taking place in the endometrium at that time.

Oestrogen promotes fleshiness of the tissues of the vagina and the labia majora and minor. It also promotes the vaginal secretions, which are particularly important for comfortable sexual intercourse.

Progesterone can be considered to be the hormone that prepares the body for pregnancy and promotes the first 3 months of pregnancy. After ovulation, the rising levels of progesterone stimulate a watery swelling of the endometrium and the production of a thick mucus. This mucus is believed to encourage the passage of the spermatozoa into the fallopian tubes, where fertilisation can take place. The changes in the endometrium provide a suitable environment for the zygote. If implantation does not occur, at about 6–8 days after ovulation the corpus luteum starts to degenerate, and progesterone levels drop. It is this drop that causes the lining of the endometrium to start to break down, culminating in menstruation at 14 days after ovulation. There are thus two distinct phases to this second half of the menstrual cycle, termed the 'secretory phase' and the 'premenstrual phase' (Figure 5.2a-VI).

Normal menstruation takes place over the course of 3–7 days. As blood, endometrial lining cells and tissue fluid are

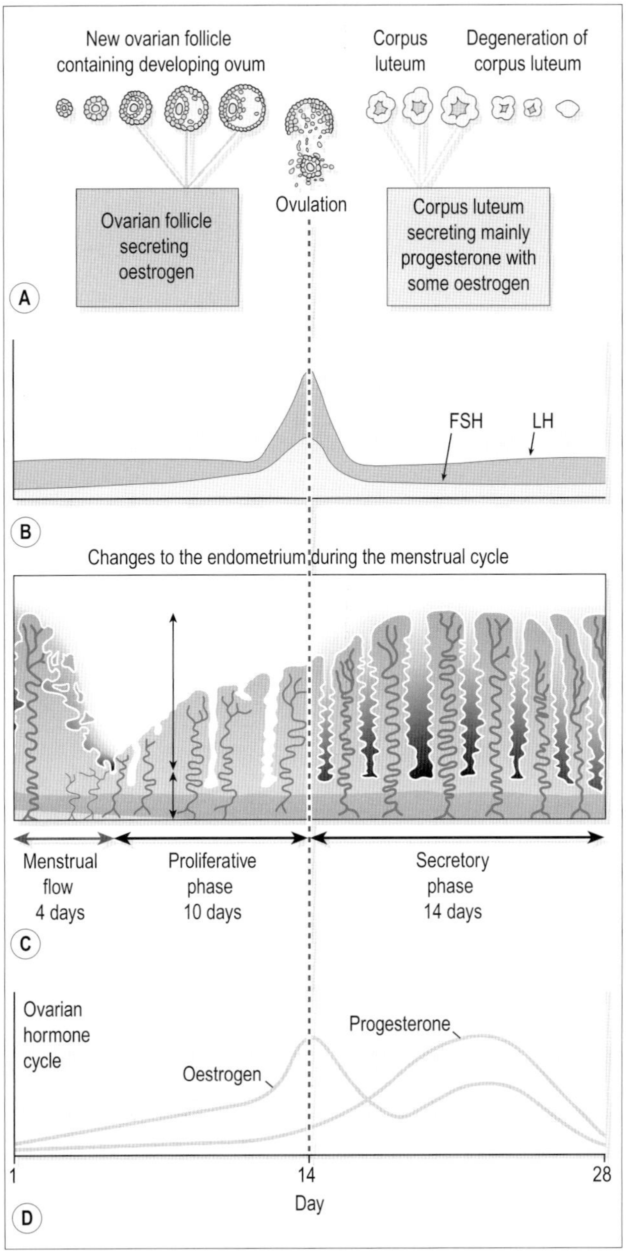

Figure 5.2a-VI • Summary of one female menstrual cycle.

shed, chemicals are released that stimulate the muscle wall of the uterus to contract, so that bleeding is minimised, and the products are effectively cleared from the uterus. This contraction is the cause of the cramping pain of menstruation. A degree of pain is therefore considered to be normal from a conventional perspective. It is important to understand that menstrual blood is not pure blood. A 'heavy' period may not necessarily indicate a large loss of blood cells, as much of the volume of what is lost may be tissue fluid.

While menstruation is occurring, the release of FSH initiates the next cycle, with the stimulation of the maturation of another ovarian follicle. This is why the first day of the menstrual bleed is conventionally considered to be the first day of the whole menstrual cycle.

The menopause

The 'menopause' is the term commonly used to describe the time in life, usually between the ages of 45 and 55 years, when menstruation ceases. Strictly speaking, the conventional use of the term menopause is to describe the precise time of cessation of menstruation. The term 'climacteric' is used to describe the period of approximately 10 years that precedes and follows this event (see Q5.2a-9).

The ageing ovaries are the cause of the onset of the climacteric. Gradually, the ovaries become less and less responsive to the pituitary hormones. This means that more and more of the menstrual cycles fail to lead to ovulation, and the production of oestrogen drops. The rate of drop in oestrogen levels varies widely between women, and this might explain why some women experience more profound symptoms than others during the climacteric.

Other features of a lack of oestrogen include a reduction in the strength of the pelvic floor muscles, with increased risk of prolapse of the vagina and uterus. Urinary problems, including urinary infections and stress incontinence, can occur because of a combination of reduced pelvic floor tone and changes in the lining of the skin around the opening of the urethra.

The notorious 'hot flushes' are a consequence of a rapid drop in oestrogen levels. The symptoms of these include bouts of profuse sweating and heat intolerance, often occurring at night. These can be accompanied by a range of bodily and psychological symptoms, which are not conventionally considered necessarily to be related to a lack of oestrogen.

A lack of oestrogen also promotes loss of calcium from the bones. This can occur very rapidly during the climacteric and can result in the symptoms of osteoporosis.

As the ovaries become less responsive to the control of the pituitary hormones, menstrual cycles become increasingly irregular. Some women experience increased frequency of periods, sometimes with excessive bleeding, for months to years, before the menopause. Usually, just before the menopause, the periods become lighter and more infrequent.

As the climacteric approaches, women become increasingly infertile as fewer and fewer cycles lead to ovulation. However, onset of the menopause does not necessarily mean that ovulation has ceased. In some women ovulation may still occur for a short time. This explains why it is that, in very rare circumstances, pregnancy can still happen after a woman's periods have ceased. Women who reach the menopause before the age of 50 years are counselled to continue to use contraception for 2 years after the menopause, and those over 50 years old are advised to continue using contraception for 1 year.

The breasts

The breasts develop in the female under the influence of progesterone and oestrogen during puberty. Each breast contains a lot of fatty tissue in which numerous exocrine glands, called 'lobules', are embedded. The lobules are responsible for milk production. During lactation milk is secreted from the lobules into ducts called 'lactiferous ducts'. Before these open out into the nipple, each duct widens into a reservoir for milk called a 'sinus'. The health of both the lobules and this fatty tissue is maintained up until the time of the menopause by oestrogen released by the maturing ovarian follicles.

The breast is prepared for milk production during pregnancy by the influence of oestrogen and progesterone. Milk production is stimulated by two pituitary hormones: prolactin stimulates the formation of milk in the lobules; and oxytocin stimulates the contraction of the ducts and sinuses, which leads to the 'let down' of milk towards the nipple. Suckling is one stimulus for the release of these two hormones (see Q5.2a-10 and Q5.2a-11).

The physiology of sexual intercourse

Sexual intercourse is necessary for natural conception to occur. It enables the meeting of the spermatozoa and the ovum in the fallopian tubes. It is, of course, also a very important aspect of bonding in human relationships.

Despite the overt differences, the physiological processes that take place during sexual intercourse are very similar in men and women. The sexual act, for both men and women, has been described as taking place in five phases, although these phases tend to merge into one another. These phases are:

- Sexual desire: the emotional/mental response to the thought, sight, touch or smell of another person.
- Sexual arousal: following sexual desire, physical changes take place in the sex organs (genitalia). The penis and clitoris become erect and the vagina becomes lubricated. The nipples can become erect. The heart rate can increase. There is a strong desire for sexual intercourse. This phase is mediated by the parasympathetic aspect of the nervous system.
- Plateau: sexual pleasure is intensified and sustained before and after penile penetration has taken place. This phase is also mediated by the parasympathetic nervous system.
- Orgasm: orgasm usually results in ejaculation of semen in men. In penile/vaginal intercourse, the semen is directed deep into the vagina, close to the entrance of the cervical canal. 90% of women are able to achieve orgasm, although only 25% will be able to reach orgasm through penile penetration into the vagina alone. There are rhythmic contractions of the perineal muscles of the women at orgasm. These contractions encourage the upward movement of the semen towards the cervix. The orgasmic phase is mediated by the sympathetic aspect of the nervous system.
- Resolution: after orgasm, both partners are relaxed, and the body gradually returns to a non-aroused state. In this phase the parasympathetic nervous system is dominant. The resolution state encourages rest, and for the woman this is the ideal state for the continued passage of the spermatozoa into the cervical canal and thence into the uterus.

Information Box 5.2.a-II

The female reproductive system: comments from a Chinese medicine perspective

From a Chinese medicine perspective, the physiology of the female reproductive system is complex. The Extra Yang Organ, the Uterus, is the central organ, but the Spleen, Stomach, Liver, Heart and Kidneys all have important roles. The four Extraordinary Vessels, the Ren Mai, the Du Mai, the Chong Mai and the Dai Mai, are important regulatory channels. Additional channels, the Bao Mai and the Bao Luo, which link the Uterus with the Heart and the Kidneys, respectively, are also important for the regulation of the female reproductive system.

Blood and Kidney Essence (Jing) are the important substances for a healthy female reproductive system. It is Heart Blood that fills and nourishes the uterus, and so the Spleen and the Liver Organs are important for the manufacture and the smooth movement of this Blood. However, Jing is required in addition to Heart Blood for menstruation to occur, as it is the basis of the menstrual Blood. In women, Jing is believed to flow in 7-year cycles. The Spleen and Jing may be the foundation of the action of oestrogen, as together they give rise to fleshy characteristics, fertility and strong bones.

The deep origin of all three of the Extraordinary Vessels (Ren Mai, Du Mai and Chong Mai) is the region of the Kidneys. These then all flow through the Uterus before reaching their more superficial pathways.

The Chong Mai, as the Sea of Blood, has a strong influence on menstruation. The Chong Mai is linked to the Stomach Channel via St 30 (Qichong). This explains how nausea can be a problem in conditions such as dysmenorrhoea and morning sickness.

The Ren Mai governs the cervix, vagina and the vulva. It also helps to provide the other Yin substances important in female reproductive physiology (Yin, Essence and Fluids), as it is the Sea of the Yin Channels. Therefore, it is important in the regulation of fertility, puberty, pregnancy and the menopause.

Because of its complex pathway, the Du Mai also influences the vagina and the vulva. The Du Mai together and the Ren Mai together can be seen as two branches of one circuit that interlinks the Uterus with the other Organs. The Dai Mai encircles the waist, and so crosses the leg Channels. In this way it influences the smooth flow of Qi in the Liver Channel and harmonises The Kidneys and the Spleen.

The relative strength of the organs and substances in the four menstrual phases correspond to the physiological phases understood in conventional terms. These are (with conventional terms in parentheses):

- Menstruation: Blood is moving, and is reliant on smooth Liver Qi and Liver Blood.
- Postmenstrual (proliferative phase): Blood and Yin are Empty and Chong Mai and Ren Mai are Empty.
- Mid-cycle (secretory phase): Blood and Yin fill up in Chong Mai and Ren Mai.
- Premenstrual (premenstrual phase): Yang Qi rises and Liver Qi moves. This phase does not occur if implantation takes place.

At the climacteric, there is a decline in the Kidney Essence and in the Qi and Blood of the Ren Mai and the Chong Mai. There is thus a general drying up of body fluids (Yin Deficiency). This culminates in the cessation of menstruation.

Self-test 5.2a

The physiology of the reproductive system

1. What is the composition of semen? Name the origin of its constituents.
2. What are the bodily effects of (i) testosterone and (ii) oestrogen?
3. How do the levels of oestrogen and progesterone vary throughout the menstrual cycle? What is the stimulus for menstruation?
4. What is one conventional medical reason why some women suffer more during the menopause than others?

Answers

1. Semen is composed of the male sex cells, the spermatozoa, and fluid. The spermatozoa originate from germ cells within the testes. The fluid contains nutrients for the spermatozoa, and provides an environment in which the spermatozoa can swim freely. The fluid originates from the seminal vesicles and the prostate gland.
2. (i) Testosterone has the following bodily effects:
    - encouragement of muscle development and increase in bone density
    - enlargement of the voice box and deepening of the voice
    - growth of facial hair, body hair and pubic hair
    - enlargement of the penis, scrotum and prostate gland
    - thickening of the skin and sebaceous glands (which produce oily secretions)
    - production of spermatozoa.

   (ii) Oestrogen has the following bodily effects:
    - enlargement of the uterus, vagina and labia
    - enlargement of the breasts
    - growth of pubic and armpit hair
    - widening of the pelvis and strengthening of the bones
    - increase in fat deposition, especially at the hips and breasts.

   All these effects begin at puberty and the changes will start to regress if testosterone and oestrogen levels drop.
3. Oestrogen is produced in increasing amounts in the first (proliferative) half of the menstrual cycle. Progesterone is produced in the first part of the second half of the menstrual cycle (secretory phase), although levels decline after about 7 days. It is the drop in progesterone that is the stimulus for menstruation.
4. The symptoms of the menopause are attributed to falling levels of oestrogen. Sudden drops in oestrogen are considered to induce more profound symptoms than a more gradual drop in oestrogen levels.

Chapter 5.2b The investigation of the reproductive system

LEARNING POINTS

At the end of this chapter you will:
- be able to recognise the main investigations used in gynaecology, andrology and genitourinary medicine
- understand what a patient might experience when undergoing these investigations.

Estimated time for chapter: 60 minutes.

Introduction

The investigation of the female reproductive system is usually carried out within the hospital speciality of obstetrics and gynaecology. The hospital specialist who deals with the all the disorders of the non-pregnant female reproductive tract is called a 'gynaecologist'. However, breast disorders are, in general, managed by a general or a specialist breast surgeon.

Disorders of the male reproductive system are often investigated within the surgical speciality of urology. In some hospitals there may be a dedicated andrology unit.

Sexually transmitted diseases are usually managed within the hospital speciality of genitourinary (GU) medicine. In the UK, in contrast to all other hospital specialities apart from accident and emergency medicine, patients can self-refer to a department of GU medicine. The content of each consultation is kept strictly confidential and is not even revealed to the patient's GP.

The investigation of the female reproductive system

The investigation of the female reproductive system includes
- a thorough physical examination, including internal examination of the uterus and ovaries
- blood tests and urine tests to assess hormone levels
- examination of samples of vaginal mucus
- cervical 'smear' (Pap smear) test
- imaging tests (in particular, pelvic ultrasound, endoscopy of the vagina and the womb, laparoscopy, and hysterosalpingography) to visualise the structure of the reproductive organs
- biopsy of the endometrium.

Gynaecological physical examination

The main part of the gynaecological examination is the internal pelvic examination. For this examination the woman has to lie on her back, with knees bent and feet apart. In the first part of the examination the doctor inserts two gloved fingers of the right hand into the vagina, whilst palpating the suprapubic area of the abdomen with the left. In this 'bimanual examination' the shape of the cervix can be assessed, and structural problems of the uterus and the ovaries may be detected. The doctor then inserts an instrument, made of metal or plastic, called a 'speculum' into the vagina. The speculum parts the soft tissue of the vaginal walls, and allows the doctor to see the cervix. A speculum is necessary to perform a cervical smear test.

If the patient can relax, these tests should not be painful. However, many patients find these procedures undignified or embarrassing. They can be very traumatic for those with a past history of sexual difficulties or abuse. The muscle tension that results from resistance to the idea of these tests can make insertion of the examining fingers or the speculum much more difficult, and potentially painful.

Blood and urine tests

Blood tests may be taken to examine the levels of FSH, LH and the sex hormones. As all these hormones vary dramatically throughout the menstrual cycle, it is important to record the time of day and the day of the cycle on which the test is taken.

Urine may also be examined for hormone levels. The most commonly performed urine test is the pregnancy test. This looks for the rising levels of HCG that appear shortly after implantation of the fertilised ovum (zygote).

Examination of vaginal mucus

A sample of vaginal mucus can be obtained by means of a swab inserted during a speculum examination. This test may be performed to investigate possible infectious disease, in which case the swab is sent to a laboratory to look for evidence of microorganisms.

Alternatively, the mucus may be examined as part of natural family planning and also in the investigation of infertility. The patient can be taught to examine her own mucus, and to look for the characteristic changes in consistency that occur at ovulation. When the mucus is at its most profuse and sticky, ovulation is occurring and fertility is at its peak.

The postcoital test is a test of the cervical mucus taken within 8 hours of intercourse and is timed to occur in the 2 days leading up to ovulation. In this test the mucus should contain sperm. The test is to examine whether or not the sperm are able to penetrate the mucus in a normal way. If they cannot, this may suggest a condition in which the mucus contains antibodies that are specific to the antigens on the sperm, and which prevent the sperm from penetrating the cervical os.

Cervical smear (Pap test)

In the cervical smear test, the opening to the cervix is visualised by means of a speculum. The cervix is then scraped gently with a spatula or brush to obtain a sample of the mucus. The end of the spatula/brush is either stirred into a fluid designed to maintain living cervical cells, or dragged over a glass microscope slide so that a 'smear' of the mucus is formed on the slide. This test should be painless.

The cell transport fluid or smeared slide is then sent to a cytology laboratory for microscopic examination. The examination looks for abnormally shaped (dysplastic) cervical cells, which may be an indication of early cancer.

The cervical smear test is offered to all women in the UK between the ages of 25 and 65 years at 3-year intervals as part of a national screening programme. However, the cervical smear is not a wholly reliable test, in that many women who have no physical abnormality will have unclear smear tests and will have to be recalled for re-examination (false-positive results), and some cervical cancers will be missed (false-negative results). There is ongoing debate over whether the cost of the programme and its inconvenience to many women are outweighed by the advantages of the early detection of cancer in a few. It has been estimated that the UK cervical screening programme saves about 3000 lives per annum by preventing the development of advanced cervical cancer.

Imaging tests

Because the uterus and ovaries are deep organs, imaging tests are very often performed to provide more information.

The pelvic ultrasound scan is a non-invasive examination which can provide very useful information. The test usually involves the use of a probe placed on the skin of suprapubic part of the abdomen. In some cases a vaginally inserted probe can give more information. Tumours and cysts of the ovaries and uterus can be visualised by means of an ultrasound examination. The formation of the Graafian follicle can be seen, and so ultrasound can give an indication of healthy ovulation.

Endoscopy of the vagina (colposcopy) is a test that requires the insertion of a vaginal speculum. A colposcope (a form of endoscope) is used to provide detailed images of the surface of the cervix, and permits the removal of cervical biopsies and treatment of the cervix. This investigation is most commonly used to provide more information and treatment after an abnormal cervical smear test.

Endoscopy of the uterus (hysteroscopy) requires the insertion of a fine endoscope into the uterus via the cervical canal. This is usually performed in an outpatient setting in a conscious patient. The test can be uncomfortable, as the cervix is very sensitive. Hysteroscopy is used in the investigation of menstrual disorders, and is the means by which samples of the endometrium may be obtained for microscopic examination.

Laparoscopy is a procedure in which a fine endoscope is inserted into the peritoneal cavity which surrounds the pelvic organs. The endoscope is inserted via a small incision made adjacent to the umbilicus. Laparoscopy can reveal the details of the external anatomy of the ovaries and the uterus. It can visualise ovarian cysts and the changes that occur in endometriosis. Laparoscopy is also the means by which some important gynaecological procedures can be performed. These include sterilisation, removal of ovarian cysts and removal of eggs for assisted-fertilisation techniques.

Hysterosalpingography is a test to examine the interior anatomy of the fallopian tubes. A 'dye' that is opaque to x-rays is injected into the cervical canal, and x-ray images taken of the pelvic area. The dye can reveal the interior shape of the uterus and fallopian tubes, and thereby whether or not the fallopian tubes are blocked.

Endometrial biopsy is performed by means of hysteroscopy. A sample of the lining of the womb is removed from a conscious patient by means of a spoon-shaped instrument called a 'curette'. The patient is likely to experience cramping pain and some bleeding after this procedure.

A less invasive method of obtaining endometrial samples is by means of a fine-ended suction instrument called a 'Pipelle curette'. This samples far less endometrium but still has a greater than 90% detection rate for endometrial cancer.

The investigation of breast diseases

The investigation of breast diseases includes

- physical examination of the breasts and armpits
- withdrawal of fluid from cysts and biopsy
- mammography.

Physical examination of the breasts

Physical examination of the breasts involves observation for lumps or asymmetry, and systematic palpation for lumps. The examination should extend into the axilla (the armpit), into which the breast tissue extends. The axillary lymph nodes are also examined.

In the UK women are encouraged to perform this examination on themselves on a regular basis. The techniques of breast self examination can be learned from a GP or practice nurse.

Fluid drainage and biopsy

Some lumps in the breast are cysts that contain fluid. This fluid can be withdrawn by means of a fine needle and syringe, and then examined under a microscope. A wider needle and syringe may be used to obtain a sample of the cells in a lump. Alternatively, a minor operation might be required to remove a small sample of tissue for a biopsy.

Ultrasound scan

An ultrasound scan is commonly used in the investigation of breast lumps in outpatients. The scan can clearly demonstrate the fluid within breast cysts, and also indicate any irregular areas of growth, which may be suggestive of breast cancer.

Mammography

Mammography is the term given to describe x-ray examination of the breasts. This test is offered to women in the UK aged 50–70 years at 1- to 3-year intervals as part of the National Health Service (NHS) breast screening programme.

Mammography is given with the intention of detecting breast cancer in an early (operable) stage. Like the cervical smear test, it is not a wholly reliable test, in that many women who have normal results will have to be recalled for re-examination (false positives), and some breast cancers will be missed (false negatives). Also, as for the cervical smear test, there is ongoing debate over whether the cost of the programme and its inconvenience to many women are outweighed by the advantages of the early detection of cancer in a few.

The investigation of the male reproductive system

The investigation of the male reproductive system includes:

- a thorough physical examination, including examination of the testes and penis
- blood tests to assess hormone levels and to look for tumour markers
- semen analysis.

Physical examination of the male reproductive system

The examination of the male reproductive system involves inspection and visualisation of the male genitalia and palpation of the scrotum. Palpation will reveal the shape and consistency of the testes, and also the spermatic cords and the epididymis. The inguinal (groin) lymph nodes are also examined. In the UK, men are encouraged to examine their own testes on a regular basis. The techniques of testicular self-examination can be learned from a GP or practice nurse.

The prostate is examined by means of digital rectal examination.

Blood tests to assess hormone levels and to look for tumour markers

Blood tests can be used to assess levels of FSH, LH and the sex hormones, although these tests are much more commonly performed in women than in men.

Testicular cancer and prostate cancers can secrete characteristic chemicals known as 'tumour markers', such as prostate-specific antigen (PSA). Blood tests may be taken for tumour markers in the diagnostic stages of cancer, but also during treatment to assess progress.

Semen analysis

A fresh sample of semen which has been obtained by masturbation can be submitted to a range of tests to assess fertility. The volume and consistency of the semen and the number (sperm count), shape and movement of the spermatozoa can be analysed and compared to the normal ranges.

Visualisation of the testes and prostate

The structure of the testes and prostate may be examined in more detail by means of an ultrasound scan. The examination of the prostate requires the insertion of an ultrasound probe into the rectum.

Biopsy of the testes and the prostate

In cases of suspected cancer, biopsy of the testes or prostate may be necessary.

The investigation of sexually transmitted diseases

The investigation of sexually transmitted diseases includes:

- physical examination
- examination of discharges
- blood tests.

Physical examination

Many sexually transmitted diseases have characteristic symptoms and signs. Physical examination of the external genitalia in men and women, and the vagina, cervix and uterus in women, may reveal some of the characteristic features of these diseases.

Examination of discharges

Samples of vaginal or penile discharges may be taken by means of a swab to examine for evidence of microorganisms and viruses. In women, often three swabs are taken, two from the cervical os and one from the vagina. The most common organisms that are isolated include *Candida, Gonococcus, Chlamydia, Trichomonas* and *Gardnerella*.

Blood tests

Blood tests can provide evidence of a sexually transmitted infection. These include the test for human immunodeficiency virus (HIV), in which antibodies to HIV are indicative of infection. Blood tests can also reveal evidence of infection by hepatitis B and C and syphilis.

GU clinics offer the HIV test on a strictly confidential basis. Because of the consequences of being tested as HIV-positive, patients will be offered pre-test and post-test counselling, irrespective of whether the test is positive or negative.

Chapter 5.2c Disorders of menstruation and the menopause

LEARNING POINTS

At the end of this chapter you will be able to:

- describe the clinical features and treatment of amenorrhoea and oligomenorrhoea
- describe the clinical features and treatment of menorrhagia and metrorrhagia
- describe the clinical features and treatment of premenstrual syndrome and dysmenorrhoea
- describe the problems that may be experienced in the menopause
- recognise the Red Flags of menstruation.

Estimated time for chapter: 120 minutes.

Introduction

The conditions explored in this chapter are:

- Amenorrhoea and oligomenorrhoea – primary amenorrhoea:
  - non-structural causes
  - congenital defects.
- Amenorrhoea and oligomenorrhoea – secondary amenorrhoea:
  - non-structural causes
  - primary ovarian failure
  - endocrine causes
  - polycystic ovarian syndrome.
- Menorrhagia:
  - dysfunctional uterine bleeding
  - uterine fibroids and endometrial polyps
  - pelvic inflammatory disease
  - hypothyroidism
  - metrorrhagia.
- Premenstrual syndrome.
- Dysmenorrhoea:

Self-test 5.2b

The investigation of the reproductive system

1. Anthea is a 35-year-old woman who has gone to her doctor with a concern that she is developing a moustache on her lip. The GP does not think that the hair growth is excessive, but offers a referral to a gynaecologist, as there are some hormone treatments that might be offered.

   He explains that in most cases of mild 'male-pattern' hair growth, no physical abnormality is found, but rarely a condition called polycystic ovarian syndrome may be diagnosed. In this condition, poorly matured ovarian follicles secrete excessive male sex hormones and cause hair growth and infertility.

   What investigations do you think Anthea might have to undergo at her first appointment with the gynaecologist?

Answers

1. Anthea will first be given a thorough gynaecological examination. This will involve examination of her skin and body hair. She will also have to have an internal pelvic examination so that the doctor can check that her ovaries feel normal in size. If she is not up to date with her smear tests, she may be offered one at this appointment.

   The doctor will perform a blood test to look for levels of FSH, LH, and male and female sex hormones.

   Anthea will then be given an ultrasound examination to clarify whether or not her womb and ovaries are normal in size and shape.

- Primary dysmenorrhoea
  - endometriosis
  - pelvic inflammatory disease.
- Problems of the menopause.

Amenorrhoea and oligomenorrhoea

Amenorrhoea is defined as total lack of menstruation. It may be primary or secondary. Primary amenorrhoea means that there has never been an onset of menstruation. This diagnosis is made if the menarche has not occurred by the age of 16 years.

Secondary amenorrhoea indicates a cessation of menstruation. This diagnosis is made when menstruation has ceased for more than 70 days. Oligomenorrhoea indicates infrequent periods with a cycle length of greater than 35 days. In general, the causes of oligomenorrhoea are the same as those of secondary amenorrhoea (see Q5.2c-1).

Primary amenorrhoea

Non-structural causes of primary amenorrhoea

In most cases of primary amenorrhoea there is no structural abnormality. There may instead be an inherited tendency to have a late onset of menstruation. There may be other factors, such as chronic illness, an eating disorder or excessive exercise, which have delayed the onset of menstruation. These inhibit the onset of menstruation by causing a reduction in the release of the pituitary hormones LH and FSH.

Congenital causes of primary amenorrhoea

More rare structural causes of primary amenorrhoea include congenital defects of the ovaries, uterus, vagina or hymen. In all but the first of these conditions, the other features of puberty will appear normally. Turner's syndrome is a relatively common chromosomal disorder in which the affected woman has underdeveloped ovaries, and often first presents with primary amenorrhoea and failure to develop the other secondary sexual characteristics of puberty.

Primary amenorrhoea is usually investigated if menarche has not occurred by the age of 16 years. A physical examination is performed, and blood tests are taken to look for FSH, LH and the sex hormones, including testosterone. Prolactin levels and thyroid function are also assessed. If it is found that the ovaries are not responding to the pituitary hormones (suggesting congenital disorders of the ovary such as Turner's syndrome), hormone (oestrogen and progestogen) replacement therapy (HRT) is prescribed. If the problem lies in factors that lead to underproduction of sufficient pituitary hormones, such as overexercise or anorexia nervosa, then ideally these factors should first be remedied. However, in some cases it may be considered best to prescribe HRT also, to prevent the problems inherent in a continued lack of oestrogen.

Secondary amenorrhoea and oligomenorrhoea

The most common cause of secondary amenorrhoea is pregnancy. This common cause may actually be a possibility that has been overlooked by the patient, but needs always to be considered in any case of absence of menstrual bleeding.

Non-structural causes of secondary amenorrhoea

In most cases of secondary amenorrhoea there is no physical abnormality, because most commonly it develops as a response to factors that affect the release of pituitary hormones. Conditions such as chronic illness, eating disorders and overexercise, already described as causes of primary amenorrhoea, can also lead to cessation of periods after a normal menarche. Less seriously, episodes of physical or emotional stress, such as exams or overseas travel, might cause amenorrhoea for a short time. Teenage girls are particularly prone to stress-related amenorrhoea. For this reason, secondary amenorrhoea is usually not investigated until it has persisted for at least 6 months.

Primary ovarian failure

This is a rare and irreversible cause of secondary amenorrhoea. In most cases the cause is unknown. In some cases there may be autoimmune damage to the ovaries. In this condition the ovaries simply stop producing follicles, and the woman enters an early menopause (defined as menopause occurring before the age of 40 years). People with primary ovarian failure are offered HRT until the age of 50 years in order to prevent the development of osteoporosis. Conception may still be possible with assisted-conception techniques.

Endocrine causes of secondary amenorrhoea

Some cases of amenorrhoea are the result of endocrine diseases, for example hyperthyroidism or excessive prolactin secretion, in which case the treatment is primarily treatment of the underlying cause.

Polycystic ovarian syndrome

In polycystic ovarian syndrome (PCOS) the ovarian follicles do not develop properly. The ovary becomes enlarged, with four or more unruptured follicles (cysts). The condition is associated with weight gain, oligomenorrhoea or amenorrhoea, excessive body hair in a male distribution and infertility. It is believed that insulin resistance and oversecretion of insulin might be the fundamental problem in PCOS.

This hormonal imbalance, which is more common in obese people, is believed to affect the LH surge from the pituitary gland (so preventing rupture of the ovarian follicles and causing infertility) as well as leading to excessive formation of male sex hormones (which cause excessive body hair and also acne). PCOS is associated with a greater than average risk of non-insulin-dependent diabetes mellitus, high blood pressure and cardiovascular disease. There is also a small increased risk of cancer of the womb and of the ovaries.

PCOS is very common. Ultrasound studies have shown that up to 20% of women have evidence of PCOS. However, only a few will exhibit the more severe manifestations of the syndrome.

In PCOS, ultrasound examination of the ovaries shows unruptured ovarian follicles and a blood test reveals an imbalance in the levels of FSH and LH, and in some cases raised levels of testosterone and prolactin.

In PCOS women are advised to lose weight, stop smoking and to increase participation in gentle exercise, as these changes can normalise insulin levels. The antidiabetes drug metformin may be prescribed, as it reduces insulin resistance, particularly in anyone who is classified as overweight according to their body mass index (BMI > 25).

If amenorrhoea is the primary problem, the combined oral contraceptive pill is prescribed to induce regular menstruation and protect the woman from endometrial cancer.

The drug clomiphene may be prescribed to induce ovulation in PCOS. If this fails to help with conception, surgical drilling of the ovaries can reduce the production of unnecessary sex steroid hormones and improve fertility rates.

Excessive male-pattern body hair in PCOS can be treated by means of medication. The oral contraceptive may be effective in reducing the hairiness. Alternatively, the drug cyproterone acetate may be prescribed. This has the effect of opposing the action of the male sex hormones.

Information Box 5.2c-I

Amenorrhoea: comments from a Chinese medicine perspective

In Chinese medicine, amenorrhoea (no periods) may be an Empty or a Full condition. Empty causes include Jing Deficiency, Blood Deficiency, Spleen and Kidney Deficiency, and Liver and Kidney Deficiency. Full causes are Cold in the Uterus, Phlegm or Qi/Blood Stagnation. Oligomenorrhoea (late periods) might indicate Blood Deficiency, Cold in the Uterus, Kidney Yang Deficiency or Qi Deficiency.

Menorrhagia

Menorrhagia is defined as menstrual bleeding that is too heavy, and specifically relates to a menstrual loss of more than 80 ml/month. However, in practice the degree of menstrual loss is very difficult to assess. Usually loss is expressed in terms of the number of tampons or towels required, and the numbers of episodes of 'flooding' (see Q5.2c-2).

The main health consequence of menorrhagia is blood loss. This can, in severe cases, lead to iron-deficiency anaemia, as the loss of iron in the menstrual blood is too great to be replaced by the diet alone. Very rarely, the blood loss is so profuse as to require emergency treatment with transfusion.

However, for most people, the main problem with menorrhagia is the inconvenience of having a prolonged and heavy period. Although many women feel tired and uncomfortable during a heavy period, they may never lose sufficient blood to become clinically anaemic.

Dysfunctional uterine bleeding

The most important and common cause of menorrhagia is functional. This means that there is no structural or readily measurable cause for the bleeding. The term 'dysfunctional uterine bleeding' (DUB) is applied to a range of syndromes, all of which involve heavy bleeding. In DUB the bleeding is usually regular. If the pattern of bleeding is chaotic, and with no predictable pattern, then the term 'metrorrhagia' is applied.

DUB is most common just after the menarche and in the years leading up to the menopause. Usually, the underlying problem is due to a defect in the maturation of the ovarian follicle or the formation of the corpus luteum. The reasons for this are usually unclear, although the root lies partly in the control of the whole process by the pituitary gland. This, of course, explains why emotional and mental factors can play an important role in the development of heavy periods.

The defective follicular development may cause the levels of oestrogen and progesterone to become subtly unbalanced, and this is the cause of the heavy bleeding. However, most women with DUB demonstrate no measurable abnormalities in the release of pituitary or sex hormones that might support this theory.

The pattern of problematic bleeding varies according to the precise underlying problem. In some cases the spotting and blood loss occurs for some days before the onset of menstruation. This bleeding may start at the time of ovulation (mid-cycle bleeding). In other cases there is slight bleeding or spotting for some days after the period.

In less common cases the underlying problem is that ovulation does not occur (anovulatory cycles), and the lining of the womb becomes thickened by excessive oestrogen production. This form of DUB is common just before the menopause. The time between periods becomes longer (up to 6–8 weeks), but when the period comes it is very heavy, and can be associated with flooding.

Another problem that can occur in the few years before the menopause is a result of fluctuating levels of oestrogen from the failing ovary. The result is more frequent periods, which may also be heavy, and flooding.

Investigation of persistent DUB is important to eliminate more serious causes (see later). If no physical cause is found, treatment is primarily directed at controlling bleeding. In women who have developed anaemia, iron tablets may be prescribed in the short term. Very rarely, a blood transfusion may be necessary to replace blood that has been lost rapidly.

Simple medications that may be used to reduce the volume of heavy bleeds include non-steroidal anti-inflammatory drugs (NSAIDs) such as mefenamic acid. Tranexamic acid is a drug that inhibits the breakdown of blood clots, and this may be used to halt a heavy bleed, but must be avoided if the patient has any risk factors for thrombosis.

DUB can also be treated by means of hormonal drugs. Contraceptive methods can be helpful for many women. The oral contraceptive pill, the progesterone-containing intrauterine device, progesterone implants or injections will all control heavy bleeding. These treatments will of course also prevent pregnancy.

In some women, withdrawal from these treatments after a few months may result in normalisation of the periods.

Norethisterone is a synthetic progesterone (progestogen) which is commonly prescribed in cases of very severe bleeding to control premature breakdown of the womb lining. This is taken daily from day 5 to day 25 of the cycle. In most women this will keep a bleed at bay until the tablets are stopped. Withdrawal of the tablets on day 26 leads to a 'withdrawal bleed'. This treatment is continued for 4–6 menstrual cycles, and may be sufficient in some women to normalise their periods.

In resistant cases, surgical treatments may be offered. Dilatation and curettage (D&C) is the surgical procedure in which the lining of the womb is scraped away with a curette. It is a low-risk procedure and can bring about a temporary (4–6 months) relief from heavy bleeding.

A more permanent approach is to remove the lining of the uterus by heat or laser via a hysteroscope. This procedure, which requires a 1–2 day stay in hospital, is called 'endometrial ablation'. This procedure causes sterility, but is less invasive than a hysterectomy. In about 80% of women who have this procedure there is either total loss of or a relative reduction in periods.

Hysterectomy is now performed less commonly for DUB because the recent developments of drug treatments and endometrial ablation are effective and are much less invasive alternatives.

Uterine fibroids and endometrial polyps

The most common structural cause of menorrhagia is the presence of one or more fibroids. These are benign tumours of the uterine muscle, and are known to develop in up to 20% of women over the age of 30 years, although very often they do not give rise to symptoms. In some women fibroids are associated with menorrhagia and dysmenorrhoea. Endometrial polyps are fleshy outgrowths of the endometrial lining, which may also be associated with menorrhagia.

Pelvic inflammatory disease

Pelvic inflammatory disease (PID) is a chronic inflammatory condition of the lining of the womb which is a long-term consequence of infection by a sexually transmitted disease. Menorrhagia can be a complication of PID.

Hypothyroidism

Hypothyroidism is an endocrine cause of menorrhagia. It must not be forgotten as a possibility, as it has profound health consequences, but is readily treatable.

Metrorrhagia

'Metrorrhagia' is the term used to describe bleeding that has no regular pattern. In some cases it may be difficult to differentiate between metrorrhagia and DUB with irregular spotting either side of a regular period.

Metrorrhagia should be investigated seriously as it may indicate a serious structural problem of the endometrium or cervix, and in particular cancer.

Information Box 5.2c-II

Menorrhagia: comments from a Chinese medicine perspective

In Chinese medicine, menorrhagia has been classified according to the pattern of bleeding. These patterns are: heavy periods, flooding and trickling, long periods and bleeding between periods. The causes of these may either be Full or Empty. Empty conditions include Qi Deficiency, Kidney (and Liver) Yin Deficiency with Empty Heat, and Spleen and Kidney Yang Deficiency. Full conditions include Qi and Blood Stagnation, Blood Heat and Damp Heat.

In Chinese medicine, metrorrhagia can been classified within the pattern of irregular periods. Causes of irregular periods include Liver Qi Stagnation, Kidney Yin Deficiency and Kidney Yang Deficiency.

Premenstrual syndrome

Premenstrual syndrome (PMS) is a functional condition that involves low mood and uncomfortable physical symptoms. PMS occurs from any time in the second half of the menstrual cycle (between ovulation and the first few days of menstruation). PMS is more common between the ages of 30 and 40 years. At the onset of menstruation, or during the period, the symptoms disappear and the woman may even feel euphoric for a few days. The symptoms of low mood and physical discomfort start again after ovulation. It is estimated that in 15% of women the mood and physical disturbances of PMS are so severe as to disturb day-to-day living and personal relationships.

The perimenstrual syndrome is a particular pattern of PMS which is described as occurring in the 2–3 days prior to menstruation.

The emotional and mental symptoms of PMS include irritability, anxiety, depression, tearfulness and confusion. Sweet cravings may be prominent in some people. Physical symptoms include abdominal bloating, breast tenderness, swelling of the ankles, headache, nausea and clumsiness.

In perimenstrual syndrome, the most common symptoms are tiredness and headache in the 2 days prior to menstruation. Migraine can occur during this time in some women. There may also be bloating and abdominal pain.

The cause of PMS is not clearly understood. Theories that propose a hormonal cause have not been consistently supported by experimental measurement of hormone fluctuations in women with PMS. A recent hypothesis is that it is how progesterone is metabolised in the brain and interacts with the GABA-A neurotransmitter receptor that determines sensitivity to the premenstrual phase.

Treatment of PMS ideally should begin with lifestyle advice. Dealing with stress is probably the most important, but in many cases this is the most difficult lifestyle factor to deal with. In some women, normalisation of diet and adoption of whole foods can be very helpful. Regular exercise can also be very beneficial for some people.

Vitamin B_6 (pyridoxine) and oil of evening primrose are two relatively 'natural' prescribed medications which can be of help for some people. The drug bromocriptine may also be useful in reducing symptoms.

For some women the regular cycle induced by the oral contraceptive pill can be helpful, presumably because it provides a regular level of (synthetic) oestrogen and progesterone.

Selective serotonin reuptake inhibitor (SSRI) antidepressants and the anxiolytic drug alprazolam (which augments GABA-A function) may also be useful in some women.

Agnus castus fruit extract is a herbal remedy which has good scientific evidence supporting the fact that it can be of help in up to 50% of people.

If the problem is very severe, some women are offered surgical treatment. The most invasive approach is to remove the womb and both ovaries and then treat with HRT. This drastic treatment approach reportedly has a 96% satisfaction rate.

> **Information Box 5.2c-III**
>
> **Premenstrual syndrome: comments from a Chinese medicine perspective**
>
> In Chinese medicine, premenstrual syndrome may result from Full or Empty patterns. The Full patterns are Liver Qi Stagnation and Phlegm Fire Harassing Upwards. The Empty patterns are Liver and/or Heart Blood Deficiency, Liver and Kidney Yin Deficiency, and Spleen and Kidney Yang Deficiency.

Dysmenorrhoea

Dysmenorrhoea is painful menstruation. This can be classified into two broad types, which may overlap. The first type, primary dysmenorrhoea, classically starts shortly after the menarche and peaks between the ages of 15 and 25 years. In primary dysmenorrhoea there are severe crampy pains, which begin after the onset of menstruation and usually last for less than 24 hours. They may be so severe as to lead to vomiting. Up to three-quarters of young women experience some form of primary dysmenorrhoea. The problem usually improves as the woman gets older, and may be markedly better after childbirth.

Secondary dysmenorrhoea, by definition, has an underlying physical cause. The most common causes are endometriosis or pelvic inflammatory disease. Fibroids may also be a cause of secondary dysmenorrhoea. Secondary dysmenorrhoea tends to begin a few days before the onset of menstruation and can continue through to late in the period. It tends to peak towards the end of the period. However, in practice, it may be difficult to distinguish primary from secondary dysmenorrhoea on the basis of symptoms alone.

Drug treatment of dysmenorrhoea involves two main approaches. Suppression of ovulation by means of an oral contraceptive may be preferred by many young women who also desire an effective contraceptive method. Alternatively, NSAIDs may be very effective in reducing the intensity of the pain. Commonly prescribed NSAIDs include mefanemic acid, and ibuprofen.

> **Information Box 5.2c-IV**
>
> **Dysmenorrhoea: comments from a Chinese medicine perspective**
>
> In Chinese medicine, dysmenorrhoea is the result of insufficient menstrual Blood or poor movement of the Blood. The patterns that give rise to dysmenorrhoea include: Qi and Blood Deficiency, Yang and Blood Deficiency, Kidney and Liver Yin Deficiency (Empty patterns); and Stagnation of Qi, Blood Stagnation, Stagnation of Cold, Damp Heat with Blood Heat, and Liver Qi Stagnation turning to Fire (Full patterns).

Problems during the menopause

The menopause is a natural physiological event, and like the menarche is a time of transition from one stage of life to another. Although it is a time in life when the body functions associated with fertility are ceasing to be active, a healthy climacteric should not be dominated by negative symptoms. Studies indicate that up to 25% of women have no symptoms during the menopause. However, 35% have mild to moderate symptoms and 40% suffer from severe symptoms.

Hot flushes (hot flashes)

Hot flushes are attributed to the response of the body to dropping levels of oestrogen. During the flush there is often a feeling of heat centred on the face, which can then spread to other parts of the body. The flush lasts for up to 3 minutes, and may be associated with a rise in temperature. At their worst, hot flushes may lead to sweating at night, with loss of sleep and tiredness in the day. Many other less specific symptoms, including aching joints, headaches, palpitations, dizziness, irritability and depression, may also be experienced.

Hot flushes can begin some years before the menopause, but peak 1–2 years before the periods stop. They may also persist for years after the menopause.

Vaginal dryness

Vaginal symptoms tend to occur later in the climacteric than hot flushes. The most usual complaint is of dryness or burning. Some women experience painful intercourse, which can have a considerable effect on intimate relationships.

The changes in the epithelium of the vagina also affect the urethra, and this can have the consequence of recurrent urinary tract infections. These changes, together with laxity of the muscles of the pelvic floor, can lead to urinary incontinence (usually stress incontinence).

Ischaemic heart disease and osteoporosis

These more long-term problems of the menopause are due to the reduction in the protective effect of oestrogen on the arteries and the bones.

Psychological effects of the menopause

Emotional symptoms, including anxiety and depression, are common during the climacteric. These are more prominent in women from westernised cultures, implying that there is a culture-based perceived threat of what will happen after the menopause. This may be a result of the emphasis in modern cultures on the importance of youthfulness and vitality, and the decreasing emphasis on the importance of the wisdom that comes with age and experience.

Studies suggest that sexual desire and drive are unchanged in most women after the menopause, but that in 20% of women they are reduced. However, this deterioration is more likely if a woman's satisfaction with her sex life was not so good prior to the menopause. In contrast, it is more likely that there is a marked change in sexual drive and sexual response of the male partner. This is the consequence of a decline in the levels of testosterone, which begins approximately after the age of 50 years.

Diagnosis of the menopause

As the menopause approaches, the ovary becomes less responsive to the pituitary hormones, and so produces less oestrogen. The pituitary response to this is to produce more FSH. As the woman approaches the menopause, the FSH levels rise to high levels, which are diagnostic of impending ovarian failure.

For this reason, many doctors will choose to test for FSH levels in order to confirm that symptoms such as hot flushes or mood swings are the result of failing ovaries. However, in most women the diagnosis is obvious from the age of the woman and the clinical picture alone. In these cases a blood test is unnecessary. It is now no longer considered good practice to encourage a woman who is approaching the menopause at the normal age range of 47–53 years to consider taking HRT.

Hormone replacement therapy

HRT used to be commonly prescribed to counteract the major menopausal symptoms, which include hot flushes and vaginal dryness, and to prevent the long-term complication of osteoporosis. These symptoms and complications result from the declining levels of oestrogen from the failing ovaries, and by providing oestrogen HRT counteracts this decline.

However, recent research into the effects of HRT in large groups of women exposed the fact that oestrogen replacement carries no cardiovascular benefits, and nor does it protect against dementia. Moreover, long-term HRT slightly increases the incidence of stroke, deep vein thrombosis and breast cancer. For this reason, HRT is no longer prescribed as a first-line treatment for the prevention of the development of postmenopausal osteoporosis. HRT may be considered as treatment for disabling hot flushes. Topical forms of HRT, in the form of oestrogen creams, are used to counteract the problems that may result from vaginal atrophy.

HRT consists of a synthetic or naturally derived form of oestrogen. As it is not healthy for the uterus to be exposed to oestrogen alone (as unopposed oestrogen can promote the development of endometrial cancer), most preparations also contain a synthetic progesterone-like compound known as a 'progestogen'. This additional progestogen is only necessary for those women who have an intact uterus. Those who have had a hysterectomy can be prescribed oestrogen-only HRT.

HRT comes in the form of tablets, skin patches or implants. In women with an intact uterus, the treatment is prescribed so that a 'period' is induced every 28 days. This bleed happens because the treatment consists of a regular daily dose of oestrogen, and a dose of progestogen to be taken on only 12 of the days of the 'cycle'. The 'period' is in fact a 'withdrawal bleed' which follows the start of the 16 days when the progestogen is not taken.

Before prescription of HRT the doctor needs to ensure that the woman is in good health. In particular, HRT is not advisable if there is any evidence of breast or endometrial cancer, liver disease or a history of recent thromboembolism. The blood pressure is checked, because in some women HRT may cause a rise in blood pressure.

Postmenopausal bleeding

An unexplained episode of bleeding (termed 'postmenstrual bleeding') is a red flag of cervical or endometrial cancer and needs to be referred for investigation. If the woman is on HRT, postmenstrual bleeding would be defined as any bleeding that occurred outside the time of the usual withdrawal bleed. The concern is that such a bleed might be a warning feature of cervical or endometrial cancer. These together are the cause of one-fifth of postmenopausal bleeds. Less worrying causes include cervical polyps (fleshy outgrowths) and inflammation of the vaginal lining. Intermenstrual bleeding in premenopausal women is much more likely to have a benign cause, but nevertheless must be referred for investigation if persistent or significant in volume.

The red flags of the menstrual disorders

Some patients with disorders of menstruation will benefit from referral to a conventional doctor for assessment and/or treatment. Red flags are those symptoms and signs that indicate that referral is to be considered. The red flags of menstrual disorders are described in Table 5.2c-I. This table forms part of the summary on red flags given in Appendix III, which also gives advice on the degree of urgency of referral for each of the red flag conditions listed.

Information Box 5.2c-V

The menopause and hormone replacement therapy (HRT): comments from a Chinese medicine perspective

In Chinese medicine, the menopause is the natural consequence of the decline in Jing which occurs in 7-year cycles in women. Hence the natural age of the menopause would be expected to be at 49 years. Studies of groups of women from diverse cultures all confirm that the median age of the menopause is 50–51 years old. The symptoms of the menopause are considered in general to be a consequence of the decline in the Jing, in its Yin and/or Yang aspect, although Kidney Deficiency may also be combined with excess patterns.

The patterns that are associated with menopausal symptoms include Kidney Yin Deficiency, Kidney Yang Deficiency, Kidney and Liver Yin Deficiency with Liver Yang Rising, Kidneys and Heart not harmonised, Accumulation of Phlegm and Stagnation of Qi, and Blood Stagnation.

HRT can benefit symptoms presumably because oestrogen is nourishing to the Spleen and to Yin (the Yin aspect of Essence), as evidenced by its beneficial effect on fleshiness and fertility. However, this effect may be suppressive, in that it may be at the expense of drawing on deep reserves of Spleen Qi, Kidney Yin and Jing. The progestogen in HRT is often blamed for the common side-effects, which include headaches, fluid retention and weight gain. This suggests that progestogens (together with oestrogens) tend to cause Accumulation of Damp and Qi Stagnation. This fits with the physiological effect they have of causing the lining of the womb to become thicker and more oedematous. It is only on withdrawal of the progestogen that breakdown of this thick lining occurs and bleeding takes place. There is also an increased risk of blood clots and breast and womb cancer with HRT, which suggest that HRT may induce Stagnation and/or Accumulation of Phlegm on a background of Kidney Deficiency.

Table 5.2c-I Red Flags 34 – menstruation

Red Flag	Description	Reasoning
34.1	**Primary amenorrhoea**: after age of 16 years	Refer any girl for investigation who has not achieved first menstruation by the age of 16 years
34.2	**Secondary amenorrhoea**: for more than 6 months	Refer if there have been no periods for 6 months
34.3	**Menorrhagia: with features of severe anaemia** (tiredness, breathlessness, palpitations on exertion)	Menorrhagia (heavy periods) can be the sole cause of significant anaemia, and merits prompt referral for investigation and treatment of the cause
34.4	**Metrorrhagia**: bleeding between periods that has no regular pattern. This includes postcoital bleeding (bleeding after intercourse)	Irregular periods are common, but bleeding that seems to fall outside the normal confines of a 2–5 day menstrual bleed might rarely signify a uterine or cervical tumour. Refer for further investigation if this happens on more than three occasions
34.5	**Postmenopausal bleeding**: any unexplained bleeding after the menopause	Predictable bleeding after the menopause is normal with HRT preparations. Otherwise it is a red flag for a uterine or cervical tumour. Refer after a single episode for further investigation
34.6	**Vaginal discharge**: after menopause	Vaginal discharge is not normal after the menopause, particularly if offensive or blood stained. Refer to exclude infection or carcinoma
34.7	**Vaginal discharge**: before puberty	Vaginal discharge is not normal before puberty, particularly if offensive or blood stained. Consider the possibility of abuse. Always refer for further investigation/treatment of infection
34.8	**Vaginal itch (if prolonged)**	Vaginal itch is a common side-effect of thrush (candidiasis) and sensitivity to soaps and bath products, so refer only if prolonged for more than 1 week and not responding to advice and treatment. Consider the possibility of atrophic vaginitis is postmenopausal women. This can respond to hormone creams. Also, rarely, itch can develop in lichen sclerosus and vulval cancer. Consider the possibility of abuse in children. Refer for investigation

Self-test 5.2c

Disorders of menstruation and the menopause

1. Hilary is a 21-year-old student. She is coming for treatment because her periods have stopped for 8 months now. She feels very well otherwise. What are the most likely causes of her amenorrhoea? What questions might you ask her to clarify the possible cause?
2. Claire is 35 years old and has been coming to see you for treatment of infertility. Over the past 5 months her energy levels have improved, although she has not conceived. Over the last few menstrual cycles she has noticed that her period has become longer. She thinks it is because it is starting earlier than it should, because it is light for a few days and then becomes heavy on the day she would have expected it. One week ago she started bleeding at what she would have expected to be mid-cycle and now is still bleeding, although not much. She is very anxious that this means there is something seriously wrong. What is the most likely cause of Claire's change in bleeding pattern? How might you manage this situation?

Answers

1. Hilary has secondary amenorrhoea. Although this has persisted for 8 months, it is always important to consider the possibility of pregnancy (she may have conceived sometime during the last 8 months). However, with this long history, a functional cause is more likely. In young women, prolonged stress can cause amenorrhoea. If Hilary is exercising to excess or undereating, these may also be contributory factors. She feels well, so a chronic illness (including hyperthyroidism) is a less likely cause. Primary ovarian failure and polycystic ovarian syndrome (PCOS) are more rare possibilities. You should refer Hilary for exclusion of these diagnoses.

   To prepare for the referral you could question her about the possibility of pregnancy, including contraceptive use if she has been sexually active during the past year or so. You might ask questions about ongoing stressors and any change in living circumstances. You need to question about exercise, diet and body image. Questions to exclude hyperthyroidism would focus around heat intolerance, changes in appetite, and weight and anxiety levels.

   In PCOS there might be a recent history of weight gain and increased body hair.
2. Claire's recent change in bleeding pattern would very likely be diagnosed as menorrhagia due to dysfunctional uterine bleeding (DUB). This is not metrorrhagia, because the period itself appears to be regular, and the change is that bleeding is occurring too early in the second half of the cycle. This pattern of bleeding is associated with ovulation, but the bleeding indicates a defect in corpus luteum development. This may well affect fertility, in that implantation is affected.

   Nevertheless, Claire is feeling better in herself, which implies that this change in bleeding does not necessarily indicate a more imbalanced state. It may be that your treatment has promoted ovulation, but that there is more imbalance to be dealt with before fertility can be achieved.

   You might wish to reassure Claire that her current pattern of bleeding does not indicate a physical problem, and may even be an indication of an improvement. If she remains very anxious, you could recommend that she go to have further investigations, but otherwise you might continue to treat for at least 3 months to see if this pattern settles down. If there is no change after this time, you should refer her to exclude physical causes such as fibroids, pelvic inflammatory disease and hypothyroidism.

Chapter 5.2d Sexual health and sexually transmitted disease

LEARNING POINTS

At the end of this chapter you will:
- understand the physical and psychological causes of the common sexual dysfunctions
- be able to describe the clinical features and treatments of the common sexually transmitted diseases
- be able to recognise the red flags of the sexually transmitted diseases.

Estimated time for chapter: 90 minutes.

Sexual health

The term 'sexual health' is used conventionally to embrace both the physical and psychological aspects of sexuality. For there to be good sexual health, sexual relationships should be physically and emotionally satisfying for both partners, and also they should carry no risk of unwanted pregnancy or transmission of disease.

Sexual dysfunctions

It is increasingly recognised that sexual satisfaction does not necessarily depend on both partners experiencing all the stages of the sexual experience as described in Chapter 5.2a. However, lack of satisfaction with sexual experience is very common. Often the problem lies in a combination of unrealistic expectations of what should happen, and a lack of communication between the partners. For example, it may be expected that the women should always achieve orgasm during penile intercourse, when in fact this is only possible for 25% of women. Other factors that can affect sexual satisfaction include low sex drive, performance anxiety, chronic illness, alcohol or drug abuse, and prescribed medication.

There are a number of specific sexual dysfunctions that may be the result of one or more of these factors. A sex therapist is a psychiatric practitioner who is skilled in the diagnosis of these dysfunctions, and who can offer treatments, which range from simple education and couple counselling to prescription of medication. However, because of embarrassment, most of these dysfunctions are not discussed with health professionals, and so many people do not have access to the support that might benefit them.

Low sex drive (lack of libido) and impotence

Sexual drive varies markedly between individuals. A low sex drive is not necessarily a sign of a dysfunction. Sex drive normally declines with age, and particularly so for men over the age of 50 years. In general, low libido is believed to affect women more than men. One estimate suggests that up to 10% of women never have sexual fantasies or desire for sexual activity.

Sex drive is influenced by psychological factors. A reduced sex drive can be a manifestation of a deteriorating relationship or depression. Traumatic sexual experiences in the past can have a great impact on sex drive.

Impotence is the inability to achieve orgasm, and often includes the inability to maintain an erection in men (erectile dysfunction). Lack of libido and impotence may go together, but not always. Isolated impotence is more likely to have an underlying physical cause.

An important physical cause of low sexual drive and impotence is chronic illness, particularly if the illness affects a part of the body that is associated with sexuality, such as the prostate, breast or the cervix. Certain chronic diseases, such as diabetes and peripheral vascular disease, can lead to impotence because they result in impairment of blood and nervous supply to the genital regions. Endocrine disease such as Addison's disease or hypothyroidism may directly affect libido by affecting the secretion of pituitary hormones. 'Recreational' drugs, including alcohol and heroin, are well known to reduce libido and lead to erectile dysfunction. It may be possible to link a recent onset of loss of sex drive with a prescription of medication. Drugs that are well known to cause low sex drive and/or impotence include diuretics, beta blockers, and the newer forms of antidepressants.

For men who have impotence, medical or physical methods may be recommended to aid maintenance of erection. A drug from the phosphodiesterase-5 inhibitor family, such as sildafenil citrate or tadalafil, may be prescribed. A single dose can be taken by mouth about 1 hour before intercourse to increase penile blood flow. Both these treatments carry the risk of inducing a painful sustained erection, which may require emergency treatment, and these treatments are not advisable in those who have coronary heart disease or who are taking nitrate medication. The phosphodiesterase inhibitor drugs are not generally available free of charge to patients under the UK NHS, but are prescribable to those with a diagnosable physical cause, including diabetes mellitus, multiple sclerosis, Parkinson's disease, prostate cancer, spinal cord injury, and those dependent on dialysis for renal failure.

A simple physical approach to erectile dysfunction is a plastic pump device which encourages erection by means of suction to a chamber held around the penis, and the erection is maintained by means of a ring applied the base of the penis. However, neither of these methods will directly improve an underlying lack of libido.

Premature ejaculation

In premature ejaculation, the man fails to sustain an erection because ejaculation occurs either before or just after penetration. This problem usually has an emotional cause, often rooted in performance anxiety, and can respond very well to sex therapy.

Dyspareunia

Dyspareunia refers to painful intercourse. It is a common condition in women, and can lead to a complete loss of sexual activity. Dyspareunia may have physical causes. Inflammation of the womb or ovaries in conditions such as pelvic inflammatory disease or endometriosis will result in pain during deep penile penetration (i.e. during thrusting). This problem, termed 'deep dyspareunia', is highly suggestive of an underlying physical problem. However, problems in the vagina, such as postmenopausal dryness and vaginal infections, can cause pain very early in penetration. This problem is termed 'superficial dyspareunia'.

Superficial dyspareunia can also result from lack of lubrication and insufficient relaxation of the perineal muscles at the time of attempted penetration. This may be because penetration has been attempted before the woman is aroused. The pain that results can cause a negative cycle of loss of sexual desire and increased tension.

'Vaginismus' is the term given to a severe form of spasm that affects the perineal muscles at the time of penetration. Vaginismus will prevent penetration totally. Factors such as lack of sexual knowledge, guilt about sexuality and a childhood sexual assault may be underlying issues in a woman who suffers from these functional causes of superficial dyspareunia.

In dyspareunia, any underlying physical cause should be treated first. Sex therapy can be effective in non-physically (functional) based dyspareunia.

Information Box 5.2d-I

Impotence: comments from a Chinese medicine perspective

In Chinese medicine, impotence is usually attributed to Kidney Deficiency. Lack of sexual drive indicates a deficiency of the Fire of the Gate of Life (Mingmen). Non-physical dyspareunia has features that suggest Stagnation of Liver Qi and Blood.

Sexually transmitted disease

'Sexually transmitted disease' (STD) is the term given to infections acquired through sexual intercourse. Increasingly, the term 'genitourinary (GU) infection' is used in preference to STD, because the term STD may be stigmatising and not all sexually transmitted diseases are acquired solely by sexual intercourse.

Since the emergence of HIV infection in the 1980s, there has been increasing emphasis on the prevention of STDs by means of safe sex practices. The first message of safe sex is that it is always possible that one or both partners may be carrying infections which can be transmitted during intercourse. Therefore, unless it is within the context of a long-term relationship, it is important always to take precautions if planning to have intercourse. Ideally, promiscuity should be minimised. Condoms are considered to be the best barrier method for protecting both men and women who practise penile, oral and anal sex. The cap, spermicidal creams and the oral contraceptive pill also carry a degree of protection, but should not be relied on solely as effective barriers to disease.

In the UK, the Department of Health coordinates the promotion of the messages of safe sex. These messages are propagated to the general public via family planning clinics, GU clinics, abortion advice centres, general medical practices, schools and the media.

The infections discussed in this section are:

- Vulvovaginal and penile infections:
  - genital herpes
  - genital warts
  - syphilis
  - infections that cause vaginal discharge.
- Infections of the internal genital organs:
  - gonorrhoea
  - *Chlamydia*
  - pelvic inflammatory disease (PID).
- General infections due to sexual transfer of body fluids.

Vulvovaginal and penile infections

Genital herpes

Genital herpes is caused by transmission of the herpes simplex virus (HSV). This is the same type of virus that causes cold sores. However, in most genital cases, the actual strain of HSV is different from the one that most commonly causes cold sores.

The first (primary) attack of genital herpes is usually the worst. In this primary infection, a crop of itchy and painful sores develop on the vulva and the vagina or the head (glans) of the penis. The patient is unwell, with a fever, and there may be tender enlarged lymph glands in the groin. Urination may be difficult.

The infection heals over the next 7 days with crusting of the spots. 30% of people experience recurrence of the attack (secondary herpes), as the virus is never fully cleared from the body. The attack is usually limited to a smaller area of the genital organs and is often progressively less painful in each recurrence. Only 2–5% of people who have had genital herpes have more than one recurrent attack. Recurrence is more common in the second half of the menstrual cycle, during periods of stress and in hot weather.

The person is only infectious during an attack and its recovery phase. Recurrent herpes is a very serious condition during pregnancy, as it can severely infect a baby during delivery. If a woman goes into labour with active herpes, a caesarean section is advised. In severe cases, antiviral drugs (including aciclovir) may be prescribed on a long-term basis to prevent attacks. However, in most cases these are not prescribed, and the recurrence subsides naturally within a few days.

> **Information Box 5.2d-II**
>
> **Genital herpes: comments from a Chinese medicine perspective**
>
> In Chinese medicine, the symptoms of genital herpes correspond to Wind Damp Heat. It primarily affects the Liver Channel.

Genital warts

Genital warts are the result of infection by certain strains of the human papilloma virus (HPV). The genital wart strains are different from those strains of HPV that cause bodily warts (which occur most commonly on the hands and knees). The virus causes a benign growth of epithelial tissue, which develops into cauliflower-shaped bumps on the vulva, vagina, cervix and penis, and also around the anus. The genital wart, like the bodily wart, is painless, and, especially in women, may not be noticed by the patient. Sometimes the patient complains of itching or burning from the area where warts have developed.

HPV infection is very common; up to 30% of sexually active adults have evidence of current or past infection. The infection is important because particular strains of HPV (subtypes 16, 18 and 33) are known to induce pre-cancerous changes in cervical cells. For this reason, a woman with warts might be offered annual cervical smear tests, so that any pre-cancerous changes can be followed up.

Warts can be treated by repeated weekly application of the drug podophyllin, which 'burns' the wart away. The patient can apply a weaker form of this drug on a daily basis in between clinic visits to maximise the chances of cure. Imiquinod cream is an alternative topical preparation which may be prescribed for self-treatment. Larger warts can be burned by means of a laser or heat probe, or frozen by means of a liquid nitrogen spray. Recurrence of the warts is common after both these treatments.

> **Information Box 5.2d-III**
>
> **Genital warts: comments from a Chinese medicine perspective**
>
> In Chinese medicine, the genital wart is viewed as a manifestation of Damp and Phlegm.

Syphilis

Syphilis is caused by infection with the bacterium *Treponema pallidum*. Probably because of access to adequate antibiotic therapy, it is now a relatively rare condition in the UK. However, it is still common in developing countries and, worryingly, its incidence is rising sharply in the developed world.

Infection with syphilis occurs in three stages. The primary stage is called a 'chancre', a thickened lump that forms in the genital area within 2–12 weeks of sexual contact with an infected person. The skin on top of the chancre breaks down, but is often painless. It is this stage that is highly infectious, but like genital warts it is often unnoticed by the patient.

After healing of the chancre there may be a delay of some weeks before the appearance of secondary syphilis. In most people there is a flu-like illness, with swollen lymph nodes, a characteristic skin rash, and the development of warty genital lumps. In some cases there might be more severe inflammation of a deep organ, such as hepatitis or meningitis.

Secondary syphilis will abate after 3–12 weeks if untreated, but can recur, due to persistence of the organism, in a more severe form as tertiary syphilis. In this stage the infection can cause large ulcerating lumps, called 'gummas', in a wide range of tissues. The heart and blood vessels can be affected, and a form of dementia (neurosyphilis) may develop. The condition termed 'general paralysis of the insane', familiar in Victorian asylums, was a result of the combined features of untreated syphilis.

These later stages of syphilis are now very rare in developed countries because the earlier stages respond well to treatment with a 1-month course of penicillin or doxycycline.

> **Information Box 5.2d-IV**
>
> **Syphilis: comments from a Chinese medicine perspective**
>
> In Chinese medicine, the formation of warty lumps in all three stages of syphilis suggests that Damp/Phlegm is a prominent feature. The recurrence of the condition in a flu-like secondary form suggests that Latent Heat is present from the primary infection.

Vaginal discharge

Vaginal discharge is a common complaint, but may be physiological rather than the result of an infection. Physiological discharge is odourless, does not cause itch and varies in quantity throughout the cycle. Nevertheless, it may be profuse and a source of embarrassment or discomfort. Benign changes of the cervix, called 'cervical erosions', and fleshy cervical polyps may be physical causes of excessive physiological discharge. Both these problems can be treated fairly simply in an outpatient procedure that involves a colposcopy.

A serious cause of vaginal discharge is vaginal, cervical or uterine cancer. In these cases the discharge is more likely to be of recent onset, varying in a way that is not related to the menstrual cycle, and may be smelly or blood stained. A discharge fitting this description should always be taken seriously, but particularly so in postmenopausal women, in whom these cancers are more common.

Candida (yeast) infection (thrush)

Thrush is the most common infectious cause of vaginal discharge. As yeasts form about 5% of the 'healthy' organisms in the vagina, a candidal 'infection' usually represents an overgrowth of these yeasts rather than a new infection. Candidal infection in women usually arises internally, but can also be sexually transmitted. In contrast, sexual transmission is a common cause of genital candidal infection in men.

Thrush develops very readily in some people, who may suffer from recurrent bouts. In susceptible people, a bout may be triggered by sexual intercourse, tight clothing, overwashing, use of a different soap or a course of antibiotics. However, serious underlying causes, including immunodeficiency and diabetes mellitus, must be excluded in people who suffer from recurrent thrush.

One complementary medical theory is that recurrent thrush is associated with the *Candida* syndrome, in which overgrowth of *Candida* is believed to be the result of excess yeasts and sugars in the diet, and to cause a wide range of physical and emotional symptoms. The *Candida* syndrome is not recognised as a medical entity by conventional medical practitioners.

Genital thrush causes itchy plaques of white discharge which may overlie red inflamed areas of epithelium. The itch can be intensely irritating, particularly in women, and may cause difficulty in urination.

Conventional treatment of thrush is with antifungal medication. In a mild case, application of a cream containing clotrimazole may be sufficient to alleviate the symptoms. In more severe cases, this drug can be administered by means of a course of vaginal tablets (pessaries). Recurrent thrush may be treated with oral antifungal medication. Fluconazole is the most commonly prescribed preparation. Some women rely on recurrent treatments with these antifungal medications to keep their symptoms at bay.

Gardnerella infection (bacterial vaginosis)

Gardnerella infection is another example of an overgrowth of 'healthy' organisms. *Gardnerella vaginalis* is a bacterium that comprises up to 30% of the normal population of bacteria in a healthy vagina. In overgrowth, this bacterium causes the discharge to become more watery, and to have a characteristic fishy smell. This condition has been termed 'bacterial vaginosis' (BV). There is usually no discomfort in BV. It is recognised that pregnant women with BV are more likely to go into premature labour, and this has led to debate about whether women with BV should be treated early in labour with antibiotics.

Treatment of BV is with a single high dose of the antibiotic metronidazole (Flagyl) and with a 5-day course of lower dose in pregnancy.

Trichomonas infection

Trichomonas vaginalis is a bacterium that comprises up to 7% of the healthy bacterial population in the vagina. *Trichomonas* 'infection' is another form of bacterial overgrowth that may also be sexually transmitted. It causes a moderate to profuse discharge, which can cause intense itching in the women. If severe, the discharge can have a green and frothy appearance.

Treatment of *Trichomonas* involves a 1-week course of metronidazole. The male partner may be advised also to take this antibiotic to prevent reinfection of his partner.

Information Box 5.2d-V

Vaginal discharge: comments from a Chinese medicine perspective

In Chinese medicine, vaginal discharge (leucorrhoea) represents Damp in the Lower Jiao. Itching, redness, and a coloured or smelly discharge all suggest Damp Heat, whereas white, watery discharges are more suggestive of Damp Cold. An underlying deficiency of Spleen Qi is possible.

Infections of the internal genital organs

Gonorrhoea

Gonorrhoea is caused by infection with the bacterium *Neisseria gonorrhoeae* (gonococcus). In women, the infection initially presents with urinary symptoms and a vaginal discharge. There is a risk of transmitting the infection to the baby during labour, in which case a severe form of conjunctivitis can result.

In men, there may also be urinary symptoms, and a slight pus-like discharge from the urethra. This condition is called 'urethritis'. Urethritis may be caused by a number of organisms in addition to the gonococcus.

In many of these initial infections, particularly in women, symptoms may be so mild that they are ignored. This means that there is high risk of transmission of the infection at this stage. The real problems of gonorrhoea come if the infection spreads. In women, the next site of infection is the cervical canal, and thence the lining of the uterus. This can lead to the chronic condition known as 'pelvic inflammatory disease'. In men the gonococcus can spread to cause a chronic infection of the prostate, epididymis and the testes. Occasionally, the infection can enter the bloodstream. A feverish illness develops, characterised by painful joints and a widespread rash. This form of gonorrhoea is more common in women.

Gonorrhoea is treated by means of antibiotics. A single dose of cefixime or ciprofloxacin is all that may be necessary in uncomplicated cases, but long courses of these antibiotics may be required to treat chronic infections. Gonorrhoea often coexists with *Chlamydia* infection, so often the patient is treated with antibiotics to cover for this infection also. Ideally, all sexual contacts should be traced and treated.

Information Box 5.2d-VI

Gonorrhoea: comments from a Chinese medicine perspective

In Chinese medicine, the symptoms of gonorrhoea would appear to correspond with Damp Heat in the Lower Jiao. In severe cases, gonorrhoea can manifest as Wind Heat on the exterior (rashes and fever) and Wind Damp (arthritis).

Chlamydia

Chlamydia trachomatis is an infection that commonly coexists with gonorrhoea. It is a very common cause of urethritis (also known as 'non-gonococcal urethritis' (NGU)). Like gonorrhoea, *Chlamydia* can ascend in the male urethra to cause prostatitis and epididymitis. In women, the infection can be a cause of discharge, but more importantly may spread via the cervical canal to be a cause of pelvic inflammatory disease. If the baby develops the infection during passage through the birth canal, conjunctivitis and pneumonia can result.

Chlamydia infections are treated with a different class of antibiotics to gonorrhoea. Azithromycin or doxycycline are most commonly prescribed to be taken by mouth between a single day and 2 weeks. Ideally, sexual contacts should be traced and treated.

Information Box 5.2d-VII

Chlamydia: comments from a Chinese medicine perspective

In Chinese medicine, *Chlamydia* infection, like gonorrhoea, would normally be a manifestation of Damp Heat in the Lower Jiao.

Pelvic inflammatory disease

'Pelvic inflammatory disease' (PID) is the term given to the syndrome that arises as a result of chronic infection of the uterus, fallopian tubes and ovaries (the female internal genital organs). It is believed that over half of these infections are caused by *Chlamydia* and a smaller proportion by the gonococcus. However, there are a number of less common organisms that may also cause PID. Commonly PID develops without any preceding symptoms.

The risk of PID is reduced by use of barrier methods of contraception and the contraceptive pill, but the risk is increased in users of the intrauterine device (the 'coil').

The most common symptoms of an acute infection include severe abdominal tenderness and pain (with deep dyspareunia), and high fever. In an advanced infection, pus may collect in a fallopian tube, leading to a severe illness akin to appendicitis. Infection may also spread to the space surround the ovaries.

In its more chronic form, PID may lead to a long-standing feeling of being unwell, and pelvic discomfort, particularly during intercourse. There may be menorrhagia or secondary dysmenorrhoea. Internally, the genital organs may become stuck together (with 'adhesions') and scarred.

A serious consequence of acute and chronic PID is infertility, as the scarring and adhesions may prevent ovulation or implantation of the fertilised ovum. Another important complication of infection is that there is an increased incidence of ectopic pregnancy in women who have had PID.

These long-term effects of untreated PID are becoming more common, as unprotected sex, particularly amongst teenagers, is increasingly prevalent.

PID is treated with combined antibiotics such as doxycycline and metronidazole, which may be given intravenously in severe acute infections. Surgery may be necessary in cases in which pus has accumulated. However, as many cases are chronic, the diagnosis may not be made until permanent damage to the internal genital organs has occurred.

Information Box 5.2d-VIII

Pelvic inflammatory disease: comments from a Chinese medicine perspective

In Chinese medicine, pelvic inflammatory disease might correspond to one or more of Damp, Heat or Qi, and Blood Stagnation in the Uterus.

General infections due to sexual transfer of bodily fluids

Although their symptoms do not affect the reproductive system, the sexually transmitted infections HIV and hepatitis B and C are most commonly transmitted through the exchange of bodily fluids during sexual intercourse. These infections are prevented by attention to safe sex practice.

The red flags of the sexually transmitted diseases

Most patients with an STD will benefit from referral to a conventional doctor for assessment and/or treatment. Red flags are those symptoms and signs that indicate that referral is to be considered. The red flags of STDs are described in the Table 5.2d-I. This table forms part of the summary on red flags given in Appendix III, which also gives advice on the degree of urgency of referral for each of the red flag conditions listed.

Table 5.2d-I Red Flags 35 – sexually transmitted disease

Red Flag	Description	Reasoning
35.1	**Vaginal discharge**: if irregular, blood stained or unusual smell	A slight, creamy vaginal discharge is usual, and tends to increase and become more elastic around the time of ovulation. An increase in this sort of discharge is normal during pregnancy If an irregular pattern of blood staining, volume, itchiness or smell develops, investigation is merited to exclude sexually transmitted disease (STD). This is of particular importance in pregnancy, as some STDs can threaten the health of the fetus If an STD is suspected, advise the patient to visit the local genitourinary department (STD clinic) for confidential advice and treatment as first port of call (rather than their GP) Thrush (candidiasis) does not necessarily merit referral, as it can subside by means of conservative measures and is not usually considered to be contagious. If recurrent and troublesome, consider referral to investigate possible underlying causes such as diabetes or immune deficiency
35.2	**Vaginal discharge**: after menopause	Vaginal discharge is not normal after the menopause, particularly if offensive or blood stained. Refer to exclude infection or carcinoma
35.3	**Vaginal discharge**: before puberty	Vaginal discharge is not normal before puberty, particularly if offensive or blood stained. Consider the possibility of abuse. Always refer for further investigation/treatment of infection
35.4	**Discharge from penis**	Always refer, as this may indicate an STD. If an STD is suspected, advise the patient to visit the local genitourinary department as a first port of call (rather than their GP)
35.5	**Sores, warty lumps or ulcers** on vagina or penis	These are very likely to indicate an STD, and rarely may be cancer. Refer to the local genitourinary department or GP for investigation
35.6	**Pelvic inflammatory disease (PID) (chronic form)**: vaginal discharge, gripy abdominal pain, pain on intercourse, dysmenorrhoea, infertility	Chronic PID poses a threat to fertility and may suggest an STD. If an STD is suspected, advise the patient to visit the local genitourinary department as the first port of call (rather than their GP)
35.7	**Pelvic inflammatory disease (PID) (acute form)**: low abdominal pain with collapse, fever	Acute PID poses a serious risk to fertility. Refer urgently for antibiotic treatment
35.8	**Outbreak of genital herpes** in last trimester of pregnancy	Refer, as there is a risk of transmission of the herpes virus to the baby during delivery
35.9	**Offensive, fishy, watery discharge** (possible bacterial vaginosis) in pregnancy	Refer for treatment as bacterial vaginosis leads to an increased risk of early labour and miscarriage

Self-test 5.2d

Sexual health and sexually transmitted disease

1. One of your patients has been troubled by a vaginal discharge for the past 3 months, which she describes as itchy, whitish and occasionally odd smelling. There is not much relationship with the menstrual cycle, although she thinks it may be slightly worse premenstrually. She is a 45-year-old teacher in a stable marital relationship.
   (i) What are the possible causes of such a discharge?
   (ii) What are the most likely causes in this woman?
   (iii) Would you refer this woman for further investigation?

Answers

1. (i) The possible causes of any vaginal discharge include:
   - physiological discharge
   - cervical erosions and polyps (excessive physiological discharge)
   - cancer
   - infections (sexually transmitted disease (STD) and overgrowth).

   (ii) The first two causes are unlikely in this woman because the discharge is itchy and has an odd smell. Remaining possibilities are, therefore, cancer of the internal genital organs, and infections including *Candida* (thrush), *Gardnerella* (bacterial vaginosis), *Trichomonas* and gonorrhoea. Although the history suggests that an STD is unlikely, there is a possibility that an unfaithful husband has passed on the infection to her. The description fits the most common of these possibilities (i.e. thrush).

   (iii) You may consider referral within 1–2 months so that this diagnosis can be confirmed. Referral does not mean the patient necessarily has to take medication, but will allow for examination to exclude more sinister possibilities, which are increasingly more common in women of this age and older.

Chapter 5.2e Contraception

LEARNING POINTS

At the end of this chapter you will:
- understand the rationale for the provision of contraception services in the UK
- be able to describe the different contraceptive methods that are currently available
- be able to recognise the strengths and limitations of the different contraceptive methods.

Estimated time for chapter: 90 minutes.

Introduction

Contraception is conventionally considered to have important health benefits. The first is the reduction in the risk of unwanted pregnancies and their unfortunate consequences, induced abortions. An indirect benefit of this is what has been euphemistically termed 'family planning'. This is the concept that, when pregnancies occur, they do so at the time when the woman and her partner are both physiologically and psychologically prepared for them. Moreover, if pregnancy can be delayed until after a woman has reached the age of at least 20 years, that pregnancy is likely to be healthier. It is also recognised that if subsequent pregnancies can be spaced by 2 years or more, the mother has a chance to regain a level of strength which will help both her and her family cope with them. The other major health benefit of certain forms of contraception is that they can be used to prevent the transmission of STDs.

However, it can be argued that it is the advent of readily available contraception that has encouraged the rise in sexual activity that has taken place since the 1960s, particularly in young people. This rise in sexual activity has been accompanied by a rise in unwanted pregnancies and STDs. Nevertheless, there is no doubt that if contraception is used appropriately, these problems can be avoided.

Contraceptive services are provided in the UK under the NHS, and are available from family planning clinics and general practices. Currently, all contraceptives, including condoms, are available free of charge to NHS patients. Nevertheless, many people choose to buy their condoms rather than attend clinics to get them free of charge.

The free provision of contraception services in the UK are a reflection of the fact that, since the early part of this century, family planning has been seen as an important mechanism to promote the control of the size of families and the prevention of unwanted pregnancies. In addition, the use of contraceptives has been increasingly promoted to encourage safe sex practices. Nevertheless, the UK has a high rate of teenage pregnancy and abortion compared with some other European countries (notably The Netherlands).

Failure rates

Failure rates are a means of expressing the effectiveness of a contraceptive method. No contraceptive method is perfect in preventing pregnancy. Usually the decision about which contraceptive to use is based on a process of weighing up the convenience of the method to the individual (or the couple) against its risk of failure.

Contraceptive failure rates can be expressed in terms of the number of pregnancies that occur in 100 women using the method for 1 year (pregnancies per 100 woman-years). If no contraceptive protection is used, the pregnancy rate is 85 per 100 woman-years (i.e. 85% of sexually active women will fall pregnant within 1 year of stopping contraception), and failure rates of contraception can be compared to this figure.

Failure rates vary dramatically according to the commitment of the user of the method. For example, natural family planning is generally not widely recommended in the NHS because of a measured high failure rate (20–25 pregnancies per 100 woman-years), but if used correctly it can be an effective and empowering method of contraception. The measured failure rates come from studies involving a broad range of users. In general, most contraceptive methods, if used correctly, are more effective than the failure rates suggest.

Failure rates are all much lower in women who are approaching the menopause, as natural fertility is declining at this time. This means that certain contraceptives (e.g. the diaphragm) may be acceptable safe methods for older women, but less reliable in women under the age of 30–35 years.

Methods of contraception

Contraceptive methods are usually grouped into the following categories (see Q5.2e-1):

- barrier methods
- intrauterine devices
- hormonal methods
- surgical methods
- natural methods.

Barrier methods

Barrier methods do not prevent the production of the spermatozoa (sperm) or the ovum, but act as a barrier to prevent their meeting. The most commonly used barriers are the condom in men and the cap/diaphragm in women.

The condom (sheath)

The condom is a latex sheath that has to be rolled onto the erect penis, ideally before any genital contact has taken place. The additional use of spermicidal cream is strongly recommended to increase effectiveness.

Failure rate: 12 per 100 woman-years.

Advantages: Simple, cheap and relatively non-invasive. Prevents fertilisation. Prevents STDs. The failure rate can be further reduced by concurrent use of spermicidal gel.

Disadvantages: Cannot be used until the arousal stage in sex, and so may be put on too late. There is a risk of the condom splitting if it is not put on correctly. Allergy to creams or latex is increasingly common. Many young people find condoms off-putting, and so do not use them.

The diaphragm and cap

These are flexible discs or cones of latex that can be inserted into the vagina up to a few hours before intercourse to cover the opening to the cervical canal. The 'cap' should then be left in place for at least 6 hours. It is only effective if used together with a spermicidal cream. The cap needs to be the correct size, and so a clinic appointment is required for a 'fitting'. This fitting should be repeated annually, and also after pregnancy.

Failure rate: 30 per 100 woman-years.

Advantages: Simple and relatively non-invasive. Prevents fertilisation. Prevents STDs. Can be inserted before sexual intercourse has started. Is usually not seen or felt by either partner. Can be cleaned easily and used again and again.

Disadvantages: A high failure rate in young women. Difficult or impossible to use for some women. Can cause thrush and cystitis in susceptible people. Allergy to creams or latex is increasingly common.

Intrauterine devices (IUDs or IUCDs) or the 'coil'

It has been known for centuries that a 'foreign body' in the uterus prevents implantation of a fertilised egg. IUDs are delicate copper-containing nylon devices which are inserted via the cervix in an outpatient clinic, and can remain in place for up to 5 years. The insertion can be uncomfortable, but does not require an anaesthetic. IUDs have nylon strings, which are left to protrude through the cervix for ease of removal. The intrauterine part of the device has fine copper wire wound around its stem.

There is an ethical issue with IUDs in that they do not prevent fertilisation. Instead they prevent implantation of the fertilised ovum. From the viewpoint of a number of world religions, this is akin to abortion, and is therefore not an acceptable contraceptive method for some people.

Failure rate: 0.22 per 100 woman-years.

Advantages: If no side-effects occur, the IUD can be completely forgotten, and remains effective for 5 years.

Disadvantages: Painful insertion. There is a risk of introduction of infection (with a risk of PID), and so it is not generally recommended in women who have not had children. Can cause heavy periods and cramping pain. Increased risk of ectopic pregnancy.

Hormonal methods

The hormonal methods use synthetic oestrogen and/or progestogens to influence fertility, either by preventing ovulation or by causing changes to the endometrium that prevent implantation.

Injectable and implantable progestogen

Both these approaches involve the administration to the woman of 'slow-release' synthetic progestogen (similar in function to natural progesterone). The progestogen is given either by injection (lasting 1–3 months) or by means of a subcutaneous implant (lasting up to 3 years). The implant is inserted under the skin by means of a minor operation, which can be performed by a GP. The high dose of progestogen that is released prevents ovulation (via inhibition of the pituitary release of LH and FSH), in the same way that progesterone released by the placenta inhibits ovulation during pregnancy.

Failure rate: 0.3 per 100 woman-years.

Advantages: A very reliable method. Prevents ovulation, and therefore no fertilisation should occur. There is no risk of forgetting to use it, or of errors in using it. Progestogens are not considered to have the serious adverse effects on health that oestrogens have.

Disadvantages: High doses of progestogens can lead to mood changes and weight gain. Acne is a less common side-effect. Usually the periods stop entirely, but some women suffer irregular and heavy bleeding. This is a particular problem in the first few months after the insertion of an implant. Once the injection has been given it cannot be reversed, and so any side-effects have to be borne for up to 3 months. If side-effects occur with implants, the implant can be removed by means of a minor operation. A major problem with the injectable progestogen is delayed return of fertility after stopping the contraceptive methods, and so it should not be used in women who are planning a family in the near future. Long-term use may be associated with a reduction in bone density (osteoporosis).

Intrauterine progesterone-only system

The intrauterine porgesterone-only system (IUS) is a form of intrauterine device designed to release a steady amount of progestogen into the uterine cavity. The IUS has the advantage over the coil in that it can be used in women who tend to suffer from heavy menstrual bleeding. In those women who tolerate this method, periods may become very light or even absent. The risk of ectopic pregnancy is lower with the IUS than with the simple IUCD.

Progestogen-only pill (POP) or mini-pill

The mini-pill contains a low dose of progestogen, and is taken daily at a fixed time of day. Low-dose progestogen inhibits the implantation of a fertilised ovum by altering the quality of the mucus in the cervix and the womb lining. It may also prevent ovulation. The dose is not sufficient to prevent ovulation reliably in most women.

Failure rate: 3 per 100 woman-years.

Advantages: Low dose, so fewer side-effects than the injection. Carries none of the serious risks of the combined pill. Can be used by breastfeeding mothers. Can reduce the discomfort of painful, irregular or heavy periods.

Disadvantages: Requires a regulated lifestyle, as the pill must be taken within the same 2-hour period every day to remain effective (with the exception of desogestrel, which can be taken within a 12-hour time window). Can have unpredictable effects on the periods: some women have no periods at all, some fall into a 28-day cycle with a light period, but many continue to have irregular bleeding. Side-effects include weight gain, acne and mood changes.

Combined oral contraceptive pill (COCP) or 'the pill'

The COCP (the 'pill') contains a combination of oestrogen and progestogen, and is usually taken for 21 days of a 28-day cycle. The 7-day gap allows a 'withdrawal bleed', which is not a true period. Some preparations include seven dummy pills to be taken during this gap to reduce the risks of forgetting to start the next course. Most preparations contain a fixed dose of hormones, but some vary the proportions of hormones throughout the cycle, in an attempt to reflect the natural pattern of hormonal change. These 'triphasic' pills are believed by some doctors to be less likely to give rise to problematic bleeding. There are a number of preparations, and this offers a choice of a range of doses of oestrogen, and type of progestogen, each of which has a different side-effect profile and risk of failure. Often it takes a few attempts to find a preparation that suits an individual woman. The COCP has a dual action, both inhibiting ovulation and also, like the mini-pill, affecting the quality of the cervical mucus.

The major health issue with the COCP is that the high dose of oestrogen increases the risk of thrombosis. It also increases the risk of cancer of the breast and cervix, but is protective against cancer of the ovary and uterus. In most women whose risk of thrombosis is very low, the additional risk from the pill is considered to be extremely low. It is often quoted that the risk of thrombosis associated with pregnancy is much higher than is incurred by taking the pill. Nevertheless, the risk is real, and may be significant in those women who have other risk factors for thrombosis. Women who are obese, who smoke, who have a family or a past history of thrombosis, those with a past history of breast cancer and those with liver disease should be advised to choose an alternative form of contraception.

As surgery increases the risk of thrombosis, women on the pill who are due to have a major operation will be advised to use an alternative method of contraception for the few weeks either side of the operation date.

An additional problem is that the progestogen in the pill tends to have an adverse effect on the lipids in the blood, and so may accelerate the development of atherosclerosis. Another circulatory side-effect, which affects about 2% of women who take the pill, is a significant rise in blood pressure. For this reason, all women on the pill should have a medical assessment that includes blood pressure measurement every 6 months.

The use of the pill is known to decrease the risk of certain cancers, but may increase the risk of breast cancer. The risk of ovarian cancer is decreased by 40% and endometrial cancer by 50%. However, breast cancer is slightly more common in women taking the pill, although current theories propose that this risk only affects a small subgroup of women who are particularly susceptible to early-onset breast cancer. For this reason, a family history of early-onset breast cancer is a reason to avoid using the pill.

There are many other less serious side-effects which can affect certain women who take the pill. For some of these side-effects a change to another preparation of the pill may resolve the problem. However, for some women the side-effects are so severe that they prevent them continuing with this form of contraception. Common side-effects of the pill include acne, mid-cycle spotting or bleeding, dry eyes, gall-bladder disease, nausea, mood changes, weight gain, increased vaginal discharge, headaches and migraine. Of all these, migraine has to be taken very seriously, particularly if it is focal in nature. Women who develop focal migraines while on the pill should be changed to another form of contraception because of a possible increased risk of stroke.

Despite all these risk and side-effects, many women find the pill improves their quality of life, over and above the sexual freedom it offers. The pill can transform the symptoms of premenstrual syndrome, dysmenorrhoea and menorrhagia. In some women the skin texture improves when on the pill. Others may report an increase in sexual desire and general well-being. Also, because of its effects on cervical mucus, it is believed to reduce the risk of pelvic inflammatory disease. The pill is the contraceptive method chosen by over half of all women in the UK under 30 years old.

One preparation of the COCP, contains in place of the progesterone a form of the drug cyproterone which acts by opposing the effects of testosterone. This has the additional effect of improving acne and male-pattern body hair, and may be prescribed for these reasons alone. However, this preparation has a particularly adverse effect on the balance of lipids in the blood, and so should not be prescribed for too long because it may accelerate the development of atherosclerosis.

Failure rate: 0.005–0.30 per 100 woman-years (very low).

Advantages: Very reliable if taken correctly. Still reliable if the pill is forgotten for up to 48 hours, so is more suitable than the POP for those with a chaotic lifestyle. Some women find problems such as premenstrual tension and painful periods are much better when taking the pill. Often, sex life improves, possibly because of freedom from fear of pregnancy. Oestrogens have been shown to protect the bones from osteoporosis. The COCP is therefore prescribed to women with anovulatory amenorrhoea to prevent osteoporosis. In combination with progestogens, oestrogens reduce the risk of ovarian and womb cancer.

Disadvantages: The COCP does require a degree of discipline to be taken correctly, and so is not suitable for some people with an irregular lifestyle. A missed pill at certain times in the cycle can lead to ovulation. Many people suffer side-effects, including headaches, nausea, lack of libido, weight gain, acne, mood changes and breakthrough bleeding. Other problems with the COCP include interactions with other medication, with the common result that the effectiveness of the pill is reduced. Antibiotics are the most commonly prescribed medication that can reduce the absorption of the pill. Women should be counselled carefully about this potential problem, and should rely on additional methods, such as condoms, when they are taking certain medications.

Information Box 5.2e-I

Hormonal contraception: comments from a Chinese medicine perspective

In Chinese medicine, the hormonal methods of contraception would be interpreted as having significant energetic effects, as evidenced by their broad range of side-effects.

The progesterone-only methods have side-effects that include weight gain, acne, mood changes and amenorrhoea. In the long term, the high-dose methods (injection and implants) may lead to osteoporosis by preventing the natural production of oestrogen. This suggests that their negative effects may be manifestations of Accumulation of Damp, Stagnation of Qi and Depletion of Kidney Qi. All three of these factors might explain their effect in reducing fertility.

The combined pill also has side-effects that suggest Accumulation of Damp and Stagnation of Qi. These side-effects include weight gain, acne, mood changes, headaches and migraine. The additional effects on the circulatory system suggest that the Stagnating effect is more powerful than with the progesterone-only methods, and the adverse effect on blood lipids suggests Accumulation of Phlegm. The increased risk of breast cancer in some women is more evidence of a tendency to cause Blood Stagnation or Accumulation of Phlegm.

There is a paradox that some women report an improvement in mood and menstrual irregularities when on the pill. This can be explained as symptoms that have been suppressed rather than transformed, as they tend to recur on withdrawal of the pill.

Emergency contraception (the 'morning-after pill')

Emergency contraception (PCP) consists of a single tablet of high-dose progesterone (levonorgestrel) given within 12–72 hours of unprotected sex. It prevents pregnancy in over 95% of cases if given within 72 hours (hence the name 'morning-after pill' is a misnomer). It is commonly offered in the case of a split condom or missed contraceptive pills.

High dose levonorgestrel works primarily by altering the nature of the cervical mucus and the womb lining to prevent implantation, but in some cases it can inhibit ovulation.

Advantages: Effective.

Disadvantages: A common side-effect is nausea, which can be problematic for absorption of the pills if vomiting occurs. In theory, it carries all the risks of the COCP, although these are minimal because of the limited time period for which it is taken. It carries the same ethical problems as the IUD and the mini-pill, because it does not necessarily prevent fertilisation.

Surgical methods

The surgical methods of contraception are very reliable, although even these have a failure rate. Patients are counselled that both vasectomy and tubal ligation ('sterilisation' by cutting and clipping the fallopian tubes) are to be considered irreversible procedures. It is conventionally believed that these procedures should only be offered to those individuals who have made an informed and considered long-term decision about not having any more children. They should only very rarely be performed in those under 30 years old or those who have never had children.

Both vasectomy and tubal ligation can be reversed surgically, but a return to fertility cannot be guaranteed. The longer it has been since the initial operation, the lower the chances are of restoring fertility.

Vasectomy

The vasectomy operation can be performed very simply as an outpatient procedure. A small incision is made in the scrotum, and each vas deferens tube is cut. The two ends of the cut tube are then stitched ('tied off'). Testosterone is produced as normal, and so, contrary to some men's fears, sex drive should not be affected. Moreover, spermatozoa are also still produced, but these get reabsorbed from the epididymis. A man who has had a vasectomy will still ejaculate, because the production of seminal and prostatic fluids is not affected by the procedure.

Failure rate: 1 in 2000 over a lifetime (very low).

Advantages: Very reliable. No need to be concerned about contraceptive methods from a few weeks after the operation.

Disadvantages: Not effective straight away. Semen samples are required at 8 and 12 weeks postoperatively to check that no sperm are present. The procedure should be considered irreversible. There is a very small risk of chronic testicular pain.

Tubal ligation ('sterilisation')

In tubal ligation, the fallopian tubes are cut and clipped ('tied off') by means of a laparoscopic operation. This is a more invasive procedure than vasectomy, and requires a general anaesthetic. There is an increased risk of ectopic pregnancy after tubal ligation.

Failure rate: 1 in 200 over a lifetime.

Advantages: Fairly reliable. There is no longer a requirement for other contraceptive methods.

Disadvantages: The procedure should be considered irreversible. There is a small risk from the surgical procedure. The risk of ectopic pregnancy is increased.

Information Box 5.2e-II

Sterilisation: comments from a Chinese medicine perspective

From a Chinese medicine viewpoint, it is possible that the surgical methods of contraception prevent a free flow of bodily fluids. Although semen is seen as Essence in a material form, and its loss is Depleting to the man, nevertheless, ejaculation may be important for preventing Stagnation of Qi in the pelvic area. The same could be said about the way in which sterilisation prevents the release of the ovum.

In recent years there has been a concern that vasectomy might be associated with an increased incidence of prostatic disease and testicular cancer, which would be consistent with this idea of vasectomy causing Qi Stagnation. However, the current view, based on long-term studies of men who have had a vasectomy, is that there is no statistical foundation for a link between the operation and these conditions.

Natural methods of contraception

Natural methods of contraception do not rely on barriers or drugs. Instead they are dependent on the couple having an awareness of the way in which conception occurs, and how fertility varies throughout the woman's menstrual cycle.

Coitus interruptus

The oldest method of contraception, coitus interruptus, is arguably the most natural method. In coitus interruptus the man withdraws from the woman just before ejaculation. This is still the favoured method for some groups of people, particularly in those for whom other methods of contraception are considered unethical. The main problem with this method is that drops of semen, containing thousands of spermatozoa, are released from the penis before ejaculation. Therefore, even if carefully practised, coitus interruptus carries a real, albeit reduced, risk of pregnancy. The failure rate is estimated to be very high, at 30–40 pregnancies per 100 woman-years.

Periodic abstinence (the rhythm method)

Periodic abstinence is the most favoured natural method. This requires the couple to be aware of the days in the cycle in which the woman is most fertile. Sexual intercourse is then avoided on those days. The fertile period is the time that spans from 5 days before ovulation to 2 days after ovulation. Ideally, a couple who plan to use this method should have guidance from an experienced teacher of the natural methods of family planning.

For a woman with a regular cycle, there are some physiological changes that allow her to predict on what day of the cycle ovulation will occur. The most reliable of these are the changes in the consistency of the cervical mucus. At the beginning of the cycle (days 1–7) there is very little mucus. Conception is very unlikely to occur during these 'dry' days. From days 8 to 14 of a 28-day cycle the mucus becomes more profuse. Initially it is cloudy in colour and thick in texture, but on the day before ovulation it becomes clear and slippery. At ovulation the mucus is clear and stringy. This change in the mucus is an indication that the woman is at her most fertile day of the cycle. To be able to rely on these changes, the woman has to be able to find her own cervix, and examine her own mucus, ideally first thing in the morning. After a few cycles, she will become aware on what day she tends to ovulate.

An additional indicator of ovulation is that in some women there can be a definite rise in body temperature just before ovulation. The temperature should be taken first thing in the morning and charted throughout the cycle. It is currently taught that temperature changes should only be used in conjunction with assessment of cervical mucus, because if used alone it is known to be quite unreliable.

Some women prefer to use fertility devices such as the Persona system to help them differentiate between fertile and infertile times. These devices rely on regular tests of early morning urine samples. The failure rate for reliance on Persona has been estimated at an impressive 6 per 100 woman years.

For those women who have a regular cycle, and who are prepared to examine themselves in this way, these methods can be very reliable. However, for those who have a very irregular cycle, this method cannot be depended upon. In these women, ovulation can happen unpredictably, occasionally even as early as during the menstrual bleed. Moreover, there are many women who do not wish to be so introspective about their own bodies and who would find the idea of examining mucus distasteful.

Also, for some couples, the idea of abstinence from sexual intercourse for 7 days is not acceptable. For this reason, some couples may generally rely on this method, but also use a barrier method on the fertile days.

Self-test 5.2e

Contraception

1. What are the important issues to discuss with a patient who is keen to start the combined oral contraceptive pill?

Answers

1. The issues to discuss might cover the following topics:
   Potential benefits:
   - very effective if taken appropriately
   - can reduce the risk of sexually transmitted disease
   - may improve the symptoms of menstrual disorders, reduce acne and increase libido
   - reduces the risk of ovarian and endometrial cancer.

   Potential problems:
   - more likely to fail if the person is not good at remembering to take tablets
   - increased risk, albeit small, of serious cardiovascular disease and cancer
   - long list of minor side-effects
   - significant adverse energetic effects from a complementary medical viewpoint (e.g. Stagnation of Liver Qi and Accumulation of Damp according to Chinese medicine).

You could also spend some time discussing the other contraceptive options, which from a complementary medical viewpoint could be seen as less energetically disturbing (the barrier methods and the natural methods).

Chapter 5.2f Infertility

LEARNING POINTS

At the end of this chapter you will:
- be able to describe the main causes of infertility
- understand the process of investigation of infertility
- be able to describe the ways in which infertility can be treated.

Estimated time for chapter: 100 minutes.

Introduction

Infertility is defined arbitrarily as the inability of a couple to conceive within 12 months, despite having regular unprotected intercourse. By this definition, infertility affects up to 15% of couples, although many of these will conceive naturally at a later date. It is only in a very few cases that the diagnosis of absolute infertility can be made.

For most couples there is a combination of factors that result in reduced fertility, but not a total inability to conceive. This is an important point from the perspective of complementary medicine, as it implies that for most couples there is scope for treatment to increase the chances of conception. By optimising the conditions for conception to take place (e.g. by Nourishing Blood and Tonifying the Kidneys in Chinese medicine), complementary medicine may encourage an improved balance of health to enable conception to occur in those with relative infertility.

In some cases of apparent infertility, it may be found that the couple are having sex on an infrequent basis, and not consistently at the woman's most fertile time. If this is the underlying problem, conception may be more likely to occur after the couple have been given advice about how to determine which are the fertile days in the woman's cycle according to the principles of natural family planning (see Chapter 5.2e). A couple will not usually be referred for investigation or treatment until after a year of having regular intercourse during the fertile times of the woman's menstrual cycle.

In about 30% of couples who are referred for investigation, no physical abnormality is detected. Despite normal ovulation and healthy semen, conception does not occur. There is no agreed conventional explanation for this problem. Some specialists suggest that this form of infertility is due to a defect in the development of the corpus luteum, which then leads to failure of implantation of a fertilised egg (see later in this chapter).

However, in 20% of cases there is some problem with the semen and in over 40% of cases the woman is found to have some abnormalities. In up to 40% of cases both partners may each have a condition that contributes to the infertility.

Investigation of infertility

Investigation of the man

The main test required is semen analysis. Even if the spermatozoa are found to be abnormal, if the couple wish to use assisted conception techniques (see later in the chapter), the woman will be expected also to undergo full investigations. This is because combined problems with infertility are not uncommon.

Investigation of the woman

Investigation of the woman involves a general physical and gynaecological examination to look for evidence of gross physical abnormalities such as endocrine disease, fibroids or pelvic inflammatory disease. A blood test may be taken in the second half of the cycle to assess the level of progesterone to determine whether or not ovulation is occurring, and to test for hormones including FSH, LH, testosterone, thyroid hormones and prolactin in the first half of the cycle to look for evidence of conditions such as polycystic ovary disease, hyperprolactinaemia, thyroid disorders or ovarian failure.

Tests to visualise the structure of the internal genital organs include ultrasound scan, laparoscopy and hysterosalpingography. An ultrasound scan will reveal gross defects of the uterus and ovaries, and can also visualise ovulation. A laparoscopy will reveal the changes of endometriosis. The hysterosalpingography can reveal whether or not the fallopian tubes are patent.

Investigation of the couple

If the results of all the tests described above are normal, a postcoital test may be performed. A positive postcoital test indicates that the man's sperm can easily penetrate the cervical mucus of his partner.

The causes of infertility

Defective semen

Although it is commonly assumed that infertility is usually a problem with the woman, in up to 40% of cases some deficiency in the quantity or quality of the spermatozoa is found. In most of these cases there is a reduced number of normal spermatozoa (low sperm count). Established causes of a low sperm count include past infection with mumps virus, late descent of the testes and treatment with anticancer drugs. It is recognised that over the past few decades the average sperm count has declined markedly. A range of dietary and environmental factors have been suggested to explain this drop, but no single cause has been proven. It is known that an individual's sperm count can vary over time, and may increase if factors such as diet and stress levels can be attended to. Moreover, in cases of reduced sperm count, normal conception may still be possible, as even if the sperm count is less than half the normal number there are still well over a million spermatozoa in an ejaculate of normal volume (2–3 millilitres).

Alternatively, the spermatozoa might be found to be abnormal in structure or movement. In these cases, assisted conception may be necessary. In rare cases, there may be total absence of spermatozoa, in which case use of donor semen is the only option available for the couple who wish to conceive.

Information Box 5.2f-I

Defects in sperm count or motility: comments from a Chinese medicine perspective

In Chinese medicine, defective semen is a manifestation of Deficiency of Kidney Essence (in its Yang aspect). Damp Heat is also considered to be a cause of male infertility in some cases.

Anovulation

Problems with ovulation are the cause of 5–25% of cases of infertility. A complete lack of ovulation is termed 'anovulation'. The causes of anovulation are the same as the causes of amenorrhoea (see Chapter 5.2c). Women who suffer from amenorrhoea are also very likely to be infertile, although this is not always the case. However, it is also possible for a woman to have a menstrual cycle that appears normal but during which there is no ovulation (an anovulatory cycle).

Anovulatory cycles are common at the extremes of a woman's reproductive years. These may be increased in frequency by factors that affect the release of the pituitary hormones, such as ongoing stress, poor diet or overexercise. A period of anovulation can follow the withdrawal from a long-term prescription of a hormone-based contraceptive. In particular, the progesterone injection can have this effect for some months after withdrawal. Other physical causes of anovulation include ovarian damage by drugs or surgery, primary ovarian failure and polycystic ovary syndrome.

Information Box 5.2f-II

Ovulatory failure: comments from a Chinese medicine perspective

In Chinese medicine, ovulation depends primarily on Blood and Kidney Essence. If one or both of these is deficient, ovulation may fail to occur. Also, lack of ovulation may be caused by a Full pattern. For example, Damp, Heat and Liver Qi Stagnation may all be contributory in the development of polycystic ovarian syndrome.

Defects in the development of the corpus luteum

As has been mentioned, some experts attribute cases of unexplained infertility to a failure in the implantation of a fertilised egg. It has been proposed that a defect in the corpus luteum may cause this form of infertility because it leads to a poorly developed endometrium in the second half of the menstrual cycle. It is suggested that a short luteal phase (less than 10 days) may be suggestive of a corpus luteum defect.

The problem with this theory is that there is no simple test available that can demonstrate reliably possible defects in corpus luteum development. Also, there are no clearly defined treatments to reverse this theoretical condition, although progesterone or HCG treatment may be prescribed. However, in common with other functional conditions, this problem is possibly amenable to complementary medical approaches.

Information Box 5.2f-III

Corpus luteum defects: comments from a Chinese medicine perspective

In Chinese medicine, the stage of the menstrual cycle in which the endometrium is being prepared for implantation corresponds to the stage in which Blood and Yin are filling the Ren (Directing) and Chong (Penetrating) Vessels. A corpus luteum defect might, therefore, correspond to Deficiency of Blood and/or Kidney Essence (in its Yin aspect). As well as nourishing Blood and the Kidneys, treatment should also involve invigorating the Ren and Chong Vessels.

The Pathogenic Factors of Cold, Damp and Blood Stasis may also prevent implantation, and so could be underlying factors in a case of infertility of no measurable physical cause.

Fallopian tube damage

The most common cause of damage to the fallopian tubes is the scarring and adhesions that result from pelvic inflammatory disease. The inflammation and damage that may result from an ectopic pregnancy can also cause permanent damage to one fallopian tube. The structural damage resulting from these conditions may impair the transport of the ovum, and so prevent fertilisation.

> **Information Box 5.2f-IV**
>
> **Fallopian tube problems: comments from a Chinese medicine perspective**
>
> In Chinese medicine, fallopian tube damage corresponds to one or more of the Full patterns which can cause infertility. Damp Heat, Toxic Heat or Blood Stagnation may be underlying Pathogenic Factors.

Structural problems of the uterus or vagina

A physical disorder of the structure of the uterus or vagina is another cause of infertility. Together, uterine and fallopian tube disorders are important factors in 15–25% of cases of infertility.

The condition of endometriosis is a common disorder of uncertain cause in which the uterine wall is distorted by the development of 'cysts' of endometrial lining within its muscular walls. Endometriosis is often associated with infertility, although whether the condition is the cause of infertility is still unclear. Fibroids, if very large, are very occasionally found to be the cause of infertility, but in most cases they do not prevent the development of a healthy pregnancy. Rarely, an inherited structural defect of the vagina or uterus is the cause of infertility. In some cases, these defects can be amended surgically.

> **Information Box 5.2f-V**
>
> **Endometriosis: comments from a Chinese medicine perspective**
>
> In Chinese medicine, endometriosis corresponds to Blood Stagnation. Fibroids also correspond to Blood Stagnation. Structural defects are usually regarded as a manifestation of Jing Deficiency.

The treatment of infertility

For some of the causes of infertility the underlying condition can be treated, and this will lead to conception. If the underlying problem cannot be remedied, the assisted methods of conception, which include in vitro fertilisation, can offer a chance of pregnancy that until a few decades ago would not have been thought possible. However, there are some forms of infertility in which it is not possible to obtain the gametes from one or both partners. In these cases, donor gametes (ova or spermatozoa) may enable a pregnancy to be achieved. Each of these approaches to the treatment of infertility is now discussed in turn.

Treatment of the underlying condition

Functional lack of ovulation may be treated by supporting the woman in making appropriate lifestyle changes, such as reducing stress levels, attaining a healthy body weight and reducing excessive exercise.

Endocrine disorders, such as hypothyroidism, and pituitary tumours, can be treated successfully by means of drugs and/or pituitary surgery. Fallopian tube blockage may be treated by means of microsurgery, although the success rate is low (within 2 years after the operation, only 20–40% of women will have conceived). Other structural disorders of the uterus and vagina, including inherited defects and fibroids, may also be treated surgically.

The symptoms of endometriosis are generally treated with a range of hormonal drugs.

In cases of anovulation that do not respond to lifestyle changes, including polycystic ovarian syndrome, drug treatment can be used to stimulate the ovary to produce eggs. The most commonly drug used is clomifene. This drug acts by stimulating a surge in FSH and LH, which in turn promotes ovulation in up to 80% of women. It is not uncommon for more than one ovum to be released with this treatment, and thus there is a risk of multiple pregnancies. More than half of all women who manage to ovulate with this treatment will fall pregnant.

The side-effects of clomifene include enlargement of ovarian cysts and the development of endometriosis. Nausea, vomiting, abdominal pain, weight gain and depression are common. There is a health concern about using such drugs for too many cycles, as they are known to increase the risk of ovarian cancer. For this reason, the drugs are generally only prescribed for fewer than six menstrual cycles. If clomifene fails to stimulate ovulation, there are a range of ovary-stimulating hormonal drugs (gonadotrophins) that have a similar effect which may be prescribed by a fertility specialist.

> **Information Box 5.2f-VI**
>
> **Ovarian stimulants: comments from a Chinese medicine perspective**
>
> From a Chinese medicine viewpoint, the induction of ovulation at a time when it would not naturally have occurred might be interpreted as Depleting of Blood and/or Kidney Essence, as these are the substances that enable ovulation to occur. The side-effects associated with the use of clomifene suggest that it also induces Liver Qi Stagnation and Accumulation of Damp/Phlegm.

New assisted techniques of conception

There are a number of methods currently used in intractable cases of infertility which enable the meeting of the parent's gametes. Apart from assisted insemination with the partner's sperm (AIH) (see below), all these techniques depend on inducing a state of 'superovulation' in the woman. This means that an ovary-stimulating drug is given to the woman to induce the development of a number of ovarian follicles at the same time.

The ovaries are 'prepared' for this stimulation by first administering a drug by daily injection or nasal spray for 2 weeks, to prevent the release of FSH and LH from the pituitary. This means that the levels of natural oestrogen drop, and a range of side-effects, including hot flushes, palpitations and sweating, develop. After 2–3 weeks, a preparation of FSH and LH is given by injection to stimulate superovulation. This causes the ovaries to swell to over twice their normal size. The development of the follicles is monitored by means of regular ultrasound scans.

When the follicles are ready to rupture, the released eggs are 'harvested' by means of a surgical technique that accesses the ovaries via the vaginal wall. The eggs are then taken to a laboratory to be examined and prepared for fertilisation. Only the healthy eggs are saved. Some of these eggs may be frozen and stored for future attempts at fertilisation or for donation to women who are unable to produce their own.

The emotional consequences to the couple of this aspect of the assisted techniques are not to be underestimated. First, the different stages of ovary-stimulating medication have a wide range of physical and psychological side-effects. While experiencing the effects of this medication, the woman has to make repeated visits to the fertility clinic for scans whilst the follicles are developing, and ultimately for the 'harvesting' operation. After all this has happened, there is a possibility that the embryos formed from the eggs generated may either be unhealthy or may fail to implant. The couple then have to decide whether or not the whole cycle should be repeated. It is estimated that one-third of women undergoing assisted conception techniques experience anxiety or depression, and one in seven becomes severely distressed.

In some health districts in the UK, limited cycles of assisted conception are funded by the NHS. In others, the couple have to pay a considerable sum for each attempt (cycle) at implantation. The cumulative cost of successive cycles is another factor that can add to the stress of a couple who have decided to opt for assisted conception.

Assisted insemination with husband's sperm (AIH)

AIH involves injection of the partner's sperm directly into the uterus by means of a fine tube inserted into the cervix. This technique is used in cases in which the sperm are unable to penetrate the cervical mucus. This technique might also be used in cases in which there are psychological or physical problems, such as erectile dysfunction or vaginismus, which may prevent normal intercourse. AIH is the least invasive of the assisted conception techniques, and carries very few risks over and above those of normal sexual intercourse.

In vitro fertilisation (IVF) and zygote intrafallopian transfer (ZIFT)

These techniques involve harvesting of eggs, and subsequent fertilisation of these with the partner's sperm in a laboratory. The term 'in vitro' literally means 'in glass', and refers to the 'test tube' (in fact a flat, lidded glass or plastic dish) in which fertilisation takes place.

Around the same time as harvesting, the partner or donor is required to produce a sample of sperm. The sperm is washed and prepared so that only fast-moving sperm cells are selected. The egg and sperm are then mixed over the next 16–20 hours. Any fertilised eggs are placed in an incubator for the next 2–6 days, after which the most healthy looking one or two embryos are selected for transfer. As this process is going on the woman is given further medication to help prepare the womb for implantation.

Up to three fertilised eggs are either returned directly to the woman's uterus, or are allowed to make a few divisions before they are returned as embryos (2–3 days) or even blastocysts (5–6 days) to the uterus via a thin plastic catheter passed through the cervix.

Successful implantation depends very much on the age and health of the woman. The success rate is nearly 40% for women under 35 years old but drops to 1.2% for those aged over 44 years. The percentage of these pregnancies that survive for the full term is lower. A significant proportion of all pregnancies end in miscarriage within the first few weeks, and this is true for pregnancies that follow from assisted conception. This means that the stress on the couple is not lifted once a successful implantation has occurred. Because two or three embryos are transferred to the uterus in each 'cycle', there is also a risk of multiple pregnancies with these techniques.

Gamete intrafallopian transfer (GIFT)

GIFT involves the direct transfer of unfertilised eggs and sperm into the fallopian tube to allow the formation of a zygote in a natural environment. This process, which can be performed directly after the eggs have been harvested, is less costly than IVF, but is not always the most suitable technique in some cases of infertility. The implantation rate of GIFT is 30–40% per cycle, which is higher than for IVF.

Intracytoplasmic sperm injection (ICSI)

ICSI involves the in vitro injection of sperm into the cytoplasm of the egg. It enables fertilisation in cases in which the sperm have a reduced ability to move or are very reduced in number. ICSI is more costly than IVF, but has a higher success rate per cycle, with implantation occurring in 50% of cycles. This high success rate may be a reflection of the fact that ICSI is used in cases in which the problem lies in defective semen, and so in these cases it is more likely that the woman has no physiological barrier to fertility. It is possible to extract sperm from the epididymis or testicle by means of minor operation, and this means that ICSI may be an option for men who suffer from total erectile failure or who have had a vasectomy.

Use of donor gametes

In some cases of infertility, one or both partners are unable to produce gametes at all. In these cases pregnancy may be possible with the use of donor sperm or donor eggs.

Donor insemination (DI) or artificial insemination (AI)

In the rare cases of total lack of sperm production, donor sperm may be used to enable conception to occur. This technique, known as donor insemination (DI), has been used successfully for decades. The semen may be donated by a friend or family member, or may be obtained from a 'sperm bank'. The samples of semen held in a sperm bank originate from paid volunteers who have been carefully screened to reduce the risk of transmission of infectious or congenital disease. The couple can select which donated sample is used according to broad characteristics of the donor such as height and skin colour. Personal details of the donor are maintained on a Human Fertilisation and Embryology Association (HFEA) register. In the UK, all children born after April 2005 have the right to find out the identity of the donor from this register should they wish to at any stage in their life.

The success rate of DI is high, with over 65% of women conceiving within a year of using DI on a monthly basis. DI carries a very small risk of the transmission of infectious disease, although this is minimised by screening of donors and also the donated semen.

Use of donor eggs

As assisted conception techniques are increasingly popular, there is greater availability of donor eggs. These eggs can be fertilised with the male partner's sperm either in vitro or within the female partner's fallopian tube (using GIFT) to enable a pregnancy to occur. As with DI, the donor may be a friend or a family member, but this is not as simple a process for the donor as it is for DI. This is because the donor's eggs have to be artificially stimulated and harvested in the same way as they are in the assisted conception techniques.

Surrogacy

Surrogacy is the method whereby the donor of the eggs also carries the pregnancy to full term after donor insemination by the male partner's semen. Commercial surrogacy is illegal in the UK, but couples may travel to countries such as the USA where it is available on a private basis, and this inevitably carries significant financial and emotional costs. The couple may experience the pregnancy 'vicariously' by keeping in regular touch with the surrogate mother. There are complicated ethical and legal issues that arise from questions about 'ownership' of the child. This is not an approach that is recommended in conventional clinics.

Information Box 5.2f-VII

Assisted conception techniques: comments from a Chinese medicine perspective

From an Chinese medicine viewpoint, use of the assisted fertility techniques raises some important questions about the long-term effects on the health of the woman and also the child. The use of drugs to induce superovulation may well be Depleting of Blood and Kidney Essence, as well as being the source of the introduction of patterns and Pathogenic Factors such as Qi Stagnation and Damp.

In Chinese medicine, the conditions of conception and the early days of embryo development are considered to be fundamental in establishing the Essence of the child to be. Ideally, the parents should be in good health and in a calm emotional state. In contrast, the stress of these techniques may mean that both partners are both physically and psychologically drained at the time of conception. In the case of in vitro fertilisation, the environment for the conception could not be more different than the very Yin qualities offered by the fallopian tube. These techniques all involve a scientifically observed conception illuminated by the bright lights of a laboratory.

Moreover, the ovum used in such a conception would not have naturally matured at that time, and in the case of intracytoplasmic sperm injection (ICSI), the sperm would not have naturally been able to penetrate the ovum. This raises questions about the health of the individual gametes, and so may have consequences on the Essence of the child to be.

Any complementary medical concerns about the energetic effects of assisted conception are speculative. There is no doubt that these techniques have enabled thousands of couples the opportunity of having a much wanted child. The positive aspects of this outcome must not be underestimated. One important role we can have as complementary medical practitioners is to be able to support couples who have chosen to take this route, so that their health and emotional state can be optimised at the time of conception, embryo transfer and during the subsequent time of pregnancy.

Self-test 5.2f

Infertility

1. A patient of yours is requesting treatment to help her conceive. She and her partner have been hoping for pregnancy for the past year since she came off the pill. When you question her you find that her periods are infrequent (once every 6–8 weeks on average), light and irregular. She considers herself very lucky to have such little trouble from her periods, and very rarely experiences any pain. However, they were 'regular as clockwork', although very light, when on the pill. She has not yet been to her GP because she does not wish to be referred for conventional fertility treatment.
   (i) What is the possible underlying problem with this woman's fertility (in conventional terms) which would also account for these symptoms?
   (ii) What are the medical conditions that might cause this particular problem of fertility?

(iii) What questions might you ask this woman to clarify which conditions might be most likely?
(iv) Would you refer this woman for conventional investigations?

Answers

1. (i) The most likely underlying problem, which also accounts for the symptoms in this case, is lack of ovulation. Irregular, light and delayed periods are more likely to be anovulatory.
(ii) The common causes of anovulatory cycles include:
   - functional changes in the release of pituitary hormones; these can result from major life events, stress, undereating, overexercise and withdrawal from hormonal contraceptives.
   - endocrine disease, such as pituitary tumours (which commonly cause excess production of prolactin) and hypothyroidism
   - polycystic ovary syndrome (PCOS)
   - primary ovarian failure (premature menopause).

(iii) The questions you might ask can be grouped in terms of the possible cause that you are trying to exclude:
   - Functional causes: ask about stress and life events, diet, possibility of eating disorders, tendency to overexercise, what her periods were like before the pill.
   - Endocrine disease: ask about visual disturbance and headaches, leaking of milk from the breasts, marked changes in energy levels, libido, tolerance of cold and heat, and unexplained weight loss or weight gain.
   - PCOS: ask about weight gain, acne, body hair.
   - Primary ovarian failure: ask about family history of early menopause, and menopausal symptoms such as hot flushes and night sweats.

(iv) The only urgent reason to refer this woman for investigation would be if you suspect a serious condition such as a pituitary tumour or hypothyroidism. However, sometimes simple investigations can be very helpful, and may inform your own approach to treatment. For example, a diagnosis of primary ovarian failure means that the infertility is irreversible, and complementary medicine would be unlikely to help. In contrast, a functional cause may well be amenable to a combination of lifestyle changes and complementary medical approaches. The diagnosis in this case could be established by means of physical examination, blood tests and an ultrasound scan. It is important that the fertility of this woman's partner is also assessed. If his sperm count is below normal, he too may benefit from lifestyle changes and complementary medical treatment.

Chapter 5.2g Structural disorders of the ovaries, uterus and vagina

LEARNING POINTS

At the end of this chapter you will:
- be able to describe the clinical features of the main structural disorders of the vagina, uterus and ovary
- understand the causes, clinical features and treatment of the cancers of the vagina, uterus and ovary
- be able to recognise the red flags of the structural disorders of the vagina, uterus and ovary.

Estimated time for chapter: 100 minutes.

Structural disorders of the female reproductive organs

The conditions studied in this chapter are those in which the underlying problem is primarily structural. The conditions studied include (see Q5.2g-1):

- Inherited defects of the female reproductive organs:
  - imperforate hymen
  - septate uterus and vagina
  - intersex disorders.
- Benign structural disorders of the female reproductive organs:
  - cervical and endometrial polyps
  - fibroids
  - endometriosis
  - ovarian cysts
  - benign ovarian tumours.
- Cancer of the female reproductive organs:
  - ovarian cancer
  - vulval cancer
  - cervical cancer
  - vaginal cancer
  - endometrial cancer.
- Prolapse of the female reproductive organs.
- Common surgical treatments:
  - hysterectomy
  - oophorectomy
  - repair operations for prolapse.

Inherited defects of the female reproductive organs

Imperforate hymen

The hymen is the thin sheet of tissue which partially closes the entrance to the vagina. Normally it has a small opening through which the menstrual blood can flow at the menarche. In rare cases, the hymen does not have this opening. Ideally, this problem is found during the medical examination of a newborn baby girl, but the condition may be missed. If the problem is not detected before the onset of puberty, at the onset of menstruation the menstrual blood cannot appear. Instead, the blood builds up within the vagina and uterus. This may not necessarily cause symptoms. The problem may actually not be diagnosed until the periods are noticed to be very late, and the girl is sent for investigations for primary amenorrhoea.

The treatment is by means of surgery, in which a small incision is made to allow the accumulated fluids to disperse naturally.

Imperforate hymen is the most common inherited defect of the vagina and uterus.

Septate uterus and vagina

Septate uterus and vagina are more rare conditions in which the structure of the vagina, uterus or both is divided into two halves by a wall (septum) of tissue. This problem may not come to light until the woman suffers from recurrent miscarriages, or when the fetus does not lie in the normal head-down position in late pregnancy.

In some cases of septate uterus, surgical removal of the septum can reduce the risk of recurrent miscarriage.

Intersex disorders

The intersex disorders are rare conditions in which incomplete development of the sexual organs has resulted in the formation of genitalia with a structure that is between that of a boy and a girl. They develop as a result of an imbalance in the hormonal environment of the fetus.

In a male fetus, normal development of the external genitalia, and also normal descent of the testes, is dependent on the secretion of hormones from the developing pituitary and adrenal glands. There are two rare conditions (congenital adrenal hyperplasia and testicular feminisation) in which these hormones are not formed properly. In these conditions, the external genitalia are either underdeveloped, or do not develop at all. In testicular feminisation the child will look like a girl. The diagnosis may only be made when this 'female' (but genetically male) child fails to menstruate at puberty.

Information Box 5.2g-I

Congenital abnormalities of the uterus and ovaries: comments from a Chinese medicine perspective

In Chinese medicine, all these inherited conditions are regarded as manifestations of Jing Deficiency.

Benign structural disorders of the female reproductive organs

Cervical and endometrial polyps

The word 'polyp' refers to a fleshy growth that develops from a thin stalk of tissue. Cervical polyps are common, benign outgrowths of the epithelium of the cervix. They usually produce no symptoms. In some cases they may lead to excessive physiological discharge. Occasionally, they may bleed irregularly, and in this way may mimic a cancer. They can be removed very easily by means of a minor operation.

Endometrial polyps are fleshy outgrowths of the endometrium in the uterus. These too can lead to irregular bleeding. They may also be a cause of menorrhagia. They can be removed by means of a curette inserted during hysteroscopy.

Fibroids (uterine myomata)

Fibroids are benign tumours of the uterine muscle and can vary in size from that of a pea to a football. They are known to develop in up to 20% of women over the age of 30 years, and are more common in women who have had either one or no children. It not unusual for a woman to have a number of fibroids of different sizes within her uterus. The fibroid is dependent on oestrogen to grow, and so will very often shrink to a small size after the menopause.

Usually fibroids do not give rise to symptoms, especially if they are small. In some women, fibroids are associated with menorrhagia and dysmenorrhoea. Very rarely, large fibroids may be associated with infertility or recurrent miscarriage. A large fibroid may also cause pelvic or back pain, dyspareunia or problems with urination.

In most cases fibroids do not need to be treated. In cases in which mild symptoms develop late in the woman's reproductive years, the best management may be simply to wait until the menopause has occurred, after which the symptoms will almost always abate.

A very large symptomatic fibroid can be treated surgically. Sometimes the fibroid alone will be removed (myomectomy), but very often the whole uterus is removed (hysterectomy). A myomectomy may lead to reduced fertility, but 40% of women who wish to conceive after this operation will still be able to do so. A hysterectomy is commonly advised for those women who are not concerned about fertility, because fibroids have a tendency to recur. The surgical approach of hysterectomy is discussed at the end of this chapter.

Uterine artery embolisation is a newer surgical technique, in which the aim is to deprive the fibroid of its blood supply. This procedure requires shorter hospital stays and has a shorter recovery time than hysterectomy, but up to a quarter of women may require further treatments to ensure symptom control.

The drugs goserilin and buserilin are LH analogues. They inhibit the release of FSH and LH, and so lead to a reduction in the natural production of oestrogen. These drugs can be useful medical options for the treatment of fibroids in people who do not wish to undergo surgery. Side-effects include menopausal symptoms of hot flushes, dry vagina and loss of bone density, a reflection of the fact that the drugs reduce the level of oestrogen in the body. It is well recognised that growth of the fibroids can recur after the course of treatment has ended.

Information Box 5.2g-II

Fibroids: comments from a Chinese medicine perspective

In Chinese medicine, a fibroid, as a substantial mass, may be seen as a manifestation of Blood Stagnation and/or Phlegm in the uterus.

Endometriosis

Endometriosis is a common disorder of unknown cause in which the uterine wall is distorted by the development of 'cysts' of endometrial lining within its muscular walls and in other sites outside the uterus. The current theory for the origin of endometriosis is that small pieces of the endometrium can separate from the uterine wall during menstruation and 'seed' in different locations. Although the uterine muscular wall is the most common location for endometriosis (in which case it may be termed 'adenomyosis'), other sites include the ovary, the bowel and the peritoneal lining that surrounds the bowel and the other pelvic organs.

This displaced endometrium is still responsive to changes in the female hormones, and will build up and break down throughout the menstrual cycle. If the location is deep in some other tissue (e.g. of the ovary or the uterus wall) then the menstrual blood cannot escape. This blood instead collects within the tissue to form what are descriptively termed 'chocolate cysts'. The formation of these miniature cysts is a source of pain, which peaks premenstrually and during the period. Endometriotic cysts can be seen during a laparoscopy, when they appear as black spots, likened to the appearance of a burnt match head, on the surface of the uterus, peritoneal wall and ovaries. If the location of the cyst is on the peritoneum, the blood can escape to the peritoneal space and can be highly irritating. Again, this pain is worst during the time of the period.

It is estimated that endometriosis is present in about 5% of menstruating women. In many cases of endometriosis, there are no symptoms. However, symptoms can be severe. They include menorrhagia, dysmenorrhoea, dyspareunia and infertility. Pain is often the most prominent symptom. In some cases it can persist throughout the menstrual cycle, but usually it is worst around the time of the menstrual bleed.

Adenomyosis and endometriotic cysts of the ovary can be detected by the relatively non-invasive test of intravaginal ultrasound scanning, but the gold standard for diagnosis is laparoscopy. Magnetic resonance imaging (MRI) may also be used to detect peritoneal deposits.

There is a range of drugs that may be used to treat the symptoms of endometriosis. NSAIDs such as mefenamic acid may be useful for suppressing pain. All the other treatments are intended to cause regression of the pain-inducing cysts. For this purpose, these drugs need to be taken for 3–12 months, after which time there may be a long-term reduction in symptoms. The drugs act by reducing the influence of oestrogen on the cysts, which then shrink in size and become permanently scarred. The choice of drug is largely based on whether or not the symptoms can be tolerated.

In some women, the combined oral contraceptive pill or a high-dose progesterone-only pill (e.g. medroxyprogesterone acetate) may reduce or eliminate symptoms. Long-acting progesterone preparations, such as the depot injection Depo-Provera, and the progesterone-containing intrauterine device (IUD) can also alleviate symptoms very effectively. However, these treatments are not suitable if infertility is the primary problem.

The LH-releasing hormone analogues buserilin and goserilin are also prescribed. These are given by means of nasal spray or a monthly depot injection over the course of 3–6 months. During this time symptoms will abate, and this effect can be sustained. These drugs reduce the release of FSH and LH, and so the levels of oestrogen drop, thus inducing a temporary menopause. Side-effects include hot flushes, night sweats and amenorrhoea. Bone loss is a potential problem and limits the time for which these medications can be prescribed.

The outcome of drug treatment depends on the initial extent of the endometriosis. In 30% of cases the disease regresses totally, in 60% there is partial regression, and in the remaining 10% there is no significant effect. In about half of those treated successfully, the disease recurs within 5 years.

Surgery is an alternative treatment for endometriosis. This is most effective if the ovaries are removed at the same time as the cysts are excised or cauterised. In some severe cases, hysterectomy may also be performed. Obviously, this radical approach is not suitable for women who still want to have children. Less radical surgical approaches, such as cautery of individual cysts, have been shown to improve fertility in the year following the intervention.

Information Box 5.2g-III

Endometriosis: comments from a Chinese medicine perspective

In Chinese medicine, endometriosis corresponds to Blood Stagnation in the uterus. The formation of blood-containing cysts may also indicate the presence of Phlegm or Phlegm Heat.

Functional ovarian cysts

A cyst is a fluid-filled swelling. In the ovary, cysts may be part of the normal follicular changes that take place in a menstruating woman, in which case they are known as 'functional cysts'. Cyst formation in the ovary is part of the natural physiology of the development of the ovarian follicle in the first half of the menstrual cycle. As the follicle matures, fluid forms within it, only to be released when the follicle ruptures at the middle of the cycle. Just before rupture, the normal ovarian follicle can reach a size of up to 2 centimetres in diameter.

The most common cause of a symptomatic cyst in the ovary is failure of this process of rupture. Instead of rupturing at mid-cycle, the ovum-containing cyst continues to enlarge as it accumulates fluid. In some cases this does not produce any symptoms, but in others the enlarging cyst continues to produce oestrogen, and this can result in menorrhagia and an irregular length of cycle. The causes of this failure are unclear, but are probably rooted in an imbalance in the release of FSH and LH from the pituitary gland.

Alternatively, failure of degeneration of the corpus luteum in the second half of the menstrual cycle can also lead to cyst formation. In this case there may be excessive production of progesterone, giving rise to the symptoms of late periods or amenorrhoea.

Polycystic ovary syndrome is the other common condition associated with benign cyst formation.

If followed by serial ultrasound scans it is seen that most functional ovarian cysts will disappear within 2–3 months. If ovarian cysts persist then the fluid within should be withdrawn by means of a minor operation so that a diagnosis of cancer can be excluded. If symptoms persist or if the cyst is irregular in shape, the cysts are surgically removed. This operation should not affect the function of the ovary.

Large ovarian cysts may cause symptoms in a number of ways. A very large cyst (more than 10 centimetres in diameter) may cause discomfort as a result of pressure on other structures in the abdomen. Occasionally, a cyst will rupture, with a release of blood-stained fluid. This can be very irritating to the peritoneum, and can present as an acute abdomen (see Chapter 3.1d), particularly if the blood loss is severe. An enlarged cyst may also cause the ovary to twist around the stalk of tissue that contains the vessels providing its blood supply. This condition, called 'torsion of the ovary', gives rise to severe pain as the ovary is threatened with infarction. Torsion may settle as the stalk untwists, but otherwise requires an emergency operation. If the torsion settles, an operation to remove the cyst will be performed to prevent recurrence.

Benign ovarian tumours

Tumours of the ovary are common, and may also be cystic in nature. 95% of ovarian tumours are benign in nature. One-quarter of these are found to be functional cysts (see above) and just under half of the remainder are growths known as 'cystadenomas'. Like functional cysts, other forms of ovarian tumour may also produce symptoms resulting from rupture, release of fluid and torsion. Some of these tumours (mucinous cystadenomas) can reach an enormous size and can cause abdominal swelling and discomfort. Others give rise to symptoms because they produce excessive sex hormones. Excessive oestrogen may give rise to irregular menstrual bleeding, whereas excessive testosterone can lead to masculinisation.

Occasionally, the tumour is only diagnosed when a routine ultrasound scan is performed in pregnancy. The mass of the tumour may cause problems in labour, and if it is large a surgical operation may be performed to remove it, ideally before the 30th week of pregnancy.

Benign tumours arising from the germ cells (immature egg cells) may also develop. These tumours are known as 'teratomas'. Teratomas may contain a range of tissues, including bone, cartilage, hair and brain. As these tumours may be malignant, they should always be removed.

If an ovarian cyst or tumour is seen by means of ultrasound scan, the clinical dilemma is whether it is benign and can be safely left alone, or whether it is malignant and needs removal. The shape of the tumour as seen on an ultrasound scan can be helpful, but is not absolutely diagnostic (an ultrasound scan will positively detect 89% of ovarian cancers). The risk that an ovarian cyst or tumour is malignant is greater if the levels of a tumour marker called CA-125 are high. Women are therefore assigned a risk score depending on age, ultrasound appearance and the CA-125 level. In younger women with a low risk score, the cyst may simply be monitored by means of regular ultrasound scans or fluid removed for examination by means of laparoscopy. Postmenopausal women with ovarian tumours are generally considered to be at greater risk of ovarian cancer. Those with a low risk score may be managed either by regular ultrasound screening or, if there is any concern, by laparoscopic removal of the ovaries only. Postmenopausal women with a high risk score are advised to have the tumour removed by means of total hysterectomy together with bilateral oophorectomy (removal of the ovaries).

> **Information Box 5.2g-IV**
>
> **Ovarian cysts and tumours: comments from a Chinese medicine perspective**
>
> In Chinese medicine, ovarian cysts and tumours might correspond to Blood Stagnation and/or Accumulation of Damp/Phlegm.

Cancer of the female reproductive organs

The most common cancers of the female reproductive organs are cervical cancer, endometrial cancer and ovarian cancer. A less common cancer, vulval cancer, accounts for about 3% of all cancers of the reproductive tract. The other cancers, which affect the vagina and the fallopian tubes, are very rare, and are not discussed further here.

Ovarian cancer

Ovarian cancers usually affect postmenopausal women. They have very few early symptoms, and so may not be diagnosed until they are at an advanced stage. First symptoms may include abdominal discomfort and swelling from accumulation of fluid (ascites) in the abdominal cavity. Other symptoms of advanced cancer, such as weight loss and loss of appetite, may also be present.

In rare cases there is a strong family history of postmenopausal ovarian cancer. It is argued that women who have a strong family history of ovarian cancer (i.e. those with two or more close relatives with ovarian cancer) should be offered the choice of surgical removal of the ovaries at the time of the menopause as a preventive treatment, as the lifetime risk of developing ovarian cancer is up to 40% in such people.

Treatment of the tumour depends on the exact type of the cancer, which is determined by means of examination of a biopsy. Extensive surgery is recommended for most ovarian cancers, although one rare type is known to respond well to radiotherapy. After surgery, chemotherapy including cisplatin and paclitaxel (Taxol) is given in 3-week cycles. Interestingly, cisplatin contains platinum, which Gascoigne (2001) suggests is a homeopathically appropriate treatment for ovarian tumours. Taxol is a drug, derived from the yew tree, which was first introduced by naturopaths. Nevertheless, these treatments in combination are highly toxic to the body, and side-effects are very common.

In those cases in which the cancer is confined to the ovary, surgery can be curative. However, in more than 70% of cases the cancer has extended beyond the ovary at the time of diagnosis, and in these cases the 5-year survival is less than 25%, despite the use of surgery and combination chemotherapy.

Vulval cancer

Vulval cancer is usually a cancer of elderly women. Itch is the most common presenting symptom, and may have been tolerated by the woman for some time before a diagnosis is made. Because the diagnosis is often delayed, in many cases metastatic spread to the local lymph nodes is also discovered at the time of diagnosis.

Treatment of vulval cancer discovered at an early stage is excision of the vulva. Radiotherapy is then given to the lymph nodes. If treated at this stage there is a very good chance of cure. If metastatic spread has occurred, much more tissue is removed, and also all the lymph nodes in the groin and pelvic area are excised. This 'radical' operation can be complicated by poor wound healing and persistent leg oedema.

Vulval cancer may be preceded by years by a chronic change to the vulval skin known as lichen sclerosus. In this occasionally precancerous condition, white plaques develop on the skin of the vulva. These may be asymptomatic or may cause intense itching over the course of many years. In some people, the atrophic patches of skin can contract to lead to painful fissures and dyspareunia. Lichen sclerosus can also affect the skin of the anus, and the foreskin and glans penis in men. It is treated by means of high-dose steroid creams and regular monitoring for cancerous change.

Vulval intraepithelial neoplasia (VIN) is a more sinister precancerous change of the vulva, which may not necessarily even itch. VIN describes a region of vulval skin that has actually begun to show cancerous change Like cervical intraepithelial neoplasia (CIN), VIN is associated with previous wart virus infection.

VIN appears as deficient white patches on the vulva, without the thickening characteristic of lichen sclerosus. In general, VIN is treated by means of regular monitoring, as the risk of full cancerous change is about 5%. More advanced cases are treated by means of excision, but this carries the risk of sexual dysfunction.

Cervical cancer

Cervical cancer most commonly develops close to the vaginal opening of the cervical canal. It almost exclusively affects women who have been sexually active. There is increasing evidence that prior infection with certain strains of the wart virus (human papilloma virus (HPV)) is associated with the development of cervical cancer. Over 80% of women with cervical cancer have evidence of wart virus infection (particularly type 16). It is believed that certain types of wart virus are carcinogenic because they inactivate tumour suppressor genes.

However, it is known that the virus can be found in the cervix without there being a history of sexual intercourse, and also that, in most cases, infection with the virus will not lead to cancer. One theory is that additional factors are required to allow a cancer to develop. These include smoking, and infection with other sexually transmitted agents, including the herpes virus.

Cervical cancer is one of the few cancers that can be detected by means of a fairly simple test at an early stage. This test is the cervical smear (also known as the Pap smear). In the very early stages of the cancer, the nuclei of the epithelial cells of the cervix undergo a characteristic change in shape. At this stage, the presence of these 'pre-cancer cells' does not necessarily mean that a cancer will develop. In fact it is now known that, in some women, these abnormal cells will disappear with time, and without the need for treatment. Nevertheless, this stage, known as 'pre-cancer', is believed to be a strong indicator of the development of an established cancer of the cervix within a time scale of 5–10 years.

The smear test can distinguish between different stages of progression of the pre-cancer according to the shape of the nuclei in the cells detected. These stages correspond to pathological changes in the lining cells of the cervix epithelium known as CIN 1, CIN 2 and CIN 3. It can also indicate the presence of active infection by the wart virus. Whereas wart virus infection carries a low risk of progression, CIN1 and CIN 2 indicate a progressively high risk of the development of cancer in the future. CIN 3 is considered to be highly predictive of the presence of a tiny tumour (carcinoma in situ).

However, up to 15% of pre-cancers or cancers will not be detected by a cervical smear (i.e. the test has a 15% false-negative rate). This is because it cannot be ensured that all parts of the cervix can be sampled evenly by the brush or spatula, even if the test is performed as carefully as is possible. There is also a false-positive rate in that not all women who have a positive smear test are destined to go on to develop cancer. Nevertheless, a positive test will usually be followed by more invasive investigations or treatment.

The smear test is now offered in the UK to all women above the age of 25 years at 3-year intervals, and is continued until the woman reaches age 65 years. The management of the woman depends on the result of the test.

The possible outcomes of a smear test are:

- *Normal (negative) test*: return for a smear test after 3 years.
- *Inconclusive result*: repeat the smear as soon as possible.
- *Wart virus infection detected*: repeat the smear at 6-month intervals until the smear is clear; then repeat the test annually for 2 years.
- *CIN 1*: *Either* examine the cervix by means of colposcopy, and biopsy the affected area of epithelium to exclude cancer. Destroy the affected area by means of laser, cold probes or heat probes. Repeat smear tests at 6-month intervals for 1 year, and at yearly intervals thereafter. *Or* repeat smear test at 6 months, and then proceed as above if CIN 1 is still found.
- *CIN 2 and CIN 3*: examine the cervix by means of colposcopy, and biopsy the affected area of epithelium to exclude cancer. Destroy the affected area by means of laser, cold probes or heat probes. This may involve the removal of a cone-shaped wedge of tissue surrounding the cervical canal (cone biopsy). Repeat smear tests at 6-month intervals for 1 year, and at yearly intervals thereafter.
- *Biopsy shows carcinoma in situ*: treat by means of hysterectomy. The cure rate is very high if the cancer is caught at this stage.

Although colposcopy is uncomfortable, most women who receive this treatment for CIN 1–3 will have normal smear-test results after 5 years of follow-up. This means that the progression to cancer is extremely rare, even in those women who are found to have abnormal smear results.

Nevertheless, colposcopy for CIN is uncomfortable and embarrassing for most women. It may be followed by a prolonged period of vaginal bleeding as the treated cervix recovers. Moreover, it may have been unnecessary in a proportion of women, as the CIN changes can resolve without the need for treatment. It is estimated that 40–60% of CIN 1 smears will regress to normal without treatment, but this figure is much lower for CIN 2 and CIN 3.

An abnormal smear test result is frightening and confusing for many women, who may interpret it as a diagnosis of cancer (which it is not). There is a conventional argument that the burden in terms of inconvenience and worry on the millions of women involved is very significant in terms of well-being. It is argued that, together with the financial cost of the national cervical smear programme, these negative factors are not outweighed by the benefit of the detection of cancer in a few women.

Although this is a powerful argument, it is difficult for a government to dismantle a cancer screening programme once it is in place, particularly if it is successful in detecting most of the early cases of a cancer. It is important to recognise that these are cases that are unlikely to have otherwise come to light until the cancer had reached a much more advanced stage (see below). There is no doubt that the early detection of cervical cancer by means of the cervical smear test prevents premature death, with an estimate of 5000 lives saved each year as a result of the UK screening programme alone.

Established cervical cancer

Established cervical cancer is most common in women aged 45–55 years, although there has been a recent trend for it to appear in increasing numbers of younger women. First symptoms include unexplained vaginal bleeding. Bleeding after intercourse is particularly suggestive of cervical disease.

If undetected, cervical cancer spreads outside the lining of the cervix, upwards to involve the uterus, and downwards to involve the vagina. Early involvement of lymph nodes is common, which means that cure of many cases of established cervical cancer is unlikely.

Treatment depends on the stage of the cancer. Radical hysterectomy (while preserving the ovaries) is very often a curative treatment for small cancers confined to the cervix (5-year survival 80–90%). In more advanced disease, radiotherapy will also be offered. This involves administering radiation from both an external and a vaginal source. In very advanced cancers, radiotherapy and chemotherapy will be combined, although cure is very unlikely if the cancer has spread beyond the cervix and the upper third of the vagina.

HPV immunisation

In the UK, HPV immunisation has recently been introduced as part of the routine immunisation programme for girls aged 12–14 years, that is before they are likely to have become sexually active. The HPV vaccine used in the UK has been developed to generate immunity to the wart virus types 16 and 18, which are most strongly associated with carcinogenesis.

Endometrial cancer

Endometrial cancer is most common in women aged 55–65 years. It is believed that the hormone oestrogen may be contributory in the causation of endometrial cancer, particularly if its effects on the lining of the womb are unopposed by progesterone. Oestrogen causes thickening of the lining of the womb. If progesterone is also produced by the corpus luteum, the womb lining will soften and break down in the second half of the cycle. If the corpus luteum does not develop properly, the endometrium continues to thicken, and this thickening may eventually progress to cancer. Preparations of HRT that do not contain progesterone, and polycystic ovary syndrome and obesity (which both lead to an altered balance of sex hormones in the body) are also associated with an increased risk of endometrial cancer for this reason.

The first symptoms of endometrial cancer are usually either a bloody vaginal discharge or frank bleeding. Because of the age range in which this cancer is most common, this symptom often occurs after the menopause, and is soon noticed by the patient as abnormal. This means that 75% of endometrial cancer is at a very early stage at the time of diagnosis.

The cancer tends to spread to affect a wide area of the endometrium before penetrating to the deeper levels of the muscle of the womb. The diagnosis is suggested by a thickening of the endometrium seen on an ultrasound scan, and confirmed by means of pipelle suction curettage or hysteroscopy and biopsy of the lining of the womb.

The treatment of early endometrial cancer is removal of the womb and ovaries (hysterectomy and oophorectomy). In some, but not all, early cases, the pelvic lymph nodes may also be removed. In premenopausal women who have no increased risk of recurrence, HRT may then be prescribed to prevent symptoms of oestrogen withdrawal. The 5-year survival in these cases is 80%.

If the tumour is considered to be deeply advanced into the muscle wall of the womb, radiotherapy or hormone treatment is also given. Radiotherapy has the disadvantage of causing scarring of the vagina, which may affect future intercourse.

In advanced cases, hormone treatment is given, involving a high dose of a synthetic progestogen. This inhibits growth of the tumour, but is a palliative, rather than curative, treatment.

> **Information Box 5.2g-V**
>
> **Cancer of the female reproductive system: comments from a Chinese medicine perspective**
>
> In Chinese medicine, cancer of the female reproductive organs corresponds to Blood Stagnation and/or Accumulation of Phlegm, on top of an underlying severe Deficiency of Kidney Yin/Yang.

Prolapse and displacements of the female reproductive organs

'Prolapse' is a term that is used medically to describe the movement of a part of the body away from its usual anatomical position. When applied to the female reproductive organs, prolapse refers to a descent of the womb and/or the vagina down towards the vulva. This usually results from the weakening of the surrounding supporting muscles and tissues of the pelvic floor. In contrast, a 'displacement' is a condition in which the position of the womb is abnormal in terms of angulation.

Uterovaginal prolapse

A degree of prolapse of the womb down into the vagina is common as women reach the postmenopausal years. Sometimes part of the vaginal wall alone may sag downwards, without any descent of the womb. These conditions are more likely to be severe if there is a history of recurrent or difficult childbirth. Obesity can also exacerbate the problem.

If it is only the vaginal wall that sags downwards, this is called 'first-degree prolapse'. The patient may then feel a lump in the vagina. An additional problem that occurs with prolapse of the anterior vaginal wall is that the bladder can also sag into the vagina (a cystocoele). This can increase the risk of bladder infections and incontinence. If it is the posterior vaginal wall that is weak, then either the wall of the rectum or a loop of bowel can drop into the vagina to form the 'lump' (a rectocoele), which is felt by the patient. This can cause difficulties in defaecation.

A second-degree prolapse is defined as a prolapse of the womb into the vagina so that it may actually project lower than the vulva if the woman strains in some way. The woman may have to push the 'lump' back in place with her fingers if this occurs. In a third-degree prolapse, the womb is permanently prolapsed. so that the cervix is always projecting outside the vulva.

All degrees of uterovaginal prolapse are a cause of persistent discomfort, particularly on urination of defecation. They may also increase the risk of urinary infections and incontinence.

Mild cases may improve with pelvic floor exercises, which can strengthen the supporting muscles of the pelvic floor. In more severe cases, one non-surgical approach to treatment is to insert a ring 'pessary' into the vagina. This polythene ring may be all that is required to hold the uterus in place in frail elderly women. The ring pessary requires an annual check-up, but in the interim period should need no other medical attention.

The surgical treatments for prolapse involve either hysterectomy with repair of the prolapsed vaginal wall, or an operation to hitch up the position of the womb.

Displacement of the uterus

Normally, the uterus is held in place above the vagina, so that it tips forwards. This means that in most women the cervix is felt on examination to point towards the back. In about 10% of women, the uterus tips backwards, and the cervix is felt to point forwards. This may simply be the way the uterus has developed, or can be a result of 'fixation' by the scarring that can develop in endometriosis or pelvic inflammatory disease.

In most cases, the uterus is mobile. A mobile backwards-facing (retroverted) uterus is not believed to be associated with any symptoms or with any problems in either conception or pregnancy.

Symptoms only occur when the uterus is fixed in a backwards position. In these cases, the woman may experience dyspareunia, chronic pelvic pain and backache. These symptoms may sometimes, but not always, be helped by an operation to correct the position of the uterus.

> **Information Box 5.2g-VI**
>
> **Prolapse of the uterus: comments from a Chinese medicine perspective**
>
> In Chinese medicine, prolapse of the uterus corresponds to Deficiency of Spleen and/or Kidney Qi. In particular, there is Sinking of the Spleen and/or Kidney Qi.
>
> A fixed retroverted uterus corresponds to Qi and Blood Stagnation in the pelvis.

Common surgical treatments

Hysterectomy

Hysterectomy is the procedure whereby the whole uterus is removed surgically. Ideally for the patient, this is performed by means of an incision made in the vaginal walls, as this procedure is less invasive than the alternative. However, if more extensive surgery is required, then an abdominal incision may be necessary. Hysterectomy performed by the 'transvaginal' route has a shorter recovery time than surgery by the abdominal route.

Simple hysterectomy is performed for a wide range of gynaecological conditions simply because, by removing the offending organ, it provides the ultimate 'cure'. However, it is increasingly appreciated that the long-term psychological and physical complications make it a less ideal option than it was previously believed to be. Therefore, fewer hysterectomies have been performed in recent years, and other approaches, including drug therapy and endometrial ablation, are increasingly chosen as the first treatment option.

The reasons for performing a hysterectomy include severe dysfunctional bleeding and dysmenorrhoea, symptomatic fibroids, endometriosis, prolapse of the uterus and gynaecological cancer. In all cases, the potential benefits of the operation have to be weighed against the risks. Although hysterectomy will alleviate the immediate symptoms of the underlying condition, it is a major operation. Therefore, it carries the risks that are associated with all major surgical procedures.

Most women require at least 6 weeks to return to usual activities, and may not feel right for 6 months or more. Hysterectomy is irreversible, and so will deny the woman the future option of having children. About 5–10% of women suffer from persisting bladder and bowel complications after the operation. There is also a possible link between hysterectomy and an early menopause (even if the ovaries are conserved), although some authorities dispute that such a link exists.

A range of psychological complications can follow hysterectomy. Conventionally, these are believed to relate, in part, to the way in which the woman was prepared for the operation, but may also result from the loss of an organ that plays an important, albeit subtle, role in sexual and general well-being. These include loss of sexual desire, inability to achieve orgasm, anxiety and depression.

Information Box 5.2g-VII

Hysterectomy: comments from a Chinese medicine perspective

There is no conventional recognition of the fact that loss of the uterus, particularly if after the menopause, may represent the loss of a vital organ, and thus loss of Blood and Qi, as would be recognised by a Chinese medicine practitioner. In Chinese medicine, there is a particular association between the Uterus and the Heart, as they are linked by the Bao Mai or Uterus Vessel (see Chapter 5.2a). Therefore, loss of the Uterus might be expected to lead to a degree of imbalance in the Blood and Qi of the Heart Organ.

Oophorectomy

Oophorectomy is the surgical removal of the ovaries. Oophorectomy alone may be performed for benign ovarian disease (usually on one side only). More commonly, oophorectomy is performed together with hysterectomy. The reasons for combined oophorectomy and hysterectomy include gynaecological malignancy, and any of the reasons for hysterectomy, particularly if they occur after the menopause. The ovaries are very often removed at the same time as a hysterectomy in postmenopausal women, because it is believed that after the menopause the ovaries are redundant pieces of tissue that have the potential of becoming cancerous.

The risks of the operation are similar to those of hysterectomy alone. In premenopausal women, oophorectomy will result in a premature menopause. In these cases, HRT is started at the same time as the operation, to prevent the dramatic effects of the sudden withdrawal of oestrogen, including loss of bone density (osteoporosis) that would otherwise occur.

Repair of vaginal prolapse

The operation that is performed to treat vaginal prolapse is called a 'vaginal repair'. In this operation, a portion of the lax vaginal wall is removed, and the prolapsed bladder wall or bowel is encouraged to return to the correct anatomical position.

These operations have been shown in long-term surgical studies to reduce the serious symptoms of incontinence. However, more recent research has shown that women's satisfaction with these operations is less than that suggested by the results reported from the surgical studies. This is possibly because many women say that they would have preferred to put up with a certain level of incontinence rather than to have gone through the trauma of vaginal surgery, even if it has resulted in a degree of improvement in the incontinence.

A vaginal repair (colporrhaphy) may be all that is needed to treat cystocoele or a rectocoele. In this operation the vaginal wall is opened and the fibrous tissue behind strengthened to prevent future prolapse of the bladder or rectum.

Uterine prolapse can be treated by means of hysterectomy and vaginal repair, but this operation is not suitable for those women who wish to have children in the future. There is an alternative type of operation in which the cervix is excised, and the uterus is held in place by means of hitching it to natural ligaments, as well repairing any additional laxity of the vaginal walls (this operation is known as the 'Manchester repair'). Although fertility is preserved, the excision of the cervix means that the chances of conception are reduced by this operation. There is also a risk of recurrence of the prolapse. Less drastic surgical techniques involve using a mesh to hitch up the vagina or uterus to fixed structures such as the pelvic ligaments or sacral bone. As with the vaginal repair, symptoms of incontinence and discomfort may improve after these operations, but may not be matched by an equivalent improvement in the woman's satisfaction with the outcome.

The red flags of the structural disorders of the female reproductive system

Some women with structural disorders of the reproductive system will benefit from referral to a conventional doctor for assessment and/or treatment. Red flags are those symptoms and signs that indicate that referral is to be considered. The red flags of the structural disorders of the female reproductive system are described in Table 5.2g-I. This table forms part of the Red Flag summary of Chapter 6.2b. This table forms part of the summary on red flags given in Appendix III, which also gives advice on the degree of urgency of referral for each of the red flag conditions listed.

Table 5.2g-I Red Flags 36 – structural disorders of the reproductive system

Red Flag	Description	Reasoning
36.1	**Primary amenorrhoea**: after age 16 years	Refer any woman for investigation who has not achieved first menstruation by age 16 years. If secondary sexual characteristics are developing normally, this might suggest an imperforate hymen or, rarely, an intersex disorder
36.2	**Menorrhagia**: with features of **severe anaemia** (tiredness, breathlessness, palpitations on exertion)	Menorrhagia (heavy periods) can be the sole cause of significant anaemia, and merits prompt referral for investigation and treatment of the cause. Menorrhagia may result from fibroids, endometriosis or an ovarian cyst
36.3	**Postmenopausal bleeding**: any unexplained bleeding after the menopause	Predictable bleeding after the menopause is normal with HRT preparations. Otherwise it is a red flag for uterine or cervical tumour. Refer for further investigation
36.4	**Metrorrhagia**: bleeding between periods that has no regular pattern, This including postcoital bleeding (bleeding after intercourse)	Irregular periods are common, but bleeding that seems to fall outside the normal confines of a 2–5 day menstrual bleed might rarely signify a uterine or cervical tumour. Refer for further investigation if this happens on more than three occasions
36.5	**Pelvic pain** or **deep pain during intercourse**	Refer if not responding to your treatment (may suggest pelvic inflammatory disease, but also endometriosis, fibroids or ovarian cysts)
36.6	**Abdominal swelling: discrete mass** in the suprapubic or inguinal region	Refer if a mass is felt (possible fibroids, ovarian cyst, tumour, pregnancy)
36.7	**Abdominal swelling: generalised**	Refer if the swelling is diffuse and increasing over days to weeks (may be fluid accumulation from a tumour (ascites)). If the patient is lying on her back, an abdomen with accumulated fluid will be dull to percussion in the flanks and resonant in the central region only
36.8	**Vulval itch or vaginal discharge** in postmenopausal women	Refer if these are persistent in premenopausal women and at any time if they occur in a postmenopausal women (usually benign, but may result from cancer of the vulva, cervix or endometrium)
36.9	**Lump in vulva**	This is usually benign (Bartholin's or sebaceous cyst) but refer to exclude vulval carcinoma or warts
36.10	**Lump in testicle/scrotum**	Most scrotal lumps are benign (varicocoele sebaceous cyst), but rarely can be testicular cancer. Refer for further investigation
36.11	Acute or chronic **testicular pain**: radiates to the groin, scrotum or lower abdomen	Refer any sudden onset of severe testicular pain (radiates to the groin, scrotum or low abdomen). This could signify inflammation of the testicle (orchitis) or a twist of the testicle (torsion). If the pain is very intense (with collapse and vomiting) refer as an emergency
36.12	Chronic dull **testicular pain**: radiates to the groin, scrotum or lower abdomen	If the pain is more of a long-lived discomfort, this could either be chronic epididymitis or varicocoele, and merits a medical examination and further tests
36.13	**Precocious puberty**: secondary sexual characteristics before the age of 8 years in girls and 9 years on boys	Refer if secondary sexual characteristics begin to appear before the age of 8 years in girls and 9 years in boys so that an endocrine cause can be excluded
36.14	**Delayed puberty**: secondary sexual characteristics not apparent by the age of 15 years in girls and 16 years in boys	Refer if secondary sexual characteristics have not started to appear by the age of 15 years in girls and 16 years in boys. Refer if menstruation has not begun by the time of a girl's 16th birthday (primary amenorrhoea)

Self-test 5.2g

Structural disorders of the ovaries, uterus and vagina

1. You are treating a 25-year-old woman for anxiety. In her most recent consultation she is obviously more anxious than normal. She explains that she has to go for a repeat cervical smear test within the next few months because her previous test has showed abnormal changes. She is in a long-term relationship and is using a barrier method of contraception. What sort of facts might you give her to allay her anxiety about her smear test result?
2. A 40-year-old patient has become aware of a lump in her abdomen. She hopes that acupuncture can help this lump to disappear. She does not believe that the lump is cancerous as it has been the same size for at least 2 years. She is otherwise well, and her periods are normal. When you examine her abdomen, there is a smooth, slightly mobile mass in the right iliac fossa (right lower quadrant of the abdomen). It is not tender, but is large. You estimate that it is about 20 centimetres in diameter. What are the possible gynaecological diagnoses? Would you refer this woman for further investigation?
3. An elderly patient describes how a lump 'comes down' when she goes to the toilet. When you question her, she describes a feeling of fullness in her vagina, which is there all the time but gets worse when she strains at the toilet or when she coughs. She has not told her GP about it because she is embarrassed. Nevertheless, she is a frequent visitor to her GP because she has recurrent urinary infections. What do you think is the cause of this woman's symptoms? Would you refer this patient?

Answers

1. The first thing you could say is that an abnormal smear test result is very common, and that usually it does not mean that there is a serious problem. The fact that the smear test is to be repeated within a few months suggests that either wart virus infection or CIN 1 changes have been detected.
   You can explain that wart virus infection is not necessarily a result of contact with an infected partner, and in most cases is not a precursor to cancer. If this is the abnormality, then repeat smear tests at 6-month intervals are all that will be required. If the abnormality suggests CIN 1, you might explain that this is a common cervical abnormality, which may progress to cancer if unchecked. Nevertheless, over half the women with this abnormality would return to having normal smear-test results even without treatment. Treatment for persistent CIN 1 requires a colposcopy. In most women the cervix returns to normal after colposcopy.
   You might summarise that, either way, the smear test result does not indicate cancer, but that treatment with colposcopy may be offered in the future to prevent the possibility of cancer developing.
2. The most likely diagnosis is that this patient has a uterine fibroid. A less likely, but possible, diagnosis is a benign ovarian tumour. The long history is not suggestive of cancer, but this cannot be ruled out. The safest course to follow is to advise the patient to see her GP so that a pelvic ultrasound examination can be performed. This non-invasive investigation will exclude the outside possibility of cancer.
3. The history suggests uterovaginal prolapse. This may well be the cause of this woman's recurrent urinary problems. As recurrent urinary infections are potentially damaging to the kidneys, it would be advisable to refer this patient. Treatment of the prolapse may then reduce the pressure on the bladder and urethra, and so could lessen the risk of urinary infection. You could reassure the patient that the treatment need not necessarily be surgical. A ring pessary alone may be sufficient to resolve both the discomfort and the urinary symptoms.

5.3

Pregnancy and childbirth

Chapter 5.3a The physiology of pregnancy and childbirth

LEARNING POINTS

At the end of this chapter you will:

- understand the physiology of conception
- be able to recognise the stages of development of the embryo/fetus
- be able to describe the physiological changes of pregnancy
- be able to describe the changes that occur in normal labour
- be able to describe the physiological changes of the postnatal period (the puerperium).

Estimated time for chapter: 140 minutes.

Introduction

Section 5.2 was dedicated to the roles of the reproductive system of both the male and the female, including the production of gametes, and the provision of an environment in which these gametes can meet to produce a zygote. This chapter explores what happens following the time of conception, which is when the gametes meet, and follows the stages of development of the embryo and fetus, together with the physiological changes that occur in the mother at this time. The chapter concludes with a description of the physiology of childbirth and of the puerperium, which is the 6-week period that follows childbirth, during which time the mother's body begins to return to its pre-pregnant state.

The formation of the embryo

Conception

'Conception' is the term used to describe the fusion of one of the millions of spermatozoa in the ejaculated sperm with the ovum, so forming a fertilised egg (zygote). In natural conception this fusion most commonly occurs in one of the fallopian tubes, within a few hours of ovulation. It is estimated that the ovum is viable for no more than 48 hours. This provides the spermatozoa with a relatively short window of opportunity to meet up with the ovum in any one menstrual cycle.

A spermatozoon reaches the fallopian tube from the vagina by means of the waving action of its flagellum (the tail-like process that projects from its cell membrane). The energy required for this feat of long-distance swimming is derived from nutrients contained in the seminal fluid (see Q5.3a-1).

The exact timing of the fertile period is unpredictable, as it depends on the timing of ovulation, which is variable even for women with regular menstrual cycles. It is recognised that women with regular cycles can ovulate earlier than day 7 and later than day 21 in a 28-day cycle. This, of course, has implications for the 'natural family planning' methods that can be used either to plan conception or to prevent pregnancy. This is why recognition of the changes in the consistency of cervical mucus is so important for the success of these methods.

Out of the millions of spermatozoa that are ejaculated, only a few hundred reach the fallopian tubes. When these spermatozoa reach the ovum, only one will be permitted to penetrate the cell membrane of the ovum. As soon as penetration has occurred, there is a change in the cell membrane that prevents the remaining spermatozoa from attaching (Figure 5.3a-I). The nuclei of the male and female gametes contain only 23 single chromosomes, rather than 23 pairs. After fusion of the ovum and sperm, their nuclei fuse to form 23 pairs of chromosomes, giving a combination of genes which is totally unique to that zygote. Within a few hours this new nucleus divides, and the zygote begins to form into the ball of cells known as the embryo.

Implantation

The tiny ball of cells of the embryo is propelled down the fallopian tube, and thence into the uterine cavity by means of the wave-like action of the ciliary epithelium of the fallopian tube. As the embryo continues to divide, a fluid-filled

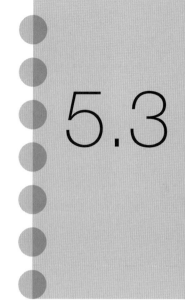

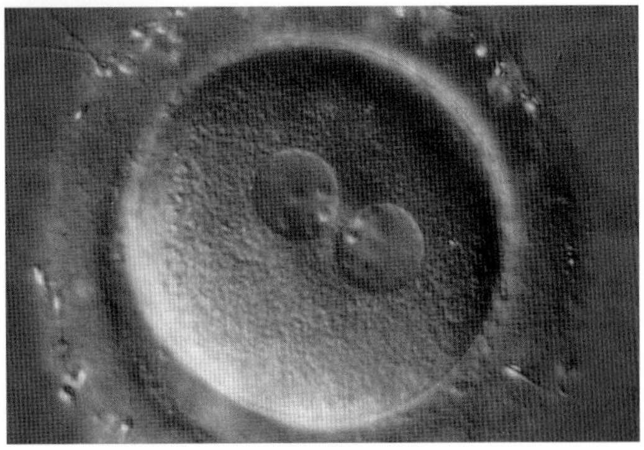

Figure 5.3a-I • A recently fertilised ovum after a single division of the nucleus • Spermatozoa that did not manage to penetrate the egg can be seen outside the cell membrane.

cavity forms in its middle. By about 7 days after fertilisation, the outer layer of the developing embryo has differentiated into cells that can penetrate deeply into the endometrial lining. It is these cells that will form the placenta. Thcsc outer cells have proteins on their surface which can 'recognise' and attach to the endometrial lining. This attachment occurs 7–10 days after conception. After attachment, these outermost embryonic cells release a hormone known as human chorionic gonadotrophin (HCG) into the bloodstream of the mother. This hormone signals to the corpus luteum in the ovary that pregnancy has occurred, and thus triggers the chain of physiological effects that are indicators to the mother of the start of pregnancy.

It is very likely that it is failure in implantation that is the reason for infertility in those couples who are shown by investigations to have no obvious physical abnormality. In these couples, despite healthy looking sperm and normal ovulation, pregnancies do not occur. Subtle defects in the formation of the corpus luteum may lead to a poorly developed endometrium in the second half of the menstrual cycle. A poorly developed endometrium may either prevent implantation from occurring at all, or may be the cause of a very early miscarriage. This problem can result from an imbalance in the production of the pituitary hormones, follicle-stimulating hormone (FSH) and luteinising hormone (LH), which in turn may be influenced by variables such as emotional stress, poor diet and tiredness.

Development of the embryo after implantation

After implantation, the identical cells forming this initially tiny hollow ball continue to multiply and differentiate. 'Differentiation' is the term given to the process whereby cells with an identical set of chromosomes become specialised to form all the different tissues of the body. At implantation, the outer portion of this ball of cells forms into the embryonic part of the placenta. Within the ensuing 14 weeks tiny blood vessels form within this tissue. This fleshy mass encourages a reciprocal development of the endometrial lining into which it penetrates. A very rich blood supply forms as this tissue develops, in which maternal and embryonic blood vessels run very close to one another. This permits an exchange of oxygen and nutrients from the mother's blood to that of the embryo, but without any mixing of the two blood supplies. However, drugs and toxins are able to cross this boundary between the mother and the embryo. It is this combination of maternal and embryonic tissue that is destined to form the placenta. The placenta will be the source of nourishment for the baby until the time of delivery.

Another portion of the hollow ball of embryonic cells is destined to become the embryo itself. This portion develops within the fluid-filled cavity. By 2 weeks there is a definite lengthening of this mass of cells, so forming the primitive spinal cord. By 3 weeks a primitive heart has formed, with vessels connecting to those of the placenta. By 4 weeks a tube has formed from top to bottom, which will later develop into the gastrointestinal system, and by 6 weeks the first features of the kidneys and sex organs have appeared. By 7 weeks all the important organs have appeared. By this time there is a distinct form to the head, with bumps for the nose and ears, and also to the limbs, with tiny buds for the fingers and toes (Figure 5.3a-II).

The sac of fluid within which the embryo develops is called the 'amniotic sac', and the fluid within this sac is called 'amniotic fluid'. The embryo is suspended in the fluid by a bridge of tissue known as the 'umbilical cord'. The blood vessels that link the embryo to the placental blood supply pass through the umbilical cord. The amniotic fluid serves as a protective space for the fetus, which, until the very last weeks of pregnancy, can permit unrestricted movement of the developing limbs. This fluid serves to keep the skin moist and nourished, and also is a space into which the first urine is excreted.

It is important to be clear that the stage of pregnancy (gestation) is dated in a different way to the actual age of

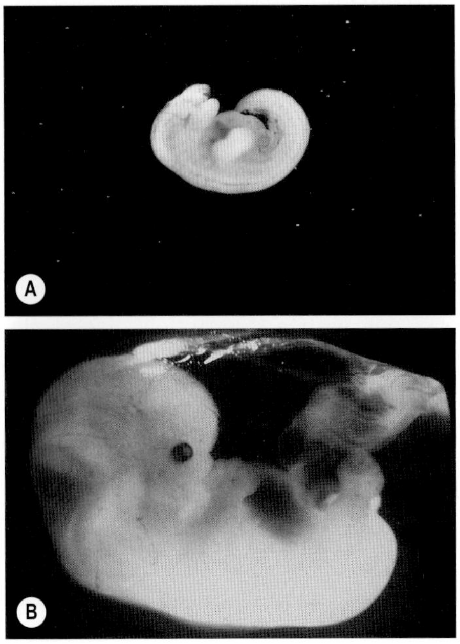

Figure 5.3a-II • The development of the embryo at (a) 6 weeks and (b) 9 weeks of gestation.

the embryo from the time of conception. 'Gestation' is the term used to describe the time elapsed since the date of the last menstrual period. This is, of course, on average 2 weeks longer than the actual time after conception. For example, in a woman who is '8 weeks pregnant', the embryo is in fact only 6 weeks old (see Q5.3a-2).

Many women will be unaware of the possibility of pregnancy for the first 8 weeks of gestation, and this is particularly the case for those women who have a light bleed at 4 weeks, despite the fact that they are pregnant. The embryo is particularly vulnerable to nutritional deficiencies, drugs and toxins in this short time. Therefore, the only way by which a woman can ensure optimum health for her developing baby is to start making lifestyle changes before she falls pregnant. This is the foundation of the practice of giving 'preconceptual advice' to couples who are planning to have a baby. The importance of giving preconceptual advice is emphasised in both conventional and alternative practice.

Preconceptual advice

From a conventional medical perspective, a couple planning to conceive should be aware that all drugs and toxins might affect the developing embryo. They will be advised to stop smoking and to avoid alcohol and other recreational drugs. A healthy diet is advised. Ideally, if possible, all therapeutic drugs should be avoided for a few weeks before conception. Women who have been taking the contraceptive pill might be advised to stop this form of contraception for at least 3 months before trying to conceive. The only nutritional supplement that is routinely advised is the vitamin folic acid. Deficiency of dietary folic acid is strongly linked with an increased incidence of spinal cord defects, including spina bifida. The advice is to take a daily supplement of this vitamin from the time of trying to conceive to at least 20 weeks of gestation. Alternative practitioners may advise a wide range of other nutritional supplements, including zinc, manganese and selenium.

Development of the fetus to the time of delivery

From about 10 weeks of gestation the embryo is termed a 'fetus'. The fetus has primitive limbs and facial features, and all the rudimentary organs in place. At this time the fetus is about 2.5 centimetres in length.

Nourishment of the fetus

The fetus obtains the nutrients it requires from the mother's circulation. It is generally believed in conventional medicine that, except in cases of extreme starvation, the fetus can obtain all it needs from the mother's bloodstream, and so will not necessarily suffer if the mother cannot have a good diet (e.g. in the case of morning sickness). Deficiency of folic acid in the maternal diet is the obvious exception to this. This is not the view held in Chinese medicine, in which the precise content of the diet of the pregnant woman is believed to have an important bearing on the health of the developing organs of the fetus.

However, the mother may suffer as her nutrients are being diverted to nourish the developing fetus and support the growth of the placenta. Deficiencies of iron and calcium are well recognised to affect women in pregnancy. These can than lead to anaemia and weak teeth. It is very likely that many more vitamin and mineral deficiencies can occur, which may partly explain the specific food cravings that many women experience during pregnancy. Although some of the foods craved may be bizarre in nature, the most common cravings are for fruit juice and dairy products, indicating a need to replace vitamins such as vitamin C and minerals such as calcium.

The main source of energy for the fetus is glucose. Glucose is also used to make the fats required by the fetus. Excessive glucose, a problem which occurs in maternal diabetes, will stimulate growth and cause excessive fat formation, and so can lead to an overlarge baby. Maternal amino acids are used to make the proteins required to build the structure of the tissues of the fetus. The wastes that the fetus produces are removed by the placenta into the maternal blood.

The fetal circulation

The circulation of the fetus has some important differences to that of a newborn baby. The blood enters the fetus through the umbilical cord, and first passes through the liver. It then is pumped through the heart, and thence to the rest of the body, before being redirected out through the umbilical cord. One major difference in this circulatory pattern is that relatively little blood is passed through the lungs, which in the fetus are filled with fluid, and are not a source of oxygen. To enable this circulation pattern to occur, the fetal heart retains a hole in its central wall, which permits the exchange of blood between the right and the left sides of the heart.

At birth, the lungs are expanded suddenly with the baby's first cry. This expansion diverts a lot of blood into the vessels of the lungs for the first time. This has the remarkable effect of altering the pressure of blood within the rest of the fetal circulation so that the 'hole' in the heart is closed by means of a flap of tissue, and the blood flow in the umbilicus diminishes markedly. Within a matter of seconds the whole pattern of blood flow in the fetus is transformed. Within a few minutes the pulsation of blood in the umbilical cord stops, and the cord can be tied off. What used to be the life source for the fetus now becomes a redundant stump, commonly known as the 'tummy button'.

The fetal digestive system

The gastrointestinal tract is relatively quiet in the fetus. As the fetus matures, it swallows amniotic fluid, which is then absorbed through the intestines and then excreted back into amniotic fluid cavity by the kidneys. By the end of pregnancy the intestines of the fetus contain a black sticky form of faeces called meconium. This is composed largely of epithelial cells that have been shed from the growing intestinal lining.

The fetal lungs

The fluid in the developing fetal lungs is in direct communication with the amniotic fluid through the mouth and nose. A circulation of this fluid is maintained by the breathing movements that occur with increasing regularity in the developing fetus. As the fetus reaches full maturity, the lungs secrete an oily substance, called 'surfactant', into the alveoli. After birth, surfactant enables the newly expanded air spaces to remain in their patent state. In premature babies, insufficient surfactant can result in a tendency for the alveoli to collapse. Deficiency of surfactant is one of the causes of the severe respiratory problems that can affect premature babies.

The fetal immune system

The immune system of the fetus begins to develop by week 20 of pregnancy. After this time the fetus is able to produce its own antibodies. Nevertheless, this response is not fully mature until some weeks after birth. The fetus gains extra protection from infection in the womb by maternal antibodies, which are able to cross the placenta. These antibodies have a life of a few weeks, and so continue to protect the newborn for a couple of months or so after the birth.

The progression of all the changes that occur in the fetus during its development are summarised in Table 5.3a-I (see Q5.3a-3).

Table 5.3a-I The stages in the development of the fetus

Age of gestation	Length of fetus	Stage of development of fetus
14 weeks	6 cm	All organs present in rudimentary form Limbs, muscles and bones all formed, baby has free movement. Sex organs developed Heartbeat strong and fast
15–22 weeks	16 cm	Hair, eyebrows, fingernails and fingerprint all formed; eyelids remain closed Baby's movement can be felt by mother
23–30 weeks	24 cm	Movement is vigorous, baby can respond to touch and sound Baby can swallow, may get hiccups Urine is formed by the kidneys Eyelids open from time to time At 28 weeks the baby has a good chance of survival if born prematurely
31–40 weeks		Fat is laid down beneath the skin of the baby, making it plump and less wrinkly At 34 weeks most babies find a head-down position, and movements become more restricted due to lack of space

The physiological changes of pregnancy

The hormones of pregnancy

The developing embryo secretes the hormone HCG into the endometrium very soon after implantation. This means that at about day 21 after the last menstrual cycle the ovaries receive a signal that implantation has occurred. HCG stimulates the corpus luteum to continue to produce oestrogen and progesterone. Without this stimulus, the corpus luteum would degenerate rapidly, and the resulting drop in oestrogen and progesterone would lead to menstruation within a few days.

HCG is produced in large amounts during the first third (trimester) of the pregnancy. It is this hormone that can be detected from a sample of the mother's urine and is used as the means of testing for pregnancy. A simple HCG test, which can be bought in the UK at a chemist, can indicate pregnancy even earlier than week 6 of gestation (2 weeks after the 'missed period').

Oestrogen is secreted in increasing amounts throughout pregnancy. This initially is produced by the corpus luteum, but is later produced by the placenta. Oestrogen brings about the increased fleshiness that is characteristic of pregnancy. The cervix becomes swollen and soft, and the breasts and nipples enlarge. Oestrogen also stimulates the increased vaginal discharge that is a normal feature of pregnancy. It also promotes an increased blood supply to all tissues. The amount of blood pumped through the heart increases, and the blood vessels dilate. In healthy pregnancies this results in a drop in the blood pressure. The healthy 'glow' commonly seen in middle to late pregnancy is a result of the effect of oestrogen on the blood supply to the skin.

Like oestrogen, progesterone is also produced initially by the corpus luteum, and then by the placenta. One important action of progesterone is to cause muscle and ligamentous relaxation. This effect is very marked on the muscular wall of the uterus, but excessive relaxation of the smooth muscle of the oesophageal sphincter, the bowel and the ureters may also occur. This effect of progesterone can result in some of the most common minor complications of pregnancy, including heartburn, constipation and tendency to urinary infections. Relaxation of the ligaments of the pelvis and lower back is important to allow for the passage of the baby during labour. However, this can lead to some of the painful musculoskeletal conditions of pregnancy, such as low backache, sacroiliac strain and pain in the symphysis pubis. Progesterone also tends to increase the body temperature. The placidity of pregnancy is attributed to a calming effect of progesterone on the brain.

Other hormones important in pregnancy include prolactin from the pituitary gland, adrenal corticosteroids and thyroid hormones. Prolactin stimulates the development of the milk-producing glands within the breast in the last 10 weeks of pregnancy. The adrenal corticosteroids are important to help the body deal with the demands of pregnancy, but in excess may lead to weight gain, high blood sugar and high blood pressure. The thyroid hormones play a role in the regulation of increased growth. Under the influence of oestrogen, the thyroid gland may enlarge to twice its normal size. Occasionally, if this enlargement is excessive, a goitre may develop.

The first symptoms of pregnancy

The first symptoms of pregnancy may be felt as early as the first 2 weeks after conception. Some women are aware of a different feeling even before the first missed period, and some may experience nausea or breast tingling at this early stage. It is more usual that symptoms are experienced at around week 6 of gestation. The most common include breast tingling or tenderness, nausea, and sensitivity to certain smells or tastes. The missed period is not a universal experience. Some women may have a painless bleed at 4 weeks, and even at 8 weeks of gestation, despite having a healthy pregnancy. As well as being a potential source of great anxiety, this form of bleeding can very much confuse the dating of the pregnancy, as the estimate of the length of the gestation normally relies on the date of the last menstrual period.

The effects of the enlarging uterus

As the embryo develops into a rapidly growing fetus, the uterus and the placenta enlarge to accommodate the growth and increasing nutritional requirements. At about 12 weeks of gestation, the amniotic sac is 10 centimetres in diameter and the uterus can be felt just above the pubic bone. At 20 weeks of gestation, the top of the uterus is at the level of the umbilicus, and by 36 weeks the uterus has reached the level of the xiphisternum. Amazingly, the remaining abdominal contents continue to function relatively normally, despite their increasingly cramped conditions.

However, certain problems can arise from the compression of the abdominal organs. In particular, compression of the abdominal aorta can lead to discomfort and faintness when lying supine (on the back) in late pregnancy. Restriction of the free flow of blood in the deep pelvic veins can contribute to the development of varicose veins, haemorrhoids and ankle swelling. Heartburn can be very severe in late pregnancy, as the uterus presses on the stomach from below. Occasionally, nerve compression can cause areas of pain and tingling. The most common site for this problem is down the front of the thigh, a result of the compression of a nerve which runs down from the crease of the groin. Rapid growth of the uterus can also lead to stretch marks and itching of the skin of the abdomen. Both these problems are compounded by the excessive weight gain that can complicate some pregnancies.

Changes in the uterus, cervix and vagina

The uterine muscle fibres lengthen markedly during pregnancy, thus allowing for the elongation of the uterus. The natural tendency for these fibres to contract becomes more pronounced. Mild contractions of the uterus start to occur from very early in pregnancy. Some, but not all, women become aware of these contractions, known as 'Braxton–Hicks contractions' from about 20 weeks of pregnancy. The sensation is usually described as a painless tightening of the abdomen, which lasts for a few seconds. Some women do describe the sensation as painful, akin to period cramps, and for this reason, Braxton–Hicks contractions sometimes can be confused with the onset of labour. Braxton–Hicks contractions increase in frequency and intensity as the time for the onset of labour approaches.

During pregnancy, the cervix and vagina respond to the increased levels of oestrogen and progesterone. The cervix becomes softer in consistency, a change that can be detected by a skilled examiner at as early as 8 weeks of gestation. This change occurs in preparation for the dilatation that has to occur during the first stage of labour. The vaginal walls also change in consistency to allow for the expansion that will be necessary to allow the birth of the baby. In addition, an odourless vaginal discharge is produced. This normal feature of pregnancy can be distressing for those women who are unprepared for its occurrence.

Changes in the maternal circulation

As pregnancy progresses, the blood vessels of the mother dilate, and an increased volume of blood circulates through them. These changes are to accommodate the increased requirements of the blood vessels in the placenta. Although the actual number of red blood cells is increased in a pregnant woman, usually the concentration of haemoglobin within them is slightly less than in the non-pregnant state. This can mean that a blood test will indicate anaemia. If this finding is mild, it need not be treated. However, many women will be offered treatment with iron tablets if the anaemia is severe, or if symptoms such as tiredness or dizziness develop.

The heart works much harder in pregnancy, as it has to pump up to 50% more blood than usual. The pulse is recognised to become more full and rapid in pregnancy, and this is accompanied by feelings of warmth. The 'slipperiness' that is a characteristic of pregnancy to a Chinese medicine practitioner is probably equivalent to this conventionally recognised pulse change.

Many women become more aware of palpitations in pregnancy. Conventionally, this symptom is not usually considered to be serious.

Changes in the respiratory, urinary and digestive systems

After about week 30 of pregnancy, the downward movement of the diaphragm becomes more restricted, and this is compensated for by an increased expansion of the ribcage during breathing. Some women will easily become breathless on exertion as this change develops.

The kidneys are more active in pregnancy, as they have to deal with the extra waste products coming from the fetus. More urine is produced. The muscles of the urinary system become more relaxed under the influence of progesterone. As previously mentioned, this can lead to an increased tendency to bladder infections. The risk of these infections spreading to involve the kidneys (pyelonephritis) is also increased in pregnancy.

The most common changes to affect the digestive system are spongy gums, heartburn and constipation. All these changes are results of the effect of progesterone. There is also an increased tendency to gum disease (gingivitis). For this reason, women are encouraged to make at least one visit to the dentist during pregnancy.

Weight gain

By the end of pregnancy, the fetus and the placenta together should weigh just over 4 kilograms. It is also normal for the mother to put on some weight as uterine muscle and breast tissue develop, and also as fat stores are laid down around the abdomen, buttocks and thighs. These fat stores will be drawn on in the first few months after birth as the mother breastfeeds. Adding up these different elements, the ideal weight gain in pregnancy is estimated to be around 11 kilograms.

However, there can be enormous variations around this ideal. Sometimes this can be because the woman herself either loses or gains weight during the pregnancy. Less commonly, abnormal weight gain may be an indication of poor fetal or placental growth, or, conversely, excessive accumulation of amniotic fluid. The most common problem with weight gain in pregnancy is that too much fat is laid down. The current advice is that a pregnant woman should eat a normal nutritious diet, and should not 'eat for two'.

Psychological changes in pregnancy

Ideally, the psychological changes of pregnancy are positive ones. Pregnant women often report feeling calm and happy in the later stages of pregnancy, an experience attributed to the effects of progesterone. However, 5–10% of women develop depression during their pregnancy. This depression seems to be more common in first pregnancies, and in women who have poor social support. Often in such cases, there may be deep unaddressed fears about the labour, giving birth to a malformed child, or coping with caring for a baby. Also, many women grieve for the loss of their figure and freedom. Women who suffer from depression in pregnancy are more likely to develop postnatal depression (see Q5.3a-4).

> **Information Box 5.3a-I**
>
> **Pregnancy: comments from a Chinese medicine perspective**
>
> According to Chinese medicine, after conception the Blood and Yin associated with menstruation accumulate in the Chong and Ren Channels to nourish the developing fetus. As a consequence, the mother becomes relatively Blood and Yin Deficient, and her Yang becomes relatively Hyperactive. This means that Heat can easily accumulate during pregnancy.
>
> The Spleen and the Kidneys are particularly important in supporting the nourishment and growth of the fetus, and so there may be a tendency to Deficiency of Spleen and Stomach Qi, with Accumulation of Damp and also Deficiency of Kidney Qi. The Liver is responsible for the smooth flow of Qi. As pregnancy is a time of accumulation of the Vital Substances in the lower Jiao, Liver Qi can easily Stagnate.
>
> All these syndromes are more likely in those women who have a pre-existing imbalance in one or more of these Organ functions. Most of the complications of pregnancy can be interpreted from a Chinese medicine perspective as consequences of these common underlying syndromes.

The physiology of childbirth

All the physiological changes of pregnancy so far described are gradual in development. In a healthy pregnancy, most women adjust well to these changes as they progress over the 40 weeks of gestation. The onset of labour is quite different. All of a sudden the woman's body is thrown into a series of profound changes, which escalate rapidly and culminate in the birth of the baby and the placenta, usually within a timescale of 24 hours.

The initiation of labour

The precise trigger for the onset of labour is not clearly understood. It is known that the uterus becomes more sensitive to the pituitary hormone oxytocin during late pregnancy. It is likely that a surge in the release of oxytocin from the pituitary actually brings about the relentless wave of contractions that are characteristic of established labour. It may be that it is a hormonal factor released from the maturing fetus, such as an adrenal corticosteroid, that actually stimulates this surge. It is recognised that external factors, such as shock, injury and fever, can stimulate early labour, and anxiety and exhaustion can delay the progression of labour.

As the time for labour approaches, the Braxton–Hicks contractions of the uterus become more frequent. Usually, at about 2 weeks before the onset of labour, the head of the baby drops into the bowl of the pelvis. This descent, known as 'engagement', often brings about a feeling of more comfort in the diaphragmatic area, as more space is created. In some pregnancies, engagement does not occur until after the onset of labour. In a few of these, this may be because the baby is not in the correct head-down, posterior-facing position.

Established labour is characterised by the onset of regular painful contractions that cause the tiny canal of the cervix to start to widen (dilate). In many women this transition between Braxton–Hicks contractions and labour contractions is not clear-cut. In these women, there may be a period of a few days in which the contractions are mildly painful and regular from time to time. Vaginal examination during this time will show that the cervix has not yet started to dilate. As cervical dilatation begins, a plug of mucus is released, which appears as an odourless blood-stained discharge called a 'show'.

Healthy established labour involves regular contractions, which gradually become more frequent and sustained. A typical pattern is that the contractions start to occur at intervals of over 15 minutes and last for only a few seconds. As the cervix gradually dilates, the interval between contractions shortens to less than 5 minutes, and the pain of the contraction lasts for 1–2 minutes. As this progression occurs, the contractions become more painful. Initially, the woman will be able to carry on usual activities between the contractions. The pain at this stage is often compared to that of period cramps. It is usually felt in the lower abdomen and low back.

In some women, the amniotic sac ruptures at this early stage, leading to a trickle or a gush of clear fluid. Occasionally, this rupture occurs before the onset of labour. This can then stimulate the onset of labour. If labour does not start within 24 hours of the 'breaking of the waters', there is a potential risk of infection, and so labour may have to be induced medically.

The first stage of labour

Labour is described in terms of three stages. The show and the onset of regular painful contractions herald the first stage of labour. This first stage is the part of labour in which the canal of the cervix dilates to a diameter of about 10 centimetres. In this stage there is only a small downward movement of the baby.

In first pregnancies, a normal first stage can last up to 36 hours, although less than 24 hours is more usual. For many women who have a prolonged first stage, for much of this period the initial dilatation of the cervix is slow and the contractions are bearable. Usually, it is only in the later part of the first stage that the contractions become very strong. In subsequent pregnancies the first stage lasts only a few hours, and the progression to very strong contractions is more rapid.

As the first stage of labour becomes established, the pain of the contractions increases markedly. As the cervix dilates to greater than 5 centimetres, the pain causes the woman to go inward, stop talking and lose eye contact with the birth attendants. The respite between the contractions shortens down to only a few seconds as the contractions last for longer and become more frequent. If this painful stage is prolonged, the woman can become exhausted. For this reason, it is now common practice to encourage the woman to continue to eat light starchy food in the early part of the first stage of labour. Glucose drinks are very often recommended by midwives in the later part of the first stage, to sustain the woman as she goes through this 'marathon'.

The transition between the first and second stages of labour

The transition time is when the cervix reaches its maximal dilatation. It is at this time that contractions are at their most painful. Very often, the woman feels totally overwhelmed by what she is experiencing. Some women experience great fear or panic, believing that they are about to die. Other women become aggressive and abusive. Some may insist that they can no longer cope with the pain, and might demand medical pain relief. However, these behaviours are often signs that labour is progressing well. This transitional time usually lasts less than 30 minutes.

Occasionally, the woman has a desire to push during the transitional stage. If this occurs, she will be advised by the midwife to avoid pushing, until it is certain that the cervix is fully dilated. This is because a premature onset of pushing can cause the cervix to tear.

It is usually around the time of transition that the waters break if they have not done so already.

The second stage of labour

The second stage of labour is the stage in which contractions of the uterus are combined with the woman voluntarily pushing her abdominal muscles. This combined action forces the baby downwards through the pelvic canal. The second stage ends with the birth of the baby. It should last no more than 2 hours.

The second stage is characterised by the experience of the urge to push. Generally, the contractions are very frequent and strong, but may be more bearable than in the first stage. This means that if a woman can be supported through the transition without resort to medical pain relief, she may not need to request it for the second stage.

The forceful downward contractions encourage the head of the baby to descend down the pelvic canal, usually with the face directed backwards. The mother begins to feel an intense pressure as the head enters the vagina. Very commonly, women panic at this stage, fearing that they are going to open their bowels. This is because the feeling of fullness can also be sensed in the rectum. The downwards descent of the head can be seen by the birth attendant a few contractions before it is actually delivered.

Once the head has reached the perineum, the surrounding tissues become very tightly stretched. At this point the woman feels an excruciating 'bursting' sensation. It is at this stage that the tissues of the vaginal wall and perineum may tear. Ideally, tearing can be prevented by controlling the force of the contractions. To enable this, the midwife will usually advise the women when to push, and when to avoid pushing, by the use of breathing exercises. The midwife will also try to control the descent of the baby's head with manual pressure. However, often, the instinctive urge to push is too great to be controlled, and tearing cannot be avoided. The practice of episiotomy, in which a cut is made in the perineum by the midwife, is now becoming outmoded. It is now recognised that most natural tears heal more efficiently than the surgical cut of the episiotomy.

Once the head has been delivered, the midwife checks that the umbilical cord is not tightly wrapped around the baby's neck. If it is, the midwife will free the cord before the rest of the baby's body is delivered. This is a common occurrence, which, if managed correctly, usually does not have serious consequences. Delivery of the rest of the baby's body usually occurs within another one or two contractions. A healthy newborn baby will make a cry within a few seconds. If there are no complications, it is common practice to hand the baby to the mother straight away to allow it to suckle. Ideally, time should be given (2–3 minutes) to allow the pulsation of blood in the vessels of the umbilical cord to stop before the cord is clamped and cut.

Once the baby has been delivered, there is usually a dramatic cessation of pain and discomfort for the mother. She often experiences a surge of renewed energy as she first sees and holds her new baby.

The third stage of labour

The third stage of labour involves the delivery of the placenta and the amniotic membranes (afterbirth). By the time of the labour, the placenta is a grapefruit-sized mass of soft tissue, with the colour and consistency of fresh liver. After the umbilical vessels have stopped pulsating, the placental blood vessels contract, so allowing the placenta to come away from the wall of the uterus without there being excessive blood loss. After about 10–20 minutes, continued contractions of the uterus force the separated placenta, amniotic membranes and remaining umbilical cord out through the vagina. A smooth third stage is enabled by the midwife, who applies pressure to the uterus, and controlled traction to the cord as the placenta passes out of the uterus.

The uterus continues to contract after the expulsion of the placenta, so that its rich network of blood vessels is encouraged to shut down. These continued contractions are encouraged by the suckling of the baby, as this stimulates a natural release of oxytocin from the mother's pituitary.

To facilitate this process, it is very common practice to administer an injection of an oxytocin-like drug called syntometrine to the mother. This ensures that the contraction of the uterus occurs rapidly so that blood loss is minimised. This injection is usually given into the mother's thigh just after the delivery of the baby's head. This treatment is known to reduce the incidence of severe blood loss by half. The main complication of syntometrine use is that the uterus may contract prematurely around the placenta, so preventing its removal. If this occurs, a minor operation is required so that the placenta can be removed manually.

The contractions of the third stage are much less painful than those of the first and second stages. Often the mother may be unaware that this stage has taken place, as she is so involved with holding and suckling her newborn baby.

After the delivery of the placenta, it is inspected by the midwife to check that it is intact, and to estimate the approximate blood loss. The amount of blood lost in an average labour is around 400 millilitres. An amount greater than 500 millilitres is considered excessive, and replacement therapy, either by means of iron or blood transfusion, may be considered necessary. If there has been a tear, this is then stitched, either by the midwife or the doctor in attendance.

The effect of labour on the fetus

During labour, the head of the human fetus experiences much greater pressure than occurs during the birth of other mammals. The soft, immature plates of bone that form the skull are often 'moulded' into an elongated shape during the passage of the head through the pelvic canal. A more normal shape is reassumed over the course of the few days after birth. Severe moulding can occur if the second stage is prolonged, or if assisted methods of delivery such as forceps have to be used.

The baby always suffers from a period of low oxygen supply during labour. This can affect the heart rate of the baby, which is monitored by the midwife. A prolonged period of abnormal fetal heart rate is taken seriously. If this occurs, it may lead to the use of medical interventions to speed up the labour, or the decision to proceed to a caesarean section.

Another response of 'fetal distress' is that the fetus opens its bowels during the course of labour. The appearance of black, sticky meconium in the leaking amniotic fluid is a warning sign of fetal distress in labour. If meconium has been released, not only does this indicate possible distress in the fetus, but there is also a risk of the meconium being inhaled by the fetus. Therefore, the release of meconium is another reason why medical intervention may have to take over the course of the labour, so that the baby is delivered as soon as possible.

There is no doubt that even uncomplicated labour is stressful for the fetus. The fetal adrenal glands are stimulated to produce excessive amounts of adrenaline and corticosteroids in response to this stress. It is believed that high levels of these hormones are important in promoting the dramatic changes that occur in the cardiovascular and respiratory systems of the baby just after birth.

Information Box 5.3a-II

Labour: comments from a Chinese medicine perspective

In Chinese medicine, labour is believed to be a time when Yang expels Yin. After 40 weeks of relative Stagnation of Qi in the Lower Jiao, a powerful and smooth downward movement of Qi leads to the expulsion of the fetus. This has been described also in terms of 'Qi moving Blood'. A healthy labour is dependent on healthy Blood and Qi. Healthy Spleen, Kidney and Liver Organs are particularly important in ensuring that a labour progresses smoothly through all three stages.

The physiology of the puerperium

The puerperium is defined as the 6-week period that follows childbirth. During this time, the uterus slowly returns to its normal size and shape. At the end of the puerperium, any trauma to the vagina and perineum should have healed completely. The puerperium is also the time when the foundations of the relationship between the mother and the baby are established.

In many cultures across the world, the time of the puerperium is a period when the woman is confined to bed-rest. This was also the practice in ancient China. This tradition allows the mother to divert all her attention into bonding with her child, to establish a pattern of breastfeeding, and to rebuild her own reserves of energy. However, in the developed world, this practice is not the norm. Many women now choose to be up and about on the day following labour, and, once at home, may resume normal activities such as shopping or housework straight away.

Immediately following a normal birth, the pelvic area of the mother is in a bruised and torn state. It is usual for there to be considerable discomfort in this area for the next few days, which can make sitting, walking and going to the toilet painful. Often it is difficult to pass urine for a few hours after labour because of pain and swelling in the region of the urethra. There is an increased risk of urinary infection at this time. Unless there has been a serious tear, these problems resolve rapidly.

For the first few weeks after birth, an odourless watery and blood-stained discharge, known as 'lochia', is usual. This discharge comes from the contracting uterus. It gradually diminishes with time, and should have stopped by the end of the puerperium.

Breastfeeding

Breastfeeding (lactation) is usually encouraged from the moment the baby is born. The suckling reflex does not have to be learned. As long as the baby is allowed to find the right position on the nipple, it will suckle efficiently. The correct positioning of the baby on the breast is absolutely essential if breastfeeding is to be problem free. Sore and cracked nipples are a very common initial experience in the first few days of feeding. This problem is worse if the positioning of the baby is not correct. This potentially preventable problem is the most common reason why many women give up breastfeeding after only a few days.

Normal milk is not produced until a few days after the birth. Until this time, a yellowish, antibody-rich fluid, called 'colostrum', is produced. This fluid is believed to be highly beneficial to the digestive and immune systems of the baby. Even if the mother has made a prior decision not to breastfeed, she may be encouraged to do so at least for the first few days, so that the baby can receive the colostrum. When the normal milk 'comes in', the breasts become engorged and uncomfortable. This discomfort is relieved over the next few days as the baby continues to suckle, when a balance is achieved between milk production and feeding.

The suckling is a stimulus for the release of two pituitary hormones. Prolactin stimulates the production of the milk from the lobules of the breast, and oxytocin stimulates the 'let down' of this milk into the lactiferous ducts, which open out into the nipple. Oxytocin also has a beneficial effect on maintaining the contraction of the uterus, which continues over the ensuing few weeks. For this reason, some women will experience mild period-like cramps in the early days of breastfeeding.

If the mother chooses not to breastfeed, it is normal for there to be period of 1–2 weeks of uncomfortable engorgement. The drug bromocriptine, which inhibits the production of prolactin from the pituitary, may be prescribed to alleviate this discomfort. Because of potentially severe side-effects of this drug, it is usually given only in situations when it is considered very important to suppress lactation, such as following the death of a baby.

Milk is usually produced according to the demand of the baby. The more the baby feeds, the more milk is produced. However, some women manage to produce much more milk than others, and can experience problems from overflow of milk at inappropriate times. It is unusual for the baby to fail to thrive because of insufficient milk production. However, illness, stress and anaemia can all contribute to poor milk supply.

Breast milk is rich in fat and sugars. It also contains all the vitamins and minerals the baby requires for at least the first 6 months. It may also contain traces of drugs and toxins that have entered the circulation of the mother. Some drugs enter breast milk more easily than others.

The breastfeeding mother requires more nutrients than a mother who chooses not to breastfeed. She will draw on her reserves of body fat, and will also require a diet rich is vitamins and minerals. It is particularly important that calcium and iron are available from the diet. If these are deficient, the mother will draw on her own reserves of these minerals. For this reason, weak teeth, thinned bones and anaemia can develop during the weeks to months of breastfeeding. It is not uncommon for the skin to dry and the hair to become lustreless and thin in this time, a result of the cumulative depleting effect of pregnancy and lactation.

Psychological changes in the puerperium

For the mother, the time following the birth is characterised by a roller coaster of emotions. There are a number of understandable reasons why these emotional changes might occur. First, a profound emotional adjustment is necessary to the arrival of the baby and the prospect of 'life never being the same again'. Second, in the first few days after childbirth, the body has to recover from an exhausting physical upheaval, and then may be expected to give more of its nutritional reserves in breastfeeding. In addition to this, there are dramatic changes in the hormone balance of the body, as the high levels of oestrogen and progesterone suddenly drop with the delivery of the placenta. The effect of these natural changes may be compounded by additional factors such as the shock of suffering a traumatic delivery, recovering from a caesarean section, or the finding of congenital defects in the baby.

However, some women are elated after the birth, and this feeling may be sustained for days to weeks. Many experience a brief period of volatile emotions, often called the 'baby blues'. This period occurs at around the third day after the birth. The mother may feel down, weepy or irritable. Normally this period of low mood should last for no more than a few days. If this state is prolonged it may be a warning sign of the more severe condition of postnatal depression.

The first 6 weeks after childbirth are characterised for most parents by periods in which the baby cries inconsolably, very disturbed nights, and anxiety for the baby's health. All these are bound to be draining, but by the end of a healthy puerperium, the mother should still feel hopeful and that she is coping.

Lack of sexual interest is normal in the first few weeks after childbirth. This may be prolonged in the breastfeeding mother. This again is normal, and is thought to be a consequence of the hormones that maintain the state of lactation. The midwife or doctor may advise the mother to refrain from sexual intercourse for the first 6 weeks after childbirth in order to give the perineal tissues a chance to heal.

In women who are not breastfeeding, fertility may return very quickly, and so contraceptive measures are advised to be used from 3 weeks after the birth. Although breastfeeding is believed to inhibit ovulation, pregnancy has been known to occur in breastfeeding mothers. Therefore, contraceptive advice is given to all women at the end of the puerperium, irrespective of their choice of feeding method.

Information Box 5.3a-III

The puerperium: comments from a Chinese medicine perspective

In Chinese medicine, it is expected that following childbirth the mother will be relatively depleted in Blood and Kidney Qi. Nevertheless, an uncomplicated labour can have very beneficial consequences, because it encourages a profound movement of Qi and so can clear Stagnation on many levels. If a woman can be supported through the puerperium so that her reserves of Blood and Qi are built up, she may actually experience an improvement in health and well-being through conceiving and giving birth to a child.

The mother's Blood and the Kidneys should be supported during the puerperium by good nutrition and rest. Any stressful factors in this time will adversely affect both the Blood and the Kidneys, and ideally should be avoided.

In Chinese medicine, breast milk is believed to be drawn from the mother's Blood and Essence (Jing). The possible negative effects of breastfeeding on the energy levels and calcium reserves of the mother accord with this interpretation. In light of this, it is understandable why certain cultures consider the 6-week confinement to be so important in protecting the mother's reserves of energy. The positive energetic effects of breastfeeding are that it enables a smooth movement of Liver Qi. In keeping with this interpretation, many women describe how breastfeeding has a calming effect. Breastfeeding can improve appetite, and yet promote the loss of the fat that was laid down in pregnancy. This suggests that breastfeeding also has a beneficial effect on Spleen Qi, and stimulates the Clearance of Damp.

After the puerperium

The puerperium is considered to be the time required for the body to return to its pre-pregnant state. Of course this is not the case for those women who continue to breastfeed. Even for those who do not breastfeed, the weeks to months following the puerperium are a time of continuing adjustment to the arrival of the baby. Most women do not feel back to their 'normal' state for up to 1 year after the puerperium.

Chapter 5.3b Routine care and investigation in pregnancy and childbirth

LEARNING POINTS

At the end of this chapter you will:

- be able to describe the structure of antenatal care as offered in the UK
- be able to describe the investigations that are performed in antenatal care
- be able to recognise the common medical interventions that may be offered during a normal labour
- be able to describe the structure of postnatal care as offered in the UK
- understand the experience of the woman receiving this care during pregnancy, labour and the postnatal period.

Estimated time for chapter: 90 minutes.

Self-test 5.3a

The physiology of pregnancy and childbirth

1. In light of your understanding about the conventional medicine understanding of the requirements for a healthy conception, what sort of advice would you give to a couple who are planning to start trying for a baby?
2. What are the broad effects in pregnancy of:
   (i) human chorionic gonadotrophin (HCG)
   (ii) oestrogen
   (iii) progesterone
   (iv) prolactin?
3. From a conventional medicine perspective, what are the main health issues that predominate in the puerperium?

Answers

1. Your advice might cover the following topics:
   - Timing: even with a regular menstrual cycle, the timing of ovulation may be erratic. Therefore regularly spaced intercourse may be more likely to result in conception than concentrating around the time of the middle of the cycle.
   - Diet: a healthy balanced diet is important for both partners, as this is known to improve the health of the sperm and may increase the likelihood of implantation. A good supply of nutrients is essential for the developing embryo. Women are advised to begin folic acid supplementation before the time of trying to conceive.
   - Drugs and toxins: some medical drugs (including the contraceptive pill), smoking and alcohol are all recognised to impair the health of the gametes, reduce the chances of conception and adversely affect the developing embryo. Ideally, these should all be stopped in the weeks leading up to the time of trying to conceive.
   - Stress: stress is recognised to impair the sperm count, inhibit ovulation and impair implantation. Any lifestyle changes that might reduce sources of stress should be advised.

   Additional advice from the Chinese medicine perspective might focus on the adverse effect of a range of internal, external and miscellaneous causes of disease. Topics such as the specific content of a nourishing diet, moderate exercise, avoidance of climatic extremes and calm emotions might be discussed.
2. (i) HCG is a hormone that is prominent in the first trimester of pregnancy. It stimulates the production of progesterone and oestrogen from the corpus luteum, and so is important in maintaining pregnancy. It may be one of the causes of nausea in early pregnancy.
   (ii) Oestrogen levels rise during pregnancy. This hormone promotes fleshiness, breast development and increased circulation of blood in the mother.
   (iii) Progesterone levels also steadily rise in pregnancy. This hormone causes muscle and ligament relaxation, and also induces a sense of calm. Adverse effects include heartburn, constipation and an increased tendency to urinary infections.
   (iv) Prolactin is produced in increasing amounts towards the end of pregnancy. This hormone stimulates the development of the milk-producing lobules within the breast.
3. The important health issues to predominate in the puerperium include:
   - the return of the uterus to its pre-pregnant state and the cessation of the lochia
   - the healing of the bruised and torn perineum
   - the establishment of a regular feeding pattern for the baby, and the encouragement of breastfeeding whenever possible
   - effective contraception from about 3 weeks after childbirth
   - ensuring adequate emotional support for the mother.

Routine antenatal care

'Antenatal' is a term which literally means 'before birth'. It is used conventionally to describe the time from conception to the onset of labour.

The rationale for routine antenatal care

The provision of routine antenatal care is known to be a very important factor in the improvement of the health of both the mother and child in pregnancy. Following the introduction of routine antenatal care in the UK in the early part of the 20th century, the numbers of deaths at the time of childbirth in both women and newborn babies (the perinatal mortality rate) dropped markedly.

Antenatal care is structured so that the common problems that are known to develop in pregnancy can be detected at an early stage and remedial action taken at that early stage. The antenatal appointments are also opportunities to encourage those aspects of life-style change which are likely to have a great bearing on the health of the pregnancy and the unborn child (see Q5.3b-1).

Antenatal care can have an impact on factors over and above physical health. During the regular antenatal visits a pregnant women will be encouraged to express her concerns and fears about the impending labour and the prospect of caring for a child. Good psychological and social support given in the context of the antenatal appointments may be very important in giving confidence, teaching parenting skills, and reducing the incidence of postnatal depression.

The structure of antenatal care

Antenatal care in the UK is usually shared between a woman's family doctor, a team of midwives that is attached to her general practice, and a hospital maternity team headed by a consultant specialist in obstetrics. The emphasis should be on the fact that pregnancy is a healthy time, and so, if all is well, investigations are kept to a minimum. In an uncomplicated pregnancy there may be no need for the woman to make any contact with the hospital department until the time when labour begins (with the exception of visits for ultrasound scans and an introductory visit to the hospital maternity wards).

In the UK, antenatal care begins at around 8–10 weeks of gestation, when the pregnant woman is encouraged to make a 'booking appointment' with either her GP or the midwife. Thereafter, she is encouraged to attend appointments, which are spaced at regular intervals and of increasing frequency as the expected date of delivery (EDD) approaches. For a healthy first pregnancy in the UK there are usually ten scheduled antenatal appointments, and seven for all subsequent pregnancies. To enable smooth communication between the different health professionals with whom she will be in contact, the mother is often encouraged to carry her own case records (maternity notes). The details of each appointment and the results of any investigations are recorded in these records.

The booking appointment

The booking appointment is made at a time when the greatest risk of miscarriage has passed (between 8 and 10 weeks). At this appointment, the general health of the mother is assessed. It is also important to clarify whether or not the pregnancy has been planned, and whether or not it is wanted. This is to gauge how happy the mother is for the pregnancy to proceed. Unplanned and unwanted pregnancies carry with them a higher risk of depression, and so in these cases the mother should receive particular support during the pregnancy.

Health factors that may adversely affect the pregnancy and labour are explored. For example, small size (reflected by height and shoe size) may be a predictor of difficult labour resulting from a small pelvis. Gynaecological problems such as ovarian cysts and fibroids may require early surgical attention. Medical problems such as hypertension, diabetes and epilepsy need careful management in pregnancy, and so the woman will need to be referred for specialist advice at an early stage.

The history of previous pregnancies will be taken, including any obstetric complications experienced by close family members, as both these may point towards potential problems in the current pregnancy.

Blood samples are taken at this stage, and tests include a full blood count (FBC), assessment of the mother's blood group and a screen for antibodies to rhesus factor. A blood test is also done to screen for antibodies to important infectious diseases that may affect the health of the fetus, including syphilis, hepatitis B and the human immunodeficiency virus (HIV). The mother is also tested for immunity to rubella (German measles).

The urine is tested for protein and glucose by means of a dipstick test.

All the information gathered at the booking appointment and the results of the blood tests are recorded in the case notes, which the mother usually is encouraged to carry. She is instructed to take these notes to every antenatal appointment she attends from then on, so that a comprehensive record of her pregnancy can be maintained.

At each subsequent appointment the growth of the baby is assessed by palpation of the size of the uterus. The fetal heart beat is assessed and the weight of the mother is measured. The mother is questioned about the movements of the baby, which should be felt after about 18 weeks. In addition, the woman's blood pressure is checked and her urine tested for protein and glucose. At about two-thirds of the way through the pregnancy, simple blood tests for anaemia and antibodies to the rhesus factor may be taken for a second time. At each antenatal appointment the doctor or midwife will also explore the particular needs and concerns of the mother.

Other routine tests made in the antenatal period

In the UK, women will be offered two ultrasound scans of the uterus during the pregnancy. These are most usually performed at 11–14 weeks and then at about 18–20 weeks of gestation. The purpose of these scans is to check for developmental defects in the growing fetus, and also to clarify the date of gestation. At 11–14 weeks, the scan will accurately confirm the age of the embryo and also reveal any gross abnormality of the spine or limbs. It will also, by means of assessment of nuchal fat (deposited at the back of the neck) suggest the possibility of Down syndrome (about 65% of Down syndrome pregnancies will be detected by means of this test, with a false-positive rate of 5%). At 20 weeks, structural problems of the fetal brain and spinal cord, heart, kidneys, genitalia, face, limbs and also the placenta can be detected.

If all appears to be well, the ultrasound scans can be a very encouraging experience for the parents-to-be, as they get their first opportunity to see their child, and in the later scans its movements, and also evidence of its sex.

Ultrasound scans are performed at later stages in a pregnancy if there are ongoing concerns about the health of the baby or the placenta. A decision to induce the labour prematurely may be made on the basis of a scan, if the baby is seen to be failing to thrive.

Ultrasound waves are believed to be totally harmless, but this is not necessarily the alternative view. Gascoigne (2001) proposes that ultrasound scans have no overall beneficial effect on the management of the pregnancy and the newborn (this is certainly not the conventional medical viewpoint), and that the effects of ultrasound waves have not been sufficiently researched to prove their harmlessness or otherwise.

Screening tests for genetic defects

There are a number of tests that may be performed to screen for genetic defects in the fetus. An ultrasound scan assessment of the physical form of the fetus as described above is one such screening test that has the benefit of not being very invasive.

Another non-invasive test involves the assessment of proteins found in a sample of the mother's blood. This blood test can give an indication of the probability of certain conditions, including Down syndrome and spina bifida. A simple form of this test, which detects two proteins, HCG and pregnancy-associated plasma protein A (PAPP-A), may be performed after the nuchal scan to increase the detection rate of Down syndrome. The results of this simple test are not definitive. An abnormal result simply suggests an increased likelihood of Down syndrome, and the woman may then be recommended to have a more invasive sampling test to confirm or exclude a diagnosis of abnormality (see below).

The most definitive prenatal tests require a sample of fetal cells, so that the chromosomes can be analysed. The two currently used methods of obtaining fetal tissue for genetic testing are chorionic villus sampling (CVS) and amniocentesis.

CVS is performed at 9–11 weeks of gestation. A needle is inserted into the mother's abdomen and guided to the placenta by means of ultrasound scanning. A sample of the placenta is sucked into a syringe from the needle. This tissue is then analysed within 24 hours. CVS carries a risk of inducing miscarriage in 1 in 100 tests. Another concern is that some evidence suggests that it may cause limb defects.

Amniocentesis can only be performed at a later stage in pregnancy. The earliest time it can be used is at 15 weeks of gestation. In this test, a needle is used to withdraw a sample of amniotic fluid from the abdomen. Amniotic fluid contains a few shed fetal cells, but not in sufficient numbers to be suitable for immediate testing. Therefore, the withdrawn sample has to be cultured for 3 weeks to allow the cells to multiply before testing can be performed. Although this may be more inconvenient for the parents, amniocentesis carries about half the risk of miscarriage as CVS.

Some genetic defects can be fairly simply detected by examining the form of the chromosomes in the fetal cells. A number of congenital conditions result from a gross defect in the shape of the chromosomes. These chromosomal defects very often lead to some degree of learning difficulty as well as characteristic physical defects. Down syndrome is the most common such chromosomal condition. The syndrome is recognised by the presence of an extra chromosome 21 (known as 'trisomy 21').

More recently, as the mapping of various genetic defects to particular places (loci) on the chromosome has advanced, increasing numbers of genetic conditions can be detected at an early stage in pregnancy. This form of genetic screening involves complex tests, which are costly to perform. Although technically it is now possible to screen for a range of conditions such as cystic fibrosis, polycystic kidney disease and haemophilia using tissue samples obtained by means of CVS or amniocentesis, these tests are only offered in special cases when the potential 'benefit' is estimated to outweigh the risks and costs of the tests involved.

All these additional screening tests are only performed in those pregnancies in which there is considered to be an increased risk of fetal abnormality. However, as the risk of having a baby with Down syndrome increases dramatically in women over 35 years old, tests such as amniocentesis are increasingly common choices (see Q5.3b-2 and Q5.3b-3).

Some women choose to refuse all screening tests, as they would never opt to have a termination, and would rather not undergo the anxiety and risks that accompany the tests. Ideally, all women are counselled by their doctor or midwife about the possible consequences of having screening tests before the tests are performed, so that they are able to make an informed decision about whether or not to go ahead with them.

Antenatal classes

As the time of labour approaches, the parents may be encouraged to attend antenatal classes. These are often offered by the local midwifery team with the aim of preparing parents for the onset of labour, what is likely to happen in labour, and the choices available for pain relief. The prospective birth partner is encouraged to attend these classes also. Basic parenting skills may also be covered in these classes. In the UK, the National Childbirth Trust also offers antenatal classes at a relatively low cost.

An added benefit of antenatal classes is that mothers to be can meet other women at a similar stage in pregnancy. It is not unusual for these meetings to lead to the formation of networks of local young mothers who continue to meet following the birth of their babies.

Routine care during labour

Assessment of the labour

The mother is encouraged to contact the midwife when she experiences the warning signs of the onset of labour. At this stage, a vaginal examination is necessary to estimate the progression of labour. If a hospital delivery is planned, the woman should be in hospital once labour is well established (when the contractions are lasting more than 1 minute and are less than 5 minutes apart).

The conventional site for childbirth in the UK is the delivery suite of the local hospital. Here, the woman is attended primarily by the midwifery team that has been overseeing her antenatal care. In most cases, doctors do not intervene unless the woman so desires, or if there are complications. The labour usually takes place in a private room, equipped with a bed, cushions and beanbags. A birthing pool may be available in some centres. Emergency resuscitation equipment and an operating theatre are always close at hand in a delivery suite.

Throughout established labour, the role of the midwife is to check that the progression of labour is smooth, to ensure that the fetus remains healthy, to make adequate pain relief available to the mother, and to encourage the mother and her birth partner(s).

Progression of labour is assessed by the frequency of contractions and by the degree of dilatation of the cervix. The maternal blood pressure is recorded at regular intervals. The fetal heart rate is monitored by means of the Doppler probe, as used in antenatal care.

If there are any concerns about the health of the fetus, the mother may be monitored more closely by means of a cardiotochograph (CTG). Taking a CTG involves placing a belt around the abdomen of the mother to assess the contractions, and electrodes on the descending head of the fetus to assess its heart rate. The CTG is used to assess whether or not the fetal heart rate responds normally to the contractions. Abnormal responses can be a sign of fetal distress. It is well known that CTG traces may indicate an abnormality when in fact all is well. This means that a woman being monitored with a CTG is more likely to have an unnecessary intervention to speed up the delivery. The CTG should, therefore, be reserved for those cases in which the health of the fetus is a serious concern.

Pain relief during labour

Increasingly, the use of techniques such as aromatherapy, massage and water birth are being accepted in delivery suites as non-medical interventions that can reduce the need for pharmacological pain relief. Transcutaneous electrical nerve stimulation (TENS) is another frequently used non-medical pain relief technique. This involves the passage of a low-intensity, high-frequency electrical current between two pads placed on the skin of the abdomen or the back. The frequency of most TENS machines is much higher than that used in electroacupuncture. TENS is believed to work by stimulating the large Aβ sensory nerve fibres, which when stimulated inhibit the thin C fibres that carry pain messages to the spinal cord (this is the 'gate' mechanism of blocking pain).

Nevertheless, very few women go through normal labour without having some form of medical pain relief. The usual options of pain relief are inhaled nitrous oxide (gas and air), injected opiates and epidural anaesthesia.

A mixture of inhaled nitrous oxide and oxygen, also known as 'gas and air' or 'laughing gas', is very commonly used during labour. It can be self-administered by the mother, and so is only used when needed, which is usually during the peak of a contraction. The pain relief wears off within about 15 seconds of inhalation, and the gas does not appear to have any adverse effects on the baby. The side-effects include nausea and drowsiness in some women.

Pethidine used to be the most commonly used injected opiate. The effects last about 3–4 hours. Side-effects include nausea, a drop in blood pressure and sweating in the mother. More seriously, the newborn may be drowsy, and can have depressed breathing as a consequence of the pethidine. More recently, another opiate, meptazinol has become increasingly used. This reportedly carries a lower risk of depression of respiration in the baby.

Epidural anaesthesia involves the injection of a local anaesthetic drug into the epidural space at the level of the third and fourth lumbar vertebrae. The epidural space lies outside the outermost (dural) lining of the spinal meninges. The roots of the motor and sensory nerves that supply the perineum, legs, low back and abdomen pass through this space. The anaesthetic temporarily numbs these nerves, so providing pain relief both from contractions and during the delivery of the baby. An epidural may also be used as the sole anaesthetic for a caesarean section. The injection is performed by an anaesthetist by means of a tiny tube. This tube is left in place so that 'top-ups' of anaesthetic may be given when required.

There is no doubt that the use of epidural anaesthesia can delay the progression of labour, and this may necessitate the need for further interventions to assist delivery, such as the use of forceps (see later). Complications in the mother include a drop in blood pressure, backache and headaches lasting up to 1 week after delivery. A misplaced epidural can have very severe consequences, but this is a very rare event.

Routine postnatal care

Postnatal care: the first 2 weeks

Routine postnatal care begins from the moment of the birth, when the mother is encouraged to bond with her newborn child. After the delivery of the placenta, the vagina and perineum are inspected for lacerations, and suturing of any episiotomy and any other significant tears is performed. Most women stay in hospital for 2–5 days after delivery, although increasingly many women opt for an early discharge back to their home.

For the first few days after birth, routine postnatal care involves at least daily visits from members of the midwifery team. In these few days it is important to ensure that a regular feeding pattern has been established, and that the baby is well nourished and hydrated. The umbilical stump is inspected, to check that it has dried up without any infection within about 1 week after birth.

In the first couple of days after the birth, the baby is given one or more oral doses of vitamin K by the midwife. This is to minimise the risk of the bleeding that can result from reduced levels of clotting factors from an immature liver. Between days 5 and 9 the baby is screened for some or all of the following inherited diseases: neonatal hypothyroidism, phenylketonuria, cystic fibrosis, sickle cell disease and medium-chain acyl coenzyme A dehydrogenase (MCAD) deficiency (a rare metabolic disorder). This involves card-testing a drop of the baby's blood, which is withdrawn by means of a heel prick (known as the 'Guthrie test'). The midwife should also examine the baby's skin for signs of neonatal jaundice in these few days.

Once it is clear that the baby is thriving, the mother is coping and the routine tests have been performed, the midwives no longer need to be involved in the future care of the mother and baby. From this stage on in the UK, postnatal care is provided by the woman's GP and a health visitor.

The 6 week postnatal check

The 6 week postnatal check marks the end of the routine postnatal care. It is often conducted by both the GP and the health visitor. At this check-up, the mother is questioned about feeding patterns, the healing of her abdominal muscles and perineum, and the presence of lochia. She is advised about contraception, and her mood is assessed for early features of postnatal depression. The baby is given its second developmental check at this appointment. The mother is given a reminder for the first immunisation at 8 weeks.

Self-test 5.3b

Routine care and investigation in pregnancy and childbirth

1. A patient of yours is about to make a booking appointment with her GP because she is 10 weeks pregnant. What aspects of antenatal care might you consider discussing with her before she attends this appointment?
2. Later in her pregnancy, the same patient is thinking about using acupuncture for pain relief during her labour, but first wants to discuss with you the sort of options she may be offered in the hospital. What are the various conventionally recommended techniques that you could explain to her?

Answers

1. You might choose to discuss the following topics:
   - The fact that antenatal care is known to be life-saving, as it aims to prevent disease and to detect serious conditions at an early stage in their development.
   - The above means that regular physical checks and screening tests of the blood and urine are performed throughout the antenatal period.
   - Recommended tests include blood tests at two or more stages during the pregnancy and two ultrasound scans, one at 11–14 weeks and one at 18–20 weeks. It is entirely within the mother's rights to refuse these tests, although conventionally they are not considered to carry any risks to the baby. One of the blood tests may be used to detect the woman's HIV status, but if this is performed it will only be with the mother's consent.
   - The combined nuchal test is a blood test performed early in the pregnancy which, together with the nuchal scan, can provide an estimate of the probability of a chromosomal defect in the fetus. If the mother is sure she does not want a termination of pregnancy, she can refuse this test.
   - More complex genetic testing is only performed in special cases, and only after informed consent has been given.
   - Antenatal classes are well worth attending to inform the woman about the workings of the hospital maternity department, and to prepare both partners for the labour and the early days of parenthood. They can also be useful in providing links with other prospective parents in the same locality.
2. You might first inform your patient that acupuncture can be performed in conjunction with any of the conventionally offered forms of pain relief (with the possible exception of the immersion stage of water births).
   - The medical techniques for pain relief on offer are inhaled nitrous oxide (gas and air), opiate injection and epidural anaesthesia.
   - TENS machines are usually available for hire, and these may provide an effective form of pain relief that is free of side-effects.
   - Non-medical techniques include massage, aromatherapy and water birth, although the provision of these alternatives will depend on the individual midwifery team and hospital centre.

Chapter 5.3c Abortion and bleeding in pregnancy

LEARNING POINTS

- At the end of this chapter you will:
- be able to define the terms 'spontaneous abortion', 'threatened abortion', 'complete abortion', 'incomplete abortion', 'missed abortion' and 'induced abortion'
- be able to describe the clinical features and treatment of spontaneous, threatened and missed abortion
- understand what a woman might experience when undergoing an induced (therapeutic) abortion
- be able to describe the clinical features and treatment of the other serious causes of bleeding in pregnancy – ectopic pregnancy, placental abruption and placenta praevia.

Estimated time for chapter: 90 minutes.

Introduction

The complications that can occur in pregnancy are studied in this and the next chapter. This chapter explores those conditions that manifest in vaginal bleeding. Chapter 5.3d looks at some of the other important conditions that can give rise to unwanted symptoms and signs in pregnancy.

The definition of abortion

This chapter begins with a discussion about abortion. This term is used medically to describe the premature expulsion of an embryo or fetus. The term is not used if the fetus is expelled after the time at which it may survive outside the womb. This time has been defined by the World Health Organization as any time after 22 weeks of gestation, or after the fetus has achieved a weight of over 500 grams.

Although the term 'abortion' is commonly used to describe medically or surgically induced removal of the fetus, it also is applied to the condition more commonly described as 'miscarriage', when the embryo or fetus is expelled as a result of a spontaneous natural process (spontaneous abortion). Medically or surgically induced abortion is known as 'induced abortion'. A more euphemistic term for induced abortion is 'therapeutic abortion'.

Spontaneous abortion or miscarriage

It has been estimated that up to 15% of diagnosed pregnancies end in miscarriage. This figure does not include those pregnancies that end at a very early stage before the pregnancy has been confirmed. Other estimates suggest that up to one-fifth of first pregnancies end in miscarriage, usually around weeks 8 or 12. It is recognised that miscarriage is more common in older women. It is also more common with successive pregnancies. Data from diagnosed pregnancies suggest that the risk of miscarriage in a third pregnancy is over twice that in first or second pregnancies.

Spontaneous abortion is considered to have two main causes:

- a congenital defect of the embryo or fetus (more common in the first 10 weeks of pregnancy or 12 weeks of gestation)
- factors relating to the health of the mother (more common at 11–20 weeks of pregnancy or 13–22 weeks of gestation).

By far the most common cause of miscarriage seems to be a failure in the healthy development of the embryo. In up to 75% of miscarriages the fetus is found either to be malformed or to have failed to implant successfully. For this reason, women who experience an early miscarriage may well be counselled that the miscarriage was probably for the best, as the fetus was very likely to have been not quite right in some way (see Q5.3c-1).

In conventional terms, miscarriage due to fetal malformation is generally seen as a quirk of nature, as it is so common, even in healthy women. After a first early miscarriage, a conventional practitioner is likely to reassure the couple that the chances are that the pregnancy will be healthy when they next conceive, particularly if they pay attention to routine preconceptual advice concerning lifestyle and diet (see Q5.3c-2).

Symptoms of spontaneous abortion

The primary symptoms of early spontaneous abortion are abdominal pain and vaginal bleeding. The pain results from uterine contractions that follow the detachment of the early placenta from the uterine lining. As the placenta detaches completely, the contractions become more efficient and the cervical canal dilates slightly to permit expulsion of the placenta and the fetus (these together are described, rather unemotionally, as the 'products of conception'). As the cervix dilates, the cramping pain can become very severe and the bleeding profuse, particularly if the miscarriage is occurring in an advanced stage of pregnancy.

There is a risk of serious blood loss in some cases of spontaneous abortion. However, in most cases, the pain and bleeding may not be too severe (comparable to a heavy menstrual period). Very often the bleeding is self-limiting over the course of a few days. Because of this, some early miscarriages may never be diagnosed. Instead, the symptoms are attributed by the woman to a late heavy period.

Complete and incomplete abortion

When all the products of conception are completely expelled, this is termed 'complete abortion'. However, there is a risk that the placental tissue is not expelled completely, a situation described as 'incomplete abortion'. The retained products of conception may lead to serious consequences, as they are a potential source of infection in the womb. Untreated incomplete abortions can result in a very severe form of acute pelvic inflammatory disease. The symptoms of an incomplete abortion would include a persistent offensive discharge, vague abdominal pain, dyspareunia and fever, all following the first few days of abdominal cramps and bleeding.

In later pregnancies, the fetus is expelled first, followed by the placenta. The uterine cramps are more like labour pains in later miscarriages, as a wide dilatation of the cervix is necessary to expel the fetus. In later miscarriages there is also a risk of retained products of conception, as the placenta can be held in the uterus after the fetus has been expelled.

Threatened abortion

Sometimes the detachment of the placenta is partial. Although some bleeding and cramping pains may result, the pregnancy may actually continue to be viable. In this situation, the pain and bleeding associated with the partial separation of the placenta is not associated with dilatation of the cervical canal. This condition is known as 'threatened abortion'.

Missed abortion

Sometimes, early death of the embryo or fetus does not stimulate uterine contractions, and so the mother may be unaware for some time that the pregnancy has terminated, as she continues to carry the non-viable products of pregnancy. This condition is termed 'missed abortion'. It is believed that in these cases, despite the death of the embryo or fetus, the placenta continues to secrete progesterone, and this maintains the semblance of pregnancy. Most cases of missed abortion end in spontaneous abortion, but some present before this happens, with less marked symptoms of vague crampy pain and a brownish discharge.

Treatment of spontaneous abortion

As a general rule, all vaginal bleeding in pregnancy should be treated as a serious condition. The only exception to this rule is the painless bleeding that can occur in healthy pregnancies at or around 4, 8 or 12 weeks of gestation. In this case, the bleeding is usually very light, and lasts for no more than 2 or 3 days. If there are any doubts as to the nature of the bleeding, the patient should be referred on the same day to a conventional practitioner for further investigations. There should be some urgency about this referral, as there is a risk that the bleeding may suddenly become excessive.

A woman who is experiencing the symptoms of a threatened or spontaneous abortion will be referred by her GP to the hospital department of gynaecology, where she may first undergo a vaginal examination to assess the degree of dilatation of the cervix. However she will usually be examined solely by means of an ultrasound scan of the uterus. This non-invasive investigation will reveal whether or not the fetus is still alive, thus distinguishing between threatened and inevitable spontaneous abortion. In established abortion, the scan will also indicate whether or not the expulsion of the products of conception is complete or incomplete.

If threatened abortion is diagnosed, the woman is advised to rest (although not necessarily in bed) until the pain and bleeding have ceased.

In the case of an inevitable abortion, the woman may be given an injection of ergometrine to promote efficient contractions of the uterus. If there are any doubts about the completeness of the abortion, the woman will be sent to the operating theatre, so that the retained products of conception can be removed by means of the surgical procedure known as 'dilation and suction curettage' (D&C). In this procedure, fine forceps may first be inserted into the womb through the cervix to remove the larger retained products. The remaining clots and tissue are then removed using a suction tube. After this operation, the bleeding usually ceases gradually over the course of 10 days. Persistent bleeding or offensive discharge after a D&C for spontaneous abortion may suggest that an infection of the womb is developing. This complication is treated with antibiotics.

If a missed abortion has been diagnosed, the usual procedure is to advise the woman to wait for up to 28 days until a spontaneous abortion has occurred, as this is considered to be a less traumatic procedure than removing the dead fetus and its placenta by medical or surgical means. If it is clear that the woman cannot bear to wait for this to happen, the expulsion of the products of conception is assisted. If the pregnancy is earlier than 12 weeks of gestation, then a D&C is performed, as was described above for incomplete abortion. If the gestation is later than 12 weeks, a medically induced labour is initiated by means of a gel inserted into the vagina. This medication contains a prostaglandin that is similar in structure to the natural prostaglandins that trigger a normal labour.

Prevention of recurrent abortion

In less than 1% of women, miscarriage is a recurrent problem. 'Recurrent abortion' is a term used to describe three or more successive miscarriages. It is recognised that women who suffer from recurrent miscarriages are also at more risk of delivering a premature baby even if they do fall pregnant. In most women who have recurrent early miscarriages the underlying cause is not clear, although uterine abnormalities and infections account for a small minority of cases.

In women who tend to miscarry after 12 weeks of gestation, physical problems of the uterus and cervix are more common, these accounting for over half of cases.

The prevention of recurrent miscarriage focuses first on the elimination of any underlying physical problem. For example, this may involve surgical removal of fibroids, or encircling a lax (incompetent) cervix with a removable suture. More general measures include advice on a healthy diet and lifestyle, and in particular cessation of smoking and intake of alcohol. Patients may be advised to abstain from sexual intercourse and travel during pregnancy. Some conventional authorities (e.g. Llewellyn-Jones 1999) advocate acupuncture as one option which may help prevent recurrent miscarriage.

Psychological effects of spontaneous abortion

A recent conventional medical study has estimated that over 90% of women experience a grief reaction following a miscarriage, and that this reaction persists for over a month in 20% of cases. It is believed that a healthy grief reaction is enabled by encouraging the woman to ask questions about why the pregnancy terminated, and what the risks are of a miscarriage happening again.

Although there is this acknowledgement that miscarriage is a disturbing event for most women, the prolonged impact on the physical and emotional state may be underestimated by many doctors. Many women feel physically drained for some weeks after a miscarriage, and may continue to suffer recurring feelings of grief or guilt about the loss of the pregnancy.

Information Box 5.3c-I

Miscarriage: comments from a Chinese medicine perspective

In Chinese medicine, a threatened miscarriage is described as 'Vaginal bleeding during pregnancy', whereas an early spontaneous abortion is termed 'Falling fetus'. The symptoms of an early spontaneous abortion are termed 'Restless fetus'. Spontaneous abortion in later pregnancy is described as 'Small labour'. The situation in which painless bleeding occurs as part of a normal pregnancy at 4, 8, or 12 weeks is termed 'Swimming menses'.

The conditions of Vaginal bleeding during pregnancy and Falling fetus are attributed to a weakness of the Directing and Penetrating Vessels, so leading to a Deficiency of Blood for nourishment of the fetus. The primary underlying pathology is a Deficiency of the Kidneys. Related pathologies include Blood Deficiency, Qi Deficiency and Sinking of Qi, and Blood Heat. Blood Stagnation may be an additional pathology in recurrent miscarriage.

The important aetiological factors for these conditions include overwork, chronic illness and fever, poor diet, emotional problems, excessive sexual activity during pregnancy, and physical shocks and trauma. All these factors are also recognised in conventional medicine.

Maciocia (1989) advises that treatment to rectify the pathology and to calm the fetus should be used in all cases of threatened miscarriage. He further offers the view that miscarriage of a seriously malformed fetus is inevitable, and will not be prevented by acupuncture.

Induced abortion

'Induced' or 'therapeutic abortion' is the term applied to an abortion that is initiated by medical or surgical means. The other very commonly used term for an induced abortion is 'termination of pregnancy', often abbreviated to 'termination'. In many western countries induced abortion is legal, but is only performed according to strict inclusion criteria. In the UK, these criteria were established through the 1967 Abortion Act. This Act was subsequently amended in 1991, during the passage of the Human Fertilisation and Embryology Bill. The amendment reduced the time limit by which most abortions could be performed, from 28 weeks of gestation to 24 weeks of gestation. This amendment was in acknowledgement of the fact that the majority of fetuses are viable at 28 weeks of gestation. Nevertheless, as has already been stated, the World Health Organization has recommended that viability could be expected to be possible after the fetus has reached 22 weeks of gestation.

Prior to the Abortion Act, abortion was illegal in the UK. This meant that some women who had an unwanted pregnancy resorted to any one of a range of risky methods for inducing a miscarriage. Some women paid out large sums of money to illegal operators to perform the so-called 'back-street abortions'. As the number of unwanted pregnancies increased in the 1960s, the serious complications of these often unsterile procedures became apparent. The Abortion Act was passed primarily to protect women from the hazards of back-street abortions, as it permitted those women who had reasonable grounds for a termination of pregnancy to have the procedure performed by skilled operators in sterile surroundings.

According to the Abortion Act, abortion may be performed for a clearly specified range of reasons. These criteria are more limiting if the pregnancy has extended over 24 weeks of gestation. Also according to the Act, two medical practitioners have to be signatories to indicate that they are satisfied that the pregnancy in question meets the criteria for abortion as defined in the Act. These criteria for legal abortion as defined in the Abortion Act are as follows:

- if continuance of the pregnancy would involve risk to the life of the pregnant woman greater than if the pregnancy were terminated
- if termination is necessary to prevent grave permanent injury to the physical or mental health of the pregnant woman
- if the pregnancy has not exceeded its 24th week, and if the continuance of the pregnancy would involve risk, greater than if the pregnancy were terminated, of injury to the physical or mental health of the woman
- if the pregnancy has not exceeded its 24th week, and if the continuance of the pregnancy would involve risk, greater than if the pregnancy were terminated, of injury to any existing children of her family
- if there is a substantial risk that if the child were born it would suffer from such physical or mental abnormalities as to be seriously handicapped.

If a woman wishes to have an induced abortion, she has to be seen by two doctors. In the UK these doctors are often either her GP or the Family Planning Clinic doctor, together with the gynaecologist who will perform the procedure.

Each doctor is legally required to complete a form indicating that they agree that the woman is entitled to a termination for one of the listed reasons. Ideally, as this process takes place, the woman is given an opportunity to think carefully about her decision to terminate the pregnancy. She should be informed about the possible physical and emotional consequences of an induced abortion, and should be given time to consider her decision.

Despite the strict inclusion criteria, it is most unusual for a woman in early pregnancy to be refused a termination. The majority of early terminations are performed for the reason that that the 'pregnancy has not exceeded its 24th week and that the continuance of the pregnancy would involve risk, greater than if the pregnancy were terminated, of injury to the physical or mental health of the woman'. Many doctors would argue that any unwanted pregnancy would probably injure the mental or physical health of the woman. Therefore, most doctors would not hesitate in advocating a termination if the pregnancy was obviously not wanted.

There are fierce opponents to this apparent laxity of interpretation of the criteria of the Abortion Act, as in practice the Act places little or no barrier to a woman who sincerely desires to terminate her pregnancy before the 24th week of gestation. The anti-abortion (Pro-Life) lobby argue that the inclusion criteria pay no reference at all to the rights of the unborn fetus before this time of gestation, despite the fact that the fetus may be viable from 22 weeks of gestation. This is a just criticism, but is at odds with the general medical opinion that the rights of the mother to make this choice for her future outweigh those of an unviable or poorly viable fetus.

The procedure of induced abortion

Most induced abortions are performed before week 12 of gestation. If the abortion is performed at this early stage of pregnancy, the risk of complications is very low. It is estimated that less than 1% of women will develop an infection following an early induced abortion, whereas the complication rate rises to 3–5% for abortions performed later than week 12 of gestation. There is no evidence that an uncomplicated induced abortion compromises the health of future pregnancies.

Early abortions can be performed by a surgical approach comparable to D&C as described earlier in this chapter. The products of conception are evacuated under anaesthetic by means of a suction tube inserted through the cervix. After this procedure, it is normal for bleeding to persist for up to 10 days. Sometimes the woman may be given a course of antibiotics to prevent infection.

The medical approach can only be used if the pregnancy is earlier than 9 weeks of gestation. This approach is considered to be the ideal because it avoids the potential risks of a general anaesthetic. It involves the oral administration of the drug mifepristone, followed 36–48 hours later by the application at regular intervals of a prostaglandin gel (as used in cases of missed abortion) in the form of a pessary inserted in the vagina.

The combination of these medications stimulates contractions of the uterus and thus expulsion of the fetus. The pain of these contractions may be severe, so that the woman may also require opioid analgesic medication. Nausea and vomiting is a common occurrence with medically induced abortion. In 10% of cases a D&C is necessary to evacuate retained products of conception.

If the pregnancy is more advanced (after week 12 of gestation), the uterus is stimulated to contract by means of a combination of prostaglandin-like drugs. The medical approach is far preferable to the surgical approach at a later stage in pregnancy, but as with earlier abortions, is not always successful. A failed late medical abortion has to be followed by a D&C, which in a more advanced stage of pregnancy is a bloody and prolonged procedure. Up to one-third of patients who have a late medical abortion will require a D&C.

After the termination has been performed, the gynaecologist is obliged to notify the Chief Medical Officer that the termination has been performed within a defined length of time. This means that accurate data about the numbers of terminations performed nationally can be collated. It is known from these data that just under 200,000 terminations are performed each year in the UK. The large majority of these terminations are for pregnancies that could have been prevented by proper use of contraceptive methods. It is well known that the termination rate in the UK is one of the highest in Europe, a fact attributed to poor use of contraception, particularly among teenagers and young single women.

The psychological consequences of induced abortion

Medical research has indicated that most women do not suffer a prolonged period of grief or guilt following a termination. An expert panel in the USA reported that 'legal abortion of an unwanted pregnancy does not pose a psychological hazard for most women'. Nevertheless, the physical effects of feeling drained for up to a few weeks are comparable to those following a spontaneous miscarriage. The fact that this physical disturbance is likely to occur may not be recognised by the patient's doctor. There is no doubt that some women do suffer from prolonged deep regret about having undergone the procedure. It is known that those who do have negative feelings after an abortion are more likely to have been ambivalent about having the procedure at the time (see Q5.3c-3).

Ectopic pregnancy

'Ectopic pregnancy', or 'extra-uterine pregnancy', is the term used to describe a pregnancy in which the fertilised ovum has implanted outside the body of the uterus. The most common site for an ectopic pregnancy is within the fallopian tube, but the zygote can also implant on the surface of the ovary, on the wall of the cervical canal and within the abdominal cavity.

It has been estimated that between 0.8 and 1.5% of all pregnancies are ectopic in location. An ectopic pregnancy is more likely to occur in women who have a condition of the uterus that might impair implantation in the uterine wall. Ectopic pregnancies are recognised to be rare complications of the use of the progesterone-only pill and the intrauterine device (IUD). This is because neither of these contraceptive methods prevents ovulation, but instead make the lining of the uterus hostile to implantation. Pelvic inflammatory disease is also associated with an increased risk of ectopic pregnancy, presumably because damage to the fallopian tubes prevents the normal passage of the zygote into the uterine cavity.

Symptoms of ectopic pregnancy

The early weeks of an ectopic pregnancy are characterised by the same symptoms as a normal pregnancy. Despite its unusual location, the invasive placenta releases the same hormones as it would if correctly located in the uterus.

In about two-thirds of cases, the ectopic pregnancy spontaneously aborts between weeks 6 and 10 of pregnancy. At the time of the abortion, the woman may not be aware that she is pregnant. The canal of the fallopian tube, the most common site for an ectopic pregnancy, is very fine, and so complete abortion from this site is very rare. Usually, the accumulation of blood and detached products of conception in the fallopian tube lead to abdominal pain, which can be very severe. The pain may or may not be associated with vaginal bleeding. In some cases the pain is not so severe initially, and thus there may be a delay before a correct diagnosis is made.

In one-third of cases, the zygote has implanted in the narrowest portion of the fallopian tube. The rapid growth of the embryo and its associated tissues causes first distension and then rupture of the fallopian tube. This may occur very early in the pregnancy, at around the time of the first missed period (4–6 weeks of gestation). In these cases, the woman will most often be unaware of the fact that she is pregnant. Rupture of the fallopian tube is a devastating event for the woman, who experiences a sudden onset of severe abdominal pain as the torn fallopian tube haemorrhages into the abdominal cavity. Often the pain is so severe as to cause collapse with fainting. A ruptured fallopian tube is a surgical emergency, as there is high risk of continuing severe internal bleeding. Again the diagnosis may be delayed because the possibility of pregnancy might not have been considered.

Very rarely, an ectopic pregnancy in the abdominal cavity may continue to progress to term, requiring delivery by surgical means. The most likely outcome of abdominal pregnancies is that the pregnancy aborts at an early stage, so causing abdominal pain due to blood in the peritoneal space. Rarely, the fetus dies at a later stage, and in most cases the fetal and placental tissue gradually get reabsorbed by the body.

An ectopic pregnancy is diagnosed in the first instance from the clinical picture, and this diagnosis is then confirmed by an ultrasound scan. A pregnancy test will be positive, even after the onset of symptoms, so this may be the first investigation to be performed if the symptoms are inconclusive.

The treatment is always surgical. In acute cases an abdominal excision is performed so that the affected fallopian tube can be removed. If the fallopian tube has not ruptured, it may be possible to excise the ectopic pregnancy by means of a 'keyhole technique'. This requires a laparoscope to visualise the fallopian tube. If the diagnosis is made very early, an alternative technique is to inject the developing amniotic sac with a cytotoxic drug. This will destroy the developing tissue, which then should be reabsorbed into the fallopian tube. The woman is then tested on a weekly basis for blood levels of HCG (i.e. a pregnancy test) to check that the pregnancy has been terminated.

It is estimated that about one-quarter of women who suffer from an ectopic pregnancy become unable to conceive naturally. For those who remain fertile, there is an increased risk of a second ectopic pregnancy.

> **Information Box 5.3c-II**
>
> **Ectopic pregnancy: comments from a Chinese medicine perspective**
>
> In Chinese medicine the pain of an ectopic pregnancy would be diagnosed as Blood Stagnation. The scarring caused by preceding pelvic inflammatory disease could be interpreted as Qi Stagnation resulting from Damp Heat in the Uterus.
>
> The energetic consequences of an ectopic pregnancy would include Blood and Kidney Deficiency. These can be severe in some cases, and could contribute to the infertility that can follow an ectopic pregnancy.

Antepartum haemorrhage

'Antepartum haemorrhage' is the term used to describe bleeding that occurs in the second half of pregnancy. Very rarely, bleeding in late pregnancy is unrelated to the pregnancy itself, instead coming from a cervical condition such as a polyp. However, most commonly the bleeding originates from the placenta, and so is a threat to the health of the fetus. Therefore, antepartum haemorrhage is always a warning feature of serious disease. The two most common causes of antepartum haemorrhage are placenta praevia and placental abruption. These are discussed in turn below.

Placenta praevia

Placenta praevia describes a placenta that is located over or close to the opening of the cervical canal. This condition is usually diagnosed, from the ultrasound scan at 20 weeks, before it is the cause of any symptoms. It is a relatively rare finding, occurring in about 1 in 200 pregnancies.

If the placenta is found to be low at the 20 week scan, a repeat scan at 30 weeks may show that there is no longer cause for concern, as the uterus has grown so that the placenta has become distanced from the cervical opening. However, if the placenta remains low, the risk of bleeding is significant.

The first symptom of placenta praevia is most often slight, painless bleeding. If this occurs, the woman should be referred immediately to hospital, where the treatment involves bed rest and repeated assessment of the pregnancy by means of ultrasound scans. There is always a risk that the bleeding will suddenly become severe. In the event of severe bleeding, the only option is to deliver the fetus by caesarean section, irrespective of its stage in development, as there is grave risk to the life of the mother.

With continued mild bleeding the treatment is more expectant, with the mother kept on bed rest under close supervision. If the placenta is so low that it completely covers the opening of the cervix, the baby will be delivered by caesarean section at 36 weeks of gestation, the time at which it is known that the chances of healthy survival outside the womb are high. If the placenta is just close to the cervical opening, normal labour may be possible, although this is likely to be induced before week 38.

Even if there has been no bleeding at all, a mother with a very low placenta should not be allowed to go into natural labour, as the dilatation of the cervix will cause catastrophic bleeding. In these cases a caesarean section is performed by week 37 or 38.

Any episode of placental bleeding is a potential risk to the fetus, but in most cases of mild bleeding, the fetus remains healthy, and perinatal mortality is low. There is an increased risk of postnatal haemorrhage for those mothers with placenta praevia who undergo a natural labour.

Placental abruption

In other cases of antepartum haemorrhage the bleeding comes from a placenta which is normally located high in the uterus. This complication affects 4 in 100 pregnancies. In the majority of cases of bleeding from a high placenta the cause is unknown, and the bleeding stops spontaneously. This syndrome has been termed 'accidental haemorrhage'. Less commonly, the bleeding occurs behind the placenta, and there is a risk that the placenta will become separated from the wall of the uterus. This is described as 'placental abruption'. In these cases vaginal bleeding may be very slight, or even absent. However, the separation of the placenta from the uterine wall causes pain, which can be severe. In these cases, on examination the uterus is found to be tense and tender. If the bleeding is severe, even though it may not be apparent vaginally, the mother can go into a state of shock resulting from the blood loss internally. This condition is a surgical emergency.

Accidental haemorrhage and placental abruption are more likely to occur in women who have had at least one baby already, and also in cigarette smokers.

In accidental haemorrhage, the mother may be discharged from hospital once an ultrasound scan has demonstrated that the fetus and placenta appear healthy, and after the bleeding has settled down.

In placental abruption there is always grave risk to the health of the fetus and, in severe cases, to the mother also. The treatment usually involves giving a blood transfusion to the mother. In severe cases, the fetus will die from blood loss, and thus a caesarean section has to be performed. If the fetus is still alive, it is delivered either by rapid induction of labour or by caesarean section.

Information Box 5.3c-III

Bleeding in pregnancy: comments from a Chinese medicine perspective

In Chinese medicine, painless blood loss from a placenta praevia may equate to Spleen Qi Sinking, with Spleen not holding Blood. This would accord with the finding of an inappropriately low placenta, which could be attributed to a combination of Deficient Spleen and Kidney Qi. In contrast, the intensely painful bleeding associated with placental abruption equates more closely to Blood Stagnation.

The red flags of bleeding and abdominal pain in pregnancy

Almost all patients with bleeding in pregnancy will benefit from referral to a conventional doctor for assessment and/or treatment. Red flags are those symptoms and signs that indicate that referral needs to be considered. The red flags of bleeding and abdominal pain in pregnancy are described in Table 5.3c-I. This table forms part of the summary on red flags given in Appendix III, which also gives advice on the degree of urgency of referral for each of the red flag conditions listed.

Self-test 5.3c

Abortion and bleeding in pregnancy

1. A 25-year-old patient telephones you to say that she is experiencing some abdominal cramps and vaginal bleeding approximately 4 weeks after a missed period. She believes that she is nearly 8 weeks pregnant. She wants to know what you advise, as she actually does not feel too bad. What would you advise her to do?
2. One of your regular patients, who is 30 weeks pregnant, has experienced a slight painless vaginal bleed, which has appeared as a slight staining of her underwear. What diagnoses might explain this symptom? How would you manage this case?
3. Why is it important to consider the possibility of early pregnancy in a woman who complains of a sudden onset of severe abdominal pain?

Answers

1. These symptoms suggest that your patient is experiencing either a threatened or inevitable abortion (miscarriage). The symptoms do not suggest a significant loss of blood, and as long as the symptoms are not progressively worsening you could advise her to rest. A calming complementary medicine treatment such as gentle acupuncture or homeopathy would be appropriate if this could be arranged at home within the next 2–3 hours. However, the patient would then need to contact her own doctor that day to arrange a scan within the next few days. The scan would indicate whether or not she was still pregnant and, if not, whether she will need surgical removal of retained products of conception.
2. Any bleed in late pregnancy should be taken seriously. The most likely diagnosis is 'accidental haemorrhage' from a normally situated placenta. Another possibility is placenta praevia, although this should have been diagnosed at the 20 week scan. A more benign diagnosis is bleeding from a cervical problem such as a cervical polyp.

   It would be advisable to refer this patient on the same day to her doctor so that an ultrasound scan of the placenta can be performed. You should advise the patient to rest quietly as much as possible until the diagnosis has been confirmed.
3. Abdominal pain without bleeding is a common presentation of ectopic pregnancy, whether or not the fallopian tube has ruptured. As the pain can occur as early as 4 weeks of gestation, the woman may not be aware that she is pregnant. Therefore this possibility should not be forgotten in the case of a sexually active woman who is experiencing a new onset of abdominal pain (even if she is using contraception).

Table 5.3c-I Red Flags 37a – pregnancy (bleeding and abdominal pain)

Red Flag	Description	Reasoning
37.1	**Bleeding: any episode of vaginal bleeding in pregnancy**	Refer all cases for investigation on the same day. Slight painless bleeding occurring at 4, 8, or 12 weeks of gestation is most likely to be physiological (i.e. benign) in nature, but nevertheless refer to exclude miscarriage Painless or painful bleeding at a later stage in pregnancy may result from placenta praevia or placental abruption, both of which seriously threaten the health of the fetus and the mother Refer as an emergency if any signs of shock are apparent (low blood pressure, fainting, rapid pulse) as internal bleeding may not be immediately apparent
37.2	**Abdominal pain: any episode of sustained abdominal pain in pregnancy**	Gripy abdominal pains (like mild period pains) are common in early pregnancy, and if they do not interfere with daily activities are not worrying Severe or worsening abdominal pain in early pregnancy may be the first indication of ectopic pregnancy, and needs to be referred on the same day Severe pain in later pregnancy may be a symptom of placental abruption, and merits urgent referral. It also can be a first sign of pre-eclampsia. It is particularly serious if any signs of shock are apparent (low blood pressure, fainting, rapid pulse), as internal bleeding may not be immediately apparent Periodic mild cramping sensations in later pregnancy (lasting no more than a few seconds) are likely to be Braxton–Hicks contractions, but if they are becoming regular and intensifying, they might signify premature labour (by definition, before week 36 of pregnancy). If in any doubt, refer for an assessment

Chapter 5.3d Other complications of pregnancy

LEARNING POINTS

At the end of this chapter you will:

- understand the clinical features, treatment approaches and warning features of the common minor disorders of pregnancy
- be able to recognise the clinical features, treatment approaches and warning features of the most important medical disorders of pregnancy
- be able to describe the common disorders of the placenta and amniotic fluid
- understand the problems that can result from pre-term labour, post-term pregnancy and prelabour rupture of membranes
- be able to define the terms 'at-risk fetus' and 'high-risk pregnancy'.

Estimated time for chapter: Part I, 90 minutes; Part II, 90 minutes.

Introduction

This chapter is divided into two parts, which are designed for study in separate sessions. Part I gives an overview of the most common minor disorders of pregnancy, while Part II is dedicated to the more serious conditions that can complicate pregnancy.

The conditions explored in this chapter are:

Part I – Minor disorders of pregnancy:

- backache
- pubic symphysis diastasis
- heartburn
- nausea and vomiting (morning sickness)
- constipation
- haemorrhoids (piles)
- varicose veins
- leg cramps
- urinary frequency and incontinence
- oedema
- mononeuropathies
- palpitations and breathlessness
- anaemia
- insomnia.

Part II – More serious complications of pregnancy:

- hypertension, pre-eclampsia and eclampsia
- maternal diabetes mellitus
- thromboembolism
- the rhesus problem
- infections during pregnancy
- abnormalities of the placenta and amniotic fluid
  - tumours of the placenta
  - oligohydramnios and polyhydramnios.
- problems in the timing of labour
  - pre-term labour and post-term pregnancy
  - pre-labour rupture of membranes.
- the 'at-risk fetus' and 'high-risk pregnancy'.

Part I: Minor disorders of pregnancy

Many of the minor disorders of pregnancy described in this first part of this chapter are conventionally considered to be normal aspects of pregnancy. Very few pregnancies are not affected by at least one of these common conditions. It will be helpful to be familiar with the theoretical basis to the physiological changes of pregnancy as described in Chapter 5.3a for full understanding of these disorders.

Backache

Backache is a very common symptom, particularly in late pregnancy. The common sites of pain are around the lumbar spine and, most commonly, the sacroiliac joints. Pain may also be referred to the buttocks and down the distribution of the sciatic nerve (sciatica). The primary cause of this pain is believed to be increased levels of progesterone, which increases the laxity of the ligaments in the lumbosacral spine. Poor posture can contribute to the discomfort. The posture of the pregnant woman can worsen as she tries to accommodate the increasing weight of the uterus.

The conventional treatment for backache during pregnancy is usually supportive. The patient may be referred to a physiotherapist who will recommend specific exercises to relieve the discomfort. Sometimes a brace may be prescribed to give support to the lower back. In most cases the problem disappears after the birth of the baby, although some women continue to suffer from recurring back problems.

Information Box 5.3d-I

Back pain in pregnancy: comments from a Chinese medicine perspective

In Chinese medicine, lumbosacral back pain may be the result of Stagnation of Blood and Qi on a background of an underlying Deficiency of Kidney Qi. Cold and Damp may also contribute to the problem.

Pubic symphysis diastasis

The pubic symphysis can also be adversely affected by the relaxing effect of progesterone on the pelvic ligaments. In pubic symphysis diastasis, the fibrous joint between the pubic bones becomes excessively lax, leading to pain in the groin and pubic area. In some women, the pain can become so severe that they are obliged to rest in bed to obtain relief. The conventional treatment of pubic symphysis diastasis includes physiotherapy, painkillers and the prescription of a supportive brace.

Information Box 5.3d-II

Pubic symphysis diastasis: comments from a Chinese medicine perspective

In Chinese medicine, pubic symphysis diastasis corresponds to Blood and Qi Stagnation. Kidney Deficiency is very likely to be an underlying factor.

Heartburn

The sensation of acid or burning in the upper chest or throat is a very common symptom of pregnancy. In many cases this discomfort is made worse after eating certain foods and by leaning forward or lying down. Heartburn during pregnancy is believed also to be the result of the action of progesterone, as this hormone relaxes the cardiac sphincter muscle that sits at the base of the oesophagus. The condition may be exacerbated as the uterus enlarges and places upwards pressure on the contents of the stomach. Iron-containing preparations, which are very commonly prescribed in pregnancy, can also irritate the stomach lining, and so worsen the discomfort of heartburn.

Conventional treatments for heartburn include dietary advice, practical measures, such as raising the head of the bed by a few inches, and antacid medication such as Gaviscon (sodium alginate with calcium carbonate). Although harmless to the baby, antacid medications may impair the mother's absorption of iron.

Information Box 5.3d-III

Heartburn in pregnancy: comments from a Chinese medicine perspective

In Chinese medicine, heartburn during pregnancy corresponds to Stomach Heat, retention of food in the Stomach or rebellious Stomach Qi. There is usually an underlying Deficiency of Spleen Qi.

Nausea and vomiting (morning sickness)

Nausea and vomiting is an almost universally experienced characteristic of the first trimester (first 12 weeks) of pregnancy. It is believed to be a bodily reaction to rising levels of either oestrogen or to HCG, and possibly a combination of both. A mild degree of nausea, beginning as early as week 4 of gestation is a very common symptom affecting up to 90% of pregnancies. It is often worse in the morning, but the term 'morning sickness' can be a misnomer, as for some women the nausea gets worse as the day goes on. Some women vomit in addition to feeling nauseated. In some, but not all, the vomiting can relieve the nausea temporarily. Morning sickness usually ceases to be a problem by weeks 12–16 of gestation.

Even without the symptom of vomiting, this condition can be extremely debilitating. The nausea can dominate the whole day, and can be accompanied by extreme aversions to everyday foods and smells. Other accompanying symptoms include extreme tiredness, food cravings and a strange taste in the mouth. In mild cases morning sickness is not believed to affect the health of the fetus. The conventional treatment of mild morning sickness is usually conservative. The mother is advised to eat small meals at regular intervals, and to avoid rich foods. Simple treatments such as drinking ginger tea or applying acupressure to acupoint PC-6 (Neiguan) by means of 'Sea Bands' may be very helpful. A regular dose of mild anti-emetic drugs, such as metaclopramide or prochlorperazine, or an antihistamine, such as cyclizine, may be prescribed.

In some rare cases the vomiting can be so severe as to lead to dehydration and exhaustion in the mother. This condition, known as 'hyperemesis gravidarum', is a serious problem, as there is a risk that liver damage may ensue when dehydration occurs in pregnancy. When the mother is in a state of dehydration, the health of the fetus is also at risk. The conventional treatment might involve hospital admission for administration of fluids and powerful intravenous anti-emetic medication, including corticosteroids and 5-hydroxytryptamine 3 (5-HT_3) antagonists such as ondansetron.

Information Box 5.3d-IV

Nausea in pregnancy: comments from a Chinese medicine perspective

In Chinese medicine, nausea in pregnancy may have a range of underlying causes. A Deficiency of Stomach and Spleen Qi is usually an important factor. Imbalances in the Liver and Kidney organs will also contribute to the symptoms.

The Chong Channel is linked with the Stomach Channel at St-30 (Qichong). If the Stomach Qi is weak, the accumulated Blood and Qi in the Chong Channel can counterflow upwards, so causing nausea and vomiting.

Deficient Kidney Yin can result in rising Yang, which can also result in a counterflow of Stomach Qi. This effect might explain the increased incidence of morning sickness in older mothers, in multiple pregnancies and in pregnancies resulting from assisted conception.

Stagnant Liver Qi can also cause the Stomach Qi to rebel upwards.

The presence of Heat, Damp or Stagnation will result in symptoms characteristic of excessive conditions, such as improvement after vomiting and worsening after eating.

Maciocia (1989) states that nausea of pregnancy may also be a result of failure of Heart Qi to descend. This is a possible reason why PC-6 (Neiguan) can be a very effective point for this condition.

Constipation

Constipation is a common symptom of pregnancy. It is believed to be the combined result of the action of progesterone on the smooth muscle of the bowel wall, and the physical obstruction caused by the enlarging uterus. The symptoms usually are not severe, and may just amount to a reduced frequency of bowel opening, dry stools and a slight degree of discomfort. Iron-containing preparations can also contribute to the symptoms.

The main treatment is the recommendation of a high-fibre diet. Non-stimulant laxatives, such as ispaghula husk and lactulose, may be prescribed.

Information Box 5.3d-V

Constipation in pregnancy: comments from a Chinese medicine perspective

In Chinese medicine, constipation can result from Deficiency of Blood and Yin, Qi Stagnation and Heat. Iron-containing preparations are Heating in nature.

Haemorrhoids (piles)

Distension of the veins in the anus is an almost universal occurrence in pregnancy. Again, the combined effects of progesterone and pressure from the uterus on the large veins in the pelvis are believed to be responsible. If severe, the distension may manifest as a bulging of the flesh at the anal margin. This can cause uncomfortable symptoms, including a feeling of fullness in the anus after defaecation, and anal itch. In some cases there may be a persistent ache or fresh bleeding from the anus after defaecation.

Haemorrhoids may also result from the straining and distension of the pelvic tissues that occurs during labour. For this reason, the symptoms may take a few weeks to abate after childbirth. In a minority of cases the condition never fully resolves after childbirth.

Conventional treatment includes reassurance that the condition usually abates in the weeks following delivery of the baby. Constipation, which can aggravate the condition, should be treated. Topical soothing preparations containing zinc oxide and bismuth subgallate may be prescribed.

Information Box 5.3d-VI

Haemorrhoids in pregnancy: comments from a Chinese medicine perspective

In Chinese medicine, haemorrhoids are usually attributed to Deficiency of Spleen Qi, with Spleen Qi sinking. Itch, discharge and bleeding may be manifestations of a combination of Damp and Heat. Blood and Yin Deficiency and Liver Qi Stagnation may contribute to the formation of Heat in the Lower Jiao.

Varicose veins in the legs

Varicose veins in the legs have the same underlying conventional medical cause as haemorrhoids. They tend to increase in size as pregnancy progresses, and may give rise to discomfort, which worsens as the day goes on.

Conventional treatment includes advice to raise the legs when resting and to wear support stockings.

Information Box 5.3d-VII

Varicose veins in pregnancy: comments from a Chinese medicine perspective

In Chinese medicine, varicose veins may reflect an underlying weakness of Zong Qi and also Spleen Qi. Discomfort and inflammation indicate that Stagnation of Blood and Qi with generation of Heat may also be contributory.

Leg cramps

The conventional understanding of leg cramps is not clear. Cramps are certainly more common in pregnancy, occurring most commonly at night and increasing in frequency as the pregnancy progresses.

Gentle exercise that involves stretching the calf muscles, such as walking and yoga, may help to prevent cramps, as can massage of the muscles before bedtime. Some women obtain relief if the foot of the bed is raised a few inches. As this is the opposite of the advice for relief of the common heartburn, this practice may not be of value to those women who suffer from both conditions at night.

Information Box 5.3d-VIII

Leg cramps in pregnancy: comments from a Chinese medicine perspective

In Chinese medicine, leg cramps reflect Blood and Qi Stagnation resulting from Liver Blood and Yin Deficiency.

Itch (pruritus) in pregnancy

Generalised itch in pregnancy is a common distressing condition affecting up to 20% of women. In most cases the cause is the changes in the skin that result from stretching and increased blood supply, and, and although uncomfortable, it is benign in nature. In up to 1.5% of cases generalised itch can be an indication of obstetric cholestasis, a condition in which the mother's liver fails to clear the bile from the bile ducts (probably a result of an inherited susceptibility to oestrogen). The build up of bile salts in the blood is the cause of the itch, and if prolonged may possibly increase the risk of stillbirth. Levels of bile can be tested simply by means of taking a blood sample. If a pregnant woman develops generalised pruritus, she should be referred to her doctor or midwife for further tests.

Benign itch in pregnancy may be relieved by simple measures to keep cool, such as turning off heating and applying ice packs to the hands and feet. Simple moisturisers can help.

Urinary frequency and incontinence

Frequency of urination is a characteristic feature of pregnancy. In early pregnancy the frequency is a consequence of increased urine production, but in late pregnancy it is the result of the decreased capacity of the compressed bladder.

A slight degree of urinary incontinence affects over half of all pregnant women, particularly in second or subsequent pregnancies. Like haemorrhoids, this symptom may also be worsened by the strain placed on the pelvic floor tissues during labour. Many women will complain of persisting incontinence of urine after childbirth, although in most cases this is relatively mild stress incontinence. Pelvic floor exercises increase the tone of the external urethral sphincter, and so can reduce stress incontinence during pregnancy. If correctly and regularly performed, these exercises are believed to prevent long-term urinary problems after childbirth.

Information Box 5.3d-IX

Urinary frequency in pregnancy: comments from a Chinese medicine perspective

In Chinese medicine, urinary frequency in pregnancy is a result of Deficiency of Kidney Qi. Incontinence in the long term after pregnancy is likely also to reflect an underlying Deficiency of Spleen Qi, leading to Spleen Qi sinking, as the underlying problem is persisting weakness of the tissues of the pelvic floor.

Oedema

A degree of accumulation of tissue fluid (oedema) is not uncommon in pregnancy. It is particularly obvious around the ankles as pregnancy advances, but may be more generalised, giving rise to swollen fingers and a sensation of bloating or heaviness. If this symptom is mild and also not associated with a rise in blood pressure, the cause is usually a combination of the effect of oestrogen and the pressure of the uterus on the veins in the pelvis.

The conventional advice is that the woman should rest with her feet elevated as much as possible. There is no place for drug treatment in mild oedema of pregnancy. However, if the blood pressure is found to be rising above the normal range, oedema may be a warning feature of pregnancy-induced hypertension or pre-eclampsia, and is treated with seriousness (see Part II of this chapter).

Information Box 5.3d-X

Oedema in pregnancy: comments from a Chinese medicine perspective

In Chinese medicine, oedema of pregnancy often results from a Deficiency of Kidney and/or Spleen Yang.

Carpal tunnel syndrome and other mononeuropathies

Carpal tunnel syndrome is a common mononeuropathy of pregnancy, which is believed to be caused by a fluid accumulation around the wrist joint. The increased pressure within the 'carpal tunnel' of the wrist affects the median nerve. This nerve follows the distribution of the Pericardium and Lung channels in the wrist and hand. The symptoms include numbness and tingling of the radial side of the hand, thumb and index finger, with weakness of grip. The discomfort may be worse at night, and may be relieved by dropping the hand by the side of the bed.

Other neuropathies may occur in pregnancy as a result of a combination of fluid accumulation and pressure from the enlarging uterus. Another common neuropathy is of the lateral cutaneous nerve of the thigh, which follows the distribution of the Stomach channel in the upper leg. When this nerve is compressed, a condition called 'meralgia paraesthetica' results. This is characterised by pain and numbness of the anterolateral aspect of the thigh.

Conventional treatment for these symptoms is supportive. Wrist splints, which prevent the wrist from flexing forward, may give relief in carpal tunnel syndrome.

Information Box 5.3d-XI

Neuropathy in pregnancy: comments from a Chinese medicine perspective

In Chinese medicine, the numbness and tingling of a neuropathy may be due to Blood Deficiency and Accumulation of Damp. The site of the symptoms will give more information about imbalances in a specific Organ and/or Channel. For example, carpal tunnel syndrome suggests an additional underlying Deficiency in the Pericardium or Lung Channels.

Palpitations and breathlessness

Both palpitations and breathlessness on exertion are common as pregnancy advances. In the majority of cases the cardiovascular and respiratory systems will be found to be normal on examination, and the patient can be reassured that these symptoms are normal features of pregnancy. In some cases treatment of anaemia of pregnancy (see below) may help these symptoms.

Very occasionally, palpitations and breathlessness may be an indication of previously undiagnosed heart disease, and so it is advisable that the patient reports these symptoms to her midwife or doctor.

Information Box 5.3d-XII

Palpitations and breathlessness in pregnancy: comments from a Chinese medicine perspective

In Chinese medicine, palpitations indicate a Deficiency in Heart Blood and/or Qi. The precise diagnosis depends on the time of onset and nature of the palpitations.

Breathlessness in pregnancy is usually most apparent on exertion. This is an indication of Blood and Lung and/or Kidney Qi Deficiency.

Anaemia

Anaemia describes a condition in which the concentration of the haemoglobin in the blood is below the normal range (below 11.5 grams/decilitre). Mild anaemia is frequently diagnosed in pregnancy through routine blood testing. In many cases mild anaemia can be attributed to the increased volume of the blood that circulates in pregnancy. As more fluid is held in the circulation, the red blood cells are diluted, and this gives rise to a measurable drop in concentration without any underlying deficiency of iron or folic acid (folate). However, depletion of iron and folic acid is not uncommon in pregnancy because of the increased demands of the growing fetus. For this reason, anaemia of pregnancy is often a combined result of physiological dilution of the blood cells together with a deficiency of iron and/or folate.

Anaemia resulting from deficiency is treated with seriousness, as it is known to be linked with increased susceptibility to infection, failure of the fetus to thrive, and increased risk of haemorrhage both before and during delivery.

The conventional approach is to treat anaemia of pregnancy only if it is quite severe (less than 10 grams/decilitre) or if symptoms such as tiredness, palpitations or breathlessness are present. An iron supplement, such as ferrous sulphate, and folic acid may be prescribed. Iron supplements are well recognised to cause side-effects such as heartburn and constipation, which can be problematic in pregnancy. Slow-release preparations of iron may overcome these potential problems. Herbal preparations of iron are often easier to digest but are less powerful sources of iron and folic acid.

Information Box 5.3d-XIII

Anaemia in pregnancy: comments from a Chinese medicine perspective

In Chinese medicine, anaemia in pregnancy is a manifestation of Blood and Qi Deficiency.

Insomnia

Insomnia is another problem that increases in frequency as pregnancy advances. Concurrent symptoms such as heartburn, palpitations, cramp and backache may impair the quality of sleep. Some women feel very uncomfortable, and even faint, when lying down in advanced pregnancy. This effect is probably because the uterus is exerting pressure on the large blood vessels that run through the abdomen. Towards the end of pregnancy, many women are wakeful at night, even without these symptoms. Some attribute this to the fact that the baby is more active at night, or that they are woken with a need to eat in the early hours of the morning.

Information Box 5.3d-XIV

Insomnia in pregnancy: comments from a Chinese medicine perspective

In Chinese medicine, insomnia in pregnancy may have diverse causes. Possible causes that are very common in pregnancy include Blood Deficiency and Deficiency of Heart and/or Kidney Yin. Worry resulting from Spleen Deficiency may contribute to the problem.

The red flags of the minor disorders of pregnancy

Some women presenting with symptoms of the minor disorders of pregnancy will benefit from referral to a conventional doctor for assessment and/or treatment. Red flags are those symptoms and signs that indicate that referral needs to be considered. The red flags of the minor disorders of pregnancy are described in Table 5.2d-I. This table forms part of the summary on red flags given in Appendix III, which also gives advice on the degree of urgency of referral for each of the red flag conditions listed.

Part II: More serious complications of pregnancy

The conditions discussed in the second part of this chapter are treated conventionally with seriousness as they pose a threat to the health of either the mother, the fetus or both.

Pregnancy-induced hypertension and pre-eclampsia

In a healthy pregnancy, the blood pressure may fall gradually by a few millimetres of mercury (mmHg) as the pregnancy progresses. However, if the blood pressure is found to be rising above the level of the measurement taken at the booking appointment, this may be a red flag of a serious condition known as 'pregnancy-induced hypertension' (PIH). If protein is also found in the urine, the condition of pre-eclampsia is diagnosed.

PIH occurs in about 5–6% of all pregnancies. Pre-eclampsia is more common in first pregnancies, of which it complicates about 1–4%. It is also more common in women who already have a pre-pregnancy diagnosis of hypertension.

In PIH, the rising blood pressure is an indication of a disturbance of placental function, the cause of which is unclear. In this condition, the placental cells release chemicals that cause the mother's arterioles to constrict, and salt to be retained in the circulation. Both these factors tend to increase the blood pressure, and to reduce the blood circulation to the placenta. Reduced circulation to the placenta then leads to a vicious cycle of events, in which there is an increased risk of blood clotting in the maternal circulation. In this situation, the circulation to the glomeruli of the kidneys can be seriously impaired.

Warning signs of kidney damage include the appearance of protein in the urine (proteinuria), rapidly worsening oedema and rising blood pressure, all features of the syndrome of pre-eclampsia. The rising blood pressure tends to worsen the condition of the placenta further. This vicious cycle can precipitate a life-threatening condition called 'eclampsia' (see below). Eclampsia can be prevented if the warning rise in blood pressure is monitored carefully, and if the blood pressure is treated as soon as it begins to rise above a certain level.

Table 5.3d-I Red Flags 37b – pregnancy (minor symptoms)

Red Flag	Description	Reasoning
37.3	**Nausea and vomiting** with **dehydration** for more than 1 day in pregnancy	Refer if unremitting (patient unable to drink freely for more than 1 day) or if there are any features of dehydration (dry mouth, low skin turgor, dizziness on standing). The patient may need hospital admission for administration of fluids
37.4	**Oedema** in pregnancy	Mild swelling of the ankles and hands is common in middle to late pregnancy Refer if extending to more than 2 cm above the malleoli, if there is facial oedema or if there is an associated rise in blood pressure of more than 15 mmHg above the usual blood pressure, or with any degree of hypertension (systolic >140 mmHg, diastolic >90 mmHg). All these suggest the possibility of pre-eclampsia. Occasionally, oedema can develop as a result of an undiagnosed cardiac abnormality
37.5	**Palpitations** in pregnancy	Usually palpitations are experienced when there is the occasional missed beat, and this is nothing to worry about. However, the increased cardiac output may lead to a previously undiagnosed heart abnormality becoming apparent Refer if the pulse rate is either rapid (>100 beats/minute), irregular or if there are frequent missed beats (more than 1 every 5 beats) Remember that palpitations may result from the added strain on the cardiovascular system that results from anaemia in pregnancy
37.6	**Pubic symphysis pain** in pregnancy	Refer for a medical assessment of the pain if it is not responding to treatment, and if the patient is obliged to remain in bed (may benefit from a brace)
37.7	**Anaemia** (tiredness, depression, breathlessness, palpitations) in pregnancy	Anaemia is common in pregnancy. The risks of bleeding during labour are higher in women with anaemia, so medical wisdom is that it should be treated with iron replacement
37.8	**Itching (severe)** especially of palm and soles in pregnancy	May result from cholestasis, which is a condition that can damage the fetus. Refer as a high priority

The most common time for these conditions to become apparent is during the third trimester (last 12 weeks) of pregnancy, although a rise in blood pressure and proteinuria may be first detected during the second trimester (from 14 to 28 weeks).

A rise in blood pressure of 30 mmHg systolic or 15 mmHg diastolic is a serious warning feature of pre-eclampsia, even if the blood pressure remains in the normal range for a non-pregnant person. For example, it would be of concern if the blood pressure was measured as 100/70 mmHg at the booking appointment, and then was found to be 125/85 mmHg at a later appointment. In a case when the blood pressure remains in the normal range, the condition is described as 'potential PIH'. If potential PIH is diagnosed, the women will be requested to return for repeated checks of her blood pressure and urine at more frequent intervals.

In mild PIH, the diastolic pressure is found to be 90–99 mmHg, the systolic pressure is below 140 mmHg and the urine is normal on testing for protein. This situation would be monitored closely, but is considered safe as long as the blood pressure rises no higher.

If hypertension is sustained above the level of mild PIH, the patient may be admitted to hospital for treatment. This involves bed rest, intensive monitoring of blood pressure and urine output, and oral antihypertensive medication. Drugs that may be used include atenolol, labetolol, nifedipine and methyldopa.

Pre-eclampsia is diagnosed if a significant quantity of protein is detected in the urine in a patient with PIH. PIH carries significant risks of widespread organ damage and is treated with seriousness. Often patients are admitted to hospital for bed rest, intensive monitoring and intravenous antihypertensive medication. The drug of choice is hydralazine. A decision may be made to perform a caesarean section if the pregnancy is at a sufficiently advanced stage.

The term 'eclampsia' comes from the Greek word for 'flash of lightning', which hints at the rapidity of the development of the symptoms. Eclampsia is the condition in which the damage to the maternal kidneys is in an established downward spiral. It is accompanied by the signs of pre-eclampsia, and also by severe headache, blurred vision and abdominal pain. Oedema is usually present. These are severe warning features of a condition characterised by signs of serious damage to the brain cells, including twitching, disorientation, convulsions and coma. The convulsions are similar in form to a grand-mal epileptic seizure, except that rapid recovery to a state of consciousness is unlikely. This state may develop either just before labour, during labour or, in just after half of all cases, just after delivery. Death may occur from either cerebral haemorrhage or from heart failure due to overload of fluids in the circulation. In those who recover, some may have persisting damage to the kidneys.

Eclampsia is treated with drugs to reduce blood pressure and drugs, such as intravenous diazepam or magnesium sulphate, to inhibit convulsions. Delivery of the fetus is considered of paramount importance. This may be effected by either caesarean section or induction of labour, depending on the state of health of the mother. With recent advances in perinatal care, the maternal mortality rate in cases of severe PIH or eclampsia is very low in developed countries. This is in marked contrast to the experience of childbirth in developing countries, in which up to one-fifth of women who develop eclampsia may die.

However, even in developed countries, the risks to the fetus in established eclampsia are much higher. The stillbirth rate is up to 30% in a pregnancy complicated by eclampsia.

Information Box 5.3d-XV

Hypertension in pregnancy: comments from a Chinese medicine perspective

In Chinese medicine, the raised blood pressure of pregnancy-induced hypertension may be attributed to Liver and Kidney Yin Deficiency with Liver Yang rising. Liver Yang rising is the cause of the rise in blood pressure. Liver Wind may then develop. This is the cause of severe dizziness, headache and convulsions. Poor diet and Spleen Qi Deficiency will contribute to the formation of Phlegm. This too will contribute to the hypertension, and, carried upwards by the Liver Wind can obstruct the Orifices of the Heart, causing unconsciousness.

Essential hypertension

If a woman with essential hypertension becomes pregnant, the pregnancy carries particular risks. First, the blood flow to the placenta can be compromised, leading to poor fetal growth. Second, there is an increased risk of the blood pressure rising further (this occurs in up to 60% of women who are hypertensive at their booking appointment). In this situation the condition is indistinguishable from PIH, and is treated as such. In such cases there is a high risk of progressing to pre-eclampsia.

The blood pressure of a woman with essential hypertension will be treated with drugs including methyldopa, beta blockers and calcium-channel blockers. She may be advised to rest as much as possible to maximise the blood flow to the placenta. If the fetal growth is shown by ultrasound scan to be slowing down, premature labour may be induced.

Maternal (gestational) diabetes

Between 1.5% and 2.5% of all women demonstrate a temporary inability to maintain their blood glucose within a healthy range in pregnancy. This condition is called 'gestational glucose intolerance' or, if the problem is more severe, 'gestational diabetes'. It appears to be an excessive response to the hormones from the placenta, which tends to counteract the effect of insulin. Although this condition usually abates after delivery, it is recognised that women who have been diagnosed with gestational glucose intolerance are more likely to develop type 2 diabetes in later life.

One important problem with raised maternal blood glucose in pregnancy is that the fetus is exposed to raised levels of blood sugar. This will stimulate the fetal pancreas to secrete excessive amounts of insulin. High levels of insulin can severely affect the development of the fetus, causing excessive body growth (i.e. large baby), impaired lung maturation and inability to control the salts in the blood. In later life, the child may develop obesity and a tendency to diabetes. Pregnancies in women who are known to be diabetic at the time of conception carry risks to the fetus, but these risks are the same in those affected by gestational diabetes.

The condition is usually diagnosed in the mother when glucose is found in the urine on routine testing. The diagnosis is confirmed by a blood test (the glucose tolerance test) and, if confirmed, the mother is referred to an endocrinologist who, in conjunction with the obstetrician, will oversee the management of the woman's blood glucose levels for the remainder of her pregnancy. The treatment is by means of attention to diet and insulin injections. Fetal well-being is monitored by means of regular ultrasound scans.

If gestational diabetes has been diagnosed, the baby will need special attention after delivery, as there is a risk of it developing a very low level of blood sugar – a result of its own excessive secretion of insulin. Blood glucose levels may have to be monitored for up to 2 days after delivery, with treatment involving intravenous nutrition and glucagon injections, until the blood sugar level stabilises.

Information Box 5.3d-XVI

Diabetes in pregnancy: comments from a Chinese medicine perspective

In Chinese medicine, the energetic interpretation of gestational diabetes is comparable to that summarised in Chapter 5.1d. The underlying deficiency is of Kidney Yin, together with accumulation of diverse pathogenic factors, including Damp, Heat, Blood Stagnation and Phlegm.

Thromboembolism

In pregnancy, there is an increased risk of diseases that result from excessive blood clotting (thromboembolism). In particular, deep venous thrombosis (DVT) is well recognised, although this serious condition is rare. Even more rarely, a life-threatening pulmonary embolus or cerebral infarction can occur. The overall rate of thromboembolic conditions is approximately 5–6 pregnancies per 10,000. It is now recognised that certain women are more at risk due to an inherited condition of the clotting factors. The risk is also increased in those women who are unable to stop smoking during pregnancy.

Information Box 5.3d-XVII

Thromboembolism in pregnancy: comments from a Chinese medicine perspective

The underlying process of thromboembolism in any part of the body would be interpreted as Blood Stagnation in Chinese medicine. The precise Chinese medicine diagnosis would depend on the part of the body affected by the blood clot.

Rhesus disease of the newborn

Rhesus disease of the newborn develops the blood group of a pregnant woman being different to that of her unborn child. This problem is only clinically important when the mother has a rhesus-negative blood group and the child is rhesus positive. Maternal antibodies to the rhesus factor can cross the placenta and damage the rhesus-factor-containing fetal red cells. This can cause severe anaemia, jaundice and sometimes death of the unborn baby.

It is recognised that maternal antibodies to the rhesus factor develop particularly in women who have already had a rhesus-positive baby, and seem to form just after the first baby is born. Usually the blood of the mother and fetus do not mix, but it is believed that a little fetal blood enters the mother's circulation during childbirth, and also during miscarriage. This can be sufficient to stimulate the mother's immune system to produce anti-rhesus antibodies. The ability of the immune system to produce these antibodies tends to persist, and so antibodies can cause problems in subsequent pregnancies.

To anticipate the problems of rhesus disease, the blood group of all women is tested in early pregnancy. In rhesus-negative women the presence of antibodies to the rhesus factor is also assayed, and this is repeated at intervals (at 28 and 36 weeks of gestation) during the pregnancy.

The development of rhesus antibodies to fetal rhesus-positive cells can be prevented. After childbirth or miscarriage, and sometimes at stages during a normal pregnancy, rhesus-negative women are given an 'immunisation' with an antibody that can destroy any rhesus-positive cells that may have entered their circulation. This allows the removal of the foreign blood cells before the mother can develop an immune memory to the rhesus factor. This immunisation has dramatically reduced the death and disability that can result from rhesus incompatibility in the newborn.

However, not all cases can be prevented. If rhesus incompatibility is suspected in pregnancy, the mother is referred to a specialist in the condition. Advanced techniques can be used to test for anaemia in the fetus and actually transfuse blood while it is in the womb. The baby may require intensive care after birth, and treatment for the jaundice that can result from the damage to its red blood cells.

Infections in pregnancy

Although, in general, a pregnant woman is no more susceptible to infectious disease than anyone else (there are exceptions to this rule), the effects of the infection on the fetus should always be of concern. For example, a prolonged high fever may induce spontaneous abortion in early pregnancy. The blood and nutrient flow through the placenta may also be affected by a fever. These are non-specific effects of infections. Specific effects of infections depend on the nature of the individual infectious agent. The important infections of pregnancy are described in turn below.

Viral infections in pregnancy

Smaller organisms are able to invade the placenta from the bloodstream with ease. This means that the fetus is usually infected with virus if the mother has a viral infection. Although most viruses (such as the rhinoviruses, which cause the common cold) are not so harmful to the fetus, there are five important droplet-borne viral infections that can have devastating effects on fetal development. The viruses that can cause significant congenital disease are rubella, cytomegalovirus (CMV), varicella zoster (chickenpox), herpes simplex (HSV) and parvovirus B19.

The fetus can also develop chronic viral infections through the placental transfer of virus, and this can lead to deteriorating ill-health in childhood. HIV, hepatitis B and hepatitis C are three viruses that are an important cause of progressive ill-health in babies born to infected women.

Rubella virus infection (German measles) used to be a very common mild childhood illness, which was contracted by just under 9 out of 10 children. Although rubella infection usually leads to lifelong immunity to the disease, about one-tenth of those who contract rubella do not obtain lifelong immunity. From these figures it can be estimated that, before the introduction of widespread immunisation to rubella, about 25% of women entered their childbearing years without immunity to rubella.

Rubella infection in the first trimester of pregnancy is known to cause damage to over 40% of fetuses. Depending on the precise stage of development, the rubella virus causes damage to the developing eye, ear, kidney and heart, as well as causing more general problems such as growth retardation and learning difficulties. This combination of abnormalities is known as 'congenital rubella syndrome' (CRS). The incidence of CRS has dropped dramatically since the introduction of widespread rubella immunisation.

Cytomegalovius (CMV) causes a mild flu-like infection in most people, although in some it can take the form of a more prolonged state of debility akin to glandular fever. It is estimated that over half of women entering pregnancy are already immune to CMV. For those women who contract CMV during pregnancy there is a small risk of the baby having a congenital abnormality, with 3–7% of babies affected in this way. CMV infection can lead to neurological problems such as deafness, epilepsy, cerebral palsy and learning difficulties. There is no way of preventing this infection.

Varicella zoster virus can affect the fetus either in the first 20 weeks of pregnancy or just before delivery. There is only a risk from this infection if the mother develops chickenpox at these stages in her pregnancy. Chickenpox during the first trimester can lead to skin, eye and neurological damage in the fetus in about 5% of cases. If the mother develops chickenpox just before or after delivery, the newborn is at risk of a severe blistering rash, which can be life-threatening. Moreover, in pregnancy chickenpox can be a particularly severe condition for the mother, with a high incidence of pneumonia. Preventive treatments for pregnant women exposed to the virus include immunisation with zoster immune globulin for the mother and, if chickenpox develops, antiviral medication (aciclovir) for the mother and also the newborn at delivery if affected.

Herpes simplex virus (HSV) is the cause of cold sores and genital herpes. This infection is only problematic if it is active in the genital area at the time of delivery, when the baby is exposed to high levels of virus during its passage through the birth canal. The consequences of neonatal infection with HSV are severe, with a high risk of neonatal death from widespread infection. For this reason, if active genital herpes is present at the time of delivery, the baby is delivered by caesarean section.

Parvovirus B19 (slapped cheek disease) is a cause of a mild childhood infection that causes fever, headache, and then, in the recovery phase, a rash like a flush appears on the cheeks. Although harmless to healthy children, parvovirus can cause a serious life-threatening condition in the fetus, called 'hydrops', if a pregnant woman contracts the infection. If a mother contracts slapped cheek disease in late pregnancy, the health of the fetus may be monitored by means of serial ultrasound scans.

Human immunodeficiency virus (HIV) infection appears to have no adverse effect on the pregnancy or the health of the fetus. However, the infection can be transmitted to the fetus from an infected mother in 20–40% of cases. This risk is substantially reduced if the mother takes antiviral drugs such as zidovudine (AZT) from week 20 of pregnancy and if breastfeeding is avoided.

Hepatitis B virus infection is readily transmitted from an infected mother to the fetus. If not treated, these babies have a high risk of developing chronic liver disease and liver cancer in later life. This risk is substantially reduced if the babies are given antibodies to hepatitis B and also hepatitis B immunisation at the time of the birth.

Hepatitis C virus, in contrast to hepatitis B infection, is only rarely transmitted to the fetus from the mother. The long-term risks of infection are chronic liver disease and liver cancer.

Bacterial infections in pregnancy

Most bacterial infections in the mother do not infect the fetus. Some may have deleterious effects on the pregnancy because of fever and general maternal ill-health.

Urinary tract infections are more common in pregnancy because of the relaxing effect of progesterone on the muscle tone of the ureters and bladder. Infections may give rise to no symptoms in pregnancy, but still can have serious consequences. This is one reason for the practice of regular dipstick testing of urine throughout pregnancy. The presence of bacteria in the urine in pregnancy is recognised to increase the risk of developing pregnancy-induced hypertension and also of having a low birthweight baby. In 30% of those women who are untreated, pyelonephritis will then develop. This severe kidney infection can cause high fever and rigors. In the long term, it can lead to reduced renal function due to chronic scarring of the kidneys. If bacteria are found in the urine in pregnancy, the mother is prescribed antibiotics such as amoxicillin, nitrofurantoin or cefalexin.

Vaginal infections can affect the health of the fetus. A flare up of *Candida* infection (thrush) is very common in pregnancy, but is harmless to the baby. In contrast, the condition of bacterial vaginosis (due to overgrowth of *Gardnerella*) can increase the risk of premature birth. If this infection is diagnosed it may be treated with antibiotics, even if symptoms are minimal.

Syphilis is a rare infection in developed countries, because of readily available antibiotic treatment. Nevertheless, all pregnant women are screened for this infection early in pregnancy because of the devastating effect it can have on the developing fetus. Congenital syphilis, a condition that leads to failure to thrive in the infant, and abnormalities of the bone and teeth, can be prevented by treating the mother during pregnancy with penicillin.

Listeria is an organism that causes a mild, flu-like illness, and very occasionally can manifest as a form of meningitis in the immunocompromised. *Listeria* originates from cattle and poultry, and so can be contracted through contact with unpasteurised dairy products, pâtés and poorly cooked chicken. Infection in pregnancy can lead to miscarriage, premature delivery or *Listeria* infection of the newborn. *Listeria* infection in a newborn can result in septicaemia, pneumonia or meningitis, and can be life-threatening. It carries a 30% mortality rate. The condition is prevented by the avoidance during pregnancy of those food products that may be contaminated with *Listeria*.

Toxoplasmosis is an infection that can be contracted from handling raw meat and from cat faeces. It can lead either to no symptoms, or to a mild, flu-like illness, which in some people can be more prolonged and debilitating. Infection in pregnancy can lead to miscarriage or to fetal deformities. In particular, the eyes and the nervous system may be seriously damaged. The condition is prevented by the avoidance of direct contact with raw meat, cat litter and garden soil during pregnancy.

Tropical diseases in pregnancy

The most important tropical disease, in terms of the risk it may pose to the fetus, is malaria. This is one of the few infections to which a pregnant woman may have an increased susceptibility compared to a non-pregnant woman. The infection affects the fetus primarily by causing profound ill-health in the mother. Occasionally, the infection is transmitted to the fetus. As many of the anti-malarial drugs are potentially harmful to the fetus, it is advisable for women to avoid travel to areas in which malaria is endemic while they are pregnant.

Abnormalities of the placenta and amniotic fluid

Tumours of the placenta (gestational trophoblastic disease)

Placental tumours are believed to be the result of 'false pregnancies', which occur either when the sperm fertilises an egg that has no nucleus, or when more than one sperm enters the ovum. The most common form of placental tumour is known as a 'hydatidiform mole'. In this condition, after the abnormal conception and implantation of the 'embryo', a large tumour develops from the placental tissue. This can almost replace the placenta. In most cases a fetus does not develop at all. Most moles are benign, but 5% may become malignant, and can metastasise to other organs (choriocarcinoma).

The first sign of a mole may be vaginal bleeding. This can be followed by a 'miscarriage' of the mole, resulting in the expulsion of fleshy, grape-like tissue. In other cases the tumour may grow without bleeding, but faster than a normal pregnancy would. In these cases diagnosis can be confirmed by means of an ultrasound scan, and the finding of very high levels of the placental hormone HCG.

Treatment of a benign mole is by means of surgical removal of the remaining abnormal tissue. The woman then will require follow-up at 2-week intervals to check that the growth is not recurring. If a malignant growth is found to be developing, the woman is treated by means of combination chemotherapy.

> **Information Box 5.3d-XVIII**
>
> **Hydatidiform mole: comments from a Chinese medicine perspective**
>
> In Chinese medicine, the development of a hydatidiform mole suggests Phlegm or Blood Stagnation.

Oligohydramnios and polyhydramnios

'Oligohydramnios' means too little amniotic fluid, and 'polyhydramnios' means too much amniotic fluid. Both may be a reflection of an underlying problem in the fetus. Also, both can cause complications in pregnancy and fetal development.

In a healthy pregnancy, the amniotic fluid is secreted by the lining cells of the placenta. It is swallowed by the fetus, and this swallowed fluid is recycled back into the amniotic fluid as it is filtered and excreted by the fetal kidneys.

Oligohydramnios may be caused by defective placental cells, but can also be an indication of a kidney problem in the fetus. If it occurs early in pregnancy, miscarriage is the usual result. Later on in the pregnancy, the fetus may suffer from the lack of adequate space and lubrication, developing problems such as weak lungs, bony deformities and dry, leathery skin.

> **Information Box 5.3d-XIX**
>
> **Oligohydramnios: comments from a Chinese medicine perspective**
>
> In Chinese medicine, the deficiency in fluids in oligohydramnios would suggest severe Deficiency of Kidney Yin or Jing.

Polyhydramnios is either due to a very large surface area of placenta, such as can occur in a multiple pregnancy, or may be an indication of an abnormality of the fetal nervous system or digestive tract (including spina bifida). Polyhydramnios can cause considerable discomfort to the mother, and can precipitate premature labour. Fluid may be removed from the amniotic sac by means of amniocentesis to relieve the discomfort. After delivery, the baby is examined carefully to exclude a poorly developed oesophagus or duodenum (atresia of the gastrointestinal tract).

Information Box 5.3d-XX

Polyhydramnios: comments from a Chinese medicine perspective

In Chinese medicine, the excessive fluid of polyhydramnios would suggest an accumulation of Damp, with an underlying Deficiency of Spleen and/or Kidney Qi.

Problems in the timing of labour

According to conventional medicine, the ideal time for the delivery of a baby is between 36 and 42 weeks after the date of the last menstrual period (LMP). The mother is given the date of the 40th week after conception as the estimated date of delivery (EDD), but in reality this date is somewhat arbitrary, as the precise length of her pregnancy of course depends on when she conceived, and not on the date of the LMP. Although the average date of conception is 14 days after the LMP, the actual timing of ovulation and conception can vary widely from just a few days after the last menstrual period to some weeks after that date in someone who is ovulating irregularly.

Nevertheless, pregnancies in which labour begins either before 36 weeks of gestation (pre-term) or after 42 weeks of gestation (post-term) are considered to carry greater risk to the fetus. For this reason, efforts are made to avoid the occurrence of both pre-term labour and post-term pregnancy.

Pre-term labour

A pre-term labour is defined as a labour that begins before the 36th week of pregnancy. The result is a pre-term or premature baby. (Also, by definition, a baby that weighs less than 2500 grams is also described as pre-term or premature. This means that a pre-term or premature baby might have been delivered at later than 36 weeks.) A pre-term baby is at risk of a wide range of problems that result from its immaturity. These problems are greater for those pre-term babies who are small not because the labour started too early, but because their growth in the womb was insufficient for some other reason.

Pre-term labour is associated with a wide range of risk factors, including: low social class, young age of the mother, multiple pregnancy, smoking, eating disorders in the mother and fetal abnormalities. In addition, various medical conditions of pregnancy may increase the risk of pre-term labour. These include any cause of placental bleeding in pregnancy, incompetent (lax) cervix, hypertension, anaemia and bacterial vaginosis.

If pre-term labour is demonstrated to be established with evidence of dilatation of the cervix, medical treatment can be given to protect the fetus and to attempt to slow the progression of labour. This may not be offered if the labour is after the 34th week, and there is a good facility for neonatal care, as a premature baby can be well cared for in an intensive care setting after this stage of development.

Otherwise the treatment given to a mother in pre-term labour first involves an injection of corticosteroids. This treatment has been shown to enhance the production of a fluid called 'surfactant' in the fetal lungs, and so prevent a serious condition called 'respiratory distress syndrome'. This treatment has to be given more than 24 hours before the birth to be effective, and so, once it is given, the mother in some cases is treated with intravenous drugs (most commonly beta blockers) that inhibit the force of the contractions. This treatment can also 'buy time' to enable the woman to be transferred to a unit that has neonatal intensive care facilities.

Caesarean section is more commonly used in the delivery of pre-term babies than term babies, because it offers a far less physically stressful passage into the outside world.

Information Box 5.3d-XXI

Premature labour: comments from a Chinese medicine perspective

In Chinese medicine, premature labour is a result of Qi and Blood Deficiency.

Premature rupture of membranes

Ideally, the membranes surrounding the amniotic sac rupture during labour, either at its onset or, most commonly, around the time of transition from the first to the second stage of labour. If the membranes rupture before the onset of labour, amniotic fluid starts to leak out through the vagina, and a potential pathway for infection of the uterus is opened. In some centres it is the practice that, if natural labour does not start within 24–48 hours following premature rupture of membranes (PRM), labour is induced in order to minimise the time during which infection might enter the uterus. However, a recent study of women with PRM after 37 weeks of gestation showed that they had no greater risk of uterine infection, even if their labour was not induced. This is probably because most of these women naturally would have progressed to labour within the next few days after PRM.

There is more of a problem with pre-term PRM, because the woman is less likely to go into labour so soon after the rupture. However, in these cases early labour is less than desirable. In such cases the risks that might result from infection and the loss of amniotic fluid have to be weighed against the potential problems of pre-term labour.

In general, the treatment in pre-term PRM is conservative. The woman is observed for signs of infection and only treated with antibiotics if these develop, or at the point when labour starts. If the membranes rupture before week 35, corticosteroids are given to the mother to protect the fetus from respiratory distress syndrome.

Post-term pregnancy

Post-term pregnancy is defined as a pregnancy that has extended past 42 weeks. This occurs in 1 in 10 pregnancies. The concern is that the perinatal mortality rate starts to rise once the pregnancy has extended into the 43rd week. This is because there are risks from the fetus 'outgrowing' the blood supply of the ageing placenta, and also of difficult labour resulting from a large baby. These risks are most marked in older women, those with pregnancy-induced hypertension, or diabetes mellitus.

The treatment of post-term pregnancy is induction of labour. This treatment can be initiated as early as the 10th day after the expected date of delivery. The onset of labour is encouraged by a stepwise introduction of treatments of increasing invasiveness. The order and range of induction techniques varies from centre to centre.

Often the first approach is one that can be performed by a midwife. This is the 'stretch and sweep', a manual procedure in which a finger is introduced into the cervix to stretch the membranes. This alone may be sufficient to initiate labour. Another manual technique is amniotomy, in which a sterile instrument is used to rupture the membranes artificially (ARM).

If these techniques are not successful, a medical approach is used. This involves the introduction of a pessary (a medication inserted vaginally) containing a hormone called a 'prostaglandin'. This will soften the cervix in preparation for the uterine contractions. The woman is then given an intravenous infusion of a synthetic form of oxytocin, the uterine stimulating hormone. As the levels of synthetic oxytocin build up in the mother's bloodstream, contractions become inevitable and will increase in intensity depending on the rate of infusion.

Medical induction is recognised to result in a labour that is rapid, more painful and, for some women, shocking in its intensity. Zita West (2001) describes the 'downward spiral of induction' in which the intensity of pain forces some women to choose opioid analgesics or epidural anaesthesia at an early stage in labour. This then can increase the likelihood of the need for interventions such as forceps and caesarean delivery.

Information Box 5.3d-XXII

Delayed onset of labour: comments from a Chinese medicine perspective

In Chinese medicine, delayed onset of labour can be the result of Blood and Qi Deficiency, Kidney Deficiency and Stomach and Spleen Qi Deficiency.

The at-risk fetus and high-risk pregnancy

The at-risk fetus

The term 'at-risk fetus' is used to describe a situation in which at any particular stage of gestation the fetus is much more vulnerable than is normal for a healthy fetus. An at-risk fetus is more likely to suffer from intrauterine death, distress during labour, death during delivery (stillbirth), and poor health in the neonatal period and early infancy. It is now recognised that this poor start to life may well be related to health problems that persist throughout childhood and even into late adulthood. A fetus may be at risk because of congenital abnormality, or because of factors that impair the environment in which it is developing. These include all the serious complications of pregnancy described above, and also the concurrent use of therapeutic or recreational drugs during pregnancy.

Intrauterine growth retardation (small-for-dates fetus)

Failure to achieve a predicted rate of growth (when the fetus is said to be 'small for dates') is the most common underlying factor that puts the fetus at risk. A wide range of risk factors are associated with a poor rate of fetal growth. For some of these the growth is slow or retarded throughout pregnancy, and for others (notably those that are to do with poor placental function) the growth rate starts off normally and then begins to decline towards the end of the pregnancy.

The factors associated with poor fetal growth throughout the pregnancy include: a previous birth of a baby weighing less than 2500 grams, previous stillbirth or neonatal death, history of urinary tract infection or kidney disease, bleeding during the pregnancy, smoking during the pregnancy and fetal malformations.

The factors that tend to affect the ability of the placenta to provide sufficient nourishment include: high blood pressure (pregnancy-induced hypertension), post-term pregnancy, eating disorders and severe anaemia in the mother, and multiple pregnancy.

Poor fetal growth may only be detected relatively late in pregnancy because the rate of weight gain in the mother or the size of her 'bump' may have little or no correlation with the size of the fetus, particularly in early pregnancy. In later pregnancy, a failure to put on weight in the later weeks, together with a lower than normal increase in girth, may be warning signs of poor fetal growth. The first accurate measurement of the growth of the fetus is usually made midway through pregnancy by means of the routine ultrasound scan.

The presence of one or more of the risk factors associated with poor fetal growth might alert the obstetrician to the possibility of poor fetal growth. If poor growth is then confirmed by ultrasound scan, the woman should receive more intensive antenatal care, particularly in the last trimester of pregnancy.

Although most at-risk fetuses demonstrate growth retardation, not all do. Some fetuses with congenital abnormalities may maintain normal growth rate, but still are more vulnerable to serious conditions than a healthy fetus. The large baby in a pregnancy complicated by diabetes is also more at risk of serious complications.

The high-risk pregnancy

A pregnancy in which the health of the fetus is at risk is termed a 'high-risk pregnancy'. High-risk pregnancies should be managed with much more attention to regular monitoring than would be normal in a healthy pregnancy. The care of a woman with a high-risk pregnancy will always be transferred from the local midwifery team and general practice to the specialist obstetric team at the local hospital.

During the last weeks of a high-risk pregnancy, tests are performed at regular intervals to assess the health of the fetus. These include counts of fetal movements, serial ultrasound scans, assessment of the blood flow in the umbilical cord and use of the cardiotochograph (CTG). As is true in labour, the use of the CTG, although very reassuring when normal tracings are obtained, may result in the use of unnecessary medical interventions when it produces an abnormal reading, when in fact all was well. This is because an abnormal pattern may, but does not always, indicate that the fetus is in distress.

If the serial assessments of a high-risk pregnancy indicate deteriorating fetal health, delivery of the baby will be expedited, either by medical induction of labour or by caesarean section. In some cases, when the health of the fetus is considered to be very much at risk, this will mean inducing a pre-term delivery.

The at-risk fetus during labour

Delivery of an at-risk fetus requires intensive monitoring, so that if any sudden deterioration in the health of the fetus is detected, delivery can be expedited (usually by caesarean section, and sometimes by forceps if the distress occurs during the second stage of labour). CTG monitoring is always used to assess the changes in the fetal heart rate during contractions. As previously mentioned, the CTG may indicate a problem when there is not actually anything to be concerned about. One consequence of a false-positive CTG trace result can be an unnecessary caesarean section. If there is doubt about how to proceed, a sample of blood may be withdrawn (via the vagina) from the scalp of the fetus. This is tested for increased acidity, which is a definite sign of fetal distress.

The at-risk fetus is more likely to require intensive care as a neonate. This need for intensive care is assessed by a paediatrician who is called to be present to examine the newborn at the end of the labour or the caesarean section.

> **Information Box 5.3d-XXIII**
>
> **The at-risk fetus: comments from a Chinese medicine perspective**
>
> In Chinese medicine, the precise energetic interpretation of the at-risk fetus and high-risk pregnancy would depend in part on the underlying causative conditions. However, it is likely that Kidney or Jing Deficiency is common to all cases.

The red flags of the disorders of pregnancy

Most women with symptoms of the serious conditions of pregnancy will benefit from referral to a conventional doctor for assessment and/or treatment. Red flags are those symptoms and signs that indicate that referral is to be considered. The red flags of the serious disorders of pregnancy are described in Table 5.3d-II. This table forms part of the summary on red flags given in Appendix III, which also gives advice on the degree of urgency of referral for each of the red flag conditions listed.

> **Self-test 5.3d**
>
> **Other complications of pregnancy**
>
> 1. A 28-year-old patient, who is in her first pregnancy, is very distressed by continual nausea. She has felt sick for the past 6 weeks,ever since the 6th week of gestation. She vomits every morning, but can manage to eat a little food for breakfast. She cannot face most food or tea or coffee, but can at least cope with water or orange juice. She is depressed and tired but not dehydrated. Do you refer?
> 2. A patient of yours, who is in the 35th week of pregnancy, is very embarrassed to describe that for the past month, whenever she coughs, she leaks urine, so much so that she has to wear a sanitary towel all the time. The problem is getting worse. How would you advise her?
> 3. How might you treat a patient who has been diagnosed with gestational diabetes, and who has started a trial of dietary therapy?
> 4. What would be the possible outcomes of a pregnancy that is allowed to go beyond week 42 of gestation?
>
> **Answers**
>
> 1. Nausea and sickness in the first trimester is common and usually benign. Your patient has no features of dehydration, and is able to keep some fluid and food down each day. Despite her tiredness and depression, there is no need to refer, particularly as the nausea wears off after week 12 (up to week 16) in most cases.
> 2. Again, mild urinary incontinence is common in late pregnancy. You could advise your patient that the problem is very likely to resolve in the postnatal period (although possibly not immediately after birth). You should strongly recommend pelvic floor muscle exercises.
> 3. In Chinese medicine, the features of gestational diabetes suggest that there is an underlying Deficiency of the Kidneys and Spleen, and Generation of Damp and Heat. You could complement the dietary advice this woman has been given with specific Chinese medicine advice about foods that are warming and nourishing to the Qi and Kidneys, and also advise about the avoidance of Damp and Cold foods. Treatment directed towards Nourishing the Kidneys and Spleen may be of benefit.
> 4. Many pregnancies that extend past week 42 may actually be absolutely normal, the late timing being a result of a relative delay in the ovulation that resulted in conception. In these cases, a labour with an onset at or just after week 42 is no more likely to be problematic than one with an onset around week 40. Nevertheless, in some cases post-term pregnancy may reflect the fact that the pregnancy really is extending past the optimum time for delivery. In these cases there is a risk that the fetus will start to outgrow the ability of the placenta to meet its needs, and may begin to suffer nutritionally. Also, continued growth of the fetus may give rise to difficult labour. It is to prevent these complications that the obstetric practice of induction of labour is implemented from the 10th day after the estimated due date (EDD).

Table 5.3d-II Red Flags 37c – pregnancy (serious conditions)

Red Flag	Description	Reasoning
37.9	**Potential pregnancy-induced hypertension (PIH)**	Refer if you find that the blood pressure has risen to 30 mmHg systolic or 15 mmHg diastolic above any measurement you have taken previously
37.10	**Mild pregnancy-induced hypertension (PIH)**	Refer as a high priority if the diastolic blood pressure is 90–99 mmHg and the systolic blood pressure is below 140 mmHg
37.11	**Moderate to severe pregnancy-induced hypertension (PIH)**	Refer as a high priority if the diastolic blood pressure is greater than 100 mmHg or if the systolic blood pressure is greater than 140 mmHg
37.12	**Features of pre-eclampsia/HELLP syndromes**: headache, abdominal pain, visual disturbance, nausea and vomiting and oedema (in mid-late pregnancy)	Headache, abdominal pain and visual disturbances can presage eclampsia even in the absence of raised blood pressure Nausea and vomiting, headache and oedema together suggest the development of the HELLP syndrome (haemolysis, liver abnormalities and low platelets) Both these syndromes, which may overlap, are absolute emergencies
37.13	**Thromboembolism**: pain in calf, swollen or discoloured leg, or breathlessness with chest pain, or blood in sputum during pregnancy	Refer any features of a thromboembolic event (deep venous thrombosis of the calf or pelvic veins, pulmonary embolus or stroke) as an emergency. The risks of these events are greater in pregnancy, and thromboembolism is currently the most significant cause of maternal death in pregnancy
37.14	**Fever**: refer in pregnancy if high (>38.5°C) and no response to treatment in 24 hours	Refer for management of the underlying cause, as a high fever may affect the embryo/fetus
37.15	**Fever with rash** in the first trimester of pregnancy	Refer suspected rubella or chickenpox so that the health of the embryo/fetus can be monitored
37.16	**Fever with rash** in the last trimester of pregnancy	Refer if chickenpox or shingles is suspected, as there is a risk of fatal fetal varicella infection
37.17	**Outbreak of genital herpes** in the last trimester of pregnancy	Refer, as there is a risk of transmission of herpesvirus to baby during delivery
37.18	**Urinary tract infection** in pregnancy	Always refer for urine testing for bacteria as if present there is an increased risk of spread to kidneys and induction of miscarriage in the first trimester
37.19	**Offensive, fishy, watery discharge** (possible bacterial vaginosis) in pregnancy	Refer for treatment, as bacterial vaginosis leads to an increased risk of early labour and miscarriage
37.20	**Any watery vaginal leakage** in middle to late pregnancy	A very watery discharge in middle to late pregnancy is amniotic fluid until proved otherwise. Premature rupture of the membranes (PRM) caries a risk of uterine infection and needs to be assessed as a high priority. Even if the pregnancy has come to term, PRM without the onset of labour carries this risk, and conventional practice is to induce labour if has not started naturally within 24 hours of PRM

Chapter 5.3e Complications of childbirth and the puerperium

LEARNING POINTS

At the end of this chapter you will be able to:

- recognise the range of complications that can affect the first and second stages of labour
- describe the three methods of assisted delivery – forceps, ventouse and caesarean section
- describe the complications that can occur in the third stage of labour and explain the treatment of these complications
- describe the complications that can occur during the puerperium.

Estimated time for chapter: 100 minutes.

Introduction

This chapter summarises the problems that can complicate the process of childbirth, from the onset of the first stage of labour, to the completion of the third stage of labour, when the placenta is delivered. In preparation for this chapter, it will be helpful to be familiar with the physiology of the three stages of childbirth and the puerperium, which is summarised in Chapter 5.3a.

The complications of childbirth discussed in this chapter are:

- Complications of the first and second stages of labour:
  - abnormal positioning of the fetus
  - prolapse of the umbilical cord

 - multiple pregnancy
 - prolonged labour and obstructed labour
 - rapid labour
 - perineal tears
 - episiotomy.
- Complications of the third stage of labour:
 - post-partum haemorrhage
 - retained placenta.
- Complications of the puerperium:
 - puerperal infection
 - thromboembolism
 - psychiatric problems.

Instrumental delivery

The term 'instrumental delivery' is used to describe a delivery in which obstetric interventions are employed to assist the delivery of a baby when labour is not straightforward. There are two instrumental techniques used to encourage the downward movement of the fetus when labour is not progressing well in the second stage: forceps delivery and delivery by vacuum extraction (ventouse). These techniques can only be used when the cervix is fully dilated, and when the head of the fetus has started its descent through the pelvis. Both require local analgesia, either epidural anaesthesia or an anaesthetic that numbs the nerves that supply the perineum. Between 5% and 12% of all deliveries in the UK involve either forceps or vacuum extraction.

Forceps delivery

Forceps delivery involves the insertion of two curved metal instruments that are designed to cup the head of the fetus and allow the obstetrician to apply downward traction on the head. The woman has to be positioned on her back with her legs held apart in 'stirrups' to allow the forceps to be inserted. After the perineal area has been anaesthetised, an episiotomy (surgical incision of the perineal tissues) is performed to widen the passageway for the descent of the head.

Although the most usual complication of forceps delivery is temporary 'moulding' of the head of the fetus, in rare cases it can result in severe physical trauma to the head of the fetus. There is also a risk of trauma to the vagina and the cervix of the mother.

Ventouse vacuum extraction

The ventouse is a cup-like instrument that is placed against the head of the fetus. Suction is then applied through the cup, so that traction on the cup will pull the head downwards. Ventouse extraction is less likely to result in vaginal and perineal damage than forceps delivery. It always leaves a temporary unsightly raised circle of swelling on the head of the baby (lasting up to 48 hours), and is more likely to damage the skin of the baby's scalp. More serious complications of ventouse extraction are rare.

Caesarean section

'Caesarean section' is the term used to describe the surgical operation to remove the baby from the womb via an abdominal incision. Planned caesarean section is performed before the natural onset of labour in order to prevent either the deterioration of the health of the fetus in the womb or the potential complications of labour. Planned caesarean section is a relatively safe operation for the mother, as there is an opportunity for her to be prepared for the procedure.

In contrast, emergency caesarean section is performed when labour has been allowed to start naturally, but then complications have arisen that threaten the health of the fetus or the mother. Emergency caesarean section is performed to expedite delivery in an ongoing labour. This is usually because labour is not progressing as smoothly as expected. Also, caesarean section may be performed if at any time the monitoring of the fetus suggests severe fetal distress. This is more likely to occur in an at-risk fetus. Emergency caesarean section is performed to enable a rapid removal of the fetus from the womb. It carries more risks to both the mother and the fetus because it is performed at a time when both are under the extreme physical stress of complicated labour.

Caesarean section is performed either under general or epidural anaesthesia. It usually involves a horizontal incision just above the pubic bone. After the operation, the mother is encouraged to be up and about within 1–2 days. Usually recovery from a caesarean section is uncomplicated, and the mortality rate is extremely low.

Nevertheless, a caesarean section will necessitate a longer stay than normal in hospital after delivery (7–10 days). As with all abdominal operations, pain from the healing wound will restrict normal activities, including lifting and driving, for the next few weeks. This can have a big impact on the experience of life with a newborn baby. Those women who have had to undergo an emergency caesarean section may take longer to recover from the physical and emotional shock of the procedure.

Between 3% and 12% of caesarean sections are affected by complications. Minor infections and bleeding from the scar are relatively common. A womb infection is a more severe complication, which will necessitate high-dose antibiotic treatment. There is a small increased risk of deep vein thrombosis after caesarean section (see Q5.3e-1 and Q5.3e-2).

The complications of the first and second stages of labour

Abnormal positioning of the fetus in the uterus

If the fetus is in a less than ideal position at the onset of labour, the smooth progression of labour may be impeded. Ideally, the fetus should have found a head-down position in the few weeks leading up to labour. In the days leading up to labour, the head should have dropped (engaged) into the bowl of the pelvis. The occiput (the posterior aspect of the crown of the head) should be the part that presses on the cervix, and which descends through the cervix foremost. If the occiput presents foremost, the head presents its narrowest diameter to the constrained passageway provided by the pelvis, and birth will be less difficult. In addition, even pressure on the cervix from a well-positioned occiput will encourage efficient and even dilatation of the cervix.

Occipitoanterior presentation

At the onset of labour the back of the fetus should be directed forwards and slightly to one side. This is termed the occipitoanterior (OA) position. In this position, the occiput is most likely to present foremost. A normally shaped healthy uterus and pelvis will encourage the fetus to 'find' this position as it grows to fill the abdominal cavity. A healthy degree of uterine muscle tone will literally squeeze the fetus into this most natural position.

It is possible for a skilled midwife to confirm the occipitoanterior (OA) position, as the body of the fetus can be palpated through the mother's abdominal wall. The smooth back of the fetus is felt to be facing outwards either to the left or the right. In addition, the shoulders can be felt just above the pubic bone, indicating that the head has indeed engaged.

Malpresentation

If the fetus is not in this ideal OA position at the onset of labour, this is described as a 'malpresentation'. A malpresentation means that the descent of the fetus is more likely to be restricted by the passageway of the pelvis, and also that the cervix is not exposed to the even pressure necessary to generate efficient contractions. The first stage of the labour is, therefore, more likely to be prolonged, the contractions more painful and the need for assisted delivery more likely. Occipitoposterior presentation and breech presentation are the two most common malpresentations. These are now discussed in more detail.

Occipitoposterior presentation

In one-tenth of pregnancies the fetus is head down, but its spine is lying against the mother's spine. This position is called the occipitoposterior (OP) position. The OP position may result either from deficient uterine tone, or from an unusually shaped pelvis. This position is commonly diagnosed before the onset of labour because of the characteristic shape of this fetal position when felt during palpation of the mother's abdomen. In the OP position the head is often unable to engage until the onset of labour, because the neck is not free to flex. Like an egg lying sideways-on in an egg-cup, the head can present a wider diameter to the pelvis, so that descent of the head becomes more difficult.

Because the head is not in the ideal position, the pressure it exerts on the cervix may be uneven, and this can result in inefficient contractions, which might start and stop. Nevertheless, the contractions can be very painful, and are often felt in the back. In about 70% of cases of OP presentation normal delivery is possible, although additional analgesia is often necessary. In about 20% of cases instrumental delivery by means of forceps or vacuum extraction may be necessary. In fewer than 10% of cases the baby is delivered by caesarean section because labour becomes too prolonged.

Breech presentation

Breech presentation means that the baby has found a head-up position in the womb. This is commonplace earlier on in pregnancy, when the fetus has a lot of freedom of movement. However, by week 35 of gestation over 90% of babies have found a head-down position. Even after this time some babies will turn spontaneously, so that only 3% of all pregnancies are breech presentation at term (40 weeks of gestation). In some of these cases there is an obvious physical reason for the malpresentation, such as an unusually shaped pelvis in the mother or placenta praevia.

If there are no obvious physical obstructions to an OA position, it may be possible for a skilled obstetrician to turn a breech baby at around week 37 of gestation by means of a procedure called 'version'. This involves manually shifting the baby's position by means of palpation through the mother's abdominal wall. The fetal heart rate is monitored throughout. There is a small risk of premature rupture of membranes or induction of labour when this technique is performed. Version is not always successful.

Breech presentation presents a problem during normal delivery because labour is inevitably more difficult. There is a 1 in 100 chance of a healthy fetus dying during delivery if it presents in a breech position, and this risk is greatly increased if the baby is premature or post-term. For this reason, 30–60% of breech presentations are managed by a planned caesarean section. Furthermore, if normal delivery is attempted, in up to 40% of cases an emergency caesarean section may be necessary.

Other malpresentations

OP and breech are the most common malpresentations. However, the fetus can present in a range of unfavourable positions at the onset of labour. These include transverse (horizontal) and oblique presentation and shoulder presentation. These malpresentations can also be diagnosed before the onset of labour by means of skilled abdominal palpation. With transverse and oblique presentations, the baby may be encouraged to find a head-down position by means of version. If this is not possible, or if there is a shoulder presentation, then planned caesarean section is usually the chosen method of delivery.

Sometimes, just the position of the baby's head can greatly complicate the progression of labour. Problems with the position of the head may not be diagnosed until labour is established. In particular, face and brow presentations can cause problems, which may necessitate a caesarean section or instrumental delivery. Occasionally, these presentations occur because of the presence of a severe malformation of the baby's head or neck.

Umbilical cord prolapse

In all the less common forms of malpresentation there is a risk that the umbilical cord will drop into the space in the uterus below the baby, and can then fall down into the vagina ahead of the baby during delivery. This complication, known as 'umbilical cord prolapse', can seriously threaten the health of

Information Box 5.3e-I

Malpresentation: comments from a Chinese medicine perspective

In Chinese medicine, a malpresentation may represent a Deficiency in the Spleen or Kidney Qi of the mother. This is particularly the case when the underlying problem is a deficiency in uterine tone, placenta praevia or an unusually shaped pelvis. If the problem is due to fetal malformation, this is more indicative of Jing Deficiency, which of course may have its foundation in a Deficiency of Kidney Qi in the mother.

the fetus because the cord can become compressed during delivery. Cord prolapse can also occur when the baby is presenting in the normal OA position, but this is a rare event, as the tight application of the occiput against the dilated cervix usually prevents the cord from dropping downwards.

If cord prolapse is diagnosed (after vaginal examination during labour), the safest option is to deliver the baby by caesarean section.

Information Box 5.3e-II

Cord prolapse: comments from a Chinese medicine perspective

In Chinese medicine, a cord prolapse is likely to reflect an underlying Deficiency of Spleen and/or Kidney Qi.

Multiple pregnancy

Multiple pregnancy occurs as a result of two distinct physiological processes. It results either from a multiple release of egg cells (ova) from the mother's ovaries, or from an early division of the cells of an embryo. The former (multizygotic) process results in non-identical siblings, and the latter (monozygotic) in apparently identical siblings.

Twins are the most common form of multiple pregnancy, occurring in approximately 1 in 90 pregnancies that reach term. Triplets occur in approximately 1 in 8100 pregnancies. The rate of occurrence of triplets, quadruplets and even larger multiple pregnancies is increasing since the introduction of assisted-fertilisation techniques.

The introduction of early ultrasound scanning has shown that twin pregnancy is more common than was previously thought. This investigation has demonstrated that it is not uncommon for one of the twins in a twin pregnancy to die in the first few weeks of pregnancy, and then to become reabsorbed into the mothers womb. This situation, described as the 'vanishing twin', will then manifest as an apparently 'singleton' pregnancy at later stages in gestation.

In a multiple pregnancy, multizygotic (non-identical) fetuses each develop with their own placenta and amniotic sac. In contrast, monozygotic (identical) fetuses share a common placenta and amniotic sac. Babies born from a multiple pregnancy are generally smaller than average, presumably because they have to draw from a single and limited source of nutrients. Monozygotic fetuses in multiple pregnancies very commonly are markedly different in size. This is because they share one placenta, and often one gets a larger proportion of the blood supply flowing through its umbilical cord.

Multiple pregnancy is more likely to be associated with complications, and so, once diagnosed, the mother will be offered more frequent antenatal care from a specialist centre. The complications that are more likely to occur in multiple pregnancies include:

- pregnancy-induced hypertension
- anaemia (due to iron and folic acid deficiency)
- polyhydramnios
- premature labour
- death of the fetus around the time of the labour.

In addition, many of the minor complications of pregnancy, such as morning sickness, backache, heartburn, haemorrhoids and poor sleep, are exacerbated in multiple pregnancies. The greater the number of fetuses, the more common are all of these complications.

Labour poses an additional problem in multiple pregnancies, partly because the incidence of malpresentation is very high. Only in 45% of cases of twin pregnancies do both fetuses present head down. There is a five times greater risk of a fetus in a multiple pregnancy dying during a vaginal delivery. This is partly a result of the risk of malpresentation, and partly because the fetus is more likely to be underweight. For this reason, caesarean section is commonly advised for the delivery of multiple pregnancies.

Information Box 5.3e-III

Multiple pregnancy: comments from a Chinese medicine perspective

From a Chinese medicine perspective, multiple pregnancies are bound to Deplete the Blood and Kidney Qi of the mother. Deficient Kidney Qi in the mother may manifest as Jing Deficiency in the fetuses; this is reflected in the low birthweight of many babies born from a multiple pregnancy.

Prolonged and obstructed labour

A normal first stage of labour should take no more than 12–24 hours in first pregnancies, and no more than 12 hours in subsequent pregnancies. A normal second stage should last no more than 2 hours. If the labour is prolonged in either of the two stages, there are increasing risks of maternal exhaustion and death of the fetus. If the fetus becomes stuck on its way through the pelvic canal, this is termed 'obstructed labour'. The end result of obstructed labour is rupture of the uterus. Rupture of the uterus is much more likely if there is a scar from a previous caesarean section.

Prolonged labour will frequently result in the use of instrumental delivery or emergency caesarean section. This is always the case in obstructed labour. Rupture of the uterus is a complication that should be avoided if at all possible, as the treatment commonly involves emergency caesarean section followed by hysterectomy.

As has been described, prolonged and obstructed labour may be a result of the position of the fetus. In malpresentation, the fundamental problem is that the presenting part of the fetus is simply too wide to pass easily through the pelvic canal. Similarly, a pelvis which is too narrow to permit the passage of the head of the fetus, even when correctly presented, will result in problems in labour. This problem, rather clumsily termed 'cephalopelvic disproportion' (CPD), is more likely to occur if the woman is of small stature, and particularly if the small stature is the result of illness or malnutrition in childhood. For this reason, CPD is much more common in developing countries than in developed nations. If it appears likely that CPD may be a problem, for example if the pregnant woman is very short, or if she has a small shoe size, the dimensions of the pelvic canal can be measured by means of a pelvic scan. A decision can then be made about whether or not the baby should be delivered by planned caesarean section.

Occasionally, if the baby is large, the head may be delivered normally, but the shoulders become stuck in the pelvic canal. This problem, known as 'shoulder dystocia', poses a severe risk to the life of the fetus. The delivery in a case of shoulder dystocia requires considerable experience on the part of the obstetrician or midwife. In this situation, tearing of the perineal tissues of the mother is not uncommon, and the baby often suffers damage to the structures in the area of its neck, such as the clavicle or the brachial plexus of nerves.

Another common reason for prolonged labour is more functional in nature, in that the presentation of the fetus is normal and the size of the pelvic canal is adequate. In these cases, the problem is attributed to an abnormality of uterine action. In some cases of abnormal uterine action, the contractions are too weak and inefficient to lead to full dilatation of the cervix. In particular, the onset of dilatation of the cervix may be very slow to start. It is now increasingly recognised that a calm and restful environment helps to encourage efficient contractions.

Any stimulus that promotes anxiety in the mother can halt the contractions and may even reverse the progression of the dilatation of the cervix. It is believed that excessive release of adrenaline in the mother can counteract the effect of oxytocin, the natural uterine stimulant. Potential stressors include transfer to an alien hospital environment, excessive pain and an anxious birth partner(s). All these may be compounded by the mother having negative expectations of childbirth, as are commonly held by women in modern societies.

Insufficient uterine activity may respond well to the provision of a calm environment for the mother. If the first stage of labour is prolonged, an infusion of synthetic oxytocin will be initiated, akin to the medical induction of labour. There is a greater than normal probability that this type of functional prolonged labour will end in a caesarean section because of failure of the labour to progress and maternal exhaustion.

In contrast, the uterus may be contracting with force, but the contractions are not coordinated, and so do not result in smooth dilatation of the cervix. In this type of functional prolonged labour, the pain of the contractions may be severe. Emotional factors appear to play an important role also in this abnormality of uterine action. Treatment of functional prolonged labour when the contractions are forceful but inefficient may also include artificial rupture of the membranes before the institution of an oxytocin infusion. There is a greater than normal probability of instrumental delivery and of emergency caesarean section with this type of prolonged labour.

In some cases the cervix ceases to continue to dilate significantly despite continued contractions. This is described as 'cervical dystocia'. If previous scarring to the cervix is the cause of the problem, it is termed 'cervical stenosis'. In this situation, there is a real risk of obstructed labour and fetal distress. If there is no response to an oxytocin infusion within a few hours, an emergency caesarean section will be performed.

Information Box 5.3e-IV

Prolonged labour: comments from a Chinese medicine perspective

In Chinese medicine, prolonged labour is often a reflection of underlying Deficiency in the mother, notably of Blood and Qi. The Deficiency may have its root in Spleen and Stomach Qi Deficiency or Kidney Qi Deficiency. Stagnant flow of Liver Qi and Blood will also contribute to the problem. Fear and tension will sink and stagnate the Qi, and so are likely to inhibit labour.

Of all the causes of prolonged labour, the problems of uterine function are those that are most likely to respond to acupuncture treatment.

Rapid (precipitate) labour

A labour that is too rapid may also cause problems. A precipitate labour is defined as one that takes less than 2 hours. In such a labour the contractions are very intense. The fetus may suffer from lack of oxygen in the womb, and from compression injuries during delivery. Moreover, the delivery is more likely to take place in an unsuitable place, and without trained birth attendants. The mother may be in a state of exhaustion and shock after a precipitate labour.

Perineal tears

Vaginal and perineal tears are very common. They occur at the end of the second stage of labour as the head and then the body of the fetus pass through the vagina and then the stretched perineum. Ideally, tearing can be minimised by controlling the speed at which the head descends through the vaginal canal. Unfortunately, this degree of control is not always possible.

In the least severe cases, these injuries will simply be superficial grazes of the vaginal and perineal epithelium. These minor tears will heal very rapidly.

More severe tears are graded as follows:

- a first-degree tear involves damage to the superficial tissues only
- a second-degree tear involves damage to the superficial tissues and the perineal muscles
- a third-degree tear extends backwards from the vagina to involve damage to the muscles of the anus also
- a fourth-degree tear not only extends to the anal muscle but also tears the lining tissues of the anal canal.

The vagina and perineum should always be inspected after delivery for tears. First-degree tears are simple to repair, and usually heal well with one or two sutures (stitches). Second- and third-degree tears require more care in their repair, but usually can be repaired well. Third- and fourth-degree tears are not common, and are most likely to occur during instrumental (forceps) delivery, delivery of a large baby or a delivery of a baby in the OP position. With a fourth-degree tear the repair requires a skilled operator. The recovery from the repair may be slow, with many women suffering from persisting incontinence of wind, and some with faecal incontinence.

Even if there are only minor lacerations, it is common for many women to suffer quite severe perineal discomfort for the first few days after delivery. Ideally, this discomfort should largely have gone by 1–2 weeks after delivery. However, it has been estimated that up to 15% of women still suffer perineal discomfort by 12 weeks after the delivery. It is not uncommon for sexual intercourse to be uncomfortable for over 20 weeks after delivery. In some cases the trauma of a perineal tear can cause profound psychological damage, and this can continue to affect a sexual relationship adversely for a much longer period.

Episiotomy

Episiotomy is a deliberate incision of the perineum performed at the end of the second stage of labour. Episiotomy is performed to ease the passage of the fetal head through the perineum. It is less commonly performed in uncomplicated labours than it used to be, because it is now appreciated that most naturally occurring tears heal just as well as an episiotomy, if not better. It is now recognised that long-term complications, including perineal pain and difficult intercourse, appear to be more common in women who have had an episiotomy. Nevertheless, in cases when the perineum appears to be overdistending and threatening to tear in a particularly damaging way, an episiotomy may be performed. In some types of forceps delivery, an episiotomy is always performed.

Complications of the third stage of labour

Postpartum haemorrhage and retained placenta

Some blood loss during and following the third stage of labour is to be expected, but is considered excessive if it exceeds 500 millilitres within the first 24 hours after delivery of the baby. If the blood loss is estimated to exceed this amount, the term 'primary postpartum haemorrhage' (primary PPH) is applied. If the blood loss occurs at some point after the first 24 hours after the birth, then the term 'secondary PPH' is applied.

Primary postpartum haemorrhage

In the majority of cases of primary PPH, the bleeding comes from a uterus that has failed to contract down sufficiently during the third stage of labour. Pre-existing conditions, including anaemia and fibroids, can increase the risk of this form of PPH. Even with the use of synthetic oxytocin (ergometrine) injection at the end of the second stage of labour, this form of primary PPH still occurs following approximately 3% of vaginal deliveries. In an additional one-fifth of cases of primary PPH, the bleed originates from a cervical or vaginal laceration.

As blood loss from the womb is prevented by efficient shrinking down of the body of the uterus, any factor that prevents this from occurring will increase the risk of PPH. Inefficient postpartum contractions may occur if the mother is exhausted after a prolonged labour, or if the uterus has been overdistended by a multiple pregnancy. Any retained blood clots or pieces of placenta in the womb will also prevent the uterus from contracting down. Finally, failure of the placenta to separate from the uterus, a situation known as 'retained placenta', will also cause PPH. Together these causes account for 80% of cases of PPH.

If there are retained blood clots or retained placenta, these have to be removed. Often, this is impossible by natural means because the uterus has contracted down around the clot or placenta, thereby preventing their release. This particular problem is exacerbated by the administration of synthetic oxytocin (ergometrine) in the second stage of labour. In this situation, if massage of the uterus has no effect, the retained products have to be removed manually while the woman is under either general or epidural anaesthesia. In this operation, the obstetrician removes the placenta from the womb using a gloved hand. After the procedure, an injection of ergometrine is given to facilitate further contraction down of the uterus.

If bleeding continues from an empty uterus, this can rapidly become an emergency situation. In such cases an intravenous drip is set up to replace lost fluids while the uterus is massaged. Then a continuous infusion of a synthetic oxytocin is administered.

The principal treatment for PPH from cervical and vaginal laceration is careful location and stitching of these tears.

Secondary postpartum haemorrhage

Delayed haemorrhage from the uterus is also usually due to failure of contraction of the uterine lining and retention of blood clots. In this case, the diagnosis can be confirmed by ultrasound scan. Most cases respond to ergometrine injection.

Occasionally, infection in the womb will manifest as secondary PPH (see below).

> **Information Box 5.3e-V**
>
> **Postpartum haemorrhage: comments from a Chinese medicine perspective**
>
> In Chinese medicine, postpartum haemorrhage is most likely to be a result of Spleen Qi Deficiency with Spleen Not Holding Blood. Excessive Heat may be contributory in some cases.
>
> Retention of the placenta suggests Stagnation of Qi or Blood in the Uterus. Blood and Qi Deficiency may be the underlying causes of this failure to generate sufficient downward movement of Qi after delivery.

Complications of the Puerperium

The puerperium is the time during which the mother's body recovers from the changes of pregnancy and the physical trauma of labour. For this reason, minor emotional and physical disturbances are common, and these are considered normal. The puerperium is also the time during which a feeding routine is established for the baby. The complications of breastfeeding, although most common during the puerperium, are described in Chapter 5.3f.

Serious complications of the puerperium are uncommon. These are summarised below.

Puerperal infection

Puerperal infection is defined as a rise in temperature to over 38°C for more than 24 hours occurring within the first 10 days after childbirth. Such a rise in temperature is usually due to either a womb infection, a urinary infection or mastitis (inflammation of the lactating breast). Very rarely, a fever may result from thromboembolism (see below). Before the advent of hygienic midwifery techniques and antibiotic therapy, puerperal infection of the womb was common, and was a major cause of perinatal maternal mortality.

The treatment of puerperal infection is administration of appropriate antibiotic therapy.

> **Information Box 5.3e-VI**
>
> **Postnatal fever: comments from a Chinese medicine perspective**
>
> In Chinese medicine, the differentiation of postnatal fever depends on the nature of the symptoms. Full conditions include invasion of Wind Cold or Wind Heat, Blood Stagnation and Food Retention. Blood Deficiency may be the underlying problem in a situation in which there is continuous low-grade fever after childbirth.

Thromboembolism

The problem of excessive blood clotting is a serious, but rare, problem during pregnancy. In fact, thrombosis is more likely to occur during the puerperium, and in particular between days 5 and 15 after the birth of the baby. Nevertheless, less than 1 in 1000 births are affected by this complication.

The most usual site for a thrombosis to occur is in the deep veins of the leg (DVT). In 1 in 6000 births a pulmonary embolus results from a DVT. This has a 1 in 5 mortality rate.

> **Information Box 5.3e-VII**
>
> **Puerperal thromboembolism: comments from a Chinese medicine perspective**
>
> Thromboembolism represents Blood Stagnation in Chinese medicine. In the puerperium, Stagnation is most likely to result from an underlying Deficiency of Blood and Qi.

Psychiatric complications of the puerperium

The two serious psychiatric complications of the puerperium are postnatal depression and postnatal psychosis.

Postnatal depression

The brief period of low mood known as the "baby blues", first described as an aspect of normal puerperium in Chapter 5.3d, affects up to two-thirds of women on day 3–5 after birth. However, in up to 10% of women a more severe form of depression can be diagnosed during the postnatal period. This is termed 'postnatal depression'.

Postnatal depression is recognised to be more common in certain groups of women. Risk factors include:

- young age at the time of the birth (<16 years)
- personal or family history of depression
- poor experience of child-rearing during childhood
- lack of positive support from husband or partner
- lack of supportive network of family or friends after the birth
- complications during pregnancy or childbirth.

In recent years there has been increased awareness of the possibility of postnatal depression amongst GPs and health visitors. Nowadays, women are asked specific questions during the 6–8 week postnatal check, the answers to which might point to a depressed state. It is believed that the best form of treatment is practical support rather than medication. In severe cases, medication or even admission to a psychiatric hospital may be necessary. Even with hospital admission, every attempt is made to ensure that the mother and baby are not separated. If possible, the mother should be admitted to a dedicated mother and baby unit.

> **Information Box 5.3e-VIII**
>
> **Postnatal depression: comments from a Chinese medicine perspective**
>
> In Chinese medicine, postnatal depression is primarily attributed to Deficiency of Blood and the effect this has on the Heart Organ. The main patterns that can underlie postnatal depression include Heart Blood Deficiency, Heart Yin Deficiency and Heart Blood Stagnation.

Postnatal psychosis

'Psychosis' is defined as a mental health disorder in which the patient loses contact with reality. It is considered to be a severe mental health condition, and is usually managed by means of a combination of hospital admission and medication with major tranquilliser drugs.

Postnatal psychosis affects 1–3 in 1000 women in the few weeks following delivery. The condition is often indistinguishable from an episode of bipolar disorder or schizophrenia. Initial symptoms include confusion, depression and anxiety. Delusions and hallucinations, often concerning the baby, are characteristic. There is a grave risk of neglect of the baby and of suicide in the mother.

Treatment usually involves hospital admission, ideally to a psychiatric mother and baby unit, where major tranquilliser medication is given. In most cases, the condition settles within weeks and the medication can be withdrawn. However, there is a significant risk that the problem will recur, either in a subsequent pregnancy, or in the form of a more chronic major mental illness. Approximately one-third of women who develop postnatal psychosis will have a recurrent form of psychosis at a later date.

Information Box 5.3e-IX

Postnatal psychosis: comments from a Chinese medicine perspective

In Chinese medicine, psychosis can be attributed to Heart or Liver Blood Stagnation or to Phlegm Fire Harassing the Heart. Underlying imbalances that may contribute to the development of psychosis include Heart and Liver Blood Deficiency with Qi Stagnation, as these can predispose to Blood Stagnation. Spleen Qi Deficiency may contribute to the development of Phlegm.

The red flags of the disorders of the puerperium

As practitioners of complementary medicine, you do not need to be familiar with the Red Flags of childbirth, as a trained midwife or doctor should be present to oversee the safety of a woman in labour. However, you do need to be able to recognise the red flags of the puerperium.

Table 5.3e-I Red Flags 38 – the puerperium

Red Flag	Description	Reasoning
38.1	**Fever in the puerperium**	Refer any case of fever developing in the first 2 weeks of the puerperium (temperature >38°C for more than 24 hours) to exclude possible uterine infection
38.2	**Postpartum haemorrhage**: refer if bleeding is any more than a blood-stained discharge	Blood-stained discharge (lochia) is normal in the early puerperium, but moderate to severe bleeding (like a heavy period or heavier) is not, and needs referral as it can herald a more serious bleed A profuse bleed of more than 500 ml or the symptoms of shock (low blood pressure, fainting, rapid pulse rate) constitute an emergency
38.3	**Thromboembolism**: pain in the calf, discoloured or swollen leg, or breathlessness with chest pain, or blood in sputum in the puerperium	Refer any features of a thromboembolic event (deep venous thrombosis of the calf or pelvic veins, pulmonary embolus or stroke). The risks of these events are greater in the puerperium
38.4	**Postnatal depression**	Refer any case of depression developing in the postnatal period that is lasting for more than 3 weeks and which is not responding to your treatment. Refer straight away if the woman is experiencing suicidal ideas, or if you believe the health of the baby to be at risk
38.5	**Postnatal psychosis**	Refer straight away if you suspect the development of postnatal psychosis (delusional or paranoid ideas and hallucinations are key features), as this condition is associated with a high risk of suicide or harm to the baby
38.6	**Insufficient breast milk**	Refer if the mother is considering stopping breastfeeding within the first few months after delivery because of apparently insufficient milk-production. In the case of poor latching on of the baby, advice from a midwife or health visitor may remedy the problem
38.7	**Sore nipples/blocked ducts** during the time of breastfeeding	Refer to the midwife (early days) or health visitor for advice on breastfeeding. Encourage the mother to keep breastfeeding despite the discomfort, as a continued flow of milk can help with healing
38.8	**Mastitis** during the time of breastfeeding not responding to treatment in 2 days	Refer only if not responding to treatment within 2 days, or if you suspect the development of an abscess (a firm mass is felt in the affected breast, and the mother feels very unwell). Encourage the mother to keep breastfeeding despite the discomfort, as a continued flow of milk can help with the healing

Some women suffering from disorders of the puerperium will benefit from referral to a conventional doctor for assessment and/or treatment. Red flags are those symptoms and signs that indicate that referral is to be considered. The red flags of the disorders of the puerperium are described in Table 5.3e-I. This table forms part of the summary on red flags given in Appendix III, which also gives advice on the degree of urgency of referral for each of the red flag conditions listed (see Q5.3e-3).

Self-test 5.3e

The complications of childbirth and the puerperium

1. What are factors which might lead to an abnormally long labour?
2. What are the different methods of instrumental delivery? For what sort of reasons might instrumental delivery be employed during labour?
3. What are the mental /emotinal complications of the puerperium?

Answers

1. An excessively long labour might result from the following factors:
   Abnormal positioning of the fetus in womb
   Abnormalities in the size or shape of the mother's pelvis (cephalopelvic disproportion)
   An abnormally large baby, as might occur in maternal diabetes mellitus (another cause of cephalopelvic disproportion)
   Abnormal function of the uterus
2. Forceps delivery and vacuum (ventouse) extraction are the two methods of non-surgical instrumental delivery.
   Caesarean section is also classified as a method of instrumental delivery.
   Instrumental delivery might be employed during labour for the following reasons:
   Forceps delivery and ventouse extraction
   (only when the cervix has dilated):
   fetal malpresentation when the head is down
   cephalopelvic disproportion
   abnormal function of the uterus leading to maternal exhaustion
   Emergency caesarian section:
   all of the above, particularly if the cervix has failed to dilate, and:
   evidence of serious fetal distress during labour
   prolapse of the umbilical cord
   difficulties in delivery with breech presentation or multiple pregnancy
   shoulder presentation
   rupture of the uterus
3. The mental emotional problems which might complicate the puerperium include:
   baby blues (mild anxiety, tearfulness and depression which peaks between days 3-5 after the delivery)
   post natal depression (a more prolonged and severe state of low mood affecting about 1 in 10 of women after childbirth)
   post natal psychosis (a rare severe mental health disturbance involving delusional ideas and hallucinations)

Chapter 5.3f Lactation and disorders of the breast

LEARNING POINTS

At the end of this chapter you will:
- understand the physiology of the breast and the process of lactation
- be able to describe the disorders of lactation
- be able to describe the disorders of the non-lactating breast.

Estimated time for chapter: 90 minutes.

Introduction

This concluding chapter of this section on pregnancy and childbirth summarises the normal physiology of the breast, and the disorders that can affect the breast. Although the principal function of the breast is to provide milk in the process termed 'lactation', for most of a woman's life the breast is not performing this role. Nevertheless, the quiescent breast tissue is vulnerable to a range of important medical conditions. It must not be forgotten that men also have a small amount of breast tissue, which can give rise to some of the breast diseases that are more commonly recognised in women.

Usually, in conventional practice, disorders of the breast are referred not to an obstetrician but to a consultant surgeon. Problems with breastfeeding are usually overseen by the woman's GP and the midwife.

The important disorders of the breast described in this chapter are:

- The disorders of lactation:
  - poor milk supply
  - sore nipples
  - blocked ducts and mastitis
  - overflowing milk.
- The disorders of the non-lactating breast:
  - benign breast disease
  - benign tumours of the breast
  - breast cancer
  - gynaecomastia.

The physiology of the breast and lactation

The breast is also known as the 'mammary gland'. It is composed of numerous exocrine glands, called 'lobules', as illustrated in Figure 5.3f-I (see Q5.3f-1 and Q5.3f-2).

Oestrogen and progesterone are important for the development of the breast tissue from puberty onwards. Oestrogen is the hormone that is released from the developing ovarian follicle in the first half of the menstrual cycle, and progesterone is released from the corpus luteum in the second half of the menstrual cycle. It is probable that it is an imbalance in the level of progesterone that is responsible for the engorgement of breasts, which is such a common feature of the premenstrual phase of the cycle.

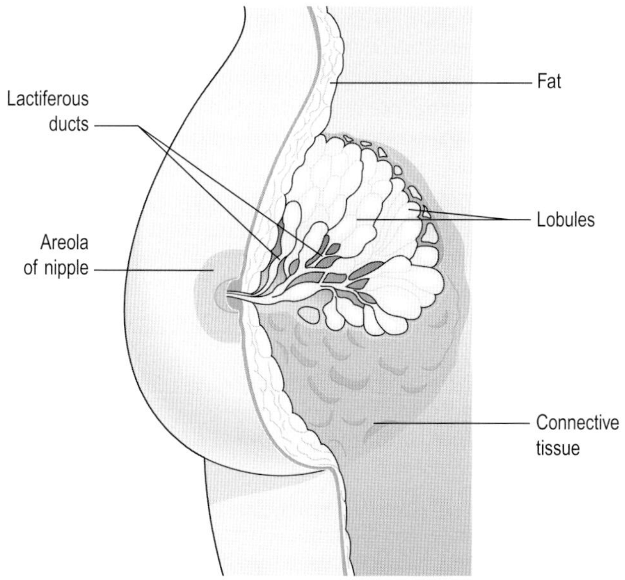

Figure 5.3f-I • The structure of the breast.

In pregnancy, oestrogen and progesterone produced in both the ovary and the placenta, are responsible for enlargement of the breast tissue and fat deposition around the breast. The lobules of the breast produce milk in response to prolactin, which is secreted by the pituitary gland. The milk produced in each lobule reaches the nipple by passing first through a lactiferous sinus and then a lactiferous duct. All the ducts converge at the nipple, from where the milk will be ejected through tiny openings. The lobules are supported and protected by fatty tissue.

After childbirth, the stimulus of suckling causes release of both prolactin and oxytocin from the pituitary. Prolactin continues to stimulate the production of milk in the lobules. Oxytocin stimulates a muscular contraction of the lining of the lactiferous sinuses, so causing a fine jet of milk to be released from the nipple (this is known as the 'let-down' reflex).

Lactation ideally should begin within minutes of delivery of the baby. A newborn will reflexively 'search' for a nipple when its cheek is stroked, and then will 'latch on' to the nipple once it is found.

Once the baby has the nipple correctly inserted in its mouth, the pinching of its jaw will stimulate the let down of milk, via the release of oxytocin. Directly after delivery, the first milk produced is a thin, watery fluid known as 'colostrum'. This has little nutritional value but is rich in maternal antibodies. Despite the production of prolactin, the production of milk is inhibited during the latter part of pregnancy by oestrogen from the placenta. As the levels of oestrogen drop after delivery, and as the nipple is stimulated by the suckling baby, milk begins to be formed. This can lead to a sudden and tender engorgement of the breasts approximately 2–3 days after delivery. At this point the milk is said to have 'come in'. The discomfort is relieved by feeding the baby, and this is a clear incentive to continue feeding.

The production of milk draws on water and nutrients from the mother's blood. Breast milk is known to contain all the nutrients required to sustain a growing baby for the first 6 months of its life. It also contains antibodies from the mother, which continue to protect the newborn from disease, including gastroenteritis. The mother's reserves of glucose, calcium, iron and fat are drawn on in particular to supply the baby's needs. Therefore, a breastfeeding mother will need to ensure that her diet is rich in nutritious, high-energy foods and calcium. It is well recognised that nutritional deficiencies manifesting in weak teeth, a reduction in bone density, anaemia, thinning of hair and weight loss can affect a woman who is breastfeeding. Many women who are breastfeeding a baby of more than a couple of months of age will describe feeling drained after feeding.

The World Heath Organization now recommends that most babies should be exclusively breastfed for the first 4 months and ideally for 6 months, either before introducing a formula milk, or before solids are introduced. This is because breast milk is considered to have a number of advantages over bottle feeding with formula milks and early weaning (supplementation with solid foods). Firstly, breast milk is recognised to be superior nutritionally to formula preparations. This is of particular significance in some developing nations in which the practice of giving over-diluted formula milks is known to be common among poorer communities. Breast milk is also protective against disease because it contains maternal antibodies. Finally, early weaning with solid food may introduce food materials that are potentially allergenic.

However, it is recognised that although many women attempt breastfeeding after childbirth, by week 6 after the birth less than 60% are still breastfeeding. This figure is much lower for women from a low socio-economic class. The reasons for stopping breastfeeding are complex, and include socially driven perceptions of acceptable behaviour, and what is best for the baby. Nevertheless, there is no doubt that some women are forced to stop feeding because the baby is not getting the nutrition it requires, or because the experience of breastfeeding is very uncomfortable for the mother. Both these problems are largely preventable, and are explored in the next section on the disorders of lactation.

Very few women in the UK will be exclusively breastfeeding by 6 months after the birth. Even for those who continue to breastfeed, many will have introduced occasional formula feeds and solid food by month 3 or 4. Women choose to supplement breastfeeding partly because it may be more convenient, but also because the baby may appear to be unsatisfied on breast milk alone.

However, current medical advice is to avoid the introduction of solid food until the baby is 6 months old in order to minimise early contact with potential dietary allergens.

If breastfeeding is stopped suddenly, either because of choice, or because of illness in the mother or the baby, the breasts will rapidly become engorged and uncomfortable. This discomfort will settle within a few days as the milk production ceases, and the stored milk is reabsorbed. In cases in which the discomfort is very distressing, the mother may be prescribed a drug that inhibits the release of prolactin (bromocriptine).

Breastfeeding is not always the best or safest option. Certain infections and drugs can be transmitted to the baby via the breast milk. In particular, HIV is known to be transmitted through the breast milk; 25% of HIV-negative babies who are breastfed by an HIV-positive mother will become HIV-positive. Recreational drugs such as nicotine, alcohol and cannabis pass readily into the breast milk. These may cause long-term developmental delay if the baby is exposed to these over a long period. Certain medications can pass into breast milk, and potentially harm the baby. If these drugs are considered necessary, the mother may be obliged to stop breastfeeding.

Information Box 5.3f-I

The breast and lactation: comments from a Chinese medicine perspective

In Chinese medicine, the Organs that have particular significance in breast diseases are the Stomach and the Liver. The Liver, in particular, is believed to control the nipple. A combination of Deficient Stomach Qi and Stagnant Liver Qi is at the root of many breast disorders. Breast milk is dependent on Blood for its formation and on healthy Qi for a smooth flow from the lobule to the nipple. Deficiency of Blood and Qi can lead to problems in lactation.

The disorders of lactation

Poor supply of milk

A baby who is not getting sufficient breast milk will, in general, be miserable, unsatisfied after feeding, and fail to gain weight as might be expected. If a baby is not contented at the breast, the mother may be too quick to assume that she has a poor supply of milk. A common consequence of this misconception is that she gives up breastfeeding and replaces breast milk with formula milk feeds.

However, a true inability to produce sufficient milk is considered only very rarely to be the underlying cause of an unsatisfied baby. Instead, most cases of problems with feeding are due to a failure in stimulation of the let-down reflex. In these cases, the milk flow can be encouraged to improve with advice about correct 'latching on' of the baby to the breast. This is because the baby needs to have a large portion of the nipple in its mouth to stimulate an adequate release of oxytocin, and this correct positioning may not always be obvious to a new mother. It is also known that stress and cold inhibits the flow of oxytocin (this is also the case during childbirth). The mother should be encouraged to breastfeed in a calm and warm setting, and be reminded that holding fears about failure may actually make the milk flow slow down.

Occasionally, the baby never adequately manages to stimulate the let-down reflex. Although milk can be expressed by means of a manual pump, the baby remains unable to obtain the milk it requires by suckling. This is more likely to occur when the baby has a coexisting developmental disorder such as cerebral palsy. In this sort of case, the use of a manual or electric pump may be a helpful short-term method for obtaining milk for the baby, but may prove too difficult and time-consuming an approach to maintain in the long term.

If the mother is very run down, stressed or chronically ill, the milk may indeed be in short supply, because her body has a need, in a stressful or depleted situation, to hold on to its nutritional reserves. In such a case the breasts would not feel engorged. In this sort of situation, it may be for the best that the baby is fed largely on formula milk, to allow the mother to regain health.

Information Box 5.3f-II

Poor milk supply: comments from a Chinese medicine perspective

In Chinese medicine, poor milk supply due to maternal depletion corresponds to Blood and Qi Deficiency. Liver Qi Stagnation can also be contributory. In this case the breasts will feel slightly distended and uncomfortable.

Sore and cracked nipples

Sore and cracked nipples are a very common complaint early in the experience of breastfeeding. The problem is attributed to poor positioning of the baby at the breast such that the nipple is only partly inserted into the baby's mouth. It may also be the result of a particularly vigorous sucking action. The pain from sore nipples can be so severe as to prevent feeding. Treatment includes the use of soothing creams and a plastic shield placed around the nipple during feeding. These treatments do not always provide satisfactory relief from the problem.

Information Box 5.3f-III

Sore nipples: comments from a Chinese medicine perspective

In Chinese medicine, sore nipples are a manifestation of local Stagnation of Qi with Generation of Heat as a result of physical trauma.

Blocked ducts and mastitis

The lactiferous ducts can easily become blocked if the production of milk in the lobules exceeds the demand made by the baby. As milk lies stagnant in the lactiferous sinuses and ducts, it can solidify. Then, a backlog of milk can build up behind the blockage, leading to pain and inflammation in the region of the lobule. A blocked duct will lead to an acutely tender, localised area in the breast, which feels warm to the touch. The skin overlying the area may appear red. A firm lump is felt in the region of the most tenderness. The treatment of a blocked duct is to encourage the baby to breastfeed as much as possible. This alone can resolve the problem. Alternatively, the mother can sit in a hot bath and massage the breasts towards the nipple. This also can encourage the flow of milk, and may even result in the extrusion of a fine worm-like cast of clotted milk as the blockage is relieved.

If not treated with speed, a blocked duct can rapidly lead to a very painful enlarging area of inflammation of the breast tissue. This condition is called 'mastitis'. The more painful the breast becomes, the more difficult it is for the mother to bear either to continue feeding from the affected breast or to massage the breast. In severe mastitis, the breast is visibly swollen and the skin is tense, red and shiny. The mother can develop a high fever and feel very unwell.

Mastitis may also be caused by bacteria entering the breast tissue from the nipple. Infectious mastitis classically occurs at the end of the first week of breastfeeding. Occasionally, this can lead to a collection of pus in the affected breast, known as a 'breast abscess'.

It is clear that mastitis is more likely to develop if the mother is tired or dehydrated. Also, a disturbance in the natural routine of feeding, such as might affect a working mother, can trigger an attack.

In all cases of mastitis the mother should be encouraged to breastfeed. In some cases the treatment as described for blocked ducts, together with bed-rest, painkillers and plenty of fluids may be sufficient to allow the condition to resolve. The conventional treatment usually includes a course of antibiotics (flucloxacillin is given because it is believed to be harmless to the breastfeeding baby). If a breast abscess has developed, it is best that this is drained by means of a minor surgical procedure.

Information Box 5.3f-IV

Poor milk supply: comments from a Chinese medicine perspective

In Chinese medicine, blocked ducts and mastitis are usually thought to correspond to Liver Qi and Blood Stagnation and the development of Full Heat. The pathology of severe mastitis and breast abscess is described as Heat and Toxic Heat affecting the Liver, Stomach and Gallbladder Channels.

Overflowing milk

Some women appear to produce milk in abundance. The milk flows not only during breastfeeding, but also at other times of the day. In particular it may be triggered by the thought or sound of the baby, an indication that these emotional responses are also stimuli for the release of oxytocin. Overflowing milk can be very inconvenient, as the women needs to wear cotton wool pads over the nipple to prevent leakage, and may need to change her clothes frequently.

From a conventional perspective, overflowing milk is not seen as a problem. Women with excessive milk production may be encouraged to express the milk by means of a manual pump, so that it can be donated for use in special care baby units.

Information Box 5.3f-V

Overflowing milk: comments from a Chinese medicine perspective

In Chinese medicine, overflowing milk is not a sign of health. In contrast, it may either be an indication of the failure of Qi to hold fluids or a result of Liver fire agitating the breast milk. The underlying imbalances are Spleen and Stomach Qi Deficiency, and Stagnation of Liver Qi, respectively.

The disorders of the non-lactating breast

Benign breast disease (lumpy breasts)

You have read how the breast tissue in a non-lactating woman undergoes a cyclical change corresponding to the consecutive peaks of oestrogen and progesterone in the first and second halves of the menstrual cycle, respectively. It is normal for the breast to enlarge slightly under the influence of progesterone in the second half of the menstrual cycle. In some women, in particular in those over 30 years old, this enlargement in the second half of the cycle is excessive. It has been suggested that this problem may be a result of an imbalance between the amount of oestrogen and progesterone circulating in the second half of the cycle.

In benign breast disease, the woman experiences uncomfortable swelling of the breasts in the premenstrual phase, and in some the breasts can feel lumpy, particularly in the outer parts of the breast tissue. Sometimes the lumpiness is confined to one portion of the breast, so giving rise to a concern that the lump represents cancer. However, the fact that the lumps become enlarged and tender premenstrually is an encouraging sign that these changes are benign, and result from fluctuations in the sex hormones.

It is recognised that benign breast disease has an emotional component. Sometimes another functional condition, such as irritable bowel syndrome, unexplained pelvic pain and premenstrual syndrome, may coexist with benign breast disease.

On examination, a tender irregular lump may be found, or there may be a general feeling of firm irregularity, with the breasts tender all over. If there is concern about the nature of the lumpiness, a sample of breast tissue cells may be withdrawn from the lumpy area by means of a fine needle and syringe (fine needle biopsy). In some cases clear or blood-stained fluid can be withdrawn from the area, indicating the formation of benign cysts. Although withdrawal of the fluid may bring about temporary relief of the problem, the cysts usually refill with fluid over the next few weeks. This test is usually combined with a simple ultrasound scan of the lumpy area. If no evidence of cancer is found, the woman is reassured that the problem is common and related to hormonal changes.

Advice includes wearing a well-fitting bra, and reducing fat and caffeine in the diet. Some women are helped by vitamin B_6 (pyridoxine) supplements and evening primrose oil (gamolenic acid). However, medical studies have suggested that these approaches have no benefit when compared to placebo treatments.

If the symptoms are very severe, drugs that suppress the release of FSH may be prescribed (danazol or gestrinone). These drugs have a range of side-effects resulting from a drop in the levels of oestrogen and an increase in levels of testosterone, the male sex hormone. Alternatively, some women may be prescribed a synthetic preparation of progesterone in the second half of the cycle, as one theory is that the problem is due to a relative deficiency of progesterone.

Although hormonally related breast disease is benign, it is now believed that women who suffer from it have a slightly increased risk of breast cancer. For this reason, a patient with this condition may be advised to have a regular mammogram examination from the age of 40 years.

Information Box 5.3f-VI

Benign breast disease: comments from a Chinese medicine perspective

In Chinese medicine, benign breast disease is primarily a result of Stagnation of Liver Qi. This might explain how functional conditions such as irritable bowel syndrome and premenstrual syndrome can coexist with benign breast disease. If the discomfort is severe, this may reflect Liver Blood Stagnation. Lumpiness and cyst formation might indicate the accumulation of Phlegm.

Benign tumours of the breast

The finding of a painless, smooth and mobile lump in the breast in a relatively young woman (often this occurs in women less than 30 years old) is indicative of a benign tumour called a 'fibroadenoma'. Sometimes the lump is extremely mobile, and may slip from under the examining fingers. For this reason it has also been described as a breast mouse. There is no link between this condition and the future development of cancer. Nevertheless, if a breast mouse is found, the woman is often advised to have it removed surgically. Removal of a breast mouse is a relatively minor operation.

Information Box 5.3f-VII

Fibroadenoma of the breast (breast mouse): comments from a Chinese medicine perspective

In Chinese medicine, the development of a breast mouse is indicative of an accumulation of Phlegm. There may be an underlying Deficiency of Stomach and Spleen Qi.

Breast cancer

Breast cancer used to be the most common form of cancer in women, although it has now been overtaken by lung cancer as a result of the increase in the incidence of smoking in women. Breast cancer affects 1 in 14 women, usually after the onset of the menopause. The cause of breast cancer is unclear, although it is recognised that it is more common in women of higher socio-economic classes, and in those who choose to have their families late in life. These factors may not be unrelated. Childbearing before the age of 30 years, which is more common in women from lower socio-economic classes, appears to be protective.

The risk of breast cancer is increased if there is a family history of breast cancer. In particular, one rare but particularly aggressive form of breast cancer is recognised to affect over 80% of first-degree female relatives. This form of cancer has been associated with a mutation in a gene called BRCA1 and BRCA2, for which genetic tests are available.

It is also recognised that long-term use of the oral contraceptive pill is associated with a slightly increased risk of breast cancer, although this risk is usually not considered to be great enough to outweigh the perceived benefits of the use of the pill. Hormone replacement therapy is also known to confer an extra risk of breast cancer.

If breast cancer is diagnosed early in its development, before any signs of spread to the axillary lymph nodes, it may be treated by a combination of surgery and radiotherapy. The aggressive approach of total breast removal, known as 'mastectomy', has now been found to be no more effective than simple removal of the tumour in early cancers. After surgery, 'adjuvant' radiotherapy is directed at the armpit, with the aim of eliminating any tiny metastases that may have formed in the lymph nodes.

If the tumour is small, but one or more of the lymph nodes is found to contain cancer cells, long-term survival is increased if the woman undergoes additional adjuvant treatment immediately after surgery. Chemotherapy, long-term treatment with anti-oestrogen drugs such as tamoxifen and anastrazole, and, in premenopausal women, removal of the ovaries, are forms of adjuvant therapy that have been demonstrated to have similar benefits in 'node-positive' breast cancer. The choice of adjuvant therapy depends partly on whether or not the examining pathologist has classified the tumour as one that may grow in response to oestrogen.

If the tumour spreads outside the breast tissue to involve either the subcutaneous tissue and skin or the underlying pectoralis muscle, it is described as 'advanced'. In an advanced cancer there may be obvious distortion of the breast contour, or puckering and a colour change of the skin over the lump. If the breast cancer is advanced, total breast removal, together with excision of the axillary nodes (radical mastectomy), is necessary. Adjuvant therapy is also used in advanced cases.

Breast cancer tends to metastasise most commonly to the bones, the brain and the liver. There is little hope of total remission once secondary spread has occurred. An increasing number of genetically engineered antibodies are available that target and cause the destruction of the protein growth factors produced by tumours. These include trastuzumab (Herceptin), which was designed to counteract a growth factor known as Her2. Her2 plays a role in the maintenance of metastatic breast cancer, and so trastuzumab may be prescribed to control the symptoms of metastatic disease.

Survival after a diagnosis of breast cancer depends on the age of the woman and the stage of progression of the tumour at diagnosis. As a general rule, a breast cancer diagnosed before age 40 years is more likely to be aggressive than one that is diagnosed after the menopause. Nevertheless, there is a possibility of prolonged remission if the tumour is diagnosed at a very early stage, whatever the age of the woman.

For this reason, early detection of breast cancer is considered to be very important. Public health campaigns focus on teaching women to examine their breasts, and to report any unusual changes quickly. Also, the national programme of X-ray imaging of the breasts (mammography) encourages women to undergo annual screening after the age of 50 years. If any abnormal changes are seen on the X-ray images, the woman is called for further tests, which may include a fine needle biopsy of the suspicious area.

Mammography carries the same problems as the cervical screening test, in that a worrying mammogram may not necessarily indicate a true cancer, and after further tests the woman can then be reassured. The mammogram is less helpful in younger women, as X-ray images of young breast tissue are much more difficult to interpret.

Information Box 5.3f-VIII

Breast cancer: comments from a Chinese medicine perspective

In Chinese medicine, as with all cancers, breast cancer is an indication of Phlegm or Blood Stagnation on the background of underlying Deficiency of Yin or Yang. In particular, imbalance of the Stomach, Spleen and Liver Organs might be expected to be present.

Gynaecomastia

'Gynaecomastia' is the medical term used to describe the development of breast tissue in men. It is a very common finding in pubescent boys, in up to 50% of whom a small amount of breast tissue may appear under one or both nipples. In most cases this tissue growth is not very visible, and will subside within a few months. If persistent, and a cause of embarrassment, it can be removed by means of a minor surgical procedure.

Gynaecomastia developing in men has wide range of recognised causes, including a response to certain prescribed medications and recreational drugs, in which case it is not serious. However, if it develops after puberty it should be taken seriously, as it can be a consequence of a hormone-secreting tumour. Once a significant amount of breast tissue has developed, it will not regress, and may need to be removed surgically.

Information Box 5.3f-IX

Gynaecomastia: comments from a Chinese medicine perspective

In Chinese medicine, the development of a painless lump in the region of the nipple in men would suggest accumulation of Phlegm consequent on an underlying imbalance in the Stomach, Spleen or Liver Organs.

The red flags of the disorders of the breast

Some patients with structural disorders of the breast will benefit from referral to a conventional doctor for assessment and/or treatment. Red flags are those symptoms and signs that indicate that referral is to be considered. The red flags of the disorders of the breast are described in Table 5.3f-I. This table forms part of the summary on red flags given in Appendix III, which also gives advice on the degree of urgency of referral for each of the red flag conditions listed.

Table 5.3f-I Red Flags 39 – breast disorders

Red Flag	Description	Reasoning
39.1	**Insufficient breast milk** when breastfeeding	Refer if the mother is considering stopping breastfeeding within the first few months after delivery because of apparently insufficient milk production. In the case of poor latching on of the baby, advice from a midwife or health visitor may remedy the problem
39.2	**Lactation/nipple discharge** but not breastfeeding	Production of milk or nipple discharge in someone who is not breastfeeding or in late pregnancy may be a sign of a pituitary disorder or breast cancer, and investigation is merited
39.3	**Sore nipples/blocked ducts** during the time of breastfeeding	Refer to the midwife (early days) or health visitor for advice on breastfeeding technique. Encourage the mother to keep breastfeeding despite the discomfort, as a continued flow of milk can help with the healing
39.4	**Mastitis** during the time of breastfeeding not responding to treatment in 2 days	Refer only if not responding to treatment within 2 days, or if you suspect the development of an abscess (a firm mass is felt in the affected breast, and the mother feels very unwell). Encourage the mother to keep breastfeeding despite the discomfort, as a continued flow of milk can help with the healing
39.5	**Inflamed breast tissue** but not breastfeeding	Inflammation of a portion of a breast is common in breastfeeding mothers (mastitis) but needs prompt assessment if it occurs in someone who is not lactating, as it may signify inflammation from an underlying tumour

Continued

Table 5.3f-I Red Flags 39 – breast disorders—Cont'd

Red Flag	Description	Reasoning
39.6	**Pain in the breast**, but no inflammation or lump	Tender breasts are common and result from periodic premenstrual hormone stimulation. This symptom can be asymmetrical. Pain is not a usual symptom of breast cancer, and an anxious patient can be reassured. It is important to question the patient to ensure the pain is not actually chest pain. Angina can present with pain that may be described as pain in the breast
39.7	**Lump in the breast**: skin dimpling, fixity or irregularity of the lump are more sinister signs	The conventional practice is now to refer all suspicious lumps in the breast for prompt assessment, as it is known that 1 in 10 breast lumps are cancerous
39.8	**Breast tissue development in teenage boys and adult men (gynaecomastia)**	Refer any case of gynaecomastia in a teenage boy or adult male. A pubescent boy can be reassured that this problem (if only confined to breast bud development) is a common feature of puberty, which should settle down, but refer nevertheless to exclude rare endocrine disorders. Adult men with this condition need investigation to exclude cancerous change and endocrine disorders
39.9	**Eczema of nipple region**	A one-sided, crusty, non healing skin disorder of the nipple may be a form of cancer (Paget's disease). Refer for investigation

Self-test 5.3f

Lactation and disorders of the breast

1. One of your patients had a baby 2 weeks ago. She is struggling with breastfeeding, and thinks that after 2 weeks of trying she is going to have to give up. She has sore nipples and feels that her baby is not satisfied with feeding. He is miserable and seems to want to suckle all the time, which makes the soreness worse. She finds it difficult to express milk for him, and believes that she is unable to produce the milk that he needs.
   (i) How might you advise this woman?
   (ii) Should you refer this problem for professional advice?
2. A 45-year-old patient has noticed a lump in her breast. She does not usually examine her breasts, but came upon an area of irregular tenderness in one breast when in the bath last night. She thinks that this is a new development, and is very concerned about breast cancer. You are treating this patient for menstrual irregularities, and you know that she suffers from premenstrual syndrome and premenstrual breast tenderness.
   (i) How might you question this patient further?
   (ii) Should you refer this woman?

Answers

1. (i) You could discuss with your patient the fact that early difficulties in breastfeeding are very rarely to do with an inability to produce milk, and more often to do with feeding technique. Simple measures that the mother might use to encourage the flow of milk include breastfeeding in a calm, warm environment after having had a hot bath. Massaging the nipples with olive oil can soothe soreness. However, these approaches will be of little help if the baby is not latching on appropriately.
   (ii) Problems with latching on can respond well to expert advice. You should encourage your patient to contact her midwife for guidance on correct feeding technique.
2. (i) You might ask about the timing of the problem in relation to the menstrual cycle. Also you might enquire whether or not there is a family history of breast disease or breast cancer. This patient may have felt the lumpiness of benign breast disease. Contrary to her understanding, lumpiness can be present for months to years in a breast before it is noticed, so this problem may not be a new development. If this tender lump has become apparent in the second half of her menstrual cycle, you can be reassuring, as this is very suggestive of a benign hormonally related area of engorgement of the breast. If this is the case, you can treat the woman with acupuncture and monitor whether there are any improvements with treatment and in the first half of the cycle.
   (ii) Nevertheless, you should refer all unexplained breast lumps to a doctor, so that further assessment by means of ultrasound scan and fine needle biopsy can be arranged.

Children's health

5.4

Chapter 5.4a Introduction to children's health

LEARNING POINTS

At the end of this chapter you will be able to:

- explain why children have special health needs
- list the special health needs of children.

Estimated time for chapter: 90 minutes.

Why do children have special health needs?

This last section of Stage 5 is dedicated to the special health needs of children and the disorders that can affect children. That children have particular health needs is reflected in the fact that in conventional medical practice the speciality of paediatrics requires further training over and above that required of a general physician. Although children may be vulnerable to many of the conditions which have already been described in this text, there is a wide range of conditions of childhood that can develop because the physiology and the susceptibility of the child are different from that of the adult (see Q.5.4a-1).

There are, of course, many conditions from which the child is protected because of its youth. These conditions are the chronic adult diseases that result from the cumulative effects of an unhealthy lifestyle and ageing. For this reason, a child is usually not vulnerable to some of the most important adult diseases such as coronary heart disease, stroke, adult cancers and the degenerative diseases of old age, such as osteoarthritis and Alzheimer's disease.

What are the special health needs of children?

Children have special health needs for two overarching reasons: first, the physiology of the child is immature; and, second, the child is in a process of rapid growth and development. These factors combine to give a third reason why children need special focus, which is that any illness developing in a growing child as a result of immature physiology may cause setbacks in growth and development, which may have lasting, even life-long, consequences. These three reasons are now explored in more detail.

The physiology of the child is immature

Immaturity of the immune system in children means that a child may be more susceptible to conditions from which adults are relatively protected. These conditions include certain infections and allergies. Also, a child who is ill is more vulnerable to extreme fever. The small size of a child means that it is more vulnerable to dehydration when unwell.

The immature nervous system of a child is more likely to be disturbed by fever or trauma, which can result in convulsions, confusion and loss of consciousness.

An immature digestive system is more likely to succumb to conditions such as colic, gastroenteritis and constipation.

Many of the common childhood cancers develop from the immature 'blast' cells, which are present in developing tissue in a small child. Blast cells are the rapidly dividing fetal progenitors of adult cells.

The physical, emotional and mental faculties of a child are immature. This means that they are more vulnerable to extremes of temperature, accidents, physical abuse (non-accidental injury), and emotional and sexual abuse.

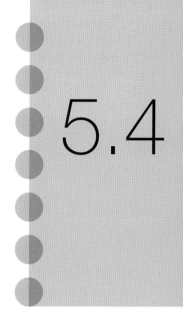

Because of the vulnerability that comes from immaturity, the child requires special protection from any noxious factors that might have the potential to damage its health.

The child is in a process of rapid growth and development

Growth requires a constant supply of adequate nutrients. Nutritional deficiencies in childhood can lead to lasting health problems.

Physical growth and the development of physical, mental and emotional skills also require a complex input of less measurable factors, including love, security, consistency, play, exercise, rest, access to education and a supportive social network. If any of these factors is deficient, the physical, mental and emotional health of the child may suffer, again with long-term consequences.

Vulnerability to setbacks in growth and development

Any disturbance in health can affect growth and development. A child with a chronic childhood illness may suffer long-term consequences of impaired growth and development as a result of the illness. In particular, the impact of congenital disease can be very significant, as it can affect growth and development from the time of the birth of the child (see Q5.4a-2).

The health needs of children are those factors that enable a child to remain healthy in the face of its immaturity and state of growth and development. Meeting these health needs is all the more important if the child has been born with a constitutional deficiency resulting from congenital disease or prematurity, or if it should later develop a serious illness.

The special health needs of children include a balanced nutritious diet, protection from injury, toxins and extremes of climate, protection from infection, freedom to play and exercise, adequate rest, love, security, consistency of care and access to a social network, access to education and protection from physical, sexual or emotional abuse.

The importance of meeting these health needs at every stage in a child's development cannot be overestimated. It is well recognised that if a child falls behind in growing and developing as might be expected, it is often very difficult for the child to catch up at a later date. Therefore, failure to meet these basic health needs during childhood can have an impact on long-term health and well-being, and so might compromise health in adult life.

The special health needs of children are considered below in detail.

A nutritious diet

A child needs an adequate supply of the basic nutrients in its diet to grow and develop healthily. The basic nutrients include protein, carbohydrate, fats, and a wide range of vitamins and minerals. All these nutrients are required to enable the tissues to form at the normal rate. If there are nutritional deficiencies, the child will fail to grow and to develop as would be expected.

Nutritional deficiency can cause problems in physical growth and development, such as the small stature and vulnerability to infection that results from protein-calorie deficiency. The high infant and childhood mortality from infection in developing countries is largely a consequence of protein-calorie deficiency. Those children who have had to subsist on too little food but who do survive to adulthood are likely to be smaller than average, and to continue to be prone to infection and problems of inadequate physical development, such as difficulties in childbirth.

It is now recognised that the long-term effects of nutritional deficiency begin in the womb. Babies who are assessed as less well nourished at the time of birth are more likely to develop a severe chronic illness such as coronary heart disease in later life.

The individual vitamins and minerals each play a role in the healthy development of the tissues. If there is a specific vitamin or mineral deficiency, this too can have a long-term bearing on health. For example, a deficiency of vitamin D in childhood can lead to the condition of rickets. Rickets leads to bony deformities, which are then set for life into the adult skeleton. Vitamin A deficiency leads to weak epithelial tissues and a vulnerability to infection, and is probably one of the most important reversible causes of infant mortality from measles in developing countries. Iron deficiency is now recognised to be common, not only in developing countries but also in the more affluent western nations, in which the food given to an infant may be plentiful, but unbalanced in nutrients. Inadequate iron in the diet of infants can have a lasting effect on mental development, leading to learning difficulties in later life.

Certain components of a child's diet may be harmful if given to the child too early or if in excess. The World Health Organization recommends that all children should be exclusively breastfed for at least the first 4 months, and ideally for the first 6 months, of life. It is increasingly recognised that certain nutrients may be harmful to the immature digestive system of the baby. It is possible that the early introduction of wheat, cows' milk, egg, nut and pulse proteins may induce long-term allergies or food intolerance. It is partly for this reason that late weaning after the sixth month is recommended, and advice is given that babies should avoid cows' milk products if possible for the first year of life. Whole foods are not considered to be so healthy for young babies and children, who may suffer from colic and diarrhoea as a result of the excess dietary fibre.

An excess of fat and refined carbohydrate will lead to obesity in children. As well as affecting the ability to play and exercise, obesity in children can lead to a long-term reduction in health and well-being. Obese babies are known to be more likely to grow into obese and inactive adults. Obesity in childhood can lead to social exclusion and being bullied. Obesity is an increasing problem in children of affluent societies, and one that carries significant consequences to health in future life.

Protection from injury, toxins, extremes of climate

Many of the important health problems of childhood are preventable, as long as the child is given adequate physical protection. In affluent countries, childhood accidents, and in particular head injuries, are the single most important cause of death in those under 14 years old. Many of the accidents which are fatal might have been prevented by the appropriate use of car restraints, cycle helmets, smoke alarms and window locks.

Poisoning is another very common cause of illness and death in children. Contrary to popular belief, the most common poisons to cause harm in children are not wild berries and mushrooms, but those found in the home, such as alcohol, cleaning fluids and prescription medicines. Again, harm would be prevented if these substances were kept out of the reach of children.

A young child is very vulnerable to extremes of heat and cold, and also to radiation from the sun. It is now recognised that sudden infant death syndrome (SIDS) can result from allowing a baby to become overheated or too cold. Children are more likely than adults to suffer from fever, dehydration, headache and confusion in very hot weather, a condition described as 'heat stroke'.

A child's skin is vulnerable to burning with very little exposure to the sun's rays. Although the discomfort of sunburn may be temporary, there is a well-established link between the incidence of sunburn in children and the development of skin cancer, including melanoma, in adult life. Sunburn is prevented by protecting the child's skin from direct sunlight by means of wearing long sleeves, sun hats and high-factor, ultraviolet light-blocking sun creams.

Protection from infection

Children can be protected from the serious childhood infections by the time-honoured method of separating an infectious child from other children. This might mean ensuring that a child has a few days of convalescence at home during and after an illness. However, this practice is increasingly less prevalent, as the pressures on parents to return to work may oblige them to return their child to school sooner than would be advisable after an infectious illness. In such situations, medications such as paracetamol and ibuprofen are commonly used to enable a child to feel well enough to return to school. Of course these medications do not cure the underlying illness.

An important medical approach for managing the risk of infection is the practice of childhood vaccination. Children in the UK are currently offered immunisations to protect them against ten childhood infections. The timing of the vaccinations in the UK immunisation schedule is summarised in Table 2.4d-I.

However, vaccines are not currently available in the UK for many of the important childhood infections. These include chickenpox, scarlet fever, tonsillitis, most forms of bronchitis and pneumonia, most forms of meningitis, herpes simplex virus, gastroenteritis, conjunctivitis and impetigo. For all these infections, exclusion of the infected child is the most important aspect of the protection of other children.

Freedom to play and exercise

It is now recognised that a child needs to be in a stimulating environment from early babyhood. Psychological studies of babies in orphanages who were given little stimulation throughout the day indicate that the mental and physical development of these babies was delayed, despite the fact that the babies appeared contented and well nourished.

If given a safe degree of freedom and stimulating objects, a child will naturally play, and through play will gradually develop physical and mental skills. A child will also naturally want to exercise. This tendency is apparent even in the womb. The routine ultrasound scan performed at 20 weeks of gestation demonstrates a fetus that is flexing its limbs and performing 'practice' breathing movements. As well as helping to develop skills of balance and coordination, exercise stimulates muscle and bone development. It also aids the proper utilisation of food and prevents obesity.

It is clear that children in affluent societies exercise far less than their parents did, and even less than their grandparents did as children. The reasons for this are multiple, and include the increased use of the car to take children to school, a reduction in allocated time for physical activity in school curricula (many children in the UK are obliged to attend less than half an hour of physical education per week) and the almost universal availability of habit-forming and sedentary methods of entertainment such as television and computer games. The impact that this decline in physical activity in today's children will have is likely to be significant. It is well recognised that children who do not exercise are even less likely to exercise when they become adults. The habit of exercise is apparently one that is most easily formed when young. Lack of activity in childhood will, therefore, contribute to problems such as heart disease, obesity and osteoporosis in adulthood.

Adequate rest

The value of adequate rest for children is emphasised in conventional guides to childcare. It is recognised that overstimulation and lack of sleep in a child will lead to poor concentration and irritability in the day. It is conventionally recognised that the development of a child can be adversely affected as a result of inadequate rest alone.

Love, security, consistency of care, and access to a social network

Although very difficult to measure, it is also well recognised that interpersonal factors, including love, a sense of security, consistency of care and access to a social network, are extremely important in the healthy mental, emotional and physical development of a child. Although it may make sense that the emotional development of a child deprived of one or more of these factors might be adversely affected, it may come as a surprise that mental and physical development can also be impaired by emotional deprivation. The effect of emotional deprivation can be so marked that the term 'psychosocial dwarfism' has been coined to describe the phenomenon of otherwise unexplained stunted growth in children in whom there is evidence of emotional deprivation. The only conventional explanation for this phenomenon is that, through the effect of emotional deprivation on the brain, the release of the hormones that stimulate growth and the development of the brain in children (including growth hormone, the thyroid hormones, insulin and, after puberty, the sex hormones) is inhibited.

Access to education

The definition of what constitutes appropriate education will vary according to the society in which the child grows up. At the very least, education should allow a child to develop skills and the confidence to be able to function as an independent adult in its society. At best, education should also enable a child to develop the skills to continue to learn and develop throughout adult life.

Theories abound about when is the best time to begin to acquire skills such as reading, playing the violin or driving a car. What is generally understood is that there is an optimum time period in the life of a child during which a skill, such as learning to read, can be acquired. Also, it is recognised that most children require a foundation of basic skills before they can progress on to learning more complex skills. For example, for most children reading will follow only after the skill of letter recognition has been mastered. A good educational system, whether it is at school or at home, will enable the child to concentrate on the skills that are most important to develop according to its particular stage in development. If the window of opportunity in childhood for learning a particular skill is missed, and reading is a good example, then it may be very difficult for the adult ever to acquire the skill with proficiency. A child may miss out on an important stage in educational development because of a long period of poor health, because of an unstable social setting or because of lack of parental support and encouragement.

Education has a significant impact on health. Not only can it enable the child to develop the skills and confidence to follow a healthy lifestyle as an adult, it also opens the door to a choice of professions. There is now no doubt that there is a strong correlation between professional status (by which the five socio-economic classes are defined) and health. For a wide range of diverse diseases, including most forms of cancer, heart disease, childhood asthma, pneumonia, and type 2 diabetes, there is a very striking correlation between the incidence of the disease and socio-economic class (of the child or parent). A person who is classified by profession into a high socio-economic class (e.g. a judge would be classified as Class I) is more likely to enjoy better health and a longer life than someone who is classified by profession to a low socio-economic class. This correlation cannot be completely attributed to differences in lifestyle between people from different socio-economic groups. So, it seems that, over and above the advantages an education might offer in terms of learning about healthy living, education (or possibly the wealth and security that tend to accompany it) also appears to protect against disease in its own right.

Protection from physical, sexual or emotional abuse

The deleterious effects that any form of abuse may have on a child are obvious. If the abuse is severe or occurs on a long-term basis, the child's growth and development will be affected adversely, probably by a similar mechanism as results from emotional neglect.

Physical abuse is also termed 'non-accidental injury' (NAI). NAI may manifest as bruises, lacerations, cigarette burns or fractures. In some cases, NAI results in wounds or fractures which would be very unlikely to occur by accident (e.g. bruising within the pinna of the ear), and so should alert the examining doctor to the possibility of abuse. Rarely, a child may be deliberately poisoned by his or her parents with alcohol or prescription medicines. Munchausen syndrome by proxy is a very rare syndrome in which the parent or carer causes or feigns illness in the child as an indirect form of attention seeking.

Physical neglect is also a form of physical abuse, and may manifest in the child as failure to gain weight, inadequate hygiene with skin infections and infestations, poor speech development and failure to attend health check-ups.

Emotional abuse includes emotional neglect and withdrawal of love, but also malicious criticism, threats and scapegoating. The child may appear withdrawn and may have speech difficulties and other features of developmental delay.

Sexual abuse may result in the features of emotional abuse and also in precocious sexual awareness or behaviour in a young child. Both physical and sexual abuse may cause the child to become vigilant and still when close to adults, a response described as 'frozen watchfulness'. A sexually abused child may present with the symptoms of a sexually transmitted disease, or may fall pregnant. There are some characteristic signs which may be found on examination of the genitalia of a sexually abused child, but the finding of these signs is not always conclusive.

Commonly, two or more of the forms of abuse may coexist. Apart from causing developmental delay, the long-term effects of child abuse on the individual's future relationships and care of future children may be serious and very difficult to remedy. It is recognised that abused children are more likely to abuse others in adulthood. Children who have been victims of sexual abuse are at great risk of suffering from psychiatric disorders and sexual dysfunction in adulthood.

The concept that parents or carers might abuse their children was only really recognised in the 1950s. In recent years there has been an increased awareness that abuse may underlie the health problems of a child, and conventional health professionals are now given specific training in recognising the warning features of abuse in a child.

If there is good reason to suspect the abuse of a child, then a conventional health practitioner in the UK is expected to report the matter to the local area Child Protection Committee. The Child Protection Committee is under the auspices of the local Social Services Department. In the first instance, a decision has to be made about whether the child should be separated straight away from the suspected abuser, either by admission to hospital or by placing the child into the care of a foster parent or a children's home. Whether or not this is done, a Child Protection Conference is convened, which will have multidisciplinary representation from a wide range of relevant professionals, including social workers, health visitors, the general practitioner, hospital doctors and nurses, police officers, teachers and lawyers. The evidence relevant to the case will be discussed and a decision will be made about:

- whether to place the child on the Child Protection Register, so that the child continues to remain at home while under the surveillance of health visitors and the social services
- whether to apply to the court for long-term protection of the child and prosecution of the possible abuser
- what sort of follow-up is required.

If, as a practitioner of complementary medicine, there are any concerns about possible abuse of a child, it is necessary to seek further advice. In the UK it would be appropriate to contact the local area Child Protection Committee. This is an example of a situation when it may be appropriate to breach the professional code of confidentiality.

Summary

How these general principles apply to particular health problems in children is explored in more detail in the rest of this section.

Information Box 5.4a-1

Children's health: comments from a Chinese medicine perspective

In Chinese medicine, children are recognised to be energetically different in nature from adults, although of course the differences become gradually less marked as the child grows older. Scott and Barlow (1999) summarise the principal differences as follows:

'Children's spleen is often insufficient'
This refers to the fact that the digestive system of a child has to work full time to ensure adequate growth and health of the Organs. For this reason, a young child is particularly vulnerable to digestive disorders. Late weaning and a balanced and regular diet consisting largely of Warm foods are extremely important for the health of the child. Accumulation Disorder (akin to the adult syndrome Retention of Food in the Stomach) and Spleen Qi Deficiency are syndromes very commonly found in young children.

'Children's yin is often insufficient'
Although the nature of children is very Yang, the Yin is immature. This can result in the tendency to high fevers and dehydration that are characteristic of children. Scott and Barlow (1999) suggest that the reason why Yin Deficiency is not seen more often in western children is that their Heat symptoms have been treated too readily with antibiotics, which are by nature cooling and damaging to the Yang.

'Organs are fragile and soft; Qi easily leaves its path' and 'Children easily become ill: their illnesses easily become serious'
These statements both refer to the fact that a slight insult from a Pathogenic Factor (such as the Heat of a hot day, or Damp Heat from over-rich food) can easily disturb the Qi and so cause illness. This can easily progress to a disturbance of the Qi of the whole body, and so lead rapidly to serious illness. Likewise, emotional disturbances can also lead to health imbalances, which can escalate into serious conditions.

'Yin and Yang organs are clear and spirited. They easily and quickly regain their health'
As a counterpoint to the preceding maxims, despite the vulnerability that arises from immaturity of the organs, the clarity of the 'Spirit' of the child's organs means that, in many cases, a child can return very rapidly to good health even after a major illness. Also, emotional disturbance in a child is often very short-lived, as long as the stress that has caused the disturbance is not maintained for a long time.

'Liver often has illness'
This statement refers to the tendency of children to succumb to Liver Wind and so to suffer from convulsions. However, health problems that result from Stagnation of Liver Qi are not so prominent in children, presumably because small children in general have not learned the tendency to restrain their emotions.

'Treat the mother to treat the child'
Health and emotional imbalances in the mother may readily be transmitted to the child, and so treatment of the mother may be important in the management of a child health problem. Conversely, a mother may become unwell in response to the health problem of her child, and her condition may only get better when the health of the child starts to improve.

This is only a brief summary of the essential points about children's health from the Chinese medical perspective. For more detail see Scott and Barlow (1999).

Self-test 5.4a

Introduction to children's health

1. Give a brief explanation of why a child may be more susceptible than a young adult to the following conditions:
   (i) diarrhoea and vomiting
   (ii) peanut allergy
   (iii) a febrile convulsion (a fit resulting from high fever)
   (iv) certain forms of leukaemia
   (v) fractures.
2. You are examining a 9-year-old child who is obviously small for his age and slight in build. His mother explains that he is not very able in either sporting activity or academic work compared with his peers at school. What sort of factors might have contributed to a delay of physical and mental development such as is apparent in this child?
3. Name the three types of abuse that can be inflicted on a child. What are the important approaches used nowadays in the management of a case of suspected abuse in a child?

Continued

Self-test 5.4a—Cont'd

Answers

1. (i) A child is more susceptible to diarrhoea and vomiting partly because of an immature digestive and immune system, and partly because a child may be more vulnerable to ingesting contaminated material if not adequately overseen.
   (ii) A child may be more likely to develop a peanut allergy as a result of exposure to peanut antigens at a time when the immune system is immature.
   (iii) A child is more likely to have a febrile convulsion because of the immature response of the nervous system to fever.
   (iv) A child is more vulnerable to certain forms of leukaemia because childhood leukaemia develops from the immature blast cells that persist in children from the time of fetal development.
   (v) A child is more vulnerable to fractures largely because of emotional and mental immaturity. A child is more likely to put itself in dangerous situations without full awareness of possible harmful consequences. A child is also less able to protect itself from physical abuse from other children or adults.
2. A delay in physical and mental development may be a result of deficiency in any one of the fundamental health needs of a child. Possible causes include:
   - inadequate diet, including vitamin/mineral deficiency
   - congenital disease (e.g. congenital heart disease, cystic fibrosis, haemophilia, Down syndrome)
   - acquired chronic illness (e.g. asthma, diabetes mellitus, childhood cancer)
   - deficiency in those factors that are important for the emotional development of the child, including love, security and consistency of care
   - sustained physical, emotional or sexual abuse.
3. The three types of abuse that can be inflicted on a child are physical, emotional and sexual abuse. Commonly two or more of these coexist in a case of child abuse.

   The first step in managing a case of suspected child abuse is that the professional concerned should report the matter to the local area Child Protection Committee. An immediate decision is then made about whether or not the child is in grave risk of continuing abuse. If there are good grounds to believe that this is the case, the child may be removed straight away to a place of safety, such as a foster home.

   A Child Protection Conference is convened, which makes the decision about whether or not the child should be placed on the Child Protection Register. The case of a child on the Child Protection Register will be subject to regular review by the range of professionals involved in the care of the child. The family of a child on the register should be offered continuing guidance and support in their care of the child.

   Serious cases may result in an application to the court for long-term protection of the child and/or prosecution of the abuser.

Chapter 5.4b Assessment of child health and development

LEARNING POINTS

At the end of this chapter you will be able to:
- explain why the assessment of child health and development is different from the assessment of health in adults
- give a definition of the term 'developmental milestone'
- recognise some of the key developmental milestones used in the assessment of child development.

Estimated time for chapter: 90 minutes.

Why does the assessment of the health of children require a specialised approach?

The assessment of the health and development of children is different from the assessment in adults, in as much as the physiology of children is different from that of adults. It should be obvious that the health of a child can only be assessed properly if there is a prior knowledge of the normal range of physiological variables in a child at that particular stage of development. Therefore, most of this chapter is concerned with what the complementary therapist can expect to be normal when examining a child at a particular age (stage of development).

Even without a specialised knowledge of how diseases manifest in children, a firm grasp of the normal physiology of childhood development will enable a more ready recognition of those situations when a child is becoming unwell.

This chapter introduces the main differences between normal children at various stages of development and adults. For the sake of clarity, the differences that might be found in the physical examination of a passive child are considered first. Then, the ways in which a child differs from an adult in terms of its interaction with its environment are discussed. These are considered within four domains: motor (movement) skills, language skills, hearing and vision, and social skills.

The child health surveillance programme

The health of a child will always be assessed when the child presents to a conventional practitioner with a particular complaint. In addition to these unpredictable points of contact with health practitioners, most children in developed countries are also offered health checks at prescribed stages in their childhood. Considered together, these health checks comprise a programme of child health surveillance.

In the UK Child Health Surveillance Programme health checks are usually offered at birth, at 6–8 weeks, 9 months and 18–24 months of age. The professionals who work together to provide a child health surveillance programme include the hospital paediatrician, the general practitioner and the health visitor (a nurse with specialist training in community health issues). For most healthy children, the only point of contact with the hospital paediatrician is likely to be during the routine neonatal examination, which should take place within the first 24 hours after birth in hospital. Thereafter, the health surveillance is overseen by the general practitioner and the health visitor. However, if a child has a serious congenital condition or chronic severe illness, the hospital or community paediatrician will be much more involved in the health surveillance programme for that child (see Q5.4b-1).

During these routine health checks important aspects (indicators) of the physical health of the child are assessed, together with certain indicators of the four domains of how the child is interacting with its environment. These four domains are motor skills, language skills, hearing and vision, and social skills.

Table 5.4b-I Median and limit ages for some developmental milestones

Developmental milestone	Median age	Limit age
Responsive smiling	6 weeks	8 weeks
Good eye contact maintained	6 weeks	3 months
Reaches for objects	3–4 months	5 months
Sits unsupported	6 months	10 months
Says single words with meaning	13 months	18 months
Speaks in phrases	24 months	30 months

Developmental milestones

Assessment of the domains of physical health, motor skills, language skills, hearing and vision, and social skills requires an understanding of how a healthy child might be expected to develop within each of these different domains as time goes on. A useful concept in the assessment of children's health over the course of time is that of the 'developmental milestone'.

A developmental milestone is a measurable attribute or skill that is attained during the course of normal development in childhood. The first smile of a baby and the ability to reach out and grasp an object, to sit unaided, to walk and to say single words with meaning are all developmental milestones that are usually attained within the first 2 years of life.

All children are unique with regard to the precise time and order in which these milestones are attained. For example, a normal healthy child might first walk unaided at any time between 7 and 15 months of age. The age by which half of all children have taken a few steps is 12 months. This is the median age for the milestone. Outside the extremes of 7 and 15 months there may be unusually early or late walkers who nevertheless continue to develop normally. There is no known link between early walking and physical prowess, despite parents' assumptions to the contrary. However, if a child is not walking by the age of 18 months, there is a significant possibility that this is an early indication of abnormality such as muscular dystrophy. Eighteen months is described as the 'limit age' for the developmental milestone of walking unaided. If a child has not achieved a milestone by the limit age for that milestone, it will be referred for specialist examination to exclude any possible underlying health problems. Median ages and limit ages for some of the important developmental milestones are listed in Table 5.4b-I.

Physical assessment of the passive child

Height, weight and head circumference

Height, weight and head circumference are measurements that are very commonly used in the assessment of the health of children. In young babies, head circumference and weight are the most frequently assessed health indicators, whereas in older children who are able to stand upright the assessment of height replaces that of head circumference.

The concept of the 'normal range' was introduced in Chapter 1.2a, and by way of illustration Figure 1.2a-I shows the normal range of birthweight according to stage of pregnancy. The normal range for a variable, such as weight, is the range of values of that variable into which the large part (usually 80% or 96% for most normal ranges) of the population will fall. When the height, weight or head circumference of a child is measured, the value is compared to charted values which indicate the normal range of that variable in the British population. The charts used by health professionals are prepared with such accuracy that the precise 'position' of the child in terms of the variable as compared to the population as a whole can be determined.

For example, a 4-year-old boy may be assessed as having a height that is on the 25th centile. This means that he just falls within the shortest quarter (25%) of the population. At the same assessment, his weight is found to be on the 33rd centile (meaning that he just falls within the lightest one-third (33%) of the population). Both these measurements are within the 94% normal range and so would be considered unremarkable by a health professional. However, if the two measurements indicated that the child was on the 2nd centile for height and weight, this would mean that he is just on the bottom edge of the 94% normal range and just falls within the shortest and lightest 2% of the population. A health professional might then take more time to assess whether or not there might be an underlying health or social issue as a cause of the short stature in that child (see Q5.4b-2).

Monitoring variables such as height and weight relative to the normal range over the course of time can be very useful. If a child is seen to 'drop in centiles' from, say, the 40th centile to the 10th centile over the course of time, this might indicate failing health. In this way a possible problem with growth can be detected long before the child can be assessed as falling outside the normal range of growth indicators (see Q5.4b-3).

However, problems can arise from repeated measurement of height, weight and head circumference. As is true for all measurements that fall outside a 'normal range', there remains uncertainty whether the measured 'abnormality' is a valid indicator of lack of health. Many health visitors will testify to the anxiety that repeated weighing of a small baby can induce. It is understandable that a mother will be concerned if her baby is assessed as not gaining weight at the same rate as an average baby (as indicated by the weight chart). Even if this is actually a healthy pattern for that child (who of course is very unlikely to be an average baby in all respects), the concern may lead to lack of well-being in the mother (which can then be transmitted to the child) or to changes in feeding behaviour, such as stopping breastfeeding in favour of formula milk.

For this reason it is important to place an 'abnormal' measured value in context against other measures of health in the child. A contented baby who is well in all other respects is unlikely to have a serious underlying health problem, even if its weight dips below the normal range. Although an abnormal finding must of course be followed up, every effort should be made to reassure the mother that it need not necessarily indicate that anything is wrong with the child.

Pulse rate

The pulse rate drops gradually over the first few years of life to assume the normal adult rate after the age of 12 years. The normal ranges for pulse rate in children are given in Table 5.4b-II.

Respiratory rate and peak flow rate

Like the pulse rate, the respiratory rate drops as the child gets older. The normal ranges for respiratory rate in children are given in Table 5.4b-III.

The peak flow rate is proportional to the height and age of the child, meaning that it increases as the child gets taller and older. The normal range for peak flow rate in children can be determined from charts such as those which usually accompany a peak flow meter when purchased.

Table 5.4b-II The normal ranges for pulse rate in children

Age (years)	Rate (beats/minute)
<1	110–160
2–5	95–140
5–12	80–120
>12	60–100

Table 5.4b-III The normal ranges for respiratory rate in children

Age	Normal rate (breaths/minute)	Rate if breathless (breaths/minute)
Newborn	30–50	>60
Infant	20–40	>50
Young child	20–30	>40
Older child–adult	15–20	>30

Heart sounds

The heart sounds of children are routinely assessed in surveillance checks to exclude the possibility of congenital heart disease. When using the stethoscope, the doctor listens for the rushing noise of a heart murmur. A murmur can be a normal finding in very young children, but is unlikely to be normal if found in school-aged children. If there is any concern, the child will be sent for a non-invasive echocardiogram to exclude defects in the structure of the heart.

Mouth, palate and anus

The mouth and palate of the newborn baby are assessed at the neonatal check to exclude hare lip and cleft palate. The anus is examined to exclude the rare condition of imperforate anus.

Abdomen and testes

The abdomen and testes are examined in newborns and children up to the pre-school years. The doctor examines the abdomen of newborns to exclude abdominal distension, enlarged liver or spleen, and abdominal masses. In this way conditions such as congenital bowel obstruction and abdominal tumours may be detected. The scrotum is palpated in boys up to the pre-school years to check for complete descent of the testes.

Hips

The movements of the hips of newborns and babies up to the age of 2 years are also routinely assessed to exclude the condition of congenital dislocation of the hip.

The skin

Benign birthmarks are common findings in newborn babies. In particular, reddened mottled patches at the nape of the neck or around the eyelids (stork marks), bluish areas of discoloration over the base of the spine and buttocks (Mongolian blue spots) and tiny white pimples on the cheeks and nose (milia) are findings that will resolve spontaneously.

The port-wine stain (a clearly demarcated, purplish patch on the face or scalp) and the strawberry naevus (a bright red, rounded lump, often the size of a strawberry) are two fairly common birthmarks that are more persistent. The port wine stain can be very prominent on the face of a growing child, but can now be treated in later childhood by means of laser therapy. The strawberry naevus tends to increase in size for the first few months of life and then often shrinks down to a negligible size. For this reason treatment is not offered unless it is a cause of physical discomfort in early infancy. Cosmetic surgery can be offered if the naevus is unsightly by the time the child reaches school age.

Tufts of hair, skin lumps or other birthmarks are taken seriously if they are found around the base of the spine, over the spine or on the skull. Rarely, birthmarks in these regions can indicate a mild form of spina bifida known as 'spina bifida occulta'.

General appearance

Finally, in the physical assessment of a passive child, the overall physical appearance of the child may indicate to a trained eye that there is an underlying congenital condition or chronic illness. Many of the genetic conditions that manifest in childhood give rise to a characteristic cluster of physical features, which in themselves are diagnostic of the condition, for example Down syndrome and achondroplastic dwarfism.

Assessment of movement (motor skills) in a child

A newborn baby should be able to make symmetrical strong movements of all four limbs when lying on its back. If supported by a hand under the abdomen it will be unable to hold up its head, but will not be too floppy (i.e. it has good muscle tone). It has a strong grip, so much so that it can support its own weight when gripping the index fingers of the examining doctor. When held upright as if standing, a newborn will make reflex stepping moves with its legs. Within 6–8 weeks the strong grip and walking reflex are no longer to be found. This is because the strong grip and walking reflex of the newborn are primitive reflexes, which later become overridden by motor nerve impulses from the developing brain.

Some of the major motor developmental milestones are listed in Table 5.4b-IV.

Assessment of language skills in a child

A newborn of course has no language, but has a characteristic cry, which is a very effective, albeit not very specific, method of achieving contact with its mother. Within the first few months the baby is able to recognise and quieten to his mother's voice. Some of the major developmental milestones of language are listed in Table 5.4b-V.

Table 5.4b-IV Some of the major motor developmental milestones

Milestone	Median age
Able to lift head when lying on abdomen	6 weeks
Sits without support	6 months
Can pass objects from one hand to another	6 months
Stands with support	7 months
Pulls to standing	9 months
Has good pincer grip of a small object	10 months
First steps unsupported	12 months
Scribbles with a pencil	14 months
Kicks a ball	20 months
Builds a tower of six cubes	24 months
Hops on one foot	3½ years
Draws a man of three parts	4 years

Table 5.4b-V Some of the major developmental milestones of language

Milestone	Median age
Babbles and says 'mama', 'dada', 'baba', but without meaning	10 months
Can understand simple commands and say one or two words appropriately	13 months
Can combine two different words	20 months
Can say first and last name	3–4 years
Can say the name of colours	3 years
Speech fully comprehensible to strangers	4 years

Speech difficulties may arise as a result of a range of reasons. The problem may be seated in difficulties in understanding speech (receptive dysphasia), either because of deafness, a global learning disability, or a specific defect in the way in which the brain processes speech. Alternatively, the actual production of words may be impaired (expressive dysphasia), despite good comprehension. For this reason, the assessment of the root of problems in language development is a complex skill.

Assessment of hearing and vision in a child

A newborn should respond to sound, and will startle or blink in response to sudden noises. It will not show any preference at this stage to particular sounds, such as its mother's voice.

The eyes of a newborn are examined to exclude conditions that are the cause of blindness, including congenital cataract and a rare congenital tumour called 'retinoblastoma'.

As the baby grows, the mother is questioned about whether or not she thinks her child reacts normally to sounds and visual images. The mother's opinion is usually an extremely sensitive indicator of whether or not there could be underlying hearing or visual defects.

Hearing is assessed in the newborn by means of objective electronic testing of the inner ear or brain to sounds focused into the baby's ear. This reliable test has in the UK largely replaced routine assessment by the distraction test, which until recently was performed by the health visitor on a baby aged 6–9 months.

By 6–8 weeks of age the eyes of the baby should be moving together (conjugate gaze), with no evidence of independent movement (squint). At every stage in the Child Health Surveillance Programme the child should be assessed informally for the presence of a squint. If there is any concern about one eye not moving as far as it should in any direction, the child is referred for a formal diagnosis by an ophthalmologist, as squint requires early treatment to prevent lifelong impairment to binocular vision.

Table 5.4b-VI Some of the major developmental milestones of hearing and vision

Milestone	Median age
Startles to a sudden noise	At birth
Looks at faces; responds to light	At birth
Stills to a sudden new noise	1 month
Eyes will follow a moving object, and will move together with no squint	6 weeks
Quietens or smiles to the mother's voice	4 months
Turns to the sound of mother's voice	7 months
Searches for quiet sounds made out of sight	9 months
Shows response to his own name and some other familiar words	12 months
Can copy a circle	3 years

Some of the major developmental milestones of hearing and vision are listed in Table 5.4b-VI.

Assessment of social skills in a child

The developing child will display increasingly complex methods of interacting with the people around it, and behaving according to expected norms. Even a newborn appears to respond to being picked up in a way that is different to its response to less social stimuli.

The assessment of the social skills domain includes the assessment of those skills, such as self-feeding and self-dressing, which are essential for the child to attain independent existence.

Some of the major milestones in social development are listed in Table 5.4b-VII.

Table 5.4b-VII Some of the major milestones in social development

Milestone	Median age
Smiles responsively	6 weeks
Can put solid food in mouth	6 months
Waves 'bye-bye'	8 months
Becomes wary of strangers	8–10 months
Drinks from a cup	12 months
Shows symbolic play with dolls, chair spoon, etc.	18 months
Can remove a garment	18 months
Feeds self with a spoon	18 months
Asserts own wishes	18 months
Washes hands and brushes teeth with help	3–4 years
Shows sympathy when appropriate	3–4 years
Vivid make-believe play	3–4 years
Will play independently with other children	3–4 years

What happens when a child fails to reach developmental norms?

In general, the failure to fit into the 'normal range' for a physical measurement such as weight or pulse rate, or the failure to have attained a developmental milestone by its limit age should be put into the context of the overall well-being of the child. If the child is otherwise well, then as has been explained regarding weight gain in babies, the mother primarily should be reassured that it is very possible that there is not an underlying health problem. Nevertheless, it is generally good practice to follow-up a child who fails an aspect of the Child Health Surveillance Programme with further tests or a referral for a specialist opinion.

Self-test 5.4b

Assessment of the health and development of children

1. (i) What is a developmental milestone?
   (ii) Explain the terms 'median age' and 'limit age'.
   (iii) What is the median age and limit age for sitting unsupported?
2. You are examining a 3-year-old boy. Which of the following features might be a cause for concern to a health professional examining the same child for the first time?
   - weight on the 50th centile
   - height on the 98th centile
   - pulse rate of 104 beats/minute
   - respiratory rate of 30 breaths/minute
   - he can say his first name but not his surname
   - his speech is unclear but he is able to say complete sentences
   - he can run but not hop.
3. A patient tells you that her small baby of 3 months has a heart murmur, but that the doctor is not sending it for any tests at the moment. She is obviously concerned about this. When you examine the child you find that the pulse rate is 130 beats/minute and the respiratory rate is 30 breaths/minute. The baby is alert, smiling in response to her mother's voice, but is unable to sit unsupported. How might you comment to the mother about the diagnosis of the murmur?

Answers

1. (i) A developmental milestone is a measurable skill or attribute that is attained throughout the normal course of childhood development.

Continued

(ii) The median age is the age when 50% of all children will have attained the milestone.
The limit age is the age at which most children would have been expected to attain the milestone. If the milestone has not been attained by a child by the limit age, the child should be referred to exclude an underlying health problem.
(iii) The median age for sitting unsupported is 6 months; the limit age is 10 months. This means that half of all children are sitting by the age of 6 months. There is only cause for concern if the child is unable to sit unsupported by 10 months, in which case a referral might be made to exclude an underlying neurological or musculoskeletal problem.

2. Actually all these features are within or just within a range that would be considered normal. The only concern is the height of the child and the weight relative to that height. A height on the 98th centile indicates that the child just qualifies as being one of the tallest 2% of children of his age. This means that he is tall, but is only bordering on what would be considered abnormal. However, such a tall child would be expected to have a correspondingly high weight relative to the average child. Therefore a weight on the 50th centile suggests that this child is relatively underweight.
3. You could say to the mother that a heart murmur can be a normal finding in small babies, and would only be of concern if it persisted past infancy. You could add that her child otherwise appears very healthy in other respects; in particular her pulse and breathing rates are normal.

Chapter 5.4c Congenital disorders

LEARNING POINTS

At the end of this chapter you will be able to:

- describe the different mechanisms by which chromosomal abnormalities, single-gene mutations and multifactorial inheritance can give rise to congenital disease
- recognise the main features of the most important congenital conditions
- describe the ways in which a preterm baby might suffer from disease
- describe the role of the clinical geneticist.

Estimated time for chapter: Part I, 70 minutes; Part II, 60 minutes; Part III, 30 minutes.

Introduction to congenital disease

Congenital diseases are those conditions which have existed in the person since birth. There are two broad categories of congenital diseases: genetic diseases and diseases of multifactorial inheritance. Genetic diseases are those diseases that result entirely from a defect in the genetic make-up of the person. In genetic conditions, the defect has either been inherited from the parent or has arisen during the division and maturation of one or both of the gametes. The genetic condition, therefore, is usually present from the moment of conception, and so will affect the genetic material of every body cell of the child with the condition. The genetic diseases can be diagnosed by testing a sample of body cells for the genetic defect. Very rarely, the genetic defect can arise as a result of an error in the early divisions of the zygote, and so will affect many, but not all, of the cells of the developing baby (this is genetic 'mosaicism'; see later in this chapter). The genetic diseases can be further divided into two subcategories: those that result from chromosomal abnormalities and those that result from single-gene defects.

In contrast to the genetic diseases, there is a broad range of congenital conditions which are described in this chapter as being of multifactorial inheritance. These conditions may have an underlying genetic susceptibility at their root, but can also result from a range of external factors which have in some way damaged the embryo or fetus during the time of its development in the womb, or during the time of labour. In these conditions, the genetic material in the cells of the body will appear to be grossly normal, and genetic testing is not usually helpful in the diagnosis of the condition, except in that it may reveal an underlying susceptibility to the condition in some cases.

The most common congenital disorders are described in this chapter. It is beyond the scope of the text to go into detail about the features and management of all these conditions, largely because most of them are rare. The aim of this chapter is to illustrate the breadth of the range of congenital conditions, and the complex ways in which they can arise.

The problems that arise from prematurity are also described in this chapter. Although a preterm baby may be entirely healthy for its stage of development, the fact that it has been born before the ideal time for delivery means that it inherits at birth a number of particular health problems which, according to the definition above, are in themselves a form of congenital disease.

This chapter is divided into three parts, which you are advised to study in separate sessions. The conditions discussed in this chapter are:

Part I: Genetic conditions

- Chromosomal abnormalities:
  - Down syndrome
  - Turner syndrome
  - Klinefelter syndrome
  - fragile X syndrome.
- Single-gene defects:
  - cystic fibrosis
  - sickle cell disease and thalassaemia
  - phenylketonuria
  - albinism
  - colour blindness
  - muscular dystrophy
  - haemophilia
  - achondroplasia
  - osteogenesis imperfecta
  - hypercholesterolaemia.

Part II: Conditions of multifactorial inheritance
- congenital heart disease
- hare lip and cleft palate
- oesophageal atresia
- pyloric stenosis
- congenital liver disease
- imperforate anus
- club foot (talipes)
- congenital dislocation of the hip
- maldescent of testes
- congenital hernia
- congenital blindness
- congenital deafness
- neural tube defects
- cerebral palsy
- congenital hypothyroidism
- inherited tendency to adult diseases.

Part III: The premature baby
- respiratory distress syndrome
- irregularities of breathing and heart rate
- temperature control
- problems with nutrition
- retinal damage
- brain damage
- jaundice
- problems after discharge from hospital.

These three parts are followed by a section on screening for congenital disease, which covers the following:

- the role of genetic counselling
- genetic screening of parents
- antenatal testing for genetic disease
- presymptomatic testing of children.

Part I: Genetic conditions

Chromosomal abnormalities

The genetic material in the human is found within the nucleus of almost all the cells of the body (the red cells and platelets are exceptions to this rule, as they lose their nucleus at a late stage in their development in the bone marrow). During the process of replication of body cells, known as 'mitosis', the nuclear material condenses into 23 pairs of elongated bodies known as 'chromosomes'. There are a total of 22 non-sex chromosomes (autosomes) and one pair of sex chromosomes (XX or XY), which make up the total complement of the non-dividing cell. The autosomes are described by a number, from 1 to 22, and the sex chromosomes by the letters X and Y. Each chromosome consists of coiled and densely packed strands of DNA (deoxyribonucleic acid). Each DNA strand is made up of chains of separate genes, which are tiny sections of DNA that direct the formation of the millions of proteins that make up the human body. Together, these strands of DNA make up what is now termed the 'human genome'.

The different genes that make up the human genome have now been mapped, and can be located to particular chromosome pairs. The function of many of these genes is now understood. For example, the gene that codes for part of the protein that forms haemoglobin is located on chromosome pair 11, and the gene that codes for the clotting factor that is deficient in haemophilia A is located on the X sex chromosome. As the chromosomes are in matching pairs, each gene is doubly represented within the nucleus.

A chromosomal abnormality is a structural problem affecting one (or more) of these 23 pairs of strands of DNA. Because a chromosomal abnormality is likely to affect a large number of the thousands of genes represented on the DNA of the chromosome, the diseases that result commonly involve multiple structural abnormalities and learning difficulties. Over 100 diseases arising from chromosomal defects have now been documented.

A chromosomal defect usually arises as a result of an error in meiosis, the process by which gametes are formed from the germ cells in the ovary or testis. In this case, the chromosomes of the parents are normal. More rarely, the defect is present in the chromosomes of one of the parents, albeit not in a form that would manifest in severe disease. In this more rare circumstance, the defect can be passed down directly to the child, and occasionally in a form that results in severe abnormalities of development of that child. In both cases the chromosomal defect may be in the form of an absent chromosome or an absent section of a chromosome (a deletion), or may involve the presence of an extra chromosome (a trisomy).

Rarely, a chromosomal defect develops after conception, during one of the first mitotic divisions of the zygote. This results in a baby who has some normal cells and some cells that carry the defect. This phenomenon is known as 'mosaicism', and often results in a condition that is a less severe form of the disease that would have arisen if all the cells had been affected.

Because chromosomal defects are often apparent simply from a study of the shape of the chromosomes (which can be seen using a simple microscope), these were the first form of genetic disease to be understood and described as such. The first three chromosomal abnormalities to be described included Down syndrome. The chromosomal defect of Down syndrome (trisomy 21) was first described in 1959, only 3 years after the normal chromosomal complement was first described.

Down syndrome (trisomy 21)

Down syndrome was first described by Dr JLH Down in 1866, but was ascribed to a chromosomal defect just less than a century later. The syndrome arises as a result of a trisomy in the chromosome pair known as 21. In 94% of cases, Down syndrome arises from an error in meiosis, and in 9 out of 10 of these cases the error has affected the ovum rather than the spermatozoon. It is well recognised that this form of Down syndrome is more likely to arise with increasing maternal age

Table 5.4c-I Risk of Down syndrome according to maternal age at delivery

Maternal age (years)	Risk of Down syndrome occurring at birth
All ages	1 in 650 births
30	1 in 900 births
35	1 in 380 births
37	1 in 240 births
40	1 in 110 births
44	1 in 37 births

(Table 5.4c-I). As will be appreciate from the table, the risk of having an affected pregnancy rises sharply after the age of 35 years, but nevertheless is a relatively unlikely occurrence (affecting less than 1 in 100 pregnancies) in women who are under 40 years old.

In a small number of cases of Down syndrome the condition arises from a defect known as a 'translocation' in the genetic material of one of the parents. If this is the case, there is risk of recurrence of the condition in a subsequent pregnancy of up to 15%.

In 1 in 100 cases of Down syndrome, mosaicism (see above) is found. This often manifests in a less severe form of the condition.

Down syndrome is the most common cause of severe learning difficulties, arising in 1 in 650 live births (see Table 5.4c-I). It is usually diagnosed at birth because of the characteristic cluster of physical features, which are apparent on examination of the newborn. These include a round 'mongoloid' face and a protruding tongue (Figure 5.4c-I), and abnormal creases on the palms and soles. The diagnosis is confirmed by means of chromosomal analysis (requiring a blood test). This test takes several days to process. At a later stage the parents will be offered genetic testing to exclude the rare possibility of a translocation.

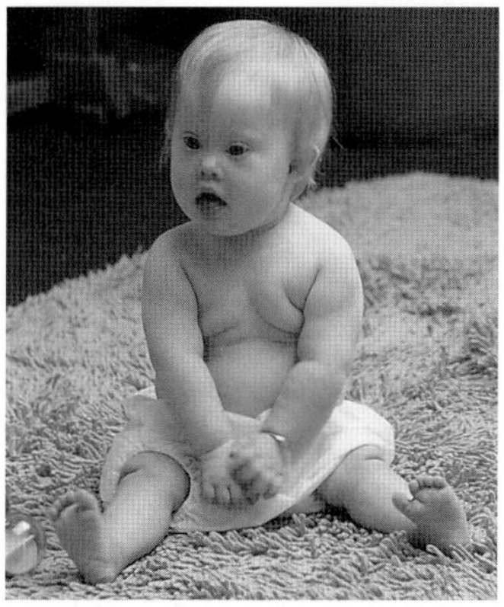

Figure 5.4c-I • Characteristic features of Down syndrome.

In addition to the external features found on neonatal examination, a baby with Down syndrome is likely to have floppy muscle tone. As the child grows, a delay in the attainment of the motor developmental milestones is likely. In addition, 40% of babies with Down syndrome have some form of congenital heart defect, often requiring surgery in infancy. Other problems that are likely to affect the child with Down syndrome include severe learning difficulties (in which difficulties in problem-solving are most prominent), a tendency to recurrent respiratory infections, glue ear and visual impairment from cataracts or squints. In later life, a person with Down syndrome is at increased risk of developing leukaemia, hypothyroidism and Alzheimer's disease.

Despite the cluster of physical and mental problems and the tendency to serious disease in middle age, a child with Down syndrome is often robust in general health and buoyant and sensitive in spirit.

Information Box 5.4c-I

Down syndrome: comments from a Chinese medicine perspective

In Chinese medicine, the underlying problem in Down syndrome is Jing Deficiency. The frequency of heart defects is an indication of a specific imbalance in the Heart Organ. This would accord with the observation that a joyful, open and warm nature is very often found in a person with Down syndrome.

A protruding tongue, and a tendency to infections and glue ear indicate that Phlegm Damp is an Excess problem in this condition. Scott and Barlow (1999) report that often the features of Phlegm Damp (including the difficulties in learning) respond very well to acupuncture given at frequent intervals before the age of 3 years, and having been cleared, may then reveal underlying Full Heat.

Turner syndrome (45 X)

Turner syndrome is a condition in which there is only a single X sex chromosome. This means that there are only 22 complete pairs of chromosomes. Babies born with Turner syndrome are always girls, as it is the Y chromosome which directs the development of the male sexual characteristics in the fetus.

It has been estimated that 95% of embryos with Turner syndrome do not survive past 8 weeks. Nevertheless, Turner syndrome is a relatively common chromosomal disorder, affecting approximately 1 in 2500 live-born baby girls. The features of the syndrome include short stature, a webbed appearance to the neck, widely spaced nipples and failure in the development of the ovaries. Intellectual development is normal. Occasionally, a congenital heart defect, coarctation of the aorta, is present. This may require surgical correction.

Diagnosis of Turner syndrome may be missed in the baby, and may only be made when it becomes apparent that the child is very short for her age, or at the time when it becomes obvious that her periods have failed to commence.

Treatment is with growth hormone (GH) therapy in childhood if short stature is a significant problem, and hormone replacement therapy (HRT) from puberty onwards. HRT, will not reverse the problem of infertility, but will enable the development of the secondary sexual characteristics, and will aid in the maturation and strengthening of the bones.

Information Box 5.4c-II

Turner syndrome: comments from a Chinese medicine perspective

In Chinese medicine, the underlying imbalance in Turner syndrome is Jing Deficiency.

Klinefelter syndrome (47XXY)

Klinefelter syndrome is the result of a trisomy in the sex chromosomes, involving the presence of an extra X chromosome (XXY). As with Turner syndrome, the abnormal complement of sex chromosomes leads to abnormalities of sexual development.

Klinefelter syndrome affects 1 in 1000 live-born males. The features of the syndrome include underdeveloped small testes, infertility, breast development in adolescence (gynaecomastia), and tall stature. Intellectual development may be normal, but there is a higher than average incidence of educational and psychological problems in boys with Klinefelter syndrome.

The main treatment is with male sex hormones in puberty, although these are used with caution in individuals who manifest behavioural problems.

Information Box 5.4c-III

Klinefelter syndrome: comments from a Chinese medicine perspective

In Chinese medicine, Klinefelter syndrome is a result of Jing Deficiency. The sexual and behavioural problems may indicate an additional imbalance in the Liver Organ.

Fragile X syndrome

Fragile X syndrome is the result of a multiplication of a small portion of the DNA in the long arm of the X chromosome. In girls, this defect can be 'balanced out' by the healthy chromosome in the pair of sex chromosomes (although the defect may give rise to mild learning difficulties in one-third of girls who carry it). However, in boys there is no additional X chromosome to perform this function. For this reason, fragile X syndrome primarily manifests in boys. The main features of fragile X syndrome are learning difficulty, large forehead, long face and protruding ears, and large testes (Figure 5.4c-II).

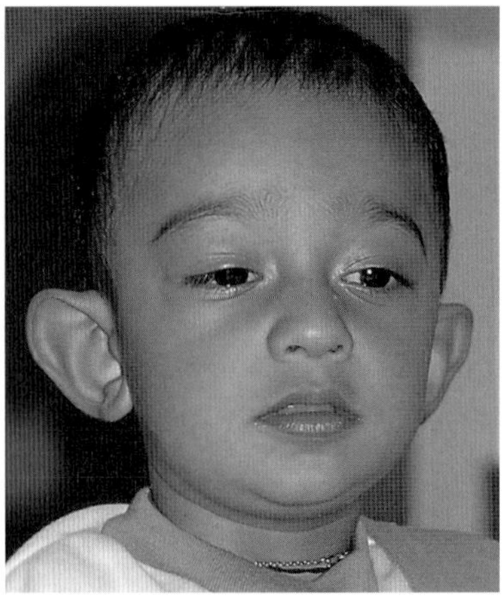

Figure 5.4c-II • Characteristic features of fragile X syndrome.

Unlike Down syndrome, fragile X syndrome is almost always inherited from the mother, who is the 'carrier' of the defect. As it affects 1 in 2000 live-born boys, this makes it the most common inherited form of severe to moderate learning difficulty (IQ ranges between 20 and 80). It is the second most common genetic cause of learning difficulty after Down syndrome.

Information Box 5.4c-IV

Fragile X syndrome: comments from a Chinese medicine perspective

In Chinese medicine, fragile X syndrome is a form of Jing Deficiency.

Genetic conditions: single-gene defects

In contrast to chromosomal defects, which can affect thousands of genes encoded within one strand of DNA, the single-gene defects are the result of a mutation in a tiny portion of DNA. A single-gene defect typically affects the production of only one of the millions of proteins that are manufactured as part of the healthy functioning of the body. Since the mapping of the human genome, gene defects can be localised to a specific area on a chromosome. For example, in 70% of cases of cystic fibrosis the condition can be attributed to a defect in a section of the DNA called δF508. This defect is located on the chromosomes in the chromosome pair 7.

A single-gene defect may arise spontaneously as a result of an error in the formation of the gametes during meiosis, or it may be transmitted from a parent who carries the defect in his or her genetic material via an affected gamete to the child.

The presence of a single-gene mutation need not manifest in overt disease. One reason for this is that the defect affects a portion of the DNA which seems not to be absolutely essential for the healthy balance of the body. In this very common scenario the mutation may have no effect, or at most make the individual different in some tiny way, but not necessarily less healthy.

Recessive gene defects

Some forms of genetic defect, even if present in a very important section of DNA, need not cause disease if the defect is not present in the corresponding chromosome of the pair. An example of this type of genetic defect is the one on chromosome 11 that leads to abnormal haemoglobin production in sickle cell anaemia.

In the case of this type of genetic defect, if there is a normal gene present on the other chromosome of the pair, this normal gene can enable the formation of the essential protein in the person who carries the defect. In this scenario, the defective gene is described as 'recessive', because it does not lead to serious disease if counterbalanced by a normal gene on the partner chromosome.

Carriage of recessive genes

In the condition of sickle cell anaemia, if only one-half of the chromosome pair 11 is affected by the genetic defect, only the mild condition of sickle cell trait manifests. However, in many of the recessively inherited conditions, the person who carries only one of the possible pair of defective recessive genes manifests no disease at all. The person who carries a single recessive gene is called a 'carrier' for that condition. The carrier state is a very common one. For example, approximately 1 in 25 seemingly healthy people carry the defective gene responsible for cystic fibrosis. It is actually very unlikely for any one person not to be carrying one or more recessive defective genes, despite the absence of any manifest genetic disease.

The fact that sickle cell anaemia is a recessively inherited condition means that the disease only becomes fully apparent if a child has inherited the sickle cell genetic defect from each of his or her parents, meaning that both of the haemoglobin genes on chromosome 11 are affected. The parents of a child with sickle cell anaemia are usually found to be carriers of the condition (if this is not the case, it implies that one or both of the gene defects in the chromosome 11 of the child arose spontaneously during formation of the gametes). The fact that both haemoglobin genes are affected means that the child has no capacity to produce a normal balance of haemoglobin proteins, and so will manifest the features of sickle cell anaemia early in life.

The inheritance of recessive conditions

Half of the gametes from a parent who carries a single recessive gene defect in one chromosome of a pair are likely also to carry that defect. This means that if the other parent does not also carry that defect, 50% of the children of those parents are likely to carry the defect. If the carrier state does not lead to manifest disease, all these children will appear as normal. The problem arises if both parents are carriers of the same defective recessive gene. This means that one-quarter of their children will inherit normal genes from their parents, half will inherit the carrier state (only one of the pair of genes is defective) and the remaining quarter will develop the recessive condition (both of the genes in the pair are defective).

The problem of 'inbreeding'

Recessive conditions are more likely to become manifest if the parents of a child are closely related to one another. This is because relatives are more likely to carry a similar pattern of recessive defective genes. 'Inbreeding', or 'consanguinity', therefore leads to an increased incidence of children who carry a matching pair of recessive genes.

Dominant gene defects

In contrast to recessive gene defects, some genetic defects will lead to disease even if only present on one of the two chromosomes of the pair. Despite the presence of a normal gene on the partner chromosome, the defective gene produces a protein that acts as if it is 'putting a spanner in the works', and leads to a recognisable syndrome. In this case, the gene defect is described as 'dominant'. Huntingdon's disease is a condition that is the result of dominant gene defect located on chromosome 4.

Dominant genes can also be transmitted from parent to child. In the case of one parent carrying a dominant defective gene (such as the one that causes Huntingdon's disease), half of the gametes produced by that parent will also carry that gene. This means that, even if the other parent is unaffected, half the children will manifest the dominantly inherited condition carried by a parent. Dominantly inherited conditions are more likely to result wholly from spontaneous mutation than are recessively inherited conditions. This is because only one of the gametes needs to be affected to give rise to a dominantly inherited condition.

X-linked recessive conditions

X-linked recessive conditions are those recessive conditions that are the result of single-gene defects of the X chromosome of the sex chromosome XY pair (rather than on any one of the remaining 22 non-sex or autosomal chromosomes). In girls, X-linked recessive conditions behave as any other autosomal recessive condition, in that the presence of a normal gene on the corresponding X chromosome of the pair will counterbalance the defect and prevent the manifestation of serious disease.

However, in boys, a gene defect on the X chromosome behaves more like a dominantly inherited defect. This is because the stumpy Y chromosome actually contains very few of the genes that are represented on the X chromosome, and so does not carry a healthy matching gene for the defective one found on the X chromosome. Therefore, all boys who inherit the gene defect in an X-linked condition will manifest the disease.

Haemophilia is one of the most well known of the serious X-linked recessive conditions. In haemophilia the carriage of the defect is always through females, and the condition is usually manifested in boys. Colour blindness is another, less serious, X-linked condition that is carried by females, and manifested usually in boys (see Q5.4c-1-Q5.4c-3).

Cystic fibrosis

Cystic fibrosis is a condition of recessive inheritance. Approximately 1 in 25 people of north European ancestry are known to carry the defective cystic fibrosis gene on one of the chromosomes in pair 7. The probability of the parents of a child both being carriers of cystic fibrosis gene is 1 in 625 (= 25 × 25). Such parents have a 1 in 4 chance of having a child with cystic fibrosis. Therefore, the incidence of cystic fibrosis is 1 in 2500 (= 25 × 25 × 4) births. Cystic fibrosis is described in more detail in Chapter 3.3d.

Sickle cell disease and thalassaemia

Both sickle cell anaemia and thalassaemia are conditions of recessive inheritance. The features of these inherited forms of anaemia are described in Chapter 3.4c.

In sickle cell disease, the condition results from a mutation in a gene on chromosome pair 11, which leads to a defect in the structure of haemoglobin. Approximately 1 in 16 people of African or Afro-Caribbean ancestry is known to carry the defective sickle cell gene (i.e. sickle cell trait). Using the principles of probability described above for cystic fibrosis, this means that there is just less than a 1 in 1000 probability of a child with sickle cell anaemia being born to parents who are both of African or Afro-Caribbean ancestry.

In thalassaemia, there are a range of genetic defects that cause problems in the rate of production of haemoglobin. One in 10 people of Mediterranean (or Asian) origin are estimated to be carriers of one of the forms of thalassaemia.

Phenylketonuria

Phenylketonuria (PKU) is a condition in which the amino acid phenylalanine cannot be handled by the body. This is the result of the absence of an essential enzyme. Without careful dietary exclusion of sources of phenylalanine (including milk), a child with PKU may develop brain damage, as excess phenylalanine in the body fluids is toxic to developing nervous tissue.

PKU can be detected at birth by means of the heel-prick (Guthrie) test. Once PKU is diagnosed in a baby, the parents are given specific dietary advice to protect the child from permanent brain damage. Although the diet is less essential for PKU sufferers in adulthood, a woman with PKU should be strict about her diet in pregnancy, otherwise the high levels of phenylalanine can damage the developing fetus.

PKU is a recessively inherited condition. The defective gene is fairly rare, being carried by 1 in 50–70 of the population. This means that the incidence of PKU is 1 in 10,000–20,000 births.

Albinism

Albinism is usually a recessively inherited condition (although there is a rare X-linked recessive form), in which there is absence of the gene that codes for the enzyme tyrosinase. Tyrosinase is essential in the manufacture of the dark-coloured pigment melanin.

There are different forms of albinism, some which affect the eye only and some which also affect the skin and hair. The most important clinical consequence of albinism comes from the lack of pigment in the eye, which affects both the iris and also the choroid layer that lies behind the retina. In albinism the iris of the eye appears pale blue. The lack of protective pigment means that the eye is unable to fix on an object because the incoming light is too bright, and so the eye flickers from position to position, with a movement called 'nystagmus'. The child learns to screw up his or her eyes to protect them from light. Without early intervention (tinted glasses or contact lenses), sight can become severely impaired.

In the form of albinism that also affects the skin, the child has very pale skin and fair hair and eyebrows. The skin is very vulnerable to sunburn, and so protection from the sun is always required.

Information Box 5.4c-V

Albinism: comments from a Chinese medicine perspective

In Chinese medicine, the Liver is the Organ that opens into the eyes (see Maciocia 1989, p. 77). The Liver Blood moistens and nourishes the eye, and gives it the capacity to see. However, Maciocia explains that many other Yin and Yang Organs affect the eye. In particular, Kidney Jing and the Heart Organ are important in maintaining the health of the eyes (Maciocia 1989, p. 80). In the case of albinism, Jing Deficiency would appear to be the fundamental problem. Squinting and flickering eye movements might suggest Wind (possibly in the Liver and Gallbladder Channels), which has built up as a consequence of Kidney Deficiency.

Colour blindness

Colour blindness is an X-linked condition. The most common form of colour blindness results in an inability to distinguish between red and green, and varying intermediate shades of brown. It is due to the absence of a particular pigment in the cone cells of the retina necessary for colour discrimination. It is common, affecting up to 1 in 50 men, and is important only in that its presence might affect eligibility for certain forms of employment (e.g. train driving).

Muscular dystrophy

Muscular dystrophy (MD) is a general term used to describe a group of congenital conditions in which the muscles undergo a process of progressive degeneration. The two most common forms of muscular dystrophy, Duchenne and Becker MD, both have X-linked recessive inheritance. The defective genes for these two distinct conditions are located on the short arm of the X chromosome.

Duchenne is the most common form of MD, affecting 1 in 4000 male infants. The clinical features of Duchenne MD are described in Chapter 4.2f.

Haemophilia

Haemophilia is a term used to describe the range of disorders of blood coagulation which result from defective production of clotting factors. The three most common forms of haemophilia are haemophilia A, haemophilia B (Christmas disease) and von Willebrand's disease.

Haemophilia A is an X-linked recessive condition, affecting 1 in 5000 of the male population. The disorder results from defective production of clotting factor VIII. The gene that codes for the production of this factor is found on the X chromosome. The clinical features of haemophilia A are described in Chapter 2.1c.

Haemophilia B is clinically very similar to haemophilia A. It too is an X-linked recessive condition, but results from the absence of clotting factor IX. It affects 1 in 30,000 males.

Von Willebrand's disease results from a deficiency of a factor that aids in platelet adherence as well as in the action of factor VIII. This rare form of haemophilia is a recessive condition because the defective gene is found on chromosome pair 12, rather than an X chromosome.

In all three conditions, the severity of the condition depends on the precise nature of the genetic defect.

Achondroplasia

Achondroplasia is a dominantly inherited condition that leads to dwarfism in the person who carries the defective gene. In 50% of cases the condition arises as a result of a spontaneous mutation. In an adult, the condition manifests with marked shortening of the limbs, a pronounced curvature of the lumbar spine, a large head and a depressed nasal ridge (Figure 5.4c-III). All these features develop as a result of defective maturation of cartilage into bone. Despite these very pronounced features in the adult, the diagnosis may not be made until early childhood.

Information Box 5.4c-VI

Achondroplasia: comments from a Chinese medicine perspective

In Chinese medicine, the underlying problem in maturation of bone in achondroplasia suggests Kidney (Jing) Deficiency.

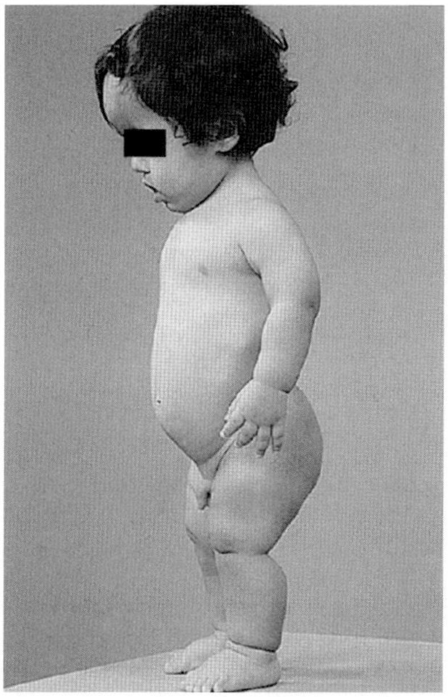

Figure 5.4c-III • Characteristic features of achondroplasia.

Osteogenesis imperfecta (brittle bone disease)

Osteogenesis imperfecta is a term, like muscular dystrophy, that is applied to a group of genetic disorders that vary in their severity. In osteogenesis imperfecta the underlying genetic defects lead to disordered metabolism of collagen, resulting in weakness of bone.

The most common form of osteogenesis imperfecta is dominantly inherited and manifests in the occurrence of recurrent fractures in childhood. If there is no prior family history, a child with the condition may be mistaken for a case of non-accidental injury. Another characteristic feature of this most common form of osteogenesis imperfecta is that the sclerae (whites) of the eyes have a bluish coloration. There is also an increased incidence of the condition otosclerosis, which leads to progressive loss of hearing in adult life.

Information Box 5.4c-VII

Osteogenesis imperfecta: comments from a Chinese medicine perspective

In Chinese medicine, the brittle bones, the blue colour of the eyes and the progressive deafness characteristic of osteogenesis imperfecta all suggest that Kidney (Jing) Deficiency is at the root of the condition.

Familial hyperlipidaemias

The term 'hyperlipidaemia' simply refers to the fact that a raised concentration of fats (including cholesterol) can be found in a serum blood sample. There are at least eight well-recognised forms of inherited hyperlipidaemia. In these conditions, an underlying gene defect, or a number of gene defects, affect the way in which lipids are manufactured in the liver.

Hyperlipidaemia is strongly associated with an increased risk of coronary heart disease (CHD). The risk of CHD associated with hyperlipidaemia depends on the precise nature of the genetic defect. Some forms of hyperlipidaemia confer a higher risk of CHD than others.

Familial hypercholesterolaemia is a common, dominantly inherited form of hyperlipidaemia, in which the most important imbalance is a raised level of cholesterol in the blood. Approximately 1 in 500 of the UK population is affected by this condition. Many adults who have familial hypercholesterolaemia may only become aware of the diagnosis through routine blood testing. However, it has been estimated that over half of men with this condition will die of a heart attack before the age of 60 years. Some, but not all, people with this condition may develop the classic skin signs of hypercholesterolaemia, the xanthoma (plural is xanthomata) and xanthelasma (plural is xanthelasmata). A xanthoma is a substantial cholesterol deposit that can appear as a yellowish nodule in the skin around bony prominences, in the tendons and on the palms. A xanthoma is a rare finding in childhood. Xanthalasmata are less substantial yellowish plaques of cholesterol, which can develop in the loose skin around the eyelids.

The treatment of most forms of hyperlipidaemia is by means of a lipid-lowering diet together with high doses of one or more of the cholesterol-lowering drugs, including the statins (e.g. simvastatin). It is known that the risk of CHD is reduced if the blood lipid levels can be reduced by this combined treatment approach.

If a person inherits a familial hypercholesterolaemia gene defect from both parents, the condition is much more serious. In these cases there is a hugely elevated cholesterol level from childhood. The natural history of this very rare condition is death from ischaemic heart disease in late childhood or adolescence.

Familial combined hypercholesterolaemia is another commonly occurring, dominantly inherited hyperlipidaemia, in which raised levels of cholesterol and also of another class of lipid, the triglycerides, are found. This form of hyperlipidaemia affects 1 in 200 of the population.

Familial hypertriglyceridaemia involves elevated levels of triglycerides alone. This condition may respond very rapidly to abstinence from alcohol.

Information Box 5.4c-VIII

Hyperlipidaemia: comments from a Chinese medicine perspective

In Chinese medicine, the finding of elevated blood lipids and the resulting development of atheroma and xanthomata suggest that Phlegm Damp is prominent in the manifestation of hyperlipidaemia. Imbalance in the Spleen and Liver Organs is likely. An underlying Deficiency of Jing is also a factor in the inherited forms of hyperlipidaemia.

Part II: Conditions of multifactorial inheritance

The genetic conditions discussed in the first part of this chapter all have an origin that can be clearly related to a defect in the structure of the genetic material. This defect will be found in the DNA contained in all the nucleated cells of an individual with the condition (with the very rare exception of mosaicism).

In contrast, the conditions of multifactorial inheritance tend to have a less clear genetic origin. In some cases of these conditions, it is well recognised that the cause is an external factor that has affected the growth of the fetus in the womb (e.g. congenital heart disease as a result of maternal rubella virus infection in the first trimester). However, in other cases of the condition there is no clear external factor. In these cases it may be concluded that the problem has arisen as a result of a combination of genetic defects (leading to a susceptibility), together with one or more of a whole host of diverse external factors that may have affected development of the embryo/fetus in the womb (e.g. malnutrition, smoking, alcohol, medication, stress). It is not unusual to find more than one congenital condition of multifactorial inheritance in the same child. For example, a child with oesophageal atresia may also be found to have congenital heart disease or a kidney defect.

In general, the risk of recurrence of these conditions in another child in the same family is low, which does suggest that environmental factors play a strong part in their origin. However, the risk is greater than it would be for an unrelated child, which does provide the evidence that genetic susceptibility is also important for these conditions to arise.

Congenital heart disease

Congenital heart disease is the single most common group of structural disorders in children. Up to 2 in every 100 children are born with some degree of cardiac malformation, although in only less than half of these is the malformation of a severe nature. Congenital heart disease may also affect the ability of the fetus to survive outside the womb, as it is known that 1 in 10 stillborn babies has a cardiac malformation.

In only a small proportion of cases can the cardiac abnormality be explained by an external factor. External factors that have been linked to congenital heart disease include maternal rubella infection in the first trimester, maternal antibodies in systemic lupus erythematosus, a high maternal intake of alcohol, and poorly controlled maternal diabetes mellitus. Congenital malformations of the heart and aorta have also been linked to certain chromosomal abnormalities such as Down syndrome and Turner syndrome.

Even in cases in which there is no obvious external or chromosomal cause of the malformation, it is recognised that the risk of the condition recurring in a second child is higher than would be expected. This suggests that there is some, as yet unexplained, genetic factor that increases the susceptibility of the developing fetus to the condition.

The most common forms of congenital heart disease, septal defect, aortic stenosis (narrowing of the aortic valve), coarctation of the aorta (narrowing of the upper arch of the aorta) and the complex abnormalities that lead to cyanotic heart disease, are explained in more detail in Chapter 3.2g.

Information Box 5.4c-IX

Congenital heart disease: comments from a Chinese medicine perspective

In Chinese medicine, Jing Deficiency usually underlies congenital heart disease. This makes sense because, if untreated, significant congenital heart disease will lead to continual ill-health and poor growth and development in the child.

According to the particular defect, Deficiency of Heart Qi, Yang and/or Yin will also be present. The bluish colour in cyanotic heart disease suggests that Qi or Blood Stagnation has developed as a consequence of severe Heart Deficiency.

Hare lip and cleft palate

Hare (cleft) lip and cleft palate affect just over 1 in 1000 babies. The problem is a failure in the normal fusion of the tissues of the lip and palate. These should grow together in the fetus in the first trimester of pregnancy. In a healthy baby the evidence of normal fusion lies in the two parallel ridges of skin that bridge the inner nostrils and the lip (the philtrum).

Most cases of cleft lip and palate arise spontaneously with no obvious external causative factor. The condition can now be diagnosed prenatally by means of the ultrasound scan done at 20 weeks of gestation.

Hare lip is the least severe of the abnormalities. In this situation the internal structure of the mouth is normal, but the philtrum is distorted and the baby has large gaps in the lip where the ridges of the philtrum should be. Although this is a very unsightly abnormality, and one that is often shocking for the parents, surgical repair of the lip can have very impressive results. Ideally, this surgery should be delayed for a few months to achieve the best outcome (Figure 5.4c-IV).

Cleft palate leaves a gaping space between the mouth and the nasal spaces. It can make breastfeeding very difficult in some cases. Cleft palate frequently, but not always, coexists with hare lip. Diagnosis is made by inserting a finger into the mouth of the neonate. Affected babies are more prone to bouts of choking and frequent episodes of ear infections (otitis media) because of distortion of the Eustachian tube. In later life speech can be affected, as the child develops a characteristic nasal quality to the voice.

Surgical correction of cleft palate is usually performed at several months of age. This also can have good results, but the child may be still be left with some degree of cosmetic, auditory and speech problems.

Oesophageal atresia

Oesophageal atresia is a rare abnormality in which the oesophagus fails to develop normally. It may first present with the accumulation of amniotic fluid (polyhydramnios) in late pregnancy, as the developing fetus is unable to swallow the fluid as does a healthy fetus. After birth, the baby will very soon start to drool saliva and choke and vomit when feeding. Once the diagnosis is made, the baby is examined for other malformations, as almost half will have at least one other congenital abnormality. The condition is treated immediately by surgery.

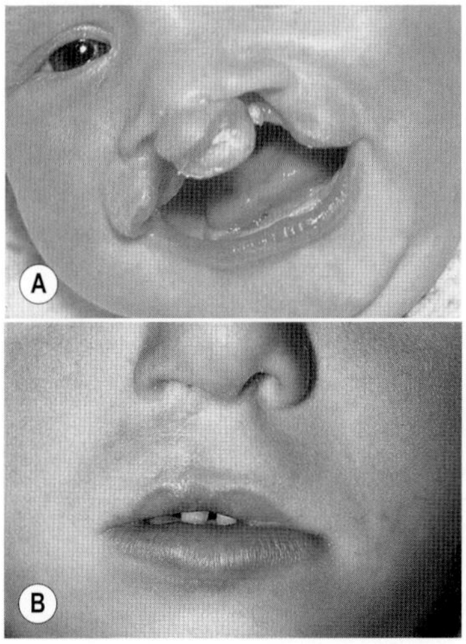

Figure 5.4c-IV • Cleft lip (a) before and (b) after surgery.

Information Box 5.4c-X

Hare lip and cleft palate: comments from a Chinese medicine perspective

In Chinese medicine, the underlying cause of hare lip and cleft palate is Jing Deficiency. The involvement of the mouth and nose suggests a more specific Deficiency in the Spleen/Stomach and Lung Organs.

Pyloric stenosis

Pyloric stenosis is another malformation that impairs the passage of nutrients through the gastrointestinal tract. In pyloric stenosis, the malformation is a thickening of the pyloric sphincter, the 'valve' that separates the stomach from the duodenum. The condition is four times more common in boys, and more common if one of the parents suffered from the condition.

The baby presents in the first days to weeks of life with vomiting of bile and undigested milk. The vomiting can be so forceful as to be projectile. The baby may be very unwell by the time of diagnosis because of loss of fluids and salts. Treatment is by means of surgery to the pyloric sphincter after the fluid and salt imbalance has been corrected.

Duodenal and small bowel obstruction is a similar, although less common, abnormality, in which the obstruction is a result of failure of the development of the passageway for food and fluids at one or more points along the bowel. These cases may take a few more days before symptoms become apparent, depending on how far down the bowel the obstruction is situated. An additional symptom is that the child may develop a very distended abdomen as the upper part of the intestine fills with wind and fluid.

Imperforate anus

In this rare malformation, there is failure in the development of the rectum and anus. If this is not diagnosed at the neonatal check at birth, the child will eventually present with similar symptoms to small bowel obstruction. Again the treatment is surgical.

Information Box 5.4c-XI

Oesophageal atresia and pyloric stenosis: comments from a Chinese medicine perspective

In Chinese medicine, abnormalities of development of the gastrointestinal tract suggest Jing Deficiency with a specific Deficiency in the Spleen/Stomach and Liver Organs. The Liver Organ is implicated because, in all forms of gastrointestinal obstruction, the symptoms suggest failure of smooth movement of Qi in the Middle and Lower Jiao.

Congenital liver disease and neonatal jaundice

Jaundice is a common finding in newborns. Over 60% of newborns become visibly jaundiced within the first few days of life. The potential problem with neonatal jaundice is that the raised bilirubin levels which cause jaundice can be very harmful to the developing nervous system, and can cause a permanent form of brain damage called 'kernicterus'.

In most cases of neonatal jaundice, the problem arises as a combined result of immaturity of the red blood cells and the liver. This condition is termed 'physiological jaundice'. Physiological jaundice becomes apparent at 2–5 days after birth, and usually resolves within 2 weeks without any need for treatment. In some babies, a temporary intolerance to breast milk may exacerbate physiological jaundice (breast milk jaundice). However, this complication is rarely so severe as to prevent continuation of breastfeeding.

The problem of raised bilirubin levels in physiological jaundice can be more severe in some babies, particularly if they are premature, in which case most will respond to phototherapy. Phototherapy involves exposing the skin of the newborn to blue light in an incubator. The light promotes the conversion of the bilirubin in the blood to a harmless pigment. In less severe cases, exposure to sunlight will perform this task. In very severe cases the baby may require a treatment called 'exchange transfusion', in which blood is withdrawn from the baby and replaced with donor blood.

Jaundice may also result from conditions that cause excessive damage to the red blood cells (haemolysis). Rhesus and other blood-group incompatibilities are the most common causes of neonatal haemolysis.

In cases in which the jaundice persists for more than 2 weeks, congenital liver disease may be the underlying problem. In these cases the jaundice is usually accompanied by pale stools and dark urine. Biliary atresia and neonatal hepatitis are the two most common forms of neonatal liver disease.

Biliary atresia (bile-duct obstruction) is a condition in which the bile ducts fail to develop normally, and so are obstructed. Unless surgical bypass of the bile ducts is performed (ideally within 2 months after birth), the baby will rapidly develop a fatal form of liver failure. Even when this operation is successful there is continued damage to the liver. The child will eventually require liver transplantation to avoid progression to cirrhosis. If the bypass operation is unsuccessful, liver transplantation has to be performed without delay.

'Neonatal hepatitis' refers to inflammation of the liver tissue at birth. The causes include congenital infections and a range of rare genetic diseases of metabolism, including cystic fibrosis. However, in many cases of neonatal hepatitis the cause cannot be clarified. Unlike in a typical case of biliary atresia, the child with neonatal hepatitis is unwell and jaundiced from birth. There may be a palpable enlarged liver and spleen. In all cases the treatment is largely supportive, and of course includes treatment to prevent rising bilirubin levels, as described above. In some cases the condition will resolve, but in others the child may develop progressive cirrhosis for which transplantation of the liver is the only treatment. There is a small risk of acute liver failure, which has a high mortality.

Information Box 5.4c-XII

Jaundice: comments from a Chinese medicine perspective

In Chinese medicine, persistent jaundice would suggest that the underlying imbalance involves Jing Deficiency, together with a specific Deficiency in the Spleen and Liver Organs.

Club foot (talipes equinovarus)

'Club foot' refers to abnormal positioning of the foot at the ankle joint. The medical term for this condition is 'talipes equinovarus'. The entire foot is inverted and the forefoot is turned outwards so that the soles of the baby's feet tend to face each other (Figure 5.4c-V). The problem is due to an imbalance in the tension of the muscles of the lower leg and foot, with consequent shortening of the tendons. A mild form of talipes is common, and results from compression of the feet in the womb. Usually this will resolve naturally, and can be helped by simple stretching exercises.

A more severe form of this condition can result in a permanent deformity of the foot, and so requires much more active management from the time of birth. Severe talipes equinovarus affects 1–2 in 1000 births, and is more common in boys. It may be a result of compression in the womb, but does also have a tendency to run in families, thus suggesting a genetic susceptibility.

The treatment of severe talipes involves stretching and strapping of the foot. Sometimes, serial plaster casts may be used to hold the foot in the correct position, so allowing the tendons to find their normal length. Corrective surgery to the tendons may be required at the age of 6–9 months.

Information Box 5.4c-XIII

Talipes equinovarus (club foot): comments from a Chinese medicine perspective

The imbalance in the tension of the muscles and tendons at the root of talipes equinovarus suggests that the underlying cause in Chinese medicine would be Jing Deficiency, with a specific Deficiency in the Liver and Gallbladder Organs.

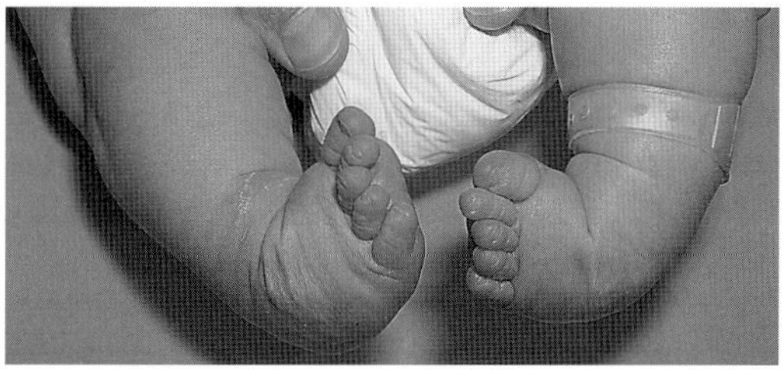

Figure 5.4c-V • Talipes equinovarus.

Congenital dislocation of the hip

The term 'congenital dislocation of the hip' (CDH) embraces a wide spectrum of disorders that involve the structure of the acetabulum which is the cup-like depression in the pelvis which cradles the head of the femur in the hip joint. In less severe cases, the curvature of the acetabulum is slightly too shallow, meaning that the head of the femur easily clicks out of place. In these less severe cases, as the child grows, the acetabulum may enlarge to cradle the femur more neatly, and the problem resolves. In more severe cases the acetabulum is very distorted in shape and, without treatment, the hip joint may never develop normally. This condition is not obviously apparent in the newborn. Before the introduction of screening for CDH in the first few months of life, undiagnosed CDH would progress to a disabling permanent condition.

CDH can be detected by a skilled examiner by the occurrence of perceptible 'clunks' from the hip joint when the thighs of the baby are moved in a certain way. The first time at which this test is performed is during neonatal screening. A specific abnormality of the hip is detected by this test in 6 out of 1000 newborns. However, most of these 'abnormalities' will resolve spontaneously. The true incidence of a problem with the hip joint is probably only 1.5 in 1000 newborns. The problem rarely may be missed initially, but then can be picked up at the 8-week examination. If missed entirely, it may not be until the child starts to walk with a limp that the possibility of CDH becomes apparent.

The degree of the problem in the newborn can be assessed by means of ultrasound examination of the hip joints. If this confirms a moderate to severe abnormality, the baby may be placed in a harness or splint for several months to hold the hips in an abducted (frog-like) position. This encourages the acetabulum to develop in a normal way. In most cases this treatment is successful in preventing a permanent deformity. If this conservative approach is unsuccessful, or if the condition is diagnosed at a later stage, surgical treatment of the bones of the joint and application of a plaster splint may be necessary.

Information Box 5.4c-XIV

Congenital dislocation of the hip: comments from a Chinese medicine perspective

In Chinese medicine, the focus of the abnormality of the hip joint suggests that Jing Deficiency, together with a specific Deficiency of the Liver and Gallbladder, may underlie congenital dislocation of the hip.

Maldescent of testes

For the production of healthy spermatozoa it is necessary for the testes to be suspended outside the abdomen in the scrotum, and infertility may result if the testis is misplaced. It is also well recognised that a misplaced testis, either in the abdomen or the groin, is more likely to become cancerous.

The testis originates in the fetus from the same embryonic tissue as the ovary. Under the influence of male sex hormones, it then descends during the third trimester through a gap in the muscles of the groin area to find its correct position in the scrotum of the fetus. In 5% of male babies this descent is found not to have occurred normally, for either one or both testes. The diagnosis is made by the examining doctor at the neonatal check, when the testes (or testis) are either impalpable, or felt higher up in the groin. The occurrence of maldescent of the testes is more common in babies born prematurely.

In some cases of maldescent of the testes the problem resolves spontaneously as the testes find their way into the scrotum during the first few weeks of life. In cases that persist beyond 3 months of age there may be little chance of spontaneous resolution. If by the age of 1–2 years the testes (testis) are completely impalpable, a laparoscopic examination is performed to assess whether the testes are either somewhere within the abdominal cavity or entirely absent.

Treatment for undescended testes is necessary to promote fertility and to prevent cancerous change. For testes that are situated in the groin area, the treatment is an operation called 'orchidopexy'. This is performed after the age of 1 year, and before the child has reached his third birthday. It is usually a straightforward procedure, in which the testes are located via an incision in the groin, and then drawn into the scrotum. It is much more difficult to move a testis that is located in the abdomen. Because of the risk of cancer, a single intra-abdominal testis will be surgically removed, and an artificial testis implanted into the scrotum at a later date (as close to adulthood as is reasonable) for cosmetic purposes. If both testes are intra-abdominal, a much more complex microsurgical technique is required to transplant the testes to their correct position.

Information Box 5.4c-XV

Maldescent of the testes: comments from a Chinese medicine perspective

In Chinese medicine, failure of the testis to descend, with the consequent risk of reduced fertility, is suggestive of Jing Deficiency. As the Liver Channel passes through the area of the scrotum, it is likely that there is also a specific Deficiency in Liver Qi.

Congenital hernia

A hernia can be defined as the movement of an internal organ outside its usual anatomical position through an area of weakness in the surrounding supportive tissue. There are three common types of hernia that can develop in adulthood: inguinal, femoral and hiatus hernias.

In adulthood, hernias usually develop as a result of prolonged strain on the supportive tissues in the area of the hernia, although in some cases there may be an underlying congenital weakness in the herniated area. In contrast, congenital hernias develop because the supportive tissue in the area is underdeveloped in some way. The three important forms of congenital hernia are the inguinal, hiatus and umbilical hernias.

Congenital inguinal hernia

Congenital inguinal hernia is related in origin to maldescent of the testes. This weakness of the muscle wall of the groin area is a result of a failure of the passageway formed in the third trimester of pregnancy by the testis (as it descends through the groin region) to close off completely. The resulting area of weakness is a site through which the abdominal contents can bulge outwards. In mild cases a lump can be felt in the groin, but in more severe cases the intestines can spill out through a gap in the muscle tissues to form a bulging mass in the scrotum (Figure 5.4c-VI). Although inguinal hernias are more common in boys, they can also affect girls. A congenital inguinal hernia is initially painless, but there is a risk that abdominal contents can become trapped and damaged as they bulge out through the opening of the hernia. The treatment is surgical repair of the weakness in the muscle wall.

If undiagnosed at birth, the hernia can present as a painful lump in the groin, which is an indication that the intestinal tissues, together with the spermatic cord, have become compressed in the tight space in the muscle tissue. It may be possible to give the baby a light anaesthetic and push this lump back into the abdominal cavity. If this is not possible, immediate surgery is required, as there is serious risk that either the bowel or spermatic cords become obstructed, or that their blood supply becomes cut off (with the risk of infarction of the bowel and loss of the testis).

Congenital hiatus hernia

In some young babies, a weakness in the lower oesophageal (cardiac) sphincter results in frequent regurgitation of partly digested milk. In mild cases this problem resolves with time, and, in the interim, may be helped by adding thickening agents to feeds. In more severe cases the repeated episodes of regurgitation can leave the child in a malnourished state. The child may be found on investigation to have a widening of the cardiac sphincter (a hiatus hernia), which is unlikely to resolve rapidly with time. Some of these cases may respond to drugs that enhance the emptying of the stomach, but in other cases surgery may be required to narrow the opening of the sphincter.

Congenital umbilical hernia

A small weakness between the two strap-like muscles that run from the anterior arch formed by the lower ribcage and xiphisternum down to the pubic bone (the rectus abdominis) is common in newborns, especially those of Afro-Caribbean descent. The result is a bulge in the area of the umbilicus. Although this is a true hernia of intra-abdominal contents, the risk of obstruction of bowel contents is very low. The condition usually resolves as the child gets older and its abdominal muscle tone increases.

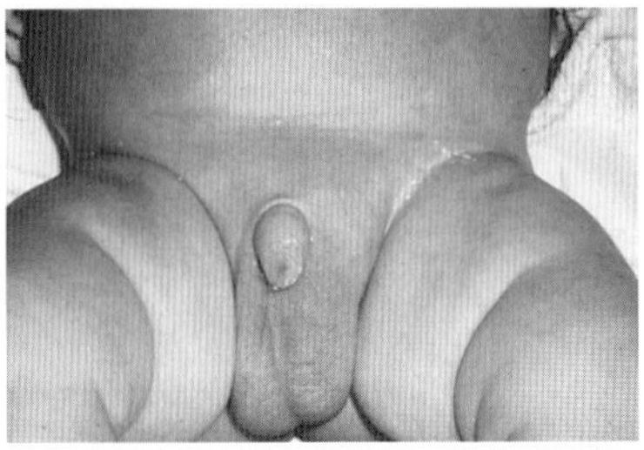

Figure 5.4c-VI • Left-sided inguinal hernia (slightly swollen left groin area).

> **Information Box 5.4c-XVI**
>
> **Congenital hernia: comments from a Chinese medicine perspective**
>
> In Chinese medicine, a congenital hernia might represent Jing Deficiency with specific Deficiency of the Spleen Organ, as it is Spleen Qi that is responsible for 'raising'.
>
> In inguinal hernia Deficiency/Imbalance of Liver Qi is also likely, particularly in view of the fact that symptoms of extreme Stagnation (obstruction and/or infarction) are a possible consequence of such a hernia.
>
> Congenital hiatus hernia presents with symptoms suggestive of Deficiency of Stomach Qi, as regurgitation is the most prominent symptom.

Congenital blindness

Severe visual impairment affects 1 in 3000 births. About 50% of these cases are genetic in origin (including albinism, congenital cataract, and a rare inherited form of tumour, retinoblastoma). Many of the remaining cases arise as a result of congenital infection such as rubella or toxoplasmosis. Another important cause of visual impairment is marked prematurity. In very premature babies (less than 32 weeks) there is a tendency for the retinal vessels to grow too rapidly, and so cause occlusion of the retina. This problem can be prevented in some cases by regular screening of the newborn baby, and by giving laser treatment to the retina if new vessel growth is detected.

Severe visual impairment is usually detected in the UK by the time the child is 6 months old. Early diagnosis by screening is of great value, as the parents of a visually impaired child will benefit from advice on how to give appropriate stimulation through speech and touch, and appropriate educational support can be arranged in advance for the child.

> **Information Box 5.4c-XVII**
>
> **Congenital blindness: comments from a Chinese medicine perspective**
>
> In Chinese medicine, congenital blindness is a manifestation of Jing Deficiency. There may also be specific Deficiencies in the Liver and Heart Organs, as these Organs, together with the Kidney, are particularly important for clear vision.

Congenital deafness

Congenital deafness affects 1 in 1000 births. The causes include hereditary malformations of the structure of the inner ear and congenital infections such as rubella, toxoplasmosis, syphilis or the human immunodeficiency virus (HIV). In many children there is no obvious cause.

In many cases the deafness is not absolute, in that the child can perceive some ranges of sound. If this is the case, it means that there is hope of improving the child's ability to hear by means of a hearing aid. If deafness is absolute, a cochlear implant (a tiny device, which includes a microphone and an electrode, implanted surgically into the inner ear; the electrode stimulates the auditory (VIII) cranial nerve in response to incoming sounds – see Chapter 6.1e) may be of great help. The early diagnosis of deafness has been much improved in the UK by the introduction of the neonatal hearing screening programme.

Electronic tools for assisted hearing work best if the diagnosis is made early so that the child becomes used to the transformed sound that they produce, and so parents and carers can be guided in the way in which they communicate with the child. It is most important that hearing aids are in use at the time when the child would be developing speech. If this window of opportunity is missed, the older child may never learn to speak clearly.

> **Information Box 5.4c-XVIII**
>
> **Congenital deafness: comments from a Chinese medicine perspective**
>
> In Chinese medicine, congenital deafness would suggest an underlying Deficiency of Jing and Kidney Qi, as it is the Kidney that is responsible for clarity of hearing.

Neural tube defects

In the early stages of its development, the nervous system begins as a flat plate of tissue, which then curves in on itself to form a tube. This tube will eventually form the brain and spinal cord. The hollow running through the centre of this tube will develop into the ventricles of the brain and the central canal of the spinal cord. These are the spaces that contain the cerebrospinal fluid (CSF). The neural tube defects result from a failure in the fusion of the tissues of the brain and spinal cord in the first few weeks of development of the embryo.

The most important neural tube defects are anencephaly and spina bifida (including meningocoele, myelomeningocoele and spina bifida occulta). Together these defects used to be the most common serious malformations detected at birth (affecting 2–4 per 1000 births in the 1960s). In developed countries the incidence has now fallen, partly as a result of improved nutrition with supplementation of food (such as breads and breakfast cereals) with the vitamin folic acid, and partly as a result of detection of the abnormality early on in pregnancy.

Anencephaly is an abnormality that always results in neonatal death or stillbirth. The baby suffers from a failure in the development of a large portion of the brain and skull bones. This abnormality is usually picked up early in pregnancy, in which case the mother will be offered a therapeutic termination of pregnancy.

'Spina bifida' literally means that the spinal bones are divided in two (bifid). In all types of spina bifida there is failure of the two arms of the spinal arch of some of the vertebrae (usually in the lumbar area) to meet together.

In spina bifida occulta, deformity of the lumbar vertebrae may be the only defect. In some cases there are no other symptoms, and the diagnosis may only be made incidentally when an X-ray image is taken of the lower back for other reasons. In other cases of spina bifida occulta, the underlying spinal cord may be distorted in some way, and this may give rise to neurological problems of the bladder and lower limbs. Occasionally, a birthmark or unusual tuft of hair may be found on the skin overlying spina bifida occulta.

A meningocoele is a fluid-filled outpouching of the spinal meninges through the gap formed by a spina bifida. A meningocoele forms a rounded swelling overlying the lumbar spine. Despite its startling appearance, the meningocoele can be repaired surgically, and may actually lead to little or no neurological deficit.

A myelomeningocoele is a more serious problem. In this condition, the tube-like structure of the lumbar spinal cord does not form, and instead the spinal cord in this region develops into a flat 'plaque' within a meningocoele. This deformity may have little or no overlying skin, and so exposes the nervous system to infection. In addition to this gross defect, babies with meningomyelocoeles also often have deformities at the level of the cerebellum that prevent a free flow of CSF out of the ventricles of the brain (see Chapter 4.1a). Without prompt treatment the result is a build up of fluid in the ventricles, and stretching and distortion of the brain tissue. The soft plates of bone of the baby's skull are stretched, so that the head enlarges. This condition is called 'hydrocephalus'.

Babies who are born with a myelomeningocoele may suffer from severe problems, including paralysis of the legs (a spastic paraplegia), sensory loss of the buttocks and legs, impaired action of the bladder and bowel, and scoliosis. Those who also suffer from hydrocephalus may suffer from intellectual impairment.

Treatment includes immediate surgery to the back to close the defect and protect the spinal cord from infection. Also, a plastic 'shunt' may be inserted at the level of the base of the brain to allow free fluid flow between the ventricles and the CSF that surrounds the brain and spinal cord.

Affected children require regular physiotherapy to prevent muscle contractures, and bladder catheterisation to prevent build up of the pressure of urine in the bladder and damage to the kidneys. The prognosis for affected children is much better now than it was even as recently as the 1970s, because of advances in surgical techniques and specialised nursing care.

> **Information Box 5.4c-XIX**
>
> **Neural tube defects: comments from a Chinese medicine perspective**
>
> In Chinese medicine, all forms of neural tube defect would be regarded as manifestations of Jing Deficiency.

Cerebral palsy

Cerebral palsy is the result of brain damage that occurs either late in fetal development, during labour or in the neonatal period. This condition is described in Chapter 4.1f.

Congenital hypothyroidism

Congenital hypothyroidism used to be one of the most important causes of severe learning difficulties. Its impact is now minimal since the introduction of the neonatal heel-prick (Guthrie) test. It is described in Chapter 5.1c.

Inherited tendency to adult diseases

Many of the most common adult chronic diseases, including coronary heart disease and cancer, have their root in a susceptibility that is congenital in origin. Sometimes this susceptibility is inherent in the genes of the affected person. In these cases, a family history of the early onset of the condition (e.g. heart attack or breast cancer) would be typical. Sometimes the susceptibility can be attributed to a less than ideal fetal environment. It is now recognised that poor fetal nutrition may predispose to conditions such as high blood pressure, type 2 diabetes and heart disease in later life. (This is the basis of the 'Barker' hypothesis; for more information about the work of Professor Barker on the long-term consequences of fetal health, see West (2001, Ch. 3)).

Currently it is only in a very few chronic adult conditions (such as some forms of inherited breast cancer) that the susceptibility to that condition can be pinpointed early in life by means of a screening test. However, with rapid advances in genetic testing, it may be possible that our individual susceptibility to a whole host of conditions may be predicted. The benefits of such screening tests might appear to be considerable, in that both appropriate lifestyle advice and treatment for the established condition can be offered at an early stage. However, the disadvantages of early screening may, for many conditions, outweigh the benefits. Early diagnosis of susceptibility to conditions such as cancer or schizophrenia may cause anxiety, stigmatisation and very practical problems in terms of reduced eligibility for work or life insurance.

Part III: The premature (preterm) baby

A preterm baby is one that is born before it has attained the maturity required for a healthy start in life. By definition, all babies born before 36 weeks of gestation are preterm. Also, whatever the stage of gestation at birth, all babies with a birthweight of less than 2500 grams are also described as preterm.

The health of the preterm baby depends on the degree to which it is of low birthweight or how much it is born before the normal time. Babies born before 24 weeks of gestation are not likely to survive. Babies born at 24–31 weeks of gestation experience the most problems, but with intensive neonatal care increasing numbers can survive the very fragile first few weeks. Nowadays, the prognosis is excellent for babies born after 32 weeks of gestation. The main problems experienced by preterm babies are described below.

Respiratory distress syndrome

Respiratory distress syndrome (RDS) is a serious condition of the lungs that results from immaturity in the production of a substance called 'surfactant'. This oily liquid is secreted by the lining cells of the lung, and is essential in enabling the full inflation of all the alveolae of the lung after birth. Without surfactant there is a tendency for the alveolae to stay in a collapsed state, thus impairing the ability of the lungs to exchange oxygen and carbon dioxide during breathing. The majority of babies born at 28 weeks of gestation have RDS, but the incidence becomes progressively lower as the age of gestation at the time of birth increases.

A newborn with RDS has a rapid breathing rate, and shows discomfort and strain when breathing. The baby may become cyanosed. Treatment is by means of oxygen at high pressure supplied to the baby by a ventilator, sometimes by mask, and sometimes by means of a tube inserted into the trachea. A recent advance is the injection of artificial surfactant into the lungs through the breathing tube. The use of artificial surfactant, which is made from extracts of animal lung or human amniotic fluid, has lowered the death rate from RDS by 40%. The administration of corticosteroid drugs to a mother at least 24 hours before delivering a preterm baby can also reduce the severity of RDS.

There is a risk of inducing a pneumothorax in a preterm baby during ventilation. This severe complication can be treated by inserting a chest drain. However, there is a greatly increased risk of mortality in a baby with RDS who develops a pneumothorax.

Babies who require a prolonged period of ventilation may develop lung damage from a combination of the high pressure of ventilation, recurrent infections and accumulated secretions. Some of these babies may require oxygen therapy in the first few months of life, and thereafter may be more prone to respiratory problems in childhood. In such babies there is an increased risk of death from respiratory problems in the first few years of life.

Irregularities of breathing and heart rate

Irregularities of breathing and heart rate, including periods during which the breathing stops entirely (apnoea), are common in babies born before 32 weeks of gestation. Therefore, the preterm baby requires constant monitoring. If episodes of apnoea are frequent, ventilation may be required.

Temperature control

A relatively large surface area compared to body weight, thin skin and low body fat all contribute to the problem of difficulty in maintaining body temperature in preterm babies. It is very important to control the external temperature of the baby at an ideal level. This is achieved by means of an incubator. The humidity of the environment within the incubator is also controlled in order to prevent excessive fluid loss from the skin.

Problems with nutrition

Babies born before 35 weeks of gestation will not be able to suck and swallow milk. Feeding has to be by means of a tube inserted into the stomach via the nose or mouth. Even in very preterm babies, breast milk from the baby's own mother is the ideal source of food, although it may need to be supplemented with vitamins, protein, calories and minerals. If the baby is very sick, a highly specialised form of nutrition may be given by vein. Blood transfusions may be required to replace blood removed for laboratory tests, to compensate for low iron stores and the immature production of blood cells.

Episodes of low blood sugar (hypoglycaemia) are more common in preterm babies. This has to be taken seriously, as prolonged episodes of low blood sugar can lead to permanent damage to the developing nervous system. Prevention involves regular blood testing and infusion of intravenous glucose solution.

A recognised very serious complication of the gastrointestinal tract in preterm babies is necrotising enterocolitis. This condition, in which the bowel becomes inflamed and then suffers tissue death, is thought to be a combination of poor blood supply to the bowel wall and invasion of the bowel tissue by bacteria. The baby develops a distended abdomen, vomits feeds and has bloody stools. Surgery for a perforated bowel may be required. About 20% of babies who develop this condition will die from shock or overwhelming infection.

Retinal damage

It has been mentioned earlier that one of the causes of congenital visual impairment is marked prematurity. The problem of new retinal vessel growth (retrolental fibroplasia or retinopathy of prematurity) is found to some degree in one-fifth of babies at 32–38 weeks of gestation. However, because of advances in screening for the condition and the use of laser treatment, the condition only causes severe visual impairment in less than 1% of preterm babies.

Brain damage

Intracranial haemorrhage is well recognised in preterm babies. It can be detected by means of an ultrasound scan. Most episodes of haemorrhage occur shortly after the birth of the baby. Brain haemorrhages are also more common in babies who suffer from RDS or a pneumothorax. The bleed commonly affects a small area of tissue around the ventricles of the brain.

Surprisingly, many babies do not seem to be affected seriously by these bleeds. However, in some cases the bleed can extend. The blood can clot and prevent drainage of the CSF in the ventricles, thus bringing about hydrocephalus. Widespread multiple areas of haemorrhage are associated with a poor developmental outcome.

Jaundice

Jaundice is a common problem of prematurity, and carries a risk because high levels of bilirubin are toxic to the developing nervous system. Premature babies will very often require phototherapy treatment to reduce the circulating levels of bilirubin. In some cases exchange transfusion will be required.

Problems after discharge from hospital

In general, preterm babies, even when they have reached the time at which the delivery should have taken place, are shorter and thinner than babies who are born at term. This discrepancy in height and weight may remain throughout childhood.

Those who have had respiratory problems may develop recurrent chest infections and wheezing episodes. Readmission to hospital in the first year of life is four times more likely in a baby who has been born prematurely.

Very low birthweight infants may develop a wide range of developmental problems. Conditions such as visual impairment, cerebral palsy, hearing loss and learning difficulty are more common in children who were born before 32 weeks of gestation. There is an increased incidence of specific learning difficulties, such as delayed language development, poor attention span and poor fine motor skills. Behavioural problems are also more common. All these problems are more marked the earlier the week of gestation at birth.

The burden on the parents of having a preterm baby in hospital for some weeks cannot be overestimated, particularly if there are older children at home to be cared for. Often, the neonatal intensive care unit is many miles away, and thus many hours each week may be dedicated to visiting the baby. Close contact and handling of the very preterm baby has to be minimised, which may have an impact on bonding. Throughout this time the mother may be expressing breast milk, which many women find a laborious and uncomfortable process.

Information Box 5.4c-XX

Preterm birth: comments from a Chinese medicine perspective

In Chinese medicine, the foundation of all the problems of prematurity would be regarded as Jing Deficiency.

The gynaecologist Chen Jia Yuan wrote in the Qing Dynasty that each lunar month of pregnancy was associated with the development of a different Chinese Organ (West 2001, p. 27). Weeks 24–32 are associated with the development of the Lungs and Large Intestine, and weeks 32–40 with development of the Kidney and Bladder.

This would very much accord with the observation that the preterm baby, by missing out on the opportunity for protected development in the womb during the period from 24 weeks of gestation onwards, carries a particular weakness in the development of the lungs and the nervous system.

Screening for congenital disease

The role of genetic counselling

If there is any concern about the possibility of congenital disease, either before conception or during pregnancy, the couple may be referred to a clinical geneticist for specialised genetic counselling. The geneticist is knowledgeable about the different modes of inheritance of the genetic congenital diseases, and will be able to advise the couple on the risks that their child (or potential child) might be carrying any one congenital disease. Potential parents are usually referred for genetic counselling if there is a personal or family history of possible congenital disease.

As techniques of DNA analysis are becoming more sophisticated, the number of disease-causing gene defects that can be detected in potential parents, and also the developing fetus, is ever increasing. The results of these tests will increase the specificity of the advice given by the geneticist (see Q5.4c-4).

Genetic screening of parents

Genetic screening through DNA analysis may be offered to parents for whom there appears to be a significant possibility that a genetic disease might be transmitted to their children. At present, there is not a specific DNA available for all the known genetic mutations that underlie the carriage of genetic diseases. However, there are many mutations that can be detected directly from a sample of bodily cells from the parent. For example, tests are possible for the carriage of some types of thalassaemia, muscular dystrophy, cystic fibrosis, sickle cell disease and Huntingdon's disease. Use of more sophisticated techniques, such as the polymerase chain reaction (PCR), can allow the detection of a genetic abnormality from a tiny sample of bodily fluid, such as is obtained in the neonatal heel-prick (Guthrie) test.

If one or both parents are found by DNA analysis to be carriers of a specific mutation, they can be given very clear unequivocal information about the risk of conceiving a child with the condition related to the carriage of that mutation.

Antenatal testing for genetic disease

In addition to testing for chromosomal abnormalities and neural tube defects, the fetal cells obtained by means of amniocentesis and chorionic villus sampling may also be tested for specific genetic defects such as cystic fibrosis or muscular dystrophy. Testing for disease in the fetus at this stage in pregnancy provides information to help the parents to make the difficult choice of whether or not to terminate the pregnancy.

Presymptomatic testing of children

DNA analysis may be used to confirm the diagnosis of a genetic disease in a child. Alternatively, the presence of a particular disease may be confirmed by means of a specific biochemical test (e.g. the amino acid assay used to diagnose phenylketonuria) or physical test (e.g. the examination of the eyes that is used to conform or exclude retinoblastoma).

Many genetic diseases vary in their severity from individual to individual. The progression of the disease in the individual may be monitored by means of repeated tests as the child grows up (e.g. repeated ultrasound scans of the kidney are performed in children and adults who are known to carry the dominant gene for polycystic kidney disease). In this way, the more severe cases of the disease may be offered early treatment, and the less severe cases be given reassurance that their own form of the disease appears to be running a more benign course.

There is an ethical debate about whether or not a presymptomatic test should be performed on an apparently healthy child, who has no say in the matter about whether or not they want to know the result of the test. For those conditions in which there is no obvious benefit of knowing the diagnosis (e.g. Huntingdon's disease), it is generally accepted that children should not be tested until the time at which they are able to give informed consent.

Self-test 5.4c

Congenital disorders

1. There are three broad categories of congenital disease as defined in this chapter. Pyloric stenosis, Klinefelter syndrome and achondroplasia are examples of congenital disease. What are the three categories of congenital disease, and into which category does each one of these diseases fall?
2. Comment on the likelihood of a second child manifesting the condition if a first child has been diagnosed with the following conditions (if you are familiar with the mathematics of probability, then predict the probability; otherwise, make a statement such as 'high risk' or 'very unlikely'):
   (i) haemophilia A (the first child is a boy)
   (ii) neural tube defects
   (iii) Turner syndrome
   (iv) type 1 diabetes mellitus.
3. What are the well-recognised ways in which a 2-year-old child who was born at 32 weeks of gestation might be more vulnerable than a child who was born at term?

Answers

1. The three categories of congenital disease are:
   - genetic disease resulting from chromosomal abnormalities (e.g. Klinefelter syndrome)
   - genetic disease resulting from a single-gene defect (e.g. achondroplasia)
   - diseases of multifactorial inheritance (e.g. pyloric stenosis).
2. (i) The chances are that the mother of this boy carries the defective haemophilia gene on one of her X chromosomes. This X chromosome will, in all probability, be passed on to 50% of her future children. Out of these, only the boys will

manifest haemophilia. Therefore, the probability of a recurrence of haemophilia in a second child is high (1 in 4 to be precise).

(ii) As the neural tube defect is a condition of multifactorial inheritance, a genetic tendency for inheritance is less marked. Although the risk of recurrence of a neural tube defect is higher than it would be for a child in the general population, the increased risk of this rare condition in a second pregnancy would still be relatively low. Environmental factors, such as nutrition, are known to be important in the causation of neural tube defects. Therefore, the risk of recurrence can be minimised further by attention to good nutrition and supplementation with folic acid.

(iii) Turner syndrome results from a chromosomal deletion. This occurs at the time of the formation of the germ cells in one of the parents. Chromosomal defects are usually not inherited, and so the risk of recurrence of this rare condition is very low.

(iv) The tendency to develop type 1 diabetes runs in families, although it is probability triggered by an environmental factor such as infection (see Chapter 5.1d). Therefore, like the risk of recurrence of a neural tube defect, the risk of recurrence is higher than it would be for a child in the general population, but is still relatively low.

3. A child who has been born prematurely might suffer from the following health problems:
   - an increased tendency to chest infections and asthma
   - generalised developmental delay and specific learning difficulties
   - increased risk of cerebral palsy
   - increased risk of visual impairment
   - increased risk of inguinal hernia and maldescent of the testes.

In addition to these specific health problems a child who has been born preterm is less likely to achieve the height and weight that might have been predicted for it (on the basis of the height of his parent) than an average child. He or she is more likely to suffer from behavioural difficulties than the average child.

The Barker hypothesis proposes that long-term health may well be the consequence of poor fetal health. On the basis of this it might be predicted that this 2-year-old may be more at risk than the average child of developing chronic adult diseases in later life, such as coronary heart disease and type 2 diabetes.

Chapter 5.4d Infectious disease in childhood

LEARNING POINTS

At the end of this chapter you will:
- be able to describe how infectious diseases can affect children in different ways to those in which they may affect adults
- be familiar with the range of infectious diseases that commonly cause illness in children
- be able to recognise the red flags of infectious disease in children.
- Estimated time for chapter: 120 minutes.

Introduction

Infections are the most common form of acute disease in children, both in developed countries and in the developing world. In the developing world, infections are by far the most important cause of death in young children, just as they used to be in more developed countries in the pre-antibiotic era. In developed countries, childhood mortality from infection has dropped markedly over the last 100 years in parallel with improvements in nutrition, sanitation, housing, and advances in medical care, including the introduction of antibiotic therapy and vaccination.

In the first months of life, the immune system of the newborn is immature. Moreover, the newborn has yet to encounter the thousands of antigens that will, in time, allow its immune system to build up an 'immunological memory' for many of the common infectious agents that will form part of its everyday environment.

For the first few weeks of life an infant relies on maternal antibodies as a protective barrier against infectious disease. These antibodies entered its bloodstream during the pregnancy, but by 3–4 months of age the antibody levels will have declined to an insignificant level. From just before the time of the birth, the fetus is able to produce its own antibodies. After birth, these will be produced in increasing quantities as the newborn is introduced to a wide range of foreign antigens, including those found on the structure of infectious agents. Gradually, the 'gap' left by the decline in the maternal antibodies will be filled by the infant's own antibodies. However, there is a period of a few months in the first year of life when the infant's blood carries relatively low levels of antibodies compared to an older child. It is during these few months that the infant is particularly vulnerable to succumbing to infection. Breast milk is one natural source of antibodies which can be transferred to the infant during this vulnerable time.

These facts inform the rationale for the introduction in the UK of the childhood vaccination programme, in which the first vaccinations are administered to babies at 8 weeks of age. Vaccination presents to the young baby a range of antigens derived from infectious agents. These are intended to stimulate the production of protective antibodies to replace, in part, the declining levels of maternal antibodies.

Even after the levels of circulating antibodies in the child have reached normal adult levels (which happens, for the large part, by the end of the second year of life), children still remain particularly vulnerable to succumbing to certain infections and, in some cases, to suffering from debilitating consequences of these infections. In many childhood infections the child's response to the disease is strong because it is the first time it has encountered the infectious agent. It also appears to be in the nature of the child's response to infection that a high fever often develops. It is not unusual for this fever to be accompanied by mental changes such as drowsiness or confusion. A febrile convulsion (fit) is a potentially serious complication of a childhood fever, which is recognised to affect over 3% of children at some point in childhood.

This chapter begins with a description of the more serious complications of fever in childhood, and then looks at some of the more important infectious diseases of childhood. The conditions discussed in this chapter are:

- Complications of febrile infections:
  - febrile convulsions
  - dehydration.
- Congenital infections (see under Infections in Pregnancy, Chapter 5.3d).
- Common respiratory infections of childhood:
  - common cold
  - sore throat and tonsillitis
  - sinusitis
  - acute otitis media
  - viral croup
  - acute epiglottitis
  - bronchitis
  - whooping cough
  - bronchiolitis
  - pneumonia.
- Other viral infections of childhood:
  - measles
  - mumps
  - rubella
  - herpes simplex virus infection
  - chickenpox and shingles
  - infectious mononucleosis (glandular fever)
  - cytomegalovirus infections
  - roseola infantum
  - slapped cheek syndrome
  - enterovirus infections
  - poliomyelitis
  - viral gastroenteritis
  - viral hepatitis
  - warts and molluscum contagiosum
  - HIV infection and AIDS.
- Staphylococcal and streptococcal infections:
  - impetigo
  - boils
  - scarlet fever
  - scalded skin syndrome
  - toxic shock syndrome
  - Kawasaki disease.
- Urinary tract infection in childhood:
  - cystitis and recurrent bacteriuria
  - reflux disease and pyelonephritis.
- Fungal infections and infestations of the skin (see under Fungal Infections of the Skin and Skin Infestations, Chapter 6.1c).
- The notifiable diseases.

Complications of febrile infections

Children have a tendency to develop a high fever when their immune system is dealing with infectious agents. Fits (febrile convulsions) and dehydration are serious consequences of the effect of fever on the immature nervous system, and of fluid loss, respectively. Conventional medicine recognises that prolonged fever can take its toll, leading to a state of exhaustion after the illness has passed.

Information Box 5.4d-I

Fever in children: comments from a Chinese medicine perspective

In Chinese medicine, fever corresponds to Heat. If prolonged this is believed to be very depleting for a child. Scott and Barlow (1999) suggest that Yin Deficiency, a common complication of fever in eastern children, is actually very uncommon in the west, possibly because of the frequent use of antibiotics. Instead, Qi Deficiency and Lingering Pathogenic Factor are two syndromes that may follow on from a prolonged fever, each requiring particular attention to enable the child to make a full recovery.

Febrile convulsions

The word 'febrile' comes from the Latin word for 'fever'. The term 'febrile convulsion', therefore, describes a fit that accompanies a fever. This phenomenon is most common in children between 6 months and 3 years of age, but can affect children up to the age of 6 years. It has been estimated that over 3% of children will suffer from this condition before they are 6 years old. A febrile convulsion appears to be most common in a viral infection in which there is a rapid rise in fever. The convulsion tends to occur in the phase during which the fever is rising most rapidly. In 10–20% of cases a first-degree relative has a history of either febrile convulsions or epilepsy, suggesting that there may be an inherited susceptibility.

The usual pattern of events is that the febrile child suffers a brief seizure, akin to a tonic–clonic seizure in generalised epilepsy. This usually lasts no more than 1–2 minutes. There is a risk of recurrence in the same illness, and overall about 1 in 3 children who have suffered a febrile convulsion will have at least one other in the future.

In a small percentage of cases (2–4%) the child will later be diagnosed with epilepsy, the febrile convulsion being the first manifestation of this chronic condition. This is more likely to be the case if the child has suffered a prolonged seizure, or has suffered recurrent fits. However, it is not believed that the febrile convulsion is a cause of epilepsy, but rather that in some cases the fact that a child has a convulsion is an early sign of underlying epilepsy.

Convulsions may be prevented by strict attention to reducing fever in early infections. The advice that is conventionally given to the parents of a febrile child includes tepid sponging, ensuring that clothing is loose and light, and the early use of medications such as paracetamol and ibuprofen. In the event of a convulsion the same advice applies. In all cases, even if the fit has settled down, a doctor should be called. If the convulsion is not settling down within 1–2 minutes, the airway of the child should be protected and the emergency services summoned, as a prolonged fit can lead to lasting brain damage.

After a seizure it is important for the doctor to visit to exclude a more serious underlying infection, such as meningitis, and to give the parents clear advice on controlling the child's temperature and the first-aid management of a future seizure. The child may be prescribed the tranquilliser medication diazepam in suppository form for the parents to administer in the case of a recurrent prolonged seizure.

Information Box 5.4d-II

Febrile convulsion: comments from a Chinese medicine perspective

In Chinese medicine, a febrile convulsion is the result of two Pathogenic Factors, Heat and Phlegm. Phlegm may be apparent in the form of a cough in the time leading up to the fever. Chinese medicine considers that Phlegm and Heat together can cause Wind, which rises up rebelliously to cause loss of consciousness, stiffness and physical convulsions. Scott and Barlow (1999) consider that fright or shock may also be an underlying factor, which leads to disturbance of the Shen, and thereby enables the turbid Phlegm more easily to cloud the sensory orifices.

Dehydration

A child is more prone to dehydration when unwell because of its small size. A consequence of small size is that the surface area of a child is much greater relative to its body weight than that of an adult. This means that fluid loss through the skin when sweating will be more likely to affect the body's fluid balance adversely. Moreover, a febrile child is more likely than an adult to suffer from a disturbance of consciousness. Confusion and drowsiness are common in otherwise benign fevers, and may mean that it is difficult to encourage the child to keep on drinking. Dehydration is of particular concern in babies and children who are suffering from vomiting or diarrhoea.

Dehydration may develop insidiously in a child. Its features include dry mouth and skin, infrequent urination and, in more severe cases, a sunken fontanelle in babies, and drowsiness or confusion. As these latter two features are also characteristic of fever, it may mean that the dehydration may pass unnoticed for some time. Severe dehydration in a child can affect the function of the brain and lead to the development of acute renal failure.

Prevention of dehydration requires vigilant attention to the fluid intake in a febrile or vomiting child. If fluid intake is impossible, hospital admission may be prudent so that the child can receive intravenous fluids.

Information Box 5.4d-III

Dehydration in infants: comments from a Chinese medicine perspective

In Chinese medicine, dehydration is seen to deplete Yin. If it occurs rapidly it can also injure both Yin and Yang. Treatment would be directed firstly at rehydration and then at supporting the Kidney function.

Congenital infections

The important infections in pregnancy that can lead to infection or developmental disorder of the unborn child include rubella, cytomegalovirus (CMV), chickenpox, herpes simplex, parvovirus, HIV, hepatitis B and C, syphilis, listeriosis and toxoplasmosis. These are all discussed in detail in Chapter 5.3d.

Common respiratory infections of childhood

Respiratory infections are common in children. A pre-school child in the west suffers from, on average, 6–8 respiratory infections per year, most of which are considered to be mild and self-limiting. Overall, 80% of respiratory infections in western children involve only the nose, throat, ear or sinuses. By definition, these are the upper respiratory tract infections (URTIs), and include the common cold, sore throat, tonsillitis, sinusitis and otitis media.

It is recognised conventionally that certain environmental factors may render a child more susceptible to developing a respiratory infection. Low socio-economic status is strongly linked to an increased risk of infection in children. This may be at least partly attributed to the fact that being poor exposes the child to independent risk factors for infection, which include large family size, exposure to cigarette smoke and atmospheric pollution, poor housing, damp environments and poor nutrition.

The health of the child is also an important factor that may determine susceptibility to respiratory infection. Respiratory infections are more common in premature infants, children with congenital heart or lung disease, and those with immunodeficiency.

The majority (80–90%) of the childhood respiratory infections are attributed to viruses. The five major classes of respiratory viruses are the respiratory syncytial virus (RSV), rhinoviruses, parainfluenza, influenza and adenoviruses. Within each class there are many different strains, which can cause several different patterns of illness. This means that a child who has developed immunity to one strain of RSV infection following an infection such as a cold, may still be prone to succumbing to another pattern of infection, such as croup, when exposed to another strain of RSV. For this reason, with the exception of the influenza vaccination, effective vaccinations for these viral infections have not yet been developed.

Viral infections do not respond to antibiotic treatment. In viral infections, antibiotics will only be effective if the infection has been prolonged and has permitted a bacterial infection to supervene. This would not be the norm in a healthy child. For this reason, the parents of children who have symptoms that are characteristic of a viral URTI in its early stages (short history of 1–4 days, clear discharges, sneezing, fever and aches) should, in general, be advised to withhold antibiotic treatment.

If the respiratory tract, including the larynx and below it, is affected, this is termed a 'lower respiratory tract infection' (LRTI). In general, LRTIs are more serious infections in children because the swelling induced can rapidly lead to life-threatening obstruction of the airways. These infections include croup, bacterial epiglottitis, bronchitis, bronchiolitis and pneumonia. Warning features suggesting that an infection is an LRTI include the development of a coarse barking cough and/or stridor and/or breathlessness.

Viral LRTIs may exacerbate an underlying tendency to asthma (see Chapter 5.4e). In this case, the cough and breathlessness may not be entirely due to infection, but instead to the bronchoconstriction of asthma. The diagnosis is crucial here. A child with virally triggered asthma may require treatment with bronchodilators and inhaled steroids, not with antibiotics.

> **Information Box 5.4d-IV**
>
> **Respiratory infections: comments from a Chinese medicine perspective**
>
> In Chinese medicine, the Lungs of a child are particularly fragile and may easily suffer from exposure to impure air (including cigarette smoke), stuffiness, dryness, too much heat or too much cold. An attack of Wind Cold can easily develop into a cough as the Lung Qi is Depleted, and the resulting impairment of dispersal of body fluids leads to Phlegm Accumulation.

Common cold

The common cold is the most common infection of childhood. As in adults, the symptoms involve a clear nasal discharge, sneezing, nasal blockage and, in some cases, a mild fever. A phlegmy (wet-sounding) cough is also a frequent additional symptom in children. Well over 100 strains of virus are recognised to be the cause of the common cold syndrome. This explains why a single child with apparently normal immunity may suffer from recurrent colds.

A child with a common cold should be treated only symptomatically. Paracetamol or ibuprofen are commonly prescribed for fever. Aspirin should never be given to a child under 12 years old because of the extremely low risk of inducing Reye's syndrome, a severe form of liver inflammation.

> **Information Box 5.4d-V**
>
> **The common cold: comments from a Chinese medicine perspective**
>
> In Chinese medicine, the common cold corresponds to an Invasion of Wind Cold or Wind Heat. A child with Lung Qi Deficiency or Spleen Qi Deficiency is more prone to these syndromes.

Sore throat and tonsillitis

The features of a sore throat (pharyngitis) include a reddened pharynx, discomfort in the throat area, and sometimes some of the more general features of infections such as fever, malaise and headache. In most cases the cause is viral. The most common bacterial cause is a penicillin-sensitive bacterium, the *Streptococcus*. This is more likely to be the pathogen in older children. In past decades, streptococcal infection carried a high risk of precipitating the serious postinfectious complications of rheumatic fever and acute nephritis (Bright's disease). For this reason, a 10-day course of penicillin was commonly recommended in the case of a sore throat. Nowadays, these complications are extremely rare, and doctors are advised not to prescribe antibiotics in an uncomplicated infection, not least because in most cases the infection is of viral origin. In most cases the infection is self-limiting and resolves within 3–5 days.

Tonsillitis is a condition that results from viral or bacterial invasion of the tonsils. In severe cases the tonsils become inflamed and enlarged, and may have yellowish patches on their surface. It is impossible to distinguish between viral and bacterial tonsillitis, although if the patient becomes more constitutionally unwell with headache, enlarged cervical lymph nodes and joint pains, this is more suggestive of a bacterial infection. Bacteria are the cause of tonsillitis in 15–50% of cases (depending on the age of the child), with *Streptococcus* being the most common pathogen. One common viral cause of tonsillitis is Epstein–Barr virus (EBV), the virus which may also cause glandular fever (see later in this chapter).

Doctors are more likely to prescribe antibiotics in tonsillitis than if the diagnosis were pharyngitis. This is despite the appreciated fact that these drugs will be totally ineffective in those cases (the majority) that are of viral origin. The tendency to prescribe is because tonsillitis can become a more debilitating condition. The malaise that accompanies tonsillitis can be profound in some cases, and the symptoms may persist for 5–7 days or more. Penicillin or erythromycin are the recommended antibiotics. It is not good practice to prescribe amoxicillin as there is a risk of inducing a rash if the infectious agent is EBV.

In some children, attacks of tonsillitis are recurrent. If a pattern of over four severe infections a year is emerging, particularly in an older child or teenager, the operation of tonsillectomy is considered to be a reasonable choice of treatment. Another indication for this operation is if the tonsils (and adenoids) have become so enlarged as to cause mouth breathing and disturbed sleep at night. This problem can have marked repercussions on daily life, as it may cause the child to be sleepy in the day. In some children the difficulty in breathing at night may be so severe as to put the heart under strain.

Tonsillectomy will often result in a marked reduction in throat infections, and almost always has beneficial results when the tonsils have impaired the ability to breathe with ease. In some cases the child who has suffered from recurrent episodes of tonsillitis might continue to suffer from repeated episodes of pharyngitis after the operation, but these are usually less severe than the original infections.

Most children make a rapid recovery from tonsillectomy, although there is a risk of severe bleeding from the root of the tonsils in the immediate postoperative period. For this reason the child requires an overnight stay in hospital, so that he or she can be carefully observed after the operation.

Information Box 5.4d-VI

Sore throat and tonsillitis: comments from a Chinese medicine perspective

In Chinese medicine, acute sore throat and tonsillitis are often manifestations of Wind Heat. In some cases of severe tonsillitis there are features to suggest that the Heat has progressed to the Yang Ming (Bright Yang) stage, with 'big fever, big thirst, big sweating and big pulse'. In some cases, Stomach Heat may be the underlying syndrome, in which case frontal headache may be prominent. Severe cases of tonsillitis, in which the tonsils are enlarged with yellow patches on them, indicate the development of Fire Poison.

In Chinese medicine, chronic tonsillitis may be a consequence of a lingering Pathogenic Factor that has never become dislodged from the throat since the first attack. The Pathogenic Factor obstructs the Qi and Blood flow in the throat area. This can lead to Phlegm accumulating in the tonsils, together with Stagnation and Heat. Scott and Barlow (1999) suggest that antibiotic treatment and immunisations can be an underlying cause of lingering Pathogenic Factor in the throat.

From a Chinese medicine viewpoint, the operation of tonsillectomy removes the route of expression of the imbalance of lingering Pathogenic Factor, but does not attend to the underlying imbalance. This means that the underlying imbalance might recur in a different form.

Sinusitis

Sinusitis is most usually a complication of a viral infection such as the common cold, influenza, measles or whooping cough.

Acute otitis media

'Otitis media' literally means 'inflammation of the middle ear'. In its acute form it is common, affecting up to 20% of all children under 4 years of age at least once a year. The middle ear, as is described in Chapter 6.1a, is, from an anatomical viewpoint, an extension of the respiratory tract. It is linked to the nasopharynx by means of the Eustachian tube, and is lined by mucus-secreting respiratory epithelium. In viral URTIs it is not uncommon for the respiratory epithelium of the middle ear to become affected also. Early symptoms may include ear pain and deafness, as excessive mucus discharge is unable to drain via the inflamed Eustachian tube. These symptoms are more common in young children. This is because blockage of this route of drainage from the middle ear is more likely to develop, a result of the anatomy of the small child's Eustachian tube.

When the middle ear cannot be drained of mucous secretions in the early stages of a viral infection, bacterial infection (often by the usual bacterial inhabitants of the healthy respiratory tract) can easily supervene, and the infection can become prolonged. In both bacterial and viral cases this can lead to severe pain in one or both ears, high fever and a red, bulging eardrum on examination. In small children, otitis media may present only with fever and confusion, and so the ears should always be examined in a child with an unexplained fever.

In some cases of otitis media the inflammation resolves through natural perforation of the eardrum. Perforation is surprisingly painless. Instead, it often results in a dramatic cessation of symptoms, as the pus is drained through the external auditory canal. A perforated eardrum usually heals within days of the resolution of the middle ear infection.

Before the advent of antibiotic therapy, severe complications of otitis media were common. It is very likely that the poor nutritional status of children also contributed to the susceptibility of these complications, which included chronic discharging ears (chronic otitis media), local bone infections (mastoiditis), meningitis and brain abscess. Although it is accepted that most cases of bacterial otitis media nowadays would resolve fully without the need for antibiotics, the spectre of this past association with severe complications has meant that it is usual practice to prescribe antibiotics (most commonly amoxicillin) in a case of acute otitis media. Also, antibiotics do reduce the severity and length of the symptoms.

The resolution of acute otitis media may be complicated by the persistence of a non-inflammatory mucous discharge in the middle ear cavity. This condition is known as 'chronic secretory otitis media' or 'glue ear'. This sticky fluid can impair the transmission of sound waves from the eardrum to the inner ear. The tendency to otitis media and glue ear is familial.

Information Box 5.4d-VII

Otitis media: comments from a Chinese medicine perspective

In Chinese medicine, otitis media may correspond to an External Invasion of Wind Heat or Wind Cold. Damp is sometimes an additional Pathogenic Factor. Also, in older children Heat can enter the Liver and Gallbladder Channels and then rise up to manifest as pain and Heat in the ear. In these children, constraint of Liver Qi might be a predisposing factor. Recurrent attacks of otitis media might suggest a lingering Pathogenic Factor.

Viral croup

Croup is the most common form of LRTI in children. It is almost always caused by a viral infection that leads to inflammation of the larynx, trachea and bronchi (also known as 'laryngotracheitis'). The affected child is usually aged 12–24 months, and suffers from symptoms that include fever, runny nose, a barking cough, and a harsh noise on inspiration (stridor), which indicate narrowing of the trachea. In severe cases there is marked obstruction of the trachea, and the child may demonstrate a rapid pulse and respiratory rate, cyanosis, and the appearance of a sucking in of the sternum and intercostal muscles on breathing in.

In mild cases the child with croup can be managed at home. Exposure to steam is believed to ease the obstructed breathing, and is often recommended. In more severe cases inhaled steroids may help to reduce inflammation, and oral steroids may also be given. In a severe case the child is admitted as an emergency to hospital, and occasionally it may be necessary to insert a stiff tube into the trachea (tracheal intubation) to keep the airway patent while the inflammation resolves.

The recovery from croup may be prolonged, with many children suffering from a recurrent coarse cough, particularly at night. In these cases it is considered important to exclude the diagnosis of virally induced asthma.

Information Box 5.4d-VIII

Croup: comments from a Chinese medicine perspective

In Chinese medicine, croup may be a result of one or more of the following: Lung and/or Spleen Qi Deficiency, Phlegm and lingering Pathogenic Factor.

Epiglottitis

'Epiglottitis' refers to acute inflammation of the epiglottis. In children this is almost always due to the bacterium *Haemophilus influenzae* type B. The epiglottis is a flap of cartilage-containing tissue that protects the larynx from the inhalation of food during swallowing. In epiglottitis the swelling of this tissue can threaten to block the opening of the larynx, an event that can be provoked by asking the child to stick out the tongue. The affected child sits upright, is breathless, drooling saliva, reluctant to speak or swallow, and may have a harsh inspiratory stridor (Figure 5.4d-I). A child with this clinical picture should be treated as an emergency and taken to intensive care facilities so that there is access to tracheal intubation. Intravenous antibiotics are given. With this intensive support, most children recover from this life-threatening condition within 3–5 days. The incidence of bacterial epiglottitis has fallen markedly since the introduction of the HiB (*Haemophilus influenzae* type B) immunisation.

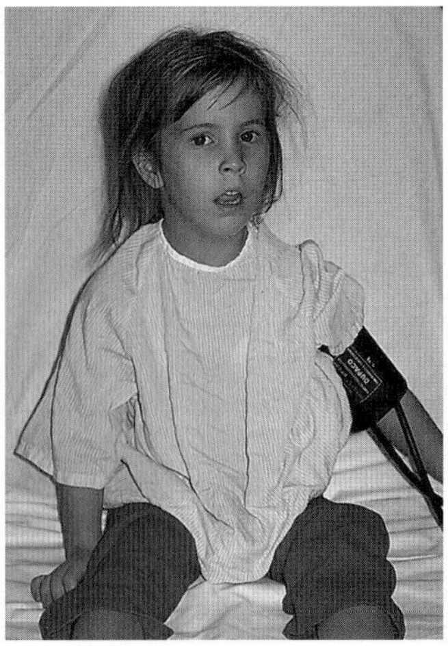

Figure 5.4d-I • Child sitting upright with acute epiglottitis.

Information Box 5.4d-IX

Epiglottitis: comments from a Chinese medicine perspective

In Chinese medicine, the rapidity of the development of epiglottitis suggests invasion of Wind Heat leading to obstruction of the Descent of Lung Qi.

Bronchitis and whooping cough (pertussis)

Bronchitis in children, unlike acute bronchitis in adults, is usually the result of a viral infection. It leads to persistent cough and fever, and does not usually respond to antibiotics.

Whooping cough is a highly infectious form of bronchitis caused by the bacterium *Bordetella pertussis*. Infections by this bacterium tend to appear in epidemics once every 3–4 years in the UK. The symptoms begin with 2–3 days of runny nose and cough, which then becomes paroxysmal (meaning involving exhausting bouts of recurrent coughing). After a paroxysm of coughing, which is usually worse and more frequent at night, a child with whooping cough characteristically will draw breath with a 'whoop'. The paroxysms may cause the child to be unable to draw breath, and may result in him or her going blue in the face. Vomiting during a paroxysm is common.

The symptoms of whooping cough can last for up to 12 weeks, during which time the child can become very drained and unwell. Complications of whooping cough include bacterial pneumonia, and long-term lung damage in the form of bronchiectasis. There is a significant risk of death from whooping cough in babies under 12 months old.

Although the infection is bacterial, antibiotic treatment does not seem to affect its course. However, antibiotics may be prescribed to prevent spread of the infection. Immunisation is strongly recommended to prevent the infection. Immunisation for whooping cough (usually given as part of the infant vaccination schedule) appears to provide protection against infection in 80–90% of those children who are immunised. Immunisation campaigns have resulted in a marked drop in the incidence of whooping cough in the community.

Bronchiolitis

Bronchiolitis is a viral infection that primarily affects babies under the age of 1 year. It is common, and affects 2–3% of babies to such a degree that they have to be admitted to hospital. The causative virus is the respiratory syncytial virus (RSV) in the majority of cases.

The symptoms begin with runny nose and cough, and then progress to breathlessness, wheeze, overinflation of the chest and a rapid pulse rate. The breathlessness is due to inflammation of the tiny airways of the lungs, the bronchioles.

A baby with severe bronchiolitis is unable to feed, and is at risk of periods of apnoea (cessation of breathing). The baby should be treated in hospital with humidified oxygen, and will be monitored for attacks of apnoea. Fluids and feeds may be given by means of a nasogastric tube.

> **Information Box 5.4d-X**
>
> **Bronchitis and pertussis (whooping cough): comments from a Chinese medicine perspective**
>
> In Chinese medicine, bronchitis corresponds to Phlegm Heat in the Lungs. The onset of pertussis is a result of an invasion of Wind Heat/Cold, which leads to impaired descent of Lung Qi. If it develops to a serious condition, it suggests that the child had a predisposition in the form of blocked Spleen Qi (Phlegm or Accumulation Disorder). The Pathogenic Heat and Phlegm can lead to rising of the Lung Qi, resulting in paroxysmal coughing, expectoration of phlegm and vomiting. Damage to the Lungs can lead to nosebleed and coughing up of blood. Phlegm Heat can obstruct the orifices of the Heart, and so cause collapse and delirium. In the long term, the condition can deplete Qi and Yin.
>
> Scott and Barlow (1999) propose that pertussis (whooping cough) may be a condition in which the child is trying to throw off a Phlegm Pathogen that has been present since the time of birth (akin to the way in which the febrile diseases of childhood are seen to allow the clearance of Heat Toxin). They suggest, with the use of alternative treatment such as acupuncture and herbs early in the infection, that a child genuinely may be strengthened through suffering from the infection. However, they do make the caveat that a child under 3 years old is at more risk from long-term damage from the copious Phlegm that is produced in the infection. They comment that many children who have recovered from whooping cough have much improved appetites as a result of clearance of Phlegm.

Many infants recover fully from the attack, although as many as 50% will suffer from recurrent episodes of cough and breathlessness in the few years following the initial episode of bronchiolitis.

> **Information Box 5.4d-XI**
>
> **Bronchiolitis: comments from a Chinese medicine perspective**
>
> In Chinese medicine, bronchiolitis corresponds to Phlegm Heat in the Lungs following on from an Invasion of Wind Heat or Wind Cold.

Pneumonia

Pneumonia results from infection reaching the air spaces of the lungs, the alveolae. In infancy, pneumonia is most commonly viral in origin, RSV being the most frequent cause. In older children, bacteria and bacteria-like organisms are the most likely pathogens. Common organisms include *Streptococcus pneumoniae*, *Haemophilus influenzae* and *Mycoplasma pneumoniae*.

The symptoms of pneumonia are similar to those experienced by an adult. Fever, cough and breathlessness, together with marked constitutional malaise are common. All these may follow on from a mild URTI. In some cases, particularly viral and *Mycoplasma* pneumonia, the symptoms may not be very severe. A child with severe symptoms of pneumonia should be nursed in hospital.

The diagnosis can be confirmed by X-ray examination of the chest. It may be difficult to obtain sputum for bacterial and viral analysis. Blood tests and fluid aspirated from the back of the nose may be required to confirm the cause of the infection.

Antibiotics are always prescribed before the results of the analysis of the infectious agent are known. Usually, a broad-spectrum antibiotic is prescribed to treat a wide range of potential organisms.

> **Information Box 5.4d-XII**
>
> **Pneumonia: comments from a Chinese medicine perspective**
>
> In Chinese medicine, pneumonia is most closely associated with the syndrome of Phlegm Heat in the Lungs. Invasion of External Wind is an important aetiological factor. However, Scott and Barlow (1999) suggest that an underlying Deficiency of Qi or Jing is also likely to have predisposed the child to such a serious condition. After recovery, lingering Pathogenic Factor, Yin Deficiency and Lung and Spleen Qi Deficiency may all persist to affect the health of the child.

Other common viral infections of childhood

There is a range of viral infections that usually manifest in a young child rather than an adult. In many of these infections the symptoms are more severe in older children or adults. With the exception of HIV infection, all the infections described below are endemic in western communities (or used to be before the advent of vaccination). Many of these infections follow a course that is characteristic of the infecting virus, and so can be diagnosed on the basis of signs and symptoms alone. In most of them the disease follows a relatively mild course, and the child recovers with lasting immunity to the infection. This is not necessarily the case if the child is weakened by a condition such as poor nutrition or congenital disease. It must not be forgotten that much of the infant mortality in some developing countries is the result of infectious disease, with 25% of premature death attributable to measles infection alone.

Measles

Measles (rubeola) is the result of infection by the measles virus. Before the widespread introduction of the measles vaccine in the 1970s, measles used to be a very common infection. However, the reported incidence of measles has dropped dramatically over the past three decades. Measles is a notifiable disease. Doctors should confirm a suspected diagnosis by means of taking saliva samples for analysis.

Measles is contracted by inhalation of infected droplets. Symptoms begin 10–14 days after exposure to an infected child. The first symptoms include inflamed eyes, cold

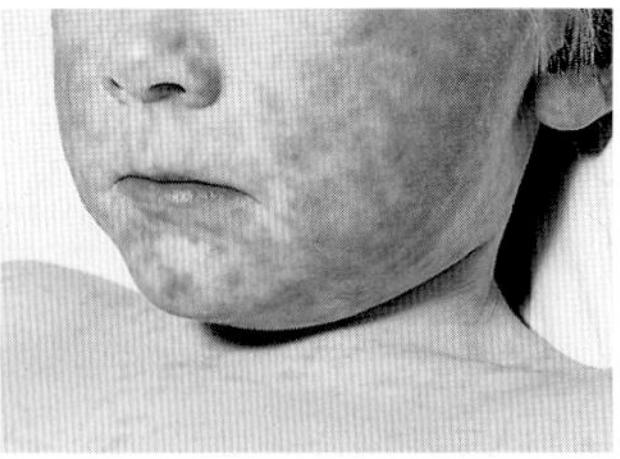

Figure 5.4d-II • Blotchy appearance of rash in measles.

symptoms, fever and a cough. The child is infectious from this stage until the cold symptoms have abated. After about 2 days, characteristic white dots, known as 'Koplik spots', appear on the inside of the cheek. It is only after 3–4 days from the onset of the cold symptoms that the measles rash appears. This blotchy, flat, non-itchy, red rash spreads downwards from behind the ears and lasts about 7 days (Figure 5.4d-II). The skin may become scaly towards the end of this time. The fever of measles peaks at around 5 days after the onset of the symptoms, and may become very high. Most children make a full recovery from measles.

Other complications of the infection have been reported to occur in 1 in 15 infections. These complications include progression to pneumonia, otitis media, febrile convulsions, diarrhoea, ulceration of the cornea of the eye and liver inflammation. All these complications are more likely in poorly nourished and chronically ill children.

In 1 in 5000 reported cases a serious inflammation of the brain, encephalitis, occurs. Over 1 in 10 children who develop measles encephalitis will die as a result. In 1 in 100,000 cases a devastating degenerative condition of the nervous system, known as 'subacute sclerosing panencephalitis' (SSPE), can develop after a delay of up to 7 years after an initial infection in a small child. SSPE is believed to be the result of delayed immune-mediated damage. It culminates in total paralysis, dementia and, eventually, death.

Conventional advice is that the child should rest in a darkened room. Vitamin A might be recommended for children who are malnourished. This is known to reduce the severity of the condition. Additional alternative advice is that the child should be allowed to rest for at least a week after the rash has subsided.

Measles vaccination is advocated conventionally because of the known risk of serious complications. These are recognised to affect preferentially those children who are seriously ill, such as those with leukaemia. There is no doubt that the incidence of serious complications has dropped since the introduction of the vaccination programme for measles.

Information Box 5.4d-XIII

Measles: comments from a Chinese medicine perspective

Scott and Barlow (1999) states that, in Chinese medicine, measles is considered to be the result of both internal and external factors. The view that measles is the result purely of release of 'Womb Toxin' is an ancient belief, dating back to the Song Dynasty (960–1279). By the Ming Dynasty (1368–1644), measles is described as a result of 'Womb Toxin combined with seasonal change', and since the Qing Dynasty (1644–1911) measles has been described as 'from Womb Toxin, change of season, warm weather and infection'.

Measles currently is viewed as a Yang toxin, which transforms into Heat and Fire deep in the Interior and which readily damages Yin and Fluids. The toxin is described as affecting a range of Yin Organs, including Lung, Spleen, Heat, Pericardium and Liver This explains the diversity of possible complications of infection. The rash is seen as a good sign, indicating that the Heat has reached the Exterior.

Mumps

Mumps also used to be a very common childhood infection, but since the introduction of vaccination it is far less common. Like measles, mumps is a viral infection spread by infected droplets. The incubation period is 2–3 weeks after exposure. The affected child then develops fever, malaise and swollen, tender parotid salivary glands. The child might complain of earache or difficulty swallowing. In most cases the symptoms subside after 3–4 days. In some children a prolonged state of tiredness and depression (lasting 6–8 weeks) can follow an attack of mumps.

In some cases the pancreas may become inflamed, and this very rarely can lead to frank acute pancreatitis. In boys, the testes may also become inflamed (orchitis). This carries a risk of the very rare complication of infertility in adulthood. In about 1 in 10 cases there are symptoms of a mild form of meningitis. As is the case in measles infection, only in 1 in 5000 cases does a more serious nervous infection, encephalitis, develop.

Information Box 5.4d-XIV

Mumps: comments from a Chinese medicine perspective

In Chinese medicine, mumps is seen as deriving in part from Womb Heat Toxin. The Pathogenic Factor is considered to be Wind Damp Heat. It is a less severe disease than measles, in that it is seen as residing in the Channels rather than the Organs. The Gallbladder Channel (Shao Yang) is affected primarily. This has an internal–external relationship with the Liver Channel, thus explaining the possibility of spread to the genitals.

Rubella

Rubella is a mild childhood disease. It is transmitted by infected droplets, and has an incubation period of 2–3 weeks. It begins with a mild fever, which is followed by the development of a fine rash that starts on the face and body and then spreads to involve the limbs. The rash is non-itchy and fades after 3–5 days. Swollen lymph nodes are common, and may be found in the suboccipital region in particular.

Complications of rubella are rare in childhood. They include persistent joint pains and encephalitis. The major concern about the infection is its effect during the first trimester of pregnancy. Widespread rubella vaccination has been followed by a significant reduction in congenital rubella syndrome (CRS).

Information Box 5.4d-XV

Rubella: comments from a Chinese medicine perspective

In Chinese medicine, rubella in the child is usually a mild condition, the manifestation of which is the result of the expulsion of Womb Heat Toxin.

Herpes simplex virus infection

The most common herpes simplex virus (HSV) infection in childhood is the cold sore. HSV can also cause more widespread infection of the mouth (gingivostomatitis), and can cause a serious complication of skin diseases in which there are broken areas of skin such as eczema (eczema herpeticum). Infection of the eye can lead to severe ulceration of the cornea. In adults, genital infection can lead to genital herpes (see Chapter 5.2d). The diagnosis of genital herpes in a child should always raise the suspicion of sexual abuse.

Very rarely, HSV can cause a very severe form of encephalitis, which has a mortality of 70%, and carries a high risk of permanent brain damage is those who recover.

There are two main types of HSV, namely HSV1 and HSV2. HSV1 is mainly transmitted through saliva, and HSV2 through a wide range of genital secretions. HSV1 is the class of HSV that is most commonly found in childhood infections. It is transmitted by close physical contact. In most children the primary infection is in the mouth. This infection may be without symptoms. In some children this primary infection can lead to the severe condition of gingivostomatitis, in which there is widespread ulceration of the lining of the mouth (Figure 5.4d-III). In a severe case the child has a high fever and is reluctant to eat or drink. In some cases hospital admission is necessary to provide intravenous fluids.

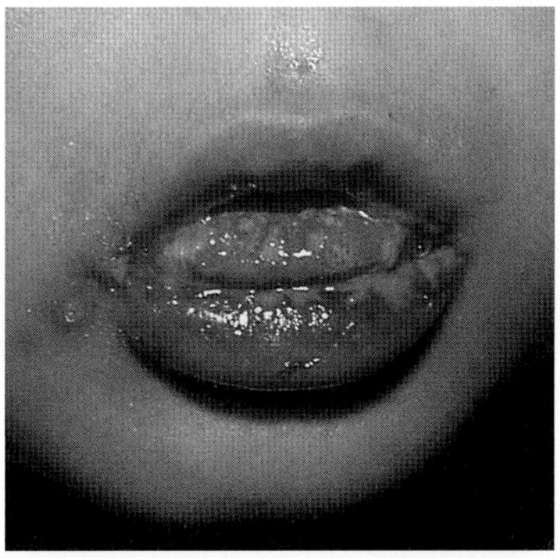

Figure 5.4d-III • Primary infection with herpes simplex virus (gingivostomatitis).

Cold sores are recurrent outbreaks of the virus that appear on the lips or the nose following a primary infection of the mouth. They are more likely to appear when the child has a fever, is run down or following exposure to intense sunlight.

In early severe cases of HSV infection the symptoms may be less severe if the patient is given the antiviral drug aciclovir. In usual practice, oral aciclovir is given only in cases of encephalitis or infections in immunocompromised children. Topical aciclovir may be prescribed for recurrent cold sores.

Information Box 5.4d-XVI

Gingivostomatitis and cold sores: comments from a Chinese medicine perspective

In Chinese medicine, gingivostomatitis corresponds to Full Heat in the Stomach and Spleen. Cold sores represent Wind Damp Heat.

Chickenpox and shingles

Chickenpox and shingles result from infection by varicella zoster virus, a virus that is related to HSV. Chickenpox is contracted by inhalation of infected droplets that originate from the mucous membranes of an infected individual, and also from the fluid-containing spots (vesicles) of the rash of chickenpox or shingles. Children are infectious up to 2 days before the onset of the rash, which usually starts on the scalp or the trunk, only later spreading to involve the limbs. In severe cases, the mucous membranes of the mouth and genitalia can be affected.

The rash is typically slightly raised (maculopapular) and consists of crops of sometimes intensely itchy, fluid-filled vesicles that enlarge, burst and then crust over. In young children severe generalised illness is unusual. However, adults can become very unwell, with fever, cough and, in severe cases, pneumonia. In both adults and children, the rash can become complicated by bacterial infection, in which case scarring due to the 'pox' is more likely. Most children recover fully from the infection, and then usually have lasting immunity to the disease.

Chickenpox encephalitis is an extremely rare complication that occurs 3–6 days after the onset of the rash.

The treatment of chickenpox is usually supportive, although in severe adult cases aciclovir may be prescribed. A vaccination does exist for chickenpox, but in the UK it is not routinely recommended in children. This is because the disease is generally so mild, and has much more severe consequences if the infection is deferred until adulthood.

The main medical concern relating to children with chickenpox is that they are infectious and may confer a risk to pregnant women with whom they have close contact. All carers of children with chickenpox should be advised of the risk of transmission of chickenpox in pregnancy, which is believed to be greatest from 2 days before the onset of the rash to 5 days after its first appearance.

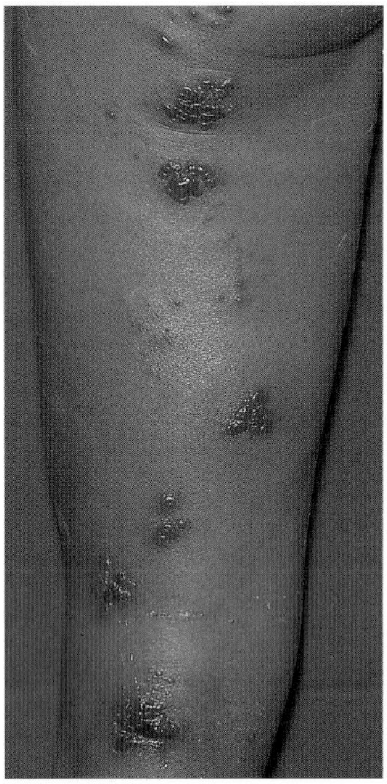

Figure 5.4d-IV • Shingles scattered on the back of the leg along the distribution of the first sacral nerve (S1) dermatome.

After infection, the varicella zoster virus can reactivate after lying dormant in the nervous system for some years. In its reactivated form, the rash of varicella zoster usually is limited to the distribution of a sensory dermatome on one side of the body. This gives rise to the localised strip of redness and crusting that is characteristic of shingles (Figure 5.4d-IV). Shingles is unusual in childhood.

Information Box 5.4d-XVII

Chickenpox and shingles: comments from a Chinese medicine perspective

In Chinese medicine, chickenpox corresponds to an invasion of Wind Heat Damp. Shingles corresponds to an invasion of the Channels by Wind Heat or Wind Damp.

Infectious mononucleosis (glandular fever)

Glandular fever is a disease that results from infection by the Epstein–Barr virus (EBV). This virus is a relation of the herpes simplex and varicella zoster viruses. The infection is contracted by droplet spread, and requires close physical contact. Most infections which are contracted through childhood and adolescence lead at most to a mild flu-like illness from which the child fully recovers. Over 90% of children will have developed antibodies to EBV by the end of their adolescence, and most of these will not have suffered from glandular fever as it is described below.

In some children the infection leads to a syndrome involving fever, malaise, tonsillitis and widespread enlargement of the lymph nodes. This is the syndrome that is diagnosed as glandular fever. In some cases the tonsils may become so enlarged as to obstruct swallowing and threaten the airway. In severe infections the liver and spleen may also enlarge and become tender. Jaundice may develop if the liver becomes significantly inflamed. In some cases there is a fine rash of reddened spots. If the child is given amoxicillin during this period (to treat suspected bacterial tonsillitis), the chances of the rash developing are greatly increased. Glandular fever is more common in older children and adolescents. It may affect a child during a time of stress, such as when taking examinations.

In severe cases the symptoms may persist for some weeks, and the child may become very tired. Glandular fever is one of the most well-recognised precursors of the prolonged syndrome currently described as chronic fatigue syndrome (CFS) (also described as myalgic encephalomyelitis (ME)). Symptoms of chronic fatigue, by definition, must have persisted for more than 6 months before the description of CFS is used.

Glandular fever is diagnosed by means of examination of a blood film, and by testing for characteristic antibodies (the Monospot test and Paul Bunnell reaction, respectively). Treatment of glandular fever is usually supportive. Rest during the symptomatic phase is recommended. Occasionally, corticosteroids may be given to reduce the inflammation of grossly enlarged tonsils. Antibiotics should only be given if a throat swab demonstrates the presence of *Streptococcus*, but amoxicillin should always be avoided.

Information Box 5.4d-XVIII

Infectious mononucleosis (glandular fever): comments from a Chinese medicine perspective

The syndrome of glandular fever as described in the text does not appear in ancient Chinese texts, suggesting that this is a condition of modern times. Scott and Barlow (1999) list three syndromes that may underlie glandular fever: Liver Qi Stagnation, lingering Pathogenic Factor and Yin Deficiency. They suggest that Stagnant Liver Qi may cause Heat and Stagnation of Fluids, and thus the formation of Phlegm in the Channels. This is the aetiology of the swollen lymph nodes and tonsils. Lingering Heat, Pathogenic Factor and Yin Deficiency may all coexist to promote the formation of Phlegm. Scott and Barlow (1999) add that, in some cases, and particularly those in which a rash is evident, the condition may also serve a function in the expulsion of Womb Heat Toxin.

Cytomegalovirus infections

Cytomegalovirus (CMV) is another close relation to the HSV, varicella zoster virus and EBV. Like EBV, CMV is a very common pathogen in children, usually leading to a very mild, flu-like illness. It is only in some cases that it can lead to a glandular-fever-like syndrome, with widespread enlargement of lymph nodes and malaise. It too can be the precursor of chronic fatigue syndrome.

CMV can cause much more serious disease in immunocompromised children and adults. As is the case in fetal infection, it can cause inflammation of a wide range of internal organs, leading to encephalitis, hepatitis, oesophagitis, colitis and inflammation of the retina. Serious CMV infection can be treated with antiviral medication.

Information Box 5.4d-XIX

Cytomegalovirus infection: comments from a Chinese medicine perspective

In Chinese medicine, the glandular-fever-like syndrome that may follow cytomegalovirus infection corresponds to the same pattern as described for glandular fever.

Roseola infantum

Roseola infantum (exanthem subitum) is a common cause of fever and rash in children caused by the human herpesvirus 6 (HHV6). The main symptom of infection is high fever lasting 2–3 days, followed in some children by a generalised red rash. Most children recover fully from the infection, although it may be the cause of febrile convulsions in some. Very rarely, the virus can cause a mild form of meningitis and encephalitis.

Information Box 5.4d-XX

Roseola infantum: comments from a Chinese medicine perspective

In Chinese medicine, the fever and rash of roseola infantum corresponds to an invasion of Wind Heat. Like rubella, it may serve a function in the expulsion of Womb Heat Toxin.

Slapped-cheek syndrome (parvovirus infection)

Slapped-cheek syndrome (erythema infectiosum) is a condition that results from infection by parvovirus B19. Infection usually leads to a very mild illness, but in some children gives rise to a syndrome involving fever, headache, muscle aches and malaise for a few days. This is followed by a characteristic facial rash during the recovery period. The rash can progress to form a lace-like reddening of the skin of the trunk and the limbs. Most children will recover fully from this infection.

Parvovirus in non-immune pregnant women is a serious infection, which can cause the death of the fetus. For this reason, children with slapped-cheek syndrome should be kept at home until they recover from the infection.

Information Box 5.4d-XXI

Slapped-cheek syndrome (parvovirus infection): comments from a Chinese medicine perspective

In Chinese medicine, the energetic interpretation of slapped cheek syndrome is similar to that of rubella and roseola infantum.

Enterovirus infections

The enteroviruses are a group of viruses that include coxsackie viruses A and B and echovirus. They are common causes of childhood infections, most of which are mild and non-specific. The viruses are spread by the faeco-oral (hand to mouth) route rather than by droplet spread. Infections are most common in the summer and autumn. This is in contrast to the viral infections described above, which are transmitted by droplet spread, and most of which peak in the winter months.

Common specific conditions that result from enterovirus infections include herpangina; hand, foot and mouth disease; and Bornholm disease.

Herpangina is a syndrome of small painful ulcers in the mouth, which may cause loss of appetite, pain on swallowing and fever. Clinically it is indistinguishable from a mild primary infection with HSV (see above).

Information Box 5.4d-XXII

Herpangina: comments from a Chinese medicine perspective

In Chinese medicine, herpangina corresponds to Heat in the Stomach and Spleen.

Hand, foot and mouth disease is not the same as foot and mouth disease. It is a mild condition in which painful, fluid-filled spots erupt on the hands, feet, mouth and tongue. It usually subsides within a few days.

Information Box 5.4d-XXIII

Hand, foot and mouth disease: comments from a Chinese medicine perspective

In Chinese medicine, hand foot and mouth disease corresponds to Heat in the Stomach and Spleen.

Bornholm disease (pleurodynia) is an inflammation of the joints between the sternum and ribs (costochondritis). The child will have a fever and complains of chest pain, which may be worse on deep inspiration (pleuritic pain). It is important to distinguish this mild condition from the more serious conditions that can also cause pleuritic pain – pericarditis and pleurisy. The child will usually recover fully within a few days.

Information Box 5.4d-XXIV

Bornholm disease: comments from a Chinese medicine perspective

In Chinese medicine, Bornholm disease may correspond to Heat and Stagnation in the Channels that have their course in the region of the pain (Kidney and Stomach usually).

Poliomyelitis

Poliomyelitis (polio) is caused by an enterovirus. The condition is very rare in developed countries, as a consequence of widespread immunisation. Poliomyelitis is discussed in Chapter 4.1g.

Viral gastroenteritis

Gastroenteritis is described in detail in Chapter 3.1c. In children, the most common cause of gastroenteritis is viral infection, rotavirus being the most common infectious agent. Viral gastroenteritis in children is highly contagious, not least because it is difficult with children to minimise close physical contact with other people, and also to maintain scrupulous hygiene.

Symptoms include vomiting, diarrhoea, abdominal pain and fever. Dehydration is the most serious concern with children, and in particular with babies. In most cases the symptoms resolve spontaneously, but in severe cases children may need to be admitted to hospital to receive intravenous fluids.

Information Box 5.4d-XXV

Gastroenteritis: comments from a Chinese medicine perspective

In Chinese medicine, the symptoms of gastroenteritis usually correspond to an Invasion of Damp or Damp Heat in the Intestines. In children, imbalances such as Stomach and Spleen Deficiency, Cold in the Stomach or Accumulation Disorder may cause the child to be susceptible to gastroenteritis.

Viral hepatitis

Viral hepatitis is discussed in detail in Chapter 3.1d. Infectious hepatitis (hepatitis A), which is now uncommon in the UK, is transmitted by the faeco-oral route. Children tend to suffer from a much more mild form of the disease, and then develop lasting immunity.

Hepatitis B is usually contracted in childhood, either from an infected mother during pregnancy and breastfeeding, or by close physical contact with an infectious family member. Although many infections contracted in childhood do not lead to inflammation of the liver, development of the carrier state puts the child at risk of chronic liver disease and liver cancer in later life. Hepatitis B infection in childhood is rare in the UK, but relatively common in countries such as Indonesia and Taiwan, in which a high proportion of the general population are carriers of the hepatitis B virus.

Hepatitis C is not as readily transmitted during pregnancy and breastfeeding as hepatitis B. In the UK, most cases of childhood hepatitis C result from receiving contaminated blood products. However, this risk has been minimised since the development of screening tests for the hepatitis viruses in blood products.

EBV infection (see under glandular fever) may also be a cause of hepatitis.

Information Box 5.4d-XXVI

Hepatitis: comments from a Chinese medicine perspective

In Chinese medicine, the symptoms of hepatitis can correspond to an Invasion of Damp Heat in the Liver, Gallbladder and Spleen.

Warts and molluscum contagiosum

Warts are due to a local infection by the human papilloma virus (HPV). Usually, bodily warts are caused by different strains of HPV to those that cause genital warts, and in particular to the strain that is implicated in the genesis of cervical cancer. Warts are common in areas such as the palms, soles and knees, where the skin is repeatedly exposed to minor trauma. A wart is a virally induced overgrowth of the cells of the epidermis.

A verruca is a wart that has developed on the pressure-bearing part of the sole. Weight bearing causes the verruca to become pressed flat into the skin of the sole. Like a stone in the shoe, the ingrowing verruca can be painful.

A wart or verruca may grow rapidly over the course of a few weeks, or may be indolent in growth, appearing slowly over a period of a few years. Warts can appear as solitary growths or in crops. They can disappear suddenly without treatment, which may be the reason for the magical qualities with which they have been attributed in folklore. This phenomenon, which can be seen to affect a whole crop of warts at the same time, is believed to be a result of an immune response which may have been triggered following minor damage to the warts.

Warts are infectious, but it is doubtful whether their removal actually reduces the transmission of the virus, as it is endemic in the community. The exception to this may be transmission in swimming pools, at which there is a general expectation that verrucae should be covered to prevent transmission of the virus.

As treatment can be inconvenient and painful, and because warts usually resolve spontaneously, it should be restricted ideally to those cases in which the wart is causing pain or has become a cosmetic problem for the child. Warts and veruccas can be treated daily by the application of salicylic acid (aspirin) paint or glutaraldehyde. They can also be damaged by a freezing spray of liquid nitrogen, but this is a painful (burning) treatment. It is likely that both these approaches work by causing sufficient damage to the wart to stimulate the natural immune response of the body.

Molluscum contagiosum is another contagious warty condition, which causes crops of pearly lumps on the skin (Figure 5.4d-V). It usually affects a very young child. The spots will usually disappear within a year. Lasting immunity is likely to follow the disappearance of the spots, as they rarely recur. Molluscum spots can also be treated by means of damage; this can be in the form of injection with phenol or the application of a spray of liquid nitrogen. However, this is not a very practical approach in the treatment of a small child with multiple molluscum spots. Most doctors recommend to leave well alone and to let the condition take its natural, albeit prolonged, course.

Information Box 5.4d-XXVII

Viral warts: comments from a Chinese medicine perspective

From a Chinese medicine viewpoint, Scott and Barlow (1999) suggest that warts will only grow in the presence of Damp. This fits with the observation that they are commonly contracted at swimming pools. The position of the warts is an indication of the location of the Damp. Warts on the hand suggest Damp in the Spleen and Lungs, and verrucae suggest Damp in the Spleen and Kidneys.

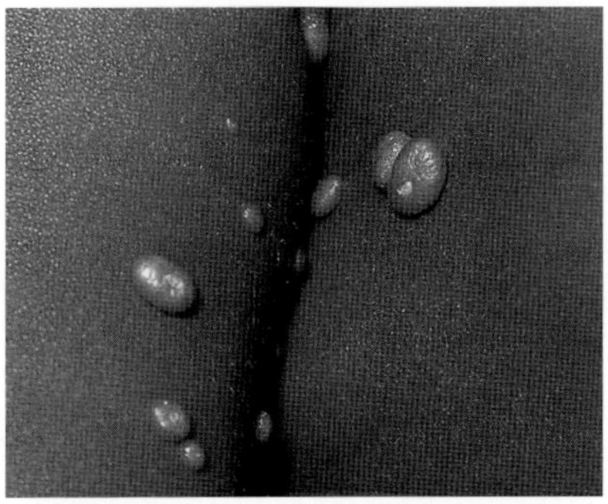

Figure 5.4d-V • Pearly papules of molluscum contagiosum on the chest and upper arm.

HIV infection and AIDS

Like hepatitis B, HIV infection in childhood is usually contracted from an infected mother, either during pregnancy or through breastfeeding. In Europe, approximately 15% of babies born to infected mothers will become infected. The infection rate has been estimated as being much higher in those developing countries in which HIV infection is endemic. In contrast to hepatitis B, transmission of HIV from an infected parent to a non-infected child is less likely to occur at a later stage.

It is now well recognised that transmission to a baby is potentially preventable if the HIV infection is diagnosed during pregnancy and the mother is first treated with antiviral medication, and then does not breastfeed the baby. HIV testing in pregnancy is now performed routinely in the UK.

Infected children may remain without symptoms for many months or years before progressing to the acquired immune deficiency syndrome (AIDS). First symptoms of AIDS include lymph-node enlargement, recurrent bacterial infections, oral thrush, diarrhoea and respiratory infections. Opportunistic infections and involvement of the nervous system are features of severe disease.

Children with HIV infection are treated in a similar way to adults with the disease. They require regular medical review, even before the development of AIDS. The management of the condition is often complicated by the fact that one or both of the parents are also HIV-positive. In established AIDS, aggressive treatment of infections is considered essential. The use of combined antiviral drugs can delay the progression of the disease, but is not curative.

Information Box 5.4d-XXVIII

HIV infection and AIDS: comments from a Chinese medicine perspective

The Chinese medicine interpretation of HIV infection, as a modern disease, cannot be drawn from the classic texts, but established AIDS has many of the features of cancer.

The initial infection has the features of an Invasion of Wind Heat Damp. The development of AIDS suggests that this Pathogen has penetrated into the Interior to damage the Organs. Immune deficiency resulting from the deterioration of the function of the white blood cells (T leukocytes) in the marrow corresponds to severe Kidney Deficiency, which is presumably a result of this initial insult. The lymph-node enlargement, infections and tumours that characterise AIDS correspond to a combination of Phlegm, Damp, Heat and Blood Stagnation, all of which may have accumulated as a consequence of the Kidney Deficiency.

Scott and Barlow (1999) admit that their experience of treating HIV infection in children is minimal. However, they report good results after treating a single child with HIV infection. Treatment principles in HIV infection would usually include clearance of Heat and Damp, and support of the Kidney Function.

Staphylococcal and Streptococcal infections

The *Streptococcus* and the *Staphylococcus* species are bacteria known as 'cocci', and are characterised by a spherical shape when viewed under the microscope. Both types of bacteria are pathogenic because they have an ability to penetrate the bodily tissues, and because they can release substances that are toxic to the tissues. They both readily induce the formation of pus, which can complicate infections, as its presence in excess may impair the full resolution of inflammation.

Nowadays, the complications of infections by the cocci are readily prevented because most strains of both types are sensitive to certain antibiotics. However, there is increasing concern that the overuse of antibiotics for both medical and agricultural reasons has promoted the development of antibiotic-resistant strains of the cocci (and, of course, other types of bacteria). Methicillin-resistant *Staphylococcus aureus* (MRSA) is an example of a strain of *Staphylococcus* that is able to multiply in the presence of all the commonly prescribed antibiotics. Infection with this strain usually would not harm a healthy individual, but can be the cause of a life-threatening and untreatable condition in someone who is immunocompromised.

Tonsillitis and pharyngitis are two consequences of infection by a strain of *Streptococcus* bacterium. Streptococcal infections may rarely be followed within 3–4 weeks by a damaging immune response to the infection. Rheumatic fever and Bright's disease are two now very rare conditions that are recognised to be post-streptococcal.

Impetigo

Impetigo is a crusting infection of the skin that may be caused by strains of *Streptococcus* or *Staphylococcus*. It is common in children, in whom close physical contact and minor injuries are features of everyday life. In many cases it presents as a small area of yellowish crusting affecting an area of cracked or damp skin (e.g. in eczema). The skin around the mouth and nostrils is a common site for impetigo. Although it can resolve without treatment, impetigo can spread to cause an enlarging area of crusting and new areas of infection on other parts of the body. It is believed to be highly contagious (Figure 5.4d-VI).

Small areas of impetigo may be treated by means of topical antibiotic creams, but a child with more extensive disease might be prescribed oral antibiotic therapy.

> **Information Box 5.4d-XXIX**
>
> **Impetigo: comments from a Chinese medicine perspective**
>
> In Chinese medicine, impetigo corresponds to Damp Heat. Accumulation Disorder is likely to underlie the development of impetigo.

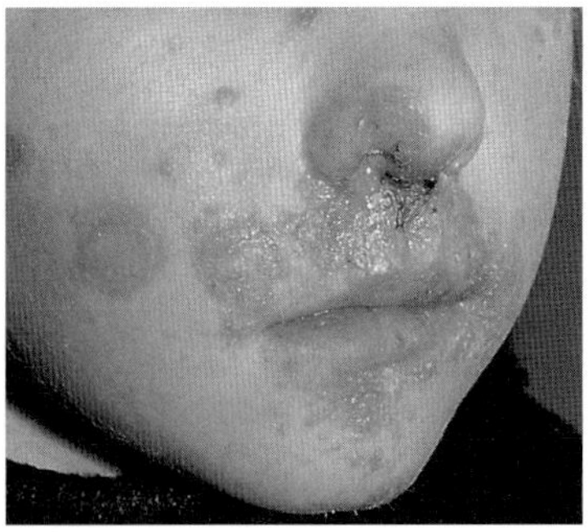

Figure 5.4d-VI • The crusting rash of impetigo.

Boils

Boils are usually the result of infection with a strain of *Staphylococcus*. It is known that this strain can be 'carried' harmlessly as part of the natural bacterial 'flora' of the skin. Recurrent boils suggest that the child is run down in some way. A diagnosis of diabetes mellitus or immune deficiency should be considered and excluded.

Boils are treated by lancing to remove the pus, and then by means of oral antibiotics.

> **Information Box 5.4d-XXX**
>
> **Boils: comments from a Chinese medicine perspective**
>
> In Chinese medicine, boils correspond to Damp Heat or Fire Poison.

Scarlet fever (scarlatina)

Scarlet fever is an unusual consequence of a streptococcal infection such as sore throat or tonsillitis. It develops 2–4 days after the initial infection, as a result of the formation of a particular toxin by the *Streptococcus*. Scarlet fever used to be a common childhood disease, and carried the risk of being complicated by rheumatic fever and glomerulonephritis (Bright's disease). However, it is far less common nowadays, and when it does develop it does not usually lead to serious complications.

The scarlet fever toxin leads to a syndrome of enlarged lymph nodes, high fever and severe malaise. Headache and vomiting are common, and so the illness may initially be suspected to be meningitis. After a day or so of these symptoms, a characteristic red rash of tiny spots appears, spreading down from the neck to involve most of the whole body, with the exception of the region around the mouth and nose, the palms and the soles. During this time the tongue develops a thick white coating, with prominent red spots on the body (strawberry tongue). Later on in the illness the white coating disappears to leave a bright red, raw appearance (raspberry tongue). After a few days, the skin starts to peel extensively. The treatment is with a 10-day course of penicillin. A patient with scarlet fever is highly contagious for up to 3 weeks after the initial infection. For this reason, children with this erstwhile dreaded disease used to be nursed in conditions of strict isolation.

Information Box 5.4d-XXXI

Scarlet fever: comments from a Chinese medicine perspective

In Chinese medicine, the symptoms of scarlet fever correspond to an acute invasion by Wind Heat. The peeled, red tongue and scaling of the skin that appear at the end of the condition suggest that the Heat has depleted Yin.

Scalded skin syndrome

Some strains of *Staphylococcus* release a toxin that causes rapid separation of the layers of the epidermis of the skin, causing the skin to appear scalded (Figure 5.4d-VII). This serious infection affects babies and infants. There is a risk of dehydration from the exposed areas of dermis. The affected child should be nursed in hospital, where it can receive intravenous antibiotics and fluids.

Information Box 5.4d-XXXII

Scalded skin syndrome : comments from a Chinese medicine perspective

In Chinese medicine, scalded skin syndrome equates to an Invasion of Wind Damp Heat.

Toxic shock syndrome

This syndrome became notorious when a number of cases resulted from the use of infected tampons in the 1970s. However, it was first described in children. It is the result of a release of a toxin from a strain of *Staphylococcus*. The primary infection may be situated anywhere in the body, including the skin. In a severe infection, the toxin causes severe systemic illness, involving fever, rash, shock and organ failure. The patient should be treated as an emergency and given intravenous antibiotics and fluids. On recovery, the skin of the palms, soles, fingers and toes can be seen to peel.

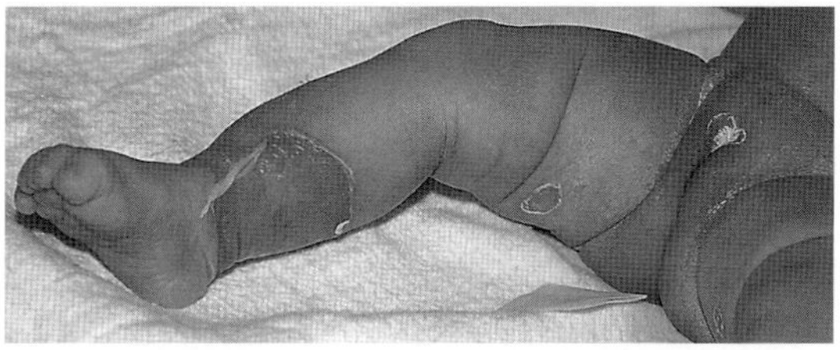

Figure 5.4d-VII • Blistering in scalded skin syndrome.

Information Box 5.4d-XXXIII

Toxic shock syndrome: comments from a Chinese medicine perspective

In Chinese medicine, toxic shock syndrome corresponds to Pathogenic Heat that has penetrated to the Interior so that it damages the Yin and the Organs. The peeling of the skin that occurs in the recovery stage is a sign of the Heat moving outwards to the Exterior.

Kawasaki disease

Kawasaki disease is a modern disease of children, first described in the 1960s. Its cause is still unclear, although it does have some similarities to toxic shock syndrome, thus suggesting that it might result from an unusual immune reaction to a bacterial toxin. Kawasaki disease is more common in children of Asian background, and it mainly affects young children between 6 months and 4 years of age.

The disease begins with fever, dry inflamed mucous membranes, conjunctivitis and enlarged lymph nodes. After a few days, a vague, blotchy rash may be seen, and then after a few further days, peeling of the skin on the hands and feet occurs, as is seen in toxic shock syndrome (Figure 5.4d-VIII). More seriously, inflammatory changes affect the large blood

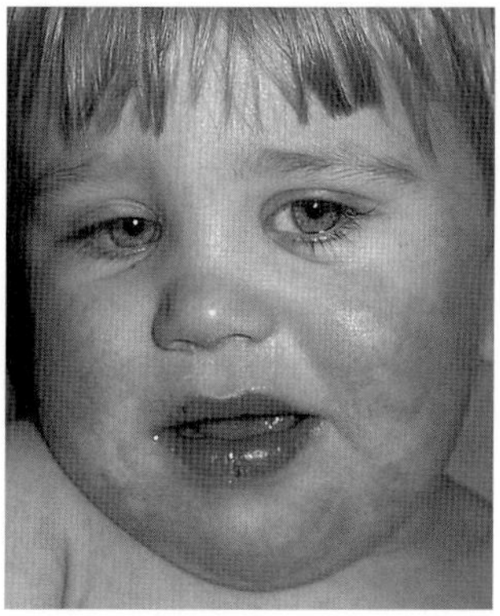

Figure 5.4d-VIII • Red cracked lips and conjunctivitis in Kawasaki disease.

vessels of the body during the course of the disease. In particular, the coronary arteries can become affected, and can develop both aneurysms and areas of narrowing. Death can then result from thrombosis and ischaemia of the cardiac muscle.

Treatment includes injections of gamma-globulin, a drug that modulates the immune response. This seems to prevent the deterioration in the structure of the coronary arteries. Aspirin is given to prevent thrombosis.

Information Box 5.4d-XXXIV

Kawasaki disease: comments from a Chinese medicine perspective

The energetic interpretation of this rare condition corresponds to that described for toxic shock syndrome.

Urinary Tract Infection in Childhood

Urinary tract infections in childhood are to be taken seriously, as they may point to a serious underlying abnormality of the urinary tract, and also can be the cause of progressive kidney disease (chronic pyelonephritis) (see Chapters 4.3c and 4.3d).

Cystitis

It is estimated that up to 3% of girls and 1% of boys have an episode of urinary infection (cystitis) before the age of 11 years. Over half of these have recurrent infections. It is important that children with urinary symptoms are referred for investigation, as up to half of these may have a structural abnormality of the urinary tract (leading to vesicoureteric reflux (VUR) disease). VUR can allow bacteria in the bladder to ascend the ureters, and damage the delicate structure of one or both of the kidneys. Cystitis is described in detail in Chapter 4.3d.

Vesicoureteric reflux disease and pyelonephritis

Vesicoureteric reflux (VUR) is a result of a relatively common congenital abnormality of the vesicoureteric junction. This abnormality tends to run in families. VUR becomes a problem in small children when the urine in the bladder is infected, as it permits passage of bacteria to the kidneys. Chronic infection of the kidneys can lead to the progressive condition of chronic pyelonephritis. Many children will grow out of the problem of VUR as their bladder enlarges with normal growth, and so early treatment in childhood can prevent long-term kidney damage. This condition is described in detail in Chapter 4.3c.

Information Box 5.4d-XXXV

Acute cystitis and vesicoureteric reflux disease: comments from a Chinese medicine perspective

In Chinese medicine, acute cystitis corresponds to Invasion of Damp Heat or Damp Cold into the Bladder. Once in the Bladder, the Pathogen usually transforms into Damp Heat.

Scott and Barlow (1999) suggest that the Pathogen may originate from the external environment, but may also originate from Damp Heat in the Liver and Damp Heat in the Stomach and Intestines.

Recurrent or chronic urinary infections (including those resulting from vesicoureteric reflux) may have one or both of Spleen and Kidney Yang Deficiency or Kidney Yin Deficiency as the underlying imbalance. Jing Deficiency would, of course, be at the root of these conditions in children with a congenital abnormality.

Notifiable Diseases

Notifiable diseases are those infections that doctors are obliged professionally to report for the purposes of nationwide disease surveillance. This requirement, which is considered to transcend any obligations on the doctor to maintain confidentiality about a diagnosis, exists because of the significant impact the notifiable diseases are believed to have on the health of the community.

Disease notifications allow the incidence of a disease and its impact to be assessed year by year. They can be very useful in the management of an outbreak of a potentially serious disease such as food poisoning. They can also help to assess the success, or otherwise, of a vaccination programme. Despite the potential limitations in terms of the accuracy and completeness of the data, it is believed that the UK has developed one of the best systems of disease surveillance worldwide.

The notifiable diseases include all those diseases that are targeted by the current childhood immunisation programme. Many of the remaining notifiable diseases are not endemic in the UK, and these include serious ‘tropical diseases’ such as malaria, typhoid fever and the viral haemorrhagic fevers.

Unlike doctors, complementary therapists are not bound by a professional code of conduct to report notifiable diseases. However, it is reasonable to propose that all healthcare workers should become aware of the features of those notifiable diseases that they are likely to encounter in their practice. If a patient is demonstrating features of a notifiable disease, the practitioner could then advise their patient to visit their doctor for a confirmation of the diagnosis (accompanied by an appropriate referral letter). In this way the diagnosis would be confirmed, and the episode reported.

Table 5.4d-I The UK notifiable diseases	
Notifiable immunisable diseases	
Measles	Viral hepatitis
Mumps	Poliomyelitis
Rubella	Encephalitis
Whooping cough	Meningitis (viral or bacterial)
Tetanus	Tuberculosis
Diphtheria	
Other notifiable diseases	
Malaria	Scarlet fever
Ophthalmia neonatorum (conjunctivitis in babies within 28 days of birth)	Dysentery and food poisoning
Leptospirosis (Weil's disease)	Cholera
Plague	Anthrax
Typhoid and paratyphoid fevers	Yellow fever
Typhus	Relapsing fever
Rabies	Viral haemorrhagic fever

It is arguable that to refer for this reason would be in the best interests of the community at large. The referral would also be a demonstration of the fact that the practitioner has respect for the values of the conventional medical profession.

Table 5.4d-I summarises the diseases that are included in the definition of notifiable diseases in the UK.

The red flags of the infectious diseases of childhood

Some children with symptoms of infectious diseases will benefit from referral to a conventional doctor for assessment and/or treatment. Red flags are those symptoms and signs that indicate that referral is to be considered. The red flags of the infectious diseases of childhood are described in Table 5.4d-II. This table forms part of the summary on red flags given in Appendix III, which also gives advice on the degree of urgency of referral for each of the red flag conditions listed.

Table 5.4d-II Red Flags 40 – childhood diseases (infectious diseases)

Red Flag	Description	Reasoning
40.1	**Maternal concern**	Any condition in which the parent is very concerned about the health of his or her child is worth referring for a second opinion. The parent is the person who will know the best if something is not right with their child, even if it is not very specific, and it is best to respect this, as small children sometimes do not generate very specific symptoms even when seriously unwell
40.2	**Inconsolable baby**: for more than 3 hours	Although this feature is very common and usually benign, consider referral if the baby is inconsolable and unexplained crying (for at least 3 hours) starts in a previously settled baby
40.4	**Any fever** in a **child less than 3 months old**	Infections in infants can become serious conditions very quickly because of their immature immune system, poor temperature control and small size. They lead easily to high fever and dehydration. The infant is at increased risk of convulsions and circulatory collapse. However, in this age group fever is common, and usually is *not* serious
40.5	**Fever >38.5°C in a child (<8 years old)** if not responding to treatment in 2 hours	High fevers can promote infantile convulsions in young children. Treatment to bring the temperature down includes keeping the environment cool, tepid sponging, acupuncture/homeopathy and, if all else fails, antipyretic medication such as paracetamol or ibuprofen suspension
40.6	**Febrile convulsion**: ongoing	Refer as an emergency if the convulsion is not settling within 2 minutes. Ensure the child is kept in a safe place in the recovery position while waiting for help to arrive
40.7	**Febrile convulsion**: recovered	Refer all cases in which the child has just suffered from a febrile convulsion (the parents need advice on how to manage future fits, and the child should be examined by a doctor)
40.8	**Dehydration in an infant (< 3 years old)**: signs include dry mouth and skin, loss of skin turgor (firmness), drowsiness, sunken fontanelle (soft spot in the region of Du24) and dry nappies	A dehydrated infant is at high risk of circulatory collapse because of their small size and immature homeostatic mechanisms. Infants who are dehydrated may lose the desire to drink, and so their condition can rapidly deteriorate

Continued

Table 5.4d-II Red Flags 40 – childhood diseases (infectious diseases)—Cont'd

Red Flag	Description	Reasoning
40.9	**Dehydration in children (>3 years old)** if severe or prolonged for more than 48 hours. Signs include: dry mouth and skin, loss of skin turgor, low blood pressure, dizziness on standing and poor urine output	Although not as unstable as an infant, a dehydrated child or adult still needs hydration to prevent damage to the kidneys. Referral should be made if the child is unable to take fluids or if the dehydration persists for more than 48 hours.
40.10	**Confusion in older children with fever**	Confusion is common and usually benign in young children (<8 years old) when a fever develops. However, it is not usual in older children, and should be referred to exclude central nervous system involvement (e.g. meningitis or brain abscess)
40.11	**Any features of a notifiable disease**[1]	All the immunisable diseases are notifiable diseases. The complementary medical practitioner should consider referral of these cases so that the GP can report the episode
40.12	**Vomiting**: refer if persistent, and either a cause of distress to the child (i.e. not possetting), a cause of dehydration or if projectile	Vomiting is common in children, and usually self-limiting. In babies, regurgitation of milk is normal and not a cause for concern if the child is contented and continuing to gain weight Refer if there are features of dehydration, or if the vomiting is projectile (a feature of pyloric stenosis in newborn babies) Food poisoning and dysentery are notifiable diseases[1]
40.13	**Diarrhoea**: if persistent, and associated with either dehydration, poor weight gain, weight loss or chronic ill health	Chronic loose stools in a child may signify the presence of an infectious organism, coeliac disease or inflammatory bowel disease Refer as a high priority if dehydration present Food poisoning and dysentery are notifiable diseases[1]
40.17	**Jaundice** (yellowish skin, yellow whites of the eyes, and maybe dark urine and pale stools)	Jaundice is always of concern in children and babies, with the exception of the mild form of jaundice that can affect the newborn. Refer all cases to ensure serious liver disease is excluded
40.18	**Any new onset of difficulty breathing** (i.e. increased respiratory rate,[21] nocturnal wheeze or noisy breathing) in a small child (<8 years old) Also if there is unexplained sudden blockage of one nostril	Always take a new onset of difficulty breathing in a child seriously and refer for medical assessment to exclude serious disease. Common causes include lower respiratory tract infections, asthma, allergic reactions, inhalation of foreign bodies and congenital heart disease A nostril may suddenly block after the unwitnessed insertion of a foreign body. This is a serious situation, as the foreign body (e.g. a pea) may then become inhaled
40.19	**Complications of tonsillitis**: severe constitutional upset not responding to treatment within 5 days	Tonsillitis is common and usually self-limiting in children. The child should be back to their usual self within 3–4 days, so refer if there is no improvement after this time period
40.20	**Complications of tonsillitis**: a single grossly enlarged infected tonsil (quinsy) in an unwell and feverish child	Quinsy is the development of an abscess in the tonsil. It carries a serious risk of obstruction of the airways and requires a same-day surgical opinion. Refer urgently if the child is experiencing any restriction in breathing (stridor may be heard; see below)
40.21	**Stridor** (harsh noisy breathing heard on both the inbreath and outbreath)	Stridor is a noise that suggests upper airways obstruction. It is a serious warning sign if it develops suddenly. It suggests possible swelling of the air passages due to laryngotracheitis, quinsy or epiglottitis. If restriction to breathing is significant the patient with stridor will be sitting very still. It is important not to ask to see the tongue, as this can affect the position of the epiglottis, and may worsen the obstruction. Exposing the patient to steam (from a kettle or running shower) can alleviate swelling while waiting for help to arrive
40.30	**Complications of acute otitis media** in a child: persistent fever/pain/confusion for more than 3–4 days after the onset of the earache (may indicate spread of the infection, e.g. mastoiditis or brain abscess)	Otitis media is an uncomfortable but self-limiting ear infection that commonly affects young children. It is now considered good practice not to prescribe antibiotics in a simple case, which will generally settle within 1–3 days, sometimes after natural perforation of the eardrum. This is a beneficial healing process. (Some sticky discharge for 1–2 days after an earache is not a cause for concern) However, persisting high fever, confusion or intense pain is not usual, and the child should be referred to exclude the rare possibility of infectious complications

Table 5.4d-II Red Flags 40 – childhood diseases (infectious diseases)—Cont'd

Red Flag	Description	Reasoning
40.32	**Persistent discharge from the ear in a child**	Chronic discharge from the ear for more than 1 week after the infection of otitis media has settled down may indicate the development of chronic otitis media, and this needs further investigation as there is a risk of permanent damage to the middle ear

[1]Notifiable diseases: notification of a number of specified infectious diseases is required of doctors as a statutory duty under the UK Public Health (Infectious Diseases) 1988 Act and the Public Health (Control of Diseases) 1988 Act. The UK Health Protection Agency (HPA) Centre for Infections collates details of each case of each disease that has been notified. This allows analyses of local and national trends. This is one example of a situation in which there is a legal requirement for a doctor to breach patient confidentiality.

Notifiable immunisable diseases	
Measles	Viral hepatitis
Mumps	Poliomyelitis
Rubella	Encephalitis
Whooping cough	Meningitis (viral or bacterial)
Tetanus	Tuberculosis
Diphtheria	Encephalitis
Other notifiable diseases	
Malaria	Scarlet fever
Ophthalmia neonatorum (conjunctivitis in babies within 28 days of birth)	Dysentery and food poisoning
Leptospirosis (Weil's disease)	Cholera
Plague	Anthrax
Typhoid and paratyphoid fevers	Yellow fever
Typhus	Relapsing fever
Rabies	Viral haemorrhagic fever

[2]Categorisation of respiratory rate in children

Age	Normal rate (breaths/min)	Rate if breathless (breaths/min)
Newborn	30–50	>60
Infant	20–40	>50
Young child	20–30	>40
Older child or adult	15–20	>30

Self-test 5.4d

Infectious disease in childhood

1. You are telephoned by a patient requesting treatment for her 3-year-old child who has had a high fever for the past day or so. The patient is concerned because the child had a strange turn about half an hour ago, during which she became very stiff, and trembled for a few seconds, but then seemed to come round. Now, as she was before the funny turn, she is alert.
   (i) What do you think is the most likely cause of the funny turn?
   (ii) Would you refer this child to a doctor?
2. A 5-year-old boy has a slight fever of 37.5°C, a sore throat, swollen glands in the neck and a runny nose. These symptoms have been present for 24 hours. The mother is asking whether or not she should take the child to the GP to get antibiotics.
   (i) What are the most likely causes of this condition?
   (ii) What would you advise the mother to do?
3. In the next 2 days the 2-year-old sister of the child in question 2 also develops a fever and a runny nose. However, she then starts to cough. This cough has been worsening over the past 24 hours, and was particularly harsh at night. She is now miserable. Her mother describes that sometimes when the child breathes in there is a harsh noise. The cough is loud and paroxysmal, and the child has retched a few times during a coughing bout.
   (i) What are the most likely causes of this condition?
   (ii) What would you advise the mother to do?
4. The mother of a 4-year-old is concerned about a cluster of lumps that has appeared under one of the child's armpits. The lumps are increasing in number, but they are painless. Occasionally, the child scratches them, and one has bled. On examination there are 10–15 circular raised pearly lumps, which vary between 1 and 3 millimetres in diameter.
   (i) What is the diagnosis?
   (ii) What should the mother do?

Continued

Self-test 5.4d—Cont'd

Answers

1. (i) It sounds like this child has suffered from a brief febrile convulsion. She has also had a fever for a day or so, although you are not told to what degree.
   (ii) The possible convulsion is a definite indication that you should recommend that this child is examined by a doctor. Also, if the fever has not responded within a few hours or so to the usual methods of bringing fever down (tepid sponging and the use of paracetamol) or to the use of alternative therapies such as homeopathy or acupuncture, this constitutes a red flag of possible repeated convulsions. In this situation, you should first ensure that the mother contacts the GP. You then could spend some time with the mother, advising her how to manage the fever and explaining the importance of maintaining a good fluid intake. You could also offer to visit to treat the child.
2. (i) This child has the features of an upper respiratory tract infection (URTI) affecting the pharynx, nose and possibly the tonsils. The fever is mild. The most likely cause of this infection is one of the hundreds of respiratory viruses, none of which would respond to antibiotic treatment. The presence of the runny nose in particular is suggestive of a viral rather than bacterial cause.
   (ii) You could explain to the mother that the child is very unlikely to benefit from a prescription of antibiotic treatment and is likely to recover naturally within the next 2–4 days. In the unusual situation of this being the result of a streptococcal infection, the long-term risks of complications are nowadays very rare, and most children will recover spontaneously. The child should be kept away from other children and allowed to rest. It is only if the fever becomes high or the child becomes generally more unwell, with headache or vomiting, that the mother should consider contacting her GP. If a rash appears over the course of the next few days, this is another indication for seeing the GP, to exclude one of the notifiable diseases such as measles, scarlet fever or rubella.
3. (i) This sounds most like a case of croup. The most likely cause of this is the same strain of virus that has affected the older brother.
   (ii) The child has a loud cough and may be now suffering from stridor. A diagnosis of early whooping cough is also a possibility. The stridor is a red flag of disease, indicating that the width of the airway is significantly narrowed. For this reason you should consider referral of this child for a conventional medical diagnosis.
4. (i) This is a description of molluscum contagiosum.
   (ii) The most usual medical advice is to do nothing about this condition, as it will spontaneously resolve in the next few months. As its name suggests, the condition is contagious, but little can be done to prevent spread to other children. You might give the mother advice about how to minimise Damp-forming foods in the child's diet and exposure to damp environments.

Chapter 5.4e Other common disorders of childhood

LEARNING POINTS

At the end of this chapter you will:
- be familiar with the common minor conditions that can affect babies and small children
- be familiar with those more important conditions of childhood that have not already been described in this book
- be able to recognise the red flags of disease in children that relate to these conditions.

Estimated time for chapter: Part I, 100 minutes; Part II, 100 minutes.

Introduction

This chapter is a summary of those common conditions of childhood that have not been described either in the earlier chapters of this stage or elsewhere in this book.

The chapter begins with a summary of the common disorders of babies and children. Although most of these conditions are not serious in terms of their impact on the long-term health of a child, they can be a source of great concern to parents. Together, they account for a significant proportion of the consultations made by parents of small children with GPs and health visitors. For many of these conditions, great benefit can result from a combination of careful explanation, reassurance and simple advice. There follows a summary of some of the more serious conditions of childhood. Note that a few of the most important childhood conditions, such as meningitis, diabetes and congenital heart disease, which are very significant in terms of their impact on children's health, are not listed here simply because they have been described in sufficient detail in other chapters.

This chapter is divided into two parts which are designed to be studied in separate study periods. The conditions discussed in this chapter are:

Part I

- Common minor problems of babies and children:
  - colic and crying
  - feeding problems
  - teething
  - toddler diarrhoea
  - constipation and soiling
  - sleep problems
  - bed-wetting
  - tantrums and disobedience
  - minor skin disorders in babies.
- Disorders of growth and puberty:
  - failure to thrive
  - short stature
  - tall stature
  - precocious puberty
  - delayed puberty

- intersex disorders.
- Disorders of the digestive system:
  - recurrent abdominal pain
  - mesenteric adenitis
  - intussusception
  - appendicitis
  - gastroenteritis
  - coeliac disease
  - inflammatory bowel disease.

Part II

- Disorders of the respiratory system:
  - asthma
  - sudden infant death syndrome.
- Disorders of the urinary system and genitalia:
  - inherited malformations of the urinary tract
  - balanitis and phimosis
  - torsion of the testis.
- Disorders of the eyes, ears and nervous system:
  - squint
  - glue ear
  - epilepsy.
- Cancer in childhood:
  - leukaemia and lymphoma
  - brain tumours
  - neuroblastoma
  - Wilms' tumour
  - bone tumours
  - retinoblastoma
  - germ cell tumours.
- Skin disorders (see Chapter 6.1c).
- Psychiatric developmental and behavioural disorders:
  - autism
  - dyslexia
  - attention deficit hyperactivity disorder
  - tics.

Part I: Common minor problems of babies and children

Colic and crying

Crying is the means by which a baby communicates its needs. Crying in a well baby may indicate hunger, physical discomfort from a wet nappy, being cold or overheated, or a need for human contact. In these cases the crying should cease when the underlying needs of the baby are met. However, all babies may cry for apparently no reason, and some do this more vigorously and more persistently than others.

An inconsolable baby can be a great source of stress to already tired parents. It is not easy for most parents, having developed a normal bond with their newborn, simply to let their baby cry, even when all obvious reasons for the crying have been excluded. The natural parental instinct is to keep on trying to find a way to settle the baby. When all attempts to provide comfort are unsuccessful, and also when this occurs frequently day after day, some parents can be driven to near breaking point. It is important for the health practitioner to be aware of the potentially serious impact that a crying baby can have on its family.

If the crying of a baby is unexplained, it is important first to check that there is no underlying illness causing the distress. This is particularly important if the crying appears as a new phenomenon in a previously settled baby. It may be wise to refer the baby for a medical opinion in this situation.

Inconsolable crying may be related to the emotional atmosphere of the baby's home. Anxiety or irritability in the parents is very easily transmitted to the baby, and may result in unsettled behaviour. However, as an inconsolable newborn can itself be a cause of anxiety and irritability in the parents, it may be difficult to untangle which problem came first.

'Infant colic' is the term given to a common condition affecting babies from 2 weeks to up to 4 months of age. It is very often diagnosed as the cause of inconsolable crying. In medical terminology, the word 'colic' literally refers to the waves of pain that result when the passageway through a tube-like organ (bowel, biliary tree or ureter) is obstructed. However, in the case of colic in young babies, there is no firm medical evidence that babies with these symptoms actually are suffering from true colic of the bowel or any other organ. The true physical cause of the symptoms is poorly understood. In some cases the symptoms may be attributed to gastro-oesophageal reflux of acid via an immature oesophageal sphincter.

The classic presentation of colic is that from a few days to weeks after birth the baby starts crying as if in pain. This pattern commonly appears particularly after feeds and towards the end of the day. The baby may draw up its knees during the bouts of crying. Sometimes, if the baby is enabled to bring up some wind, this brings temporary relief. Some breastfeeding mothers find that particular dietary constituents, such as dairy products, spicy foods or oranges, make the symptoms worse. Babies who are fed formula milk may be more settled after the type of formula has been changed, and occasionally if cows' milk formulas are excluded.

Conventional advice is that the baby should be allowed to feed in a calm environment and should be allowed to bring up wind at regular intervals during the feeds. Thickening of food, which has the aim of preventing reflux of acid into the oesophagus, can be of benefit in some cases. Dimeticone is a medication described in the British National Formulary as an 'antifoaming agent'. It is commonly used for colic, despite a lack of firm evidence that it is of true benefit. In more serious cases, a preparation such as Gaviscon Infant may be prescribed, again to mitigate the effects of acid reflux. Parents should be reassured that the symptoms rarely persist beyond 6 months of age, and usually have subsided within 3 months.

Feeding problems in babies

Ideally, according to guidance from the World Health Organization, babies should be fed entirely on breast milk at least until 6 months of age. However, over and above the cultural

Information Box 5.4e-I

Infant colic: comments from a Chinese medicine perspective

In Chinese medicine, the symptoms of colic may be ascribed to Cold. This can be either External in its origin (e.g. from foods that have a cold energetic nature or cold weather), or it may result from Deficiency of the Organs, in particular the Stomach and Spleen. Cold stagnates Qi, and this causes intense pain.

Another cause of colic is irregular feeding and overfeeding, which can then lead to Accumulation Disorder, a very common 'Full' condition of childhood. Too much food blocks the Middle Burner, obstructs the flow of Qi, and thus causes pain.

forces that might act against the continuation of breastfeeding, often potentially preventable difficulties in producing milk or discomfort in feeding can lead a mother to choose to stop breastfeeding.

Formula-milk feeding is the alternative to breastfeeding. Unmodified cows' milk is not suitable for babies under 1 year old. A cows' milk formula is based on cows' milk protein (casein), but has a more appropriate balance of salts, added nutrients and whey protein. Soya protein formulas are available for babies who demonstrate intolerance to cows' milk protein. It is not advisable for these to be used unless there is proven cows' milk intolerance, as soya itself is quite allergenic in young babies. Also, the regular use of soya formula is associated with lower levels of protective antibodies in the baby.

As formula milk is heavier in nature than breast milk, a formula-fed baby may appear more 'satisfied' after a feed, and may fall into a deeper sleep after feeding. Formula-fed babies tend to have a greater weight gain than do breastfed babies. This factor should be taken in to account when interpreting predicted weight gain for a breastfed baby from charts that demonstrate average predicted weights. It should be remembered that these averages will have been calculated from a population of babies, the bulk of whom would have been formula fed.

Current advice is that solid foods should not be introduced before the age of 4 months. The baby can then be given small amounts of pureed simple grains and vegetables, such as baby rice, carrots and cooked fruit. Added salt and sugar are not necessary, and should be avoided for as long as possible in the child's life. More lumpy foods, and also meat and eggs, can be introduced after 6 months, when the baby begins to be able to chew.

New foods should be introduced one day at a time so potential intolerances to a particular food can be isolated. Currently, it is advised that pulses are not introduced until 9 months of age, and cows' milk not until 12 months of age, because of both their indigestible and their potentially allergenic nature.

Although many parents will experience difficulties of one sort or another in feeding their babies and small children, feeding should only be considered a medical problem if the child is failing to receive the nutrition it requires for healthy growth and development. In many cases of apparent feeding difficulties it is evident that the child is well, and is gaining sufficient weight for its stage in life. In these cases the parents should be reassured that, although the child may appear to be refusing milk or fussing at the breast, it is obviously getting sufficient nutrition for its needs.

However, there are cases in which difficulties with feeding do lead to nutritional deficiency and poor weight gain. A small baby, and particularly one that is premature, is particularly vulnerable to the effects of a poor dietary intake. This is because a small baby has not had the opportunity to build up sufficient reserves of fat, proteins, minerals and vitamins to tide it over lean times.

The measurements of weight in babies and height in older children are very frequently-used indicators of healthy development. Sometimes it is when a baby or a small child is found to be consistently dropping below a previously satisfactory centile measurement for weight or height that problems with feeding are exposed.

Infant colic is one cause of problematic feeding. The unsettled baby may be reluctant to take feeds, or may start feeding with willingness, only to stop after a few minutes apparently because of pain or discomfort. This problem usually subsides by the time the baby is 3 months old.

Vomiting of part of a feed (also known as 'possetting') is a normal phenomenon and affects most babies, often towards the end of a feed. In most cases, the baby brings up a small proportion of the feed, usually together with some wind. Usually, this form of vomiting in otherwise healthy babies is effortless, and does not seem to cause them distress. Formula-fed babies may tend to vomit larger amounts of more strong-smelling milk than breastfed babies. Possetting does not lead to nutritional deficiency. If possetting is very frequent, thickening of the milk may be helpful, but in breastfed babies this will require the mother first to express the milk.

Vomiting that appears as a new phenomenon in a previously easily fed baby suggests that either an infection or an intolerance to a new food may be the underlying problem. Infection that has its focus anywhere in the body, such as otitis media or cystitis, can lead to vomiting in an infant. If the cause is not clear, and the vomiting is persisting, the baby should be referred to a doctor for investigation.

Forceful (projectile) vomiting in a small baby is a serious warning feature, and may be an indication of pyloric stenosis. Projectile vomiting can lead rapidly to an imbalance of the salts and fluids in the blood in small babies, and should be referred for medical diagnosis and treatment.

Refusal of feeds is a problem that is much more prevalent in toddlers than in smaller babies. A common pattern is that a child who previously accepted a wide range of solid foods when a baby becomes very fussy after the age of 18 months and refuses all but the smallest range of foods. This problem can persist well into the school years, and can be very trying for parents. The general approach of health practitioners is to reassure parents that most children, despite having bird-like dietary tendencies, do seem to manage to put on weight and develop well. Children tend to respond adversely to emotional issues at mealtimes, and so parents should be advised to try not to make the food refusal an issue, which can easily escalate into a three-times-a-day losing battle.

Vitamin and iron supplements may be offered if there are concerns that the child who is refusing food is not receiving the basic nutrients that it requires.

Information Box 5.4e-II

The infant digestive system: comments from a Chinese medicine perspective

A Chinese medicine view is that the 'child's Spleen is often insufficient'. The child's digestive system has to work full time to provide the nutrients required for growth and development, and so can easily become taxed by inappropriate food, lack of food, excessive food, eating at the wrong times and eating when surrounded by an unhelpful emotional atmosphere.

Accumulation Disorder (comparable to the adult syndrome of Acute Retention of Food in the Stomach) and Spleen Qi Deficiency are syndromes very commonly found in young children.

Accumulation Disorder is a Full condition, which results from stagnation of food in the child's system. It results from a combination of overfeeding, at the same time as the Spleen function is being taxed. Stagnating food leads to Heat, which manifests as irritability, insomnia, foul-smelling stools and red cheeks. Fluids can then dry up to form Phlegm, and so lead to thick nasal discharge, glue ear and a phlegmy cough.

Spleen Qi Deficiency is an Empty condition, and is a very common imbalance in western children. It can also be a consequence of long-term Accumulation Disorder, and so can present as a mixed condition. The features of Spleen Qi Deficiency include a pale complexion, and a weak, lacklustre disposition. The child might be sleepy in the day, but then does not sleep well at night (because Qi and Blood are weak). The stools may not smell bad but can be loose, or alternate with constipation. The child is prone to Phlegmy illnesses and is picky about its food.

Scott and Barlow (1999) advise that, from a Chinese medicine perspective, babies ideally should be fed breast milk and offered solids at no earlier than 2 months of age. The child should not be demand fed, but instead an interval of 2 hours should be left between feeds. The breast milk can be affected by the mother's emotions, and can cause abdominal pain if the mother is not relaxed. They state that cows' milk protein formulas are Phlegm forming in newborns. Overfeeding of any type of food can lead to diarrhoea and digestive disturbances.

The nature of the food given to the baby is very important. Wholefoods (such as wholemeal bread) might be too indigestible for a baby, even though they are considered 'healthy' foods as part of an adult diet. Cold energy foods (e.g. bananas and yoghurt) can cause particular problems in a child of a cold disposition, and hot foods (red meat and spices) can cause problems in one who tends to heat. Physically cold foods straight from the refrigerator can be particularly damaging.

Poor or picky appetite in babies or small children suggests Spleen Qi Deficiency.

Vomiting in small children might simply be a result of Retention of Food and Milk as a result of overfeeding a healthy child. If it is recurrent, it might suggest the development of Accumulation Disorder. In less healthy children who suffer from recurrent vomiting, Deficiency of the Stomach and Spleen is usually the underlying problem. The Deficiency may be complicated by Interior Cold, Phlegm or Heat.

Teething

'Teething' is the term used to describe the process of the eruption of the milk teeth in babies. The first teeth to appear are the lower incisors (cutting teeth), which erupt at the front of the mandible. These usually are 'cut' after the age of 5–6 months. By 9–10 months all eight incisors (four upper and four lower) have appeared in most babies. The four canines (tearing teeth) and the first four molars (chewing teeth) do not usually appear until after the first birthday. The second molars make their appearance after another delay, at some time between 20 and 24 months of age.

A child can become quite unsettled just before a new tooth appears. This is more common with the appearance of the molars, and in particular the second molars. Before the eruption of the tooth, the child may be irritable, and even may have a slight fever. A common sign is reddening of the cheek on the affected side of the mouth. Also, during teething the stools may become loose, and nappy rash can develop. All these symptoms indicate that teething can lead to a temporary generalised constitutional upset in the child.

The teething child may obtain some comfort from chewing on a hard toy or food, such as a rusk. Some parents find that anaesthetic gels or oil of cloves rubbed onto the gums can be of help, although rubbing of the gum alone may in itself be therapeutic. An infant preparation of paracetamol is commonly used to ease the distress of teething. The homeopathic remedy Chamomilla may also be of benefit.

Information Box 5.4e-III

Teething: comments from a Chinese medicine perspective

Interestingly, teething is not a recognised pattern in Chinese medicine. Scott and Barlow (1999) suggest that, although this may be the result of a racial difference in susceptibility, cultural and dietary factors could be just as important in explaining the fact that Chinese babies do not seem to suffer from this common western problem. He suggests that teething is primarily a digestive problem, which develops only if Accumulation Disorder is already present.

The eruption of teeth is dependent on Kidney Qi. However, as teeth push through the gums, they influence the flow of Qi through the Stomach and Intestines. This can cause stagnation of Qi in these Channels, and can cause the manifestation of the Full symptoms of a previously mild case of Accumulation Disorder. For this reason, it would make sense to advise the parents to lighten the baby's diet when teething, to offer only simple foods, and especially to avoid meat and high-protein foods.

Toddler diarrhoea

Toddler diarrhoea is the most common cause of persistent loose stools in young children. As its name suggests, it is a functional condition that primarily affects otherwise well children. The stools vary between being soft but formed, and explosive and loose. Undigested food may be seen in the stools (peas and carrots syndrome), suggesting that the food has made a very rapid transit through the gastrointestinal tract.

From a medical viewpoint, toddler diarrhoea is usually not serious. As long as food intolerances (e.g. coeliac disease), other causes of malabsorption (e.g. cystic fibrosis) and chronic infection (e.g. *Giardia*) have been excluded by means of stool tests, the parents will be reassured that their child should grow out of this condition.

In older children, the passage of loose stools and slight faecal incontinence may be a manifestation of overflow diarrhoea, a problem that paradoxically results from constipation. It is very important in these cases that the correct diagnosis is made (see below).

> **Information Box 5.4e-IV**
>
> **Chronic diarrhoea: comments from a Chinese medicine perspective**
>
> In Chinese medicine, chronic diarrhoea in a small child suggests that either Accumulation Disorder or Deficiency of Spleen Qi is an underlying problem. The precise diagnosis depends on the symptom pattern in the child.

Constipation and soiling

Difficulty passing stools is a common problem in young children. In some children, the passage of a hard stool after a period of straining can lead to pain, and even a shallow anal tear. This is more likely to occur after a short period of illness during which the child has taken in much less food or drink than usual, so causing the stools to become dry. Pain during the passage of a stool can in some cases lead to a vicious cycle, as fear inhibits the passing of later stools. Negative emotions associated with defecation, perhaps a result of forceful potty training, can also cause this vicious cycle to be set up.

In most children, a change in diet, increased fluids and sometimes a dose of a mild laxative can relieve the problem. In more serious cases the rectum can become impacted with hard stool. Involuntary soiling of stool may then occur, as liquid faeces seep past this solid mass and leak out. This can generate a social problem for the child, who is usually of pre-school or early school age, as he or she then becomes vulnerable to embarrassment and teasing.

It is important in a case of constipation to exclude medical causes, such as hypothyroidism and a rare congenital abnormality of the bowel called Hirschprung disease. In this condition the autonomic nerve supply to the bowel is not sufficient. For this reason, children with constipation and overflow diarrhoea may be referred to a paediatrician for correct diagnosis and management.

In cases in which impacted faeces have accumulated, it is important to manage the child with care. Ordinary laxatives may only serve to worsen the problem of overflow diarrhoea. The child is first treated for a fortnight with stool-softening laxatives (lactulose or docusate), and only then is given a large dose of a stimulant laxative over the course of the next few days. This regimen should induce expulsion of the impacted stools in liquid form. Some children may require brief hospital admission so that an enema can be given to aid bowel emptying.

However, the treatment is not complete at this stage. The child often then needs to relearn the habit of regular bowel emptying, as the normal bowel-emptying reflexes are commonly disrupted during the period of impaction. This can be a laborious process, often requiring prolonged treatment with reducing doses of laxatives and a reward system (such as a 'star chart') to encourage daily bowel opening.

Soiling of the underpants or bed with faeces (encopresis) is most commonly an involuntary result of stool impaction. However, it can occur in children are not constipated and who were previously continent. In these cases the problem is often one of emotional distress. For those children who soil despite having an empty rectum, psychiatric advice may be sought.

> **Information Box 5.4e-V**
>
> **Constipation: comments from a Chinese medicine perspective**
>
> In Chinese medicine, constipation may be a manifestation of Accumulation Disorder or Spleen Qi Deficiency. As is the case for diarrhoea, the precise diagnosis depends on the symptom pattern in the child.

Sleep problems

A healthy newborn baby will wake between 2 and 4 times a night to be fed and changed. Usually one of these feeds is before midnight, and the others spread between midnight and 5.30 a.m. Each feed, together with a nappy change, may require 20–60 minutes until the baby is settled again, and this is even if the child does not start crying for some inexplicable reason. It is no wonder that parents of newborns can become exhausted so rapidly.

Many babies lose this pattern of regular nocturnal waking after a short time, some 'sleeping through the night' from as early as 2 months of age. However, others continue to wake and demand food or comfort for over a year, with some persisting well into the pre-school years. This means that some parents, and particularly those who go on to have more children, may continue to have recurrent broken nights for a period of few years. The impact on the health and the emotional state of the parents, not to mention the child, can be significant.

Getting the baby to fall asleep can also become a big problem. Most young babies initially will require to be held and comforted while they drop off to sleep in the early evening. This is normal. Many will later settle down very quickly after being put down in the cot following a bedtime routine. However, others loudly continue to demand the presence of a parent if left in the cot. The parent's choice is either to stay with the child to keep the peace, or to let the child cry itself to sleep. The latter is an option which is not the most natural one for many modern parents. The problem is that staying with the child until it falls asleep can become an ingrained habit. Bedtime can thus become a gruelling marathon, involving reading stories, getting drinks, stroking a small head for half an hour, and then creeping out of a darkened room only to be called back in within minutes by agonised cries from the 'abandoned' child.

Most doctors and health visitors will advise behavioural methods described as 'sleep training' to help with the problems of getting off to sleep and nocturnal waking. The basic principle behind sleep training is that the child is educated in a gradual way that crying at night will not generate the rewards of unlimited comfort that it previously did.

The advice given to the parents of a child who cannot fall asleep on its own is that, after a brief but consistent bedtime routine (e.g. pyjamas on, teeth brushed, one story, cuddle), the parent says a clear goodnight and leaves the child. The child is allowed to cry for a short time (say 2 minutes), and then the parent returns to reassure the child that they are still there, but that they are going to leave them to sleep again. Then the child is allowed to cry for a little longer (say 5 minutes) before the parent returns. This process of returning for reassurance after increasingly longer intervals is repeated until the child falls asleep. The first few nights of sleep training may be gruelling, but a surprisingly high percentage of babies and children respond very rapidly (within days) to this approach, so that within 1–2 weeks they no longer cry when left at bedtime. A similar approach is used for nocturnal waking. The parent appears to give reassurance, but neither stays with the child nor offers a sweet drink or food. After leaving with a clear goodnight they should only reappear after allowing increasing time intervals for crying.

These simple techniques are pleasing in theory, but actually require strong willpower on the part of the parents in practice, particularly in the early hours of the morning. Some doctors might prescribe the child sedatives to give the parents a couple of nights of respite before they tackle sleep training.

Some children wake at night having suffered from nightmares. If this is the case, sleep training is not appropriate. The child will require comforting. As long as the nightmares are not occurring more than once a week, most doctors would be reassuring about their occurrence.

Night terrors can be a disturbing experience for parents of children aged 3–6 years. In a night terror, the child appears to wake suddenly in a disorientated or terror-struck state, but actually does not respond to being comforted. The child might push the parents away or seem to look right through them. He or she often then will fall back off to sleep after a few minutes. In some cases the child may actually get out of bed and sleep walk. In the morning the child has no recollection of the episode. Night terrors tend to recur at the same time in the night. They can indicate, in some cases, that the child has been shocked or unsettled in some way in their day-to-day life.

Information Box 5.4e-VI

Difficulty in sleeping in children: comments from a Chinese medicine perspective

In Chinese medicine, digestive disturbance is common in children who have difficulty sleeping. Spleen and Heart Deficiency may underlie a pattern of Qi and Blood Deficiency in a child who is not sleeping well. These children will wake frequently in the night. Cold foods, in particular, can lead to a Cold Spleen and a colicky pain, which can cause the child to wake at night in a disturbed state. Also, Heat in excess can cause restless sleep and early waking.

Excessive overstimulation by computer games, TV or strong parental emotions and unexpressed fright can be held in a child's body, and then can lead to disturbed sleep. In these cases the child can wake with nightmares or night terrors.

Bed-wetting (enuresis)

Children usually become dry by day a little earlier than they become dry by night. Most children learn to use the potty by day at some point during their third year of life. Girls often become potty trained a little earlier than boys.

However, most children will not be dry by night until at least some point during their fourth year. For a few months after a child has learned to be dry by night, still the occasional wet bed is to be expected, particularly if the child's daily routine has been disrupted or if it is under stress in some way. Occasional bed-wetting continues to affect a few children as they enter their school years. It is estimated that 15% of 5-year-olds, 7% of 7-year-olds and 1% of young adults still wet the bed on occasion. A pre-school child is usually unconcerned about bed-wetting, but as a child enters the school years the problem can become an increasingly potent source of shame and embarrassment.

An established pattern of bed-wetting (enuresis) is more common in boys and first borns. It also seems to run strongly in families. It is very rare for there to be any underlying physical abnormality, such as spina bifida occulta or recurrent urinary infections, which might account for the problem, but these causes need to be considered. However, coexistent constipation is a more common treatable cause, and if this is a problem it needs to be addressed by dietary change, increasing fluids and possibly prescription of gentle laxatives. Also, it is not unusual to find that the child who continues to wet the bed is suffering from emotional distress of one form or another, and this possibility needs to be explored and addressed.

Parents may try a range of simple treatments for the problem, most of which are not considered in current medical practice to be very effective. Fluid restriction can help in those cases in which the child was drinking excessively before bedtime, but this is not the case for most bed-wetters. Lifting the sleeping child to the potty in the night prevents the consequences of bed-wetting on the bedding, but does not treat the problem. Bribes and punishment of the child do not work.

Other treatments need not be offered before the child has reached 5 years of age, as the majority of bed-wetters will stop spontaneously before their fifth birthday. For older children, a simple reward system such as a star chart (praise and a star given in the morning after every dry night) can be a very effective behavioural technique. Over 50% of bed-wetting children will become dry by using this method alone. In children over the age of 7 years, a bed-wetting alarm is considered to be the most effective method. A moisture-sensitive pad is placed under the child's bedding. This sounds a bell when the child begins to urinate in the bed. Although a positive response may take up to 8 weeks, most children are deterred from the habit of bed-wetting by this apparatus. The alarm is kept in use until there has been at least 1 month of dry nights, and then is removed. Success is more likely if there are no underlying psychological triggers for the problem. If the child relapses from this treatment more than twice (as occurs in 20–40% of cases), the child may be referred to a psychologist so that any underlying emotional factors can be explored more carefully.

Drugs are available to prevent bed-wetting, but these suppress rather than cure the problem. They should be restricted to those occasions, such as overnight visits, when the bed-wetting might become problematic socially. The drugs that are currently used include a low dose of the antidepressant imipramine, and a synthetic form of antidiuretic hormone (ADH), known as desmopressin. Desmopressin is administered via nasal spray.

> **Information Box 5.4e-VII**
>
> **Enuresis (bed-wetting): comments from a Chinese medicine perspective**
>
> In Chinese medicine, there are four main patterns associated with enuresis. These are Kidney Qi Deficiency ('weakness in the lower gate'), Spleen and Lung Qi Deficiency, Damp Heat in the Liver Channel, and Lingering Pathogenic Factor. In the last three of these patterns there will also always be some underlying Kidney Deficiency.

Tantrums and disobedience

A tantrum is an expression of fury, which becomes more prevalent from the age of 2 years. It is believed that by the age of 2 years the child begins to want to exert its independence, but at the same time has to be very much under the control of its parents. This paradox is the cause of the frustration, and the mounting extreme anger that is experienced can induce great fear in the child.

Typically, a child who is having a tantrum is consumed by the rage, and enters a state of screaming, hitting out and kicking, which can persist for some minutes. When in the state of a tantrum, it can be very difficult for the child to be calmed down. It sometimes seems as if any approach to the child simply exacerbates the anger. Some children can scream so much in a tantrum that they may actually vomit or go blue in the face. Some hold their breath until they almost lose consciousness. Although these behaviours can be disturbing for the parents to witness, they are very rarely a cause of physical harm to the child.

Some children resort to this route of expression of their anger more readily than others. Many parents find the third year of their child's life an exhausting time, as they struggle with the management of a child who might explode into uncontrollable anger whenever thwarted. This is why this period has been termed the 'terrible twos', although some children may continue to have tantrums well past their third birthday. In contrast, some children never really experience explosions of anger that are not readily soothed by appropriate parental responses.

Current advice is that a child having a tantrum cannot be reasoned with. Rewards or appeasements offered during a tantrum may simply reinforce the behaviour. Parents may be advised either calmly to walk away from the child (as long as it is safe) to let the tantrum burn out, or to take the child to a particular room or corner where it is left to have 'time out'. Neither of these techniques is very practical if the tantrum begins by the checkout queue at the supermarket, but can be helpful in reducing the occurrence of tantrums if practised with calmness in the home.

A child who is wilfully disobedient can be a source of extreme frustration to the parents. The temptation to hit a child who is ignoring all other forms of control can be very strong. Smacking is no longer advocated as a valid method of control of a disobedient child. Although it can be effective in the short term, it is now believed that it can reinforce in the child the idea that violence is the way by which things can be achieved.

Current advice for dealing with disobedience centres around some basic principles. First, the parent should not display or react with emotion that is out of control (e.g. extreme anger), and second, the parent should be consistent with regard to any rules that may have been set. If a rule (such as 'You do not throw food') is broken, the child is treated in the same way every time this occurs.

In the case of food throwing, the response might be a reprimand and removal of the plate of food. If there is a repeat performance, the next step might be to remove the child and calmly place him or her in the bedroom for 5 minutes of 'time out'. If this occurs every time, most children will learn that it is not worth their while breaking the rule. However, if a few episodes of the behaviour are overlooked (and this usually occurs because of parental exhaustion), this inconsistency can strongly erode the potential effectiveness of the method.

In summary, with difficult behavioural patterns in children, the basic principles are the same; make rules, stick to them, keep calm and cool, do not give in (i.e. be consistent once the rules have been established) and take the child to a separate place to have 'time out' if necessary.

> **Information Box 5.4e-VIII**
>
> **Tantrums: comments from a Chinese medicine perspective**
>
> From a Chinese medicine viewpoint, excessive tantrums are not considered to be a healthy expression of anger. Perhaps surprisingly, the underlying patterns that Scott and Barlow (1999) describe do not relate to Stagnation of Liver Qi, which they believe is not usual in small children. Instead, they attribute the extreme physical manifestations of anger in children to patterns of underlying Heat, Phlegm Heat and Hyperactive Spleen Qi Deficiency.

Minor skin disorders in babies and small children

There are a number of common skin complaints of young children that are not related to infection and which tend to resolve as the child gets older. These include neonatal urticaria, milia, cradle cap and nappy (diaper) rash.

Neonatal urticaria is a painless rash that can appear in newborns within a few days of delivery. The spots are tiny white pimples (papules) surrounded by a reddened halo, and come and go from different sites, particularly on the trunk. This rash usually resolves after a few days.

Milia are tiny painless pimples that appear on the face of a newborn and can persist for some weeks. The name comes from the Latin word for 'millet seed', and this very much describes their appearance. Milia also resolve spontaneously without any need for treatment.

Many small babies will develop transient blotchy red patches, particularly on their face, which can come and go with surprising rapidity. In some cases their occurrence may be related to feeding. The cause is poorly understood. Most children will grow out of this skin reaction as they reach toddler age. In some children these blotches can be a precursor of the development of eczema (see later in this chapter).

'Cradle cap' is the popular name for a condition medically described as 'seborrhoeic dermatitis'. This first appears on the scalp of babies at about 8 weeks of age, when it appears as a non-irritating scaling of the scalp. In mild cases moisturising creams can be sufficient to treat the scaling. In more severe cases the scales heap on top of each other to form the waxy thickened layer described as the cradle cap.

In some babies, the rash can spread to the skin behind the ears and to the skin creases of the limbs. This may appear like eczema, but the rash of seborrhoeic dermatitis is not itchy. However, it can be very unsightly. Although this problem will always resolve within a few months, most parents will want treatment for cradle cap. If moisturising creams are insufficient, olive oil can help to dissolve the waxy coat of the cradle cap, and the scales can then be removed by gentle friction. Some doctors will prescribe a corticosteroid cream or a mixture of topical sulphur and salicylic acid, both of which are effective treatments.

Information Box 5.4e-IX

Minor skin disorders in children: comments from a Chinese medicine perspective

From a Chinese medicine viewpoint, the fact that the mild skin complaints resolve spontaneously suggests that many of them are manifestations of Pathogenic Factors, such as Heat and Damp, which are being cleared. Some of these factors may have been present from before the time of birth (e.g. Womb Heat), and in other cases they may result from inappropriate dietary constituents. This implies that their presence should be welcomed and, particularly as the child is not distressed by them, they should not be treated with topical suppressive creams unless absolutely necessary.

Nappy (diaper) rash affects most babies at some point in the first year of life, but some are afflicted more seriously and persistently than others. This problem has been less prevalent since the introduction of disposable nappies. The most common cause of the rash is irritation of the skin which is in prolonged contact with urine and/or faeces. The rash usually affects the buttocks, perineum and the top of the thighs, and often is absent from the skin creases. In severe cases the skin can appear scalded and ulcerated. Most children tend to stop succumbing to nappy rash after the first year of life, presumably because the skin matures and becomes less sensitive to the effect of external chemicals, including those found in urine.

The severity of the problem can be reduced by the regular use of barrier creams and frequent changing of nappies. If it is possible to leave the child without a nappy, this can also help allow the rash to heal. In very severe cases the doctor might prescribe a short course of a topical corticosteroid cream.

Candida infection (thrush) can complicate severe nappy rash. In this case, the rash may appear more brick red, and often spreads to involve the skin creases. The treatment for *Candida* infection is a topical antifungal cream such as clotrimazole.

Information Box 5.4e-X

Nappy rash: comments from a Chinese medicine perspective

In Chinese medicine, the symptoms of nappy rash correspond to Heat, or Damp Heat. External Pathogenic Factors originating from the diet or the climate are often the cause. As is the case with teething, during which nappy rash can develop more often, Accumulation Disorder may underlie the problem.

Part I: Disorders of growth and puberty

Failure to thrive

'Failure to thrive' (FTT) is a term used to describe a case in which the child is consistently failing to achieve the expected developmental milestones for weight and growth. In addition, the child who is failing to thrive will not appear to be in full health, although any features of illness may be non-specific. Typical non-specific features include an irritable disposition, a poor appetite and loose stools. The plotting of serial measurements of weight and height is crucial in the diagnosis of FTT. FTT is a very common reason for referral to a paediatrician. In all cases the treatment should be directed at treating the underlying cause, whether it be organic (physical) or non-organic (psychosocial).

There is a wide range of physical (organic) causes of FTT. These include those disorders that prevent the child from obtaining the nutrients it requires for normal growth, such as feeding problems, diarrhoea and vomiting, malabsorption and food intolerances. Chronic illness can also be a cause of FTT, even if the diet is adequate and the digestive processes of the child are normal. Conditions such as severe eczema, asthma, cystic fibrosis, congenital heart disease, chronic renal failure, hypothyroidism and childhood cancer may all result in poor growth and development in a child.

'Non-organic FTT' is one term used to describe the poor growth and development that occurs in a child exposed to psychosocial deprivation. This might be the result of, for example, maternal psychiatric illness, parental learning difficulties or chronic child abuse. 'Psychosocial dwarfism' is one term that has been coined by doctors to describe the poor growth apparent in non-organic FTT.

Information Box 5.4e-XI

Failure to thrive: comments from a Chinese medicine perspective

In Chinese medicine, failure to gain weight and to grow can reflect a Deficiency in Kidney Qi and, more particularly, the Essence. This would be the case for some of the children who have chronic illness and also in congenital disease.

A lingering Pathogenic Factor (which can cause a condition such as chronic cough) can also impair the production of Qi, and so also may be the cause of failure to thrive in chronic illness.

A previously healthy child may fail to thrive if it is unable to produce the Qi it requires from its environment. This would be the case if the diet is poor or if the child is emotionally deprived in some way. In both cases the Spleen Qi in particular will be weak, and the child can benefit from Tonification of Qi.

Short stature

Short stature is usually defined as height below the 2nd or 3rd centile. However, because of the vagaries of defining normality (as discussed in Chapter 5.4b), most of the children so labelled will actually have no other health problems. They are short simply because that is the height that has been determined by their genetic constitution. However, in a small proportion of short children an underlying physical or emotional problem may be found as a cause of poor growth. Failure to thrive (FTT) is an all-embracing term for the various pathological conditions that can result in short stature. FTT usually manifests with additional features of ill-health (see above).

Chromosomal disorders such as Down syndrome or Turner syndrome are often associated with short stature. As the child is often otherwise well, the failure to grow to a height that is within the normal range would not be classified as FTT.

There are endocrine causes of short stature in which the child may otherwise be in good health. This is in contrast to the child who is failing to thrive. Growth-hormone (GH) deficiency is the most important of these disorders. This can occur with no other apparent physical problem. It may result from pituitary damage (e.g. from birth trauma or a brain tumour). Diagnosis is problematic, as GH deficiency is notoriously difficult to distinguish from constitutional growth delay (a 'normal' cause of short stature). Even if the underlying cause cannot be established for certain, the affected child can respond well to regular injections of genetically engineered growth hormone. Before 1985, GH was extracted from human pituitaries at post-mortem examinations. The use of nervous tissue from cadavers is now known to increase the transmission of prion diseases, including Creutzfeldt–Jakob disease. The use of cadaveric GH before 1985 unfortunately did result in a few cases of this fatal condition.

Information Box 5.4e-XII

Short stature: comments from a Chinese medicine perspective

In Chinese medicine, short stature, if not associated with any other form of ill-health, is not in itself a sign of energetic imbalance. Any underlying physical cause, such as a chromosomal disorder or growth hormone deficiency, would point to a relative Deficiency in Kidney Essence.

Tall stature

Tall stature is less commonly considered to be a medical problem, as in western cultures it is socially more acceptable to be relatively tall. In most cases of tall stature the underlying cause is the genetic constitution of the child. It is only in rare cases that a physical abnormality is the cause. The most notorious cause of tall stature is the very rare endocrine condition of gigantism, in which there is excess growth hormone secretion as a result of a pituitary tumour. In this case the affected child can, by adulthood, reach a height of over 2.10 metres (7 feet). Other causes include hyperthyroidism and Klinefelter syndrome.

Precocious puberty

Precocious puberty is defined as the premature development of secondary sexual characteristics before the age of 8 years in females and 9 years in males. It is most common in females. As in most cases of short stature, the most common cause in females is familial tendency, and the condition is therefore not associated with any other form of ill-health. However, as puberty heralds the final stages of bone growth and the ossification of the epiphyses, a child with precocious puberty may only attain a relatively short stature by adulthood. In boys, the most common cause is a pituitary-hormone-secreting brain tumour. This serious problem can also affect girls. There are also rare congenital conditions that can lead to precocious puberty in both sexes.

A child with precocious puberty should be investigated for the rare possibility of a physical cause, which then should be the focus of treatment. Drugs to suppress the effect of the sex hormones may be used to reduce the speed of skeletal maturation. The child may need specialised psychological support to enable him or her to adjust to the potentially stigmatising changes that are occurring to their body.

Information Box 5.4e-XIII

Premature puberty : comments from a Chinese medicine perspective

In Chinese medicine, although premature puberty manifests in early development of sexual characteristics, the end result is short stature because of premature bone maturation (even in familial cases). The underdevelopment of the bones as a result of the premature puberty suggests that in such cases there is Deficiency of Kidney Essence.

Delayed puberty

Delayed puberty is defined as the absence of pubertal development by the age of 14 years in females and 15 years in males. Delayed puberty is more common in boys, and is usually a result of a familial tendency, rather than any underlying physical cause. An affected child will have delayed growth relative to his or her peers, and may be the focus of teasing, but is likely to 'catch up' in height once he or she enters puberty, albeit at a late stage.

Other underlying causes that can affect both boys and girls include chronic physical disease and emotional deprivation (akin to FTT). Causes that more specifically affect the release of the pituitary hormones, luteinising hormone (LH) and follicle-stimulating hormone (FSH), include anorexia nervosa, excessive physical training, hypothyroidism, pituitary tumours and Klinefelter syndrome.

Information Box 5.4e-XIV

Delayed puberty: comments from a Chinese medicine perspective

Although it depends on the cause, in most cases delayed puberty is very likely to suggest a relative Deficiency in Kidney Essence.

Intersex disorders

There is a range of intersex disorders that result in a child in whom the external sexual characteristics do not match its genetic sexual identity. In general, these disorders result from a failure in the sexual differentiation of the genitals and gonads that occurs in the fetus during the first trimester of pregnancy. These disorders are mentioned briefly in Chapter 5.2g.

Part I: Disorders of the digestive system

Many of the childhood digestive disorders correspond directly to their adult counterparts. The following conditions are either characteristic conditions of childhood, or follow a different course to that which is usually followed in adulthood.

Recurrent non-organic (functional) abdominal pain

Recurrent abdominal pain of sufficient intensity to interrupt day-to-day activities is a very common complaint affecting children of school age. Episodes of pain, recurring over a period of at least 3 months, are estimated to affect up to one-tenth of all school-age children. In the bulk of these cases there will be no clearly definable physical cause. In other words, the pain is non-organic or functional. For those children in whom no obvious physical cause can be identified, the nature of the recurrent pain may have some typical features: it is often located around the umbilicus, it is worse on waking, and may be associated with a family history of migraine, travel sickness or irritable bowel syndrome. In many of these children the symptoms are worse with stress.

In the management of recurrent abdominal pain, first it is important to exclude the more common physical causes of abdominal pain, which can explain about 10% of cases. The physical causes of functional abdominal pain include mesenteric adenitis (see below), appendicitis (see below), inflammatory bowel disease (see below), peptic ulceration, urinary tract infection or urinary stones (see below), and gynaecological disorders.

Once a physical cause has been excluded, it is important to reassure the parents and the child that the pain is most likely to be due to an abnormality of the sensitivity of the bowel to the normal bowel movements. This explanation, which is akin to the conventional explanation for the pain of irritable bowel syndrome, is supported by scientific evidence. This evidence, based on studies that correlated pain with the pressure within the contracting bowel, also suggests that anxiety increases the pain by increasing the frequency of the bowel movements.

In about one-half of children with non-organic recurrent abdominal pain, referral to a paediatrician and reassurance can result in rapid resolution of the pain. Of the remainder, one-half have partial resolution, and the other half go on to experience irritable bowel syndrome in adulthood.

Information Box 5.4e-XV

Abdominal pain in children: comments from a Chinese medicine perspective

In Chinese medicine, abdominal pain in children can be a feature of a wide range of patterns, of which External Cold (usually from Cold foods), Accumulation Disorder, Interior Cold from Deficiency, Retention of Phlegm Damp, and Lingering Pathogenic Factor are the most common. Qi Obstruction and Stasis can explain some of the more serious forms of abdominal pain, which would be more frequently seen in hospital departments.

Mesenteric adenitis

'Mesenteric adenitis' is a term used to describe abdominal pain that arises from inflammation of the abdominal lymph nodes. In small children, this cause of abdominal pain can accompany upper respiratory tract infections and other more generalised illnesses.

On examination, there may be tenderness on palpation, which can be localised to one particular region of the abdomen. Clinically, if the pain is severe it can be difficult to distinguish mesenteric adenitis from appendicitis (see below). Although mesenteric adenitis is not a serious condition, the child might have to undergo surgical exploration to exclude appendicitis if the pain is severe and persistent.

> **Information Box 5.4e-XVI**
>
> **Mesenteric adenitis: comments from a Chinese medicine perspective**
>
> In Chinese medicine, the pain of mesenteric adenitis might correspond to any of the patterns listed above for recurrent abdominal pain.

Intussusception

Intussusception is the most common cause of bowel obstruction to affect young children, particularly those under the age of 1 year. The obstruction is the result of one segment of the bowel folding inside itself, so obstructing the flow of faeces, and causing compression of the blood vessels that supply that segment. There is often no obvious underlying cause of this problem. The most popular explanation is that viral infection has caused swelling of the lymphoid tissue of the bowel lining, which can then form the 'lead point' of the infolding of the bowel tissue. If intussusception occurs in an older child, a more substantial physical cause may be found (e.g. a polyp or bowel tumour).

The obstruction causes severe pain, which causes a baby to draw up his legs and scream. The baby may vomit or pass small amounts of blood-stained stool. The abdomen distends and a sausage-shaped mass may be felt in the abdomen. The child, if not too shocked, may be treated by means of pumping air gently into the rectum. In many cases this can help the bowel to unfold. If the child is very unwell, surgical treatment is required.

> **Information Box 5.4e-XVII**
>
> **Intussusception: comments from a Chinese medicine perspective**
>
> In Chinese medicine, the acute abdominal pain of the intussusception corresponds to Qi and Blood Obstruction, and Stasis.

Appendicitis

The appendix is a blind-ended, worm-like tube that projects outwards from the first part of the large intestine (the caecum). It sits in the region of the abdominal cavity described as the 'right iliac fossa'. The lining wall of the appendix contains a dense concentration of lymphoid tissue.

Appendicitis is a term that refers to the fact that the appendix has become inflamed. This is a relatively common occurrence in children aged 3–16 years. In children, the lymphoid tissue in the gastrointestinal system readily swells in reaction to exposure to new antigens found within the intestinal contents. Because the hollow of the appendix is very narrow, just a slight swelling of its lining wall will cause the passageway to become blocked, thus causing faecal material to become retained within the appendix. This situation can then rapidly lead to inflammation, as the stagnant faeces start to irritate the lining of the appendix.

The early stages of inflammation of the appendix present as deep pain in the centre of the abdomen. The child may be reluctant to move, and may vomit. A low-grade fever is common. In some cases this pain can fluctuate in intensity over the course of days to weeks, and may even settle down. This is the so-called 'grumbling' appendix.

In more severe cases, the pain can intensify as the inflammation spreads to affect the complete width of the appendix wall. Then, as the lining layer of the peritoneum becomes involved, the pain can move downwards and to the right, becoming localised in the right iliac fossa. If this progression occurs, the child can become very unwell, with severe pain and vomiting. If the progression is very rapid, the appendix may rupture and so lead to the serious condition of peritonitis. In this case, the child's condition will deteriorate rapidly and shock can ensue. This is a surgical emergency.

Diagnosis of an early case of appendicitis is not straightforward. Functional abdominal pain is common in children, and also mesenteric adenitis can readily mimic the classical features of appendicitis. In very young children the features of appendicitis can be very non-specific, sometimes only becoming apparent in the form of fever and irritability. However, because the complication of peritonitis is so devastating, early surgical exploration of suspected cases is considered good practice, particularly as the operation is a simple and relatively safe one to perform. The operation of appendectomy involves locating the appendix via a small incision in the right iliac fossa, and then removing the whole of the appendix, whether or not it is obviously inflamed. In conventional practice it is not believed that the loss of the appendix is detrimental to the health of the child. The child would be expected to make a rapid recovery over the course of the next few days.

> **Information Box 5.4e-XVIII**
>
> **Appendicitis: comments from a Chinese medicine perspective**
>
> From the conventional understanding of the pathology of appendicitis, it would be expected that the Chinese medicine interpretation would embrace Qi Stagnation and Heat. Scott and Barlow (1999) describe a pattern that corresponds to appendicitis as Qi Obstruction and Blood Stasis. This Obstruction could be preceded by Exterior Cold or Accumulation Disorder. Early cases of appendicitis may be resolved by acupuncture treatment alone, although referral to a conventional practitioner would be advised in all suspected cases.

Gastroenteritis

Gastroenteritis is described in detail in Chapter 3.1c. The most important point to bear in mind with a case of gastroenteritis in a small child is that the risk of dehydration is much greater than that in a previously healthy adult.

Coeliac disease

Coeliac disease is described in detail in Chapter 3.1e as one of the most common causes of the malabsorption syndrome. Coeliac disease in children will often present with failure to thrive. Although loose stools are one of the cardinal features of malabsorption, this symptom may not be a prominent feature, even in a case of sufficient severity to cause delayed attainment of developmental milestones in a child. For this reason, coeliac disease should always be considered in a case of unexplained poor growth in a child (Figure 5.4e-I).

Inflammatory bowel disease

'Inflammatory bowel disease', a term which embraces Crohn's disease and ulcerative colitis, is described in detail in Chapter 3.1e.

Crohn's disease is a condition which, for a reason that is unclear, has been increasing in incidence since the 1950s. This increase has been particularly marked in children. About one-quarter of patients with Crohn's disease first present in childhood or adolescence. However, Crohn's disease is rare in children under the age of 10 years. Suggestions that this increased incidence may be attributed to the introduction of the measles–mumps–rubella (MMR) vaccination are hotly contested by the medical establishment. The scientific evidence that has been used to support this possible link with the MMR vaccine is not at all conclusive when considered from a conventional viewpoint.

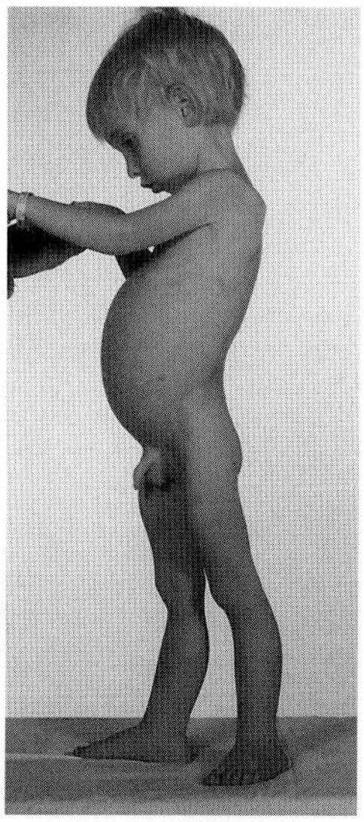

Figure 5.4e-I • Coeliac disease, causing muscular wasting together with distension of the abdomen.

In children, Crohn's disease can present with the characteristic features of diarrhoea, weight loss and the passage of mucus. Failure to thrive and delayed onset of puberty are common. In some children, loss of appetite and weight may be more prominent than the symptom of loose stools, so much so that the condition may be confused with anorexia nervosa. In general, the long-term outlook for children with Crohn's disease is good, with most being able to lead a normal adult life, albeit with occasional bouts of recurrent disease.

In contrast to Crohn's disease, the incidence of ulcerative colitis has not altered over the past few decades. The presentation of ulcerative colitis in children is similar to that in adults. As with Crohn's disease, failure to thrive and delayed puberty are common features in severe cases in children.

Part II: Disorders of the respiratory system

The most common disorders of the respiratory system in children are the infectious diseases of the respiratory tract, which are described in detail in Chapter 5.4d. This chapter, describes asthma, the most common non-infectious respiratory disease of childhood, and the relatively rare but very important condition of sudden infant death syndrome. All the other important respiratory disorders of childhood, such as cystic fibrosis, are discussed elsewhere in this book.

Asthma

Asthma is the most common chronic respiratory disorder to affect children. Recent studies suggest that up to 15% of schoolchildren in the UK have been given the diagnosis of asthma at some point in their lives. Moreover, asthma now accounts for up to 20% of acute paediatric hospital admissions. Although the condition is rarely of a very severe nature in children, nevertheless asthma accounts for a great deal of restricted activity and school absenteeism in affected children. The incidence of asthma in children has been increasing in recent decades for reasons that are unclear. Young boys are affected twice as commonly as girls, but by adolescence equal numbers are affected.

The pathology of asthma is described in detail in Chapter 3.3d. Children almost always develop the extrinsic form of asthma, in which there is a tendency for the child to be oversensitive (allergic) to a wide range of environmental allergens, and in which a family history of atopy is common. One-third of children with asthma suffer also from eczema, and up to one-half have the features of allergic rhinitis, including a persistently stuffy nose and nasal discharge. Common triggers for childhood asthma include animal dandruff, house-dust-mite faeces, pollen and moulds, and certain foods, including wheat, milk and eggs. It is well known that other environmental factors, such as damp living conditions, atmospheric pollution and cigarette smoke, can exacerbate the symptoms of asthma in children.

The diagnosis is based on a history of wheeze, cough and breathlessness or, in pre-school children, nocturnal cough.

The diagnosis can be confirmed in children over the age of 5 years by means of serial peak-flow measurements. In some children the symptoms may only occur in brief bouts, sometimes precipitated by a respiratory infection. Less commonly, the symptoms are more chronic. Unless the asthma is very severe, the health of the affected child is usually otherwise unaffected. However, in severe cases there may be evidence of failure to thrive, with poor attainment of developmental milestones.

The aim of treatment is to enable the child to lead a normal life, and to prevent deterioration of the symptoms to a serious, potentially life-threatening condition. The management of asthma by means of inhaled and oral bronchodilators and prophylactic (preventive) medication is similar in principle to the management strategy that conventional practitioners are advised to follow for adults and which is described in Chapter 3.3d. The main difference is that in young children a new anti-inflammatory medication, called montelukast, or a form of theophylline may also be prescribed in tablet form in addition to a corticosteroid such as beclometasone. Even small babies can be administered inhaled medication by means of a plastic 'spacer' device, with a mask or a 'nebuliser' pump if large doses are required. From the age of 5 years many children become competent in the use of dry-powder inhalers.

Most asthmatic children (about 70%) have less than four episodes a year. In these children the symptoms can be controlled by means of intermittent use of a bronchodilator inhaler such as salbutamol. Severe episodes may require the additional use of nebulised bronchodilators or a brief course of oral steroids, but with the expectation that the child can be weaned off these medications after a few days.

About 25% of children have asthmatic symptoms at least once every 2–4 weeks, but also have some periods of complete respite from symptoms. These children will be prescribed a regular dose of a prophylactic medication, such as beclometasone.

The remaining 5% of asthmatic children have persistent symptoms. Most of these will be prescribed regular doses of inhaled corticosteroid and bronchodilators. These are children who may also be prescribed oral theophylline or montelukast. In severe cases, oral corticosteroids may also be prescribed. These children may be supervised by a hospital consultant, and will require regular monitoring of their general health and growth, particularly if they are on oral steroid medication. Because of judicious use of preventive medication, severe uncontrollable exacerbations of asthma are uncommon in children; in the UK, 20–30 children die of status asthmaticus per year.

Information Box 5.4e-XIX

Asthma: comments from a Chinese medicine perspective

In Chinese medicine, asthma is known as Xiao Chuan (meaning wheezing and breathlessness or gurgling). In general, the underlying patterns found in children are Deficiency of Lung, Spleen and Kidney Qi, together with Accumulation of Damp and Phlegm. Invasion of External Pathogenic Factors or a Lingering Pathogenic Factor can exacerbate these patterns. In the acute attack, Liver Qi insulting the Lungs (described by Scott and Barlow (1999) as 'spasm'), Phlegm or Heat are the principal causes of the difficulty in breathing. Scott and Barlow (1999) propose that medication, including repeated prescriptions of antibiotics, will only serve to worsen these imbalances in the long term. Inhaled bronchodilator and corticosteroid medication tend to weaken the Qi of the Lungs and Kidneys, and corticosteroids can cause accumulation of Damp and Heat in the Lungs.

Predisposing factors in the aetiology of asthma include an inherited Deficiency, repeated infections with prescription of antibiotics, Phlegm-forming foods and additives in the diet, and weakening of the Spleen from irregular and inappropriate feeding of the small child. Scott and Barlow (1999) also suggest that excessive use of TV and computer games, lack of exercise, poor posture and emotional trauma (particularly when a state of fear or panic is induced) can also be very important contributors to the development of asthma.

Sudden infant death syndrome (cot death)

Sudden infant death syndrome (SIDS) is defined as the sudden and unexpected death of a child for which no adequate cause is found at post-mortem examination. This tragic event most commonly occurs in babies aged between 2–4 months. SIDS is the most common cause of death in babies aged between 1–12 months. It is believed that the underlying cause of death is cessation of breathing (apnoea), primarily as a consequence of immature respiratory reflexes. It is believed that the small baby is relatively insensitive to the build up of carbon dioxide in its bloodstream, which is normally a potent trigger for more rapid and deeper respirations. It is recognised that an ongoing respiratory infection and environmental cigarette smoke both increase the risk of SIDS.

The incidence of SIDS in the UK has fallen dramatically over the past few years since the introduction of a national campaign that has advocated three cardinal principles. These are:

- the child should not be laid to sleep on its front (i.e. not face down)
- the child should not be allowed to overheat when sleeping
- the child should not be exposed to cigarette smoke.

In the event of SIDS, the family will require sensitive support to enable them to comprehend what has happened and to move on from their bereavement. It is believed that it is very important for the family to be allowed hold the dead child. In all cases the coroner has to be informed of the death and a post-mortem performed. The family will have to be interviewed by the police in all cases. The family needs to be prepared for this, and it is essential that it is explained to them that this does not imply that they are under any suspicion. Written information about the nature of SIDS should be given to the parents, together with the details of bereavement support agencies such as Child Death Helpline or CRUSE. When the results of the post-mortem are known, the parents should be offered an explanatory interview and, when relevant, genetic counselling.

Part II: Disorders of the urinary system and genitalia

The most important conditions to affect the urinary system in children include the inherited malformations of the urinary tract, urinary infections (which are often associated with inherited abnormalities), glomerulonephritis and tumours of the kidney. Of these, only the inherited deformities are discussed below, as urinary infections and glomerulonephritis have already been discussed in detail in Chapters 4.3c and 4.3d. Tumours of the kidney are described later in this chapter.

The most important disorders of the genitalia in children are those that affect boys. Of these, maldescent of the testis and congenital inguinal hernia have been discussed in Chapter 5.4c. Germ-cell tumours of the testis are described later in this chapter. Only the important disorders of the foreskin, phimosis and balanitis, and torsion of the testis are discussed below.

Inherited malformations of the urinary tract

The widespread use of antenatal ultrasound screening of the 20-week-old fetus has allowed the early demonstration of gross abnormalities of the urinary tract. These abnormalities are detected in 1 in 400 of fetuses, indicating that a malformation of the urinary system is a relatively common occurrence. However, not all these malformations will lead to manifest disease in the child.

Abnormalities that often do not lead to serious symptoms include a 'horseshoe kidney', in which the two kidneys are fused together and the ureters descend to form the resulting horseshoe-shaped organ, and a 'duplex system', in which one or both kidneys give rise to two ureters. However, in some cases both these abnormalities may give rise to an obstruction of the flow of urine through the unusually situated ureters. This can lead to back-pressure of urine in the kidney, and thus progressive kidney damage, increased risk of repeated kidney infections, and chronic pyelonephritis. Vesicoureteric reflux (VUR) is also more common with a duplex system, and is an important cause of chronic pyelonephritis.

Obstruction to the flow of the urine in one or both ureters, usually due to a malformation of the ureter itself, can also be detected by means of ultrasound scans. Obstruction to flow can also occur at the neck of the bladder in boys, as a result of a flap of tissue known as a 'posterior urethral valve'. In cases of severe obstruction, the affected kidney may appear dilated or shrivelled, even at this early stage of fetal development. Both kidneys will be affected if a posterior urethral valve is the cause of the obstruction. In severe cases the child can be born with permanently damaged renal function, which will then lead to chronic renal failure in early childhood. Detection of bilateral kidney damage would be a reason to induce labour as early as possible (35 weeks) so that the obstruction can be relieved by means of immediate surgery, and the progression of damage to the kidneys halted.

> **Information Box 5.4e-XX**
>
> **Urinary tract malformations: comments from a Chinese medicine perspective**
>
> In Chinese medicine, inherited malformations of the urinary tract would normally indicate Deficiency of Kidney Essence.

Balanitis and phimosis

The foreskin of a baby boy is usually prevented from retracting and exposing the glans of the penis by fibrous adhesions that join its inner surface to the surface of the glans. As the child gets older these adhesions break down, so that in the majority of 6-year-old boys the foreskin has become retractile. By the age of 16 years only 1% of boys are unable to retract their foreskin.

'Phimosis' is the term used to describe a non-retractile foreskin. Phimosis is normal in very young boys. Phimosis that persists, but causes no symptoms, is not usual, but is not a cause for concern. Phimosis only becomes a problem if the foreskin becomes inflamed or damaged. This can occur if there have been repeated forceful attempts of retraction of the foreskin, or if there have been episodes of infection of the space between the foreskin and the glans, a condition known as 'balanitis'. An episode of balanitis is usually treated by means of oral antibiotics.

A damaged foreskin can become scarred and thickened. This can restrict the normal flow of urine, and can predispose to recurrent bouts of balanitis. A scarred and thickened foreskin is considered to be an indication for circumcision. This operation, when necessary for health reasons, is always performed under anaesthetic.

> **Information Box 5.4e-XXI**
>
> **Balanitis and phimosis: comments from a Chinese medicine perspective**
>
> From a Chinese medicine perspective, asymptomatic phimosis probably does not represent any underlying imbalance. However, in cases in which balanitis and scarring occur, this suggests the Pattern of Damp Heat in the Liver overlying an underlying Kidney Deficiency or Liver Disharmony, as both these Organs relate to the penis.

Torsion of the testis

Torsion of the testis is a condition that primarily affects the young child or adolescent, but it may occasionally occur in young men. It is believed that the problem, which involves the testis twisting around the root that provides its blood and nerve supply, is much more likely if there is a slight congenital abnormality of one or more of the position, orientation or shape of the testis. The ovary can also undergo torsion, although this problem almost always occurs in women of childbearing years. In women, the presence of an ovarian cyst will predispose to torsion of the ovary.

A testicular torsion will present as a sudden onset of severe pain in the lower abdomen and scrotum. The affected scrotum becomes swollen and inflamed. The child may vomit with the pain. If the torsion affects an undescended testis, the pain will be localised to the abdomen and groin, and may mimic a strangulated hernia. In some cases, the acute episode may have been preceded by a few episodes of partial torsion, in which less severe warning pains in the groin region were felt for short periods of time.

Torsion requires emergency surgery to prevent gangrene of the testis. This has to be performed within a few hours, at most, of the onset of the symptoms if the function of the testis is to be preserved. If the testis can be saved, it is anchored surgically to the surrounding tissues. This procedure is usually repeated for the unaffected testis. A gangrenous testis has to be removed (orchidectomy), and the unaffected testis is surgically anchored in place. When the child reaches late adolescence he will be offered an operation to implant a prosthetic testis in the empty side of the scrotum.

Information Box 5.4e-XXII

Torsion of the testes: comments from a Chinese medicine perspective

In Chinese medicine, acute pain in the scrotum might correspond to Stagnation of Blood and Qi or Cold in the Liver Channel. As there is a congenital predisposition to torsion of the testis, this suggests that there is an underlying Deficiency of Kidney Essence.

Part II: Disorders of the eyes, ears and nervous system

The conditions of the eyes and ears will be studied in detail in Chapters 6.1d and 6.1e. This chapter introduces only the two most important of these conditions which primarily affect children, namely squint (strabismus) and glue ear (chronic secretory otitis media).

Squint (strabismus)

Squint, or strabismus, is primarily a disorder of the external ocular muscles (the muscles that control the coordinated movements of the eyeballs within the orbits of the skull) rather than an internal problem of the eye itself. However, if uncorrected, a squint can lead to a long-term underdevelopment of the nerve pathways that are responsible for depth (or stereoscopic) vision, a condition known as 'amblyopia'. For this reason, squint is one of the conditions that should be excluded through the routine child health surveillance checks of the pre-school years.

In health, the eyes should both be directed towards the object that is the focus of the gaze. If the object moves, the eyeballs move so that they each remain directed towards the object. Because the eyes are not in exactly the same place in relation to the object, each receives a slightly different image. As the nervous system develops during the pre-school years, the brain learns to use the differences in these images to recognise how far away the object is in relation to other objects in the field of vision. This is stereoscopic vision. Stereoscopic vision is an important faculty that enables the judgement of distance and the controlled and accurate movement of the limbs or body. It is of particular importance for the correct performance of delicate manual tasks, such as needlework, and also for all forms of sport that require the judgement of distance, such as ball games.

In the form of squint that is most common in childhood, the direction of the eyes in relation to each other is misaligned so that the eyes do not receive corresponding images of the viewed object. In some children this misalignment is obvious, in that one eye always appears to be gazing slightly in the wrong direction. In other children, the misalignment is more prominent when the child is tired.

If this sort of misalignment were to occur suddenly in an adult (most commonly as a result of a mononeuropathy of one of the cranial nerves that supply the eye muscles), the result would be unremitting double vision. One way for the adult to cope with this problem is to place a patch over one eye in order to suppress the confusing image from the affected eye.

However, in the developing nervous system of the small child, double vision does not occur. Instead, the image from one of the eyes is suppressed internally by nerve impulses from the brain. This means that far less confusing information is received, and a clear image of the object can be generated, albeit without the added information required to judge its distance. If this suppression occurs for long enough, the ability of the nervous system to perceive a clear image from the affected eye is permanently lost. Although the child does not become blind in the affected eye, when both eyes are used it is as if only one eye is active in generating the image that is perceived by the brain. This is amblyopia, or as it is more commonly known, 'lazy eye'. In a case of established amblyopia, if the good eye is covered, it is evident that the affected eye is able to receive only very vague visual information as compared with the good eye. This is a problem that cannot be corrected at all by wearing glasses.

Squints are relatively common. They are even more common in children who have other neurological problems that have been present from birth. In rare cases, the inability to focus one eye on the object may be due to a very severe refractive error (a problem in the ability to focus the lens of the eye), a congenital cataract (clouding of the lens) or an intraocular tumour (retinoblastoma). For this reason, when a squint is detected, the child should be referred for expert opthalmological diagnosis.

Once serious underlying causes have been excluded, the child is treated by means of glasses to correct any refractive error, and by the use of patches to cover the good eye for defined times of the day. This stimulates the affected eye, and enables the nerve pathways that radiate from the eye to the visual centres of the brain to continue to develop. This treatment should be initiated as long as possible before the child's seventh birthday, after which there is little hope for further improvement. In cases when there is very obvious divergence or convergence of the eyes, the child may be offered a surgical operation to correct the squint. This is of value for cosmetic reasons, but is recognised not to be an effective treatment for the prevention of amblyopia.

Information Box 5.4e-XXIII

Strabismus (squint): comments from a Chinese medicine perspective

From a Chinese medicine perspective, Scott and Barlow (1999) suggest that the manifestation of a squint may be the result of Womb Heat. This has become lodged in the Channels that relate to one or more of the extraocular muscles (Liver, Gallbladder and Bladder). In this case the squint is present from birth, and is often quite pronounced in appearance.

Alternatively, if the squint develops after the time of birth, it may be the result of the Depletion in energy of the eye muscles resulting from an Invasion of Full Heat or a lingering Pathogenic Factor in the Channels. Scott and Barlow (1999) also suggest that the internal (empty) Heat generated from overstimulation or overexcitement of a child can, in the same way, deplete the Qi in the Channels that relate to the eye muscles. These forms of squint may vary in severity according to the nervous state or level of tiredness of the child.

Scott and Barlow (1999) report that significant improvement can result from acupuncture treatment of squint, particularly if initiated before the fifth birthday. Treatment principles include Clearing of Heat from the Liver, Gallbladder and Kidney Channels, and Tonification of the Kidney Qi.

Glue ear

Glue ear is the aptly descriptive common term for the condition of chronic secretory otitis media (CSOM) (also termed 'otitis media with effusion' (OME)). CSOM can be a complication of an attack of acute otitis media, the infectious inflammation of the middle ear which is known to affect up to one-fifth of all children under 4 years of age within any one year. The tendency to develop a persistent, thick but non-infective discharge in the middle ear runs strongly in families. It is believed that it is a combination of a particular anatomical structure of the Eustachian tube in children (inherited) and susceptibility to upper respiratory tract infections that causes the susceptibility to this condition. CSOM affects up to one-third of children at some point in their lives. The condition is most common in children between the ages of 2 and 9 years.

There need not be a history of acute otitis media for CSOM to develop. Secretions in the middle ear originate from the respiratory epithelium that lines this cavity. Normally these secretions drain away to the throat via the Eustachian tube. Anatomical abnormalities of the Eustachian tube, the presence of enlarged adenoids, and a cleft palate are all recognised to be associated with CSOM, because they lead to impaired drainage of the middle ear. Factors that lead to increased secretions in the middle ear, such as infections, allergic rhinitis, damage to the eardrum during air travel and cigarette smoke, can also promote the development of CSOM.

The primary symptom of CSOM is deafness in one or both ears. This 'conductive deafness' is a result of the fluid in the middle ear impairing the transmission of sound waves from the eardrum through to the nerve endings in the inner ear. If the deafness is not recognised, the child may appear to be dreamy, or in a world of their own. The child may also develop low-grade discomfort in the affected ear, tinnitus or unsteadiness, but these complications are relatively rare. CSOM is a significant problem in young children, because it can have a marked impact on their interactions with the people around them, and on their development of speech and language.

CSOM gives rise to a characteristic appearance of the eardrum, and so its presence may be suspected by the GP after simple visualisation of the eardrum (otoscopy). The diagnosis can be confirmed by an audiologist by means of a non-invasive test called 'impedance audiometry'. This test assesses the degree to which sound is absorbed by the eardrum, and also the springiness of the membrane of the eardrum.

Most cases of CSOM will resolve spontaneously, although, if there is a susceptibility, the condition may recur several times in the early life of the same child. Current medical opinion is that a period of watchful waiting should be allowed before treatment is offered for CSOM. The decision to treat should be based not on test results, but on how the condition is affecting the child. Simple medical treatment includes the prescription of short courses of antibiotics if infection is suspected, antihistamines in cases of allergic rhinitis, and mucolytics (drugs intended to reduce the thickness of secretions, the benefit of which is very uncertain). Surgical treatment is considered if hearing loss persists for some months, if the child is demonstrating negative social or educational consequences of intermittent deafness, or if there are symptoms such as pain or dizziness.

The surgical treatment of CSOM involves piercing the eardrum, aspiration of the fluid from the middle ear and the insertion of a tiny tube-like structure known as a 'grommet' into the hole formed by the piercing. The tube of the grommet has a widened margin at each of its ends, and stays in place as a result of this structure. However, the grommet will eventually be pushed out of the eardrum into the outer ear canal as the epithelium of the eardrum turns over. This takes an average of 6 months. The grommet is intended to permit free drainage of fluid from the middle ear. It should not adversely affect hearing, and the eardrum usually appears completely normal after its extrusion. Insertion of grommets conventionally is considered to be a relatively non-invasive operation.

In some children the CSOM recurs after the extrusion of the grommets, and in these cases it may be considered necessary to repeat the operation.

Epilepsy

The various forms of epilepsy are described in detail in Chapter 4.1f.

Childhood epilepsy is fairly common, affecting 5 in 1000 school-aged children. In 70–80% of cases of childhood epilepsy there is no obvious underlying cause. Intrauterine infections, brain damage from birth trauma, intracerebral bleeds in

Information Box 5.4e-XXIV

Chronic secretory otitis media (glue ear): comments from a Chinese medicine perspective

In Chinese medicine, otitis media is considered to be a Channel problem, and thus chronic secretory otitis media can respond well to acupuncture treatment. It may correspond to Lingering Pathogenic Factor. This can result in the build up of Phlegm and the Obstruction of Qi in the ear cavity. The child may also suffer from a pre-existing depletion of Spleen Qi. This can contribute to the accumulation of Damp and Phlegm.

Alternatively, and less commonly, depletion of Liver and Kidney Yin may lead to undernourishment of the ear. This would lead to a sticky fluid on the eardrum rather than a profuse phlegmy discharge. In these cases the Depletion may be a result of overstimulation, and may result in a slightly hyperactive child.

prematurity, and brain tumours are the most common of the known structural causes in children.

In addition to tonic–clonic epilepsy, which usually presents in later childhood, there are some particular syndromes that are characteristic of childhood epilepsy. These are considered briefly here.

West syndrome is a form of epileptic spasm that affects children from the age of about 4–6 months. The diagnosis may be delayed, as the spasms may not be recognised as such for some time. In many cases there is an underlying physical abnormality of the brain. In later childhood, many affected children show developmental delay and can suffer from forms of epilepsy more characteristic of adulthood, such as tonic–clonic epilepsy.

Absence (petit mal) seizures affect 1–2% of children with childhood epilepsy. The age of onset is 4–12 years of age. The affected child will momentarily go pale and stare for up to about 30 seconds. The child will regain consciousness as if nothing has happened, but may look puzzled if they become aware that they have missed something during the absence. In most children the absences cease before adulthood. Frequent absence attacks may interfere with concentration, and so can affect school performance.

Benign rolandic epilepsy is a partial epilepsy of childhood in which the seizures almost always stop by the mid-teens. Seizures often affect one side of the body only, but may become generalised tonic–clonic in form if they occur during sleep.

As in adult epilepsy, diagnosis is established by means of electroencephalogram (EEG) examination. Computed tomography (CT) or magnetic resonance imaging (MRI) may be used to exclude focal brain pathology if the age of onset is less than 5 years.

Seizures in children may be provoked by diverse factors, including deep sleep, lack of sleep, excitement, anxiety, menstruation and rapid withdrawal of anticonvulsant medication. In some cases seizures may be provoked by exposure to rapidly flashing light sources (photosensitive epilepsy). Children with photosensitive epilepsy will be advised to watch television only in a brightly lit room, and to avoid stroboscopic lighting.

Children who are prone to unpredictable seizures in the daytime are in need of protection against injury. They are advised to avoid swimming unless under very close supervision, and also other activities such as cycling or climbing, during which a seizure could place them in great danger.

Anticonvulsant medication is prescribed with caution in children, and may not be used at all in some cases. The anticonvulsant drugs that are prescribed are the same as those prescribed in adult epilepsy. In a very few cases the seizures may be relieved by surgical removal of the physical focus of the fits from the brain.

Information Box 5.4e-XXV

Epilepsy: comments from a Chinese medicine perspective

A grand mal seizure is seen in Chinese medicine as Liver Wind stirring upwards and causing Phlegm to Obstruct the Orifices of the Heart. Other seizures that manifest in muscular twitching would also be diagnosed in terms of Liver Wind. In absence seizures, the prominent pathology would appear to be Phlegm impeding the functions of the Shen.

The sudden onset is again indicative of Wind. There is usually an underlying Deficiency in all forms of epilepsy, including Deficiency of Liver and Kidney Yin, which predispose to the Stirring of Liver Wind, and Spleen Deficiency, which predisposes to the Accumulation of Phlegm.

Scott and Barlow (1999) suggest that epilepsy that suddenly becomes apparent in childhood does so as a progression from an earlier deeply rooted imbalance. They suggest that three primary factors may underlie the development of epilepsy in children: weak Yuan (source) Qi, Phlegm Obstructing the Orifices and Blood Stasis (brain injury). They go on to describe that weak Yuan Qi will predispose to Liver and Kidney Yin Deficiency, and also instability of the Qi of the Heart and the Liver.

Scott and Barlow (1999) list the External factors that may contribute to the development of childhood epilepsy as repeated febrile convulsions, immunisations, sudden shock, brain injury, a severe attack of diarrhoea and inappropriate (Cold) medication. They explain that the first three of these factors contribute to Depletion of Yin, and the last two promote the development of Phlegm by Depletion of Spleen Qi.

Part II: Cancer in childhood

Cancer affects 1 in 650 children under the age of 15 years. Over one-third of these cancers are leukaemias, the cancerous growth of the immature white blood cells. Lymphomas, cancers of the mature white blood cells, account for a further 10% of childhood cancer. The other important childhood cancers, in order of frequency of occurrence, are brain tumours (the cause in over 20% of childhood cancer cases), kidney (Wilms') tumours (7%), nerve-cell tumours (7%), bone tumours (6%), muscle tumours (5%) and tumours of the retina of the eye (3%).

The range of cancers known to affect children is different to that recognised in adults. The hopes for survival in childhood cancer are greater than in most forms of adult cancer.

Over 60% of children diagnosed with cancer will be alive 5 years after diagnosis, and many of these can be considered cured. The survival rate in childhood cancer has improved dramatically over the past 30 years. Much of this improvement can be attributed to modern approaches in chemotherapy and radiotherapy.

It is believed that in most cases of childhood cancer the underlying cause is a combination of individual susceptibility and exposure to adverse environmental factors such as radiation or viruses. In many childhood cancers, a structural change in the genetic material of the cancer cell can be detected, and some of these changes can be linked to an inherited chromosomal or genetic abnormality. In childhood cancer, the condition may present either as a localised growth, or with features of more generalised disease, such as recurrent infections, or bruising and bleeding, or both.

When cancer is diagnosed in a child, the treatment ideally should be managed from a dedicated cancer centre at which multidisciplinary supportive care can be offered to the child and the family. Children need particular support in dealing with the side-effects of treatment and its long-term effects. Both the child and the family need to be supported as they struggle with the prospect of a potentially fatal illness. Practical issues that need to be surmounted include education and social stimulation for the sick child, and finances for the family to cover the expenses of transport to numerous hospital appointments, time off work for the parents and child-care for siblings.

It has been estimated that currently about 1 in 1000 young adults in the UK are survivors of treatment for childhood cancer. These young people are likely to have residual problems resulting from recurrent cycles of chemotherapy and radiotherapy, including poor growth and infertility, and the consequences of reduced access to education. There is also an increased risk of secondary tumours in children who have been exposed to cancer therapies.

Leukaemia and lymphoma

Leukaemia and lymphoma have been described in detail in Chapter 3.4e. Although leukaemia and lymphoma are rare in adults, they are two of the most common forms of cancer in children and young people.

Leukaemia accounts for about 35% of childhood cancer. In four-fifths of these cases the cause is a form of acute leukaemia known as 'acute lymphoblastic leukaemia' (ALL). As is the case in adults, affected children present with symptoms of rapidly worsening bone-marrow failure (susceptibility to infections, bruising and bleeding, and anaemia). The treatment depends on the precise diagnosis of the leukaemia. Nowadays, up to 65% of cases of ALL will be cured by chemotherapy regimens, the success depending in part on how extensive the tumour is at diagnosis. Treatment for ALL may often extend over a course of over 2 years. For the remaining forms of leukaemia, the prognosis is less favourable (e.g. the cure rate is below 50% in acute myeloid leukaemia).

Lymphoma can be categorised into various types according to the type of white blood cells involved. Hodgkin lymphoma is the form that is recognised to be particularly frequent in young adults and teenagers. However, in young children, the other forms of lymphoma (generally termed 'non-Hodgkin lymphoma' (NHL)) are more common.

The treatment for NHL depends on the nature of presentation. Some forms present very similarly to ALL and are treated in the same way as ALL. The prognosis for survival is similar. The form of NHL that most often presents in the form of enlarged head or neck lymph nodes is treated with relatively short courses of chemotherapy and has a very good prognosis. However, the types of NHL that present with nodes in the abdomen are often at an advanced stage at diagnosis, and the prognosis is less good.

The treatment for Hodgkin lymphoma depends on the stage of the disease. Localised disease (in one lymph-node site) can often be cured by radiotherapy alone. Otherwise, combined chemotherapy and radiotherapy is used. Hodgkin lymphoma has a relatively very good prognosis, with 80% of children who are treated being cured.

Brain tumours

In children, brain tumours are almost always primary (rather than metastatic as is the case for most brain tumours in adults). The most common childhood brain tumours are malignancies of the glial cells. They most often develop in the cerebellum or the brainstem, and can present with symptoms such as headache, vomiting, squint, double vision and dizziness.

The outcome of the treatment of a childhood brain tumour depends very much on the type of the tumour and on how closely the tumour is located to vital areas in the brain. Treatment usually involves surgery and radiotherapy, together with chemotherapy in some cases. The combination of damage from the growing tumour, surgery to a delicate area of the brain, and the effect of radiotherapy can cause the very few surviving children to suffer from long-term complex difficulties, such as poor growth, physical disability, epilepsy and educational problems.

Neuroblastoma

Neuroblastoma is a tumour of primitive nerve cells. It most commonly arises in the adrenal medulla or in the chain of sympathetic nerves that run either side of the spinal cord. It usually presents in a child of less than 5 years of age as an abdominal mass. Often, by the time of diagnosis, the disease has metastasised to the bones or bone marrow.

Non-metastatic disease has a relatively good prognosis, with many children being cured by surgery alone. However, if the disease has metastasised, the prognosis is not at all good. The disease is then treated with a combination of surgery and high-dose chemotherapy. Less than 30% of children with metastatic disease will be cured.

Wilms' tumour (nephroblastoma)

Wilms' tumour is a tumour of primitive kidney cells. It is a tumour that is associated with a genetic susceptibility, and its development has been linked to a deletion in chromosome 11. In most cases the disease presents in a child under 5 years of age as an abdominal mass.

In 15% of cases of Wilms' tumour, metastases are found, most commonly in the lung. Other problems that can complicate treatment result from the tumour bulk, particularly if it is compressing the major vessels of the abdomen, such as the renal arteries or the inferior vena cava.

Treatment is by means of surgical removal of the mass, followed by chemotherapy. In advanced disease, radiotherapy may be given also. Overall, about 80% of children will be cured of the disease.

Bone and muscle tumours

Malignant bone tumours are rare in children before puberty. Malignant osteosarcoma is the most common form of childhood bone tumour. This tumour primarily affects the long bones of the limbs. Ewing sarcoma is a less common bone tumour that also mainly affects the limbs.

Both forms of bone tumour are difficult to treat. However, the prognosis has improved in recent years as a result of the use of combination chemotherapy before surgery. Radiotherapy can also be of value in controlling the growth of Ewing sarcoma.

The rhabdomyosarcoma is a tumour that originates from primitive muscle tissue. It most commonly arises in the head and neck region or the genital region. In 15% of cases metastatic spread to the lung, liver, bone or bone marrow has occurred by the time of diagnosis. Only in the minority can the tumour be excised completely, in which case the prognosis is favourable. Otherwise, the disease requires treatment with combination chemotherapy and radiotherapy, and has a poor prognosis.

Retinoblastoma

Retinoblastoma is a tumour of primitive retinal cells that arises within the posterior chamber of the eye. It is usually first detected in a child under the age of 2 years through routine eye checks, when it manifests either as a squint or in difficulty of the examiner in obtaining a view of the retina.

In about one-third of cases the condition arises as a result of an inherited mutation of a gene on chromosome 13. This gene is known to control retinal differentiation. In some cases of inherited retinoblastoma, tumours are found to be developing in both eyes. In the non-inherited cases, the mutation of the gene has occurred in one of the cells within the developing embryonic retina.

Treatment by means of radiation or laser therapy may be sufficient to treat small tumours, but in advanced cases the eye needs to be removed (enucleation). In hereditary cases there remains a significant risk of a second tumour developing (osteosarcoma being the most common form). For this reason, in hereditary cases there should be regular screening of affected children and their siblings for retinal and other tumours.

Germ-cell tumours

Germ-cell tumours arise from the immature germ cells which in the fetus are destined to mature within the gonads. These rare tumours develop either in the sacrococcygeal region, and so become apparent as a mass close to the anus, or in the gonads themselves.

Even the malignant forms of these tumours are very sensitive to chemotherapy, and there is generally a good prognosis with treatment.

Information Box 5.4e-XXVI

Childhood cancer: comments from a Chinese medicine perspective

Most of the childhood tumours arise from primitive cells that were present in the embryo. In health, these rapidly dividing primitive cells are destined to be the basis of more mature cells in the growing child. The fact that these growing and developing cells are defective suggests that, from a Chinese medicine perspective, Deficiency of Kidney Essence is likely to be a prominent imbalance in childhood cancer. As in all forms of cancer, the substantial manifestation of the disease corresponds to Stagnation of Blood and/or Accumulation of Phlegm. In cancer, both these imbalances develop as a consequence of a severe underlying Deficiency.

Part II: Skin disorders

The most important skin disorders of children, including infantile eczema, will be described in detail in Chapter 6.1c.

Part II: Psychiatric developmental and behavioural disorders

Chapter 6.2b describes how mental health disorders are classified. In childhood psychiatry the psychiatric disorders can be broadly classified into developmental, behavioural and emotional disorders. In the two most respected systems of classification of psychiatric disorders, the International Classification of Diseases, tenth revision (ICD-10), and the Diagnostic and Statistical Manual of Mental Disorders, fourth revision (DSM-IV), the developmental disorders of childhood are defined as embracing autism (pervasive developmental disorder), and the language, speech and reading disorders (including the dyslexias). In DSM-IV, mental retardation is also classified as a developmental disorder of childhood. The important behavioural and emotional disorders of childhood are classified into a range of categories that include disruptive behaviour or hyperkinetic disorders (including attention-deficit hyperactivity disorder (ADHD)), tic disorders (including Tourette's syndrome), anxiety disorders and elimination disorders (encopresis, or soiling, and enuresis). Eating disorders are classified in DSM-IV as a disorder of childhood and adolescence, and in ICD-10 under adult disorders.

This chapter considers only the following important psychiatric conditions of childhood: autism, the disorders of spelling and reading (dyslexias), ADHD and tics. Anxiety disorders of childhood and eating disorders are described in Chapter 6.2d.

Autism

Autism is a diagnosis that falls under the broader diagnosis of pervasive development disorder (PDD). PDD is a relatively uncommon spectrum of disorders (affecting up to 15 children per 10,000 births), and is characterised by disturbance in communication skills, difficulties in social interactions, and problems in imaginative and play activities and behaviour. It is often associated with impaired intellectual capacity.

Autism is the most common form of PDD. Asperger syndrome is a form of PDD in which language and intellectual skills are better developed. Both these forms of PDD are 4–8 times more common in boys than in girls.

PDD classically presents before the age of 3 years. Features that are noticeable at this age include impaired speech development, poor eye contact, aloofness, treatment of people as objects, ritualistic behaviour, intolerance of change and limited creative play. In some children odd movements, such as flapping of the hands, spinning or walking on tiptoe, may also appear by this age.

There is evidence that in some cases there is a genetic predisposition to PDD, suggesting a biological basis for the condition, although no consistent abnormalities of the brain have been identified to account for the symptoms. In up to 20% of cases epilepsy is a concurrent problem, which is further evidence of a structural biological basis. Occasionally, the condition can follow on from episodes of organic brain disorders such as encephalitis. Claims that autism can result from the MMR vaccine are not substantiated by conventional analyses of the statistics of the incidence of autism. However, such analyses cannot absolutely disprove such an association. There is no evidence to suggest that the condition results from emotional trauma or poor parenting.

The long-term outlook for a child with PDD is improved if the child can be integrated into a specific educational and behavioural programme from an early age, usually within the setting of a special school. Such a setting should also become an invaluable source of support for the families of affected children. Although PDD cannot be cured, about 10% of children with autism will develop a capacity for independent living. A further 50% might be able to achieve semi-independent supported community living. The prognosis is better for those children who, from an early age, have higher scores on IQ (intelligence quotient) testing and more advanced development of speech.

Information Box 5.4e-XXVII

Autism: comments from a Chinese medicine perspective

Scott and Barlow (1999) emphasise that autism can respond well to acupuncture. They describe the common patterns that underlie autism as extreme Qi Deficiency, Lingering Pathogenic Factor (particularly Heat and Phlegm), Kidney Weakness and Disturbances of the Spirit. They also describe brain damage as a separate pattern. Scott and Barlow (1999) suggest that in some cases an extreme fever or immunisation can cause the Shen to be unable to rest in the Heart, either because of extreme Depletion of Qi, or because of Residual Heat in the Heart. In contrast to the conventional view that the social influences on a child have no impact on the development of autism, Scott and Barlow (1999) believe that both shock and the imploded anger that can follow abuse or neglect can also lead to an autistic state.

Dyslexia

'Dyslexia' is a term used to describe a range of distinct conditions all of which have the consequence of difficulty in learning to read despite adequate intelligence and teaching.

Disorders of reading are common, affecting up to 10% of children, and are up to four times as common in boys than in girls. They are more common in children from disadvantaged families. They are associated with disruptive behaviour and other psychiatric disturbance, although these problems may be a result of the educational difficulties and stigmatisation that the child with a disorder of reading very often experiences.

In some children, the main problem appears to be a problem in processing language, and in others the problem lies more in the realm of visual perception. In some cases there may be other developmental problems, such as clumsiness (motor dyspraxia) or hyperactivity. In a very small number, a problem with eye dominance can be demonstrated, and in this minority the child may benefit from the occlusion of one eye for several months.

There is general assent that some cases of dyslexia may have at their root a problem with the communication of information from one side of the brain to another. Scott and Barlow (1999) note that dyslexia is not a significant problem in China, and suggest that there is some evidence to support the fact that Chinese script (which is composed of ideograms) is easier to process by the brain than Roman script. They explain that this is because ideograms allow a word to be identified by its shape rather than by its sound, and so less right-to-left processing is required of the brain.

However, there is no agreed classification system for dyslexia, and no proven medical treatment. The general approach for a child with a disorder of reading is to offer intensive reading support. In most cases the child will learn to read, but difficulties with spelling may persist.

Attention-deficit hyperactivity disorder (ADHD)

Attention-deficit hyperactivity disorder (ADHD) is a disorder of disruptive behaviour, which usually presents in children aged 5–12 years. It is up to four times more common in boys than in girls. Overall, it may affect up to 5% of children, depending on exactly how the condition is defined.

> **Information Box 5.4e-XXVIII**
>
> **Dyslexia: comments from a Chinese medicine perspective**
>
> From a Chinese medicine perspective, Scott and Barlow (1999) describe four imbalances, each of which may be a factor underlying dyslexia. These are; Heat, Phlegm, Qi Deficiency and Kidney Weakness. They explain that with Heat the words all come tumbling out too fast, whereas with Phlegm it seems as if there is a fog inside the head. In the deficient conditions it is as if the child has no energy to string the words together in the correct way.

> **Information Box 5.4e-XXIX**
>
> **Hyperactivity: comments from a Chinese medicine perspective**
>
> From a Chinese medicine perspective, Scott and Barlow (1999) describe four patterns that might account for hyperactivity in a child. These are Heat, Heat and Phlegm, Weakness in the Middle Burner, and Kidney Deficiency. Heat can originate from immunisations, food additives and Toxic Womb Heat.

ADHD is characterised by inappropriate degrees of inattention, impulsiveness and overactivity. On questioning, parents will often say that the child has been restless and a poor sleeper ever since he or she was a small baby. Children with ADHD are accident prone. They become notorious in the nursery or at school for their inability to complete set tasks and their ability to disrupt other children. Language delay and learning difficulties often accompany ADHD.

Some theories suggest that an important contributing factor to ADHD may be food additives in the diet. The Feingold (additive-free) diet is acclaimed by some parents, although there is little conventional evidence to support its proposed benefits. Inconsistent parenting, unrealistic parental expectations and poor housing have also been suggested to be contributing factors.

Treatment should involve meetings with a child psychologist, who might work around family issues and behaviour modification. Reduction of sugar, caffeine and other additives from the diet may be helpful in some cases. Increasingly, children over the age of 7 years are referred to a child psychiatrist for consideration of the prescription of a stimulant drug (most commonly methylphenidate) for a period of 1–2 years. The stimulant drugs paradoxically help the child to focus his or her energies, and can very much improve behaviour and compliance at school. They can help the child to benefit from the behaviour modification as advised by the child psychologist. However, the stimulant drugs do have serious potential side-effects, including growth retardation, insomnia, irritability, headache, thought disorders and the development of tics. On withdrawal of the medication, depression and worsened hyperactivity can develop.

The long-term outlook for children who have been prescribed Ritalin to support them in behaviour-modification programmes is as yet not well understood. Before the introduction of such regimens, affected children tended to continue to do poorly at school and could drift into truancy and antisocial activities.

Tics

A tic is a repetitive movement of a part of the body, usually the head or neck. The tic apparently appears to be purposeful, in that the child has a degree of control over the movement, and it can be repeated by the child on request. However, if the child is asked to refrain from the movement, this can result in mounting discomfort. Common tics include blinking, frowning, sniffing and head flicking. Tics appear to be more frequent when the child is inactive, and can also become more prominent when the child is anxious. They tend to disappear if the child is busy concentrating on performing a task. In most cases the tics are minor and will pass with time. The parents should be reassured, and advised not to draw too much attention to the tic.

A more serious tic disorder is Giles de la Tourette syndrome (Tourette's disorder), in which the child is rarely free of performing a diverse variety of tics and involuntary vocalisations, including hoots, grunts and swear words. This disorder can be extremely embarrassing and socially disabling. Tourette's disorder is very strongly associated with obsessive–compulsive disorder. In a severe case the child may be prescribed major tranquilliser medication.

> **Information Box 5.4e-XXX**
>
> **Tics: comments from a Chinese medicine perspective**
>
> A possible Chinese medicine interpretation of muscular tics could be Wind developing upon a Liver imbalance such as Liver Yin Deficiency. In Tourette's disorder, the imbalance is more profound. The involuntary vocalisations suggest that, in addition to Wind and Liver imbalance, a disturbance involving obstruction of the Heart Orifices such as Phlegm or Heat might also be a factor.

The red flags of the common non-infectious diseases of childhood

Some children with symptoms of non-infectious disease will benefit from referral to a conventional doctor for assessment and/or treatment. Red flags are those symptoms and signs that indicate that referral is to be considered. The red flags of the non-infectious diseases of childhood are described in Table 5.4e-I. This table forms part of the summary on red flags given in Appendix III, which also gives advice on the degree of urgency of referral for each of the red flag conditions listed.

Table 5.4e-I Red Flags 40b – childhood diseases (common non-infectious diseases)

Red Flag	Description	Reasoning
40.1	**Maternal concern**	Any condition in which the parent is very concerned about the health of his or her child is worth referring for a second opinion. The parent is the person who will know the best if something is not right with their child, even if it is not very specific, and it is best to respect this, as small children sometimes do not generate very specific symptoms even when seriously unwell
40.2	**Inconsolable baby**: for more than 3 hours	Although this feature is very common and usually benign, consider referral if the baby is inconsolable, or if unexplained crying (for at least 3 hours) starts in a previously settled baby
40.3	**Childhood cancer**. Red flags include progressive symptoms: weight loss, sweats, poor appetite, an unexplained lump or mass or an enlarged unilateral lymph node (>1.5 cm diameter), recurrent infections, bruising, anaemia and bleeding	Refer any case in which there is a short history of new unexplained symptoms that have arisen within the past weeks to months and which are progressive. Also, refer as a high priority if there are warning features of bone marrow failure
40.12	**Vomiting**: refer if persistent, and either a cause of distress to the child (i.e. not possetting), a cause of dehydration or if projectile	Vomiting is common in children, and is usually self-limiting. In babies, regurgitation of milk is normal, and is not a cause for concern if the child is contented and continuing to gain weight Refer if there are features of dehydration, or if the vomiting is projectile (a feature of pyloric stenosis in newborn babies) Food poisoning and dysentery are notifiable diseases[1]
40.13	**Diarrhoea**: if persistent, and associated with either dehydration, poor weight gain, weight loss or chronic ill-health	Chronic loose stools in a child may signify the presence of an infectious organism, coeliac disease or inflammatory bowel disease Refer as a high priority of dehydration present Food poisoning and dysentery are notifiable diseases[1]
40.14	**Soiling with faeces** (in underwear or bed)	Always refer for diagnosis if persistent and appearing in a previously continent child (could signify constipation with faecal overflow, a developmental problem of the bowel or emotional disturbance)
40.15	**Recurrent or constant intense abdominal pain**: if pain is associated with fever, vomiting, collapse and rigidity and guarding on examination	All these features are signs of the acute abdomen, which in children is most commonly due to appendicitis or a form of bowel obstruction (from a twist or obstruction in a hernia). Urgent surgical assessment is required. All these conditions can spontaneously resolve, but recurrence is likely. Refer for treatment or assessment
40.16	**Recurrent mild abdominal pain**	Features of abdominal pain in children that suggest a more benign (functional) cause include mild pain that is worse in the morning, location around the umbilicus, and pain that is worse with anxiety
40.17	**Jaundice** (yellowish skin, yellow whites of the eyes and maybe dark urine and pale stools)	Jaundice is always of concern in children and babies, with the exception of the mild form of jaundice that can affect the newborn. Refer all cases to ensure serious liver disease is excluded
40.18	**Any new onset of difficulty breathing** (i.e. increased respiratory rate[2]), nocturnal wheeze or noisy breathing) in a small child (<8 years old) Also if there is unexplained sudden blockage of one nostril	Always take a new onset of difficulty breathing in a child seriously and refer for medical assessment to exclude serious disease. Common causes include lower respiratory tract infections, asthma, allergic reactions, inhalation of foreign bodies and congenital heart disease A nostril may suddenly block after the unwitnessed insertion of a foreign body. This is a serious situation, as the foreign body (e.g. a pea) may then become inhaled
40.22	**Features of severe asthma**: at least two of the following: • rapidly worsening breathlessness • increased respiratory rate[2] • reluctance to talk because of breathlessness • need to sit upright and still to assist breathing • cyanosis is a very serious sign	Severe asthma is a potentially life-threatening condition and may develop in someone who previously had no history of severe attacks Urgent referral is required so that medical management of the attack can be instigated. Keep the child as calm as possible while you wait for help to arrive Cyanosis describes the blue colouring that appears when the blood is poorly oxygenated. Unlike the blueness from cold, which only affects the extremities, central cyanosis from poor oxygenation can be seen on the tongue

Continued

Table 5.4e-I Red Flags 40b – childhood diseases (common non-infectious diseases)—Cont'd

Red Flag	Description	Reasoning
40.23	**Bedwetting**: if persisting over the age of 5 years	Consider referral if the child is over 5 years of age, so that physical causes can be excluded and so parents can have access to expert advice
40.24	**Features of vesicoureteric reflux disease (VUR) in a child**: any history of recurrent episodes or a current episode of cloudy urine or burning on urination in a prepubescent child	Urine infections are common in young children but need to be taken seriously, particularly if there is a history of recurrent infections. The small child is more vulnerable to VUR, which means that when the bladder contracts some urine is flushed back towards the kidneys. In the case of infection of the bladder, VUR can lead to infectious organisms causing damage to the delicate structure of the kidney. Sometimes this damage occurs with very few symptoms, but if cumulative and undetected can lead to serious kidney problems and high blood pressure in later life For this reason it is wise to refer all prepubescent children with a history of symptoms of urinary infections to exclude the possibility of VUR
40.25	**Acute testicular pain**: radiates to groin, scrotum or low abdomen	Refer any sudden onset of severe testicular pain (radiates to groin, scrotum or lower abdomen). This could signify inflammation of the testicle (orchitis) or a twist of the testicle (torsion). If the pain is very intense (with collapse and vomiting), refer as an emergency
40.26	**Precocious puberty**: secondary sexual characteristics before the age of 8 years in girls and 9 years in boys	Refer if secondary sexual characteristics begin to appear before the age of 8 years in girls and 9 years in boys so that an endocrine cause can be excluded
40.27	**Delayed puberty**: secondary sexual characteristics not apparent by the age of 15 years in girls and 16 years in boys	Refer if secondary sexual characteristics have not started to appear by the age of 15 years in girls and 16 years in boys. Refer if menstruation has not begun by the time of a girl's 17th birthday (primary amenorrhoea)
40.28	**Epilepsy**: refer any child who has suffered from a suspected blank episode (absence) or seizure	Epilepsy most commonly first presents in childhood, and is more common in children who have experienced febrile convulsions. Early diagnosis is important so that early management can help prevent deleterious effects on education and social development
40.29	**Squint or double vision**: in any child if previously undiagnosed	Refer any child who demonstrates a previously undiagnosed squint. In young children this usually results from a congenital weakness of the external ocular muscles, but needs ophthalmological assessment to prevent long-term inhibition of depth vision. If appearing in older children it may signify a tumour of the brain, pituitary or orbital cavity
40.31	**New onset of difficulty hearing in a child**: lasting >3 weeks	Refer if prolonged, if interfering with social interactions and education, or if associated with pain in the ear or dizziness. Most likely cause is glue ear, a chronic accumulation of mucoid secretions in the middle ear
40.33	**Features of autism**: slow development of speech, impaired social interactions, little imaginative play, obsessional repetitive behaviour	Remember that mild degrees of autism may not be diagnosed until the child reaches secondary school age. Refer if you are concerned that the child is demonstrating impaired social interactions (aloofness), impaired social communication (very poor eye contact, awkward and inappropriate body language) and impairment of imaginative play (play may instead be dominated by obsessional behaviour such as lining up toys or checking), as early diagnosis can result in the child being offered extra educational and psychological support
40.34	• **Sexual or physical abuse:** • unexplained or implausible injuries • miserable withdrawn child • frozen watchfulness • overtly sexualised behaviour in a prepubescent child • vaginal or anal discharge or itch	All these features may have a benign explanation, but if you have any concerns you should take the situation very seriously. In the UK you can start by seeking confidential advice from the NSPCC helpline. If you need to report a case, this should be done via the Child Protection Committee, which is part of the local services team. This is definitely a situation in which you should break your professional obligation of confidentiality.

Table 5.4e-I Red Flags 40b – childhood diseases (common non-infectious diseases)—Cont'd

[1]Notifiable diseases: notification of a number of specified infectious diseases is required of doctors as a statutory duty under the UK Public Health (Infectious Diseases) 1988 Act and the Public Health (Control of Diseases) 1988 Act. The UK Health Protection Agency (HPA) Centre for Infections collates details of each case of each disease that has been notified. This allows analyses of local and national trends. This is one example of a situation in which there is a legal requirement for a doctor to breach patient confidentiality.

Notifiable immunisable diseases	
Measles	Viral hepatitis
Mumps	Poliomyelitis
Rubella	Encephalitis
Whooping cough	Meningitis (viral or bacterial)
Tetanus	Tuberculosis
Diphtheria	Encephalitis

Other notifiable diseases	
Malaria	Scarlet fever
Ophthalmia neonatorum (conjunctivitis in babies within 28 days of birth)	Dysentery and food poisoning
Leptospirosis (Weil's disease)	Cholera
Plague	Anthrax
Typhoid and paratyphoid fevers	Yellow fever
Typhus	Relapsing fever
Rabies	Viral haemorrhagic fever

[2]Categorisation of respiratory rate in children

Age	Normal rate (breaths/min)	Rate if breathless (breaths/min)
Newborn	30–50	>60
Infant	20–40	>50
Young child	20–30	>40
Older child or adult	15–20	>30

Self-test 5.4e

Other common disorders of childhood

1. (i) What are the most important causes of feeding problems in babies under the age of 1 year?
   (ii) If you are treating a baby who is not feeding well, how might you determine whether or not the problem is of a serious nature?
2. An 8-year-old girl has been complaining of recurrent bouts of abdominal pain, which are particularly bad just before she goes to school in the morning. Her mother thinks that the pain started after an episode of flu, for which the child was off school for 3 days. The child says she feels sick with the pain, and that it feels worse around her tummy button. She has had 4 days off school in the past 3 weeks since the pain started. On examination she is reluctant for you to press in the region of the umbilicus, but there is no rebound tenderness.
   (i) Are there any red flags of serious disease in this case history?
   (ii) What are the possible causes of this pain?
3. You are called in the evening by a mother of an 8-year-old boy who you have been treating for asthma for the past few months. Over the past few hours, since a horse ride in the country, the child has been more wheezy and has been coughing frequently. Now the mother says that, despite numerous puffs of the salbutamol inhaler, the child is still having difficulty breathing with ease. He is reluctant to move from the chair, where is he sitting upright. His mother thinks his respiratory rate is over 10 inhalations in 15 seconds (over 40 breaths/minute). She wants you to make an emergency visit. How would you respond?
4. One of your patients telephones to ask if acupuncture could be of any help for her 3-year-old boy. He has been complaining of a sore penis for the past 2–3 days. She describes that now there is a yellowish discharge coming from under the foreskin, and the region of the glans is swollen.
   (i) What is the diagnosis?
   (ii) How would you manage this case?

Answers

1. (i) The most important reasons for feeding problems include:
   - sore nipples, poor milk supply, blocked ducts and mastitis
   - infant colic
   - a neuromuscular problem in the child which affects suckling (rarely)
   - pyloric stenosis (rarely).

   (ii) Although feeding problems can be frustrating for the mother, they are only to be considered a cause for concern if the child is failing to receive the nutrition it requires for healthy growth and development. If the child is miserable or sickly, or is failing to keep up with predicted weight gain or developmental milestones, then you should consider that the feeding problem is of a serious nature.
2. (i) This child has a history that is most consistent with either functional abdominal pain or mesenteric adenitis. There are no warning features of serious disease.
   (ii) Other possible causes that could be borne in mind are constipation and grumbling appendicitis, although you would only consider referral for the latter if her condition worsened significantly, or if fever or vomiting occurred.
3. This child has features of severe asthma. Red flags include the rapid respiratory rate and the need to sit still and upright. Failure to respond to salbutamol is another warning feature. You should insist that the mother call the emergency doctor straight away, as this child is in an unstable state, and should receive emergency medical support (oxygen, nebulised salbutamol and corticosteroid medication) and possibly referral for hospital supervision of treatment. If you wish to visit to support the child with acupuncture, this would be acceptable, but emergency medical support is the priority.
4. (i) This child is suffering from balanitis, which means inflammation of the mucous membranes that underlie the foreskin. In its early stages it is not in itself a reason for referral.
   (ii) Medical management of balanitis is by means of oral antibiotics. From a Chinese viewpoint, this is a case of Damp Heat affecting the Liver Channel, and possibly with an underlying Kidney Deficiency. The child may well benefit from acupuncture to clear Damp Heat and to boost Kidney Qi, while at the same time regularly bathing the region under the foreskin with warm sterile salt solution. You should be particularly alert for progression of the infection if the foreskin is still non-retractile, as this will hinder clearance of the infection. In all cases refer if there is no improvement in 48 hours.

Diseases of the skin, the eye and the ear

6.1

Chapter 6.1a The physiology of the skin, the eye and the ear

LEARNING POINTS

At the end of this chapter you will be able to:

- describe the structure of the layers of the skin and list the functions of the skin
- describe the structure of the eye and explain how it responds to the stimulus of light
- describe the structure of the ear and explain how it responds to the stimuli of sound and altered bodily position.

Estimated time for chapter: 90 minutes.

Introduction

This chapter focuses on the physiology of three of the sensory organs of the body: the skin, the eye and the ear.

The skin is considered as a physiological system in its own right, also known as the 'integumentary system' (a term derived from the word 'integument', which means 'skin'). In conventional practice, diseases of the skin are managed within the medical speciality of dermatology.

The eye and ear are, technically speaking, complex sensory organs that form part of the nervous system. However, in conventional practice the diseases of the eye and the ear are managed within distinct specialities. Eye diseases are managed within the medical speciality of ophthalmology, and ear diseases are managed within the surgical speciality of otorhinolaryngology (meaning the study of the ear, nose and throat). This speciality embraces diseases that relate to two overlapping systems: the nervous system and the respiratory system.

For clarity, in this section the diseases of the skin, eye and ear are considered in separate chapters as if each is an individual system.

The physiology of the skin (the integumentary system)

The functions of the skin

The skin is often described as the largest organ of the body. It may not be obvious immediately that the skin, like many of the deep organs, has a range of complex functions (see Q6.1a-1). The functions of the skin include:

- Protection of the body: the skin provides a mechanical barrier that protects the deeper tissues from mechanical injury, toxins in the environment and radiation from the sun.
- Regulation of body temperature: the skin contributes to the homeostasis of body temperature by means of mechanisms including sweating in the heat and erection of body hair in the cold (goose pimples). The blood vessels in the skin also are very responsive to body temperature – they dilate in the heat and contract in the cold.
- Formation of vitamin D: the skin is the main source of vitamin D, which is essential for the maintenance of the health of the bones. Vitamin D prevents rickets and osteomalacia. It is manufactured in the skin (from a steroid precursor chemical) as a response to the action of sunlight.
- Sensation: the skin forms the boundary between the external environment and the internal environment of the body. The nerve endings in the skin are adapted to sense light, touch, deep pressure, pain and temperature. In this way the skin can communicate to the internal tissues what is going on in the outside world.
- Excretion: the skin is able to excrete unwanted substances through the sweat. It is also able to secrete aromatic chemicals, which give each person a unique smell that contributes to the non-verbal communication between individuals.

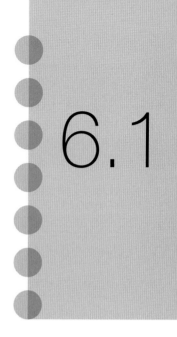

- Absorption: although this function is believed conventionally to be limited, the skin can absorb substances from the external environment. This can be interpreted as another aspect of the sensory role of the skin, allowing the body to respond to what is happening in the outside world.

The structure of the skin

The skin is composed of two thin layers known as the 'epidermis' and the 'dermis'. Throughout the body these two layers rest on a deeper layer of subcutaneous fat. The fascia, which is considered part of the musculoskeletal system, is the silvery fibrous connective layer that underlies the subcutaneous fat and separates it from underlying muscles and bones. This is the tissue that is seen when the skin of animals is removed in the process of food production.

The epidermis is an example of stratified squamous epithelium, whereas the thicker dermis is made up of loose (areolar) and fatty connective tissue. Figure 6.1a-I illustrates the structure of these two delicate layers of the skin and how they rest on the underlying fat. The upper part of the dermis forms folds called 'papillae', and it is these that give rise to characteristic skin markings such as the fingerprint. The bumpiness prevents easy separation of the epidermis and dermis.

Figure 6.1a-II is a more detailed image of the stratified structure of the epidermis. The cells of the epidermis continually multiply from the germinative layer and grow upwards in layers. As they progress upwards the cells become progressively more hardened with the protein keratin. The uppermost layers, the stratum corneum and lucidum, consist of lifeless keratin-stuffed cells, which have a vital protective function. This layer thickens in response to repeated trauma, such as continually occurs to the palms of the hands and soles of the feet. As dead epithelial cells are shed from the skin they are replaced by new cells growing upwards from the germinative layer.

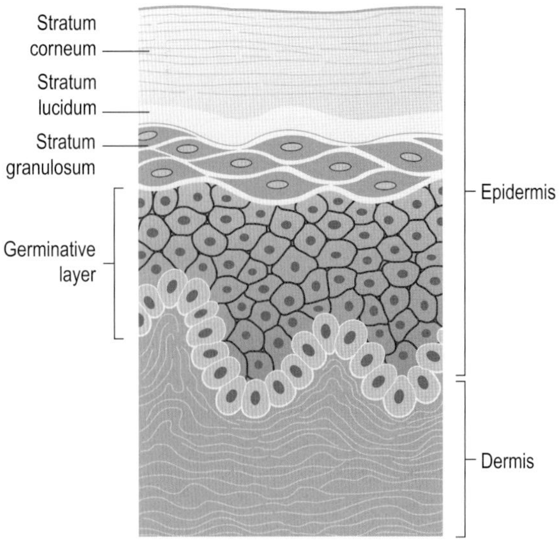

Figure 6.1a-II • The epidermis, illustrating the stratified squamous epithelial nature of this tissue.

The pigment called melanin (dark brown), also produced by the cells of the epidermal layer, gives the skin its colour. Clusters of deeply pigmented germinative cells form moles and freckles.

The sweat glands and the sebaceous glands originate in the looser areolar tissue of the dermis. The sweat glands are shaped like a coiled tube. They excrete a watery fluid onto the skin via a duct that passes through the epidermis. The watery fluid contains waste products. However, the most important function of the sweat is temperature control rather than excretion of wastes.

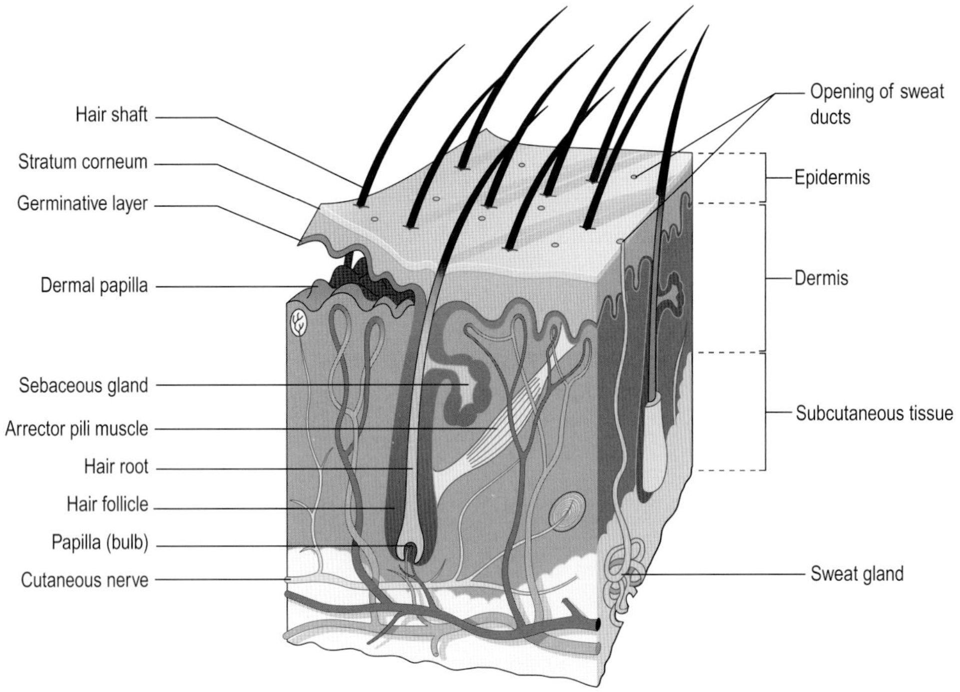

Figure 6.1a-I • A section of the skin, showing how the epidermis rests upon the dermis, which in turn rests on a layer of subcutaneous fat.

The sebaceous glands secrete an oily substance into the hair follicles and thence onto the skin. The sebum has a protective role in that it waterproofs the skin and hair, and helps to keep them soft and pliable. It is also believed to help keep skin infections at bay.

The hair follicles are specialised tubules of germinative epithelium that generate the cells and the protein keratin, which will form a strand of hair. A hair develops at the base of a hair follicle, where numerous keratin-containing skin cells are compacted together. As the skin cells die, the keratin remains and this is pushed out of the follicle to form a single hair. The arrectores pilorum muscles are tiny smooth muscle structures that attach the base of a hair follicle to connective tissue fibres in the dermis. When the muscle contracts, the hair becomes erect and 'stands on end'.

The nails are also composed of keratinised dead skin cells. They grow out of the nail bed, which is an area of tissue lined with the rapidly dividing epidermal skin cells of the germinative layer.

The dermis is also richly supplied with nerve endings and blood capillaries. A healthy blood supply gives the skin a reddish pink glow. Bile salts (yellow/green) from the liver and carotenes (red/yellow) obtained from the diet also contribute to skin colour (see Q6.1a-2-Q6.1a-4).

The role of the skin in the control of temperature

It is vital that the body maintains a steady temperature because the complex metabolic processes of the body work best within a very narrow temperature range. If the temperature rises, the metabolic processes speed up, and if it drops they slow down. If the metabolic rate becomes too fast or slow, the fine balance between the different chemical reactions in the body can be lost and ill-health will result, as evidenced in someone suffering either from a prolonged high fever or from hypothermia.

The skin plays only a minor role in heat production. The main heat-producing tissues are the skeletal muscles, the liver and the digestive organs. Nevertheless, the contraction of the arrectores pilorum muscles in the skin does also generate a certain amount of heat. These tiny but numerous muscles also cause the body hair to stand on end, a response which will tend to conserve heat in a furry animal.

However, the most important physiological mechanism for heat conservation in the human is the constriction of the capillary network in the skin. This is mediated by the sympathetic nervous system. When vasoconstriction occurs, the blood is held deep in the body, and the skin will start to feel cold, and look pale or even blue. A similar response occurs in acutely frightening or stressful situations.

The role of the skin in the loss of heat is also very important. By far the largest proportion of body heat is lost from the skin. This heat loss is minimised by vasoconstriction and the erection of body hair. Body fat and layers of clothing also reduce this loss of body heat. In contrast, the loss of heat is increased by the physiological responses of vasodilatation and sweating.

Dilatation of the blood vessels in the skin raises the surface temperature of the skin, and so heat loss to the outside environment is increased. Vasodilatation is mediated by the parasympathetic nervous system, and is controlled by the hypothalamus. Sweating, which occurs when the body temperature rises by a fraction of a degree, causes the skin to become moist. Moisture requires energy (heat) to evaporate, and thus in hot, dry weather the evaporation of the sweat has a cooling effect (see Q6.1a-5 and Q6.1a-6).

Information Box 6.1a-I

The skin: comments from a Chinese medicine perspective

In Chinese medicine, the skin and body hair are considered to be controlled by the Lungs, and sweating by the Heart. Other Chinese Organs play a part in the healthy function of the skin as it is conventionally understood. The Spleen is attributed to the control of healthy flesh and muscles. Temperature control depends on a healthy balance of Yin and Yang. This function of the skin might be attributed to the Kidney (in particular the Ming Men) and Triple Burner Organs. The production of vitamin D would seem to correspond to a function of the Kidney Organ.

The physiology of the eye

The eye and the optic nerve pathways in the brain

The eyes are sensory organs that are specialised to respond to the stimulus of light. The eyes contain the cell bodies and nerve endings of the sensory nerves known as the 'optic nerves' (second cranial nerves). Optic nerve fibres carry visual messages to the brain to a control centre in the thalamus. From here the information is taken further back via connector neurons to the visual areas in the occipital lobe at the back of the brain. Here the complex processing necessary for visual perception takes place. Before the optic nerve fibres reach the thalamus, some of the fibres cross to the opposite side. This crossing point, known as the 'optic chiasm', is adjacent to the site of the pituitary stalk (overlying the sphenoid bone of the skull). This explains why pituitary tumours often result in visual disturbance. Figure 6.1a-III illustrates the optic nerves and their pathways from the eyes, which cross before they reach the occipital lobe of the brain.

Although the eyes are situated at the front of the head, the information that they sense is processed at the back of the brain. Because of the optic chiasm, information from each eye is sent to each half of the occipital visual area. This allows for the 'binocular vision', the facility that gives what we see an appearance of depth.

The structure of the eye

The eye has a very specialised structure that allows it to perform the function of focusing and sensing visual images. This structure is illustrated in simplified form in Figure 6.1a-IV.

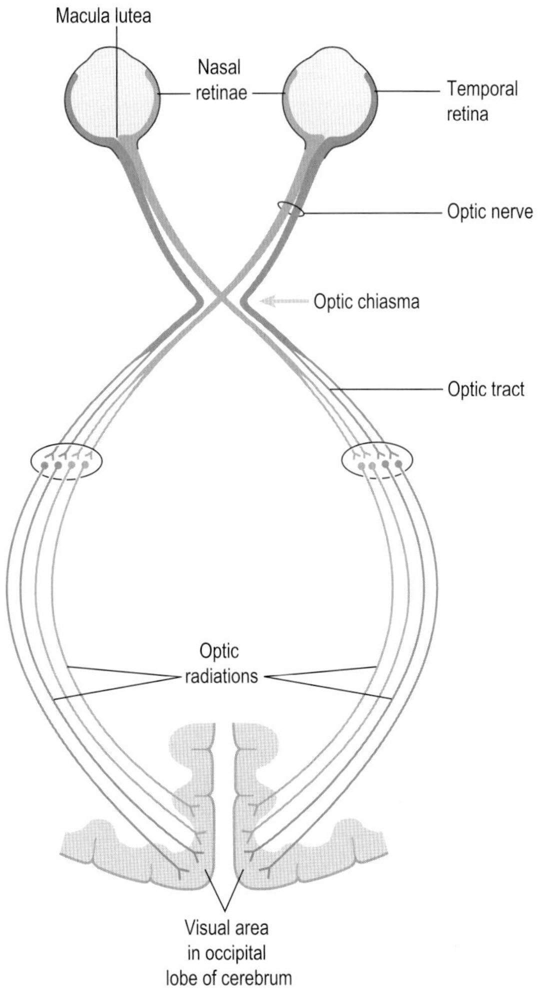

Figure 6.1a-III • The optic nerves and their pathways.

The outer lining of the eye is composed of three distinct layers. The outermost layer, the sclera, is dense and glistening white in colour. The sclera becomes transparent anteriorly; this clear area is called the 'cornea'. The next layer, the choroid, is dark in colour. This blends into the ciliary body and the iris at the front of the eye. The deepest layer is the light-sensitive retina. The retina is not present anteriorly, as it stops at the border of the ciliary body. The lens in the eye is responsible for focusing the light that enters the cornea so that it forms an 'image' on the retina, akin to the way a camera lens focuses light onto a film. The space that lies between the lens and the cornea is called the 'anterior chamber'. This chamber contains a watery fluid called the 'aqueous humour' (in this situation the term 'humour' means 'fluid'). The space in the body of the eyeball behind the lens is called the 'posterior chamber'. This chamber contains a jelly-like fluid called the 'vitreous (glass-like) humour'.

The ciliary body is responsible for suspending the lens in the correct position in the eye. The smooth muscle of the ciliary body controls the stretching and relaxation of the lens. This muscle control of the curvature of the lens enables the eye to alter its focus so that both distant and close objects can be seen clearly.

The iris controls the amount of light that enters the eye, in a similar way to the aperture of a camera. The smooth muscle fibres in the iris contract and relax to vary the diameter of the pupil, the central hole in the iris. The pupil tends to contract in response to bright light, and also when the eye is required to focus on a close object. The colour of the iris depends on the amount of brown and green pigment it contains. The amount and composition of these pigments is genetically determined.

The retina contains specialised sensory nerve cell bodies called 'rods' and 'cones'. These contain a light- and colour-sensitive pigment which alters in structure in response to light of different wavelengths. Each rod and cone has a long nerve axon, which sweeps backwards and leaves the eye within the optic nerve. The rods play an important role in the vision of low-intensity light, and it is thus the rods that enable night

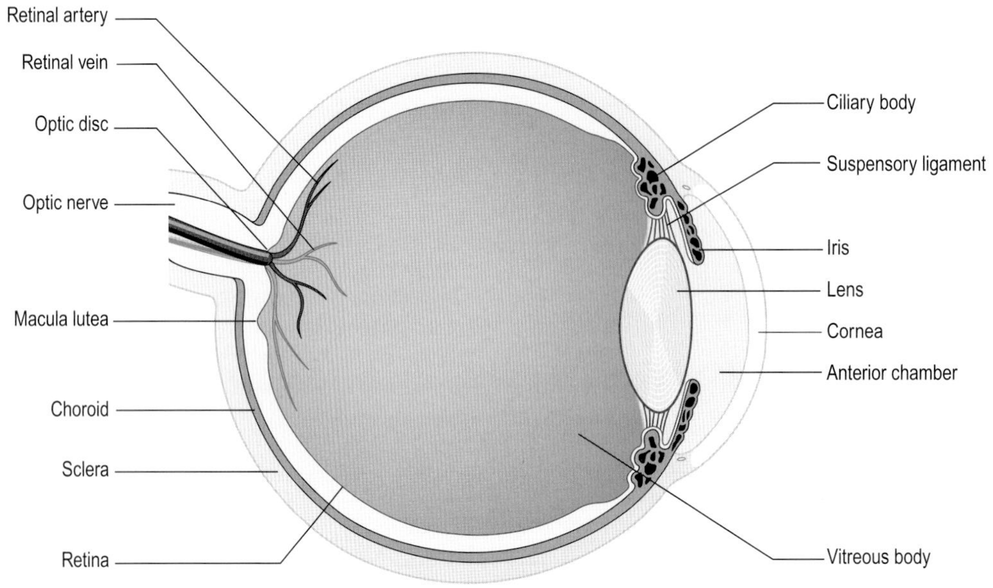

Figure 6.1a-IV • Cross-section of the eye, showing the three layers to its wall and the lens.

vision. They are not sensitive enough to distinguish between lights of different wavelengths (i.e. of different colour).

The cones are sensitive to different colours of light, but do not respond to light of low intensity. This is why it is not possible to distinguish colours in a darkened room.

The blind spot (optic disc) is the point at which all these nerve fibres converge to form the optic nerve. It is a tiny area of the retina that is devoid of rods and cones. Therefore, it is literally a blind spot, as it cannot respond to the light that falls on it. The macula lutea (yellow spot) is the region of the retina that holds the most dense concentration of sensory cell bodies and is the region that responds to light coming from the centre of the field of vision. It is at the macula where fine detail and bright clear colours are distinguished.

The globe of the eye sits embedded within fatty tissue in the bony orbit. The optic nerve extends from the back of each eye to pass posteriorly through the sphenoid bone towards the optic chiasm (optic nerve crossing) within the skull. Six strips of muscle extend from the walls of the orbit to attach to the sclera of each eye. These are the extrinsic or extraocular muscles of the eye. All these structures hold the eye in place (Figure 6.1a-V).

In thyroid eye disease, the eyes become pushed forward so that the eyelids appear to retract. In severe cases, the eyelids can no longer fully close. This is the result of excessive growth of the supportive fatty tissue in the orbit, which is stimulated by an autoantibody that appears in some cases of Graves' disease (see Q6.1a-7-Q6.1a-10).

The physiology of sight

The lens enables an 'image' of the outside world to fall on the retina. For this to be possible for all objects in the field of vision, whether they be close or distant, the lens has to alter

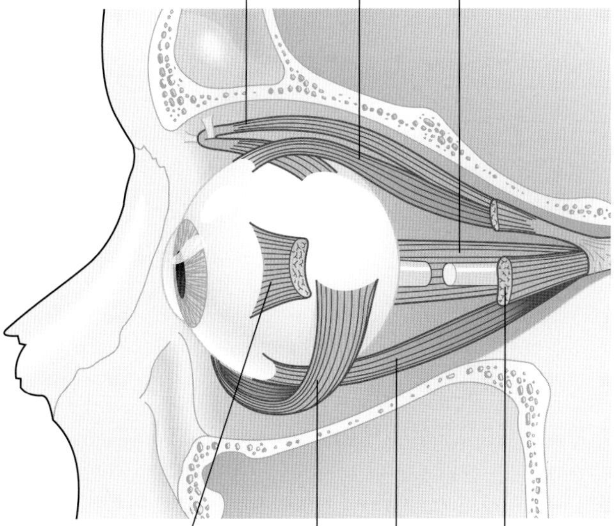

Figure 6.1a-V • The extrinsic muscles that hold the eye in the bony orbit.

in shape to allow a clear image of the viewed object to be formed at the retina. Simply speaking, the lens needs to be fat (bulging) in shape to focus a near object and thin (stretched) to focus a distant object. In a healthy eye, when the ciliary muscle is relaxed, the lens is stretched so that it can focus on distant objects without any effort. The ciliary muscle has to work to contract so that the bulging lens can allow the eye to focus on close objects, and this is why close work can tire the eyes.

The eye has to make two other adjustments to enable close vision. First, constriction of the pupils takes place. This reaction enables only a thin beam of light to pass through the lens. This aids the focusing of the image because a narrow beam of light is easier to focus. This principle is used in a pinhole camera. Secondly, the eyeballs converge inwards when viewing a close object. When extreme, convergence causes the viewer to appear cross-eyed. Convergence allows the image of the object being viewed to fall onto the centre of each retina. Without convergence the viewer would experience double vision.

In distance vision (objects more than 6 metres away) constriction of the pupils and convergence are not necessary, and also, as mentioned, the ciliary muscle becomes fully relaxed. It follows from this that the most restful aspect of vision is distance vision (e.g. when gazing on a countryside scene), as none of the three adjustments for close vision are required.

Each eye receives slightly different images, and the differences are more pronounced for close objects. The visual centre of the occipital lobe of the cerebrum is important in the interpretation of the two slightly different images that come from each retina, thereby giving the viewer an appreciation of the distance of a viewed object. The ability to visually appreciate distances is called 'stereoscopic vision' (see Q6.1a-11).

The extraocular muscles and accessory organs of the eye

The six strips of skeletal muscle that form the extrinsic muscles of the eye guide the coordinated movements of the eyeballs (see Figure 6.1a-V). These movements, which are upwards, downwards, sideways and rotatory, are usually coordinated so that the two eyes move together. Figure 6.1a-VI illustrates the extrinsic muscles of the eye in the orbit and the muscles which control the movements of the eyelids. One of these muscles, the levator palpebrae, lifts the eyelid when it contracts, while the other muscle, orbicularis oculi, because its fibres run circularly around the eyelids, closes the eyelid when it contracts. Figure 6.1a-VI also shows how the conjunctiva forms a protective sac behind the upper and lower eyelids (see Q6.1a-12).

The eyebrows, eyelids and conjunctiva are adapted to provide mechanical protection for the eye. The lacrimal gland is a specialised organ for producing the tears. Tears are constantly produced by this gland (Figure 6.1a-VII) to lubricate the conjunctiva. Tears drain away via tiny channels called 'canaliculi' to the nasolacrimal duct (tear duct), and thence to the nose. This is why a watery discharge from the nose frequently accompanies an episode of crying (see Q6.1a-13).

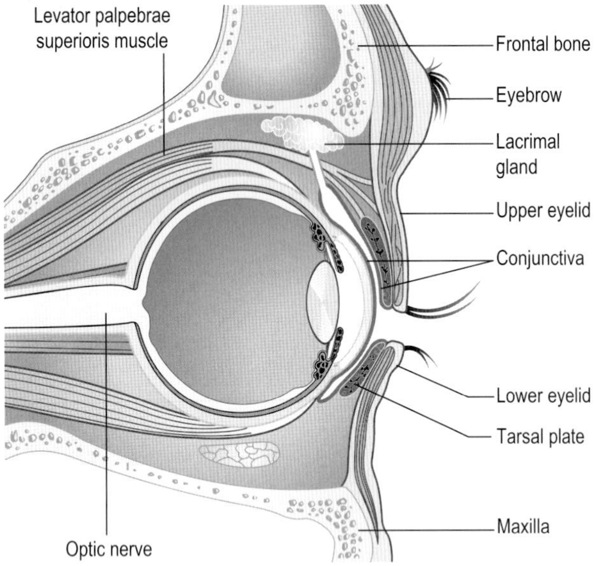

Figure 6.1a-VI • The position of the eye in the orbit and the accessory structures of the eye.

Information Box 6.1a-II

The eye: comments from a Chinese medicine perspective

In Chinese medicine, the Liver is the Organ that opens into the eyes. The Liver Blood moistens and nourishes the eye and gives it the capacity to see. However, Maciocia (1989) explains that many other Yin and Yang organs affect the eye. In particular, Kidney Essence and the Heart Organ are important in maintaining the health of the eyes.

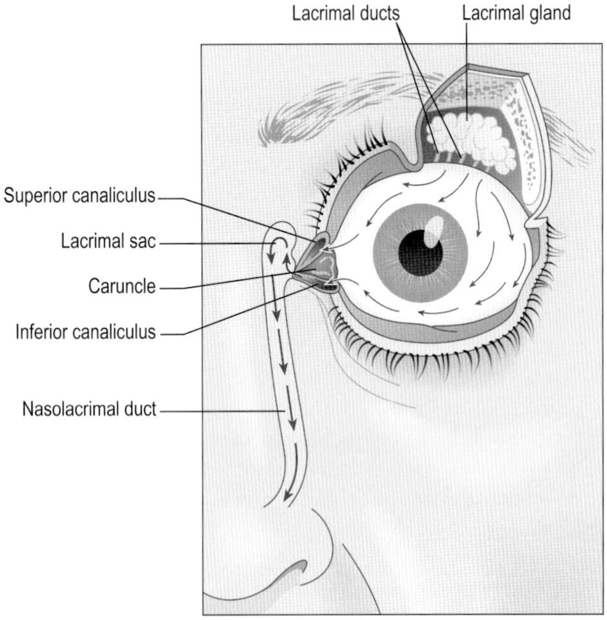

Figure 6.1a-VII • The position of the lacrimal gland and the tear duct.

The physiology of the ear

The functions of the ear

The ear is the sensory organ responsible for hearing. The ear is also an important sensory organ in the control of balance. The nerve impulses leave the ear via the auditory or vestibulocochlear nerve (eighth cranial nerve), which passes from the ear to the brain through a tiny hole in the temporal bone of the skull. Impulses from this nerve are transmitted via control centres in the brainstem and the mid-brain to the auditory area of the cerebral hemispheres (for the perception of sound) and the cerebellum (for the control of balance).

The structure of the ear

The structure of the ear can be considered in three parts: the outer, or external, ear; the middle ear; and the inner ear. This structure is illustrated in Figure 6.1a-VIII.

The external ear consists of the pinna (auricle), the auditory canal (acoustic meatus) and the tympanic membrane (eardrum). The main purpose of the external ear is to provide a protective opening for the delicate inner structures of the ear. The hair- and wax-lined auditory canal protects the eardrum from trauma, foreign bodies and infection. The pinna also plays a role in directing sound waves into the auditory canal, although it is more obviously adapted for this purpose in species such as dogs, cats and rabbits.

The middle ear is a chamber lined with respiratory epithelium, which contains three tiny interlinked bones (ossicles), known as the malleus (hammer), incus (anvil) and stapes (stirrup). The ossicles provide a link between the eardrum (tympanic membrane) and another membrane that separates the middle from the inner ear (the oval window). The purpose of the ossicles is to transmit the sound vibrations that strike the eardrum through to the cochlea of the inner ear. Tiny movements of the oval window lead to vibrations within the fluid (perilymph) that bathes the membranous cochlea (Figure 6.1a-IX). The largest ossicle, the malleus, can be seen through the eardrum when the eardrum is visualised by means of the hand-held otoscope (Figure 6.1a-X).

From the perspective of the development of the ear in the embryo, the link that the middle ear has with the respiratory system becomes more clear. In the embryo, the middle ear forms from an upward pouching of the nasopharynx, whereas the inner ear develops outwards from the primitive nervous tissue. The middle ear and the interlinked mastoid air cells are lined with ciliated respiratory epithelium. The air that they contain is in direct communication with the air in the nasopharynx. This explains why respiratory infections can so readily involve the middle ear and lead to deafness and earache.

The spaces of the inner ear contain two interlinked fluid-filled membranous sacs which, like the middle ear, are safely protected, being bathed in fluid (perilymph) within bony cavities in the temporal bone of the skull. The first chamber, the

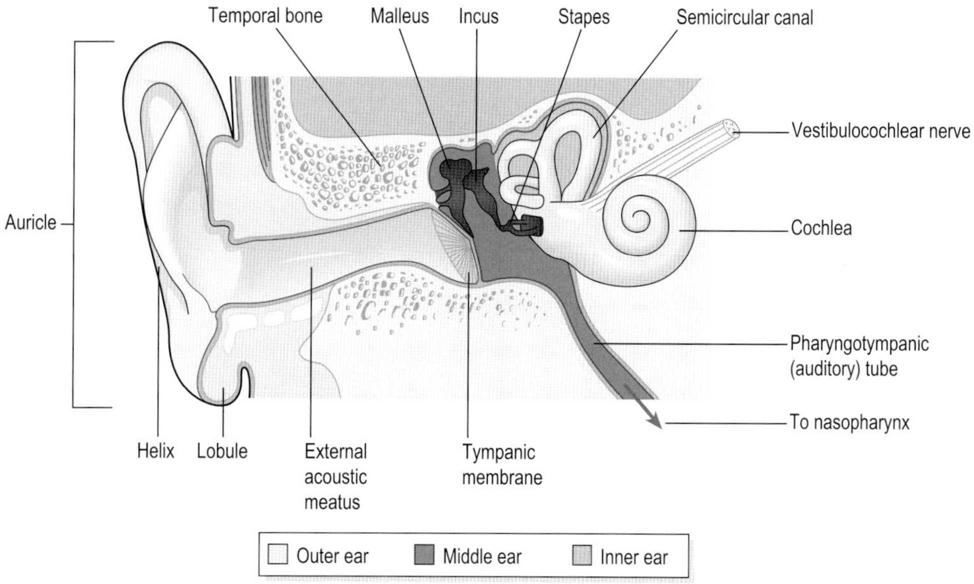

Figure 6.1a-VIII • The structure of the three parts of the ear.

cochlea, is spiral in form and contains fluid called 'endolymph'. The cochlea is responsible for the interpretation of sound vibrations (Figure 6.1a-XI).

Within the cochlea, the spiral organ of Corti lies along its length and is fully immersed in endolymph fluid. This tiny structure consists of a side-by-side arrangement of sensory nerve bodies, which are able to respond to sound vibrations. Messages are sent via nerve axons to auditory centres in the brain, where they can be interpreted as sound. Sound waves of different frequencies (corresponding to sounds of different pitch) stimulate different cells, and so pitch can be distinguished by the ear. Therefore, the organ of Corti is to the ear and hearing as the rods and the cones are to the eye and sight.

The second chamber of the inner ear consists of three semicircular canals, which sit in three different planes at right angles to each other. The semicircular canals are in direct communication with the cochlea, and, like the cochlea, also contain a membranous sensory organ, which is bathed in perilymph fluid. Movement of the head leads to fluid waves in the endolymph within the semicircular canals which are interpreted to allow perception of the head's position in space.

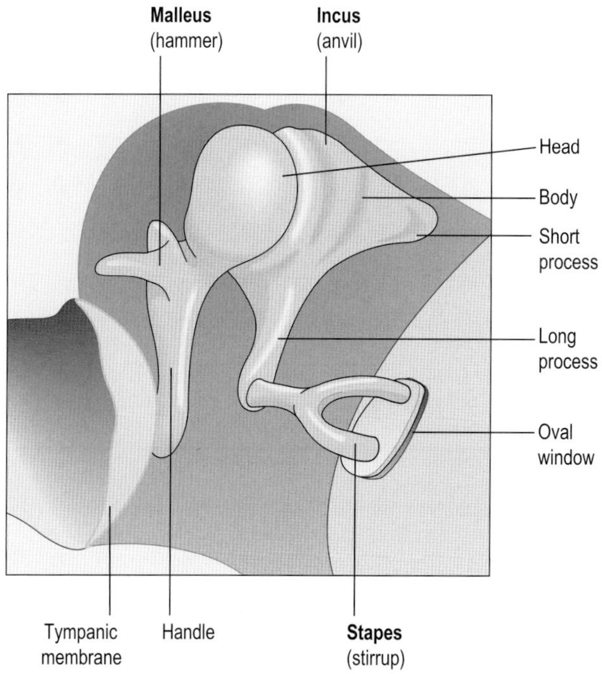

Figure 6.1a-IX • The structures of the middle ear.

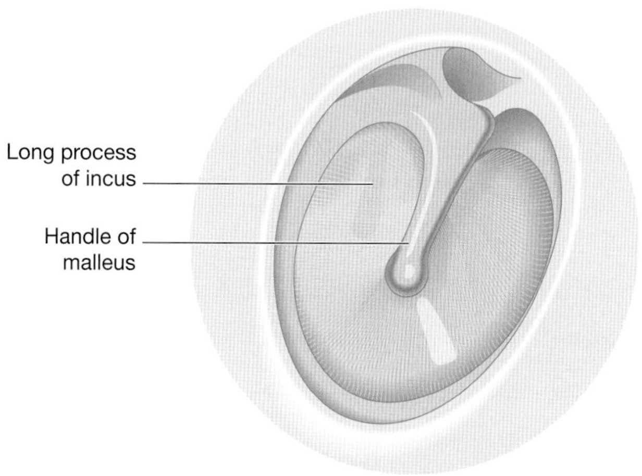

Figure 6.1a-X • Otoscopic view of the eardrum, showing the handle of the malleus and a shadow formed by the incus.

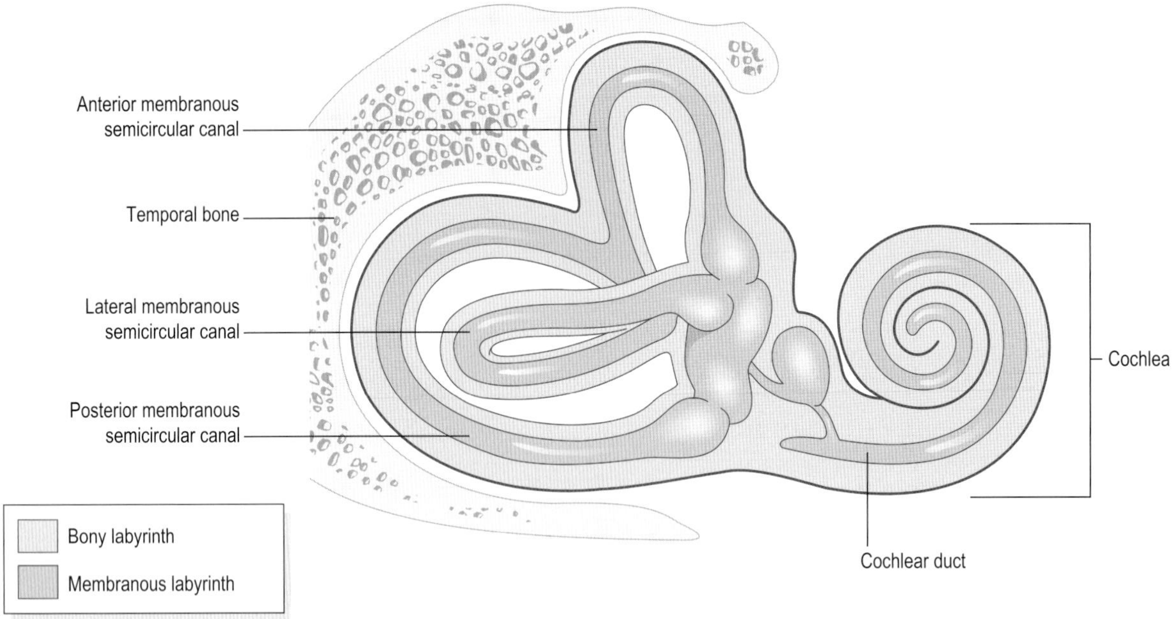

Figure 6.1a-XI • The structures of the inner ear.

The semicircular canals provide important sensory information to aid the maintenance of balance. This information is processed, together with visual information and sensory information from the large joints of the feet and leg, in the cerebellum. As the head moves into a new position, particular waves of fluid movement are set up in the three canals, which are then sensed by sensory cells in the dilated ends of the semicircular canals. This sensory information can be interpreted in the brain in terms of the position and rate of movement of the head (see Q6.1a-14-Q6.1a-19).

Information Box 6.1a-III

The ear: comments from a Chinese medicine perspective

From a Chinese medicine perspective, the Kidney Organ opens into the ears. Maciocia (1989) states that, if the Kidneys are weak, hearing may be impaired and there may be tinnitus (ringing in the ears). He also describes that the Heart has an influence on hearing, with some types of tinnitus resulting from Heart Qi Deficiency.

Self-test 6.1a

The physiology of the skin, the eye and the ear

1. Describe the role of the skin in:
   (i) temperature regulation
   (ii) the health of the bones
   (iii) protection against disease.
2. What are the three layers of the eye? Describe how each of these layers is modified anteriorly to enable the eye to focus the light that enters it.
3. What are the three parts of the ear? Describe how sound waves travel through these three parts to lead to a sensory stimulus in the nerve fibres of the vestibulocochlear (auditory) nerve. Describe how a change in head position will also give rise to a sensory stimulus in the nerve fibres of this nerve.

Answers

1. (i) The skin contributes to temperature regulation in three main ways: conservation of heat (provision of a fatty layer, vasoconstriction and erect body hair), production of heat (piloerection) in the cold, and loss of heat (vasodilatation and sweating) in the heat.
   (ii) The skin contributes to the health of the bones because, in the presence of sunlight, it is the site of manufacture of vitamin D, which is an essential vitamin in calcium metabolism.
   (iii) The skin protects against disease by being a physical barrier against trauma. toxins, microorganisms and radiation. The stratified squamous keratinised epithelium is specialised to protect against wear and tear. The waxy coating of sebum has an additional fungicidal and bactericidal effect.
2. The three layers of the eye are the sclera, the choroid and the retina.
   The sclera forms the cornea anteriorly. This is the transparent window of the eye.
   The choroid forms the ciliary body and the iris anteriorly. The ciliary body suspends the lens between the anterior and posterior chambers of the eye. By contraction and relaxation, it can vary the accommodation of the eye. The iris provides a variable aperture to control the amount of light that enters the eye.
   The retina is discontinued anteriorly, stopping just behind the ciliary body.

3. The three parts to the ear are the external ear, the middle ear and the inner ear.
   Sound waves are funnelled into the external ear by means of the pinna. The sound travels down the short external auditory meatus to the eardrum. Vibration of the eardrum is transmitted and amplified by the three ossicles in the middle ear to the membrane of the oval window. Vibration of the oval window sets up fluid waves in the perilymph of the cochlea. This, in turn, causes vibration of the endolymph, which bathes the organ of Corti. The organ of Corti contains sensory nerve cells, which transform these fluid movements into sensory messages, which are then sent down the vestibulocochlear nerve.
   Movements of the head cause fluid movements in the perilymph and endolymph of the semicircular canals. These movements stimulate sensory nerve endings, which also respond by sending sensory messages down the vestibulocochlear nerve.

Chapter 6.1b The investigation of the skin, the eye and the ear

LEARNING POINTS

At the end of this chapter you will:

- be able to recognise the most important tests that are used for the investigation of diseases of the skin, the eye and the ear
- understand what a patient might experience when having to undergo any one of these tests.

Estimated time for chapter: 40 minutes.

Introduction

The diseases of the skin, eye and ear are managed within the distinct specialties of dermatology, ophthalmology and otorhinolaryngology (ear, nose and throat), respectively.

Investigation of disorders of the skin includes:

- a detailed inspection of the skin rash, including exposure to a Wood's light
- culture and examination of samples taken by swab from the area of the rash
- examination of skin scrapings and nail clippings
- examination of a skin biopsy
- patch testing for allergies
- a physical examination to exclude underlying medical conditions
- blood tests to exclude underlying medical conditions.

Investigation of disorders of the eye includes:

- examination of visual acuity using Snellen charts
- examination of the visual fields
- examination of colour vision
- examination of the eye movements
- examination of the structure of the eye by means of a hand-held ophthalmoscope
- examination of the structure of the eye by means of a slit lamp
- examination of the intraocular pressure by means of a slit lamp and tonometry
- examination of the blood flow to the retina using fluorescein angiography
- imaging tests, including ultrasound, computed tomography (CT) and magnetic resonance imaging (MRI)
- electrophysiological tests
- culture and examination of samples taken by swab from the eye.

Investigation of disorders of the ear includes:

- visual inspection of the external ear and eardrum
- clinical assessment of hearing
- testing of hearing by means of audiometry
- testing of the flexibility of the middle ear by means of impedance tympanometry
- electrophysiological tests.

These investigations are considered below briefly in turn.

Investigation of skin disorders

Inspection of the skin rash

Pattern recognition is crucial in the assessment of skin disorders. A skilled dermatologist will be experienced in the recognition of the variety of ways in which skin disorders can manifest. Some skin disorders have such a characteristic appearance that once the rash is seen in a patient the doctor can be sure of the diagnosis. A physical sign that points to only one possible diagnosis is described as 'pathognomic' (meaning that the sign itself leads to the knowledge of the underlying pathology).

Inspection of the skin should be thorough and systematic. All parts of the body should be examined to look for aspects of the rash that may not have been discovered by the patient. The skin may then be viewed under a hand-held microscope called a 'dermoscope', which can reveal subtle changes to the skin markings not clearly visible to the naked eye. The rash may also be illuminated using ultraviolet light from a Wood's lamp. This light causes some rashes to fluoresce, and can allow pigmented rashes to be viewed with more clarity.

Culture and examination of samples taken by swab

If the cause of the rash is believed to be infective, the rash, or its discharge, may be swabbed, and the swab sent for microbiological analysis.

Examination of skin scrapings and nail clippings

Skin scrapings and nail clippings are samples that can be obtained painlessly. Microbiological examination of these samples can reveal fungal infection and infestation by scabies mites.

Examination of a skin biopsy

Skin biopsy is a very important technique in the diagnosis of skin disorders. If the problem is small and localised (e.g. a worrying mole), a biopsy can both treat the condition by removing it and generate a sample for examination. This approach, known as 'excisional biopsy', ideally is performed in such a way that the diseased area is completely removed, with no portion left remaining. A wide excision may be required to ensure full removal of a suspected skin cancer such as a melanoma. If only a small ellipse of skin is removed, the wound can be sutured so that the resulting scar is almost invisible. However, a wide excision may require a graft of skin from another part of the body (usually the outer thigh) to permit full healing of the area from which the section of skin was removed.

If the skin rash is more extensive, an incisional biopsy can be performed to remove a long ellipse of skin from the edge of the rash. As is the case with excisional biopsy, the resulting wound will require closure by sutures. Examination of the incisional biopsy should reveal both normal and affected skin, and thus allow comparison of the two.

A punch biopsy removes a fine column of affected skin by means of a tubular hollow sampling blade. This leaves a tiny hole, which may require a single stitch to stem bleeding.

Patch testing for allergies

Patch testing is used to test for the sensitivity to various allergens that can result in contact dermatitis (contact eczema). The test involves holding diluted samples of a battery of common allergens against a flat area of skin (usually the back) for up to 48 hours by means of an adhesive strip of 'patches'. The development of a thickened red area of skin under one of the patches is indicative of a sensitivity to that allergen. Allergens that commonly cause positive reactions in the patch test include nickel, rubber and colophony (a common constituent of sticking plasters).

Patch testing is a specific test for contact eczema. The aim is to exclude a delayed allergic reaction (type 4 hypersensitivity) which manifests in dermatitis/eczema (redness, localised swelling and itch) after 2 days or more of exposure to the allergen.

Prick or scratch tests are allergy tests that are aimed at excluding the more immediate allergic reaction that leads to urticaria, oedema and asthma (type 1 hypersensitivity). In prick or scratch testing, a diluted sample of allergen is allowed to penetrate under the epidermis via the prick or the scratch, and the skin is examined for the appearance of a characteristic wheal. This reaction tends to develop within seconds to minutes if the test is positive. Allergens that are commonly found to lead to positive reactions in prick or scratch testing include animal dandruff, pollen, and dietary constituents such as egg and nuts.

Physical examination to exclude underlying medical conditions

Dermatologists have a thorough grounding in clinical medicine. If a rash is found that indicates a possible medical condition as the underlying cause, the dermatologist will proceed to examine the patient for other features of that disease.

Blood tests to exclude underlying medical conditions

Blood tests may be ordered to exclude a suspected underlying medical diagnosis. For example, the blood may be tested for autoantibodies if an autoimmune condition such as systemic lupus erythematosus (SLE) is suspected as the cause of the rash.

Investigation of eye disorders

Often, eye disorders are first picked up during examination by an optician. The optician routinely tests for clear, unrestricted sight by means of tests for visual acuity, the integrity of the visual fields, colour vision and the eye movements. The optician will also examine the internal structure of the eye by means of a hand-held ophthalmoscope.

A hospital ophthalmologist will also perform these investigations, but also has access to other powerful tools of examination, including the slit lamp, tonometry, fluorescein angiography and imaging tests.

Examination of visual acuity

'Visual acuity' (acuteness) is the medical term used to describe the ability of the eye to see a clear image of the viewed object. A normal level of acuity depends on the health of the cornea, lens, vitreous humour, retina and the optic pathways. However, even in a healthy eye, acuity is always limited by the size of the image that lands on the retina. It makes sense that the smaller the image is, the less clearly its features can be seen. This is because the different aspects of an image that falls on the retina simply cannot be distinguished if they are smaller than the size of single cones on the retinal surface.

Acuity can be tested simply by means of the Snellen chart, probably the most familiar test associated with the optician. The Snellen chart consists of rows of letters (or pictures for those patients who are unable to read) of progressively decreasing height. The patient is placed at a fixed distance from the chart and is asked, for each eye in turn, what is the smallest size of letter that he or she can read with confidence. This is then compared with what is known to be a normal and healthy level of acuity.

The optician will then proceed to explore to what extent correcting the vision by means of a lens will improve the acuity. The degree to which a lens can correct the vision depends on the exact cause of the impairment in acuity. If the problem is due totally to a problem in the focusing of the image by the lens in the eye, glasses or contact lens should be able to offer the patient a return to normal visual acuity. If, however, the problem is due, for example, to cataract or retinal damage, glasses may not be able to improve vision very much.

Examination of the visual fields

The 'visual field' is the term used to describe the extent of the view from each eye when the person is looking straight ahead. In health, even when looking straight ahead, movement that occurs almost to the side of the head can be detected because of the extent of the visual field. The visual field is less extensive to the medial side of the eye because the bridge of the nose gets in the way. However, objects can be seen when they are held almost at a right angle to the direction of the gaze on the lateral side of the eye.

There is a small area of the visual field, slightly lateral to the area on which the eye focuses, in which the image of the object becomes less distinct. This area is the blind spot, and corresponds to the area on the retina overlying the origin of the optic nerve, known as the optic disc.

Mapping of the visual fields and the blind spot can reveal restrictions that are characteristic of certain diseases, including chronic simple glaucoma and damage to the optic nerve chiasm by pituitary tumours.

Examination of colour vision

Colour blindness can be diagnosed by means of pictures that are made up of many dots of different colours. Colour blindness will prevent an observer from distinguishing certain aspects of the pictures.

Examination of the eye movements

The eye movements are assessed by asking the patient to follow a moving object in the field of vision while keeping the head still. During the test the examiner watches for divergence or convergence of the eyes, and questions the patient about any episodes of double vision. This examination can reveal the presence of a squint (strabismus).

Examination of the structure of the eye by ophthalmoscope

The ophthalmoscope is a hand-held instrument through which the examining practitioner can focus on the various internal structures of the eye, ideally with the patient in a darkened room. The ophthalmoscope should allow inspection of the cornea, the iris and lens, the vitreous and aqueous humours, the pattern of vessels on the retina, and the optic nerve head (the disc).

Ophthalmoscopic examination of the retina is the only means by which the neurologist can make a direct, but non-invasive, inspection of part of the nervous system. In addition to visualisation of the optic nerve head, examination with an ophthalmoscope can reveal the characteristic changes that occur in a wide range of eye diseases, including cataract, vitreous detachment, retinal detachment, diabetic retinopathy and the changes that result from high blood pressure.

Examination of the structure of the eye by means of the slit lamp

The slit lamp (or biomicroscope) allows the examining practitioner to obtain a high-quality view of the external and internal structures of the eye. Prior to a slit lamp examination, a few drops of a mydriatic (a drug that causes widening of the pupils) are placed into the patient's eyes. This can have the effect of causing blurred vision until the drug wears off, and so the patient is advised not to drive until this side-effect has faded. Once the mydriatic has taken effect, the patient sits in a chair in a darkened room and, to ensure immobility, places his or her head against a headrest attached to the slit lamp. The magnifying lens of the slit lamp can then be focused on the various structures of each eye in turn. A specialised 'dye' called fluorescein can be instilled into the eye to reveal scratches and ulcers on the corneal surface. These damaged areas fill up with fluorescein, and so fluoresce green when viewed through the slit lamp.

Examination of the intraocular pressure by means of the slit lamp and tonometry

The fluid contents of the healthy eye are maintained at a steady level of pressure, which ensures that the tension of the lining of the eye is of a sufficient degree to maintain its spherical shape, but is not so high that the delicate nerve endings of the rods and the cones are damaged. 'Glaucoma' is the name of the sight-threatening condition that results from excessively high intraocular pressures.

The intraocular pressure can be assessed by means of a sensitive pressure gauge called a 'tonometer'. The measurement of the pressure can be made during a slit lamp examination during which the tonometer is held against each of the corneas in turn. This non-invasive examination, which takes a matter of seconds, is uncomfortable but not painful.

Examination of the blood flow to the retina using fluorescein angiography

Fluorescein angiography is a more invasive technique, which involves the injection of fluorescein into the circulation. The retina is then illuminated with blue light, which causes the fluorescein flowing through the retinal arteries to fluoresce with a bright green light. A photograph of the fluorescing vessels is then taken by means of a specialised camera. This examination can reveal more detail about the damage to the retinal circulation that can result from conditions such as chronic diabetes mellitus or atherosclerosis.

Imaging tests including ultrasound, CT and MRI scans

The ultrasound scan is a frequently used tool in ophthalmology to assess the health of the vitreous humour, the retina and the posterior coats of the eye. It is particularly useful when a cataract in the lens prevents slit lamp examination of the structures behind the lens.

CT and MRI are of value in assessing the shape of the orbit and the pathways of the optic nerves as they pass from the optic nerve head to the brain.

Electrophysiological tests

Specialised electrophysiological tests can be used to assess the responses of the nerves in the retina, optic nerve pathways and the visual cortex (at the back of the brain) to visual stimuli (such as flashing lights) presented to the eyes.

Culture and examination of samples taken by swab from the eye

Infections of the conjuctiva can be investigated by means of culture and examination of samples taken by means of swab from the conjunctival secretions.

Investigation of ear disorders

Visual inspection of the external ear and eardrum

The external ear (the pinna), the external ear canal and the outer aspect of the eardrum can be assessed by means of a hand-held instrument called an 'auriscope' (or otoscope). The auriscope provides illumination of the external ear canal by means of a fibre-optic light source. The auriscope is inserted painlessly into the outer ear by means of a plastic conical 'speculum'. The examining practitioner places gentle traction on the pinna of the ear to enable straightening of the external ear canal and so to permit visualisation of the eardrum (see Figure 6.1a-X).

Examination of the external ear and external ear canal can reveal the changes caused by otitis externa and the excessive accumulation of earwax. Visualisation of the eardrum will demonstrate certain problems affecting the middle ear, including acute otitis media, chronic secretory otitis media (glue ear), perforated eardrum and cholesteatoma.

Clinical assessment of hearing

As deafness is one of the major symptoms that accompany diseases of the middle and inner ear, clinical assessment of hearing can provide very useful diagnostic information. Voice and whisper tests are 'rough and ready' methods of assessing the hearing in each ear. While simple to perform, they can be very useful in certain patient groups, young children in particular.

A more specific test involves the use of a tuning fork. A large tuning fork is used, which when percussed will produce a note of low pitch. The vibrating tuning fork is placed close to the external ear canal, and then held with its foot touching the central area of the forehead (close to the acupuncture point Yintang). The patient is asked to compare the volume of sound produced by both positions, and to say where they 'hear' the sound when it is placed against the forehead. If the hearing problem is located in the middle ear (e.g. in glue ear), the sound conducted by the bones of the head, when the fork is placed on the forehead, will be louder than that produced when it is held close to the affected ear (in health the tuning fork will be loudest when placed close to the external ear canal). This is because bone conduction of sound bypasses the blocked middle ear, and will be 'heard' by a healthy inner ear.

If the hearing in the inner ear on one side is compromised, the sound of the tuning fork when placed against the forehead will sound as if it is closer to the unaffected side.

Testing of hearing by means of audiometry

The audiometer is a machine that produces pure tones of sound at varying frequencies and varying intensities. The sound is fed to the patient either through earphones or via a vibrator held against the mastoid process (the prominence of bone that sits posteroinferiorly to each ear). In this way air conduction of sound (to the middle ear) can be compared against bone conduction (directly to the inner ear).

The audiogram is a chart of hearing produced as a result of audiogram testing. This chart reveals the threshold of hearing for varying intensities of sound at different frequencies for each ear. Different hearing problems result in characteristic audiograms. For example, the damage to hearing that results from exposure to excessive noise results in impairment of hearing at high frequencies (high-pitched sound).

Speech audiometry is a variant of audiometry in which a recorded word list, rather than pure tones, is presented to each ear.

Testing of the flexibility of the middle ear by means of impedance tympanometry

Impedance tympanometry is a less patient-dependent non-invasive test which assesses objectively the degree to which the eardrum reflects the pure tones with which it is presented by an audiometer. This is a very useful test in assessing the degree to which glue ear is compromising hearing in babies and young children.

Electrophysiological tests (electric response audiometry)

The nerve responses to a sound wave that reaches the inner ear can be tested by means of a similar method to that used to test the nerve responses in the visual pathways. In electric response audiometry, a sound stimulus is applied to the outer ear. The response to this stimulus in the nerves that originate in the inner ear, and which travel via the auditory nerve to the auditory cortex in the brain, can be assessed by means of

Self-test 6.1b

The investigation of the skin, the eye and the ear

1. A patient is referred to the ophthalmology department by his optician because the optician suspects that a cataract (cloudy opacity) is developing in the lens of one eye. What investigations do you think this patient might expect to undergo when he attends his appointment?
2. How do you think that a child with an onset of reduced hearing following a cold 2 months ago might be investigated? (Before you answer this question, you might wish to reread the section on glue ear in Chapter 5.4e.)
3. A patient is referred to the dermatology department with an unexplained itchy red rash affecting the palms of both hands. Describe how you think the dermatologist will investigate the rash.

Answers

1. The optician should have already tested the visual acuity in each eye by means of the Snellen chart, the visual fields by means of confrontation with a moving object, and the eye movements. Evidently, reduced visual acuity was found affecting the eye in which the optician suspects cataract formation. Ophthalmological examination will then have revealed a cloudy obscurity in the lens, which will have prevented clear visualisation of the retina.

   These tests might have been repeated at the appointment in the ophthalmology department (eye clinic), but the additional test that the patient should expect is slit lamp examination. First, his pupils will be dilated by means of mydriatic drops, and then he will be asked to sit in front of the biomicroscope in a darkened room. The examining doctor will probably also want to assess the intraocular pressure by means of tonometry, as well as examine the cataract. If surgery to the cataract is considered, an ultrasound scan of the eye may be arranged to assess the structure of the eye posterior to the cataract.
2. In the first instance, the child is likely to be investigated by the GP or health visitor. With young children, simple distraction tests can be used to assess hearing loss. The child is distracted by means of an entertaining event while sounds are made or words whispered behind each ear in turn. A child with healthy hearing will normally turn from the entertainment to investigate the origin of the noise.

   With an older child, a tuning fork assessment may give useful information, and in the case of glue ear confirm that the deafness is conductive (i.e. the location of the problem is in the middle ear).

   Examination with an auriscope (otoscope) might reveal the characteristic dull appearance of the eardrum in a case of glue ear.

   A more detailed assessment can be made after referral to an audiologist, who can generate an audiogram for each ear and perform impedance tympanometry.
3. The most important aspect of dermatological assessment is pattern recognition. The experienced dermatologist might have a good idea of the diagnosis in this case simply by detailed inspection of the rash and its pattern of distribution.

   If fungal infection or scabies infestation is suspected, skin scrapings might be taken for microbiological analysis, and a Wood's lamp might be used to view the rash. If a bacterial or viral infection is a possibility (unlikely in this sort of distribution of rash), swabs might be taken of any fluid exuding from the rash. If the rash appears to be eczema, patch testing might be used to investigate whether or not the patient is allergic to any one of the common environmental allergens known to precipitate contact dermatitis.

   Although unlikely to be performed in a first appointment, skin biopsy might be used to exclude the possibility of conditions such as psoriasis or pemphigus (a blistering condition).

sensory electrodes placed against the bones of the middle ear, the base of the neck and the skull.

Because this non-invasive technique requires no response from the patient, it can be used in babies and young children, and also, by dint of its objectivity, in cases of litigation for industrial deafness.

Chapter 6.1c Diseases of the skin

LEARNING POINTS

At the end of this chapter you will:

- be familiar with the most important conditions that can affect the skin
- be able to recognise the red flags of the diseases of the skin.

Estimated time for chapter: Part I, 120 minutes; Part II, 120 minutes.

Introduction

The skin is recognised conventionally to react rapidly to a very wide range of triggers. Known triggers for skin disease include genetic susceptibility, degeneration from ageing, infectious agents, physical trauma, allergic reactions, light, heat, cold, psychological stress and self-harm. However, in many cases of skin disease the underlying cause is never clarified. It is recognised that any one trigger can lead to a diverse range of manifestations of skin disease. From a conventional perspective it is often not very clear exactly why one person under stress develops itch and another psoriasis, or why antibiotics in one person will cause a painful blistering reaction and in another a rash of red spots.

From a more holistic perspective, it is generally appreciated that the skin, as it is the most superficial organ, might readily express symptoms and signs as an indication of a deeper imbalance. These symptoms and signs would be the result of a combination of both internal and external factors, which would begin to explain the diversity of skin diseases.

The aim of this chapter is to introduce the wide range of ways in which the skin can manifest symptoms, and also the common treatment approaches used in dermatology. This chapter is split into two parts, which are designed to be studied in separate study sessions.

Generalised diseases in which the skin can be involved include peripheral vascular disease, diabetes mellitus, thyroid disease, Cushing's syndrome, Addison's disease, rheumatoid arthritis, chronic liver disease and a wide range of infectious diseases. As all these diseases have already been described in some length in earlier chapters, their skin manifestations (with the exception of some of the important infectious skin diseases) are not mentioned further in this chapter (see Q6.1c-1).

The conditions discussed in this chapter are:

Part I: Infectious diseases and the skin

- Bacterial infections:
  - cellulitis and erysipelas
  - boils and carbuncles
  - impetigo
  - scalded skin syndrome
  - leprosy.
- Viral infections:
  - warts
  - molluscum contagiosum
  - rashes in generalised viral infections
  - herpes simplex
  - herpes zoster
  - hand, foot and mouth disease.
- Fungal infections:
  - tinea (athlete's foot and ringworm)
  - candidal (yeast) infections
  - pityriasis versicolor.
- Skin infestations:
  - scabies
  - head, pubic and body lice
  - fleas and papular urticaria.
- Acne:
  - acne vulgaris
  - acne rosacea.
- Eczema:
  - exogenous eczema (primary irritant eczema; allergic contact eczema)
  - endogenous eczema (atopic eczema; discoid eczema; varicose eczema; asteatotic eczema; seborrhoeic eczema (dermatitis)).
- Psoriasis:
  - plaque psoriasis
  - scalp psoriasis
  - guttate psoriasis.
- Erythroderma.

Part II

- Moles and other naevi:
  - freckles and melanocytic naevi (common moles)
  - stork marks and blue spots in newborns
  - strawberry naevi
  - port wine stains
  - Campbell de Morgan red spots
  - spider naevi.
- Skin tumours – benign lumps:
  - seborrhoeic warts (keratoses)
  - skin tags
  - dermatofibromata
  - epidermal cysts and lipomas
  - milia
  - keloid scars.
- Skin tumours – malignant skin tumours:
  - solar keratoses
  - basal cell carcinoma
  - squamous cell carcinoma and Bowen's disease
  - Paget's disease of the nipple
  - malignant melanoma
  - Kaposi's sarcoma
  - lymphoma and the skin.
- Connective tissue disorders:
  - systemic lupus erythematosus
  - dermatomyositis
  - scleroderma.
- Disorders of hair growth:
  - excessive hair growth
  - scalp hair loss.
- Other common skin conditions:
  - urticaria and angio-oedema
  - prickly heat (miliaria)
  - polymorphic light eruption
  - chilblains
  - xanthelasmata
  - lichen planus
  - pityriasis rosea
  - pruritus
  - skin ulcers
  - reactions to drugs.

Part I: Infectious diseases and the skin

Many of the common infectious diseases cause symptoms in and signs on the skin. Most of these conditions have been referred to earlier in the text. The following section of this chapter on infections and the skin will serve as a summary of these diseases.

Bacterial infections and the skin

Cellulitis and erysipelas

Cellulitis is a rapidly spreading streptococcal infection of the subcutaneous and deeper tissues. 'Erysipelas' is a term given to the most superficial forms of cellulitis, but clinically there is no clear distinction between the two conditions. Both conditions manifest as a spreading redness and swelling of the skin and underlying tissues, and are accompanied by fever, malaise and enlarged local lymph nodes.

The conventional treatment is with oral or systemic antibiotics (penicillin in most cases).

Boils, carbuncles and folliculitis

The pathology and energetic interpretation of boils and their treatment are described in Chapters 2.2b and 5.4d.

Information Box 6.1c-I

Cellulitis and erysipelas: comments from a Chinese medicine perspective

A Chinese medicine interpretation is that the cellulitis or erysipelas is a manifestation of Wind Heat. The infection is usually on a background of Depletion of Blood/Yin and/or Internal Heat.

'Furuncle' is another term for a boil. A carbuncle is a large boil (a collection of pus within inflamed subcutaneous tissue), which is often centred on a hair follicle. Folliculitis is a condition in which a number of tiny boils develop, each centred around a hair follicle (often on the anterior thighs). The treatment of furuncles and carbuncles ideally should involve lancing to drain the pus. Antibiotics may also be prescribed. Folliculitis is treated with oral antibiotics.

Information Box 6.1c-II

Boils: comments from a Chinese medicine perspective

In Chinese medicine, a boil represents Damp/Damp Heat, or Fire Poison. Internal factors are important in the causation of the accumulation of these Pathogenic Factors.

Impetigo

The pathology and energetic interpretation of impetigo (Figure 6.1c-I) and its treatment are described in Chapter 5.4d.

Scalded skin syndrome

The pathology and energetic interpretation of scalded skin syndrome and its treatment are described in Chapter 5.4d.

Leprosy

The pathology and energetic interpretation of leprosy and its treatment are described in Chapter 4.1g.

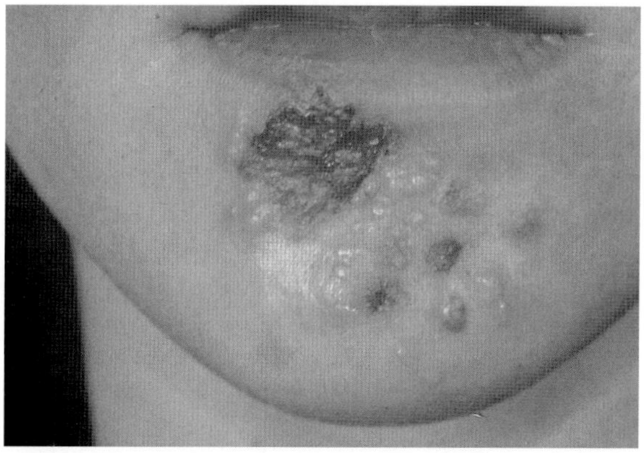

Figure 6.1c-I • The crusting rash of impetigo.

Viral infections and the skin

Warts

The pathology and energetic interpretation of warts (Figure 6.1c-II) and their treatment are described in Chapter 5.4d.

Molluscum contagiosum

The pathology and energetic interpretation of molluscum contagiosum and its treatment are described in Chapter 5.4d.

Rashes in generalised viral infections

A number of generalised viral infections can manifest with a rash of pink blotches or flat spots (macules). These so-called 'viral exanthems' (Figure 6.1c-III) are common in childhood, and usually are not serious. The most well-described viral infections that present with a rash include measles (rubeola), German measles (rubella), slapped-cheek disease and roseola infantum (exanthem subitum). The pathology and energetic interpretation of all these infections are described in Chapter 5.4d.

There is a wide range of respiratory and faeco-orally transmitted viruses that can lead to the development of a rash. It is not uncommon for a child to suffer from a rash

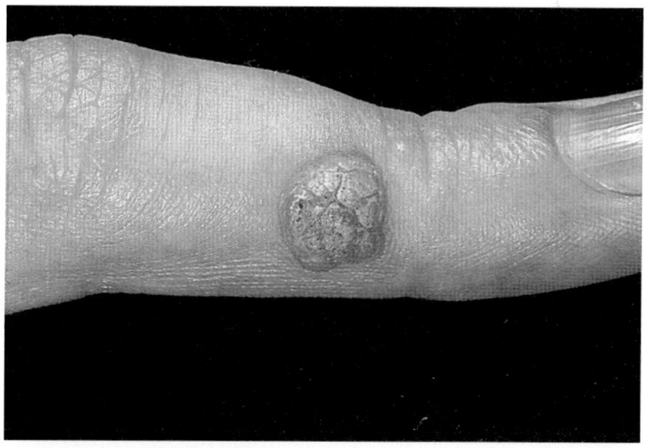

Figure 6.1c-II • A viral wart.

Figure 6.1c-III • The rash of rubella (German measles), a typical viral exanthem.

accompanied by features of a generalised viral infection such as fever and/or runny nose and sore throat and/or diarrhoea and/or joint aches, while the precise diagnosis remains unknown.

The common viral infections that cause a vesicular rash (fluid-filled blisters), rather than macular rash (flat pink spots), are described below.

Herpes simplex infections

The pathology and energetic interpretation of herpes simplex infections and their treatment are described in Chapter 5.4d.

Herpes zoster infections (chickenpox and shingles)

The pathology and energetic interpretation of chickenpox and shingles (Figure 6.1c-IV) and their treatment are described in Chapter 5.4d.

Hand, foot and mouth disease

The pathology and energetic interpretation of hand, foot and mouth disease and its treatment are described in Chapter 5.4d.

Fungal infections and the skin

In a healthy person it is rare for fungal infections to cause symptoms anywhere else in the body other than the skin, nails and hair. Although deep fungal infections are rare, fungal infections of the skin and mucous membranes of the mouth and genitalia are very common.

Tinea (including athlete's foot and ringworm)

The fungi that infect the epidermis of the skin are known as 'dermatophytes'. The word 'tinea' means 'gnawing worm', and is a general term used to describe dermatophyte infection.

The manifestation and description of tinea infections is based on the site. Tinea pedis is infection of the foot, more commonly known as athlete's foot. Tinea corporis is infection of the body skin, more commonly known as ringworm. Tinea cruris (Figure 6.1c-V) is infection of the inguinal region, a problem that is more common in men than women.

The main symptoms of tinea infection are itch, scaling of the affected skin and very often a red, well-demarcated border to the infected area. The infection is often asymmetrical, a feature that is not common in other skin diseases.

Tinea unguium (Figure 6.1c-VI) is a fungal infection that has penetrated the nail bed. The affected nail becomes yellowed and thickened, and may split into flakes at its distal margin.

The diagnosis of these tinea infections can be confirmed by the microscopic examination of skin scrapings and nail clippings, although most infections have a characteristic appearance, which means that this investigation usually is unnecessary.

Treatment of tinea pedis, corporis and cruris involves primarily the regular application of local antifungal drugs such as clotrimazole. For more persistent infection, oral antifungal medication such as terbinafine and griseofulvin may be prescribed for up to 4 weeks in skin infections, and for as long as 12 weeks in toenail infections. These medications carry a risk of headaches, digestive disturbance, rashes and disturbed liver function.

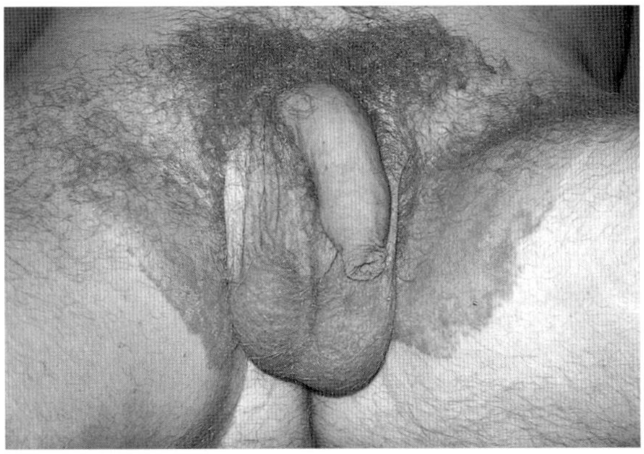

Figure 6.1c-V • Tinea cruris: ringworm of the groin.

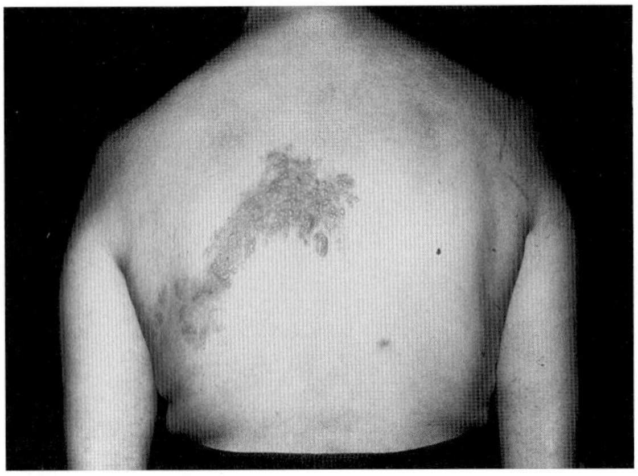

Figure 6.1c-IV • The rash of shingles affecting a thoracic dermatome.

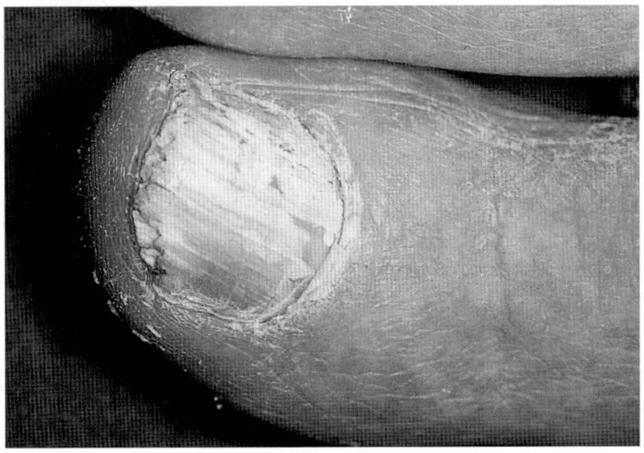

Figure 6.1c-VI • Tinea unguium: fungal infection of the toenail.

Information Box 6.1c-III

Tinea: comments from a Chinese medicine perspective

In Chinese medicine, a tinea infection would suggest Damp or Damp Heat. The location of the infection would be significant in making a more precise energetic interpretation of the condition.

The antifungal medications evidently clear Damp Heat, but the side-effects suggest that they can induce Spleen/Liver disharmony and perhaps Accumulation of Heat.

Candidal (yeast) infections

Candida is a yeast that is a normal resident of the gastrointestinal tract and the vagina. The candidal infections of oral thrush, genital thrush and a certain form of nappy rash are a result of abnormal overgrowth of this yeast. The term '*Candida* syndrome' is used to describe a constellation of symptoms that are attributed to overgrowth of *Candida* in the gastrointestinal and reproductive tracts. This syndrome is not recognised as an organic (as opposed to functional) condition in conventional medicine.

All the common presentations of *Candida* are described in Chapters 2.4b (*Candida* syndrome), 3.1c (oral thrush), 5.2d (genital thrush) and 5.4e (candidal nappy rash).

Candida will only develop on the skin in healthy people in areas in which the skin is perpetually moist (e.g. the nappy region in babies, and between folds of flesh in obese people). Candidal infection of the skin is much more common in people on long-term antibiotic therapy, in those with immune deficiency and people with diabetes mellitus. The skin infection is characterised by a brick-red rash with a clearly demarcated border. There may be tiny circular 'satellites' of rash clustered close to the margins of the affected area (Figure 6.1c-VII). Often the moist rash will have a yeasty or offensive odour.

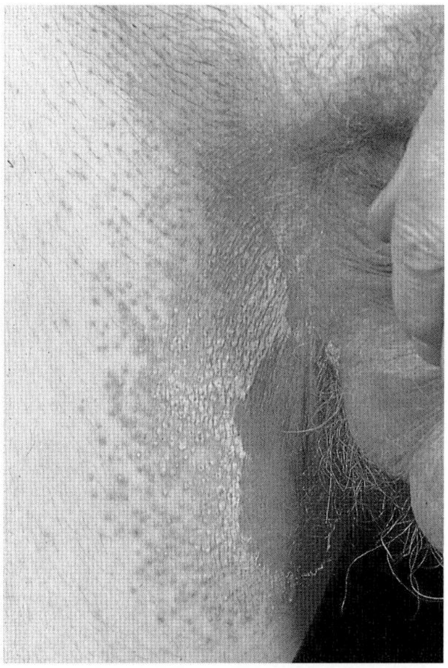

Figure 6.1c-VII • Candidal rash of the groin, showing satellite lesions.

Information Box 6.1c-IV

***Candida*: comments from a Chinese medicine perspective**

In Chinese medicine, *Candida* of the skin would be a manifestation of Damp Heat. Candidal nappy rash in babies might indicate Accumulation Disorder.

Pityriasis (tinea) versicolor

Pityriasis versicolor is an overgrowth of another yeast that is a normal resident of the hair follicles of the skin. Under certain conditions, the yeast multiples to cause scattered, light-brown macules on the trunk and upper arms. In pigmented skin, the affected areas may become depigmented.

The treatment of pityriasis versicolor involves application of selenium sulfide shampoo or an antifungal cream. Oral antifungal agents may be prescribed in resistant cases.

Information Box 6.1c-V

Pityriasis versicolor: comments from a Chinese medicine perspective

In Chinese medicine, the development of pityriasis versicolor is probably a manifestation of Damp.

Skin infestations

Skin infestations are infections by parasites that inhabit the surface of the skin. In the majority of infestations occurring in the developed world, the symptoms result from biting and burrowing by the parasites (usually lice, ticks, insects or mites), and the problem that results is primarily one of discomfort rather than a serious threat to health.

However, the invading parasites can be carriers of disease. Typhus is a serious disease of undernourished populations that is transmitted via body louse infestation. The features of typhus include high fever, headache, meningitis and a bruising rash. Lyme disease is a generalised infection that can lead to a range of symptoms, including fever, arthritis, meningitis and a skin rash. This disease is transmitted via tick bites (from sheep and deer ticks), and is well recognised to occur in temperate climates.

Scabies

Scabies is an infestation by the scabies mite. Transmission occurs by close physical contact, and therefore it is more common in children and young adults. The infestation often begins in the hands or genital regions, from where the mite burrows into the skin. After a few weeks, a sensitivity to its faeces builds up, and this results in intense itch in the skin, which is characteristically worse at night. The rash of scabies consists of clusters of tiny red bumps (papules), particularly in the armpits, on the thighs

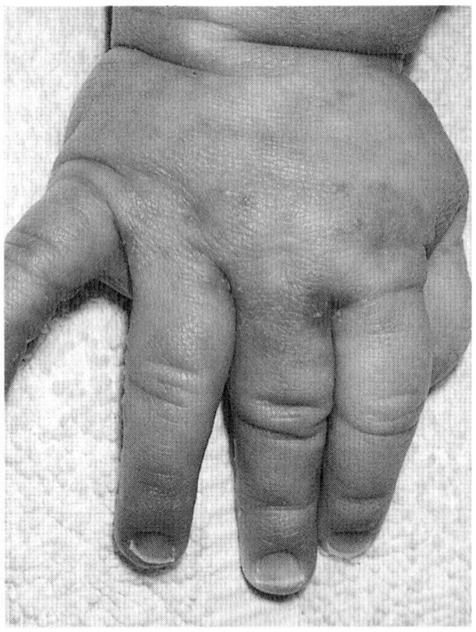

Figure 6.1c-VIII • Typical scabies rash around the web spaces between the fingers.

and on the abdomen. Tiny tracks, which are the burrows of the mite, may be found on the fingers, in the web spaces, and on the wrists, palms, soles and genitalia (Figure 6.1c-VIII).

Scabies is usually diagnosed from the clinical appearance, but can be confirmed by examination of the mites and eggs obtained by taking scrapings of a burrow.

The treatment of scabies involves painting the whole body (from the neck down) of the patient, and also family members, with a preparation of an insecticide such as benzyl benzoate, lindane or permethrin. All these chemicals are toxic, and should be used with caution. Itching will resolve 2–3 weeks after successful treatment.

> **Information Box 6.1c-VI**
>
> **Scabies: comments from a Chinese medicine perspective**
>
> In Chinese medicine, scabies could be interpreted as an invasion of Wind Heat. It is more likely to occur in undernourished or chronically ill people, which suggests that an underlying Deficiency (of Wei Qi/Kidney) is likely to be present in severe cases.

Head, pubic and body lice

There are three broad families of lice that use humans as their host. The head louse favours head hair, eyebrows and eyelashes, the pubic louse ('crab' louse) lives in the pubic regions, and the body louse lives on unwashed clothing. All three forms of human louse derive their nourishment from human blood, and cause itching when they bite through the skin.

The head louse is about 2–3 millimetres long and is transmitted by close head contact with an infected person. Children are the most likely hosts in developed countries, although they can readily pass on their lice to adult family members. The female louse lays eggs which firmly adhere to the hair roots. These 'nits' are diagnostic of an established infestation, and herald the emergence of increasing numbers of lice. Head louse infestation can be prevented by regular combing with a fine-toothed comb. Once nits have been laid, twice-daily combing for at least 2 weeks is necessary to remove the lice as they emerge from the eggs.

The pubic louse is transmitted by sexual contact. It cannot colonise scalp hair, but can affect eyelashes, beards and armpits, as well as the genital region. As is true for head lice, when the eggs are laid they adhere to the shafts of the hair in the pubic regions.

Both head and pubic lice can be treated by chemical means. The insecticides carbaryl, malathion and permethrin in a lotion or shampoo preparation are prescribed. Two treatments are recommended. The second treatment should be given 1 week after the first in order to eliminate any lice newly hatched from the more resistant egg cases.

The body louse is only really seen in conditions of poverty or poor hygiene. The body louse lays its eggs in clothing or bedding. Both the body lice and its eggs are killed readily by laundering.

> **Information Box 6.1c-VII**
>
> **Headlice: comments from a Chinese medicine perspective**
>
> In Chinese medicine, the itch and inflammation from louse infestation would represent Invasion of Wind Heat. Internal Heat might also be a contributory factor.

Fleas and papular urticaria

In healthy populations the flea does not use the human as its host, but fleas resident on pets or birds can lay their eggs on furnishings and multiply within the home. Flea bites are characteristically found below the knee, an indication of how high the fleas can jump from floor level. In most people the bites are insignificant, and may result only in transient itch. Some individuals develop sensitivity to the flea proteins injected into the skin through biting, and so can become prone to developing firm, itchy, red papules at the site of flea bites. In some people, sensitivity can be of such a degree that the papule can enlarge to form a significant blister. A number of bites can lead to a rash-like appearance (usually on the lower legs), a condition termed 'papular urticaria'.

The most appropriate treatment for papular urticaria is to 'de-flea' the offending host and its surroundings.

Acne

The term 'acne' (a corruption of the Greek word meaning 'point') is used to describe the skin condition in which the formation of papules (firm, red spots) and pustules (papules that have come to a head with a point of yellow pus) is prominent. There are a number of variants of acne, but the most

Information Box 6.1c-VIII

Papular urticaria: comments from a Chinese medicine perspective

In Chinese medicine, papular urticaria might be described as Wind Heat with an underlying Deficiency of Wei Qi or Kidney Qi. Internal Heat may also be a contributory factor in a severe case.

common by far is acne vulgaris, which is experienced in some form by up to 80% of adolescents in the UK. 'Acne rosacea' is the term used to describe a flushing condition of the facial skin in which pustules can occur.

Acne vulgaris

Acne vulgaris is characterised by papules, pustules and blackheads (comedones), often on the background of greasy skin (Figure 6.1c-IX). As the pustules involve some inflammation, scarring of the skin can occur as they resolve. In a severe case, multiple scarred pits are permanent reminders of adolescent acne. Acne vulgaris most commonly affects the most sebum-rich areas of skin, including the nasal region, the chin and the forehead. In severe cases, wider areas of the face, and the neck, shoulders and chest can be affected.

Acne vulgaris most commonly first appears as the sebum of the skin alters its composition at the time of the pubescent surge in male sex hormones (androgens). A surge in the levels of androgens affects girls as well as boys, but obviously is more pronounced in boys. The excessive sebum leads to blockage of the sebaceous ducts, and the formation of blackheads, and also to the small bumpy papules known as 'whiteheads'. This results in inflammation of the duct as a normal skin bacterium becomes trapped within the sebaceous gland and overgrows. The blackhead then becomes a papule, and ultimately a pustule. In severe cases, deep cyst-like areas of inflamed tissue and pus can develop at the site of a blocked sebaceous duct. Most conventional doctors would disagree with the commonly held view that factors such as diet, poor hygiene or sexual behaviour play any role in the development of acne.

Acne vulgaris is a cause of intense emotional distress for many teenagers. Doctors are well aware of this, and a wide range of powerful treatments may be prescribed to alleviate the anguish that is a very common accompaniment to the development of spots in adolescence.

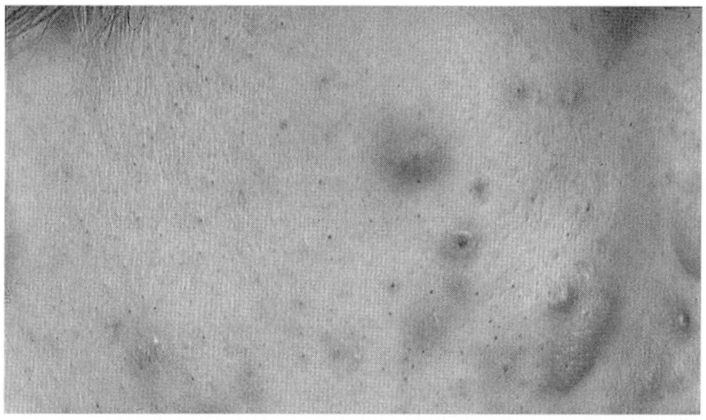

Figure 6.1c-IX • Blackheads and pustules in acne vulgaris.

The first stage of treatment is with topical lotions containing benzoyl peroxide, an irritant, or retinoic acid, a derivative of vitamin A, both of which cause the core of the blackheads to break down. These lotions should be applied regularly for optimal effect. Topical antibiotic preparations may also be useful. In more resistant cases, oral antibiotics (tetracycline, oxytetracycline or erythromycin) may also be prescribed for a period of at least 3 months, and often longer. Some girls can respond positively to a particular preparation of the oral contraceptive pill that contains an anti-androgen called 'cyproterone acetate'. In very severe cases, an oral derivative of vitamin A called 'isotretinoin' may be prescribed.

Isotretinoin carries a risk of causing quite marked dryness and inflammation of the skin, joint aches and liver toxicity, and carries a high risk of damage to an embryo in the event of pregnancy. For this reason, it is generally only prescribed under the supervision of a hospital clinic. A course of over 4 months of isotretinoin will usually have a positive effect on symptoms and, in the majority of cases, can lead to a long-term improvement in the symptoms of acne.

Information Box 6.1c-IX

Acne vulgaris: comments from a Chinese medicine perspective

In Chinese medicine, the symptoms of acne would normally be regarded as a manifestation of Damp Heat. Heat in the Stomach is likely to manifest in the facial region, and so, contrary to conventional wisdom, modification of diet would appear to be crucial in the treatment of acne. Scott and Barlow (1999) suggest that the Heat very commonly has its origin in pent-up anger, which makes the condition rather difficult to treat in western children.

The anti-acne treatments evidently serve to clear Heat and Damp. Side-effects suggesting Heat/Depletion of Yin (skin irritation and dryness) are common with both topical and oral treatments. The serious potential side-effects of isotretinoin suggest that Liver Disharmony and damage to the Blood can result from this long-term medication.

Acne rosacea (rosacea)

In contrast to acne vulgaris, acne rosacea is a condition that usually first appears in middle age, and is more common in women than men. The initial symptoms are that the skin of the cheeks, forehead and nose tends to flush, a feature that is more prominent after alcohol consumption or exposure to the sun. In long-standing cases, broken veins can appear and pustules can develop (Figure 6.1c-X). The skin takes on a permanent flushed appearance. In men, overgrowth of the tissues around the sebaceous glands can lead to a coarseness and thickening of affected areas of skin, particularly the nose. In severe cases the nose can appear bulbous and malformed, a condition known as 'rhinophyma'. Blackheads are not a feature of acne rosacea. Some patients report that they also suffer from migraine.

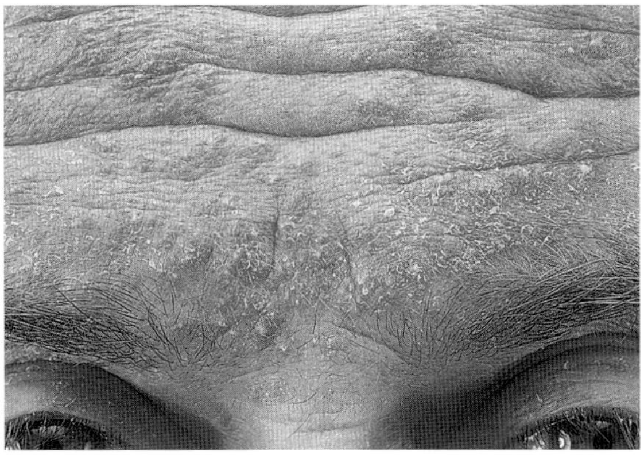

Figure 6.1c-X • Papules and pustules in acne rosacea.

Treatment is by means of long-term oral antibiotics. Topical antibiotic or salicylic acid creams may also be prescribed.

> **Information Box 6.1c-X**
>
> **Acne rosacea: comments from a Chinese medicine perspective**
>
> In Chinese medicine, the symptoms of rosacea could represent Stomach and/or Lung Heat and Damp, although the effect of Damp is less prominent than in acne vulgaris. The increased incidence of migraine in sufferers, together with the worsening with alcohol consumption, would suggest that Liver Stagnation/Yang Rising may also have a part to play in the aetiology.
>
> The development of rhinophyma is suggestive of Phlegm.

Eczema (dermatitis)

'Eczema' is a general term used by dermatologists to describe a skin reaction in the acute stages of which itching, redness, some swelling, damp oozing of the skin, and tiny fluid-filled areas (vesicles) may be seen. The itching can be so intense as to provoke scratching that leads to bleeding.

In more chronic cases, dryness and thickening of the skin is more prominent. In a severe case of chronic eczema painful fissures may develop in the skin close to joints. Eczema is typically symmetrically distributed.

'Eczema' is a term derived from the Greek word meaning 'to boil over'. The term 'dermatitis', meaning 'inflammation of the skin', is used interchangeably with the word eczema. It is important to appreciate that the terms eczema and dermatitis both describe a reaction of the skin, and not a disease in its own right. There is actually a wide range of causes of eczema.

Eczema is categorised according to whether the cause is seen conventionally as external (exogenous eczema) or internal (endogenous eczema).

Treatment of eczema

The treatment of eczema first involves identifying any triggers of the problem. These may be external irritants or allergens, or may be dietary in origin. The diagnosis of the triggers is described below according to the type of eczema. Once identified, the triggers should be avoided if at all possible. This may mean that the person has to make a significant change in lifestyle, such as leave a current job, get rid of a pet or follow an exclusion diet. However, very often dietary change is not strongly advocated in conventional dermatology, as a general belief prevails that dietary change often has little effect on eczema.

Emollient preparations

The least energetically disturbing treatment of eczema is the use of emollient (moistening and softening) preparations. Skin that is already dry and cracked will be more vulnerable to irritation by external triggers, and so regular use of an emollient can help keep eczema at bay. Preparations that are commonly prescribed include aqueous cream and emulsifying ointment, both of which contain white soft paraffin. These provide a waxy layer on the skin surface and so prevent further drying. Some emollients may contain potential allergens such as lanolin (derived from wool) and peanut oil, and so the response to the emollient must be monitored carefully.

Zinc, icthammol and coal tar all have antiscaling and anti-inflammatory properties, and may be combined with emollients in a case of chronic eczema.

Topical corticosteroids

If the eczema is severe, it is generally considered wise practice to apply a corticosteroid cream to the affected areas. The corticosteroid creams are produced in a range of potencies, of which hydrocortisone (0.5% and 1%) is the least potent, clobetasone butyrate is moderately potent, and betametasone valerate and clobetasol propionate are very potent.

It is well recognised by doctors that corticosteroids simply suppress symptoms, and that very often symptoms can recur rapidly after discontinuing use of the cream. Also, it is well known that long-term high doses can have adverse affects on both the skin and general health. Corticosteroids can cause general thinning of the skin and subcutaneous tissues, and can precipitate a reddening of the skin (especially of the face) akin to acne rosacea. They should not be used alone in infective conditions and acne. This is because they can inhibit the local immune response to infection, and so worsen the condition (although combined corticosteroid and antibiotic/antifungal preparations may be prescribed if an infection has led to an eczematous-type response). Also, it is known that corticosteroids applied over the long term to large areas of skin will lead to the general side-effects of systemic steroids, and may suppress growth in young children.

For these reasons, the decision to prescribe a corticosteroid cream should not be made lightly. The risk of potential side-effects should always be balanced against the adverse effects of the eczema. Moderate- to high-potency creams should never be applied to the delicate skin of the face. Nevertheless, it is conventionally understood as good practice to apply a high-potency cream from the outset to a moderately severe case of eczema in order to get control of the symptoms, and then rapidly to reduce the dose once control has been gained. This is similar in principle to the guidance given to doctors about the management of an attack of acute asthma.

In very severe cases of eczema, emollients and corticosteroid creams may be held in place against the skin by means of overnight bandaging (wet wraps).

Other treatments used for eczema

Antihistamine medications may be prescribed at night for sedation and inhibition of itch. Exposure to ultraviolet light can be helpful in some cases. Oil of evening primrose may inhibit eczema, although the clinical evidence for this is not strong.

> **Information Box 6.1c-XI**
>
> **Eczema: comments from a Chinese medicine perspective**
>
> In Chinese medicine, the redness, vesicles and oozing of eczema correspond to Wind Damp Heat. The root of this is commonly internally generated Damp Heat, and the Wind may be external or internal in origin. Itch may be a result of Wind or Stagnation of Qi (due to Heat, Phlegm Damp under the skin, or suppressed emotions). Underlying Wei Qi (and/or Jing) Deficiency will predispose the patient to Wind Invasion.
>
> The thickened and dry skin in chronic eczema is an indication of underlying Blood Deficiency, as Blood nourishes the skin. Blood Deficiency can predispose to the accumulation of Wind Damp Heat on the surface of the body.
>
> Dry flaky skin in atopic eczema in children may be a manifestation of Phlegm (and accumulation syndrome).
>
> Some patients say that scratching the eczema until it bleeds can provide some sort of relief. This may be because bleeding can lead to clearance of Heat in Chinese medicine terms.
>
> Most of the medical approaches to eczema are suppressive in nature, in that they target the symptoms rather than the root cause of Deficiency of the Wei Qi, Kidneys and/or Blood. One exception might be oil of evening primrose, which may act by nourishing the skin, and so might be interpreted to work by strengthening one of the root Deficiencies.

Exogenous eczema (dermatitis)

Exogenous eczema results from direct contact with environmental triggers. The terms 'primary irritant' and 'allergic contact' describe whether or not the resulting reaction is mediated by an allergic response to the contact. However, a patient who suffers from endogenous eczema can be more prone to both these forms of exogenous eczema, so in practice it can be difficult to be specific about the cause of a case of eczema.

Primary irritant eczema (dermatitis)

Primary irritants physically damage the skin. Irritants that are well recognised to cause eczema include acids, detergents, petroleum products, and also exposure to extremes of cold and wind. The hands are a very common site for this form of eczema. Primary irritant eczema can become a significant problem in many occupations in which the person is continually exposed to an irritant. For example, a hairdresser might develop primary irritant eczema as a result of repeated hair-washing with detergent-containing shampoos and conditioners.

In most cases the offending trigger is clear. The main treatment for primary irritant eczema is to avoid the trigger. The use of barrier creams and gloves may be sufficient to protect from primary irritant eczema, but in severe cases the patient may be forced to change occupation.

Allergic contact eczema

Allergic contact eczema is a delayed immune reaction to exposure to an environmental allergen. The range of potential allergens is very wide. The allergens that are most commonly implicated in allergic contact eczema include nickel (in cheap jewellery, watches, studs in clothing and metal clips on bra straps), colophony (a component of sticking plaster), rubber (in gloves and shoes), chromate (in cement), hair dye, topical medications and plants (particularly the primula family in the UK).

Allergic contact eczema is diagnosed primarily on the basis of the history and the distribution of the rash, although often, because of the delay in the development of the rash, the cause may not be clear (Figure 6.1c-XI). Patch testing using a standard battery of the most usual allergens will expose which are the primary triggers for the eczema. If the eczema is severe, it may be treated first with potent steroids, as the test can in itself trigger a generalised attack of eczema.

This form of eczema is treated by means of avoidance of the triggers and, if severe, with emollients and steroid creams.

Endogenous eczema

Endogenous eczema can manifest in a range of forms, of which the syndrome of atopic eczema is the most significant in terms of frequency and severity of symptoms.

Atopic eczema

'Atopy' describes an inherited tendency to be susceptible to allergic conditions such as asthma, eczema and seasonal rhinitis (hay fever). Atopic eczema is a very common condition of childhood, which often first presents in the first year of life. In most cases the eczema resolves before the onset of puberty, but it may persist into adult life.

In early childhood the eczema may be generalised over the body, but later on in childhood takes on a characteristic

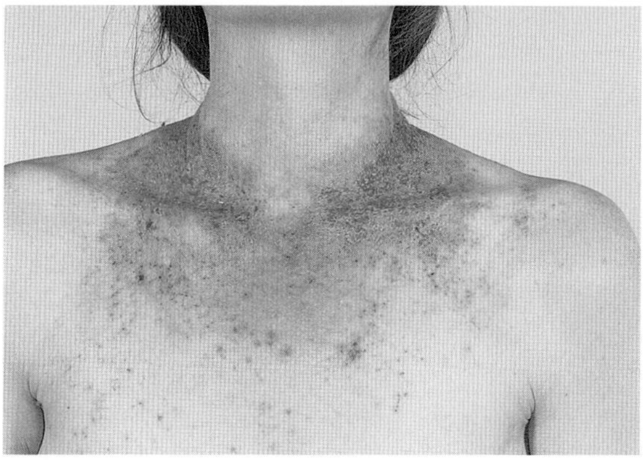

Figure 6.1c-XI • Dry inflamed eczematous skin resulting from contact with perfume.

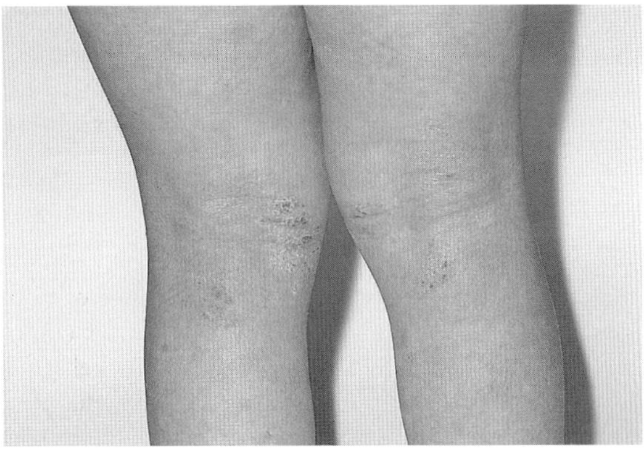

Figure 6.1c-XII • Cracked and thickened skin in atopic eczema.

distribution in which it can be found on the neck, the flexural skin creases of the elbow and knees (antecubital and popliteal fossae), the wrists and the dorsum of the feet (Figure 6.1c-XII). In many cases, environmental triggers (e.g. animal dandruff, grass pollen), dietary constituents (e.g. egg, cows' milk) and also emotional stimuli (especially anxiety and frustration) are well recognised to cause a rapid flare-up of symptoms.

Secondary infection of the eczema is a common complication. Impetigo is more likely to occur in a child with eczema. Children with eczema are also more likely to suffer from viral warts and molluscum contagiosum.

Eczema herpeticum is a very serious manifestation of herpes simplex virus infection which can spread rapidly across the skin of a child with severe generalised eczema.

The life of a child with generalised atopic eczema can be severely disrupted by chronic itch, disturbed sleep, associated conditions such as asthma, and also the stigma that comes with a disfiguring skin condition. It is recognised that severe eczema can inhibit the growth and general well-being of the child. In a severe case, the routine of the whole family will be adversely affected by having repeatedly to apply topical treatments, avoid environmental triggers and the experience of broken nights' sleep.

For these reasons, the symptoms of eczema in children are often treated aggressively, meaning that strong treatments are used from the outset. Emollients should always be used, but potent steroid creams may also be prescribed to inhibit symptoms, although the duration of the course is limited to the absolute minimum possible. Medicated bandages (wet wraps) containing zinc, icthammol or coal tar can be applied to areas of severe eczema on the limbs. Sedative antihistamine tablets may enable uninterrupted sleep in some children.

Discoid eczema

This is a disorder in which scattered circular patches of eczema develop on the trunk and limbs. The cause is unknown. Discoid eczema is usually treated with potent steroid creams and can resolve spontaneously after months to years.

Varicose eczema

This term applies to areas of eczema in the region of varicose veins. It is probably the result of chronic accumulation of toxins in the regions where the blood flow away from the tissues is less than efficient. Interestingly, secondary spread of the eczema to the forearms is well recognised in varicose eczema.

Information Box 6.1c-XII

Atopic eczema: comments from a Chinese medicine perspective

From a Chinese medicine viewpoint, atopic eczema in children has been described as a result of Accumulation of Phlegm and Damp under the skin, Heat obstructing the flow of Blood to the skin, Qi and Blood Deficiency, Accumulation Disorder and Lingering Pathogenic Factor. Damp, Phlegm, Heat and unbalanced emotions can all lead to Stagnation of Qi under the skin and so to intense itch.

Atopic eczema very often first appears at the time when the child is introduced to a bottled or solid foods, which is a time when the Spleen is being overtaxed and when Damp and Phlegm can accumulate. It may also erupt after an infectious disease or immunisation, suggesting in these cases that Lingering Pathogenic Factor is a cause.

Dietary advice is crucial in the management of eczema. Scott and Barlow (1999) recommend the elimination of Phlegm-forming foods in all cases (e.g. cows' milk, peanut butter, oranges, bananas), and a careful consideration of possible food allergies.

Asteatotic eczema

Asteatotic eczema is a form of eczema seen in old age, when the oil content of the skin decreases. When this state is advanced, the skin can develop a slightly shiny 'crazy paving' pattern. Itching usually begins on the legs, but may also affect the trunk and arms. Emollients are often all that is needed to provide relief, and if not, topical steroids may be prescribed.

Seborrhoeic eczema (dermatitis)

Seborrhoeic dermatitis is usually classified as a form of eczema, although it is currently theorised that the cause may be an allergic response to a yeast that is a normal inhabitant of the skin. The condition presents usually in young men, with patches of itchy diffuse redness and scaling of the skin in the region of the scalp, forehead, eyebrows, nasolabial folds and beard area (Figure 6.1c-XIII). Patches can also develop on the chest and upper back.

In infancy, seborrhoeic dermatitis is very common, and patches mostly appear on the scalp, although the neck and

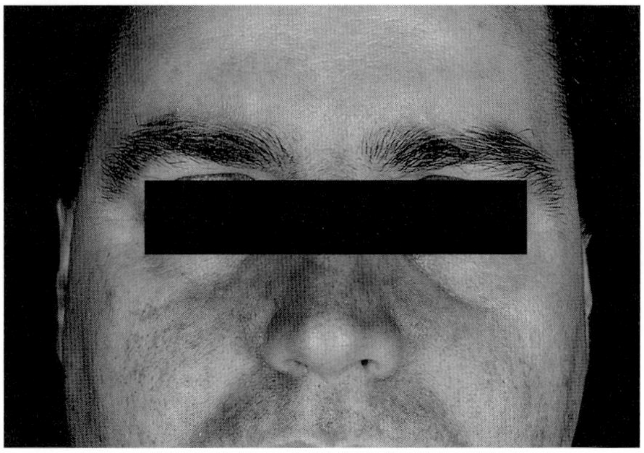

Figure 6.1c-XIII • Seborrhoeic eczema affecting the cheeks and nasolabial folds.

trunk can also be affected. If severe, a waxy layer can develop over the whole scalp, a condition termed 'cradle cap'. However, the child remains symptom-free, and the parents should be reassured that this condition will resolve as the child grows older. In old age, seborrhoeic eczema can progress to affect widespread areas of the body.

Current treatments for seborrhoeic eczema in adults involve the use of emollients, mild steroid creams and tar shampoos. Antifungal creams and shampoos may also be of help. In infancy, the patches can be 'treated' by gentle cleaning with olive oil.

The development of seborrhoeic dermatitis is a common complication of acquired immune deficiency syndrome (AIDS), which is evidence that the cause is related to the immune system. It is also more common in patients with Parkinson's disease.

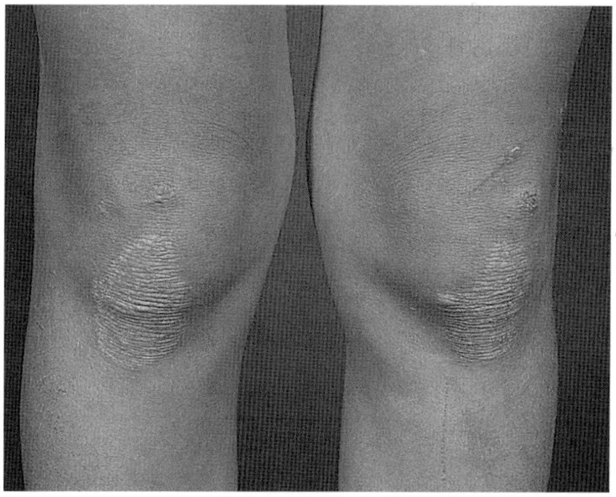

Figure 6.1c-XIV • Plaque psoriasis affecting the knees.

Information Box 6.1c-XIII

Seborrhoeic eczema: comments from a Chinese medicine perspective

The Chinese medicine interpretation of seborrhoeic eczema would be similar to that of eczema, with Heat and Phlegm/Damp as a prominent aspect of the diagnosis.

Psoriasis

Psoriasis is an inflammatory condition of the skin that affects about 1.5% of the western population. For most people affected, the most significant symptom of psoriasis is distress because of its cosmetic appearance, although excessive skin scaling and itch can also become severe problems. As psoriasis is a condition which, once it has appeared, often remains in some form for the whole of the patient's life, it is a significant cause of disease in the population.

The microscopic examination of psoriasis indicates that the epidermal layer of the skin undergoes marked thickening, and inflammatory cells accumulate in the affected areas. These cellular changes manifest in patches of skin that are thickened and have an underlying redness, but which are covered in a layer of silvery scales that flake off very readily.

Psoriasis is classified according to the pattern in which these patches appear. Plaque psoriasis is the most common form, in which large rounded areas of affected skin develop, primarily on the extensor surfaces of the limbs, the trunk and the scalp (Figure 6.1c-XIV). In scalp psoriasis the affected skin is confined to the scalp. Guttate psoriasis frequently develops after a respiratory infection. In this form of psoriasis, there are numerous tiny patches on the affected areas of skin that first appear as a bodily rash. All forms of psoriasis have a tendency to develop at the sites of trauma or scarring.

A form of generalised inflammatory arthritis develops in up to 8% of cases of psoriasis. The most common presentation is of pain and deformity in the distal interphalangeal joints. In severe cases this arthritis is aggressively deforming, and can affect the large joints and also the sacroiliac joints. In many ways, psoriatic arthritis is akin to rheumatoid arthritis.

Information Box 6.1c-XIV

Psoriasis: comments from a Chinese medicine perspective

In Chinese medicine, it would appear that Phlegm and Heat are important Pathogenic Factors in the development of psoriasis. The thickened plaques and scaling, and redness suggest Phlegm and Heat, respectively. Local Qi Deficiency and Qi Stagnation may play a role in the aetiology, particularly in view of the fact that psoriasis can develop at the sites of trauma or scarring. The deforming arthritis is also suggestive of Damp/Phlegm and Heat. The location at the distal interphalangeal joints is also suggestive of accumulation of Heat, as these joints are close to the location for the Jing-Well (Heat clearing) points on the Channels of the limbs.

Nails are commonly also involved, and can develop widespread pitting. These nail changes are almost always present if arthritis has developed. Nail involvement suggests Liver Disharmony.

Like eczema, psoriasis is usually treated by the application of creams and pastes. Emollient creams containing white soft paraffin may be sufficient to control scaling in mild cases. Preparations containing salicylic acid and/or tar can also reduce scaling.

Corticosteroid creams will suppress the formation of plaques, but are not recommended by all dermatologists because of the risks of long-term use, and also because in some cases they can trigger a change of plaque psoriasis into a more unstable scaling condition called 'brittle psoriasis'.

Dithranol is a potent suppressor of the plaques of psoriasis, although the mechanism of this action is unknown. It is applied in paste form to plaques on a daily basis, and can completely clear the skin within 3 weeks. However, it can burn the skin and can cause staining of both the skin and clothing. Calcipotriol is a drug derived from vitamin D that can be effective when applied regularly to the plaques, and is generally free of side-effects.

Ultraviolet light therapy (UVB) can be very effective in reducing the formation of plaques. The patient is exposed 2–3 times a week to a dose that is sufficient to cause mild redness, but not full sunburn. Although there is a theoretical concern about the risk of skin cancer, in reality very few patients with psoriasis develop this complication from UVB therapy.

In severe cases of psoriasis the patient will be prescribed oral medication. Psoralens are drugs that cause inhibition of plaques on the skin when it is exposed to UVA light. The treatment, known as PUVA, therefore involves oral psoralen medication together with regular exposure to UVA. Unlike exposure to UVB alone, PUVA carries a significant risk of inducing cancerous skin changes.

Other oral drugs prescribed in very severe cases include cytotoxic medications, retinoids (which are similar in structure to isotretinoin which is used in acne), systemic corticosteroids and the immunosuppressants such as methotrexate, leflunomide and ciclosporin. All these drugs have a wide range of potentially toxic side-effects, and so should be prescribed with great caution.

> **Information Box 6.1c-XV**
>
> **Treatment of psoriasis: comments from a Chinese medicine perspective**
>
> The conventional treatments for psoriasis are either Moisten Dryness, Clear Heat or Clear Phlegm. They are all suppressive in nature. Chinese medicine treatments for psoriasis in adults are often not very effective. However, Scott and Barlow (1999) suggest that, in children, psoriasis may have a significant emotional component, and can respond well to acupuncture.

Plaque psoriasis

Plaque psoriasis is characterised by large, rounded areas of thickened skin which are symmetrically distributed on the extensor surfaces of the body, the scalp, the trunk and back. Elbows and knees are very commonly affected. The most effective treatment for the majority of people is dithranol or calcipotriol creams.

PUVA and the other potent oral treatments are reserved for cases when the plaques are extensive, or when there is significant emotional distress resulting from the cosmetic appearance.

Scalp psoriasis

In scalp psoriasis, the thickening and scaling is confined to the hairy portion of the scalp and its borders. In severe cases there may be temporary hair loss.

Tar shampoos can work well in keeping scalp psoriasis at bay. Tar gels and corticosteroid lotions are also used if thick plaques develop.

Guttate psoriasis

Guttate psoriasis involves the rapid development of a number of tiny plaques (about 1 centimetre in diameter) scattered symmetrically over the body. The rash often appears in young people as a response to a streptococcal infection. These slightly itchy plaques can resolve very rapidly, but a few may persist and enlarge to develop into chronic plaque psoriasis.

Guttate psoriasis may respond well to a combination of a tar-based ointment and UVB therapy.

Erythroderma

Erythroderma (exfoliative dermatitis) describes a generalised condition of the skin in which the whole skin surface is inflamed, and so the whole body surface appears red, hot and scaly. It results most commonly either from an extreme allergic reaction to a medication, or from severe extensive eczema or psoriasis. Rarely, it can be a manifestation of lymphoma of the skin.

Erythroderma is a medical emergency, because when the skin is inflamed in all parts it loses its heat- and water-retaining properties. In addition, the metabolic rate rises and the body rapidly consumes its stores of energy. The patient becomes vulnerable to dehydration, heart and kidney failure, and hypothermia.

A person with erythroderma will require intensive nursing and fluid replacement. The underlying cause has to be treated with systemic drugs (corticosteroids in the case of eczema, and antipsoriatic drugs in the case of psoriasis).

> **Information Box 6.1c-XVI**
>
> **Erythroderma: comments from a Chinese medicine perspective**
>
> Erythroderma is a condition of Heat leading to collapse of Yin.

Part II

Moles and other naevi

'Mole' is a commonly used term that describes a discrete area of the skin in which there is a concentration of altered but benign growth of the skin cells. In many moles there is an excess of melanin-producing cells, and in some there is thickening from excessive fibrous tissue in the dermis. The term 'naevus' literally means 'birthmark', but is a term used more broadly in dermatology to embrace moles and other localised benign changes in the skin, as well as birthmarks.

Freckles and melanocytic naevi (common moles)

A freckle consists of a benign cluster of epidermal skin cells that contain a higher concentration of the pigment melanin than in surrounding cells. It is believed that these cells in freckled skin are over-responsive to ultraviolet radiation, and so freckles become more apparent after sun exposure. The structure of the skin within a freckle is otherwise normal. In the area of the freckle the skin retains its usual texture and smooth surface. Freckles are common in people who have pale skin, and particularly in those of Celtic origin. The most common sites for freckles are the face, upper body and arms.

A mole (melanocytic naevus) is different to a freckle in that it consists of a cluster of melanin-producing cells, either in the deeper layer of the skin (the dermis) or at the junction between the dermis and the epidermis. The life history of most moles is that they originate at the dermoepidermal junction and then migrate downwards in the dermis. They tend to start their life as deeply pigmented circular spots, after which they then can grow in size, sometimes significantly. Growth can cause the mole to be palpable as a smooth bump in the skin. Then, in later life (after 40 years of age) moles gradually lose the depth of the pigmentation as they mature and migrate downwards. This explains why elderly people have relatively few visible moles of this type.

The clinical significance of moles is that, very rarely, malignant change can occur in the melanin-producing cells, and so lead to the development of a malignant melanoma (see below). Rapid growth of a mole is not usually an indication of malignant change, as long as the growth is regular (i.e. maintaining a circular or ovoid contour). In some cases deep moles can take on a slightly bluish appearance. In other cases an immune response to the mole can cause a halo of pale skin to develop around the mole, which then may become red and then disappear. Both these developments in moles are benign in nature.

A congenital mole is found in about 1% of newborns. In some cases a large area of skin is affected, over which there may also be increased body hair growth. Congenital moles are clinically significant because the risk of malignant change, particularly in giant hairy congenital moles, is much higher than for acquired moles. For this reason, parents might be advised that a large congenital mole is removed surgically.

Stork marks and blue spots in newborns

A stork mark is a flat area of pink skin commonly seen in newborns. One of the most common sites for these regions of dilated capillaries is at the nape of the neck, hence the name. Usually the pinkness of these patches fades over time, and so they are rarely a cosmetic problem for the child.

A Mongolian blue spot is another common benign finding in newborns, and in this case is usually located at the base of the spine. The blue spot is a diffuse blue-black patch resulting from an excess of melanin-producing cells in that area of skin. The appearance of the patch may be confused with that of bruising.

Strawberry naevus

A strawberry naevus becomes apparent very shortly after birth, and may enlarge rapidly over the first few months of life (Figure 6.1c-XV). The principal underlying abnormality is a cluster of enlarged capillaries in the area, which means that the naevus can bleed profusely if damaged. The naevus is often a deep red in colour and has a raised spherical or ovoid border. It is usually perceived as very unsightly, and so the parents have to be reassured that very often the lump becomes paler and less prominent over the first few years of childhood. In about half of cases there is total resolution of a strawberry neavus by the age of 5 years. Only if the naevus is close to the eye, or if it is persistent beyond the age of 10 years, is surgical removal advised.

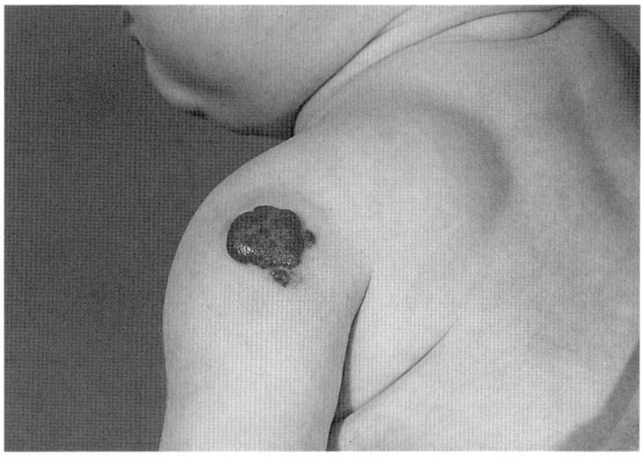

Figure 6.1c-XV • A strawberry naevus in an infant.

Port wine stains

A port wine stain is a flat region of deep violet coloration of the skin resulting from dilated capillaries deep in the dermis. The surface of the port wine stain can be bumpy because of irregularities in the pattern of the enlarged capillaries. Although the nature of the underlying problem is similar to that of the stork mark, port wine stains are much more of a cosmetic problem, and also do not tend to fade with time.

Rarely, a port wine stain may be associated with vascular abnormalities in the brain, and in these cases a mental health disorder, fits and paralysis may become apparent.

Information Box 6.1c-XVII

Moles and naevi: comments from a Chinese medicine perspective

From a Chinese medicine perspective, the fact that a naevus of one form or another has developed may reflect a degree of Deficiency in that particular region of the body, as most naevi reflect abnormal development of the skin and subcutaneous tissues. This means that the precise location of naevi may hint at a specific energetic imbalance. For example, a large mole on the anterolateral border of the shin might suggest an Imbalance or Deficiency in Stomach Qi.

Multiple naevi scattered over diverse regions of the skin might indicate an underlying imbalance of Lung and/or Jing, as the Lungs dominate the skin and Jing is the foundation of the healthy development of tissues. The tendency to develop multiple naevi is commonly inherited.

Information Box 6.1c-XVIII

Strawberry naevus: comments from a Chinese medicine perspective

A Chinese medicine interpretation of a strawberry naevus might be that there is an underlying Deficiency of Jing, together with Heat in the Organ associated with the site of the naevus.

Port wine stains can now be treated cosmetically by means of laser therapy to the skin. Prior to the development of this expensive technique, the only treatment was the use of camouflaging cosmetic creams.

Information Box 6.1c-XIX

Port wine stain: comments from a Chinese medicine perspective

The Chinese medicine interpretation of a port wine stain might be similar to that as described for the strawberry naevus. The deeper colour might suggest that Stagnation of Qi as well as Heat is more prominent in the diagnosis.

Campbell de Morgan red spots

Campbell de Morgan spots are the cherry red, mole-like spots that are very commonly found on the limbs and body of adults, particularly after 40 years of age. These are benign, and are the result of a cluster of abnormal blood vessels in the dermis or subcutaneous tissues, known as an 'angioma'.

Spider naevi

A spider naevus is more correctly termed a 'telangiectasis'. A telangiectasis is a cluster of thread-like vessels that appear to radiate from a central vessel in the skin, akin to legs from a spider's body. The usual spider naevus (which is not really a naevus at all) is less than 5 millimetres in diameter, although they can reach sizes of up to 1 centimetre.

Spider naevi are of clinical significance, as they can be associated with an underlying medical condition, particularly if more than five are found. The most common underlying problem is chronic liver disease, in which the 'spiders' commonly form on the face, neck, upper limbs and upper body.

Skin tumours: benign lumps

A naevus has been defined as a mole, birthmark or other benign minor skin change. All the other benign conditions that present as lumps in the skin can be categorised as skin tumours. The various forms of benign skin tumours are described below.

Seborrhoeic warts (keratoses)

A seborrhoeic wart is an almost universal finding on the body of an elderly person. In some cases there can be over 100 of these brown, patch-like areas of skin, scattered particularly over the back, abdomen and chest (Figure 6.1c-XVI). The usual size of a seborrhoeic wart is 0.5–3 centimetres in diameter. The colour varies from pale to deeply pigmented, and the surface has a slightly greasy and warty texture.

Seborrhoeic warts appear to be the result of a benign overgrowth of the deep cells of the epidermis. In some cases, friction (e.g. from a bra strap) seems to stimulate their development.

The main clinical problem with seborrhoeic warts is that they can be perceived as unsightly, and in some cases they may be confused with malignant growths. They can be removed by surgery, cautery or cryotherapy.

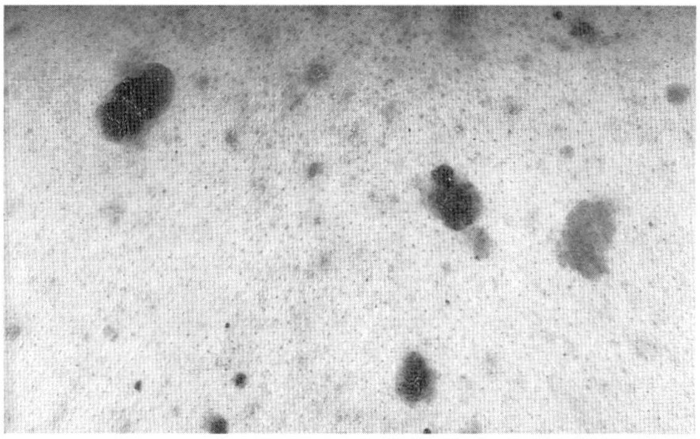

Figure 6.1c-XVI • Seborrhoeic warts on the skin of the back.

Information Box 6.1c-XX

Seborrhoeic warts: comments from a Chinese medicine perspective

From a Chinese medicine perspective, the thickened, waxy appearance of seborrhoeic warts suggests that Phlegm Damp may be an underlying Pathogenic Factor.

Skin tags

Skin tags are tiny fleshy outgrowths of the skin that commonly appear to be on a stalk. They form around the neck, inner arms and armpits, particularly in obese and elderly people. Skin tags are entirely benign and can be easily removed by means of cautery.

Information Box 6.1c-XXI

Skin tags: comments from a Chinese medicine perspective

In Chinese medicine, the structure of skin tags would suggest that they are manifestations of Phlegm.

Dermatofibromata

A dermatofibroma appears as a painless, lentil-sized lump in the dermis, with a slightly pigmented appearance. Dermatofibromata are usually found on the legs, and may result from minor trauma such as an insect bite. They consist of fibrous tissue and blood vessels.

Dermatofibromata cause concern because they may be confused with a melanoma. For this reason doctors may be very ready to excise them, although this procedure is unnecessary in most cases.

Epidermal cysts, milia and lipomas

Epidermal cysts and lipomas can both present as large, smooth lumps under the skin. They can cause considerable concern to the patient when they are first discovered, but both are benign in nature.

Information Box 6.1c-XXII

Dermatofibroma: comments from a Chinese medicine perspective

A dermatofibroma may well be a manifestation of Phlegm.

Epidermal cysts (which include sebaceous cysts) contain a broken down form of keratin that is cheesy in consistency. They are attached to the overlying skin and so move with it when palpated. They usually feel smooth, and the larger ones have a rubbery texture. They are common on the scalp, neck and trunk. Milia are tiny, millet-seed-sized keratin cysts that most commonly appear around the eyelids. They should be no cause for concern.

A lipoma is an overgrowth of adipose (fat) tissue and is found in the dermis and subcutaneous layers. It is readily distinguished from an epidermal cyst because it is not usually attached to the overlying skin (it moves freely over the underlying muscle) and because it has a very soft consistency.

Keloid scars

The pathology and energetic interpretation of keloid scars are described in Chapter 2.1b (Figure 6.1c-XVII).

Information Box 6.1c-XXIII

Epidermal cysts and lipomata: comments from a Chinese medicine perspective

Both epidermal cysts and lipomas suggest the presence of Phlegm Damp.

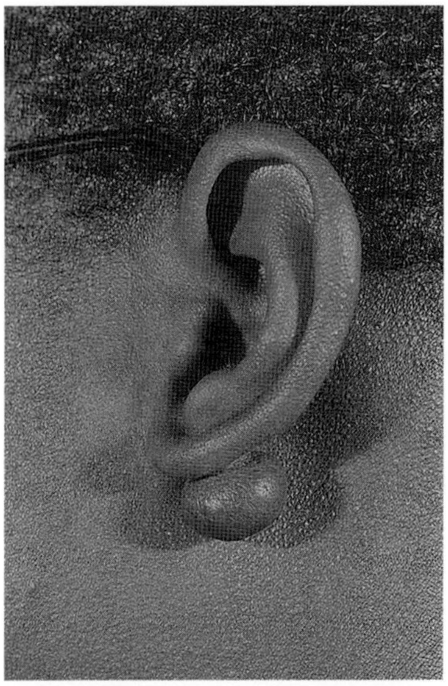

Figure 6.1c-XVII • A keloid scar resulting from ear piercing.

Malignant skin tumours

Although the term 'malignant' describes the disordered pattern of growth that is characteristic of cancer, many malignant skin tumours are slow growing. For this reason, the majority of malignant skin tumours are readily treatable if diagnosed at an early stage in their development.

Information Box 6.1c-XXIV

Skin cancer: comments from a Chinese medicine perspective

In Chinese medicine, the development of skin cancer suggests a marked underlying Deficiency of Vital Substances (in particular Lung Qi and Jing) and the accumulation of Phlegm (and/or Blood Stagnation). Exposure to sun and other environmental toxins is common in the history of skin cancer. It would make sense that sun exposure, as it involves burning, is likely to induce local Yin Deficiency, so participating in creating the background Deficiency recognised in the pathology of cancer. Heat is also likely to be important in the aetiology of sun-related skin cancers.

Solar keratoses

Solar keratoses are reddened, scaly patches of skin that occur in chronically sun exposed areas such as the scalp, bridge of the nose and forearms (Figure 6.1c-XVIII). They consist of regions of the skin in which there is chaotic growth of epithelial tissues, but their size can wax and wane over time, and they may even regress fully. However, they can progress to a more established form of skin cancer, and so may be removed by cryotherapy or treated by means of a cream containing 5-fluorouracil (a chemotherapeutic agent) if they seem to be persistent or are growing relentlessly.

Basal cell carcinoma (rodent ulcer)

The basal cell carcinoma (BCC), or rodent ulcer, is a slow-growing tumour that tends to develop in sun-exposed regions of the skin (e.g. scalp, nose, behind the ear) in the

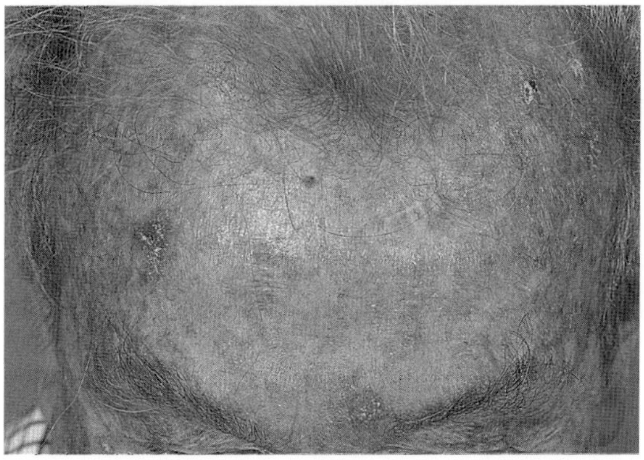

Figure 6.1c-XVIII • Solar keratoses on the sun-exposed forehead.

elderly (Figure 6.1c-XIX). It usually first appears as a smooth, raised nodule that then grows outwards with rolled edges, leaving a slight central depression. If the growth is unchecked, the central area can ulcerate (i.e. lose its epithelial surface layer). Fine, thread-like vessels can be seen on the edges and the surface of the tumour, and these cause it to bleed readily with minor trauma. Although growth is slow, the BCC can extend downwards into bony tissue, at which stage it is much more difficult to halt its destructive growth pattern.

Small tumours are treated with cryotherapy or topical cytotoxic creams, and large tumours with excision and/or radiotherapy.

Squamous-cell carcinoma and Bowen's disease

A squamous-cell carcinoma (SCC) is another epidermal skin cancer that has a predilection for sun-exposed areas. The least invasive form of this cancer, known as Bowen's disease, involves a spreading of cancerous cells in the epidermis. This leads to a flat, red, scaly patch with an irregular border, and is a fairly common finding in elderly people.

Treatment for Bowen's disease is given to prevent progression, although this eventuality is fairly rare. Treatment involves local cryotherapy to small areas, and radiotherapy if the skin changes are extensive.

Invasive SCC can take on a range of appearances, from an irregular, scaly lump (akin to a large solar keratosis), a fleshy tumour, or a non-healing ulcer (Figure 6.1c-XX). Physical trauma, such as a burn or repeated exposure of the lips to cigarettes, can promote the development of an invasive SCC.

Treatment is by means of surgical removal or radiotherapy.

Paget's disease of the nipple

This is a specific variant of Bowen's disease, which develops in the region of one nipple. It should be taken seriously, as Paget's disease often reflects the presence of an underlying breast tumour.

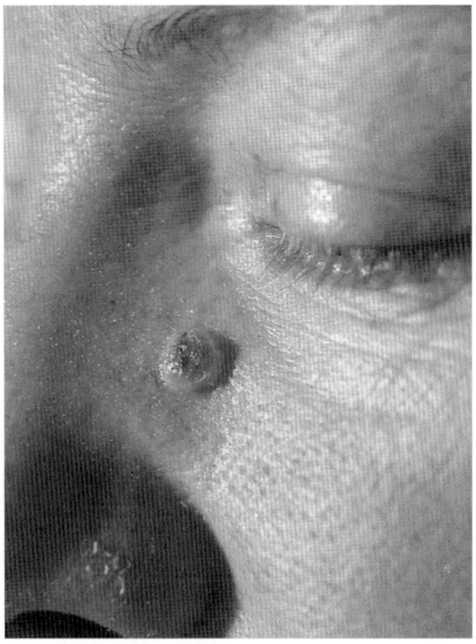

Figure 6.1c-XIX • A basal cell carcinoma on the cheek.

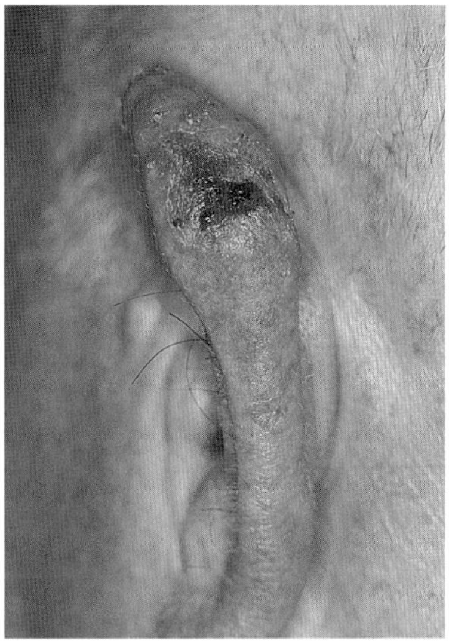

Figure 6.1c-XX • A squamous-cell carcinoma on the earlobe.

Malignant melanoma

The malignant melanoma is the most dangerous of the malignant skin tumours and, in contrast to the BCC and SCC, tends to affect a younger population. The incidence is rising rapidly, and this is believed to be attributable to increased sun exposure in sun-seeking westerners on holiday, and also to a general increase in the levels of solar radiation that reach the Earth because of changes in the composition of gases in the atmosphere. A history of sunburn of the skin is of particular relevance in the development of melanoma, and it is known that the cumulative effects of episodes of sunburn in childhood are particularly dangerous.

The malignant melanoma has a range of appearances, of which the superficial, spreading form carries the best prognosis. In this form, the tumour appears as a fairly flat, brown-black patch with irregular areas of depth of pigmentation and also irregular borders. In contrast with the BCC and SCC, common locations are the upper leg and trunk. Unlike a melanocytic naevus, the surface of the malignant melanoma is unstable, and so it may itch or bleed easily. These are all warning features of its potential invasiveness. The more rare and rapidly growing nodular melanoma tends to have a more full growth both outwards and also inwards to deeper tissues.

In both forms of melanoma the prognosis depends on the depth to which the tumour has penetrated. Good prognosis (over 90% cure rate) is associated with a depth of less than 1.5 millimetres. However, if the tumour has extended to a depth of more than over 3.5 millimetres, the cure rate drops to below 40%. This is because the malignant melanoma very readily metastasises, and the chances of this are increased as the tumour grows deeper into the dermis.

The most effective method of treating malignant melanoma (after minimisation of sun exposure) is public education so that suspect 'moles' are brought to medical attention as soon as possible. Ideally, suspect tumours can be removed immediately and sent for pathological analysis. This may be the only treatment required to 'cure' a malignant melanoma that is small and non-invasive.

In the case of a large malignant melanoma, surgery is still the preferred treatment, and a wide excision may be advised. To date, radiotherapy and chemotherapy seem to have very little effect in malignant melanoma that has metastasised.

> **Information Box 6.1c-XXV**
>
> **Malignant melanoma: comments from a Chinese medicine perspective**
>
> From a Chinese medicine perspective, the development of a malignant melanoma, as with all skin tumours, suggests chronic Depletion of Vital Substances, in particular Lung Qi and Jing. The dark black colour might indicate that Blood Stagnation as well as Phlegm is important in the diagnosis.

Kaposi's sarcoma

Kaposi's sarcoma is a once rare tumour of blood vessels that has been more widely reported in recent decades as it appears in an aggressive form in people with AIDS and other forms of immunosuppression. Kaposi's sarcoma presents as a number of purplish plaques and nodules in the skin. It is treated by means of radiotherapy.

Lymphoma and the skin

Lymphoma rarely can either spread to the skin, or may originate in the skin. It leads to red, scaly irregular patches, which may be confused with psoriasis or eczema. It is also the most rare cause of erythroderma. Treatment includes radiotherapy, chemotherapy and PUVA (see under Psoriasis).

Connective tissue disorders

The connective tissue disorders are a form of multisystem (or rheumatic) autoimmune disease. This means that, in these conditions, diverse tissues are affected by an autoimmune disease process. In the connective tissue diseases, so called because the autoimmune damage is focused on various types of connective tissue, the skin is very often involved.

Systemic lupus erythematosus and discoid lupus erythematosus

Systemic lupus erythematosus (SLE) has been mentioned briefly in earlier chapters of this book as a multisystem connective disuse disorder that can cause arteritis, glomerulonephritis and arthritis. Also, psychiatric disorders are common in SLE as a result of arteritis of the vessels in the brain. SLE typically affects women of childbearing age. It usually progresses in a series of relapses separated by remissions. In most cases the outlook is good, but in severe cases SLE can be fatal. The most common cause of death in SLE is glomerulonephritis and consequent kidney failure. Discoid lupus erythematosus (DLE) is a variant of SLE in which the skin only is affected.

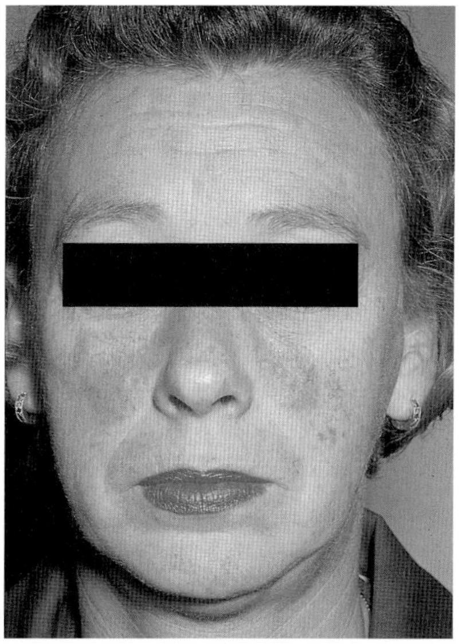

Figure 6.1c-XXI • The butterfly facial rash in systemic lupus erythematosus.

A butterfly-shaped rash affecting the cheeks and bridge of the nose is common in SLE (Figure 6.1c-XXI). Sunlight provokes the development of this butterfly rash. Additional skin problems result from arteritis in the vessels of the dermis, and can manifest as itching and purpura (tiny areas of bruising).

In DLE the skin changes are slightly different. Light-exposed areas are affected principally, most usually presenting with a reddened, scaly appearance. In severe cases, large areas of the skin can become disfigured by scarring. The scalp can be affected, leading to areas of permanent hair loss (Figure 6.1c-XXII).

SLE is confirmed by means of assays of the serum for autoantibodies. DLE is diagnosed by means of skin biopsy.

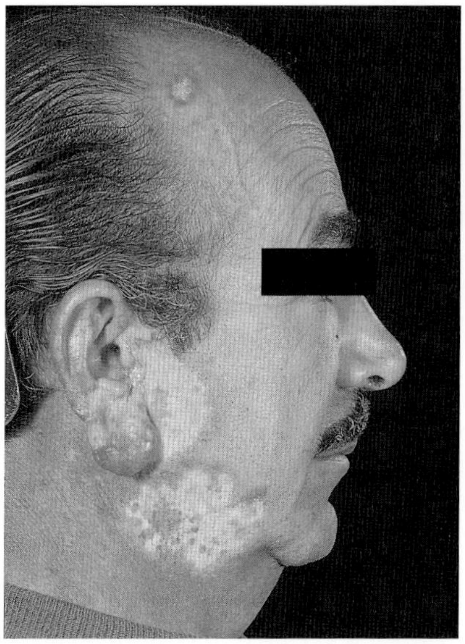

Figure 6.1c-XXII • The scarring rash of chronic discoid lupus erythematosus.

Mild SLE can be treated with non-steroidal anti-inflammatory drugs (NSAIDs) or disease-modifying antirheumatic drugs (DMARDs). Severe relapses may require steroid injections and immunosuppressant medication. DLE is treated with corticosteroid creams and sunscreens.

> **Information Box 6.1c-XXVI**
>
> **Systemic lupus erythematosus: comments from a Chinese medicine perspective**
>
> In Chinese medicine, the features of systemic lupus erythematosus, in common with all multisystem autoimmune diseases, suggest that Heat and Phlegm might account for the most florid symptoms of rash, arthritis and psychosis. The underlying problem is autoimmune, indicating that a profound Deficiency in Kidney Qi and Essence is the basis of the accumulation of Heat and Phlegm.

Dermatomyositis

Dermatomyositis is an autoimmune condition of the skin and muscles that can occur in both childhood and adult life in slightly different forms. In the adult form of the disease there may be an association with an underlying cancer.

The skin is affected by a purple-red rash affecting the face, neck and hands, together with puffiness of the skin around the eyes. There can be profound muscle weakness in some cases, typically of the thighs and upper arm muscles.

The treatment involves exclusion of cancer, and treatment of this if it is found to be present. Oral corticosteroids and immunosuppressants are used to control the inflammatory symptoms.

> **Information Box 6.1c-XXVII**
>
> **Dermatomyositis: comments from a Chinese medicine perspective**
>
> From a Chinese medicine perspective, the violaceous rash in dermatomyositis might suggest that Stagnation of Qi is an additional Pathogenic Factor to Heat. The weakened muscles also are suggestive of an imbalance of Liver Qi. All these have occurred against a background of Deficiency of Kidney Qi and Essence.

Scleroderma and morphoea

'Scleroderma' literally means thickening of the skin, and is a term used to refer to a process of uncertain cause in which there is progressive formation of fibrous tissue in the skin. If scleroderma develops without any other medical features it is called 'morphoea'. In systemic sclerosis, scleroderma occurs as part of a multisystem disorder.

In morphoea, rounded areas or strips of skin undergo a process of thickening, which begins with the appearance of patches of a purplish hue. These then become white, shiny and inelastic. Impairment of limb movement and breathing can develop in severe cases. In most cases morphoea will gradually resolve. There is no known treatment.

In systemic sclerosis the scleroderma results from a vasculitis of the skin. Thickening and tightening of the skin of the digits leads to reduced circulation to the fingers and toes, which manifests in Raynaud's phenomenon (white finger). Ulceration of the fingertips can develop. Other features of systemic sclerosis include pinching of the facial skin, difficulties in swallowing and digestion (due to thickening of the lining of the oesophagus and bowel), respiratory impairment, mild kidney failure, biliary cirrhosis, cardiac muscle impairment, arthritis and leg ulcers. It can be appreciated that systemic sclerosis is a true multisystem disorder. However, the progression of the condition is usually slow, and so the prognosis is fairly good in most cases.

There is no satisfactory disease-modifying treatment for either morphoea or systemic sclerosis. Symptomatic treatment is the mainstay of medical therapy.

> **Information Box 6.1c-XXVIII**
>
> **Systemic sclerosis: comments from a Chinese medicine perspective**
>
> In Chinese medicine, the main features of thickening and loss of elasticity indicate Phlegm and Deficiency of Qi and Yin. Qi and Blood Stagnation is suggested by the impairment of the normal peristaltic action of the bowel and the severity of the Raynaud's phenomenon. Because of the similarity to the autoimmune multisystem disorders, a profound Deficiency of Kidney Qi and Essence may underlie the development of these diverse imbalances, although the cause is not obviously autoimmune in nature.

Disorders of hair growth

Excessive hair growth

Excessive hair growth is a problem because of its cosmetic consequences. For this reason, the problem mostly affects women. It has to be remembered that the development of excessive facial or body hair does not usually constitute a medical problem, but rather a distortion of what western society has come to appreciate as normal or beautiful.

It is normal for many western women to have visible body hairs on the legs, lower back, the pubic region and the skin close to these regions (the bikini line), around the nipples, and on the upper lip and chin. The density and thickness of these hairs can increase throughout the childbearing years. The visibility of body hair varies very much with family patterns of hair growth and also racial origin. It can be particularly marked in women of Mediterranean extraction.

It is also normal for there to be a great variation in the density of body hair in men, and again for this to be related to family patterns of hair growth. Hairiness in men has been seen as a marker of Samson-like manliness and strength. However, in some western cultures excessive body hair in men has become less desirable.

There is also a marked variation of the degree of distress experienced by a person with a particular density of body hair growth. This can strongly reflect the cultural influences to which the person has been exposed. If the distress appears to be out of proportion to the actual amount of hair growth (when put into the context of the patient's culture), this can be a manifestation of dysmorphophobia (a condition in which the person perceives a normal body feature to be grotesque in some way).

Most western women and men who perceive their body-hair pattern to be unacceptable in some way will seek methods of removing the hair. Shaving, depilation creams and waxing are commonly used techniques, all of which lead only to a temporary cessation of the problem. Electrolysis, a technique in which the hair follicle is damaged by a combination of heat and electricity delivered by a pinpoint probe, is a method for bringing about a more permanent reduction in body hair.

In some cases excessive body hair may indicate an underlying medical problem. If the body hair distribution is in the usual distribution seen in men, the term 'hirsutism' is applied. If the hair growth is more generalised, it is termed 'hypertrichosis'. The most common underlying causes of hirsutism in women are disturbances in the production of the sex hormones. Polycystic ovary syndrome is the most well recognised cause of secondary hirsutism in women. Anorexia nervosa can also lead to an increased density of very fine body hair (lanugo). Cushing's disease is a far less common, but more sinister, cause of excessive facial and bodily hair.

Some medications, including those that contain one of the steroid family of drugs, can lead to excessive body-hair growth. The drug minoxidil, developed for the treatment of severe hypertension, was found to have the side-effect of hirsutism. This property has since been utilised for 'benefit', as minoxidil is now marketed in the form of a topical fluid that can be applied to prevent male-pattern baldness.

Information Box 6.1c-XXIX

Excessive body hair: comments from a Chinese medicine perspective

From a Chinese medicine perspective, distribution of body hair in the normal range would not indicate an energetic imbalance. Generalised excessive body hair growth might indicate a specific imbalance in Lung Qi, as the Lung is the Organ that manifests in the body hair. Hirsutism, which follows a male pattern of hair distribution, might in women represent an excess of Yang. As the Liver and Kidney Organs are associated with sexuality, one might expect imbalances in the Qi of these Organs to be present also.

The treatments of shaving, depilatory creams and waxing have few obvious side-effects. However, depilatory creams (which literally dissolve the protein of the hair) are toxic to the skin. They can cause temporary redness and dryness of the treated skin, and so are Heating in nature. It might be expected that waxing may lead to a degree of shock to the skin as numerous hair follicles are stripped of their hairs simultaneously.

Electrolysis is obviously Heating, as it produces its effects by burning and scarring of the hair follicles. This is likely to induce Yin Deficiency, and may lead to deeper imbalances (possibly in the Qi of the Lungs, Liver and/or Kidneys) as the treatment is suppressive of growth.

Abnormal scalp hair loss (alopecia)

The diagnosis of scalp hair loss (alopecia) depends on whether or not the pattern of loss is diffuse or patchy. Scalp hair loss may be accompanied by a more generalised loss of body hair, but this feature is very rarely seen to be a problem by the patient.

Male pattern baldness

The most common pattern of diffuse scalp hair loss is male-pattern baldness (androgenetic alopecia), in which the hair thins progressively from the temples and the crown, so leading to the very commonly seen 'receding hairline' and 'bald pate'. In most cases this is a normal response to male sex hormones in genetically susceptible individuals. Normal male-pattern baldness runs very strongly in families, and the extent and pace of the developing baldness is also strongly familial.

As is the case with normal visible body hair growth, male-pattern baldness can be a cause of acute distress because of its perceived cosmetic effects, and so can lead the patient to seek a solution to the 'problem'. Male-pattern baldness can also affect a minority of women, in which case the cosmetic effects are usually much more significant for the patient.

The available treatments for male-pattern baldness include minoxidil lotion and surgical transplant of tiny portions of hair-producing scalp into the balding regions. Minoxidil appears to have some effect in slowing the progression of the baldness.

Information Box 6.1c-XXX

Male-pattern baldness: comments from a Chinese medicine perspective

In Chinese medicine, the scalp hair is the manifestation of flourishing Kidney Essence. Shiny, strong and springy hair suggests healthy Kidney Qi and Essence, and weak, brittle, lacklustre hair would indicate a Depletion in these substances. Male-pattern baldness does not necessarily indicate a problem in Kidney Qi, as long as the remaining hair is healthy in nature.

Diffuse alopecia

Hairdressers recognise that flourishing hair growth is an indication of health, and thin, lacklustre, brittle hair can mean that the individual is run down in some way. More specifically, gradual thinning of hair over time can indicate a nutritional deficiency (especially iron deficiency), a generalised medical problem such as thyroid disease, SLE or a response to certain drugs (e.g. corticosteroids and cytotoxic drugs).

The hair, or a large amount of it, can literally fall out over night (or at least over the course of a few days) approximately 3 months following an experience of emotional or physical stress (e.g. childbirth, an operation, a car accident, major illness). This dramatic reaction is called 'telogen effluvium', and is a delayed response to the sudden cessation of the growth of many hairs. In the natural pattern of hair growth, when the growth of a hair has ceased it takes some weeks before the hair actually falls out, hence the delayed response. If the patient already has some grey hairs, a preferential loss of dark hairs can cause the appearance of 'going grey overnight'. The normal consequence of telogen effluvium is that new hairs begin to grow immediately, but may temporarily have a different texture to the lost hairs.

> **Information Box 6.1c-XXXI**
>
> **Diffuse alopecia: comments from a Chinese medicine perspective**
>
> Diffuse alopecia represents a Depletion of Kidney Qi and Essence. Shock is particularly damaging to the Kidney Qi and Essence, and it makes sense that it can result in telogen effluvium.

Alopecia areata

Alopecia areata is the consequence of an immune reaction in the skin, leading to patches of total hair loss which expose a normal-appearing, rounded area of scalp skin. Most patches regrow after a few weeks, but this does not always occur. In severe cases the scalp might acquire a moth-eaten appearance, or the alopecia may be total (and also include body hair).

There is no satisfactory treatment for alopecia areata, although steroid injections might be used.

> **Information Box 6.1c-XXXII**
>
> **Alopecia areata: comments from a Chinese medicine perspective**
>
> In Chinese medicine, alopecia areata equates to Kidney Deficiency.

Hair loss with abnormal scalp skin

Diseases that affect the scalp skin, such as psoriasis, seborrhoeic dermatitis and tinea capitis (all mentioned earlier in this chapter), can manifest in patchy hair loss from the affected areas.

Other common skin conditions

Urticaria and angio-oedema

The term 'urticaria' is derived from the Latin word for 'stinging nettle'. It is used to describe the skin reaction in which there is a rapid development of wheals, akin to the rash that develops after a nettle sting. A wheal is an area of raised skin that initially appears more pale than the surrounding skin. It may itch or sting. Wheals always resolve within minutes to hours, but they may be replaced by the formation of successive wheals in different body sites (Figure 6.1c-XXIII).

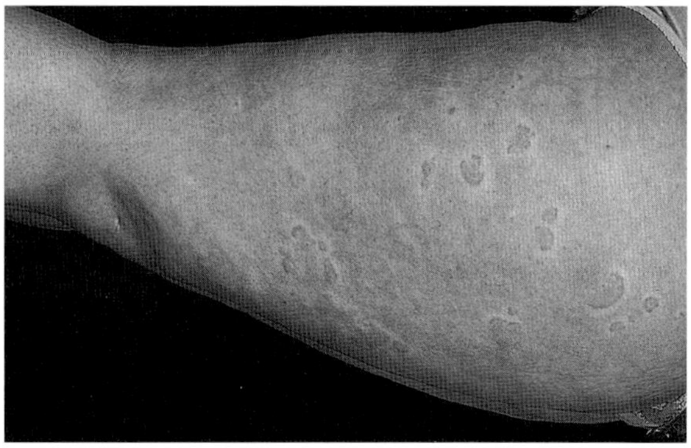

Figure 6.1c-XXIII • Wheals on the arm in urticaria.

Urticaria results from a rapid dilatation of the dermal blood vessels, which then permit excess fluid to pass from the blood into the surrounding skin tissue (oedema). The chemical histamine, released from the mast cell (a form of tissue-based lymphocyte), stimulates this reaction. In the case of the stinging nettle, a histamine-like chemical is introduced into the dermis from tiny prickles on the nettle leaf and stem.

'Angio-oedema' is a term that describes the extension of the oedema of urticaria to the subcutaneous tissues. This can result in an alarming swelling of the loose tissues around the eyes, lips and the airway in the pharynx. Angio-oedema can also be accompanied by asthma, which is another histamine-mediated allergic reaction.

Both urticaria and angio-oedema can be the result of a generalised anaphylactic reaction as a result of exposure to an allergen. Common causes of acute urticaria and angio-oedema include skin contact with plants, animal fur or foods (e.g. milk, egg white), ingestion of certain foods (e.g. milk, shellfish, egg, nuts) and ingestion of drugs (e.g. penicillin). People with atopy are more prone to allergic urticaria and angio-oedema.

Urticaria can also develop in response to pressure to the skin, heat, sweating, sunlight and cold, in which case its course is often chronic. In some cases of chronic urticaria there is no obvious trigger.

Acute urticaria often responds well to antihistamine tablets. If the allergic response is acute and severe, intravenous steroids, adrenaline and inhaled bronchodilators may also be used to control the reaction and prevent worsening of the airways obstruction. Chronic urticaria is less responsive to medication, and the treatment often depends on avoidance of the triggers, if these can be identified.

> **Information Box 6.1c-XXXIII**
>
> **Urticaria: comments from a Chinese medicine perspective**
>
> In Chinese medicine, the symptoms of urticaria correspond to Wind Heat Invasion, and angio-oedema to Wind Water Invading the Lungs. In both there will be an underlying Deficiency of Wei Qi. Wei Qi Deficiency results from Lung Qi Deficiency and/or Kidney Deficiency.

Prickly heat (miliaria)

'Prickly heat' (miliaria) is the medical term used to describe the tiny, itchy heat bumps that develop as a result of obstruction of the sweat ducts in hot, humid conditions. The condition is aggravated by anything that stimulates sweating. Prickly heat can contribute to heat stroke because it inhibits the cooling benefits of sweating.

The treatment is avoidance of triggers to sweating, and application to the skin of emollient lotions.

Information Box 6.1c-XXXIV

Prickly heat (milaria): comments from a Chinese medicine perspective

In Chinese medicine, prickly heat is usually seen as a manifestation of Damp Heat.

Polymorphic light eruption

Polymorphic light eruption (PLE) is a common disorder which is commonly misdiagnosed as prickly heat. It is an abnormal reaction to sunlight, not heat, and so primarily affects light-exposed areas. The manifestation of PLE is as tiny red spots, and sometimes blisters.

Sunscreens and sun avoidance will prevent PLE in most cases.

Information Box 6.1c-XXXV

Polymorphic light eruption: comments from a Chinese medicine perspective

In Chinese medicine, polymorphic light eruption is a manifestation of Heat (and underlying Yin Deficiency).

Chilblains

Chilblains are painful areas of inflammation that develop in response to cold. They can develop on the fingers, toes and the fleshy aspect of the upper legs. Treatment of chilblains is simply avoidance of extremes of temperature.

Information Box 6.1c-XXXVI

Chilblains: comments from a Chinese medicine perspective

In Chinese medicine, chilblains are a result of Cold Stagnation leading to Heat. Zong Qi Deficiency can underlie the development of chilblains, as it is Zong Qi that is responsible for the even flow of Qi and Blood to the extremities.

Xanthelasmata and xanthomata

Xanthelasmata (singular is xanthelasma) are small (1–5 millimetres in diameter), yellowish plaques (the name is derived from the Greek word for 'yellow') that form in loose areas of skin, in particular around the eyelids. They sometimes develop in association with some of the various forms of hyperlipidaemia.

Xanthomata (singular xanthoma) are a less common finding. These are more substantial cholesterol deposits, which appear as nodules in the skin around bony prominences, in the tendons and on the palms. Xanthomata are much more closely associated with hyperlipidaemia, and so are a warning feature of atherosclerosis.

Treatment is not usually offered for these cholesterol deposits, as they are rarely a cosmetic problem.

Information Box 6.1c-XXXVII

Xanthelasmata: comments from a Chinese medicine perspective

In Chinese medicine, cholesterol deposits are a physical manifestation of Phlegm Damp.

Lichen planus

Lichen planus is an immune-related skin reaction of unknown cause, in which the skin erupts with numerous itchy, purplish, flat-topped papules. The papules most commonly appear on the wrists, ankles and small of the back (Figure 6.1c-XXIV).

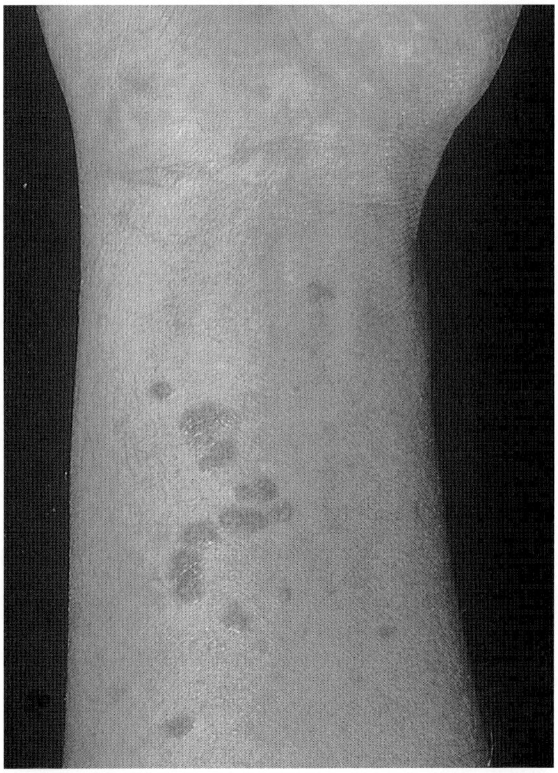

Figure 6.1c-XXIV • Papules on the forearm in lichen planus.

Changes can also be found in the mucous membranes of the mouth and genitalia.

In most cases the eruption settles within a few months, although some cases can be persistent. If the rash and itching are severe, steroid creams and even corticosteroid tablets may be prescribed.

Information Box 6.1c-XXXVIII

Lichen planus: comments from a Chinese medicine perspective

The purplish colour and the itch are suggestive that lichen planus is an expression of Heat and Stagnation of Qi.

Pityriasis rosea

Pityriasis rosea is a mysterious self-limiting condition that primarily affects apparently otherwise well children and young adults. It may well be a delayed response to a viral infection. The rash begins with a so-called 'herald patch' of red, scaly skin on the trunk or upper arm. Then, within a few days, this herald is followed by an eruption of small, pink, oval patches on the back, abdomen, upper arms and thighs.

The patches in pityriasis rosea are slightly scaly and may be a cause of slight irritation. The rash clears up spontaneously within 6–8 weeks. Usually no treatment is needed.

Information Box 6.1c-XXXIX

Pityriasis rosea: comments from a Chinese medicine perspective

In Chinese medicine, this rash would appear to result from an invasion of Wind Heat. The scaling is suggestive of Phlegm Damp.

Pruritus

'Pruritus' is a general term used to describe itching in the absence of an underlying skin disorder. Any cause of pruritus will lead the patient to scratch, and so initially will lead to the appearance of excoriated or bleeding skin. Chronic pruritus can cause the skin to become thickened and dry (lichenified), as can also occur in chronic eczema. Lichenified skin is more likely to itch, and so a vicious cycle of itch–scratch–itch is set up. If severe and chronic, pruritus can be a very distressing condition.

Itching has a wide range of causes, many of which have already been described in this chapter. Any possible underlying skin disease (e.g. scabies) has to be excluded before a diagnosis of pruritus can be made.

Localised pruritis may manifest in the form of a patch of lichenified skin, often in an overstressed or anxious individual. Common sites are the back, neck, shins and, distressingly for the patient, the perianal and vulval regions. Itchy skin nodules can also develop in addition to the thickened itchy patch of skin. Good hygiene, especially of the perineum, is important in the treatment of pruritis. Ideally, the patient's level of stress should be addressed. High-dose topical steroids may be used to inhibit the inflammation and so break the cycle of itching and scratching.

Generalised pruritus is a very unpleasant disorder that is recognised to occur in a wide range of generalised medical conditions (e.g. iron deficiency, obstructive jaundice, chronic renal failure, thyroid disease, cancer). In pregnancy, generalised itch can in some cases be a serious indication of obstetric cholestasis, a condition in which the mother's liver fails to clear the bile from the bile ducts (probably a result of an inherited susceptibility to oestrogen). The build up of bile salts in the blood is the cause of the itch, and is a warning feature of serious damage to the unborn baby. If a pregnant woman develops generalised pruritus, she should be referred to her doctor or midwife for further tests.

In the management of generalised pruritus, first the underlying cause should be treated, and then symptoms may be controlled by use of topical steroids and oral sedative antihistamine tablets. In elderly people, pruritus of unknown cause may simply be the result of dry, poorly nourished skin. In this case emollient creams can be of help.

Information Box 6.1c-XL

Pruritus: comments from a Chinese medicine perspective

In Chinese medicine, itch may be the result of Wind or Qi Stagnation. In the case of pruritus, Qi Stagnation may have developed on a background of emotional stress and/or Depletion of Vital Substances.

Skin ulcers

'Skin ulcer' is the term used to describe any breach in the epithelial lining of the skin. Chronic skin ulcers are areas of skin in which this breach persistently fails to heal over (Figure 6.1c-XXV). The cause, features and Chinese medicine interpretation of chronic skin ulcers have been described in some depth in Chapter 2.1b.

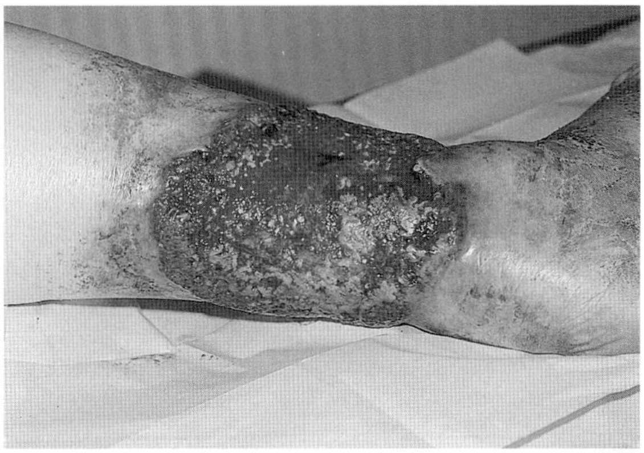

Figure 6.1c-XXV • A chronic venous skin ulcer on the lower leg.

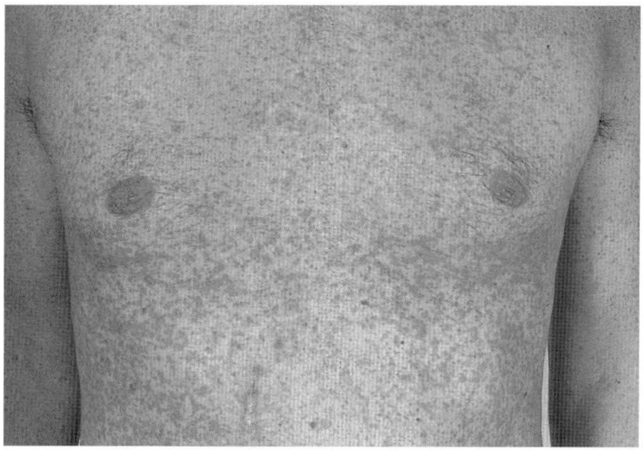

Figure 6.1c-XXVI • A typical rash resulting from penicillin allergy.

Reactions to drugs

The skin can manifest a wide range of clinical features as side-effects to prescribed medication. A scan through the side-effect summaries for the diverse drugs in the British National Formulary will reveal that 'rash' is very commonly listed. The drugs that are most commonly implicated in adverse skin reactions include antibiotics, NSAIDs and tranquillisers (Figure 6.1c-XXVI).

The commonly recognised skin reactions to drugs are:

- itchy red rashes (exanthems)
- urticaria and anaphylaxis (see earlier in this chapter)
- inflamed scaliness (exfoliative dermatitis)
- vasculitis (inflammation of the tiny blood vessels that supply the skin)
- lichen planus
- acne-like rashes
- abnormalities in hair growth
- changes in pigmentation
- blistering
- light sensitivity
- SLE-like reactions
- worsening of pre-existing skin disease.

It can be appreciated that drugs can induce all manner of skin disease, and so when a skin disease suddenly appears it is wise to take a good drug history. The ideal treatment for all these reactions is to withdraw the medication.

The red flags of the diseases of the skin

Some people with diseases of the skin will benefit from referral to a conventional doctor for assessment and/or treatment. Red flags are those symptoms and signs that indicate that referral is to be considered. The red flags of the diseases of the skin are described in Table 6.1c-I. This table forms part of the summary on red flags given in Appendix III, which also gives advice on the degree of urgency of referral for each of the red flag conditions listed.

Table 6.1c-I Red Flags 41 – diseases of the skin

Red Flag	Description	Reasoning
41.1	**A rapidly enlarging patch(es) of painful, crusting or swollen red skin**	Crusting, spreading skin disease suggests erysipelas or severe impetigo. If spreading rapidly, antibiotic treatment should be considered Refer with some urgency if this occurs in someone with eczema, as it can rapidly become a serious condition (or it may indicate herpes infection of the broken skin: eczema herpeticum)
41.2	**A rapidly advancing region or line of redness tracking up the skin of a limb** (following the pathway of a **lymphatic vessel**)	This suggests the deep spread of infection from a distal site (cellulitis and/or lymphangitis), and antibiotic treatment should be considered
41.3	**Pronounced features of candidal infection** (thrush) of the **skin** or **mucous membranes of the mouth**	Widespread candidiasis suggests an underlying chronic condition, such as immunodeficiency or diabetes mellitus. Refer to exclude underlying disease
41.4	**The features of early shingles**: intense one-sided pain, with an overlying rash of crops of fluid-filled, reddened and crusting blisters The pain and rash correspond in location to a neurological dermatome The pain may precede the rash by 1–2 days	Shingles is an outbreak of the chickenpox virus (varicella zoster) that has lain dormant within a spinal nerve root since an earlier episode of chickenpox. It tends to reactivate when the person is run down, exposed to intense sunlight and in the elderly Warn the patient that the condition is contagious and advise that immediate treatment with the antiviral drug aciclovir has been proven to reduce the severity of prolonged pain after recovery of the rash (in this way you are allowing the patient the opportunity of making an informed decision about choosing conventional treatment) Shingles that affects more than one dermatome might be a feature of underlying HIV/AIDS infection

Continued

Table 6.1c-I Red Flags 41 – diseases of the skin—Cont'd

Red Flag	Description	Reasoning
41.5	**Generalised itch**	Generalised itch (not eczema) suggests an underlying medical cause (e.g. cholestasis), iron deficiency or cancer. It may also result from scabies. Refer for diagnosis if persistent over days
41.6	**Itching (severe)** especially of the palms and soles during pregnancy	May result from cholestasis, a condition that can damage the fetus. Refer as a high priority
41.7	**Large areas of redness affecting most (>90%) of the body surface (erythroderma)**: refer because of the risks of dehydration and loss of essential salts	Erythroderma can develop in severe cases of eczema and psoriasis and as a reaction to some medications. It can become a medical emergency, as the cardiovascular system can become under strain from the massively increased blood flow to the skin that results
41.8	**Generalised macular rash (flat red spots)**	Refer if you suspect the possibility of a notifiable disease (i.e. rubella, measles or scarlet fever) NB: Chickenpox is not a notifiable disease and there is no need to refer if there are no other red flags.
41.9	**Purpura or bruising rash (non-blanching)**	A rash which contains areas of non blanching or bruising suggests a bleeding disorder or vasculitis. Refer as an emergency if the patient is also acutely unwell with headache/fever or vomiting (possible meningococcal infection)
41.10	**Any lumps/moles with features suggestive of malignancy: irregularity**, a **tendency to bleed**, **crusting**, **>5 mm in diameter**, **intense black colour**	Skin tumours include basal-cell carcinomas, squamous-cell carcinomas and malignant melanomas. Premalignant skin tumours are often in associated with changes due to sun damage (on the scalp, temples and the backs of the hands), and appear as spreading flat areas of dark pigmentation, or irregular scabs that never seem to heal. If you have any doubt, it is always worth referring for early diagnosis
41.11	**Progressive swelling of the soft tissues of the face and neck (angio-oedema)** and/or **urticaria (nettle rash)**	Angio-oedema can result from acute allergic reaction and can precede life-threatening asthma. Refer urgently if there are any features of respiratory distress (itchy throat/wheeze)
41.12	**Hirsutism (unexplained hairiness)**	Refer any unexplained increase in body hair in middle life, as this may indicate an endocrine disease or, in women, polycystic ovary syndrome

Self-test 6.1c

Diseases of the skin

1. A child is brought to you with a 3-week history of itchy hands, wrists, armpits and abdomen. The itch has been getting progressively worse, particularly at night. Emollients and a mild steroid cream prescribed by the GP a week ago have not been much help. The mother points out to you that the rash consists of tiny bumps, but she has noticed a few bumps on the child's hands that seem like tiny raised lines in the skin.
   (i) What is one possible diagnosis that might explain why this rash has not responded to the usual treatment for eczema?
   (ii) Would you refer this patient back to the GP?
2. A teenager is seeking alternative advice for treatment of acne. She has tried over-the-counter topical treatments (benzoyl peroxide) with little success, but is reluctant to try the options of oral antibiotics or the combined contraceptive pill, which have been offered by her GP. When you examine her skin the acne is clearly severe, in that pustules and comedones (blackheads) are extensive over her nose, chin and forehead.
   (i) Was her GP giving appropriate advice in recommending the medications?
   (ii) What other oral preparation for acne might the GP have mentioned to her?
   (iii) Would you advise her to take any of these medications at this stage?
3. An elderly patient of yours has extensive psoriasis, which appears to be getting worse despite your treatment. Now it seems like the patches of psoriasis are extending, so that most of her skin is becoming dry and scaly.
   (i) What condition might be developing?
   (ii) What features of the rash might make you consider referring this patient to a doctor?
4. Another elderly patient has developed a painless, scaly and raised irregular patch of skin on the side of his nose. The patch, which is of usual skin colour, occasionally itches and occasionally bleeds and scabs over, but usually is no problem to the patient. What are the possible diagnoses that might merit referral?

Answers

1. (i) The diagnosis that most readily fits this case history and description is scabies.
   (ii) As scabies is highly contagious, it would be advisable to refer any case to a doctor for appropriate topical treatment.
2. (i) Yes, the GP was recommending the usual next steps in the medical management of acne, although consideration might also have been given to a topical preparation of retinoic acid or antibiotics before oral preparations were used.
   (ii) The other oral preparation that might have been mentioned is isotretinoin, which is usually only prescribed after referral to a dermatologist.
   (iii) However, there is no need to recommend oral treatment at this stage. Acne may respond very well to a combination of dietary change, stress reduction and acupuncture/herbs.
3. (i) This patient's psoriasis appears to be progressing towards the state of erythroderma.
   (ii) You might consider referral at this stage because there has been no good response to your treatment and because established erythroderma carries considerable risks of dehydration, heat loss and organ failure.
4. From this brief description, this patch of skin might be one of the fairly commonly consequences of long-term exposure to solar radiation: a solar keratosis, a basal cell carcinoma or a squamous cell carcinoma. As all these may well progress, but may readily regress with local cryotherapy, then early referral for diagnosis is advisable.

Chapter 6.1d Diseases of the eye

LEARNING POINTS

At the end of this chapter you will:

- be familiar with the most important conditions that can affect the eye
- be able to recognise the red flags of the diseases of the eye.

Estimated time for chapter: 120 minutes.

Introduction

Eye diseases are managed medically within the discipline of ophthalmology. However, many people with eye disorders may never encounter an ophthalmologist, and instead will rely on the diagnosis and treatment offered by an optician. Opticians are non-medical specialists who are trained in the field of optics, and in the appropriate correction of problems in focusing. Problems in focusing are by far the most commonly experienced eye conditions in adults. However, the optician is trained to recognise and refer on any eye conditions that may merit specific medical treatment (e.g. chronic glaucoma or acute conjunctivitis) or that may be red flags of serious underlying medical disease (e.g. diabetes or hypertension) (see Q6.1d-1).

The conditions discussed in this chapter are:

- Optics – problems in focusing images:
  - myopia (short-sightedness)
  - hypermetropia (long-sightedness)
  - astigmatism
  - presbyopia (long-sightedness of old age).
- Conditions of the conjunctiva, cornea and sclera:
  - infective conjunctivitis
  - allergic conjunctivitis
  - infections of the cornea (keratitis)
  - episcleritis
  - scleritis
  - corneal surgery.
- Conditions of the orbit, extraocular muscles, eyelids and tear-duct system:
  - orbital cellulitis
  - chalazion
  - stye
  - blepharitis
  - dry eyes
  - blocked tear ducts
  - ptosis (drooping eyelid)
  - exophthalmos
  - squint.
- Conditions of the internal structures of the eye (lens, ciliary body and retina):
  - cataract
  - uveitis
  - glaucoma
  - age-related macular degeneration
  - diabetic retinopathy.
- Conditions of the optic nerve:
  - optic neuritis.

Optics: problems in focusing images

Optics is the science of the behaviour of light. With regard to clinical medicine, the term 'clinical optics' refers to the study of how light is refracted (focused) by the eyeball to produce a clear image of the viewed object on the sensitive 'screen' of the retina at the back of the eyeball. The cornea and the lens are the two parts of the eyeball that contribute most significantly to its refractive power (ability to focus).

Short-sightedness (myopia) and long-sightedness (hypermetropia) are both conditions in which the ability of the eye to focus an image normally is impaired. In refractive conditions such as these, either the lens of the eye is not structured or functioning correctly, or the position of the retina with respect to the lens is not ideal (the eyeball is too long or too short).

Myopia (short-sightedness)

In myopia the lens of the eye tends to focus an image too far in front of the retina. In other words, for the patient's length of eyeball, the focusing power of the lens is too high. A patient with myopia will find it easier to focus on an object that is held very close to the eye, whereas all objects at a distance from the eye will be blurred. It is conventionally understood that the most usual cause of myopia is an inherited tendency for the eyeball to be too long in shape. This theory is used to explain why there can be a marked exacerbation of short-sightedness during the growth spurt in the mid-teens.

A contrasting alternative viewpoint is that myopia results from overstrain of the ciliary muscle of the eye through excessive use of the eyes in close-up activities, such as reading and looking at television and computer screens. Moreover, conventionally prescribed corrective concave (negative) lenses are believed to exacerbate the problem, as they permit a child to continue to use the eyes in excessive close work while the accommodating muscles are under strain. According to this theory, the answer to the prevention of myopia lies in reducing the amount of close-up work that is done in childhood, and using visual aids such as pinhole glasses to minimise the degree to which the eye muscles have to accommodate during close visual work.

The Bates method, which was proposed by Dr William Bates over a century ago, is another alternative approach to myopia. The method is based on exercises that teach the eye to move while maintaining relaxation of the external eye muscles. Proponents of the Bates method claim that the approach can be beneficial not just for myopia, but for all types of refractive error.

Myopia is corrected conventionally in the first instance by means of spectacle lenses or contact lenses that are concave in structure. This form of lens counteracts the focusing power of the eye (Figure 6.1d-I). Refractive surgery is a more permanent approach to the treatment of myopia. In this approach, the ability of the cornea to contribute to the focusing of light is modified. Radial keratotomy and laser keratoplasty are procedures that lead to flattening of the central cornea by means of surgery and laser therapy, respectively.

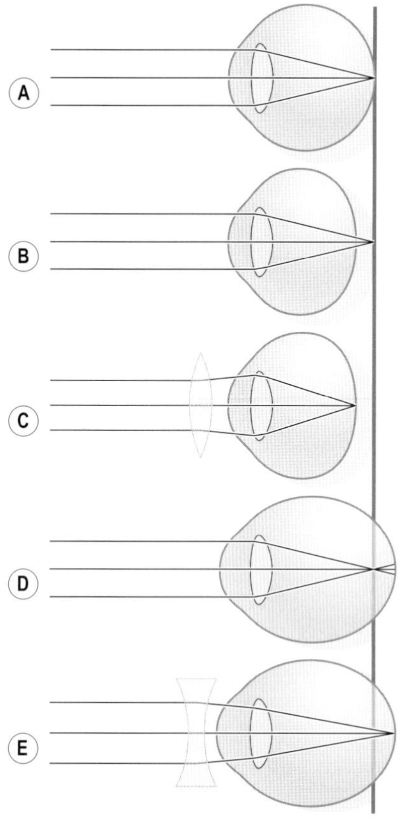

Figure 6.1d-I • The common refractive errors of the eye with and without corrective lenses. • The images illustrate how light is focused by the lens of the eye. In the normal eye (A) the light is focused on the retina. In the short-sighted (myopic) eye (D) the light is focused in front of the retina, and in the long-sighted (hypermetropic) eye (B) the light is focused behind the retina. Corrective lenses (C) and (E) enable the light to be focused in the correct place for clear vision.

Hypermetropia (long-sightedness)

In hypermetropia (long-sightedness), the eye fails to focus the image on the retina. It is most usually a result of a relatively short eyeball. It can also result from the removal of the lens, which is part of a cataract extraction, which results in an extreme form of hypermetropia. A patient with hypermetropia will find it easier to focus on objects at a distance than on those that are close to the face.

Hypermetropia can be corrected by means of concave lenses (see Figure 6.1d-I) and also by laser keratoplasty.

Astigmatism

'Astigmatism' is a term used to describe a condition of the lens or the cornea in which there is an uneven (cylindrical) curvature of the lens, rather than the even curvature that would be akin to a section from a sphere. This means that only part of an image might be focused with clarity. A patient with astigmatism might have particular problems in focusing an image that consists of lines at right angles to each other, such as a grid or a musical score.

Astigmatism often coexists with either myopia or hypermetropia, and is corrected by means of cylindrical concave or convex lenses, respectively.

Presbyopia (long-sightedness of old age)

The long-sightedness that develops in old age (but which may become apparent as early as the mid-40s) is not, strictly speaking, hypermetropia. Rather, it results from a weakening of the ability of the lens to accommodate for near objects (i.e. to fatten in response to constriction of the ciliary muscle).

The patient with presbyopia is still able to focus objects at a distance, but has trouble in seeing close objects with clarity. In presbyopia reading is aided by holding the book at arm's length.

Presbyopia is corrected by means of convex lenses within bifocal spectacles that are designed specifically for the condition. Bifocals have a stronger lens inserted at the bottom of the field of vision so that reading (when looking down) is aided, but usual vision (when looking ahead) need not be modified at all. The lenses in varifocal spectacles have a more gradual transition of power from the usual vision to the reading section of the lens. However, many people with presbyopia prefer to have two pairs of glasses, one for usual vision and one for reading.

Information Box 6.1d-I

Refractive errors: comments from a Chinese medicine perspective

From a Chinese medicine viewpoint, all the refractive errors might be explained in terms of Deficiency of Liver and/or Kidney Qi, or a general Deficiency of the Qi and Essence which flow in the Yang Channels which nourish the eye.

Presbyopia, appearing as it does very often at the end of the fifth decade of life, is very likely to be the result of decline in Kidney Essence.

Scott and Barlow (1999) explain that in children the cause of myopia is insufficient flow of Qi to the eyes. In a child there may be an inherited weakness, but this can be overlaid by the effects of eye strain, illness, rapid growth and emotional distress.

Conditions of the conjunctiva, cornea and sclera

The conjunctiva is the protective epithelial membrane that lines the inner surface of the eyelids and the anterior portion of the eyeball (the anterior sclera and cornea).

Infective conjunctivitis

The conjunctiva is very commonly involved in minor infections due to either bacteria or viruses. Conjunctivitis is diagnosed very often in children. The infections are transmitted either by droplet spread or by direct contamination with infection-laden discharges from an affected eye. Hand-to-eye contact is very common, and particularly so in children, and so conjunctivitis is very contagious. A particular form of conjunctivitis can be contracted by the newborn during childbirth, this being a result of infection with the sexually transmissible organisms *Chlamydia* and *Gonococcus*.

The symptoms of conjunctivitis are redness and slight swelling of the conjunctiva, discomfort and itch of the eye, and discharge. The discharge is more likely to be thick and sticky in bacterial infection, and watery in viral infections. Usually both eyes are infected, but one may become symptomatic up to a few days before the other. (If there is severe pain conjunctivitis is not a likely diagnosis and another explanation such as episcleritis or iritis should be excluded.)

Trachoma is the consequence of recurrent conjunctival infections, and occurs almost exclusively in developing countries. Trachoma takes a much more serious course in that the surface of the eye can become permanently scarred. Trachoma is the most common cause of blindness in the world. The infectious agent is the bacteria-like organism *Chlamydia*, which is transmitted by hand-to-eye contact and also possibly by flies. The tragedy is that infections can be entirely prevented by means of an appropriate prescription of antibiotics.

Most cases of conjunctivitis will settle down spontaneously with gentle cleansing with salt water. Conventional treatment is to exclude the affected child from his peers for the course of the infection and to encourage the regular application of antibiotic drops (in the UK most often chloramphenicol). Treatment with antibiotics is advisable in the newborn, immunocompromised or undernourished.

Information Box 6.1d-II

Infective conjunctivitis: comments from a Chinese medicine perspective

In Chinese medicine, infective conjunctivitis could correspond to an invasion of Wind Heat. It can also be attributed to a rising of Heat and Damp in the Channels local to the eye, or to Liver and Gallbladder Heat.

Allergic conjunctivitis

The eye can also become inflamed as a result of an allergic reaction to particles that have entered the eye. Common allergens in susceptible people include grass and tree pollens (in hay fever), animal dander, house dust mite, and foods such as egg, milk and wheat.

The symptoms are similar to those of viral conjunctivitis, although itch and periorbital swelling may be much more prominent. In severe cases the conjunctiva can become so congested with fluid that its (temporary) appearance is that of a mass of clear jelly.

The allergic reaction can become chronic if exposure to the allergen is repeated. In this case, a characteristic appearance of seed-like bumps of inflammatory tissue may be seen on the inner surface of the conjunctiva.

Treatment of allergic conjunctivitis is by means of antihistamine or sodium chromoglycate eye drops. Both these drugs act to inhibit the excessive immune response to the offending allergens. Oral antihistamine may be prescribed for chronic allergic conjunctivitis, or in cases in which there are other symptoms of hay fever (allergic rhinitis).

Information Box 6.1d-III

Allergic conjunctivitis: comments from a Chinese medicine perspective

In Chinese medicine, the syndromes in allergic conjunctivitis would be similar to those described for infective conjunctivitis (see above), although Heat may be more prominent and Damp less prominent. An underlying Kidney imbalance may also be part of the aetiology of the condition.

Infections of the cornea (keratitis)

Normally the conjunctiva and the tears protect the deeper portions of the eyeball from infectious organisms. Infection of the cornea (keratitis) is serious because it can lead to scarring, and thence to permanent impairment of sight.

The cornea can become infected by bacteria if the protective barriers to disease are deficient, as can occur in eye trauma, or if the production of tears is impaired, as can occur in autoimmune diseases such as rheumatoid arthritis (see below). Bacterial keratitis first presents with redness around the cornea, dislike of light (photophobia), discharge and intense pain. Intensive treatment with antibiotics is required to prevent progression of the condition. The lid may be taped over the affected cornea to aid healing.

Viral keratitis can occur without prior damage to the conjunctiva or the lacrimal system. Herpes simplex virus keratitis can be contracted by hand-to-eye contact or droplet spread from an infected person. Herpes zoster virus keratitis can develop if shingles erupts from the branches of the trigeminal nerve that supply the conjunctiva. In both cases, the symptoms are similar to those found in bacterial keratitis, although the risk of permanent scarring is not as great. The treatment is with antiviral creams and closure of the lid over the affected cornea.

Information Box 6.1d-IV

Keratitis: comments from a Chinese medicine perspective

In Chinese medicine, the initial infection of keratitis may be described as an Invasion of Wind Heat, although, as this is a deep condition, an underlying imbalance of Liver Heat or Kidney Deficiency may be considered to have predisposed a person to the infection.

Episcleritis and scleritis

Episcleritis is a superficial inflammation of the sclera that presents as persistent patchy redness and discomfort of the white of the eye. There is no discharge, and so episcleritis should be easy to distinguish from conjunctivitis. Episcleritis is rarely serious, but when present the deeper condition of scleritis should be excluded (see below).

In scleritis there may be an underlying autoimmune disease such as rheumatoid arthritis. Scleritis is a penetrating inflammation of the sclera in which there is patchy, deep redness and weakening of the sclera, accompanied by intense pain. The sclera is at risk of perforation. Perforation of the eye is an ophthalmic emergency. The iris may also be involved (uveitis; see below), in which case there is a risk of scarring of the lens of the eye (cataract).

The condition is treated by means of high doses of steroid or immunosuppressant medication.

Information Box 6.1d-V

Scleritis: comments from a Chinese medicine perspective

From a Chinese medicine perspective, the intense pain and seriousness of scleritis indicates a deep condition of Full Heat in the Liver with Kidney Deficiency. Episcleritis is also an indication of Heat in the Liver.

Corneal surgery

Scarring of the cornea can follow from the chronic inflammatory conditions of trachoma, keratitis and scleritis, and if severe will result in impairment of vision and even blindness. The scarred cornea can be replaced by a donor graft by means of a relatively straightforward operation. In most cases the donor graft is not rejected because this part of the eye is relatively protected from the immune system.

Unlike all other transplant operations, in which long-term immunosuppressant medication is necessary, the patient does not usually require any more than a short course of steroid eye drops in order to prevent rejection.

Donor corneas are obtained from the cadavers of people who have permitted their eyes to be used for donation, and can be stored in controlled sterile conditions in corneal banks until the time when they can be used.

Conditions of the orbit, extraocular muscles, eyelids and tear-duct system

Orbital cellulitis

Orbital cellulitis is a spreading infection of the tissues that surround the eye, and originates most commonly from a sinus infection. The symptoms are a swollen and painful eye and lids and difficult eye movements in a very unwell patient. There is serious risk of the infection spreading inwards to form a brain abscess, and so the patient should be referred immediately for intravenous antibiotic therapy.

Chalazions and styes

A chalazion is a blocked meibomian gland (oil gland) in the eyelid, which usually appears as a painless, rounded swelling of the lid margin (Figure 6.1d-II). This cyst, which comprises accumulated sebaceous secretions, can become infected, in which case the lump will enlarge and become painful. A chalazion can be treated by surgical excision if unsightly or infected.

A stye is an infected eyelash follicle. It appears like a boil, the head of which is on the lid margin. When examined carefully, it can be seen that a lash is protruding from the centre of the head of a stye. Most styes will discharge or settle down spontaneously. Conservative treatment involves bathing the affected area with hot salt water. Nevertheless, antibiotic creams (and sometimes oral antibiotics) are commonly prescribed.

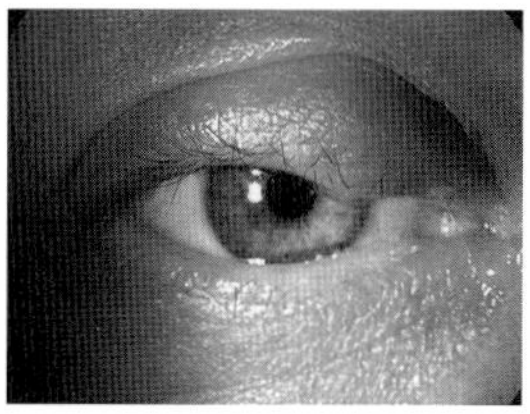

Figure 6.1d-II • A chalalzion of the eyelid.

> **Information Box 6.1d-VI**
>
> **Chalazion: comments from a Chinese medicine perspective**
>
> From a Chinese medicine perspective, an uncomplicated chalazion would suggest Damp/Phlegm and also an imbalance of the Liver. Infection of a chalazion could be described as Damp Heat. A stye has a similar interpretation, although, as it can appear rapidly, a possible diagnosis would be Wind Damp Heat.
>
> The development of an infected chalazion or a stye (although these are considered to be minor conditions) is an indication that the patient may be quite run down or stressed (the Heat developing as a result of Yin Deficiency or Stagnation of Liver Qi).

Blepharitis

Blepharitis describes a longstanding inflammation of the eyelids that manifests as crusting of the lids and consequent irritation of the eyes. There may be scaling of the lid margins. In severe cases the eyes themselves can become inflamed.

Blepharitis is associated with seborrhoeic dermatitis, atopic eczema and acne rosacea, and is believed to originate in an imbalance of the formation of the waxy secretions from the meibomian glands in the eyelids. It is a difficult condition to treat, although topical antibiotics and gentle cleansing of the scales with warm salty water may relieve the symptoms.

> **Information Box 6.1d-VII**
>
> **Blepharitis: comments from a Chinese medicine perspective**
>
> In Chinese medicine, blepharitis would correspond to Damp Heat with an underlying Liver imbalance (e.g. Deficiency of Liver Blood and Yin).

Dry eyes (keratoconjunctivitis sicca) and Sjogren's syndrome

The medical condition of dry eyes (keratoconjunctivitis sicca (KCS)) results from disease of the tear-forming lacrimal glands. The usual cause of KCS is a poorly understood degenerative process of ageing, although it is well recognised as a feature of autoimmune diseases such as rheumatoid arthritis. KCS associated with dry mouth (xerostomia) is suggestive of Sjogren's syndrome, a connective tissue disease.

The symptoms of KCS include grittiness and tiredness of the eyes and dislike of light (photophobia). These symptoms are often worse in the evening. The eyes may become reddened and prone to attacks of conjunctivitis and keratitis (see above).

KCS is treated by means of 'artificial tears', which can be instilled into the eyes by the patient whenever needed. Shielded spectacles can ensure that the environment around the eyes stays as humid as is possible.

> **Information Box 6.1d-VIII**
>
> **Dry eyes: comments from a Chinese medicine perspective**
>
> In Chinese medicine, dryness of the eyes suggests Liver Blood and Yin Deficiency.

Blocked tear ducts (epiphora)

If the nasolacrimal tear duct of the eye (which drains from the inner canthus) is blocked, tears cannot drain into the tear duct, and so will accumulate and eventually spill over (epiphora). The duct is commonly blocked in newborns, a result of the fact that the developing tear duct normally achieves patency only very close to the time of delivery. In this case, the problem almost always resolves with time. If blocked tear ducts are persistent up to the end of the first year of life, a minor surgical probing of the duct can be performed to clear the blockage.

In adults the passageway through the tear duct can become blocked by an inflammatory or degenerative process (Figure 6.1d-III). The main symptom of blockage is epiphora, but also a persistently sticky eye may result. The symptoms are usually on one side only, and the sclera of the eye remains white, so distinguishing the problem from conjunctivitis.

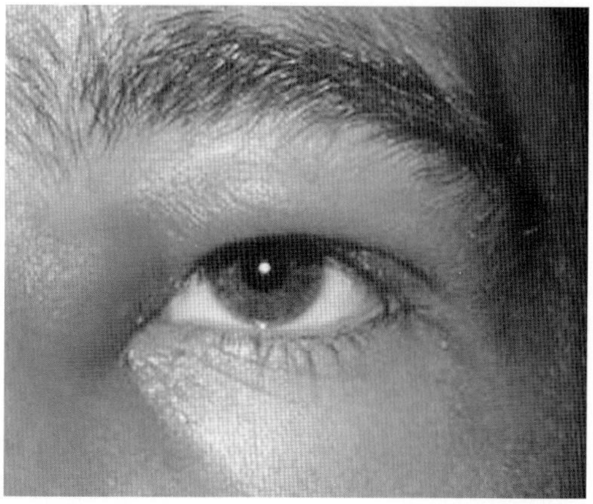

Figure 6.1d-III • Acute inflammation of the lacrimal sac: dacrocystitis.

Treatment is by surgically opening the upper portion of the tear duct into the nasal cavity (dacrocystorhinostomy). This operation involves the removal of a small portion of the intervening nasal bone.

Information Box 6.1d-IX

Epiphora: comments from a Chinese medicine perspective

From a Chinese medicine perspective, an interpretation of epiphora probably would be one of general Deficiency, and in particular of Kidney Essence.

Ptosis (drooping eyelid) and paralysis of the lid

A drooping eyelid (ptosis) can be a congenital abnormality. If uncomplicated, ptosis usually causes little other than a cosmetic problem, as it rarely leads to occlusion of the pupil. In those congenital cases that cause cosmetic or visual problems the lid can be slightly lifted by means of a minor surgical operation.

A ptosis that develops in later life may be a warning feature of nerve damage. In very rare cases, and as a consequence of the complex anatomy of the nerves that supply the eyelid, this damage may result from a developing tumour of the apex of the lung or of the brain. Ptosis can also develop as part of myasthenia gravis, the disorder of muscle fatigability. For this reason the patient with a recent onset of ptosis should be referred for further investigations.

A one-sided (unilateral) paralysis of the lid can occur in Bell's palsy, in which case it appears as part of a generalised paralysis of the facial nerve. In a facial nerve paralysis, the nerve can be so severely affected that the lid cannot close at all, in which case the eyeball is at risk of damage (ulceration of the conjunctiva) through drying out. In the majority of cases the paralysis recovers fully within 3 months, but in longer-standing cases the lid may need to be partially closed by means of a minor operation (tarsorrhaphy) so that the eyeball can remain lubricated and protected.

Information Box 6.1d-X

Ptosis: comments from a Chinese medicine perspective

In Chinese medicine, a weakness of the eyelid muscle in ptosis might indicate a Spleen or Liver Blood Deficiency that has become manifest in the Channels of the face. Facial palsy is considered to be the result of a Wind Invasion of the facial Channels.

Exophthalmos

'Exophthalmos' (also known as proptosis) is the medical term used to describe the bulging outwards of an eyeball from the orbit. It is most commonly observed in Graves' disease (when it is described as thyroid eye disease) as a result of an antibody-stimulated accumulation of fatty tissue behind the eye. In Graves' disease, exophthalmos usually affects both eyes, although very often it can be more prominent in one eye. Exophthalmos can also develop on one side only (unilaterally) as a result of a tumour in the orbit, although this is very rare.

Exophthalmos becomes apparent as a staring look in the eye(-s). If severe, the white of the eye can be seen both above and below the sclera. This is not a usual feature of a relaxed face.

Even in the early stages of exophthalmos, an examining doctor will be able to confirm that the movement of the lid is slowed over the eye as the patient is asked to look down (a sign known as 'lid lag'). As the condition progresses, the patient may develop sore, red eyes, double vision or loss of clear vision.

The primary risk to the eye from exophthalmos is that the eye will eventually be unable to close fully and so will suffer the results of dryness in the same way as the eye affected by facial paralysis (see above). In thyroid eye disease there is added danger to the eye, as the accumulating soft tissue can start to compress and damage the optic nerve. The soft tissue can also affect the external muscles of the eye and lead to squint (see below). Treatment of the underlying thyroid disease may slow the progression of the exophthalmos, but cannot reverse the process. The main medical treatment is corticosteroid injections. Surgical treatments include removal of the accumulated soft tissue and, as is used to treat paralysis of the eyelid in Bell's palsy, partial closing of the eyelid (tarsorrhaphy).

Information Box 6.1d-XI

Exophthalmos: comments from a Chinese medicine perspective

From a Chinese medicine perspective, the staring look seen in exophthalmos (the 'four whites') is a feature of extreme Kidney Deficiency. In hyperthyroidism the primary Deficiency is of Kidney Yin (with Full Heat). The inflammation of the eye (also suggestive of Heat) and muscle paralysis of the external ocular muscles suggests that Liver pathology is also a feature of thyroid eye disease.

Squint (strabismus) and double vision

Congenital (non-paralytic) squint is described in Chapter 5.4e. In infancy, the brain suppresses the images received from a divergent or convergent non-dominant eye so that the child can see clearly without double vision. If not treated before the age of 7 years at the latest, this developmental response has the deleterious consequence of amblyopia (permanent loss of depth vision).

Congenital squint usually is the result of an inherited imbalance in the functioning of the external muscles of the eye. More rarely it may follow from an inability of the eye to receive clear visual information, such as can occur in congenital cataract. The effects of the squint may be subtle, and so it may remain undetected until it is too late for treatment.

In contrast, the development of a squint in an adult becomes very obvious very quickly, as the patient develops disabling double vision. The most usual cause of a squint in an adult is a paralysis of one or more of the cranial nerves that supply the external muscles of the eye. For this reason, this form of squint is termed 'paralytic strabismus'. Orbital tumours and the accumulation of the soft tissue that occurs in thyroid eye disease can also hinder the action of these muscles and so lead to the double vision of paralytic strabismus, although these are much less common causes of double vision.

Any cause of a mononeuropathy can lead to a paralytic squint resulting from damage to the third, fourth or sixth cranial nerves. Common causes of cranial mononeuropathies include diabetes, vascular disease and compression by brain tumours. Head injuries and raised intracranial pressure can also be complicated by damage to the cranial nerves that supply the eye muscles. For these reasons the development of double vision should be treated as a warning feature of serious disease.

Ideally, the cause of the paralytic squint can be treated rapidly to reverse the double vision, but often the damage that has occurred to the cranial nerves is irreparable. Urgent diagnosis and treatment of the underlying cause of the paralysis is always necessary.

If a permanent paralytic squint cannot be prevented by early treatment, the simplest treatment is to patch the affected eye. Spectacles containing prism lenses may also be used to realign the images of viewed objects that fall on the two retinas. Surgical correction of the extraocular muscles may also prevent double vision in cases in which the paralysis is permanent.

Information Box 6.1d-XII

Squint: comments from a Chinese medicine perspective

Scott and Barlow (1999) suggest that a congenital squint may be the result of Womb Heat which has become lodged in the Channels that relate to one or more of the extraocular muscles (Liver, Gallbladder and Bladder). In this case, the squint is present from birth, and is often quite pronounced in appearance.

Alternatively, if a congenital squint becomes apparent after the time of birth, it may be the result of the Depletion in energy of the eye muscles resulting from an Invasion of Full Heat or a Lingering Pathogenic Factor in the Channels. Scott and Barlow (1999) also suggest that the Internal (Empty) Heat generated from overstimulation or overexcitement of a child can, in the same way, deplete the Qi in the Channels that relate to the eye muscles. These forms of squint may vary in severity according to the nervous state or level of tiredness of the child.

A sudden onset of paralytic squint in an adult suggests that Wind is an underlying Pathogenic Factor that has triggered the condition. Again the Gallbladder, Liver and Bladder Channels are those which are affected. Underlying vascular disease, diabetes or cancer might indicate that Phlegm and Heat are also lodged in the Channels, which may have become vulnerable because of longstanding Deficiency in the associated Organs.

Conditions of internal structures of the eye (lens, ciliary body and retina)

Cataract

'Cataract' is the medical term used to describe opacification of the lens of the eye. It is the commonest cause of treatable blindness worldwide. In the west, ageing is the most common cause of cataract (age-related cataract), and a long history of sun exposure is known to increase the risk of its development. Medical causes of cataract include diabetes mellitus and long-term use of corticosteroid medication.

A patient with significant bilateral cataracts will experience increasing difficulty in focusing which cannot be corrected with glasses. Bright light can make the symptoms worse for some patients who are troubled by glare.

The principal treatment for cataract is surgery. Surgical treatment is usually offered in the UK as soon as the cataract is recognised to be significantly affecting the patient's quality of life. There are two surgical techniques. The first involves an incision at the edge of the cornea and then removal of the clouded lens from its supporting capsule. The second surgical technique (phacoemulsification) involves liquefaction of the lens induced by an ultrasound probe inserted into the eye via a similar incision. In both cases the lens is replaced by an artificial lens implant, which is designed to allow the eye to focus for distance viewing. Usually only one eye is operated on at a time.

Cataract extraction is considered a minor procedure, and carries very few risks even for frail elderly people. After the operation the patient is prescribed a short course of steroid and antibiotic drops to reduce inflammation and minimise the risk of infection. In the vast majority of patients there is a significant improvement in visual acuity.

However, in approximately 20% of patients clouding of the remaining lens capsule can lead to a reduction in acuity over the months following the operation. This complication can be treated by means of laser therapy as an outpatient procedure.

Information Box 6.1d-XIII

Cataract: comments from a Chinese medicine perspective

In Chinese medicine, a gradual deterioration in vision such as occurs with the slow development of a cataract has been attributed to Deficiency of Liver and Kidney Yin, Deficiency of Qi, and Blood and Stagnation of Liver Qi.

Uveitis

Uveitis describes inflammation of the iris, ciliary body and the choroid layer of the eye (also known as the uveal tract). Depending on which of these three structures is predominantly affected, uveitis may also be termed iritis, cyclitis, choroiditis or posterior uveitis.

Uveitis can develop for no obvious reason, but in approximately half of cases it is associated with a more generalised disease, the most common of these being ankylosing spondylitis, juvenile arthritis, inflammatory bowel disease and chronic infections including those of cytomegalovirus (CMV), toxoplasmosis and human immunodeficiency virus (HIV).

Uveitis is a condition that can flare up and then settle down (a relapsing–remitting condition), but there is a significant risk of permanent damage to the eye during an attack as a result of the inflammation. For this reason, a case of uveitis is treated with urgency in conventional medicine.

The patient with uveitis will experience intense pain in one eye, and the eye may appear red, with the redness particularly marked around the iris. This is in contrast with the redness and discomfort of the more benign condition of conjunctivitis, in which the redness is usually bilateral and affects the whole of the conjunctiva. In uveitis there will be blurring of the vision and a dislike of bright light.

The patient with uveitis will be examined by means of slit lamp. In an established case this will reveal inflammatory cells collecting in front of the iris, and may indicate that the iris is distorted, as there is a tendency for it to adhere to the lens as a result of the inflammation. If this is the first attack, the patient may well be offered a number of investigations to exclude a more generalised underlying condition.

The treatment of uveitis involves dilatation of the pupil by means of mydriatic eye drops (containing a drug such as atropine or cyclopentolate). This treatment prevents the iris from adhering to the lens, and so prevents scarring of these delicate tissues. Corticosteroids are applied in drop form to reduce the inflammation.

The risks of uveitis are that recurrent attacks can promote the development of cataracts and glaucoma (see below).

Information Box 6.1d-XIV

Uveitis: comments from a Chinese medicine perspective

From a Chinese medicine perspective, an attack of uveitis would appear to correspond either to an Invasion of Wind Heat or to Rising of Liver Fire.

Glaucoma

'Glaucoma' is a term used to describe any condition in which the pressure of the fluid within the eyeball (intraocular pressure) is raised. The problem with glaucoma is that, over time, the increased pressure will damage the retina and the head of the optic nerve, and so will affect visual acuity. If the rise in pressure is sudden (acute glaucoma) the condition can be very painful.

The intraocular pressure depends on the production of the aqueous humour, the fluid inside the body of the eye, and also on the rate of its removal. In glaucoma, the pressure becomes raised because the fluid is not removed at the same rate at which it is produced. Aqueous humour normally drains from the eye through a meshwork of tissue situated in the angle between the iris and the cornea in the anterior chamber of the eye.

In those people who have an inherited tendency to glaucoma, this meshwork appears to become increasingly resistant to the outflow of fluid, and so the pressure in the eye rises slowly and painlessly. This is known as 'primary open angle glaucoma'. It is a relatively common condition, being present in 1 in 200 people over the age of 40 years. The prevalence of the condition rises with age, so that 10% of the over-80s are known to have developed this form of glaucoma.

In some people the meshwork becomes blocked because of a condition that has developed in later life, such as uveitis or the damage that results from a traumatic bleed in the anterior chamber. In this case the condition is known as 'secondary glaucoma', and may develop fairly suddenly or slowly, depending on the cause.

Acute closed-angle glaucoma results from a sudden blockage of the angled area in which the meshwork is situated, and tends to occur in people who have a naturally narrow angle to the anterior chamber of their eyes. The acute attack is triggered in such people by administration of pupil-dilating medication (mydriatic drops).

In slowly developing chronic glaucoma of whatever cause, the patient will initially be unaware of the presence of the condition. Unless it is picked up early by an optician, undiagnosed glaucoma can lead to progressive damage to the optic nerve, and ultimately to loss of visual acuity. Classically, a patient with untreated chronic glaucoma will experience 'tunnel vision' as it is primarily the periphery of the field of vision that is affected.

Chronic glaucoma is diagnosed and assessed painlessly by means of slit lamp tonometry. During this procedure both the intraocular pressure and the angle of the anterior chamber of the eye can be measured, and the optic nerve head can be examined.

Treatment for chronic glaucoma includes medication to reduce the production of aqueous humour. For example, beta blockers such as timolol are commonly prescribed in drop form to be administered twice daily on a long-term basis. Laser treatment to the meshwork may offer temporary relief of the intraocular pressure, but it often starts rising again after a short respite. Surgical opening of the anterior chamber to the space that lies under the conjunctiva (trabeculectomy) is very often the preferred option.

Acute closed-angle glaucoma presents as an emergency, with excruciating pain in the tense eyeball. The pain is often so severe as to be associated with vomiting. The patient may also complain of distorted or lost vision. Urgent treatment is required, not only to reduce the pain, but also to prevent permanent damage to the vision. In an acute attack the eye is red and the cornea may appear cloudy. The pupil may be fixed and dilated.

Treatment involves the administration of painkillers, drugs that inhibit the formation of the aqueous humour (intravenous acetazolamide and topical beta blocker drops), and a drug to constrict the pupil and so open the angle of the anterior chamber of the eye (topical pilocarpine drops). Subsequent attacks are prevented by the surgical operation of iridectomy, in which a small hole is made in the iris.

> **Information Box 6.1d-XV**
>
> **Acute glaucoma: comments from a Chinese medicine perspective**
>
> From a Chinese medicine perspective, acute glaucoma is clearly a Full condition. The intensity of pain suggests Heat. Possible diagnoses include Liver Fire and Liver Blood Stagnation. Chronic glaucoma presents in a similar way to cataract, in the form of steady loss of visual acuity, and so the Chinese diagnoses may include Liver and Kidney Yin Deficiency, Deficiency of Blood and Qi and Liver Qi Stagnation (see under glaucoma). The fact that fluid is accumulating does, of course, suggest that Damp is an additional Pathogenic Factor.

Age-related macular degeneration

The macula lutea, also known as the 'yellow spot', is the name given to the part of the retina onto which the centre of the field of vision is focused. If the macula is damaged, the affected eye will never be able to generate a clear image of a viewed object.

Degeneration of the delicate cells of the retina with old age is a well-recognised phenomenon, and is the most important cause of irreversible visual loss in the west. An affected patient will experience blurring of vision and may also describe distorted vision. As peripheral vision is retained, the condition will not progress to total blindness. Cigarette smoking is a known risk factor for age-related macular degeneration (ARMD), and zinc and antioxidants (such as might be obtained from tomatoes and leafy vegetables) are thought to be protective.

ARMD can be diagnosed on the basis of the reduction in vision and the characteristic retinal changes that can be detected by means of the ophthalmoscope.

For most patients there is no known curative treatment. In a minority, with the more rapidly progressive 'wet' form of ARMD, laser therapy can help impede the progression of the degeneration. Injections directly into the eye of a monoclonal antibody drug (ranibizumab), which prevents overgrowth of epithelial cells, have also been shown to slow the progression of wet AMRD. All patients can be helped by means of magnifying aids.

Diabetic retinopathy

The retina is dependent on a rich and consistent blood supply for optimal function. In diabetes, because of sugar-related damage to the retinal capillaries, there are three important ways in which the retina can become damaged. First, tiny leaks of blood and fat-containing fluid can be deposited outside the vessels and progressively damage the retina. Second, clots in the vessels can lead to infarcts in the retina. Although these are also tiny, as they accumulate, more and more of the field of vision becomes impaired. Finally, as the retina is starved of a rich supply of oxygen, its vessels are stimulated to sprout new branches. Although this is a healthy response in most of the body, in the eye this neovascularisation crowds the retina with branching capillaries that literally block out the field of vision.

The first warning features of retinopathy can be detected by ophthalmoscopic examination even before the patient experiences any visual loss. If the characteristic changes are detected, the patient can be referred for preventive laser treatment to the retina. This outpatient procedure prevents leaks and also reduces neovascularisation. The patient will also be counselled about the need to be very attentive to blood sugar levels, as the progression of diabetic retinopathy appears to be directly related to how often the blood sugar is poorly controlled. Smoking and poor control of blood pressure are also risk factors.

Diabetes is also associated with the development of cataract and glaucoma. Because of the seriousness of retinopathy and the other ocular complications, all patients with diabetes should undergo an ophthalmoscopic examination at least once a year.

Conditions of the optic nerve

Optic neuritis

'Optic neuritis' is the term used to describe inflammation of the optic nerve and optic nerve head, the point at which the optic nerve meets the retina. In many cases the cause of an episode of optic neuritis is unclear, although such an episode very often (in 40–70% of cases) turns out to be the first in a series of neurological episodes in a case of multiple sclerosis.

Optic neuritis is characterised by a sudden deterioration of vision, and pain on movement of the eyes (as eye movements lead to traction of the optic nerve). The deterioration in vision can then progress over the course of the next few days.

On ophthalmoscopic examination, the blind-spot area (optic disc) of the retina may appear swollen (papilloedema), and tests of acuity will demonstrate impairment in both acuity and colour vision.

Usually no treatment is offered, although in a severe attack a short course of intravenous corticosteroids may be prescribed. After a period of days to weeks normal vision is resumed, although acuity is often never as sharp as it was before. A skilled examiner will notice that after the attack the optic disc appears more pale than it should.

> **Information Box 6.1d-XVI**
>
> **Optic neuritis: comments from a Chinese medicine perspective**
>
> Optic neuritis leads to a sudden deterioration of vision, which very commonly occurs in the context of multiple sclerosis (MS). In Chinese medicine, MS is a form of Atrophy Syndrome. Maciocia (1989) attributes the visual symptoms of MS to the Kidney–Liver Deficiency that is characteristic of the condition. The sudden onset of optic neuritis is an indication of Wind Invading the Channels of the eye, presumably on a background of more longstanding Deficiency.

The red flags of the diseases of the eye

Some people with diseases of the eye will benefit from referral to a conventional doctor for assessment and/or treatment. Red flags are those symptoms and signs that indicate that referral is to be considered. The red flags of the diseases of the eye are described in Table 6.1d-I. This table forms part of the summary on red flags given in Appendix III, which also gives advice on the degree of urgency of referral for each of the red flag conditions listed.

Table 6.1d-I Red Flags 42 – diseases of the eye

Red Flag	Description	Reasoning
42.1	**An intensely painful and red eye**	A painful red eye could result from iritis, choroiditis, acute glaucoma, corneal ulcer or keratitis. All these are serious conditions, and the patient should be advised to attend the nearest emergency department for early assessment
42.2	**Painful red and swollen eyes and eyelids**; the patient (often a child) is very unwell	If the eye and the surrounding tissues are intensely painful and swollen this could be a spreading infection of the soft tissues of the eye, orbital cellulitis. Refer urgently to the nearest emergency department
42.3	**A painful eye with no obvious inflammation**; eye movements are painful	Pain that is deep and intense, and exacerbated by eye movement, is characteristic of optic neuritis or choroiditis. Refer as a high priority to the nearest emergency department
42.4	**Discharge from the eye**; if severe, prolonged and painful, or if in the following vulnerable groups: • the newborn • the immunocompromised • malnourished people	Discharge from the eye(s) is usually the result of acute allergic, bacterial or viral conjunctivitis, and as such is usually self-limiting, and will not necessarily require antibiotic treatment. Advise the patient that he may be very contagious while the eye is discharging Only consider referral if the discharge continues for >5 days or if there is any pain
42.5	**Sudden onset of painless blurring or loss of sight in one or both eyes**	Loss of sight or blurring in one or both eyes may be due to thromboembolic disease, optic neuritis, retinal tear or corneal ulcer. Some of these conditions require high-priority treatment to prevent blindness, so refer as high priority to the nearest eye casualty department Floaters and blurring alone in middle age is usually the result of the benign condition of vitreous detachment. Nevertheless, referral is advised to exclude the more serious possible causes
42.6	**Sudden onset of painless blurring or loss of sight in one or both eyes accompanied by one-sided headache**	Loss of sight accompanied by a headache in an older person (>50 years old) may represent temporal arteritis. This is more likely to occur in someone who has been diagnosed with polymyalgia. Urgent treatment with corticosteroids may prevent progression to blindness. Refer urgently to the nearest emergency department
42.7	**Gradual onset of painless blurring** or **loss of sight in one or both eyes**	Refer for assessment, as treatment of the causes of gradual loss of sight may prevent progressive deterioration of the sight. Causes include refractive error, cataract, glaucoma and macular degeneration
42.8	**Squint: in any child,** if previously undiagnosed	Refer any child who demonstrates a previously undiagnosed squint. In young children this usually results from a congenital weakness of the external ocular muscles, but needs ophthalmological assessment to prevent long-term inhibition of depth vision. Squint appearing in an older child may signify a tumour of the brain, pituitary or orbital cavity
42.9	**Recent onset of double vision in an adult**	Double vision suggests a physical distortion of the orbital cavity or damage to a cranial nerve. Refer as a high priority

Table 6.1d-I Red Flags 42 – diseases of the eye—Cont'd

Red Flag	Description	Reasoning
42.10	**Recent onset of drooping eyelid (ptosis)**	Possible damage to the nerve by a tumour or muscle-wasting disease. Refer for investigation
42.11	**Features of thyroid eye disease**: staring eyes (whites visible above and below pupils), inflamed conjunctivae, symptoms of hyperthyroidism (tremor, agitation, weight loss, palpitations)	Thyroid eye disease results from specific antibodies that are generated in Graves' disease. If severe it can threaten the health of the eyes as soft tissue builds up in the orbit, pushing the eye forward and putting pressure on the optic nerve
42.12	**Inability to close the eye**	The eye may not close fully in thyroid eye disease and also in Bell's palsy; this can rapidly lead to serious damage of the conjunctiva and cornea (which rely on the moistness of tears to remain healthy). A simple treatment is to keep the affected eye shut with medical tape until medical advice has been sought
42.13	**Foreign body in the eye**	If there is a foreign body that cannot be removed, gently keep the lid closed by means of a pad and medical tape and arrange urgent assessment at the nearest emergency department

Self-test 6.1d

Diseases of the eye

1. A 55- year-old female patient has mentioned gritty and tired eyes over the past few weeks. She says that the margins of the lids of her eyes have been a bit dry and scaly over this time, but recently the eyes themselves feel uncomfortable and sore. When you examine her you notice that the lids are slightly reddened with scaly margins, and that the conjunctivae appear slightly bloodshot. There is no obvious discharge. The patient's vision is normal.
   (i) What are the causes of red eyes?
   (ii) Does this patient present a red flag of disease?
   (iii) What is one possible cause of these symptoms and signs?
2. An elderly patient is complaining of increasingly poor vision over the past months.
   (i) What are the most likely causes of deterioration of vision in a person over 70 years old?
   (ii) Would you refer this patient for a conventional diagnosis or treatment?
3. A 30-year-old patient who is under a lot of stress at work discovered a lump in her eyelid about 2 weeks ago. Over the past 2 days the lump has become tender, more swollen and the skin overlying it is slightly inflamed. When you examine the eyelid you note that the lump is about 4 mm in diameter and seems to be coming to a head like a boil at the root of an eyelash.
   (i) What are the common causes of lumps in the eyelid?
   (ii) What is the most likely cause in this patient?
   (iii) Will you refer this patient for conventional diagnosis or treatment?
   (iv) Name a possible underlying Chinese medicine syndrome.

Answers

1. (i) The causes of red eyes include allergic and infective conjunctivitis, corneal ulcer, keratitis, episcleritis and scleritis, orbital cellulitis, blepharitis, dry eyes, uveitis, and acute glaucoma.
   (ii) Of these, the serious conditions that would merit referral are the painful conditions of uveitis (iritis and choroiditis), acute glaucoma, corneal ulcer, keratitis and orbital cellulitis. Conjunctivitis only merits referral if the discharge is severe and prolonged. This patient's symptoms and signs do not fit any one of these diagnoses, so there are no red flags presenting in this case.
   (iii) Grittiness of the eyes may be experienced in dry eyes, conjunctivitis and also blepharitis. In this case the time scale of the symptoms does not fit with conjunctivitis, and the scaling of the eyes is more suggestive of blepharitis.
2. (i) The causes of progressive loss of vision in an elderly person include presbyopia (usually becomes apparent in the sixth decade of life) cataract, macular degeneration, diabetic retinopathy, ischaemia of the retina (a result of arteriosclerosis) and chronic glaucoma. A sudden loss of vision might be attributed to an occlusion of one of the retinal blood vessels (akin to a stroke); occipital transient ischaemic attack or stroke, or a retinal tear.
   (ii) Only the former diagnoses might apply to your patient as the onset of the loss in vision is gradual. If the loss in vision is undiagnosed, you should urge the patient to make an appointment with an optician in the first instance.
3. (i) The common causes of lumps in the eyelid are stye (infected eyelash follicle), chalazion (blocked meibomian gland) and xanthelasmata (small, painless accumulations of cholesterol-containing matter indicative of raised blood lipids).
   (ii) The most likely cause in this patient is a stye.
   (iii) Styes will usually settle down of their own accord, often as a result of discharge of the pus. You would only consider referral if the patient was generally unwell because of the infection or if the condition appeared to be spreading or not resolving within 5 days.
   (iv) Possible underlying Chinese medicine syndromes include Liver Fire, Damp Heat in Liver and Invasion of External Wind Damp Heat. An underlying condition of Liver Qi Stagnation, Yin Deficiency or Full Heat, all of which can be the result of stress, can predispose to the manifestation of a stye.

Chapter 6.1e Diseases of the ear

LEARNING POINTS

At the end of this chapter you will:

- be familiar with the most important conditions that can affect the ear
- be able to recognise the red flags of the diseases of the ear.

Estimated time for chapter: 120 minutes.

Introduction

Most of the important diseases of the ear are managed within the conventional surgical speciality of otorhinolaryngology, which is the Latinised term for the study of the ear, nose and throat. This speciality falls into the domain of the surgeons, because much of the management of the serious disease of the ear, nose and throat requires surgical treatment of one form or another.

Those conditions of the nose and throat that require medical management are managed within the broader speciality of respiratory medicine, or within general practice if fairly minor (e.g. chronic sinusitis, pharyngitis). Most of the medical management of ear conditions occurs in general practice in the UK (e.g. treatment of otitis externa or otitis media) (see Q6.1e-1 and Q6.1e-2).

The conditions described in this chapter are:

- Deafness.
- Conductive deafness:
  - wax
  - acute otitis media
  - chronic secretory otitis media (glue ear)
  - chronic otitis media
  - otosclerosis
  - otitis externa and furunculosis.
- Sensorineural deafness:
  - congenital deafness
  - deafness of old age (presbycusis)
  - noise-induced deafness
  - Menière's disease
  - acoustic neuroma
  - deafness due to drugs and infections.
- Earache:
  - dental and mandibular causes
  - pharyngeal and laryngeal causes
  - cervical spondylosis.
- Tinnitus – local causes:
  - wax and serous otitis media
  - Menière's disease
  - presbycusis (see under deafness)
  - otosclerosis (see under deafness)
  - noise related.
- Tinnitus – general causes:
  - fever
  - disease of the nervous system
  - anaemia
  - drugs and alcohol abuse.
- Vertigo:
  - vestibular neuronitis
  - benign paroxysmal vertigo
  - central causes of vertigo.

Deafness

The causes of reduced hearing and deafness can be broadly categorised into two groups: those that result from disease of the external and middle ear, and those that result from damage to the sensory apparatus in the inner ear and the neural pathways which conduct nervous impulses resulting from sounds to the auditory centres in the brain.

Deafness resulting from the first group of causes is described as 'conductive', so called because it is the result of a problem in the conduction of sound waves to the inner ear. Deafness resulting from the second group of causes is termed 'sensorineural', because in this case it is the sensory apparatus or the neural pathways that are at fault. A simple tuning fork test can be used to distinguish between the two causes of deafness, although a more accurate assessment can be made by means of audiology tests.

If the cause of the deafness cannot be treated, for example in deafness of old age, a hearing aid will be considered. Most hearing aids currently prescribed are worn behind the ear, and are attached to a mould fitted into the patient's ear. A more sophisticated form of this sort of aid has all the electronics built into the mould, so obviating the need for a behind-the-ear component to the aid. Some patient groups, for example children, will be more suited to an aid that is held in a pocket attached to the clothing, and linked to the mould by means of a flexible wire. In all these forms of aids the principle is simple amplification and then redirection of the amplified sounds directly into the auditory canal. This is a less than perfect solution for sensorineural forms of deafness, as there can be a very narrow threshold between sound that can be heard and sound that is too loud to be tolerated. Many modern hearing aids are fitted with a loop inductance system to facilitate the use of the telephone.

More recently, bone-anchored hearing aids have been developed that direct amplified sounds via a surgically implanted titanium screw through the temporal bone towards the inner ear. These aids are of value in patients who have disease of the outer or middle ear, which would prevent the use of the usual forms of hearing aid.

The cochlear implant involves the insertion of range of electrodes directly into the cochlea (inner ear). The electrodes receive sound information from an externally situated microphone, and convert this information into impulses within the auditory nerve. This technically very complex device is only suitable for those who have absolute hearing loss, as the information that they generate in the auditory nerve is of a different quality to that generated by sound. Nevertheless, for those who were profoundly deaf, the brain can learn to process the nerve impulses to enable lip reading, speech and, in some cases, the ability to converse by telephone. Cochlear implants are now available for small children. The long-term benefits and risks of these devices are not clear, as they have only been in widespread use since the 1990s.

Lip reading is a valuable skill for the hearing impaired, and one that can be taught by skilled instructors. It is easier to acquire this skill while there is some residual hearing, so in a case of progressive hearing loss the patient should be urged to get instruction in lip reading as early as possible.

Information Box 6.1e-I

Deafness: comments from a Chinese medicine perspective

From a Chinese medicine viewpoint, impairment of hearing may be the result of a Full condition or a Deficient condition, or a combination of the two. Possible Full conditions include Phlegm and Damp obstructing the Shao Yang Channels (Gallbladder and Triple Heater), and Liver and Gallbladder Fire Rising. Deficient conditions include Kidney Qi Deficiency and Heart Qi Deficiency. As Deficiency of Kidney Yin can predispose the Flaring Up of Liver Yang and Fire, it may be appreciated that deafness can be a mixed condition.

Conductive deafness

Obstruction by wax

Earwax is a protective secretion which is produced by modified sweat glands in the outer ear canal. It contains antibodies and is sticky, which enables the trapping and removal of dirt and foreign bodies from the canal. Some people produce more wax than others, but the generally held view of impaction of the external ear canal by wax is that it is the result of misguided attempts to clean the ear by the insertion of a hard object such as a cotton bud. Frequent immersion of the ears in water can also precipitate impaction by wax, as saturated wax tends to expand as it absorbs water.

Impacted wax can be the cause of pain, vertigo and deafness, but can easily be removed by syringing. If the wax is likely to be hardened, the application of olive oil or sodium bicarbonate drops nightly for 1 week can facilitate the syringing process. The syringing procedure involves the direction of a jet of warm salt water along the roof of the auditory canal, by means of either a manual or an electric syringe.

Information Box 6.1e-II

Earwax: comments from a Chinese medicine perspective

In deafness resulting from obstruction by wax, the most likely Chinese medicine diagnosis would appear to be Phlegm Damp obstructing the Shao Yang Channels.

Acute otitis media

Acute otitis media (AOM) is the result of bacterial or viral infection of the middle ear. It can cause temporary deafness, and can predispose to the development of glue ear or chronic secretory otitis media, an important cause of hearing impairment in children under 10 years of age (see Chapter 5.4d).

Information Box 6.1e-III

Acute otitis media: comments from a Chinese medicine perspective

In Chinese medicine, acute otitis media may correspond to an External Invasion of the Shao Yang Channels by Wind Heat or Wind Cold. Damp is sometimes an additional Pathogenic Factor. Also, in older children Heat can enter the Liver and Gallbladder Channels, and then rise up to manifest as pain and heat in the ear. In these children constraint of Liver Qi leading to Heat might be a predisposing factor. Recurrent attacks of otitis media might suggest a Lingering Pathogenic Factor.

Chronic secretory otitis media (glue ear)

Chronic secretory otitis media (CSOM) (also termed 'otitis media with effusion') is a very important cause of conductive deafness in children (see Chapter 5.4e).

Information Box 6.1e-VI

Chronic secretory otitis media: comments from a Chinese medicine perspective

In Chinese medicine, chronic secretory otitis media may correspond to Lingering Pathogenic Factor. This can result in the build up of Phlegm and the Obstruction of Qi in the ear cavity. The child may also suffer from a pre-existing Depletion of Spleen Qi. This can contribute to the accumulation of Damp and Phlegm.

Alternatively, and less commonly, Depletion of Liver and Kidney Yin may lead to undernourishment of the ear. This would lead to a sticky fluid on the eardrum rather than profuse phlegmy discharge. In these cases the Depletion may be a result of overstimulation, and may result in a slightly hyperactive child.

Chronic otitis media

Chronic otitis media (also known as 'chronic suppurative otitis media') is a confusingly named, long-term consequence of acute otitis media (AOM). It has to be distinguished from chronic secretory otitis media, which is the non-infective condition of childhood also known as 'glue ear' (see above). Chronic otitis media is much more common in undernourished or immunocompromised children.

In chronic otitis media there has been failure of resolution of the infectious process of acute otitis media. This means that there is an ongoing infective process with the production of damaging pus. Although the eardrum normally heals over after the perforation that can occur in AOM, in chronic cases the continued production of pus prevents this healing process, and the eardrum retains its perforation and the ear continues to discharge pus.

If the infection simply affects the lining of the middle ear and the eardrum, there is good chance of healing with the combined treatments of meticulous cleaning of the ear by means of delicate suction and mopping, along with appropriate antibiotic therapy.

The condition is much more serious if the infection has spread to the delicate bony structures within the ear or into the bony walls of the middle ear and the mastoid process. In this sort of case, surgery is required to clear away any infected material and bony regions. Mastoidectomy is one of the operations performed for bony chronic otitis media. The surgery required for middle-ear damage is extremely delicate, and may involve refashioning of the eardrum and ossicles in order to preserve hearing.

The presence of chronic infection in the middle ear can also predispose to other deep serious conditions, including meningitis, acute mastoiditis (an acute pus-forming infection of the air cells in the mastoid process), brain abscess and paralysis of the facial nerve (this presents like Bell's palsy).

Information Box 6.1e-V

Discharging ear: comments from a Chinese medicine perspective

From a Chinese medicine perspective, the chronic production of pus indicates Damp Heat against a background of chronic Deficiency, and in particular of the Spleen and Kidneys. Progressive erosion of the bony walls of the middle ear as a consequence of chronic infection suggests Phlegm and Kidney Yin Deficiency.

Otosclerosis

Otosclerosis is a hereditary condition in which there is a progressive development of deafness as a result of abnormal bone growth around the base of the stapes, the stirrup-shaped ossicle of the middle ear. This growth can be worsened in pregnancy, and so the condition is more common in women. The operation of stapedectomy involves replacing the affected end of the stapes with a steel implant, but carries a small risk of total loss of hearing. If successful, and performed early in the progression of the condition, normal hearing can be regained.

Information Box 6.1e-VI

Otosclerosis: comments from a Chinese medicine perspective

Because of its progressive and hereditary nature, otosclerosis would suggest a Chinese medicine diagnosis of Jing Deficiency.

Otitis externa and furunculosis

'Otitis externa' is the term given to any condition in which there is inflammation of the epithelium that lines the external ear canal. Common causes include fungal and bacterial infections, and contact eczema resulting from sensitivity to environmental substances. The symptoms and signs include itching, crusting, and sometimes intense discomfort of the ear canal and the pinna of the ear. It is important to ensure that the crusting and discharge do not in fact originate from a discharging middle-ear infection, so an otoscopic examination is advisable.

The condition can be triggered by persistent dampness of the ear canals, such as might affect frequent swimmers, and also sensitivity to environmental substances such as shampoo, and medical treatments such as antibiotic ear drops. Trauma to the ear canal as a result of attempts to scratch or clean the affected area can exacerbate the condition.

Treatment would include avoidance of immersion of the ears and of any potential skin sensitisers. A piece of cotton wool coated in Vaseline can prevent water entering the ears when showering, and ear plugs can be of use when swimming. Medical treatments include careful cleaning of the ears (dry mopping) and syringing. In severe cases dressings soaked in antibacterial, antifungal and corticosteroid medication can be inserted into the ear on a daily basis, and if less severe the patient can self-administer a combination of antibiotic and steroid ear drops.

'Furunculosis' describes the tendency for small boils to form at the base of hair follicles in the external ear canal. Because the skin in this area is tightly apposed to the bony cavity through which the ear canal passes, furunculosis can be extremely painful. It is more common in people who suffer from diabetes, so this diagnosis should be excluded. Medical treatment includes insertion of a wick soaked in icthammol to help the boil come to a head, and antibiotics by injection if the condition is severe.

Both conditions can be a cause of deafness resulting from occlusion of the ear canal.

Information Box 6.1e-VII

Otitis externa: comments from a Chinese medicine perspective

In Chinese medicine, otitis externa could represent an invasion of Wind Damp Heat, or simply Damp Heat if the condition is chronic. Likewise, furunculosis would seem to be consistent with a manifestation of Damp Heat.

Sensorineural deafness

Congenital deafness

Congenital deafness is recognised to affect 1 in 1000 children. Early diagnosis is considered essential, and so in the UK there is now a routine neonatal hearing screening programme.

Deafness of old age

Deafness of old age, also termed 'presbycusis', is the most common cause of sensorineural deafness. In this case the deafness is simply the result of a gradual degeneration of the delicate structure of the cochlea and the vestibular nerve. The onset is characteristically gradual, and the deafness is more marked for sounds of high frequency (the range of female voices). The usual treatment for presbycusis is the prescription of a hearing aid.

A sudden onset of deafness in old age would be most likely the result of a vascular stroke or a viral infection on the vestibular nerve.

> **Information Box 6.1e-VIII**
>
> **Presbycusis: comments from a Chinese medicine perspective**
>
> In Chinese medicine, presbycusis would be a manifestation of declining Kidney Qi failing to nourish the ears.

Noise-induced deafness

Noise-induced deafness can be a component of presbycusis. In this case the deafness to high-frequency sounds is more marked because of trauma to the sensory cells of the cochlea from exposure to high-intensity sounds. Usually, for the deafness to be long term, the exposure to the sounds has to have been repeated over a prolonged period.

Noise-induced deafness is a recognised risk in some occupations, such as in the construction industry, and in this case it is the duty of the employer to ensure that exposed employees are provided with suitable protective ear muffs. Affected employees may be eligible for compensation.

Menière's disease

In Menière's disease, the fluid-filled labyrinth of one or both cochleas becomes waterlogged with excessive fluid. Onset is usually after 40 years of age. The cause is unknown.

The symptoms of Menière's disease include disabling vertigo, deafness and tinnitus, each of which typically appear in bouts, although the tinnitus and slight deafness can become persistent. In an acute attack the vertigo often will cause prostration and vomiting, and emergency treatment with an injection of a sedating antiemetic medication such as prochlorperazine can be helpful.

Advice for the prevention of attacks includes fluid and salt restriction, and avoidance of coffee, alcohol and smoking. Betahistine hydrochloride and cinnarizine are commonly prescribed drugs to be taken on a regular basis to reduce the frequency of attacks.

Surgical options for Menière's disease are available but carry the risk of inducing deafness on the operated side, and so are usually offered only in severe cases or in those cases in which deafness is already established.

> **Information Box 6.1e-IX**
>
> **Menière's disease: comments from a Chinese medicine perspective**
>
> Menière's disease has the characteristics of a Full condition. A possible Chinese medicine interpretation would be Phlegm and Damp obstructing the rising of Qi on a basis of underlying Depletion of Kidney Qi.

Acoustic neuroma

An acoustic neuroma is a benign, slow-growing tumour of the vestibular (acoustic) nerve. The tumour typically presents with the gradual onset of one-sided deafness and/or loss of balance. The diagnosis can be confirmed by MRI. Early diagnosis can maximise the chances of a safe operative removal of the tumour, although surgery is unlikely to restore normal hearing on the affected side.

> **Information Box 6.1e-X**
>
> **Acoustic neuroma: comments from a Chinese medicine perspective**
>
> As it is a tumour, in Chinese medicine the symptoms of an acoustic neuroma may correspond to Phlegm and/or Stagnation on the basis of an underlying state of Depletion of Kidney Qi.

Deafness due to drugs and infections

Some prescribed medications, including certain antibiotics, aspirin, some diuretics and beta blockers, can in rare cases lead to deafness. In most cases the hearing impairment will abate on the withdrawal from the medication.

Certain infections can cause inflammation of the vestibular nerve, and so cause sudden deafness. This is a medical emergency that merits immediate referral. Mumps, herpes zoster virus, meningitis and syphilis are all recognised to be causes of deafness.

Earache

Earache can result from a number of the diseases of the ear already discussed. These include otitis externa and furunculosis, mastoiditis and acute and chronic otitis media. There is also a range of other conditions that lead to referred pain in the ear. This is because branches from four of the facial nerves and also the nerves emerging from the C1 and C2 levels of the cord also lead to the ear. Although in these conditions the seat of the pain is elsewhere, acupuncture or electroacupuncture focused on points close to the ear, the site of the pain, can be effective.

Dental and mandibular causes of earache

Impacted wisdom teeth and dental caries of the molars (back teeth) can lead to pain in the ear. Excessive tension or arthritis of the temporomandibular joint (TMJ) can also lead to referred ear pain. With TMJ dysfunction, there is commonly also a trigger point in the masseter muscle which is worth treating by means of acupuncture.

Pharyngeal and laryngeal causes of earache

Pain from tonsillitis, quinsy and disease of the base of the tongue may also refer to the ear because a branch of the glossopharyngeal nerve also supplies the eardrum. Cancer of the larynx or pharynx can lead to sustained unexplained earache, and so if this is mentioned by a patient it should be referred for investigation.

Cervical spondylosis

Rarely, pain from cervical spondylosis can be felt in the ear.

> **Information Box 6.1e-XI**
>
> **Earache: comments from a Chinese medicine perspective**
>
> From a Chinese medicine perspective, pain felt in the ear is in all cases a reflection of Stagnation of Qi in the Channels associated with the ear. The underlying cause of this Stagnation will relate to the underlying cause of the pain.

Tinnitus

'Tinnitus' is the term used to describe the sensation of noises in the ears. Tinnitus may be unilateral or bilateral, high pitched or low pitched, intermittent or constant. Tinnitus is generally more troubling in quiet environments, as external noise can serve as a distraction from the internally generated sounds. Tinnitus, if persistent, can markedly affect quality of life. If the cause is unknown or cannot be treated, then hearing-aid-like tinnitus maskers, which are designed to produce white noise, can make the tinnitus less obtrusive. Sometimes a radio playing in the background can provide the patient with relief from the noise.

In many cases the cause of tinnitus cannot be explained. Tinnitus may be the result of disease within the ear itself or can result from more general disease.

Local causes of tinnitus

Tinnitus can result from wax in the external ear canal and fluid in the middle ear, such as develops in chronic secretory otitis media (glue ear). It is also a well-known complication of Menière's disease and otosclerosis. It is also associated with the development of presbycusis and noise damage to the ears.

General causes of tinnitus

Tinnitus can also result from more generalised conditions. For example, it is well recognised as a transient symptom of fever. It may also accompany a diagnosis of anaemia and some degenerative diseases of the nervous system (e.g. multiple sclerosis). Certain medications (including aspirin) and alcohol abuse are toxic causes of tinnitus.

Vertigo

The medical definition of vertigo is the experience of movement, often manifesting as a spinning sensation. When patients describe a sensation of dizziness this need not mean vertigo, as this term is often used to describe a feeling of faintness or light-headedness. Vertigo can only be ascribed if the patient describes a moving sensation (as if they had just got off a boat or a roundabout).

Sustained vertigo is most unpleasant, and is often accompanied by sweating and vomiting. It is an absolute contraindication to driving. Patients who suffer from vertigo should be advised not to drive until they are free from episodes of dizziness.

Tranquillising drugs such as prochlorperazine, chlorpromazine and cinnarizine can all be effective in reducing the severity of the symptoms of vertigo. These are the same type of drugs that are prescribed to prevent motion sickness.

Vertigo originates either from a disorder of the semicircular canals of the inner ear, or from the brainstem.

> **Information Box 6.1e-XII**
>
> **Vertigo: comments from a Chinese medicine perspective**
>
> In Chinese medicine, the symptom of vertigo is a manifestation of Liver Wind Rising and/or Turbid Phlegm. Wind is implicated if the episodes are sudden in onset.

Vestibular neuronitis (labyrinthitis)

Vestibular neuronitis is probably the most common cause of sustained vertigo in young people. This presumed viral infection often accompanies the onset of a cold, and leads to a sudden onset of severe vertigo, which may then be episodic. In most cases there is full recovery, although this can be very gradual and may take a few weeks.

Benign paroxysmal vertigo

This episodic form of vertigo manifests in brief episodes of dizziness, which are triggered by a postural change to the head. It is the result of a mild degenerative change in the semicircular canals of the ears.

Central causes of vertigo

Damage to areas of the brainstem, such as can occur in strokes or the demyelination of multiple sclerosis, can result in loss of balance and vertigo. In such cases the vertigo is usually fairly short lived (lasting no more than a few weeks), but if the damage is significant, the loss of balance may persist.

The red flags of the diseases of the ear

Some people with diseases of the ear will benefit from referral to a conventional doctor for assessment and/or treatment. Red flags are those symptoms and signs that indicate that referral is to be considered. The red flags of the diseases of the ear are described in Table 6.1e-I. This table forms part of the summary on red flags given in Appendix III, which also gives advice on the degree of urgency of referral for each of the red flag conditions listed (see Q6.1e-3).

Table 6.1e-I Red Flags 43 – diseases of the ear

Red Flag	Description	Reasoning
43.1	**Vertigo** in young person: lasting for more than 6 weeks, or if so severe as to be causing recurrent vomiting, or if there is increased risk of thromboembolic disease (e.g. in pregnancy)	The most likely cause of a sudden onset of dizzy spells in a young person is an inflammation of the inner ear (labyrinthitis). This usually settles down completely within 6 weeks. Medical treatment is to prescribe antisickness medication, so only refer if the sickness does not respond to your treatment Rarely, a sudden onset of dizziness is the consequence of a stroke or multiple sclerosis. Consider referral if there has been any previous episode of neurological disturbance (e.g. blurred vision, numbness) or if there is an increased risk or history of thromboembolic disease
43.2	**Vertigo** in older person (>45 years old)	Refer so that the patient can have investigations to exclude the possibility of stroke (dizziness can result from brainstem or cerebellar stroke)
43.3	**Complications of acute otitis media**: persistent fever/pain/confusion for >3–4 days after the onset of the earache (may indicate spread of the infection, e.g. mastoiditis or brain abscess)	Otitis media is an uncomfortable but self-limiting ear infection that commonly affects young children. It is now considered good practice not to prescribe antibiotics in a simple case, which will generally settle within 1–3 days, sometimes after natural perforation of the eardrum. This is a beneficial healing process (so some sticky discharge for 1–2 days after an earache is not a cause for concern) However, persisting high fever, confusion or intense pain is not usual, and the child should be referred to exclude the rare possibility of infectious complications
43.4	**Persistent discharge from the ear**	Chronic discharge from the ear for more than 1 week after the infection of otitis media has settled down may indicate the development of chronic otitis media, and this needs further investigation as there is a risk of permanent damage to the middle ear
43.5	**Features of mastoiditis**: fever, with a painful and swollen mastoid bone	Mastoiditis is a now rare complication of otitis media and usually affects children. It is a serious condition, as it is a bone infection and can be difficult to treat with antibiotics. Refer as a high priority
43.6	**New onset of difficulty hearing in a child**: lasting for >3 weeks	Refer if prolonged, if interfering with social interactions and education, or if associated with pain in the ear or dizziness. The most likely cause is glue ear, a chronic accumulation of mucoid secretions in the middle ear

Continued

Table 6.1e-I Red Flags 43 – diseases of the ear—Cont'd

Red Flag	Description	Reasoning
43.7	**Sudden onset of absolute deafness** (one-sided or bilateral)	Absolute deafness suggests damage to the acoustic nerve or auditory centres of the brain, and requires high priority/urgent assessment
43.8	**Gradual onset of relative deafness in an adult** for >7 days	A degree of hearing loss is common after a cold, but has usually subsided within a week. If hearing loss is slow and progressive, referral for audiometric assessment is advised to exclude the rare, but treatable, slowly growing acoustic neuroma Earwax is probably the most common cause of relative hearing loss, so it is useful to possess an otoscope to check for this treatable possibility (the wax can be softened by administering 5 drops of olive oil in each ear every night for a week)
43.9	**Tinnitus if progressive or if associated with hearing loss**	Tinnitus (ringing or buzzing in the ear) is usually a benign finding, and remains fairly constant, or may increase in times of stress. It is not normally progressive or associated with hearing loss, and if it is this may suggest a progressive disorder of the ear or the auditory nerve. Refer for audiometric assessment
43.10	**Earache in an adult for >3 weeks**	Earache is common after a cold, but should subside within a week or so. If persistent (>3 weeks) and unexplained, referral is merited as it is a red flag for cancer of the nasopharynx

Self-test 6.1e

Diseases of the ear

1. You are telephoned by a 28 year old patient of yours who is off work because she has been overcome by a bout of dizziness. She describes how the room is spinning round and round, and if she lifts her head off the pillow she feels extremely nauseated. The attack came on suddenly late last night. She explains how she would prefer to try natural treatment rather than visit the GP.
   (i) What is the most likely explanation of what has happened to this patient?
   (ii) Would it be advisable to refer her?
   (iii) What other advice might you offer to this patient?
2. An elderly patient mentions that she is increasingly hard of hearing.
   (i) What are the most likely causes of deafness in an elderly lady?
   (ii) Would you refer this patient for a conventional diagnosis or treatment?
3. A 65 year old patient of yours mentions that he has been suffering from earache for some weeks. His hearing is unaffected and he has not been suffering from discharge, tinnitus or vertigo. The pain is deep in his right ear and feels "boring" in quality. On examination you can find no abnormality local to the ear, although there is some discomfort over the right temporomandibular joint (TMJ) and tension in the body of the right masseter muscle.
   (i) What are the causes of unilateral earache?
   (ii) What are possible causes in this gentleman?
   (iii) Would you refer this patient?

Answers

1. (i) This patient is most likely suffering from a bout of vestibular neuronitis (viral labyrinthitis). The sudden and severe onset is characteristic of this condition.
   (ii) The GP can offer only symptomatic treatment so there is no need to refer straight away. You can mention that the GP can prescribe tranquillising medication for the vertigo, but offer to treat first with acupuncture.
   (iii) You might also advise the patient that these symptoms will start getting better within a few days but may not actually disappear for a few weeks.
   You should also be very clear that she must not drive in the period whilst she is experiencing attacks of vertigo.
2. (i) The causes of progressive deafness in an elderly person may be categorised as conductive or sensorineural. The most likely cause of conductive deafness in this age group is obstruction of the external ear canal by ear wax, although congestion of the middle ear following a cold is a possibility.
   Of the sensorineural causes presbycusis is the most likely cause is the deafness is bilateral. If the deafness affects one ear only then stroke or acoustic neuroma are possible causes.
   (ii) Whatever the cause of the deafness, this lady would benefit from a referral. Firstly treatable causes such as earwax and acoustic neuroma can be excluded. Secondly, even if the deafness is not treatable, the prescription of a hearing aid can be discussed.
3. (i) The common causes of earache can be categorised into ear diseases and causes of referred pain. The ear diseases include otitis media and otitis externa and furunculosis. Referred pain can originate from disease of the teeth, temporomandibular joint, larynx, pharynx and cervical vertebrae.
   (ii) In the absence of other abnormalities in the affected ear, this suggests that the pain in this case might be referred. The symptoms in the right TMJ are suggestive that this is the source of the pain.
   (iii) Unexplained persistent earache is a warning feature of disease as it can point to undiagnosed malignant disease in mouth or throat. In this case it is worth treating the TMJ dysfunction as this is likely to be the source of pain, but consider referral if there is no response to treatment.

Mental health disorders

6.2

Chapter 6.2a Introduction to mental health disorders

LEARNING POINTS

At the end of this chapter you will:

- be able to describe the conventional medical interpretation of the mind
- be able to describe the conventional medical definition of mental illness
- understand the biopsychosocial model of the causation of mental illness.

Estimated time for chapter: 100 minutes.

Introduction and definitions

This section is dedicated to the study of the mind and its related diseases. The mind is unlike all other physiological systems, in that its physical structure and functioning cannot be scientifically measured and described as can the anatomy and physiology of a system such as the skin or the blood. However, in many ways the mind and its related diseases are studied within conventional medicine by means of a very similar approach to that used in the study of the more physically defined systems.

In conventional medicine the diseases of the mind are termed 'mental health disorders'. The mental health disorders are managed within the medical speciality of psychiatry and the non-medical clinical speciality of psychology.

The medical speciality of psychiatry is a relatively young discipline in the history of conventional medicine. The term is derived from the Greek words 'psyche' (meaning 'mind') and 'iatros' (meaning 'doctor'). Psychiatry is the speciality dedicated to the medical treatment of the mental health disorders.

'Psychology' is a term used to describe the academic and clinical disciplines that are based on the study of the workings of the mind. A clinical psychologist is a therapist who has gained a degree in psychology, and then undergone further training in the practical application of psychology in the clinical situation.

Psychotherapy (literally meaning treatment for the mind) is a term which describes any approach which involves the use of the formal and systematic clinical relationship between the therapist and the client as a therapeutic tool. Psychotherapy may be utilised by psychiatrists and clinical psychologists but also by practitioners who have undergone specific training in one (or more) particular form(s) of therapy. The different types of psychotherapy will be explored in more detail in Chapter 6.2c.

The aim of this chapter is to introduce the general approach by which mental health disorders are understood conventionally. These disorders are classified by psychiatrists and psychologists in a quasi-systematic way, but unlike most of the diseases studied within the other medical specialities, the two classification systems currently used are largely based on the manifestation (symptoms and signs) of the disorder rather than on its physical cause(s).

The chapter begins with a brief exploration of how the mind is generally seen from a medical perspective as a distinct entity with respect to the other physiological systems. This is despite increasing scientific evidence that the mind is inextricably linked with (and may well even be rooted in) the function of these other systems. The chapter then goes on to consider the conventional understanding of the causation of mental illness (see Q.6.2a-1).

Mental health and the mind–body divide

The very existence of the disciplines of psychiatry and psychology indicates the depth to which the mind has in recent medical history been recognised as a separate entity to the other physical systems of the body, such as the cardiovascular or the urinary systems, and even the central nervous system.

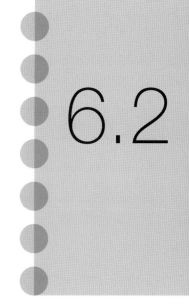

A dictionary description of the mind describes it as 'the seat of awareness, thought, volition and feeling ... concentration (and) memory'. This description does not strongly imply that the mind has any physical basis, even though most psychiatrists would agree that the mind springs from the workings of the brain. Moreover, the structure and known workings of the brain are embraced within the medical speciality of neurology. Although modern psychiatrists have a robust foundation of neurology as part of their training, the converse is not necessarily true of neurologists. This reflects the fact that, although conventional practitioners generally believe that mental health problems must originate in the physical brain, as yet the precise links between the workings of the physical brain and mental health disorders have not been adequately explained.

The link between the mind and the brain is a relatively recent phenomenon in western culture. In contrast, the idea that the mind and its disorders are rooted in the bodily humours and their imbalances was a much more prevalent and prevailing view that persisted in Europe well into the third and fourth centuries AD (this perspective is comparable to the Chinese medicine Organ perspective). Thereafter, in the west, the influence of the monasteries strengthened the concept that mental illness resulted from a possession of the spirit by devils, and the mentally ill were taken for treatment to monks and priests. It was only as the healing role of the medical profession became distinct from that of the priesthood in the late 17th century, and mind was seen as distinct from the body (Cartesian dualism), that mental illness began to be viewed more as a medical disorder, and, specifically, insanity as a disorder of the mind.

Until very recent decades, there was a tendency for doctors to attribute many psychiatric conditions to a problem stemming purely from the mind, with absolutely no physical basis. This is in keeping with the Cartesian perspective of the body, in which the mind and body are seen as separate entities, rather like a driver is separate from her car.

However, more recently, in the last two to three decades, a more holistic 'biopsychosocial model' has begun to replace the outmoded mind/body medical model as the theoretical basis of psychiatric practice. This model proposes that psychiatric conditions arise as the result of a combination of biological, psychological and social factors. In this way their origin is seen as linked not only to the mind, but also to physical changes in the body and to factors in the social environment of the patient.

There is an increasing body of scientific evidence that strongly links some mental health disorders with certain chemical imbalances of neurotransmitters in the brain, and, more controversially, with levels of the hormones that circulate throughout the whole body. In conventional practice, this is the realm of neuropsychiatry, a rapidly expanding discipline in which the focus is on how disease of the chemical structure of the brain might manifest as mental illness.

From a holistic perspective, neuropsychiatry offers a conventional description of an undeniable link between mind and body (i.e. the physical structure of the brain). Moreover, as it is increasingly recognised that there is a significant overlap between the diverse neurotransmitters of the central nervous system and the hormones of the endocrine system, it becomes possible that this mind–body link need no longer be confined strictly to the brain. Instead, as a product of the subtleties of hormone expression, the changes that appear to spring from the mind might have their origin in diverse sites throughout the body.

Exciting though the potential for holism in these conventional explanations may be, the concept of the mind–body divide does not really seem to have been eroded significantly in conventional medical practice. Currently, many patients of conventional hospital practitioners will experience their mental and physical problems being treated as if they have no relationship to each other (with the exception of those well-described diseases of the nervous system that are recognised to result in mental health dysfunction, such as multi-infarct dementia).

For example, it is a common experience for a specialist within in a medical speciality (such as cardiology, respiratory medicine or gastroenterology) to be referred patients whose physical symptoms are directly related to an imbalance in their mental or emotional state. For example, the tachycardia, hyperventilation and diarrhoea that can accompany chronic anxiety are very commonly seen in general medical hospital clinics. However, the explicit task of the specialist in this sort of case is to exclude a measurable physical basis for symptoms such as these. In the patient with chronic anxiety, the task is to exclude conditions such as a structural heart abnormality, asthma or ulcerative colitis. Once this has been done, the patient is discharged back to the care of the GP, and thence, if the resources are available, to a mental health specialist.

To conclude, the mind is currently seen in conventional medicine as a body system that obviously does have a relationship with the other physically described systems, but this relationship is more tenuous than those all the other physiological systems share with each other. Although the mind–body split paradigm is necessarily being eroded as a consequence of scientific study into the causation of mental illness, in current practice this paradigm frequently prevails.

The definition of a mental health disorder

The American Psychiatric Association (APA) offers the following definition of mental health disorder:

> each of the mental disorders is ... a clinically significant behavioural or psychological syndrome ... that is associated with present distress or disability or with a significantly increased risk of suffering death, pain, disability or an important loss of freedom ... Whatever its original cause, it must be currently considered a manifestation of a behavioural, psychological or biological dysfunction in the person.

In this definition, the mental health disorder is defined as a characteristic cluster of behaviours, or psychological symptoms and signs (behavioural or psychological syndrome), which are associated with negative consequences for the individual (distress, disability, risk of death, pain or loss of freedom). Although for any one mental health state the first part of this definition, which embraces the syndromes, may be defined with a degree of objectivity, the second part is necessarily subjective and difficult to classify. What might appear as distress or loss of freedom to the diagnosing doctor might not be so interpreted by the patient or within their culture of origin.

This definition is useful in explaining how mental health professionals interpret mental health states, and also what they believe to be the root cause of mental health disorders (i.e. a 'behavioural, psychological or biological dysfunction in the person'). The definition reflects the biopsychosocial model of thought, which has been increasingly embraced within modern psychiatry.

The causation of mental health disorder: the biopsychosocial model

As implied by the APA definition of mental health disorder, the diverse mental health disorders are generally considered to have a multifactorial basis for their origin. Many psychiatrists would subscribe to this biopsychosocial model of mental illness. The term 'biopsychosocial' refers to the understanding that a combination of inherited and acquired physical factors (biological factors), factors related to the emotional development of the individual (psychological factors) and factors related to the cultural environment of the individual (social factors) are all relevant in the development of a mental health disorder in an individual. Ideally, in every case presenting to a psychiatrist or psychologist, biological causes, psychological causes and social causes need to be considered.

Biological factors in mental health disorders

A biological theory of the causation of mental illness proposes that physical changes/illness are at the root of the development of the illness. The biological perspective is supported by the fact that many diseases or conditions that are known to involve physical changes in the brain can manifest with mental disturbance (e.g. Alzheimer disease, traumatic head injury, alcohol intoxication). Moreover, the fact that certain conditions tend to run in families is strongly suggestive of a genetic inheritance, and thus physical basis, of a condition.

Adoptive studies, which demonstrate that children who have been adopted shortly after birth appear to carry the risk of developing mental health disorders apparent in their blood relations, are very strongly suggestive of the genetic inheritance of mental illness. Studies of twins who have been separated at birth and adopted by different families offer even more powerful evidence of the inheritance of mental health disorders. Conditions such as schizophrenia, manic depression, simple depression, anxiety and panic disorder, obsessive–compulsive disorder and alcoholism have all been shown by these sorts of studies to have an inherited component in their causation. This means that a child of someone with one of these conditions is more likely than the average person to develop that condition.

The neuropsychiatric explanation offered for an inherited tendency to mental health disorders is usually given in terms of an inherited neurochemical makeup. For example, it is recognised that in schizophrenia there is increased activity of those brain systems that involve the release of the neurotransmitter dopamine. It is possible that the increased tendency for schizophrenia to run in families is due, in part, to an inherited tendency for these physical systems to be overactivated. This chemical basis for the genesis of schizophrenia is further supported by the fact that dopamine-stimulating drugs, such as amphetamines and cannabis, can trigger a psychosis similar in form to schizophrenia. Moreover, the drugs discovered originally by chance to be of benefit in schizophrenia, the major tranquillisers (first developed as anaesthetic agents), are now known to act by blocking the action of dopamine.

Similarly, the tendency to develop depression may be, in part, a result of an inherited reduction in the expression of monoamine neurotransmitters such as noradrenaline and serotonin (5HT). This is supported by the fact that the various classes of antidepressant drugs all seem to increase the levels of monoamines in the brain. It is increasingly recognised that some of the addictive recreational drugs (e.g. nicotine, ecstasy) may induce a release of serotonin after their use, which is then followed by a more long-term depletion of this neurotransmitter in the brain. Because of this, use of the drug forces the user to face a long-term state of low mood if they choose to withdraw from the drug, particularly if the use of the drug has been prolonged over a period of months to years.

However, an inherited tendency to a condition does not in itself destine a child to develop that condition. It is clear that other factors are usually required to force the expression of a condition such as schizophrenia or depression. These other factors are considered to be either psychological or social in nature.

Psychological factors in mental health disorders

The psychological explanation of mental illness rests on the principle that experiences during childhood and early adulthood can have a profound bearing on a person's mental and emotional health. This is such a commonly accepted principle that few would argue against the suggestion that a shocking experience or a period of deprivation in childhood would have long-term psychological repercussions. However, it is only in fairly recent years that studies of traumatic events in childhood have clearly demonstrated a link between certain forms of childhood deprivation and long-term mental ill-health. One of the earliest studies (by the psychologist John Bowlby in the 1950s) demonstrated that prolonged or recurrent absence of a consistent mother figure in early life was associated with difficulties in forming emotional bonds and a tendency to anxiety and depression in later life.

Since that time, psychological studies have shown that diverse factors in the family environment, including expressed angry discord, maternal depression, divorce, bereavement, overprotection, lack of parental authority, physical and sexual abuse, unremitting criticism, and taunting and inconsistent discipline, can all be risk factors for misbehaviour in children and mental health disorders in later life.

Even theories that propose psychological mechanisms for the causation of mental illness are only just over a century old. Sigmund Freud, now considered the founder of psychoanalysis, first proposed that there are both conscious and unconscious aspects to the mind. He theorised that unconscious forces deriving from deeply ingrained value systems originating from parents or society (the superego), or instinctive drives (the id) could, together with pressures in one's external life, challenge and cause conflict with the conscious self (the ego). The conscious self was considered by Freud to develop to its healthy adult form in distinct stages throughout childhood. Freud proposed that the healthy child has to progress appropriately through oral, anal, phallic, latent and genital phases in order to mature as a healthy adult, and problems encountered in any of the stages could result in lasting psychological disorder. For example, he proposed that the anal stage was when the toddler ideally achieves a sense of separateness and becomes independent in terms of toilet training and feeding. Problems in this phase might appear in adulthood as a fear of losing control, obsessional traits or depression because of not living up to expectations.

Freud's theories and their rigid distinctions are less accepted nowadays, but his beliefs that the psyche undergoes progressive development throughout childhood, and that unconscious 'material' originating from episodes scattered along the course of that development can persist to lead to mental illness, still very much influence modern psychotherapeutic practice.

The concept of defence mechanisms, proposed first by Freud and later developed by his daughter Anna Freud, is one that is still very much recognised in modern psychology. 'Defence mechanism' is a term used to describe any mental response used by a person to protect himself from psychological pain such as guilt, anxiety or shame. The naming of the various defence reactions has entered common usage. Commonly described defence reactions include denial, repression, regression, rationalisation, displacement, projection, introjection, sublimation and reaction formation.

Defence mechanisms can be healthy, and responses such as distraction (e.g. looking for the positive, use of humour) are likely to be used by people who enjoy good mental health. However, mechanisms such as repression of unpleasant feelings (such as might follow an episode of severe abuse), or denial of what has really happened (e.g. an inability to take in a diagnosis of cancer), may actually lead to long-term problems in mental health. The theory is that these sorts of defence mechanisms simply shift conscious mental pain into the unconscious, where the pain may still be felt in the form of depression or anxiety, but from where it is much harder to treat the pain at its root. With this perspective on causation, a psychotherapist works to enable the patient to arrive at a place where this unconscious material is made conscious and the roots of the pain can be understood, and so transformed.

The cognitive–behavioural psychological perspective on the causation of disease is based on the idea that the patient has learned inappropriate responses to the world around them because of negative past experience. The cognitive–behavioural model interprets unhelpful behaviours in the light of the incorrect thoughts that underlie them. For example, a child who was shocked by the barking of a dog might then tend to be fearful whenever a dog comes close. A behavioural response of avoidance, and maybe even a physiological response of palpitations and sweating, might then persist into adulthood. The cognitive–behavioural interpretation of this problem (termed a 'simple phobia') is that, because of the childhood experience, the belief that 'dogs will make me frightened' has been learned, and the inappropriate reaction to dogs has become ingrained as a result of that belief.

Anxiety disorders, eating disorders and depressive disorders are examples of disorders that can be analysed according to cognitive–behavioural theory. The negative responses to the world expressed in these disorders can be related in cognitive–behavioural theory to unhelpful learned patterns of thought.

Social factors in mental health disorders

A social perspective on the causation of mental illness necessarily overlaps with the psychological perspective, because it sees factors in the social environment as impacting on the developing psyche. Social theories of the causation of mental illness are particularly bound up in the studies of cultural factors common to communities. Studies on the incidence of mental illness in communities have identified that mental illness can relate to variables such as gender, age, marital status, social support and economic status. For example, there is a recognised link between depression in men and being divorced, a link that is far less pronounced in women who are divorced.

The study of the effect of life events, such as marriage, birth, divorce, emigration and bereavement, falls into the remit of understanding the social causation of mental illness.

Predisposing, precipitating and perpetuating factors in mental illness

A psychiatrist or psychologist seeks to understand the evolution of mental illness in terms of three factors of causation: predisposing, precipitating and perpetuating factors. Ideally, the factors that have predisposed to the condition, those that have precipitated the condition and those that might be perpetuating the condition need to be clarified if the most appropriate treatment is to be chosen.

Predisposing factors are those factors that might have led a person to have become more at risk of developing a mental illness before the illness became apparent. For example, if one looks at the case of schizophrenia appearing for the first time as the sudden onset of a paranoid psychosis in a 22-year-old male student, the predisposing factors might include a family history of serious mental illness (grandfather was in an asylum for 10 years and mother had an episode of postnatal psychosis after the birth of his younger brother). There might also be volatile emotional environment in the family home (mother and father have frequent arguments, and mother often breaks down in tears when stressed). As a child, this student was recognised to be withdrawn and awkward socially.

Precipitating factors are those factors that have triggered a particular episode of illness. In this case these might include the stress of leaving home for the first time, and the inability to fit into a supportive network of people at college. A recent history of experimenting with ecstasy and frequent use of cannabis could also be included as precipitating factors.

Perpetuating factors are those factors that might prevent the resolution of the mental illness. In this case these could include the lack of social support, continued drug use and self-neglect (see Q6.2a-2).

The biopsychosocial model and the choice of treatment

Although there is a general appreciation amongst conventional practitioners that there are diverse factors at play in the generation of mental illness, psychiatrists and psychologists vary in their treatment approaches as a direct result of the way in which they might emphasise the importance of one factor in the causation of mental health problems over any other. For example, for a patient with a mental health issue, a hospital psychiatrist might favour medical drug treatments (biological causation of illness), whereas a psychoanalyst might concentrate on enabling the patient to explore primitive emotional reactions experienced in a relationship which started to emerge in childhood (psychological causation of illness) (see Q6.2a-3). The diverse approaches to the treatment of mental health disorders and their relationship to the perceived underlying cause of the disorder are explored in more detail in Chapter 6.2c (see Q6.2a-4).

Information Box 6.2a-I

Mental health disorders: a Chinese medicine perspective

The mind (Shen) is seen in Chinese medicine as a fundamental aspect of Qi. Therefore, any imbalance or disturbance in the flow of Qi will have a manifestation at the level of the Shen. All Chinese medicine patterns, therefore, may include signs and symptoms of a mental and/or emotional nature. Unlike conventional medicine, in Chinese medicine mental health is not seen as a distinct speciality, but instead as one aspect of health as a whole. Psychiatric or psychological diseases are described in Chinese medicine as Jing Shen Bing (Essence Spirit diseases).

There are many terms used in Chinese medicine texts associated with the mind, but Shen (Spirit) and compound terms that include the term Shen, such as Jing Shen (Spirit Essence), are those that are used most commonly. In Chinese medicine the Shen, together with Qi and Jing (Essence), are described as the 'three treasures'. These three substances are the interdependent manifestations of Qi. The Shen is classically the most insubstantial and rapidly moving form of Qi, and is specifically associated with the mind. Shen is mainly associated with Heart Qi, and the Heart is said to 'house the Shen'. Spirit, in the Chinese sense, has many layers of meaning, but when used from the perspective of the psychological diseases it embraces the outward manifestation of life, together with consciousness, thinking and feeling.

The 5 Shen

The Chinese considered the Shen to consist of the five spiritual aspects of a human being, each of which is associated with a Yin Organ. The five aspects are the Hun (Liver), the Yi (Spleen), the Zhi (Kidney), the Po (Lung) and the specific spiritual aspect of the Heart Organ, also given the name Shen. To minimise confusion, in this text this last particular aspect of the Shen will be called 'Heart Shen'.

Each of the five aspects of the Shen is recognised to have particular characteristics, as described below.

The mind/spirit (Heart Shen)

The Heart Shen is that aspect of the spirit which specifically resides in the Heart, but which also embraces the other four Shen. It is considered to be responsible for consciousness, intelligence, thought, insight, the generation of ideas and memory.

The Heart Shen is also important for the ability to fall to sleep easily and to have sleep that is deep and refreshing. 'Shen' is also used to describe the quality of liveliness that is inherent in someone who is emotionally very healthy.

The Heart Shen gives the capacity to have insight and to feel the emotions. The ability to form healthy relationships and to feel love and joy is a characteristic of the Heart and Pericardium, which must in turn be related to their spiritual aspect, the Heart Shen.

A healthy Heart Shen also confers wisdom, which is the ability to respond to knowledge and challenges with discernment.

The ethereal soul (Hun)

The Hun was thought to be that part of the spirit which leaves the body after death. It is rooted in the Liver Yin, from where it enables a sense of purpose, vision and direction in life. It is also linked with the courage required to face life's challenges, and the ability to make decisions.

If the Hun is well rooted, sleep is normal and dreams are few. However, the ability to gain inspiration, be intuitive and have dreams is a characteristic of the Hun. The Hun can make images, archetypes and symbols accessible to the conscious mind, and has a link with the 'universal mind' (comparable to the collective unconscious as described by Jung).

The ability to move easily between introspection and relationships with other people has been attributed to the Hun. A balanced Hun prevents the emotions from becoming excessive, so underlying a healthy emotional life.

The corporeal soul (Po)

The Po was thought to be that part of the spirit which is linked to the body, and which remains with the body after death. The Po enables the body to move, and gives the skills of agility, balance and coordination.

The Po was also seen to be very important in enabling appropriate movement of the Jing (Essence), and so is involved in the first physiological processes after birth (such as the perception of the senses and the onset of breathing).

The Po is also important for the acuity of the senses. The Po is responsible for the experience of grief and for crying. It is also closely linked to breathing, and so can be calmed if the breath is regulated.

While the Hun is important for relationships with other people, the Po is more important for the establishment of internal integrity and protection from external psychic influences.

The intellect (Yi)

The Yi was thought to reside in the Spleen, and is responsible for clear thought. The ability to study, concentrate, assimilate new ideas and retain facts, and to work things out are all functions of the Yi. Memory will be good if the Yi is healthy, and this particularly relates to the memory of facts and ideas.

The will (Zhi)

The Zhi was thought to reside in the Kidneys, and is also important in the function of memory. The Zhi appears to be linked with long-term retention of facts and ideas, whereas the Yi is related to the laying down of memory of facts and ideas.

The Zhi is also linked to the drive and determination required to follow through with an idea. It also has the characteristic of tenaciousness in following an idea through to its conclusion. The Zhi is also characterised by the courage required to stand up to the challenges that life presents and which threaten to prevent success in one's endeavours.

Continued

Information Box 6.2a-I—Cont'd

The pathology of the Shen

There are three general patterns described in Chinese medicine that result from imbalance of the Shen: Deficient Shen, Disturbed Shen and Obstructed Shen. The general patterns of pathology of the Shen are:

Deficient Shen	Dullness Apathy Lack or spirit or vitality Lack of joy
Disturbed Shen	Insomnia and dream disturbed sleep Forgetfulness Anxiety and propensity to startle Poor memory
Obstructed Shen	Confusion and dull depression Clouded consciousness Unconsciousness

These patterns describe general imbalances that are seen in all manner of mental illness. However, each of the five Shen have their own characteristics, which when out of balance may be discerned in mental illness. The characteristics of imbalance of the five Shen are:

Aspect of the Shen	Associated Organs	Characteristics of imbalance
Shen (mind/spirit)	Heart, Small Intestine, Pericardium, Triple Burner	Low intelligence, unclear thought, lack of clarity of ideas Poor memory for events Difficulty falling asleep and disturbed sleep Dull and lifeless personality and lack of joy Confusion and lack of consciousness Lack of experience of emotions or oversensitivity to emotions Problems in interpersonal relationships Unwise life decisions
Hun (ethereal soul)	Liver, Gallbladder	Lack of purpose, vision and direction Timidity and indecisiveness Dream disturbed sleep and out-of-body experiences Lack of inspiration and intuition, and a sterile inner life Marked emphasis on the intuitive and 'second sight' (e.g. connection with the spirit world, seeing ghosts, clairvoyance) Excessive emotional outbursts; in particular anger
Po (corporeal soul)	Lung, Large Intestine	Difficulties with movement, clumsiness and lack of coordination Weakening of the senses and uncomfortable sensations (e.g. itching) Excessive grief and crying, or inability to feel grief Breathing difficulties, hyperventilation and shallow breathing A poor sense of self, and vulnerability to external influences and 'vibes'
Yi (intellect)	Spleen, Stomach	Dull intellect, slow thinking, poor memory for facts Overthinking Difficulty in concentration
Zhi (will)	Kidney, Bladder	Poor long-term memory Lack of drive and initiative, ideas and dreams do not reach fruition Excessive fearfulness

The organ syndromes and mental–emotional problems

As described earlier, the Shen is simply an aspect of Qi. If Qi is out of balance when an Organ pattern is being expressed, it is to be expected that there will be some accompanying imbalance of the Shen. For example, in a state of Qi Deficiency one might expect Shen Deficiency, and in Qi Stagnation one might expect some degree of Shen disturbance. As Qi is a Yang substance, the same applies to any pattern in which Yang is out of balance. In Yang Deficiency one might expect Shen Deficiency, and when Yang is Rising one might expect Shen Disturbance.

Similarly, a disorder of the Shen can be expected if there is an imbalance of Blood, as Blood is not only directly related to Qi as the 'mother of Qi', but is also said to House the Shen. If Blood is Deficient, Shen might be expected to be Deficient, but also Disturbed as it can no longer be properly rooted. As Blood is a Yin Substance, a deficiency of Yin might also be expected to be accompanied by a Deficiency and Disturbance of the Shen.

In Full Patterns it is also possible to predict the effect that certain Pathogenic Factors might have on the Shen. One might expect Heat and Wind to disturb the Shen, and Phlegm and Damp to Obstruct it. Empty Heat simply disturbs the Shen, but Full Heat can affect consciousness and thus can Obstruct as well as disturb the Shen.

The disorders of the Shen and their overlap with the main pathologies in Chinese medicine are as follows:

Shen pathology	Chinese medicine pathologies
Deficient Shen	Qi Deficiency
	Blood Deficiency
	Yin Deficiency with Empty Heat
	Yang Deficiency
Disturbed Shen	Blood Deficiency
	Yin Deficiency with Empty Heat
	Empty Heat
	Qi Stagnation
	Blood Stagnation
	Full Heat
	Phlegm/Fire
	Wind
Obstructed Shen	Blood Stagnation
	Phlegm
	Full Heat
	Phlegm/Fire
	Damp

It is possible to use these correspondences to understand more about the mental–emotional disturbances described in the particular Organ Syndromes. Even more insight will be gained if the mental–emotional correspondences of the five Shen are also used to inform an interpretation of a particular Organ Syndrome.

For example, in the Syndrome of Spleen Qi Deficiency, some features of deficient Shen and also some features of imbalance of the Yi might be expected. It is no surprise then that tiredness, lassitude and overthinking are features of this pattern, which reflect Shen Deficiency, but with a particular 'flavour' associated with imbalance of the Yi. On this basis, difficulties in thinking, generation of ideas and memory for facts might also be expected to be features of Spleen Qi Deficiency, and these are indeed familiar symptoms seen in patients in clinical practice.

Summary

In conclusion, using the approach described above it is possible to describe what sort of mental–emotional features might be apparent in a presentation of any particular Chinese medicine Syndrome. This aspect of the Chinese medicine interpretation of mental health symptoms and signs has been elaborated in some detail, as it will provide a foundation for the Chinese medicine interpretation of conventional descriptions of mental illness in subsequent chapters in this section.

Self-test 6.2a

Introduction to mental health disorders

1. (i) What are the characteristics of the mind according to a conventional medical definition?
   (ii) What is the seat of the mind according to conventional medicine?
2. What are the characteristics of a mental health disorder according to a conventional definition?
3. For each of the three possible categories of the causation of mental illness, describe two forms of evidence that are strongly suggestive that mental illness can indeed result from factors within each category:
   (i) biological causation
   (ii) psychological causation
   (iii) social causation
   (This question is intended to test your understanding of the biopsychosocial model of the causation of mental illness.)

Answers

1. (i) The characteristics of the mind according to a conventional definition include awareness, thought, volition, emotions, concentration and memory.
   (ii) Until very recently, the mind was presumed to be a product of the neurochemical activity of the brain. Increasingly, it is recognised that what we recognise as the mind may also be an expression of elements in the body outside the brain, such as the peripheral and autonomic nervous systems and the endocrine system.
2. According to the American Psychiatric Association, a mental health disorder is a constellation of behavioural or psychological symptoms and signs that is associated with negative consequences for the individual. In other words, it represents a way of performing or reacting to the world which is not helpful for the patient. Also, a characteristic of a mental health disorder is that it is a manifestation of dysfunction in one or more of the biological, psychological or social realms.
3. (i) Evidence for biological causation to the neurochemistry of the brain (as caused by degenerative disease, infections and drugs) includes:
   - an increased tendency to mental illness can be inherited (as demonstrated by adoptive and twin studies)
   - the symptoms of mental illness can respond to physical treatments such as medication.

   (ii) Evidence for psychological causation includes:
   - psychological trauma in childhood has been shown to be associated with mental ill-health in adult life (e.g. separation from mother, bereavement, physical and sexual abuse).

   (iii) Evidence for social causation includes:
   - mental illness can be shown to be related to variables such as gender, age, marital status, social support and economic status
   - mental illness can result from the stress of experiencing significant life events.

Chapter 6.2b Classification of mental health disorders

LEARNING POINTS

At the end of this chapter you will be able to:
- describe the benefits and limitations of the psychiatric systems of classification
- define some of the key terms used in psychiatric classification
- correctly assign some common psychiatric conditions to their appropriate diagnostic category.

Estimated time for chapter: 70 minutes.

Introduction

In conventional medicine, the mental health disorders are classified in a systematic way. Superficially, this is comparable to the classification of diseases of any one of the more readily measurable physiological systems. However, the diseases of the mind are classified according to their symptoms and signs, rather than according to the underlying pathological process. For example, the various phobias are classified according to the nature of the phobia, rather than what precisely is going on in the nervous system in these disorders. This is in contrast to the basis on which the diseases of systems such as the cardiovascular or gastrointestinal systems are classified.

The process of classification in psychiatry involves sorting episodes of mental illness into diagnostic groups on the basis of common clinical features. For example, two episodes of depression might be very different, in that one might be triggered by a bereavement, and so be characterised by extreme sadness, and the other might occur in the postnatal period, and so be characterised by feelings of guilt. However, both episodes will be recognised by a psychiatrist as cases of depression because of the common features of pervasive low mood, poor sleep, altered appetite and the presence of suicidal ideas.

The systematic classification of psychiatric diseases is recognised to be of benefit for the purposes of communication about the condition, for facilitation of research and also for developing treatment protocols. Thus is because once a condition can be assigned a category, it can be compared readily with other cases diagnosed to fall within the same category. The responses to different treatments for people with the same sort of condition can be compared. Moreover, a new patient suffering from a condition from a recognised category can be offered treatment which has been shown to benefit other people diagnosed with the same sort of condition (see Q6.2b-1).

Potential problems with classification of mental health disorders

However, the benefits of psychiatric classification and its corollary, the labelling of patients with a diagnosis of mental illness, are the subject of debate. The psychiatrist Kendell, when writing about the role of diagnosis in psychiatry, stated 'in the last resort, all diagnostic concepts stand or fall by the strength of the diagnostic and therapeutic implications they embody' (Bloch and Singh 1994). What Kendell means is that a classification system is only of value if the diagnostic categories actually enable a truly therapeutic outcome for the majority of people who fall into each of the categories.

It can be argued that the diagnostic categories used in modern psychiatry are too simplistic. For example, consider a person who has a unique make-up and who is exposed to unique and diverse stressors in his life. At a point of crisis he has a mental breakdown, which likewise has its own very unique characteristics. No other person has ever before experienced the same pattern and range of troubling thoughts and disability as this person, and yet a psychiatrist might focus in on a few key characteristics of this man's disorder and give him the diagnosis 'paranoid schizophrenia'.

First, we need to question whether the diagnostic category of schizophrenia is appropriate. Although this man may share some clinical features in common with other patients, is it really right to group him together with these patients for the purpose of choosing treatment? On the basis of his diagnosis, this man might be hospitalised against his will, and forced to be treated with the most widely accepted therapeutic option for acute schizophrenia, drugs from the major tranquilliser group. These drugs may lead to a wide range of side-effects, including sedation, confusion, weight gain, parkinsonian (i.e. akin to the stiffness seen in Parkinson disease) muscle stiffness and restless movements (tardive dyskinesia). It is important to be sure that these side-effects are 'worth' the hoped-for benefit of improved mental health.

The problem of choosing one treatment to fit all members of a diagnostic category has raised earlier in this text. Just because the majority of people in a clinical trial of treatment for, say, hypertension, respond positively to a given drug, this does not guarantee that every individual with hypertension will respond positively. One drug does not necessarily fit all cases of hypertension. It is arguable that this issue is of even more significance in psychiatry, in which the clinical presentations of two people with the same diagnosis can be very different. Is it reasonable to expect one drug to fit all cases of depression or panic attack?

In the case of schizophrenia, it is not always clear whether or not the therapeutic option has conferred a benefit. In many cases, after a first episode of schizophrenia there is a prolonged period of up to a few years in which the patient may not regain his previous level of functioning in society. Some of this disability may well result from the side-effects of hospitalisation and drug treatment. Can we be sure that this treatment option was the best for this man in his unique situation?

The diagnosis of schizophrenia is undoubtedly one that is stigmatising in western culture. The label provokes the memories and images that western culture associates with the term. Most of these will not be positive, and importantly may actually be irrelevant to the person's individual situation. The label carries consequences, not just in terms of the treatment that is offered, but also may affect the person's self-image and the way in which he will be able to integrate back into his community.

To summarise, the classification of mental health disorders, as well as offering benefits in terms of communication, and aiding in research and the design of treatment protocols, can also carry some negative consequences. Being assigned to a diagnostic category may oversimplify an individual case of mental illness. Being assigned to a category may imply that only a certain recommended treatment path is suitable for a particular patient (e.g. antidepressants in diagnosed depression), when this might not be the case at all. Moreover, categorisation may actually lead to harm as a result of the application of a label that is perceived to be stigmatising to a patient.

There are two widely accepted systems of the classification of mental health diseases: the International Classification of Diseases (ICD), a system drawn up by the World Heath Organization (WHO); and the Diagnostic and Statistical Manual of Mental Disorders (DSM), designed by the American Psychiatric Association.

The international classification of diseases (ICD 10)

The most recent revision of the International Classification of Diseases, ICD 10, was drawn up in 1992. ICD 10 consists of a number of chapters, each dedicated to a different physiological system or disease group. By means of this system, each disease category can be ascribed a unique numerical code, which can be useful for the purposes of studying the epidemiology of disease. Chapter 5 of ICD 10 is dedicated to the mental health disorders.

In ICD 10, the mental health and behavioural disorders are subdivided into ten categories, as summarised in Table 6.2b-I (see Q6.2b-2).

Definitions of some of the terms used to describe these ten categories are as follows:

Definition of "Organic"

This is a term which is used in all aspects of conventional medicine to describe a condition which has a measurable physical basis. From a psychiatric perspective, the organic mental health disorders include Alzheimer disease and other forms of dementia, and any mental health disorders which result from brain damage, brain tumour or generalised disease.

Table 6.2b-I The ten categories of mental health disorder according to the Tenth International Classification of Diseases (ICD 10) (Chapter 5)

- Organic, mental disorders
- Mental or behavioural disorders due to psychoactive substance use
- Schizophrenia, schizotypal and delusional disorders
- Mood (affective) disorders
- Neurotic and stress-related and somatoform disorders
- Behavioural syndromes associated with physiological disturbances
- Disorders of adult personality and behaviour
- Mental retardation
- Disorders of psychological development
- Behavioural and emotional disorders with onset usually in childhood or adolescence

Definition of "Psychoactive"

Psychoactive describes something which has an effect on the functioning of the mind, and in the context of ICD 10 refers to substances such as alcohol, sedatives, recreational drugs and caffeine.

Definition of "Affective"

The term affective literally means relating to the mood. In psychiatry, the term affect is used almost interchangeably with the word mood. This category includes all the depressive disorders and also the condition of mania which manifests as periods of elevated mood.

Definition of "Neurotic"

Neurotic is an adjective which is derived from the term used in psychiatry to describe a minor mental health disorder, a neurosis. By definition the neuroses are those conditions in which there is mental health disturbance but that the patient's insight into the fact there is a mental health disturbance is maintained. By this definition, any person with a neurosis would readily admit that that was their problem. For example, minor depression and phobias are examples of neuroses in that the patient suffering from these conditions would be prepared to agree with the doctor about the nature of their problem.

N.B. The formal definition of a neurosis given in ICD 10 is as follows: "a mental disorder in which the patient may have considerable insight and has unimpaired reality testing, in that he does not easily confuse his morbid subjective experiences and fantasies with reality".

In contrast the psychoses (singular psychosis) are those mental health conditions in which the patient has lost insight into the fact they have a mental illness. A psychosis is characterised by a degree of denial that there is any thing wrong, and possibly by a reluctance to admit that treatment is necessary. Broadly speaking this technical term corresponds to the commonly used words insanity and madness. Psychotic is a term which in psychiatry describes a state of mental health in which insight is lost. It might be used, for example, to describe a case of acute schizophrenia. It does not in any way imply dangerousness which is the unfortunate common misunderstanding of the term.

N.B. The formal definition of a psychosis given in ICD 10 is as follows: "a mental disorder in which impairment of the mental function has developed to such a degree that interferes grossly with insight, ability to meet some ordinary demands of life or to maintain adequate contact with reality."

Definition of "Somatoform"

Somatoform literally means a condition in which a mental health disorder is largely experienced as physical discomfort and attributed by the patient to a bodily problem. Somatisation is the term used to describe the tendency to experience recurrent functional disease (such as headache, irritable bowel disease, and dysmenorrhoea) when the medical interpretation of the root of the problem is a mental illness such as depression or anxiety.

Definition of "Personality disorder"

Personality disorder is a term defined in ICD 10 as "deeply ingrained and enduring behaviour patterns manifesting as inflexible responses to a broad range of personal and social situations". What this means is that person diagnosed with a personality disorder has emerged from childhood as an adult with what the psychiatrist would consider an abnormal and often unhelpful way of responding to the world.

A tendency to mood swings, "cyclothymia", a tendency to low mood "dysthymia" and a tendency to negatively interpret the intentions of the others "paranoia", are all examples of ways of responding to the world, which, if extreme, could be classed as personality disorders. Using these examples, a person markedly exhibiting these tendencies might be diagnosed as having respectively a cyclothymic, dysthymic or paranoid personality disorder.

The diagnostic and statistical manual of mental disorders (DSM IV)

The American Psychiatric Association's fourth revision of the Diagnostic and Statistical Manual of Mental Disorders (DSM IV) classifies the mental health disorders under five 'axes'. This system explicitly avoids classification on the basis of known pathology, but rather categorises purely on what can be gleaned from the clinical features (symptoms and signs) of the condition. This system also introduces lists of diagnostic criteria, which are lists of features that have to be present in order for a diagnosis to be made. These criteria were designed to increase the reliability of forming a psychiatric diagnosis.

Axis I of DSM IV embraces all the currently recognised mental health disorders, but excludes personality disorders and learning disability. These two categories are conditions that have long-term and enduring mental aspects, and are included in Axis II. General medical conditions that might manifest in mental health disturbance are listed in Axis III. Axis IV embraces problems that result from environmental or social factors, and Axis V is a summary of the psychiatric clinician's opinion of general functioning. What this means is that a patient who receives a diagnosis according to DSM IV will have a clinical label (Axis I), a description of whether or not there is an enduring mental health problem (Axis II), a description of any coexistent medical psychological and social factors (Axes III and IV), and a summary of how their condition impacts on their skills of daily living (Axis V). Table 6.2b-II gives the clinical categories listed under Axis I of DSM IV.

The structure of DSM IV reflects the biopsychosocial model of the causation of mental illness. A DSM IV diagnosis allows for separate assessment of the various factors that might have contributed to the development of an episode of mental illness (see Q6.2b-3–Q6.2b-4).

Definitions of some of the terms used to describe these sixteen categories are as follows:

Table 6.2b-II The 16 categories of mental health disorder listed in Axis 1 of the American Psychiatric Association Fourth Diagnostic and Statistical Manual (DSM IV)

- Disorders usually first evident in infancy, childhood or adolescence (e.g. autism, attention deficit disorder or dyslexia)
- Delirium, dementia and other cognitive disorders
- Mental disorders resulting from a general medical condition
- Substance-related disorders
- Schizophrenia and other psychotic disorders
- Mood disorders
- Anxiety disorders
- Somatoform disorders
- Factitious disorders
- Dissociative disorder
- Sexual and gender, and identity disorders
- Eating disorders
- Sleep disorders
- Impulse-control disorders not otherwise classified
- Adjustment disorders
- Other conditions which might be the focus of clinical attention

Definition of "delirium"

Delirium is a state in which although there is consciousness, it is clouded and the level of consciousness may fluctuate. Delirium is characterised by restlessness and the tendency to experience visual hallucinations. It is commonly seen accompanying severe medical conditions such as septicaemia and liver failure, and is much more likely to develop in elderly people and children. Delirium tremens (the "DTs") is a well known form of delirium resulting from acute withdrawal from alcohol.

Definition of "cognitive"

The term cognitive simply means relating to thought (cognitions). Cognitive disorders are those disorders in which the ability to think clearly is impaired.

Definition of "factitious"

Factitious is an adjective used in conventional medicine to describe those conditions which do not really exist, but instead have been wilfully staged by the patient. In other words the factitious disorders are not what they seem to be in that the evidence for them, the symptoms and signs, have been exaggerated or falsified by the patient. A factitious disorder is not the same as malingering in which the pretence of illness is for some obvious gain such as financial compensation. It is presumed that the gain from factitious illness comes in the form of the care given to a person in the sick role. Munchausen syndrome is a well known factitious condition in which the patient self harms to generate the symptoms of illness.

Self-test 6.2b

Classification of mental health disorders

1. What are the benefits of having a classification system for the mental disorders?
2. What are the problems inherent in psychiatric classification?
3. What are the broad distinctions between psychoses and neuroses?
4. The following lists of conditions can be sorted so that neighbouring conditions come from the same diagnostic category in both ICD 10 and DSM IV. Sort the lists so that conditions from the same category are next to each other.

specific phobia	schizophrenia
delirium	attention-deficit disorder
brief psychotic disorder	generalised anxiety disorder
nicotine addiction	Alzheimer disease
tic disorder of childhood	acute alcohol intoxication

Answers

1. The potential benefits of a system of psychiatric classification are that it enables communication about the mental disorders, and it enables the study of psychiatric conditions and the development of treatment protocols (as patients with a common diagnosis can be recognised and then studied as a group).
2. The problems associated with psychiatric classification include that it may simplify diagnoses and force the grouping together of cases which perhaps should not be treated as similar entities. Following on from this, if disease outcome and treatment protocols have been developed on the basis of a patient group that is not necessarily representative of other people assigned a similar diagnosis, then future patients may be given misleading psychiatric labels and offered inappropriate treatment. Also, psychiatric diagnoses, even if reliable, can be very stigmatising because of inaccurate public perceptions of the mental disorders.
3. Broadly speaking, neuroses and psychoses are distinguished by the fact that in a neurosis a significant degree of insight into the problem is maintained by the patient. In a psychosis it would seem that the patient has lost some contact with reality, and is without insight that this is the case. The person with a neurosis would not generally be seen as 'mad', whereas a person exhibiting a psychosis might easily be labelled as such.
4. The sorted lists is as follows:

specific phobia	generalised anxiety disorder
delirium	Alzheimer disease
brief psychotic disorder	schizophrenia
nicotine addiction	acute alcohol intoxication
tic disorder of childhood	attention-deficit disorder

Phobias and anxiety disorders are categorised as anxiety disorders.
Delirium and Alzheimer disease are categorised as organic disorders.
Brief psychotic disorder and schizophrenia are categorised as schizophrenia and other psychotic disorders.
Acute alcohol intoxication and nicotine addition are categorised as substance-related disorders.
Tic disorder and attention-deficit disorder are categorised as disorders usually first diagnosed in infancy, childhood or adolescence.

Definition of "dissociative"

Dissociative is a term used in psychiatry to describe those conditions in which there is a "partial or complete loss of the normal function of identity, memory and consciousness".

In the dissociative disorders it appears as if an aspect of memory or personality has been split off from normal consciousness. A sudden loss of personal memory in response to psychological trauma (dissociative amnesia), and depersonalisation (a recurrent sense of being cut off from reality) are forms of dissociative disorders. Multiple personality disorder is another very rare but well publicised example.

Definition of "adjustment disorders"

An adjustment disorder is a psychological syndrome which has developed in response to an understandable stressor and which has persisted for no more than six months. An episode of depression resulting from the shock of witnessing a car crash would be an example of an adjustment disorder. Adjustment disorders can manifest in diverse forms including depression, anxiety, panic attacks, confusional states and antisocial behaviour. If the condition is only short lived but still clinically significant, then the reaction is termed an acute stress reaction.

Chapter 6.2c Assessment and treatment of mental health disorders

LEARNING POINTS

At the end of this chapter you will be able to:
- describe the broad stages of the assessment of a psychiatric patient
- describe how treatment is chosen for a mental disorder
- list the different types of treatment used in psychiatry.

Estimated time for chapter: 100 minutes.

The assessment of mental health disorders

The assessment of the mental health disorders in conventional medicine usually begins with a formal psychiatric examination. Ideally, the assessment will be in the form of an interview with the examining psychiatrist, lasting for about an hour. As is the case for the other physiological systems, the assessment follows the stages of questioning (history taking), examination and clinical investigations. However, in psychiatry, although physical examination may be relevant in the case of organic disease, the most important aspect of the examination is of the 'mental state'. The mental state is assessed primarily also by questioning.

The psychiatric history

In psychiatry the questioning to elucidate the history of the mental disorder includes not only the development of the presenting problem, but also the family history of mental disorder, a detailed history of childhood development and family relationships, an educational, occupational, medical and psychiatric history, and details of the patient's current social situation. In this way, the psychiatrist builds up a picture of all the factors that may have contributed to the development of the current condition. By questioning in this way, the psychiatrist is reflecting a training in the biopsychosocial model of the causation of mental illness.

The mental state examination

As with the routine of the physical examination, the examination of the mental state is structured and follows clearly defined stages. These stages are:

- assessment of appearance and behaviour
- assessment of speech (especially rate, articulation, quantity and form)
- assessment of mood
- assessment of the content of the thoughts
- assessment of abnormal beliefs
- assessment of abnormal experiences
- assessment of cognitive state (i.e. orientation, memory, attention, concentration and intelligence)
- assessment of insight.

Systematic examination of all the aspects of mental functioning reflected in the mental state stages is intended to reveal patterns of thought, mood and behaviour that are characteristic of particular mental health disorders.

Physical examination and investigations

The psychiatrist may conduct a brief physical examination and perform relevant investigations to exclude any possible organic causes of mental health problems (e.g. hypothyroidism, substance misuse or withdrawal, raised intracranial pressure).

The treatment of mental health disorders

Having formed an initial diagnosis through the history, mental state examination, physical examination and investigations, the psychiatrist will then consider the treatment options. As is the case for the diseases of the other physiological systems, a precise diagnosis is central to the process of choosing treatment. As is also true in general medicine, treatment ideally is chosen on the basis of high-quality research or well-established professional medical opinion.

Although in the majority of cases of minor mental health disorder drug treatment may be unnecessary, for many psychiatric diagnoses there are recognised pharmacological treatments for the condition. Drugs exert their effects primarily in the physical realm. Other physically directed treatment options include electroconvulsive therapy and psychosurgery.

In accordance with the biopsychosocial perspective, many patients will be also recommended a treatment that is intended to exert its effects in the psychological domain, such as cognitive therapy, behavioural therapy or psychodynamic psychotherapy.

In addition, referral for social support, or a recommendation for couple counselling or grief counselling might be chosen to ameliorate any social factors that are seen to be perpetuating the mental health disorder.

An important added aspect of the choice of treatment is whether or not treatment should be offered to the patient within a hospital setting or as an outpatient. Hospital may be appropriate for some patients, as their mental illness may be preventing adequate self-care or attention to treatment plans. Ideally, the patient is willing to be admitted to hospital for psychiatric assessment and treatment, and fortunately this is usually the case. At best, in hospital a patient with a mental illness will have all their bodily needs attended to, constant supervision of their mental state, supervised regular drug therapy if necessary, and be offered easy access to other therapies and social support.

In the situation in which a patient is not willing to be admitted to hospital for assessment or treatment of a mental health disorder, in the UK the psychiatrist may choose to exert powers as specified under various of the sections of the England and Wales Mental Health Act 1983 to make admission to hospital compulsory. These powers should only be exerted in cases when such treatment would be considered necessary either to protect the patient's own well-being or for the safety of others.

Biological therapies for psychiatric disorders

There are six classes of commonly prescribed medications used in mental health disorders: the hypnotics, anxiolytics, antipsychotics, mood stabilisers, antidepressants and drugs used in Alzheimer disease (see Q6.2c-1).

Hypnotics

The hypnotic drugs are prescribed to induce a state of sedation or to treat insomnia. They generally have a duration of action in the region of a few hours, and this is suitable for the purpose of enabling a full night's sleep.

The hypnotics include the benzodiazepines (e.g. temazepam) and the benzodiazepine-like drugs (e.g. zopiclone), which are believed to act on the same receptor in the brain as benzodiazepines, antihistamines (e.g. promethazine) and the drug chlormethiazole. All these drugs cause sedation and drowsiness, and in excess would lead to unconsciousness.

The benzodiazepine-like hypnotics are known to act at a receptor in the brain which, when bound by the drug, affects the action of a neurotransmitter known as GABA (gamma-aminobutyric acid). GABA is known to be an inhibitory neurotransmitter, and its action includes the calming of overactive nerve pathways in the brain.

Side-effects include prolonged drowsiness the next day, confusion and unsteadiness, and in some cases inhibition of breathing. Rarely, in some people, these drugs can lead to an unstable mental state, with aggression and thought disorder. The most important complication of benzodiazepine use is that they induce the state of dependence on the drug, and this is more pronounced if used for a long time. This means that the patient will experience a withdrawal syndrome, involving restlessness, anxiety, sleeplessness and possibly aggression, on stopping a regular dose of medication. For this reason, the UK Committee on the Safety of Medicines (CSM) recommends that benzodiazepines are only used for insomnia if the insomnia is 'severe, disabling or subjecting the individual to severe distress'.

The antihistamines are chemically related to the drugs which are used for control of psychosis (see later in this chapter under Antipsychotic Drugs). They are known to affect the action in the brain of a range of neurotransmitters, including dopamine, acetylcholine, histamine, serotonin and noradrenaline. It is thought that the action of inhibition of dopamine contributes most significantly to the sedating action of these drugs. Promethazine is the antihistamine most widely for sedation because it has a relatively low risk of adverse side-effects, and also does not usually induce dependence. Side-effects of promethazine include prolonged drowsiness, difficulty in urination, dry mouth, blurred vision and digestive disturbances.

Chlormethiazole is a sedating drug that is used in the care of the elderly and to help with the management of the state of acute alcohol withdrawal. However, if used over a prolonged period, it is well recognised to induce a state of dependence, and so should be prescribed with care.

The barbiturates are a class of drug which was once used widely for sedation, but are now not recommended for use in the management of psychological conditions. Phenobarbitone is a barbiturate used principally in the control of epilepsy.

The older antidepressants, such as amitriptyline, may also be prescribed in low doses, principally for their sedating effects. They are of particular use when insomnia is accompanied by low mood or chronic pain.

Anxiolytics

Anxiolytics are drugs prescribed for the purpose of reducing anxiety.

Short- to medium-acting benzodiazepines (see above under Hypnotics), including diazepam and lorazepam, are the most commonly prescribed anxiolytics in the UK. As described above, these are believed to act by promoting the action of the inhibitory neurotransmitter GABA in the brain. The action of these drugs is fairly rapid and short lived, which makes them appropriate for treating anxiety that might be short lived (e.g. the fear of a plane flight) and to control a panic attack or a reaction to acute trauma. Long-term prescription of these highly addictive drugs is not considered by the UK CSM to be good practice. Side-effects of the short- to medium-acting benzodiazepines include drowsiness, confusion, unsteadiness, increase in aggressiveness and, occasionally, headache, digestive disturbances, urinary problems and blood disorders. As described for the hypnotics, the benzodiazepines readily induce a state of dependence and so are highly addictive. After withdrawal from a long-term prescription an unpleasant withdrawal syndrome may become apparent.

Buspirone is a non-benzodiazepine anxiolytic that is considered to be a less-addictive alternative to the benzodiazepines. It is believed to act at the serotonin ($5HT_{IA}$) receptor. The response to buspirone is delayed and may take up to 2 weeks to take effect, which means it is less likely to be prescribed in cases of acute overwhelming anxiety. Side-effects of buspirone include nausea, dizziness, palpitations and dry mouth.

Beta blocker drugs, such as propranolol, may also be prescribed for their anxiety-reducing action. The beta blockers act by blocking the action of the neurotransmitter hormones adrenaline and noradrenaline. For this reason, the beta blockers may be particularly effective if physical symptoms such as palpitations and tremor are the primary problems for the patient (such as might affect stage performers or musicians).

Side-effects of beta blockers include slow heart rate, cold extremities, impotence and dream-disturbed sleep.

Information Box 6.2c-I

Hypnotic drugs: comments from a Chinese medicine perspective

From a Chinese medicine perspective, the induction of drowsiness and sedation could be described in terms of Obstruction of the Shen. The side-effects of these drugs are manifest primarily in the realm of the mind and spirit, and may be described in terms of Qi Stagnation and Phlegm which Obstructs the Orifices of the Heart.

Gascoigne (2001) states that the benzodiazepine drugs are Cooling in nature and exert their effect by 'calming the spirit', which he explains will in the long term lead to depression (through Stagnation). He goes on to explain that the features of the withdrawal syndrome are due to flaring of Heart Fire. This does suggest that the 'Cooling' action is a form of Suppression, rather than Clearing, of Heat.

The side-effects of the antihistamines manifest more prominently in the physical realm, and some of the more common side-effects such as dry mouth and difficulty in urination suggest that these drugs can be Heating and may affect Kidney Yin. These side-effects might also be described in terms of a manifestation of Suppressed Heat.

Information Box 6.2c-II

Anxiolytic drugs: comments from a Chinese medicine perspective

From a Chinese medicine perspective, the anxiolytics have a similar action to the hypnotics. The reduction in anxiety can be described as a Calming of the Shen (Cooling), but if they cause confusion or drowsiness then this is a manifestation of Obstruction of the Shen (possibly by Phlegm or Stagnation).

Antipsychotic drugs

The antipsychotic class of drugs are also known as 'neuroleptics' and 'major tranquillisers'. They may be used to manage patients who are acutely disturbed for a range of underlying causes. In the long term they are prescribed to manage the symptoms of thought disorder, hallucinations and delusions, which are characteristic of the psychoses (including schizophrenia and bipolar disorder). They also may be prescribed in the long term to patients who manifest long-term symptoms of mental disturbance as a result of an underlying chronic mental health disorder (such as can develop in Alzheimer disease).

The antipsychotics are usually administered in tablet or liquid form, but may be given by intramuscular injection for rapid sedation in an acutely disturbed patient. For some of the antipsychotics a slow-release form of the drug (depot medication) is available. Depot medication may be offered to patients in the community who are considered to be less likely to take tablets on a regular basis. The depot injections are usually given every 2–4 weeks by a community psychiatric nurse.

The antipsychotics are recognised to block the dopamine D_2 receptors. They may also act on a range of other peptide receptors, including the acetylcholine, adrenaline, histamine and serotonin (5HT) receptors. Interference of the dopamine systems in the brain is believed to be the mechanism that underlies the antipsychotic action of these drugs. However, for some of the older antipsychotic medications this interference carries the well-recognised negative consequence of a 'Parkinsonian syndrome', including muscle stiffness, poverty of spontaneous movement and coarse tremor.

The important side-effects of the antipsychotic medications are summarised in Table 6.2c-I.

There is a large number of antipsychotic drugs, each of which has its own characteristic range of side-effects. For example, the more sedating drugs (such as chlorpromazine) may have less pronounced neuromuscular side-effects than the less sedating drugs (such as fluphenazine).

The more recently developed antipsychotics (the atypical antipsychotics), which include risperidone and olanzapine, are currently more widely prescribed because they appear to be associated with a reduced range of side-effects, although they do have the unfortunate tendency to induce metabolic syndrome (weight gain, raised blood sugar and lipids and hypertension) in many people.

The National Institute for Health and Clinical Excellence (NICE) guidelines (June 2002) recommend that these new

Table 6.2c-I Side-effects of the antipsychotic drugs (major tranquillisers)

Category of side-effect	Specific side-effects
General side-effects	Drowsiness and sluggishness: these are very common and can contribute to the state of dullness or vacancy that can be characteristic of a person on antipsychotic medication Confusion and agitation Weight gain: this is very common, particularly with the newer major tranquillisers Raised blood sugar and diabetes (in association with weight gain) Acne and rashes: acne is common and sensitivity to sunlight is well recognised Drop in blood pressure and arrhythmias Disturbances in temperature control (rarely, life-threatening hyperthermia) Jaundice (disturbed liver function)
Antimuscarinic side-effects (resulting from the effect of the drug in inhibiting the action of acetylcholine)	Dry mouth Constipation Difficulty in urination Blurred vision
Extrapyramidal symptoms (movement disorders resulting from neurochemical changes in the extrapyramidal nerve pathways in the brain)	Parkinsonian symptoms: muscle stiffness and tremor can appear gradually after a few days, but can progress to become both disabling and stigmatising. These symptoms will reverse if the drug is withdrawn. Drugs such as trihexiphenidyl (Benhexol) may be prescribed concurrently to counteract the parkinsonian side-effects Dystonia and dyskinesia: these terms describe acute states of muscular tension and bodily distortion which are rare but tend to affect young people after just a few doses of drug Akathisia: this term is used to describe a state of muscular restlessness in which the patient feels an irrepressible urge to shift position, move their limbs and walk around. All these manifestations can add to the visual stigma associated with major mental illness Tardive dyskinesia: this is a state of abnormal muscle movement which usually appears after long-term treatment with antipsychotic medication. The patient will experience involuntary movements which particularly affect the muscles of the face (e.g. lip smacking, pouting and chewing movements). Again these side-effects are stigmatising, and of the four muscle-associated side-effects of the antipsychotic drugs are considered the most serious as they may not resolve on withdrawal of treatment

drugs should be the first choice of medication for new episodes of schizophrenia. However, one of these atypical antipsychotics, clozapine, carries a significant risk of depleting the white blood cells (agranulocytosis), and so is only prescribed if the patient can have regular blood tests and if two other antipsychotics have not proved acceptable.

Because of the range of disabling and stigmatising side-effects, the prescription of antipsychotic medication should be one that is made only after deep consideration. Ideally, the prescription and monitoring of these potent and potentially dangerous drugs should be supervised by a consultant psychiatrist.

Sudden withdrawal from antipsychotic medication is not advised because a recurrence of psychosis is a possible serious consequence. Ideally, withdrawal is supervised and gradual, and the patient is supported throughout the withdrawal process.

Information Box 6.2c-III

Antipsychotic drugs: comments from a Chinese medicine perspective

The Chinese medicine interpretation of the antipsychotics is complex. The principal therapeutic action is sedation and calming of agitated thoughts. The condition treated with these drugs is often the form of mental disorder known in Chinese medicine as Dian Kuang (see Chapter 6.2e). This is, in very general terms, a manifestation of Phlegm, and Heat Obstructing the Orifices of the Heart, often on the background of long-term Deficiency of, for example, Spleen, Heart and/or Lung Qi.

Because of this, the effect of the antipsychotics might be interpreted as Cooling, in a similar way as the hypnotics and anxiolytics are seen as Cooling. It could also be said that these drugs Move Phlegm. However, the drowsiness, confusion, sluggishness and dullness that result from these drugs all suggest that they cause a marked Obstruction of the Shen. Weight gain and acne imply the generation of Damp Heat and Phlegm, and rashes, dry mouth, constipation and hyperpyrexia all imply Heat. The extrapyramidal side-effects of stiffness, tremor and involuntary muscle movements imply Stagnation of Liver Qi and Liver Wind. Jaundice suggests Damp Heat in the Liver.

The wide range of side-effects is testimony to the potency of these drugs, and from an alternative perspective would speak very strongly of Suppression of the expression of Pathogenic Factors characteristic of psychosis (Heat and Phlegm) so that they manifest instead in the physical form of these sometimes very severe side-effects.

Mood stabilisers

The mood stabilisers (or antimania drugs) are medications that have been found to prevent the profound swings of mood that are characteristic of bipolar disorder (manic–depressive psychosis). The most commonly prescribed mood stabiliser is lithium carbonate (usually known as 'lithium'), but some of the antiepileptic preparations may also be used with some effect if lithium is not helpful. The antiepileptic drugs that are used are carbemazepine, sodium valproate and lamotrigine. The atypical antipsychotics, such as onlanzapine, may also be prescribed for their mood-stabilising effects.

The action of lithium was discovered entirely by chance in the late 1940s. Even now the mechanism of the mood-stabilising drugs is not clearly understood, although it has been recently clarified that lithium seems to damp down the activity of secondary messenger systems within nerve cells. These systems are those that are set in action within a cell when a peptide binds to a membrane receptor.

Lithium is a toxic drug, and its levels have to be monitored carefully (every 3 months), even when the patient is on a steady dose. Because lithium is particularly toxic to the kidneys and may induce hypothyroidism, both renal and thyroid function blood tests should be performed before the patient commences treatment. Side-effects include digestive disturbances, weight gain, thirst, excessive urination, tremor and fluid retention. If the levels of lithium become too high the patient can experience confusion, severe tremor, slurred speech and vomiting. This is a life-threatening situation and requires rehydration and hospital management.

In the long term, lithium has been associated with impairment of memory, thinking and thyroid disorders. Although the side-effects in the short term are less disabling and stigmatising than those associated with the antipsychotics, nevertheless the mood-stabilising drugs are powerful preparations. They should not be prescribed without careful consideration of the balance of the potential risks and benefits.

Information Box 6.2c-IV

Mood-stabilising drugs: comments from a Chinese medicine perspective

From a Chinese medicine perspective, the primary action of lithium of stabilising mood might be also be interpreted as Cooling and Clearing of Phlegm and Stagnation. However, the side-effects of lithium are very different to those of the antipsychotic drugs. Thirst and excessive urination suggest Depletion of Kidney Qi, with Deficiency of Yang and Yin becoming manifest. Hypothyroidism is primarily a condition associated with the features of Yang Deficiency and accumulation of Damp Phlegm. Long-term damage to thinking, memory and thyroid function all suggest Kidney and Jing Deficiency. Tremor suggests Liver Wind. Weight gain suggests Damp Phlegm, and digestive disturbances suggest Disorder of the Spleen/Stomach Qi.

Some of these diverse side-effects can be explained in terms of Suppression of Heat (thus damaging Kidney Yin) and Phlegm.

Antidepressants

The antidepressant drugs are used to treat episodes of moderate to severe depression and also states in which there is chronically depressed mood. Ideally, brief periods of mild depression should not be treated with antidepressants.

There are four broad classes into which most prescribed antidepressants fall: the tricyclics (amitriptyline and clomipramine), the monoamine oxidase inhibitors (MAOIs), the selective serotonin reuptake inhibitors (SSRIs) and the newer serotonin and noradrenaline reuptake inhibitors (SNRIs).

The MAOIs are far less frequently used since the advent of the SSRIs because they can result in a dangerous syndrome when the patient consumes food containing the substance tyramine (e.g. cheese, pickled fish, yeast extracts). However, these drugs may still be prescribed in a specialist setting in the case of severe intractable depression.

The tricyclics and SSRIs appear to have a similar profile of effectiveness in depression, but differ in terms of their side-effects. The side-effects of dry mouth, constipation, difficulty in urination and blurred vision are all more common with the tricyclics, but the safety of these drugs is well established. The SSRIs may have fewer long-term side-effects than the tricyclics, but concern about safety (in terms of increasing the risk of aggressive outbursts and suicide) may affect prescribing choices. SSRIs are also more associated with nausea and other digestive disturbances, although often these side-effects diminish after a few weeks of treatment.

Antidepressants take 2–6 weeks to have an effect on mood, although side-effects will become apparent straight away. The patient needs to be informed of this so that they do not give up on the treatment before it has had the time to take effect. After this time interval, the patient often feels more optimistic and able to get on with life in a way that may have formerly seemed impossible. Observant onlookers may report that the personality of the patient may appear slightly blunted, as if a degree of sensitivity to the vagaries of life has been lost.

Sometimes the dose needs to be increased gradually for the optimum effect on mood to be obtained. In some cases a change in the type of antidepressant may effect a more beneficial change. The general recommendation is that the minimum length of prescription is 6 months.

Antidepressants are not addictive in the way in which the hypnotics and anxiolytics are. A patient will not crave his dose should he have to miss one or two. However, it is becoming increasingly recognised that antidepressants do induce a form of dependence in that a risk of relapse to a state of depression is more likely if withdrawal from the drug is abrupt. Also, some patients experience a withdrawal syndrome, which includes symptoms such as anxiety, nausea, vomiting, diarrhoea, dizziness and headache, on abrupt withdrawal from the drug. For this reason it is advised that if a long course of treatment is followed, the withdrawal should be gradual and carefully monitored by the prescribing doctor.

St John's wort (*Hypericum perforatum*) is a herbal preparation that has established benefits in mild to moderate depression, although there is no proven benefit in major depression. The mode of action is unclear, but it is considered likely that St John's wort acts in the body in a similar way to the SSRIs. For this reason it is not recommended that St Johns wort is taken concurrently with any other antidepressant. Furthermore, because there are known interactions of St Johns Wort with a range of prescribed medications, it should not be commenced by someone on other medication without first consulting the prescribing doctor. St John's wort is not currently available in the UK on NHS prescription.

Dietary supplements such as tryptophan and 5-hydroxytryptophan (5-HTP) are also claimed to improve mood in some people, and demonstrate a rapid rather than delayed effect on mood. These supplements are both precursors of the manufacture of serotonin in the body, and so it would make sense that they could in theory help to lift mood by leading to a rise in serotonin levels. Tryptophan is an amino acid that is found in a range of high-protein foods, including warmed milk products, turkey, beef, chicken, eggs, yeast, nuts, seeds and bananas. 5-HTP is a naturally occurring relative of tryptophan that is prepared from the African herb *Griffonia simplicifolia*.

Drugs used in the treatment of Alzheimer disease

There is a class of drugs that has recently been demonstrated to show benefits in terms of memory and concentration in up to about half of patients with mild to moderate Alzheimer disease. These drugs, which act at a brain enzyme called acetyl cholinesterase, should only be prescribed under specialist supervision, and should be reviewed after 3 months of treatment to see if the benefit of taking the drug outweighs the problems that might have resulted from the side-effects of the drugs (these include digestive disturbance, fatigue and dizziness). The drugs include donezepil, galantamine and memantine.

Information Box 6.2c-V

Antidepressant drugs: comments from a Chinese medicine perspective

In lifting depression, the primary Chinese interpretation of the therapeutic effect of antidepressants would be that they help to move the Liver Qi Stagnation that often is very apparent in depression. The brighter outlook, ability to act on plans and feelings of hope that can result from treatment are all testimony to a movement of Liver Qi. The return of feelings of emotional warmth would also relate to a movement or boosting of Heart Qi.

The tricyclic antidepressants often cause dry mouth, thirst, constipation and rapid pulse rate, which could be all be attributed to Heat. On rare occasions they can cause heart arrhythmias and rashes, and are also recognised to trigger episodes of mania, confusion or psychosis. The rapid arrhythmias may be a manifestation of Heat in the Heart, and the mental complications may be due to Heat and/or Phlegm Obstructing the Orifices of the Heart.

Side-effects of selective serotonin reuptake inhibitors (SSRIs) include initial digestive disturbances, dry mouth, rashes and problems in sexual function. They can also trigger aggressive outbursts, suicidal ideas and episodes of mania. The digestive disturbances can be described in terms of Liver Qi invading Stomach and Spleen (nausea, vomiting, diarrhoea and abdominal pain). Sexual dysfunction (commonly an inability to achieve orgasm) can also be described in terms of an imbalance of Liver function, as can aggressive outbursts. The risk of mania might be related to the tendency of the drugs to lead to Obstruction of the Orifices of the Heart by Stagnation, Heat or Phlegm.

The side-effects of the common antidepressants indicate that there is a possibility that these drugs might be shifting the imbalance of depression to a different level of expression in the body. The side-effects of the tricyclics speak strongly of release of Heat, perhaps created as a consequence of longstanding repressed emotions, whereas the side-effects of the SSRIs suggest that these drugs have led to a re-expression of an imbalance in the flow of Liver Qi.

Information Box 6.2c-VI

Drugs used in Alzheimer disease: comments from a Chinese medicine perspective

From a Chinese medicine perspective, the action of the drugs used in Alzheimer disease could be interpreted as Boosting Kidney Jing (Essence), but possibly at the expense of Depleting Qi at a deeper level.

Electroconvulsive therapy (electric shock therapy)

Electroconvulsive therapy (ECT) was first considered when the observation was made that the incidence of schizophrenia in people who suffered from epileptic fits appeared to be low. For this reason, the practice of inducing epileptic fits in schizophrenic patients (initially by intravenous administration of insulin, and later by application of an electric current to the temples) was introduced in the 1930s. Within 20 years ECT was being used to treat a wide range of psychiatric conditions. Despite the link between epilepsy and schizophrenia being later discredited, ECT was found to bring about an improvement in mood in some patients. Currently, ECT is used almost exclusively to treat severe intractable mood disorders. Studies have demonstrated that up to 80% of patients show an improvement in mood after treatment.

The administration of ECT prior to the 1950s was very basic, and patients frequently suffered from severe complications. Anaesthetics were not given, and so the patient had to be strapped down prior to the shock. Poor control of the fit meant that severe injuries could be sustained. In current practice, the patient is given an anaesthetic and a muscle relaxant prior to the treatment, so that the induced fit is less traumatic and dangerous. It has been discovered that application of the electrode to one temple only, rather than both, maintains the effectiveness of the treatment, but reduces the incidence and severity of memory loss and confusion afterwards. The risks of the procedure are now similar to those of giving a general anaesthetic alone.

ECT is administered by a psychiatric doctor with an anaesthetist in attendance in a hospital setting. Usually a course of 6–10 treatments is given over the period of 2–3 weeks, each of which is expected to lead to a stepwise improvement in mood. The negative aspect of ECT is that it causes a cumulative impairment in memory, which is the reason why ideally the maximum number of treatments given to any patient should not exceed ten.

Information Box 6.2c-VII

Electroconvulsive therapy: comments from a Chinese medicine perspective

From a Chinese perspective, an epileptic fit is usually described as a Stirring of Phlegm by Liver Wind. This term embraces the loss of consciousness and the tonic–clonic muscle contractions that occur in a generalised fit. This is possibly how one could describe the immediate action of the controlled ECT convulsion. The lifting of the state of profound low mood would suggest that this extreme stimulus has led to the movement of Phlegm and Liver Qi. However, as has been suggested in the interpretation of the electric shock of cardioversion, the shock is a Yang stimulus, and as such will be inherently Depleting of Yin. The cumulative memory loss that results from this treatment may be evidence of an insidious Depletion of Kidney Qi, and possibly Jing.

Psychosurgery

Brain surgery is now only a very rarely recommended treatment for psychiatric disease, although it was an option chosen much more often in the 1930s to 1960s. The operation of lobotomy, which involves the severing of the fibres that link the frontal lobes to the other parts of the brain, was first introduced in the late 1930s in an attempt to treat schizophrenia. Marked change in personality and the development of epilepsy were serious outcomes of this crude procedure.

Nowadays, the psychosurgical approaches are far less crude, and involve surgical destruction of very tiny and precisely located areas of the brain. These operations are exclusively used to treat severe intractable obsessive–compulsive disorder and depression.

Information Box 6.2c-VIII

Psychosurgery: comments from a Chinese medicine perspective

By its very nature, the removal of a portion of the brain has to be interpreted as Depleting of Qi and Jing. A positive outcome from the perspective of obsessive–compulsive disorder or depression would have to correspond to a movement of Liver Qi and/or Phlegm, but this will have been at the expense of a Depletion of Vital Substances.

Psychological therapies for psychiatric disorders

A number of 'talking therapies' have emerged for treating the psychological roots of mental health disorders. Most of these therapies involve the patient undergoing change as a result of talking with a therapist, or as part of a therapist-guided group. The talking therapies are also described as 'psychotherapies', and range in approach from simple supportive counselling to intensive psychoanalysis.

The talking therapies are characterised by some common features:

- the therapist–patient relationship is the therapeutic tool
- rapport and trust are essential for the effectiveness of the therapy
- change often occurs because the interaction provides the patient with new knowledge which helps him to make sense of his situation

- the interaction between therapist and patient enables new ways of thinking and behaving which ideally are beneficial for the patient.

The talking therapies differ from the help that might be offered by a supportive friend in that the therapist maintains a distinct role as a compassionate but detached professional, rather than an equal, and the therapist works in a systematic way from a series of previously defined psychological principles.

'Counselling' is a term that is often used interchangeably with psychotherapy, but strictly speaking refers to an approach in which the explicit aim is to help the patient through the development of increased insight into their situation in order to make important decisions about specific aspects of their lives. Counselling may be tailored to diverse situations such as marriage guidance, grief management, dealing with terminal illness and making career choices.

Other therapies focus on encouraging the patient to make positive changes through certain activities. Art therapy, music therapy and participation in exercise programmes are examples of these. The talking therapies are summarised in Table 6.2c-II.

Most of these therapies, and in particular short courses of cognitive–behavioural therapy, are accessible to patients in

Table 6.2c-II The different forms of psychotherapy

Therapy type	Description
Behavioural therapy	Focuses primarily on helping the patient to create changes in unhelpful behaviours. It is based on the theory that, because all behaviour is learned, maladaptive behaviours can be unlearned and new more helpful behaviours can be acquired. Different forms of behavioural therapy can be used to treat phobias, obsessional behaviour, poor social skills and sexual deviance. Techniques used in behavioural therapy include: • graded exposure to an object of fear (e.g. a spider) in the treatment of phobias • flooding – the sudden exposure to an object of fear to enable the patient to realise that the anxiety will not overwhelm them (also for the treatment of phobias) • modelling – the patient is encouraged to model the therapist's behaviour in order to learn new patterns of acting (used to treat phobias and obsessional behaviour such as excessive hand-washing) • Social skills training
Cognitive therapy	Focuses primarily on helping the patient to modify unhelpful thought patterns. It can be used to treat depression, anxiety, phobias and eating disorders. The psychologist Beck proposed that negative patterns of thought may actually cause and maintain the state of depression, and so developed techniques to challenge these thought patterns and encourage more positive ways of thinking. The techniques used by a cognitive therapist include helping a patient to recognise and name their negative thoughts and then to challenge them. For example: 'Do you think that it is really true that you get things wrong all the time?' or 'Is it really possible that everybody hates you?' The therapist will also explore with the patient the roots of these thought patterns (often by uncovering negative experiences and relationships experienced in childhood) in order to help the patient understand their origin. The patient may be prescribed exercises to do at home, such as keeping a diary of negative thoughts and repeating positive affirmations
Individual analytical psychotherapy	Focuses on uncovering the deep psychological roots to a psychological problem. Often individual psychotherapy involves regular sessions one or more times a week, and may continue for several years. Ideally, the insight gained by the patient is the trigger for positive change. Techniques such as free association, dream analysis and recognition of projected feelings between the therapist and the patient (counter-transference and transference) are used to help point to the underlying psychological issues. There are a number of approaches to individual psychotherapy, which reflect their underlying psychological theories (e.g. Freudian, Jungian, Rogerian, Reichian and transactional analysis)
Brief focal psychotherapy	Uses a range of approaches to meet a clearly defined goal (e.g. the management of anger outbursts) within a defined number of sessions
Group psychotherapy	Used to uncover deep psychological roots to problems, particularly problems that may manifest in the patient's interpersonal interactions. In group therapy the therapist facilitates the social interactions that occur within a 'safe' group of people in order to help the individuals arrive at a deeper insight about themselves and the way in which they interact with other people. Safety is achieved by stressing the importance of confidentiality and clear boundaries for the group (e.g. group members will be advised against meeting socially outside the time of the sessions while the therapy is in progress)
Family therapy	Used to facilitate insight into the nature of the dynamics between the members of a family unit. The intention is to deal with dysfunctional family patterns or difficult behaviour in one of the family members
Couples therapy	Focuses on the particular issues that can develop within intimate relationships. Ideally, both individuals involved in the relationship attend for most of the sessions with the therapist. Relate is a national organisation in the UK which both trains therapists in couples work and offers subsidised therapy sessions for couples
Sex therapy	A particular form of couples therapy focused on sexual problems rather than relationship problems. It is not appropriate in those cases where the sexual problem is a manifestation of an underlying relationship problem. The sex therapist is likely to use a

Table 6.2c-II The different forms of psychotherapy—Cont'd

Therapy type	Description
	combination of cognitive and behavioural techniques to help deal with problems in the formation of a satisfying sexual relationship between partners
Art and music therapies	Often used in a group context to allow patients to express more unconscious aspects of their thought processes. The therapist can then, if it seems appropriate, enable the patient to learn to interpret what they have expressed, and so to gain insight into deep psychological issues. The expression of unconscious material through music and art can be seen as cathartic and therapeutic in itself. Both music and art therapy can be of particular help in working with children and people with learning difficulties
Supportive psychotherapy	Involves therapy sessions that enable the patient to manage life issues which would otherwise overwhelm them. If the issues are acute in onset (e.g. following a sudden trauma or bereavement), the term 'crisis intervention' may be used. If the issues are of longstanding, the supportive psychotherapy can be compared to a medication used to control a chronic medical condition. In some situations the psychological problems are so longstanding and disabling that the patient requires regular supportive input literally to keep going. In such cases, dealing with the deep roots of the problem may be an unrealistic, or at the least only a very long-term, goal

the UK through the NHS, but provision can be sporadic and often does not meet the demand. Faced with long waiting lists, patients may self-refer for private counselling or psychotherapy, without a clear understanding of their particular needs or whether or not the approach of their therapist is one that is suited to these needs. It is also often the case that GPs are not fully cognisant of the strengths and weaknesses of the wide range of therapies on offer through the NHS and also from local private practitioners. For this reason it is worth advising patients to do some personal research to increase their own understanding of the different types of psychotherapy before they elect to undergo a particular form of therapy.

Social interventions for psychiatric disorders

Occupational therapy in the treatment of psychological problems involves teaching patients skills of daily living such as cooking, shopping and organising daily activities. Finding a satisfying recreational activity is also an aim of occupational therapy, and so arts and crafts workshops and yoga classes may fall under the remit of the provision of occupational therapy in hospitals and outpatient clinics. Finally, skills such as word processing or gardening can be taught, which might enable a patient to find employment. Sheltered workshops are establishments in the community that preferentially employ people who have experienced mental health problems in order to enable them to develop skills that would be relevant to more independent employment in the future.

'Rehabilitation' is a term used to describe the process whereby a patient is enabled to return to as normal a life as possible after an episode of illness, be it physical or psychological. In the context of mental health problems, the process of rehabilitation of a patient requires multidisciplinary support from psychiatric nurses, occupational therapists, social workers and the patient's doctors. In the UK this

Information Box 6.2c-IX

Psychotherapy: comments from a Chinese medicine perspective

From a complementary medical perspective, any therapy that enables the patient to move towards a more balanced and less dependent state could be described as curative in nature. In an ideal world all therapies would deal with the root causes of psychological imbalance, and so by definition would be effecting cure.

However, the root cause is not always immediately apparent, and many therapies, for pragmatic reasons, are not designed to target the root of the problem. For example, the behavioural therapies focus on modification of behaviour, and so may not directly address the root causes of the unhelpful behaviour patterns. If they do so, they may actually be suppressive in nature and, although symptoms may improve, a deep imbalance may persist after therapy has been concluded. The problem of long-term dependence on therapy is well recognised (and can of course also apply to Chinese medicine consultations), a clear indication that whatever is being offered is not actually attending to the root cause.

In chronic severe psychological problems, a state of dependence on the therapy, as would apply in cases of supportive psychotherapy, could be the most that could reasonably be expected to be achieved. For this reason, a state of dependence on the therapist must not be seen as necessarily negative, particularly if it is enabling a patient to cope from day to day in a way that would have been impossible without the support offered by the therapy.

However, when dependence is recognised, the question needs always to be asked whether the patient could be offered something different that might enable them to move from their static position. Sometimes the addition of an entirely different approach to healing, such as hypnosis, acupuncture or other forms of body work, may be what is required. This may then move the patient on from a place of dependence to a place from where they can allow the insights gained in therapy to generate significant internal changes.

Therapies can, of course, also carry the risk of side-effects. An unhelpful therapeutic relationship may actually compound emotional problems or, at worst, if abusive in some way, may even cause new imbalances.

multidisciplinary approach is mediated by community mental health teams (CMHTs), which support the patients who live in a particular locality.

Sheltered and supported housing ideally provide a supportive home in the community, where a person with mental health problems can find both social support and a sense of community. Often this is in the context of a group home, which is either overseen by a trained member of staff or regularly visited by members of the local community mental health team.

Psychiatric social workers play a crucial role in the support of a person with severe mental illness, both in hospital and in the community. The social worker can advise the patient on their legal rights and also on access to financial support, such as housing and sickness benefits. As part of the CMHT, the social worker will function as a member of the team supporting the patient in the process of rehabilitation into the community.

The 'approved' social worker is a professional who has been recognised to have the training appropriate for making recommendations that patients be admitted to hospital for assessment and/or treatment according to the various sections of the England and Wales Mental Health Act 1983. The approved social worker plays a key role in relation to the practical application of the sections of the Mental Health Act as they apply to individual patients, as will be explored presently.

The England and Wales Mental Health Act 1983

The England and Wales Mental Health Act 1983 (MHA) summarises the legislation that has been designed principally to protect the rights and enable the safe treatment of people suffering from specific mental health disorders. Section 1 of the act attempts to provide a legal definition of those mental heath problems that the MHA is intended to cover (i.e. mental health disorders), and also specifies that the term 'mental health disorders' should not be applied 'by reason of promiscuity or other immoral conduct, sexual deviancy or dependence on alcohol or drugs'.

Sections 2–5 of the MHA specify the conditions under which a patient can be compulsorily admitted to or held in hospital for assessment and/or treatment. The verb 'to section', as it applies to patients with mental illness, derives from these sections of the act, and is often used to describe this process of admitting patients to psychiatric hospital against their will. Statistics from the charity MIND reveal that in a single year (2000–2001) over 40,000 people in England and Wales were detained in hospital under one of these sections of the MHA.

Section 2 of the MHA describes the conditions for admission for 'assessment'. This applies to a period of no longer than 28 days. For a patient to be compulsorily admitted to hospital under Section 2 of the Act he needs to have a recognisable mental disorder as specified under Section 1. In addition, the admission has to be formally recommended by two medical practitioners, one of whom has been previously 'approved' (according to Section 12 of the Act) to make psychiatric assessments.

An approved social worker or the nearest relative in the patient's family is entitled under the terms of the Act to apply for the admission of the patient. It is usually best for the social worker to make this application rather than the relative, in order to protect the relative from the implications of being the one who caused the admission to hospital.

Section 2 of the Act may be applied to a patient in whom the actual diagnosis of the mental disorder is unclear and where there is a need for an inpatient assessment of the mental health condition. Once in hospital under a Section 2 assessment order, the patient is not permitted to leave the ward at will. If the patient is considered to be at risk of absconding they may be placed in a locked unit, and if they are considered at risk of self-harm they may be placed under close nursing supervision.

Section 3 of the MHA describes the conditions for 'admission for treatment'. This applies for a period of no longer than 6 months. In the case of Section 3 of the Act, the patient needs to have a recognisable mental health disorder which would be expected to respond to treatment, and which requires inpatient admission for the treatment to be administered.

Section 3 can be renewed by formal application by the responsible psychiatric doctor, and thereafter at yearly intervals. The patient has a right to appeal against the decision to a Mental Health Review Tribunal within 6 months of admission.

The responsible psychiatric doctor, the hospital managers and the patient's closest relative all have powers under Sections 2 and 3 of the Act to discharge the patient, although the responsible doctor can override any decision to discharge if they feel the patient or those around them would be put at risk if discharge were permitted.

Once in hospital under a Section 3 treatment order, a patient is not permitted to leave the ward at will and is obliged to comply with prescribed treatment. If treatment is refused by the patient, the doctors and nursing staff are legally entitled to enforce the treatment on the patient. This might involve the use of 'control and restraint' techniques, during which the patient might be held down whilst an injection is administered.

Section 117 of the MHA specifies that the medical team has a responsibility to set up adequate aftercare arrangements for patients discharged from an admission to hospital under Section 3 of the Act. In this Section a multidisciplinary approach to care is emphasised. The Mental Health (Patients in the Community) Act 1995 follows this Section of the Act and controversially describes the conditions for supervised discharge for certain patients. In supervised discharge, the patient is obliged to follow certain requirements after discharge, which include living at an agreed place and attending for the administration of recommended treatment such as medication and occupational therapy. The patient also has to agree to permit access to a doctor or approved social worker when this is requested. This Act stops short of requiring patients to take medications against their will (see Q6.2c-2).

Self-test 6.2c

Assessment and treatment of mental health disorders

1. What are the stages that would be followed by a psychiatrist in the assessment of a mental health disorder?
2. List three biological therapies used in the treatment of:
   (i) anxiety
   (ii) depression.
3. What sort of psychological therapies might be of value to a person suffering from:
   (i) anxiety
   (ii) depression?

List at least three types of therapy for each disorder.

Answers

1. The stages in the assessment of a mental health disorder are broadly the same as those that would be followed by a physician assessing a patient with a physical condition.
   The first stage is questioning about the current symptoms, history of the complaint, medical and psychiatric history, family and social history, and use of drugs and medication.
   The next stage is examination, but this is largely focused on examination of the mental state. A physical examination for the features of relevant organic disease is also conducted.
   Finally, biological tests may be conducted to confirm or exclude the presence of measurable organic disease.
2. (i) Biological therapies used in the treatment of anxiety include the hypnotic drugs (e.g. nitrazepam, temazepam and zopiclone) and the anxiolytics (e.g. diazepam, buspirone and the beta blockers).
   (ii) Biological therapies used in the treatment of depression include the antidepressants (e.g. amitryptiline, fluoxetine and sertraline). The mood stabilisers lithium and carbemazepine may be used if there are pronounced mood swings or bipolar disorder.
   In very severe psychotic depression electroconvulsive therapy may be prescribed.
3. (i) Anxiety can take diverse forms. It may be generalised or may be focused on particular triggers, as occurs in phobias or obsessive–compulsive disorder.
   The psychological treatment approach that is most commonly prescribed for anxiety disorders is cognitive–behavioural therapy (CBT), in which the content of negative thought patterns and habitual problematic behavioural responses are challenged.
   Group therapy may be appropriate for individuals whose anxiety is focused on social situations.
   Individual analytical therapy may be of value in exploring the roots of anxiety disorders, but would rarely be prescribed for this reason within the UK NHS.
   (ii) Depression is a state of chronic low mood, and is usually characterised by patterns of negative thinking. For this reason cognitive therapy, in which negative thoughts are challenged, may be prescribed as a suitable therapy for patients with long-term depression.
   If depression is severe and is affecting the patient's ability to cope with day-to-day activities, supportive psychotherapy may be an appropriate choice of treatment. Individual analytical therapy may be of value in exploring the roots of chronic depression, but would rarely be prescribed for this reason within the UK NHS.

It is important to clarify that the purpose of the Mental Health Act (1983) and the Mental Health (Patients in the Community) Act (1995) is simply to protect the patient with a mental health disorder by means of ensuring that they can be held when necessary in a place of safety and medical treatment can be given. These acts have nothing to do with whether or not the patient may have the mental capacity to make a decision about treatment. The UK Mental Capacity Act (2005) is concerned with ensuring the best interests of people who may not have the mental capacity to make the best judgements about living circumstances, finances and medical treatment.

Chapter 6.2d Anxiety, depression, somatoform and eating disorders

LEARNING POINTS

At the end of this chapter you will:
- be familiar with the following mental health conditions: anxiety disorders, depression, somatoform disorders and eating disorders
- be able to recognise the red flags of these mental health disorders.

Estimated time for chapter: Part I, 100 minutes; Part II: 100 minutes.

Introduction

This chapter is dedicated to those mental health disorders in which it is generally agreed that personality is intact and a degree of insight into the condition is retained by the patient. In all these disorders it would be possible to say that normal communication could be maintained between the patient and another person, and in general the patient would be seen as troubled rather than 'mad'. The term 'neurosis' can be used to describe a mental health disorder such as these in which a degree of insight into the condition is retained by the patient.

The conditions discussed in this chapter are:

Part I: Anxiety disorders
- Panic disorder
- Agoraphobia
- Social phobia
- Simple phobia
- Obsessive–compulsive disorder
- Post-traumatic stress disorder
- Generalised anxiety disorder.

Part II
- Depression:
  - clinical depression
  - bereavement and grief.
- Disorders manifesting in bodily functions:
  - malingering
  - factitious disorder
  - conversion disorder

  - hypochondriasis
  - somatisation disorder
  - neurasthenia
  - dissociative disorders
  - psychosomatic disorders.
- Eating disorders:
  - anorexia nervosa
  - bulimia nervosa.

Part I: Anxiety disorders

The syndrome of anxiety

The term 'anxiety', derived from the Latin word for 'choking', is used to describe a very commonly experienced syndrome. The term 'syndrome' is appropriate for anxiety, as the full experience of anxiety is not just a fearful emotion but also involves a cluster of physiological changes and characteristic changes in thinking. Most people will be more than familiar with these features, as anxiety is one of the normal human responses to frightening situations. In the short term, anxiety serves a useful purpose in preparing the body for the fight-or-flight response to a threat. It is when anxiety becomes overwhelming or ingrained as a chronic (i.e. long-standing) response that it becomes debilitating and disabling. Here we explore what the syndrome of anxiety entails in terms of symptoms and signs, and then describe the different forms in which maladaptive anxiety can manifest.

The clinical features of anxiety

As mentioned above, the syndrome of anxiety has three distinct components: the emotional experience, characteristic changes in thinking, and physiological symptoms and signs.

The emotion associated with anxiety is a sense of foreboding or dread, and can be as extreme as a fear of impending doom.

In the state of anxiety the thoughts might appear to speed up or slow down, and there can be unusual perceptions of light, sound and reality. The anxious person can become overvigilant and irritable, and very commonly sleep is disturbed.

The physiological changes associated with anxiety include a rapid heart beat, raised blood pressure, chest pain, rapid breathing, tremor, muscle tension, dizziness, tingling, sweating, a sensation of choking, nausea, loss of appetite, altered bowel movements, frequency of urination and tendency to a pronounced startle response.

Of course, not everyone who experiences anxiety will experience all these symptoms and signs, although in severe chronic cases it is not uncommon for a person to experience a large proportion of these clinical features.

If the degree of anxiety intensifies, it can develop into an overwhelming syndrome known as 'panic' or 'panic attack'. In panic the emotion is one of intense fear, and often specifically a fear of dying. The physical symptoms intensify, leading to symptoms such as a racing heartbeat, thumping palpitations, pressure in the head, chest pain, difficulty breathing and shaking.

The rapid breathing or hyperventilation that develops in panic can lead to reduced levels of carbon dioxide in the blood. This causes a biochemical change which triggers involuntary muscle spasm and numbness of the extremities. Hyperventilation can also lead to dizziness and confusion.

The experience of these intense symptoms is, in itself, a trigger for more fear, and a vicious cycle of fear–symptom–fear develops, and this prevents the panic attack from subsiding rapidly.

In all forms of anxiety, the patient very often becomes absorbed in complex behavioural patterns in which the trigger for the anxiety is avoided. When this occurs, as it very commonly does, not only is the anxiety unpleasant and disabling, but the behaviour that results from its avoidance can seriously impact on the patient's well-being and freedom (see Q6.2d-1 and Q6.2d-2).

The causation of anxiety

The causation of anxiety can be considered using the biopsychosocial model of disease. Biological theories of the generation of anxiety are increasingly popular, and are supported by the fact that the tendency to develop anxiety disorders runs very strongly in families. It is known that a tendency to anxiety is associated with abnormalities in serotonin levels, and that serotonin-modulating antidepressants (such as the SSRI antidepressant paroxetine) are of specific benefit in certain anxiety disorders. This supports a physical basis of the condition.

However, commonly a trigger event or situation can be traced as the cause of a case of anxiety. This indicates that psychological and social factors are also important in the development of maladaptive anxiety. For example, it is not uncommon for chronic anxiety to develop after a sudden shocking episode of illness such as a heart attack. The high level of anxiety in populations who have survived the trauma of living in a war zone or in groups who have experienced chronic abuse is clear evidence that chronic anxiety can be induced by extreme adverse events impacting on individuals or even whole communities.

Anxiety is a feature of a number of distinct conditions known as the 'anxiety disorders'. These are considered below in turn.

Panic disorder and agoraphobia

Panic disorder is a condition is which panic attacks are common. The attacks may appear to develop without an obvious trigger, although there may be a background level of generalised anxiety present for most of the time. In some cases the panic is very specifically associated with leaving a safe place, usually the patient's home. In this case the condition is known as 'agoraphobia' (from the Greek meaning 'fear of the marketplace'). This pattern may have originated with the experience of a particularly disabling or embarrassing panic attack in a public place, and this has then led to the development of fear of a repetition of this event. The affected patient might thereafter prefer to stay at home whenever possible, and become acutely anxious when having to leave home. In agoraphobia, anxiety might become particularly acute in crowded places such as cinemas, supermarkets or tube trains, where the 'escape route' is not always close by.

In agoraphobia the avoidant behaviour is one of withdrawal, although not necessarily into a hermit-like state. In mild cases, the affected person may simply avoid crowded places, or situations in which they are 'hemmed in'. In a more severe case the person with agoraphobia becomes housebound and may be dependent on friends or family to run errands.

In all cases, when panic attacks are recurrent the treatment is first one of education about the bodily changes that occur in anxiety and panic attacks. The patient commonly feels that the symptoms are warning features of madness or heart disease, and very often can be reassured by a clear explanation of the vicious cycle of 'symptom–fear–symptom. There should also be an explanation of how hyperventilation leads to muscle spasm, numbness and dizziness. The patient then can be taught practical methods of relaxation, how to calm the breath and the use of rebreathing into a paper bag, all of which can help to abort a developing panic attack.

Ideally, cognitive–behavioural therapy is offered to help the patient address the excessive fear of losing control in a public place, and the patient can be given graded exercises that help him or her face a seemingly fearful situation rather than avoid it. The idea is that, if the patient can learn that he or she can prevent a panic attack occurring in a public place, the fear of that situation will become extinguished over time.

In some cases, anxiolytic medication is prescribed for use only in acute situations, with the rationale that it can offer the patient the security of knowing that they will be able to get the situation within their own control.

Social phobia

Social phobia is a syndrome in which the patient is less concerned about crowds but instead with social encounters. In social phobia there may be fear of talking, shaking, blushing or vomiting in a social situation. The patient demonstrates excessive concern about what other people might think about his or her behaviour. Like agoraphobia, social phobia can be characterised by avoidance of any situation that would stimulate the anxiety, and in this case situations such as parties, visits to the pub or having to talk to shop assistants might be avoided. Social phobia tends to develop at an earlier age than agoraphobia, and often has its roots in early adolescence.

Social phobia is often accompanied by depression. Ideally, the patient is offered cognitive–behavioural therapy. The patient may benefit from analytical psychotherapy if the roots of the condition appear to have arisen in early childhood.

Simple (specific) phobia

In simple phobia the patient demonstrates an intense, but very specific, fear of a single trigger. Anxiety may otherwise not be a prominent part of that person's life. Typical triggers for simple phobias include subjects that tend to be generally seen in a negative or dangerous light by modern society, such as spiders, wasps, large dogs, snakes, heights, air travel and lightning. Fear of needles is a very common phobia, which has a particular impact on the practice of acupuncture. The 'rationale' for some phobias is less obvious; for example, fear of cats, birds, feathers and wind are not uncommon.

Simple phobias can have their origins in very early childhood, and do appear to run strongly in families. One theory is that there may be an inherited tendency in some people to have an excessive fear response, which when experienced in an overwhelming way in early childhood becomes internally linked to the original source of the fear response. As is the case for the other phobias, the core problem does not seem to be what the feared object can do in terms of harm, but rather that the resulting panic will become overwhelming. The phobia is again characterised by avoidance of trigger situations. Although described as 'simple', this sort of phobia can have an overwhelming impact on a person's day-to-day existence, particularly if the trigger, such as cats or dogs, is one that is a normal part of modern life.

Simple phobias can respond remarkably well to a cognitive–behavioural approach, in which the patient is encouraged by the clinical psychologist to face up to increasingly close contact with the feared object. This approach, called 'graded exposure', is accompanied by education about the nature of the panic response, and encourages the patient to learn that he or she need not become overwhelmed by the fear.

Obsessive–compulsive disorder

Obsessive–compulsive disorder (OCD) is a more complex anxiety disorder in which the avoidance of becoming overwhelmed by fear also a plays a part. However, in OCD the trigger for the fear is often a thought or an idea about a situation, which seems to intrude into the patient's mind in such a way that the patient tends to find a behaviour that will give them some relief from the anxiety induced by the thought. The intrusive, recurrent thoughts are termed 'obsessions' in psychiatric language. They are often seen as senseless and futile by the patient, who nevertheless finds it impossible to resist them appearing. 'Compulsion' is the term used to describe the behaviour that is chosen to relieve the anxiety induced by the obsessions.

For example, a patient with OCD might be plagued by the thought that, having left their house, they might have left it unlocked. This very commonly experienced doubt can lead to anxiety. A normal response would be to return to the house to check the lock. However, in OCD, having checked once, the doubt recurs and recurs, so much so that the patient may find himself checking the locks over and over again. In this case, the obsessive thought is 'the house is unsafe' and the compulsive behaviour is the checking. In this sort of situation the person can be so disabled by the OCD that he may choose not to leave the house, rather than be trapped in the exhausting cycle of anxiety and checking.

Another common obsessive pattern of thought in OCD concerns fears of contamination. In this sort of case a patient might be plagued by concerns that germs or other dangerous influences are affecting their body or environment. The compulsive behaviour in such a case is repetitive and excessive cleaning and disinfecting, and avoidance of potentially contaminated objects. This too can become exhausting and disabling, as the patient spends so much time in washing and cleaning, and may avoid normal social situations.

Sometimes the obsessive thoughts have a slightly 'magical' or superstitious quality, in that only by performing a behaviour in a certain way will 'everything be alright'. In this form of OCD, the affected patient might need the objects in their environment to be ordered "just so", or they may find themselves indulging in behaviours such as having to count as they go up the stairs, or always touching a certain gatepost as they walk to the shops. This sort of behaviour is a very common and normal aspect of early childhood, but can become disabling and stigmatising if it persists into adulthood.

OCD is a more complex problem to treat in conventional psychiatry, as the obsessive thoughts seem to pervade a person's values and ideals in a more profound way than is found in the phobias. A person with OCD might have deep beliefs about personal security, or health and hygiene, or the interrelationship of events, all of which need exploring in much more depth than might be needed in the treatment of someone with a simple phobia. Often, the OCD will significantly affect all aspects of the person's life and cannot be easily avoided. Depression is very commonly found to be a complicating feature of OCD.

Ideally, OCD is treated with psychological approaches, including cognitive–behavioural therapy. Analytical psychotherapy may be of benefit in certain individuals. It is believed that the SSRI antidepressants, such as paroxetine, can be of particular benefit, and so these may be prescribed, even if depression does not appear to be marked. Severe OCD is one of the rare examples of a mental health disorder in which psychosurgery may be of benefit. In OCD surgical approaches such as leucotomy, in which specific tracts of interconnecting nerve fibres in the brain are severed, may be performed, but this is done only as a last resort.

Post-traumatic stress disorder

Post-traumatic stress disorder (PTSD) is another anxiety disorder in which there is a deep fear of being overwhelmed by panic and avoidance, but in this case the trigger for the anxiety is a memory of a traumatic event. Typical events include physical or sexual abuse, involvement in a road traffic accident, witnessing a death or being involved in armed combat. It is known that PTSD develops in over 50% of rape victims.

The patient with PTSD may avoid any behaviour that might trigger the intrusion of the memory, and may develop panic symptoms if they begin to be reminded of the event. It is typical in PTSD for the patient to experience powerful 'flashbacks' of the event, which can disturb sleep or interrupt normal life, as they can lead to overwhelming waves of fear, guilt, anger or grief. The affected patient can become watchful, nervous and can startle easily. They may report a general sense of feeling numbed to life. Avoidant behaviour can involve use of drugs and alcohol, which can greatly complicate the recovery from the initial trauma. Depression is also a very common aspect of PTSD.

Psychological treatment for PTSD ideally involves a cognitive–behavioural approach to dealing with the panic. Cognitive–behavioural approaches can greatly speed up recovery from PTSD, although not all cases will respond to treatment. The approach of encouraging the patient to face up to the memory in great detail, a technique known as 'flooding', is now largely outmoded, as in some cases it appeared to worsen the condition.

Generalised anxiety disorder

In contrast to each of the previously described anxiety disorders, in generalised anxiety disorder (GAD) there may be no specific trigger for the anxiety. Instead, in GAD the anxiety is a pervasive aspect of the way in which the person experiences the world. A person with GAD will be known as a 'worrier'. They might appear as nervous and jumpy, and may suffer from physical symptoms such as tremor, muscle tension, digestive disturbances, sweating and frequency of urination.

GAD is common. It has been estimated that GAD is present in 8% of people who visit the GP, although it probably affects just less than 3% of the general population. It is twice as common in women as in men. In general practice, GAD is likely to present as recurrent concerns about bodily symptoms, and so may not initially be diagnosed.

As GAD is a pervasive problem, the treatment is not straightforward. The patient might benefit to some degree from some simple cognitive–behavioural approaches, but analytical psychotherapy might be more appropriate for dealing with the deep roots of this condition.

Information Box 6.2d-I

Anxiety disorders: comments from a Chinese medicine perspective

From a Chinese medicine perspective, all the anxiety disorders are manifestations of the diverse Chinese syndromes that demonstrate Shen Disturbance. These include: Blood Deficiency (Heart and Liver), Yin Deficiency (Heart, Liver, Lung, Kidney, Stomach and Spleen), Empty Heat, Liver Qi Stagnation, Blood Stagnation (Liver and Heart), Full Heat, Phlegm Fire and Wind.

Each of the anxiety disorders has its own 'flavour' of Organ imbalance depending on the nature of the individual symptoms. For example, the prominence of intrusive thoughts in obsessive–compulsive disorder suggests that Spleen pathology will be prominent. As worrying is a component in generalised anxiety disorder, a Spleen disorder might again be predicted. It could be expected that the trauma preceding post-traumatic stress disorder (PTSD) might have had an impact on Heart and Kidney Qi, and thus these Organs may be more prominent in the differential diagnosis of cases of PTSD.

More specifically, Flaws and Lake (2001) describe the Chinese disease categories of 'Anxiety and Thinking' (Shan You Si), and also 'Susceptibility to Fear and Fright' (Shan Kong and Shan Jing). Shan You Si includes diseases characterised by Spleen pathology, including Spleen Qi Deficiency with Liver Qi Stagnation, Heart and Spleen Qi Deficiency, and Lung and Spleen Qi Deficiency.

Shan Kong and Shan Jing are characterised by Kidney, Gallbladder and Heart pathology, including the Empty/Mixed patterns of Kidney Jing Deficiency, Qi and Blood Deficiency, Heart and Gallbladder Qi Deficiency, Liver Blood Deficiency with Qi Stagnation, and Kidney Deficiency. Phlegm Fire and Heart Fire can also lead to a susceptibility to fear, startling and palpitations.

Part II: Depression and related syndromes

The syndrome of depression

Although in common usage the term 'depression' describes a range of emotional states, from a medical perspective it is a syndrome with a number of defined characteristics. According to the range and intensity of these characteristics, depression can be graded as mild, moderate or severe (according to ICD 10), as or minor or major (according to DSM IV). The grading of depression has important consequences in how treatment is chosen.

The features of a depressive episode include characteristic emotions and thought patterns, which include:

- low mood
- inability to feel enjoyment
- poor attention and concentration
- ideas of guilt and worthlessness
- lowered energy and tiredness
- a belief that life is not worth living.

In severe depression, biological changes in body and brain function can occur. These include:

- loss of appetite, or abnormal appetite
- significant change in weight (usually loss, but can be gain)
- marked daily variation in mood, with it often being worse in the morning
- poor sleep, with early morning wakening
- physical agitation or, conversely, slowing down of movements.

According to DSM IV, if at least five of the above features (including low mood or inability to feel enjoyment) have been present every day for a 2-week period, a diagnosis of a major depressive episode can be made. The ICD 10 diagnosis of severe depression is similar to this. This carries clinical weight because it is recognised that the risk of suicide is much higher in severe depression (occurring in up to 15% of patients with a major depressive episode) than in the less severe forms of depression. It is also important to note that the syndrome of major depression is common, affecting up to 26% of women and 12% of men in their lifetime.

Minor depression is characterised according to DSM IV by low mood but with less than five of the above listed features present. According to ICD 10, in mild depression normal daily functioning is only slightly impaired, and in moderate depression daily functioning is more significantly impaired.

Depression is recognised as an episodic condition from which people can recover. After recovery, there is a 40–60% chance of relapse, but this need not necessarily occur. However, in some people a state of depression, even if mild, seems to be an ongoing condition. The diagnosis of dysthymia is made if a person experiences low mood for most of the time over a 2-year period or longer. If the only abnormal mood change that the patient experiences is towards depression, this is known as a 'unipolar mood disorder'.

If the episodes of depression alternate with episodes of elevated mood (a state known as 'mania'), this is the condition of bipolar mood disorder. This less common condition is explored in Chapter 6.2e.

In certain groups of patients, depression may be present but may not appear with the usual syndrome as described above. In children, depression might appear in the form of behavioural disturbance, poor academic performance or sexual promiscuity. In elderly people, depression can manifest in the form of memory loss, and difficulty in concentration and thinking. In this way it may appear to be like an early form of dementia (known as 'pseudo-dementia'). It is of utmost importance to the patient that this reversible condition is differentiated from a dementia, because, of course, depression is treatable with appropriate support and antidepressant medication. Alternatively, depressed elderly people might not admit to a low mood but might instead develop symptoms such as constipation, weight loss and excessive concern about their bodily symptoms.

The causation of depression

It is clear that the tendency to depression can be inherited, and this suggests that there is a biological basis to depressive symptoms. It is currently believed that depression can result directly from reduced levels of certain neurotransmitters in the brain, including serotonin (5HT), and chemicals known as the amines. This theory is supported by the fact that drugs that are known to reduce levels of these neurotransmitters are also recognised to cause depression.

There are also well-founded psychological theories for the causation of depression. For example, it is recognised that negative life events in childhood, such as loss of a parent or the experience of sexual abuse, are associated with an increased risk of depression in adult life.

Research into the immediate triggers of depression has revealed that, in many cases, recent stressful life events led up to the onset of an episode (as is true for the onset of a wide range of psychological conditions). Bereavement (see later in this chapter) is one example of a stressor that is well recognised to carry a high risk of depression. Childbirth is another major life event that can be followed by depression in one or both parents. While it is very likely that biological factors, such as changes in hormone levels, physical debility and loss of sleep, must play a part in postnatal depression, it is likely that the psychological impact of the arrival of a new baby also will play a part in the causation of this syndrome.

It is also well recognised that a number of physical illnesses are associated with depression. For example, it is known that the incidence of depression is much higher in hospitalised patients than in the general population. As is the case in postnatal depression, there may be a number of biological reasons why physical illness could manifest in depression. However, it also has to be appreciated that illness has social and psychological consequences, which could also contribute to the causation of depression. The stress of constant pain or discomfort, and the fear of loss of health and livelihood are psychological factors that may contribute to depression in the context of chronic illness.

It is also clear that personality factors play a part in the development of depression. What might be a depression-causing stressful event in one person, might leave another relatively untouched. It is recognised that those people who can be described as having obsessional, dependent or histrionic personality types are more likely to develop depressive symptoms (see Chapter 6.2e).

Treatment of depression

Before treatment is begun, the degree of depression needs to be evaluated fully. Questionnaire scoring systems such as the Beck Depression Inventory or the Hamilton Rating Scale for depression may be useful in providing an objective measure of severity. Ideally, the medical practitioner should grade the symptoms into minor or major (DSM IV grading) or mild, moderate or severe (ICD 10 grading) depression, and in particular should explore the possibility of suicidal ideas and plans.

Suicidal ideas are common, particularly in major depression, but certain features indicate a greater risk that the patient might actually go on to attempt suicide in a serious way. In general, people who are solitary, male and elderly are more likely to attempt suicide and not survive the attempt. People who suffer from chronic illness or a substance-misuse disorder are also at increased risk. Any evidence that the patient has made concrete plans for the attempt (e.g. purchased tablets, acquired a hosepipe for the car exhaust, made provision for family members who will be left behind) should be taken as extremely serious features.

According to the biopsychosocial model, ideally all the three domains (biological, psychological and social causes) should be attended to in the treatment of depression.

Medical treatment with antidepressant medication need not be the first line of action in minor or mild depression. In these less severe cases, ideally more conservative physical approaches, such as attention to healthy diet, sufficient sleep and regular exercise, should be recommended in the first instance. Any biological triggers, such as ongoing medication or recreational drug use, should be explored. Psychological and social causes may be attended to by means of appropriate counselling or psychotherapy.

In many cases cognitive–behavioural therapy might be considered the most appropriate form of psychotherapy. In cognitive–behavioural therapy the therapist will encourage the patient to assess his or her own negative thought patterns, and then challenge the patient about the validity of these thought patterns. The patient might be encouraged to keep diaries of negative thought patterns, and be recommended exercises in which they experiment with different ways of responding to stressful situations.

In moderate to severe depression, the patient may be considered unlikely to be able to respond to psychotherapy alone. One reason for this is that lifestyle change and engagement in psychotherapy are both dependent on the patient being able to focus and have the drive to generate change. Both these skills may be significantly impaired in more severe cases of depression.

If the severely depressed patient is not considered to be acutely at risk of a suicide attempt, they are likely to be offered a prescription of antidepressants. In this sort of case, the most commonly prescribed type of antidepressant is a SSRI (e.g. citalopram).

If the depression is so severe that the patient is failing to take care of themselves adequately, or if there appears to be a very high risk of suicide, admission to a psychiatric unit may be considered to be the most appropriate option. In such cases it may be considered necessary to admit the patient under a section of the Mental Health Act. In situations in which urgent treatment is considered necessary, a brief course of electroconvulsive treatment (ECT) may be administered, because of the recognised delay in action of the antidepressants.

Most patients however (60–70%) will respond to antidepressant medication, although some may need more time to find which type is best for them. Some patients might only respond to a prescription of two or more antidepressants, although this combined prescribing is usually only practised by a psychiatrist with specialist experience.

Ideally, the improvement in symptoms will be such that the drug can be withdrawn, gradually, after a period of 6–9 months. Some patients may find that they need to remain on a long-term prescription to keep negative symptoms at bay. In addition, some patients with profound mood changes might be prescribed lithium or one of the other mood-stabilising drugs on a long-term basis to prevent further relapses.

Bereavement and grief

Bereavement is not considered to be a psychiatric diagnosis. Instead it is a recognised and normal reaction to loss. In the long term it may lead to acceptance of the loss in such a way that the bereaved person may be stronger and more mature as a result. The process of grief after bereavement has been clearly described by various psychologists in terms of certain key stages.

One of the most well known descriptions of the stages of grief originates from the writings of the Swiss-born psychologist Elisabeth Kübler-Ross. In her book *On Death and Dying* (1969) she describes five responses that a patient might go through on being given the news of terminal illness. These are:

- denial
- anger
- bargaining
- depression
- acceptance.

These stages are frequently seen in the process of developing acceptance of any type of loss, and they can be a useful model for those involved in grief work. It is recognised that no one has to systematically progress through all these stages in order to arrive at acceptance of the loss.

However, these stages do not describe many of the commonly experienced responses to acute loss, including numbness, acute physical and mental pain, intrusive thoughts, guilt over what was not done, a sense of injustice and mood swings. It is also a normal response for someone who has been suddenly bereaved to experience hallucinations of the lost loved one, either in the form of seeing them or hearing their voice.

Normal bereavement leads to negative emotions, but these do not strictly equate to depression. Although it may be normal to have periods of sadness at the memory of the loss after bereavement, in normal bereavement the person is likely to have moved on from experiencing a continuous state of painful emotions within a year or so.

In abnormal or pathological grief the bereavement leads to a decline in physical or mental health. There might be little or no apparent emotional grieving, but instead the development of bodily symptoms might occur. Alternatively, an excessively extreme grief response might develop into severe depression, with biological symptoms. In some cases grief might manifest in the form of a psychotic illness, with features of thought disorder (see Chapter 6.2e).

Normal grief is a gradual process, and a healthy progression to acceptance and reinvestment in life without the lost person can be enabled by supportive counselling. Grief counselling is a specialist discipline. In the UK access to grief counsellors can be facilitated through contact with a GP or through the charity CRUSE.

> **Information Box 6.2d-II**
>
> **Depression: comments from a Chinese medicine perspective**
>
> In Chinese medicine, the symptoms of low mood and depression would generally fit in the category of diseases described as 'Frequent Sorrow' or Shan Bei. These diseases have Lung pathology in common, and the patterns include Lung and Heart Qi Deficiency, Liver Qi Stagnation with Fire Invading the Lungs, and Heart Qi Deficiency and Lung Fire. Flaws and Lake (2001) suggest that the Lung pathologies in Frequent Sorrow might result from excessive grief, overwork and chronic disease. Internally generated Heat resulting from Stagnant Liver Qi can flare upwards to damage the Lungs.
>
> However, depression commonly overlaps with symptoms of 'Anxiety and Overthinking' (Shan You Si in Chinese medicine), in which case Spleen pathology would be recognised to coexist with the previously listed patterns.
>
> It can be seen that depression might be a manifestation of either Empty or Mixed patterns.

Part II: Disorders manifesting in bodily functions (somatoform disorders)

The somatoform disorders are those conditions that are considered to have a root in a mental/emotional imbalance, but which manifest in physical symptoms as if they had originated in physical disease. In somatoform disorders the patient is not considered to have any wilful control over the symptoms, which are believed to be generated unconsciously.

Malingering and factitious disorder

Malingering and factitious disorder are two conditions in which physical symptoms are wilfully created by the patient. Therefore, these are not somatoform disorders. In malingering, illness is feigned so that the patient can have some sort of material gain, such as leave from work duties or financial compensation. In factitious disorder there can also be feigning of symptoms, or even systematic and secretive self-harm (in which case the disorder is also known as 'Munchausen's syndrome'), but in these disorders the gain for the patient from feigning illness is less obvious. It may be that the gain for the patient is the medical attention these symptoms attract. Munchausen's syndrome by proxy is a sinister variant of factitious disorder in which the systematic harm is inflicted on a third party, usually a vulnerable person such as a child or an elderly person.

> **Information Box 6.2d-III**
>
> **Somatoform disorders: comments from a Chinese medicine perspective**
>
> In Chinese medicine, the physical basis, or otherwise, of a symptom does not have the relevance that it carries in conventional medicine. In all the somatoform disorders it would be the symptoms, the pulse and the tongue characteristics, rather than their physical roots, which would point to the underlying patterns.

Conversion disorder

A conversion disorder is one in which there appears to be a loss or change of physical functioning that would ordinarily result from physical disease. However, on examination there are no signs of physical disease, and all tests reveal normal function. The symptoms in conversion disorder commonly mimic those of neurological disease (e.g. paralysis, loss of the voice, blindness, fainting, epileptiform fits).

The term 'hysteria' has been used to describe a condition in which an emotional disorder becomes manifest in the physical realm. This term, which originates from the Greek word for 'womb', is now largely outmoded because of its pejorative associations. Freud suggested that hysterical symptoms were the result of the conversion of emotional distress into a bodily symptom, which itself had symbolic significance for the patient. Psychological theory proposes that the development of the symptom somehow serves a purpose by diverting the anxiety of an emotional conflict for the patient.

The French psychiatrist Janet described patients with 'hysteria' who appeared relatively unperturbed by their developing a symptom, such as paralysis, which in most people would have led to distress. This so-called 'la belle indifference', a happy state of indifference to the symptom, can be a feature in some cases of conversion disorder, but is by no means characteristic.

It is now recognised that, in a number of cases of conversion disorder, a true physical disease such as stroke or multiple sclerosis is subsequently diagnosed, and so the diagnosis of a conversion disorder must be made with great circumspection.

True conversion disorder generally tends to resolve with time, often spontaneously. Psychoanalysis may be of value in exploring the roots of the origin of the symptoms, and a hypnosis-like treatment known as 'abreaction' may also prove to be effective.

One subtype of conversion disorder is persistent somatoform pain disorder, in which the patient complains of persistent chronic pain for which no medical basis can be found. Common sites of the pain include the lower back, the head and, in women, the pelvic area. Persistent somatoform pain disorder is is a very difficult condition to diagnose with confidence, and also to treat, without making the patient feel that the severity of their condition is being denied. Patients with chronic pain suffer considerable disability, and depression is very commonly part of the patient's experience. In some cases the pain can respond to a prescription of antidepressant medication.

Hypochondriasis

'Hypochondriasis' is a term now used specifically for the tendency of the patient to worry that they may be suffering from one or more serious underlying diseases such as cancer or human immunodeficiency virus (HIV) infection. The patient might focus unduly on particular bodily symptoms, and may be unready to accept reassurance that these are benign. These patients might request medical tests and referrals to specialists, but still may not be reassured.

The condition is characterised by anxiety, and can respond to cognitive–behavioural therapy. Hypochondriasis differs from somatisation (see below) in that the central cause of distress to the patient is the worry about the cause of the symptoms, rather than the symptoms themselves.

Body dysmorphic disorder (BDD) is a specific type of hypochondriasis in which there is excessive concern about a perceived defect in appearance, such as a wrinkle, a cleft in the chin, or the shape of the breasts. This can lead to social withdrawal, or the decision to undergo cosmetic surgery. Some authorities consider BDD to be a subtype of obsessive–compulsive disorder, in that it is characterised by persistent negative thoughts and the compulsion to act to alter or cover the affected body part. BDD also can respond to cognitive–behavioural therapy and also SSRI antidepressant medication.

Somatisation disorder

'Somatisation' is the medical term used to describe the pervasive tendency to experience mental or emotional distress as a physical symptom. Often, patients who somatise will tend to seek help for their symptoms, which can for them be a source of long-term distress.

'Somatisation disorder' is used to describe the long-term tendency for a patient to frequently attend their doctor complaining of a range of recurrent physical symptoms. This is possibly the most disabling of the somatoform disorders, in that its repercussions on the life of the patient may be lifelong, and also it is very resistant to psychological treatment. Typical symptoms in somatisation include those listed in Table 6.2d-I. Although these symptoms are all common, at least eight have to be complained of before a diagnosis of somatisation can be made.

Table 6.2d-I Somatisation: typical symptoms experienced (eight or more need to be present for a diagnosis to be made)

- Pain during urination
- Headaches
- Shortness of breath
- Palpitations
- Chest pain
- Dizziness
- Amnesia
- Difficulty swallowing
- Vomiting
- Abdominal pain
- Nausea
- Bloating
- Diarrhoea
- Pain in the arms or legs
- Back pain
- Joint pain
- Vision changes
- Paralysis or muscle weakness
- Sexual apathy
- Pain during intercourse
- Impotence
- Painful menstruation
- Irregular menses
- Excessive menstrual bleeding

Patients who tend to somatise may be referred inappropriately to a number of specialists for further investigations. All the symptoms tend to be functional in nature, and so medical tests often show no abnormalities. The symptoms generally tend to be resistant to medical treatments. Somatisation is currently understood to be a manifestation of underlying unhappiness or depression, and is believed to have its roots in early childhood when patterns in illness behaviour are formed.

Patients may experience their doctors losing patience with their frequent consultations. Doctors often find somatisation frustrating, as the cause of the problems is often elusive and medical treatments fail to benefit the patient. This frustration is expressed in the term 'heart-sink patient', which has been used by doctors to describe patients with somatisation disorder.

Benefit might be achieved by means of cognitive–behavioural therapy, which enables the patient to make links between their emotional feelings and their bodily symptoms. However, it is commonly found that patients with somatisation disorder tend to resist exploration of the possible psychological roots of their symptoms.

Neurasthenia

Neurasthenia is a condition that was first described over a century ago. The term embraces the syndrome of excessive fatigue, especially after mental effort or physical exertion, difficulty in concentration, and diverse symptoms including dizziness, headache, muscle pains and digestive disturbances. Although originally considered to be a somatoform disorder, and so one with a psychological basis, neurasthenia does carry a remarkable similarity to the chronic fatigue syndromes.

Dissociative disorders

The dissociative disorders are, like the conversion disorders, conditions in which emotional distress is not directly experienced by the patient. However, instead of the distress manifesting in the physical realm, in the dissociative disorders the condition manifests in terms of a problem of identity, memory or consciousness.

Total psychogenic amnesia is a rare dissociative disorder in which the patient suddenly loses the ability to remember essential personal information. The most usual trigger is extreme trauma. The amnesia may be total, or limited to a period of time surrounding the traumatic event. It may be selective so that only portions of the traumatic event can be remembered.

A psychogenic fugue is a very rare state. In such a state, a patient might travel and continue normal activities although he or she has lost some touch with the reality of who they are.

Multiple personality disorder is considered to be a rare form of severe dissociation.

The underlying reasons for both psychogenic amnesia and fugue can be explored by means of hypnosis and abreaction (a form of chemically induced hypnosis using the drug sodium thiopental).

Psychosomatic disorders

The term 'psychosomatic' is commonly used with pejorative overtones, with the implication that a person's illness is 'all in their head'. However, the precise medical use of the term is quite different. The psychosomatic illnesses are those very physically rooted conditions which also appear to have a strong interrelationship with intercurrent stress. Examples might include migraine, peptic ulcer, asthma and eczema, inflammatory bowel disease and rheumatoid arthritis.

Although the precise mechanisms of how the effects of stress are mediated in these very physical forms are unknown, the fact that stress can manifest in measurable physical illness is fully accepted by the conventional medical community.

Part II: Eating disorders

The eating disorders anorexia nervosa and bulimia nervosa have some similarities with body dysmorphic disorder, in that the primary issue for the patient appears to be an excessive focus on and dissatisfaction with bodily form. However, these two discrete disorders have so many features in common that they are considered to be in a category of their own. For this reason they are not classified as somatoform disorders. In ICD 10, the eating disorders are classified as behavioural syndromes associated with a physiological disturbance, and in DSM IV they are classified as developmental disorders (i.e. appearing first in infancy, childhood or adolescence).

Anorexia nervosa

Anorexia nervosa is a condition that generally appears in teenage girls, although it is increasingly recognised to affect boys, and also to have a later onset in adulthood in some cases. The primary concern for the patient is a fear of fatness and an excessive dissatisfaction with the amount of fat on their body. The concern is out of keeping with what would be considered an acceptable body shape by the general population, although it may be supported by similar concerns expressed in the patient's peer group or influence group.

The fear of fatness and concern for a certain body form drives the patient with anorexia to restrict food intake, and in particular to avoid fattening foods. There may also be a drive to overexercise and to misuse laxative medication. Low levels of nutrition and overexercise will readily manifest in amenorrhoea (cessation of the periods) in young women.

Anorexia nervosa is diagnosed if there has been a weight loss of over 15% of the normal body weight, if the patient demonstrates a fear of becoming fat and has a distorted body image, and also, in women, if there is amenorrhoea for more than three consecutive periods. 'Anorexia' is a misnomer in this condition as the term literally means 'loss of appetite'. However, in anorexia nervosa, although the patient tends to avoid eating, it is often clear that there is excessive focus on and interest in food, an interest that can appear almost obsessional. It has been noted that, as a child develops anorexia nervosa, he or she may become more serious and introverted and less argumentative.

If anorexia persists, some characteristic physical changes appear, including dry skin and hair, downy body hair (lanugo), low body temperature, slow pulse rate and poor sleep. In the long term there is risk of death from starvation or heart failure. There is a high risk of suicide in patients with anorexia nervosa.

Psychological theories for the causation of anorexia suggest that the problem is more likely develop on a background of low self-esteem. By achieving an 'ideal' body weight, the anorexic patient can bolster a poor sense of self-worth. In addition, it is postulated that the anorexic finds some degree of control in their eating patterns, and this can provide a sense of comfort, particularly in the setting of a family in which expectations of performance are high. As anorexia progresses, there are marked similarities with obsessive–compulsive disorder, in that the controlled eating behaviour can pacify a welling anxiety regarding loss of control of weight.

The problem in treating anorexia nervosa is that it is often a hidden condition, and one that the patient may be reluctant to address. Some success may be achieved by forms of counselling that focus on self-esteem. If family dynamics are considered to be important in the causation, family therapy may be of value. Behavioural therapy, in which rewards are negotiated in response to adopting more normal eating patterns, can also be effective. Dietary advice is usually necessary. In some cases antidepressant medication can be of profound benefit.

In extreme cases of near starvation or suicide risk, hospitalisation may be deemed necessary, ideally in a dedicated unit.

Bulimia nervosa

Bulimia nervosa is also a condition in which there is an excessive concern with fatness, but in this condition the eating patterns are more chaotic. The patient experiences urges to binge on food, particularly on carbohydrates, and then finds relief by inducing vomiting, or 'purging' with diuretics, laxatives or enemas. At the time of the binge the patient experiences an overwhelming desire to keep eating, and has a sense of being out of control. In between binges a person with bulimia might achieve stringent control over their diet, in a form akin to anorexia nervosa. Some cases of anorexia nervosa can progress to bulimia.

Although patients with bulimia tend to be of average weight, nevertheless they can suffer profound health consequences. The female patient with bulimia might also develop amenorrhoea. The teeth can be eroded by the gastric acid, and the hands can develop sores from manual induction of vomiting. The salts in the blood can become imbalanced by the vomiting of fluids, and there is risk of death by heart attack.

Bulimia also primarily affects women, but is also fairly common in men, who account for up to a quarter of cases.

Patients with bulimia are more likely to seek help for their condition, as the sense of failure and guilt that accompanies the pattern can be overwhelming. However, this often comes after years of an ingrained pattern of eating, and so the condition may be very resistant to treatment.

It is considered that advice on proper nutrition and the medical consequences of vomiting and purging is an essential part of treatment. Psychotherapy for this condition focuses on issues of low self-esteem. Behavioural approaches can also be effective in the management of bulimia. Antidepressant medication can be effective for some people.

Summary

The eating disorders carry one of the highest risks of ill-health and death of all the psychiatric diagnoses. There is undoubtedly a very strong social component in their causation. It is likely that these disorders will continue to cause a heavy burden of ill-health until such a time as the popular adulation of excessive thinness in models, dancers and athletes can be successfully challenged.

Information Box 6.2d-IV

Eating disorders: comments from a Chinese medicine perspective

From a Chinese medicine perspective, the underlying psychological factors in the eating disorders point clearly to different elements in the Five Element system of diagnosis. Low self-esteem and a sense of needing to aspire to an ideal hint at imbalance in the Metal Element. Overconcern with food relates to an imbalance of the Earth Element. Excessive need for control suggests an overactive Wood Element.

Hence, in anorexia nervosa there might be a primarily Deficient pattern of Lung and Spleen Qi or Yang Deficiency, together with Blood Deficiency. Liver Qi Stagnation could also be present.

In bulimia nervosa, however, there may be a more Mixed pattern. In addition to Deficiency of Blood and Yin, there may also be a build up of Heat, Phlegm and Stagnation from overeating and induction of vomiting.

The red flags anxiety, depression, somatoform and eating disorders

Some people with anxiety, disorders of mood or one of the other neuroses will benefit from referral to a conventional doctor for assessment and/or treatment. Red flags are those symptoms and signs that indicate that referral is to be considered. The red flags of anxiety, and depression, and the somatoform and eating disorders are described in Table 6.2d-II. This table forms part of the summary on red flags given in Appendix III, which also gives advice on the degree of urgency of referral for each of the red flag conditions listed.

Chapter 6.2e Psychoses, personality disorders and learning disability

LEARNING POINTS

At the end of this chapter you will:

- be familiar with the following mental health conditions: schizophrenia, bipolar disorder, the organic psychiatric conditions, personality disorders and learning disability
- be able to recognise the red flags of these mental health disorders.

Estimated time for chapter: Part I, 90 minutes; Part II, 90 minutes.

Introduction

The first half of this last chapter on mental health disorders considers the psychoses and organic conditions. These are disorders in which a profound disorder of mental function and insight can be apparent. Both these categories of disorder affect a patient in such a way that normal communication with another person may be severely disrupted. This disruption results from either thought disorder or clouded consciousness. Very often a patient suffering from one of these conditions in its acute form would be seen as either insane or very confused.

As stated in the previous chapter, the term 'neurosis' is used to describe a mental health disorder in which a degree of insight into the condition is retained by the patient. In contrast, a psychosis is a condition characterised by a loss of insight by the patient.

There are two broad categories of mental disorder that involve a psychosis and in which the underlying process of disease is not yet clearly understood. These are schizophrenia and bipolar disorder (manic–depressive disorder). Because the underlying process of disease is poorly understood, these conditions are sometimes known as the 'functional psychoses' or 'idiopathic psychoses'.

In contrast to the functional mental health disorders, the organic disorders are those in which the underlying cause is clearly rooted in a measurable physiological change in the function of the brain. Brain function can be affected by specific degenerative changes (the cause of the dementias), by drugs and toxins, and also by a wide range of bodily responses to

Table 6.2d-II Red Flags 44a – mental health disorders: anxiety, mood disorders and other neuroses

Red Flag	Description	Reasoning
44.1	**Suicidal thoughts**: with features that suggest serious risk – old age, male sex, social isolation, concrete plans in place	This symptom may not be volunteered by a person suffering from depression. It is alright to ask something like 'Have you ever thought life is not worth living?' Such a thought does not necessarily signify serious risk, but if present should lead you to question further about features that will suggest seriousness of intent and a high-risk social situation. High-risk factors include old age, male sex, isolation or marital separation, and plans in place about how to do it If you have any concerns that your patient is at a serious risk of suicide you should discuss your concerns with the GP. This is a situation when it may be appropriate to breach your normal practice of confidentiality
44.5	**Severe depression/obsessive–compulsive disorder or anxiety**: if not responding to treatment and seriously affecting quality of life	In certain cases of minor mental health disorder the symptoms of depression, obsessive thoughts or anxiety can be so overwhelming as to be disabling. Referral needs to be considered for psychiatric or psychological support if these symptoms appear to be seriously affecting quality of life (e.g. the patient is unable to leave their home)
44.6	**Severe disturbance of body image**: if not responding to your treatment, and resulting in features of progressive **anorexia nervosa** or **bulimia nervosa** (e.g. progressive weight loss, secondary amenorrhoea, repeated compulsion to bring about vomiting)	Severe forms of eating disorder can result in progressive ill-health that can be so severe as to be life-threatening. If the symptoms are not responding to your treatment you should consider referral for professional psychiatric support. This may be met with resistance. Referral in such a situation may result in the serious outcome of the patient being detained against their will in hospital under a section of the Mental Health Act. As this may be a situation in which you may need to breach patient confidentiality, you may wish to seek prior advice from your professional body about how to proceed
44.8	**Postnatal depression**:	Refer any case of depression developing in the postnatal period that has lasted for >3 weeks and which is not responding to your treatment. Refer straight away if the woman is experiencing suicidal ideas, or if you believe the health of the baby to be at risk

Self-test 6.2d

Anxiety, depression, somatoform and eating disorders

1. List five different anxiety disorders.
2. List three psychological, one emotional and eight physical features that are characteristic of the syndrome of anxiety.
3. Name some of the features of severe or major depression (list three mental or emotional features and three biological features).
4. Suicidal ideas are common in depression. What sort of additional features might point to an increased risk of a serious suicide attempt?
5. Match the following terms
   - hypochondriasis
   - malingering
   - somatisation
   - conversion disorder
   - dissociative disorder
   - factitious disorder

   with the following definitions of somatoform disorders:
   - the expression of emotional distress in the form of a physical symptom, often of a neurological nature
   - the long-term tendency for emotional distress to be experienced in multiple physical complaints that are the source of distress for the patient and which can lead to recurrent medical consultations
   - the tendency to develop anxiety about minor bodily symptoms because of overconcern that they might relate to a severe underlying illness
   - the expression of emotional distress in the form of a disorder of memory, identity or consciousness.

   Two of the terms do not have matching definitions because they are not somatoform disorders. What are the two conditions, and why are they not classified as somatoform disorders?

Answers

1. In this chapter you have studied seven discrete anxiety disorders: panic disorder, agoraphobia, social phobia, simple phobia, obsessive–compulsive disorder, post-traumatic stress disorder and generalised anxiety disorder.
2. Psychological features of anxiety include: thoughts appear to speed up or slow down; there may be unusual perceptions of light, sound and reality; there may be an overvigilant state, irritability and sleeplessness.

   Emotional features of anxiety include: fear of impending doom, and a sense of foreboding or dread.

Self-test 6.2d—Cont'd

Physical features of anxiety include: rapid heart beat, raised blood pressure and chest pain; rapid breathing and hyperventilation; tremor; muscle tension; dizziness and tingling; sweating; a sensation of choking; nausea or loss of appetite; altered bowel movements; frequency of urination; and a pronounced startle response.

3. Severe or major depression is characterised by pervasive low mood and/or inability to feel enjoyment (every day for more than 2 weeks), together with three or more of: poor attention, poor concentration, ideas of guilt, low self-worth, lowered energy and tiredness, and a belief that life is not worth living.

   Biological features are particularly indicative of a severe episode, and include: loss or change in appetite, significant change in weight, marked daily variation in mood (often with a worsening in the morning), poor sleep and early morning wakening, and physical agitation or slowing down.
4. Features that suggest increased suicide risk in the case of expression of suicidal ideas include male sex, old age, solitary social status, intercurrent drug or alcohol abuse, and chronic illness. The description of a clear and concrete plan for the suicide attempt is also a serious feature.
5. The correct definitions are as follows:
   - Hypochondriasis: the tendency to develop anxiety about minor bodily symptoms because of overconcern that they might relate to a severe underlying illness.
   - Somatisation: the long-term tendency for emotional distress to be experienced in multiple physical complaints that are the source of distress for the patient and that can lead to recurrent medical consultations.
   - Conversion disorder: the expression of emotional distress in the form of a physical symptom, often of a neurological nature.
   - Dissociative disorder: the expression of an emotional distress in the form of a disorder of memory, identity or consciousness.

Malingering and factitious disorder are not somatoform disorders because the physical symptoms in these conditions are wilfully generated by the patient.

disease. For example, the states of fever, uraemia in kidney failure and hypoglycaemia all have an impact on brain function. The organic disorders can result in a profound change in the mental function, as they very often lead to confusion or altered consciousness. In this way they are more akin to psychoses than neuroses.

The second half of this chapter focuses on those conditions that seem to be clearly rooted in a person's constitution. These conditions are either congenital or develop very early in childhood. They include the personality disorders, and the various causes of learning disability. The important developmental and behavioural disorders of childhood have already been summarised in Chapter 5.4e.

The conditions discussed in this chapter are:

Part I
- Schizophrenia and bipolar disorder:
  - schizophrenia
  - bipolar disorders
  - other psychotic disorders.
- Organic psychiatric disorders:
  - dementia
  - confusional states and delirium.

Part II
- Disorders of adult personality:
  - paranoid personality disorder
  - schizoid personality disorder
  - schizotypal personality disorder
  - antisocial personality disorder
  - borderline personality disorder
  - histrionic personality disorder
  - narcissistic personality disorder
  - avoidant personality disorder
  - dependent personality disorder
  - obsessive–compulsive personality disorder
  - passive–aggressive personality disorder.
- Learning disability.

Part I: Schizophrenia and bipolar disorder

Schizophrenia and bipolar disorder are two categories of functional psychoses. In both DSM IV and ICD 10 they are classified as separate conditions, because bipolar disorder is classified, together with depression, as a mood disorder. However, there are some strong similarities between the clinical features of these two forms of psychosis, and also similarities in how they are treated medically.

Schizophrenia

The term 'schizophrenia' is derived from the Greek words meaning 'split' and 'mind'. The name points at the lack of integration between thoughts, emotions and will that can be so apparent in schizophrenia. However, the term is commonly a source of confusion and stigmatisation, as it is easily misinterpreted as meaning 'split personality', and, for some, conjures up images of an unpredictable Jekyll and Hyde character. This is totally erroneous in the case of schizophrenia. It is misunderstandings such as these that have led to inappropriate fear and avoidance of those given this diagnosis. Schizophrenia is a relatively common condition. One in 100 people in the UK will experience a schizophrenic breakdown in their lifetime.

As schizophrenia is a condition that tends to first develop in the late teens or early twenties, and then may persist in a disabling form for years, its impact on the health of a population is significant, and rivals the impact of the more physically based diseases of coronary heart disease or cancer. Although it is true that in 25% of cases a person will make a full recovery after an episode of schizophrenia, in two-thirds of cases symptoms will relapse and remit over the course of many years. In about 10–15% of cases there will be long-term disability as a direct result of the condition.

The symptoms of schizophrenia can be grouped into the more striking 'positive symptoms' and the less remarkable, but arguably more disabling, 'negative symptoms'.

The positive symptoms of schizophrenia include:

- delusions
- hallucinations
- incoherence and loosened associations.

Delusions. A delusion is, simply speaking, a false belief. In contrast to religious beliefs (which some might argue are erroneous), a delusion is not a belief that is understandable in the context of the person's culture, and nor is it one that can be shaken in the light of evidence which strongly suggests it is misguided. Delusions in schizophrenia are often paranoid in nature, and can involve beliefs that the person is somehow being watched or systematically harmed. Beliefs that the television is the source of a mechanism of surveillance of one's thoughts, or that poison has been secretly inserted into one's food, are examples of typical delusions in schizophrenia. Paranoid delusions can make life unbearable, and can lead the sufferer of such beliefs to withdraw socially. In severe cases they can drive the person to suicide.

For others, the delusions relate to their perception of the nature of their personality, and these can include the well-described 'delusions of grandeur' (e.g. believing that one is the Prime Minister). Delusions that thoughts are being interfered with, transmitted, inserted, blocked or removed are particularly characteristic of schizophrenia. The delusional perception, a sudden appreciation of a delusional idea which seems to appear out of the blue after a sensory experience, is also very characteristic. An example of a delusional perception might be that, just after a thunderclap has been heard, it suddenly becomes clear to the patient that aliens are in control of the armed forces.

Hallucinations. A hallucination is a sensory perception that has not been triggered by a physical stimulus. Any sound, sight, smell, taste or bodily feeling is a hallucination if it is experienced with no obvious physical explanation. Auditory hallucinations (sounds) of voices are the most common hallucinations in schizophrenia. To the patient, the voices seem as if they are coming from an external source. Brain scans have proved that these voices are not 'figments of the imagination', as they are associated with increased brain activity in the region of the brain that deals with speech.

Incoherence and loosened associations. Another feature of schizophrenia is that thoughts may seem to ramble and not be related to thoughts which have gone before (loosening of associations). Speech can be difficult to follow (incoherence). Totally new words (neologisms) can appear, and strange patterns of speech or word play might be observed.

The negative symptoms of schizophrenia include:

- catatonic behaviour
- flat or inappropriate affect (emotional responses).

Catatonic behaviour. 'Catatonic' is a term which describes behaviour that tends to total inaction. This can appear insidiously in the onset of schizophrenia. The affected person tends to withdraw from social contact, may neglect personal hygiene and basic bodily functions, and loses all volition.

Flat or inappropriate affect (emotional responses). In schizophrenia the emotions may appear 'blunted', with a narrowing of the normal range of emotions, a state described as 'flattening of affect' ('affect' is a technical term meaning mood). There can also be the unprompted inappropriate expression of emotions in the form of outbursts of laughter, tears or anger.

The diagnosis of schizophrenia is not one to be made lightly. By definition, it is only made if there have been persistent symptoms for at least 6 months of markedly reduced function in areas such as work, social relationships and self-care, together with at least 1 week's experience of two of the positive or negative symptoms listed above. If there are either particularly bizarre unshakeable delusions, or auditory hallucinations of voices talking to each other or commenting on the person's activity (e.g. 'Now he is going into the shop'), these alone are almost diagnostic of schizophrenia.

The onset of schizophrenia most commonly occurs in the late teens or early adulthood. There may be a period of gradual deterioration of function which precedes the appearance of more positively diagnostic features. In this period the person might tend to withdraw socially and their behaviour might seem increasingly more bizarre. Speech can become vague and difficult to understand. Odd beliefs might become apparent. However, in other cases the onset may be quite abrupt.

It is clear that there can be an inherited vulnerability to schizophrenia. The identical twin of someone with schizophrenia has a 50% chance of developing the condition, even if raised in a totally different environment. Siblings have a 15% chance. It is suggested that the inherited vulnerability might lie in the function of the serotonin–dopamine pathways in the brain, or in the structure of certain nerve membranes, as these are aspects of brain function that are known to be different in people with schizophrenia.

However, it is recognised that other triggers are required in addition to an inherited vulnerability. There are also theories that an early source of brain damage, such as birth trauma, head injury in childhood or viral infection, might also lead to a vulnerability. For all these potential triggers there is epidemiological evidence to support the theory that they are relevant in the causation of schizophrenia.

There is no doubt that drugs can promote the development of schizophrenia. Cannabis use in early teens is increasingly implicated in the development of psychosis in young people. Amphetamines, hallucinogens and ecstasy may also be associated with the causation of psychosis. For this reason it is of utmost importance that these triggers are avoided after a psychotic breakdown.

It is also known that extreme stress can lead to a schizophrenic breakdown, and can also be implicated in a relapse in someone who has recovered from schizophrenia. Studies of Afro-Caribbeans in the UK have shown that the incidence of schizophrenia is much higher in those who have moved to the UK than in Afro-Caribbeans who remained in Trinidad and Barbados. The risk is even higher in second-generation immigrants. The implication of such studies is that the loss of cultural identity, social isolation and systematic racial abuse which are most likely to affect second-generation immigrants can be a very significant factor in the causation of schizophrenia in this group of people.

The UK National Institute for Health and Clinical Excellence (NICE) has published guidelines for the management of schizophrenia. It emphasises that the management of the condition requires a detailed assessment of social, cultural, emotional and physical needs, thus involving a coordinated multidisciplinary approach. Treatments should be chosen with the consultation of the patient and any carers involved, and wherever possible informed consent for treatment should be obtained.

The recommended treatment for an acute episode of schizophrenia is an initially low dose of an atypical antipsychotic drug. The recommended range of drugs includes amisulpride, olanzapine, quetiapine, risperidone and zotepine. These drugs all have a markedly lower incidence of the more disabling side-effects recognised to occur with the older antipsychotic drugs such as chlorpromazine.

The dose is gradually increased, and the drug is only changed if there is no significant response in 6–8 weeks. In this case a second atypical antipsychotic drug is prescribed. Only if two of the recommended atypical drugs fail to have sufficient effect is the drug clozapine prescribed. Although it is one of the most effective drugs available, clozapine carries the risk of inducing a dangerous drop in the white blood cells, and so the patient needs to be monitored with regular blood tests.

Most people will experience a reduction in both positive and negative symptoms with the first prescription of one of the newer antipsychotic medications. The current recommendation is that the drug is continued for 1–2 years and then withdrawn very gradually only if symptoms have resolved. The patient is then monitored for at least 2 years more. Approximately 1 in 5 people will suffer no further relapse with this treatment approach. Current practice is to treat an acute episode, or an acute relapse, of schizophrenia as a matter of urgency.

If the patient is failing to care for himself adequately and if he is refusing to take medication, a decision may be made to admit the patient to a psychiatric inpatient unit. This admission may be made compulsory according to Sections 2 or 3 of the Mental Health Act 1983. It is not unusual for a first hospital admission for an acute psychosis to last for weeks to months. Ideally, while in hospital, and also after discharge, the patient is offered a range of psychological and social therapies. In particular, cognitive–behavioural therapy may be of benefit.

A patient who has suffered an acute psychotic breakdown may remain in a very vulnerable state for weeks to months. They will need a safe and stable environment in which to live and may require a lot of support to cope with the routine activities of daily living.

Following the breakdown, a patient may need to be encouraged to avoid potentially stressful situations and recreational drugs, both of which are known to inhibit recovery. Because their condition often places them outside normal cultural norms of behaviour, a patient who has suffered a schizophrenic breakdown may become victim to prejudice and physical abuse.

For all these reasons, whether the patient is in hospital or in the community, ideal care should involve the coordinated support of a team of mental health professionals, including the psychiatrist, community psychiatric nurses, occupational therapists and social workers. For some, placement in sheltered housing overseen by residential carers may be the most appropriate living environment in the medium to long term.

Bipolar disorder (manic–depressive psychosis)

Bipolar disorder is a long-term condition characterised by episodes of elevated and depressed mood. A period of markedly elevated mood (by definition lasting for more than 1 week) is termed 'mania'. 'Hypomania' is the term reserved for a period of elevated mood lasting for more than 4 days which does not quite meet the criteria for mania (see below). If there is no history of an episode of either mania or hypomania, the diagnosis of bipolar disorder cannot be made.

Like schizophrenia, bipolar disorder is common, affecting 1% of the adult western population in any one year. It, too, has a peak age of onset in the late teens and early adulthood. Unlike schizophrenia, bipolar disorder is more likely to be a lifelong condition, and as time progresses the episodes of abnormal mood, which initially may be separated by long periods of normal mood, tend to become more prolonged and closer together. Also, as time progresses, periods of depression tend to predominate over the periods of elevated mood.

Mania is characterised by a prolonged period of 'high' mood, and this is associated with three or more of the following features:

- increased energy, drive and restlessness
- racing thoughts
- rapid speech
- distractibility (the train of conversation may move rapidly from one topic to another, but the speech is never as disorganised as can be seen in schizophrenia)
- reduced need for sleep (less than 3 hours a night may seem sufficient)
- irritability
- an unrealistic perception of one's own abilities and powers, which may be so extreme as to be delusional (e.g. believing oneself to be the Messiah or the President of the USA)
- indulgence in extreme behaviour that may be ultimately harmful (e.g. spending sprees, unwise sexual encounters, making foolish business investments)
- denial that anything is wrong with one's beliefs or behaviours
- hallucinations may also be experienced in some cases.

Although, by definition, these features have to be present for 7 days consecutively, often an episode of mania will last for weeks to months, with 4 months being the average duration.

Hypomania is characterised also by high mood and driven behaviour, but does not qualify for the diagnosis of mania as the indulgence in unwise behaviour, and the experience of delusions and hallucinations, are not present.

The depressive episodes in bipolar disorder meet the same criteria as for unipolar depression, and by definition have to be present for 14 days consecutively. Psychotic features may become apparent in these episodes in the form of delusions of extreme low worth, poverty or illness, and the development of catatonia (extreme inactivity).

The episodes of mood disorder in bipolar disorder can be very disabling. In a state of mania personal and work relationships can break down, and there can be extreme financial and other material loss as a result or unwise behaviour. The person can become both sexually and physically vulnerable. Once the episode has passed, the patient can experience deep embarrassment and remorse about what has happened during the episode. The patient may become out of work and isolated as a result of their behaviour during the manic period.

The periods of depression, which can become increasingly common, can be severe, and the risk of suicide may be significant.

In 50% of cases of bipolar disorder there is a family history of psychosis (either bipolar disorder or schizophrenia), thus suggesting a biological basis to the condition and also some overlap in causation with schizophrenia. As in schizophrenia, stress and illicit drug and alcohol abuse may precipitate a relapse.

The aim of medical treatment for bipolar disorder is to stabilise mood. The atypical antipsychotics olanzapine and quetiapine, the anticonvulsant drugs, such as carbemazepine and sodium valproate, and also lithium are all currently recommended as first treatments for bipolar disorder. All these drugs seem to inhibit the cycling of mood that is characteristic of the disorder, but each has its own unique but significant side-effect profile. Antidepressants are not recommended as first treatment in bipolar disorder, even for a depressive episode, as it is well recognised that they can precipitate mania. However, they may be used with caution if a depressive episode is not responding fully to the mood-stabilising drugs and if there is no known sensitivity to the drugs.

Ideally, mood is stabilised within 6–8 weeks of starting the mood-stabilising drug. As is the case in acute schizophrenia, in both acute mania and profound depression a hospital admission may be considered necessary to ensure the patient is in a safe environment in which basic needs of daily living can be attended to. Often, it may be necessary to make this admission compulsory according to Sections 2 or 3 of the Mental Health Act, as denial that there is anything wrong is characteristic of mania. If there is an incomplete response to the medical treatment, a second mood-stabilising drug may be added. If either the depression or mania is extremely severe or disabling, a course of electroconvulsive therapy (ECT) may be considered as a treatment option.

In the long term, continuous treatment with mood-stabilising drugs may be the treatment of choice, and this is particularly the case if there have been two or more manic episodes, or if suicidal behaviour is prominent. In both these cases the risks of a relapse are considered to outweigh the problems caused by the treatment. It is not currently considered appropriate to prescribe antidepressants in the long term for a person with bipolar disorder.

As is the case for schizophrenia, a person who has experienced an acute episode of bipolar disorder may well need support from a range of professionals, including the psychiatrist, community psychiatric nurse, social worker and occupational therapist. It is recognised that structured psychological counselling, such as cognitive–behavioural therapy, may be of benefit.

Other psychotic disorders

In some cases of functional psychosis the symptoms do not clearly fall into the categories of schizophrenia or bipolar disorder. Schizoaffective disorder is a condition in which the diagnostic features of schizophrenia are present together with a significant and episodic appearance of a mood disorder. As in bipolar disorder, the psychosis can be episodic. It is treated with either antipsychotic drugs or mood stabilisers, and may have a relatively good prognosis.

'Brief psychotic episode' or 'brief reactive psychosis' describes a period of psychosis that often comes on suddenly but which, by definition, does not last for more than 1 month. It most often occurs in people aged 20–30 years as a response to an acute shock or ongoing stress. This is the usual diagnosis in postnatal psychosis, which only rarely lasts for more than 30 days. The usual treatment is with antipsychotic medication.

Schizophreniform disorder is akin to schizophrenia, but does not meet the diagnostic criterion of lasting for more than 6 months.

Delusional disorder is a condition which tends to appear in slightly later life, and in which non-bizarre delusions, including a belief of being followed, harmed and conspired against, are persistently held despite evidence to the contrary. Delusions of jealousy, in which the person suspects that they are being betrayed by a loved one, can be particularly damaging, and have been known to be the cause of a violent vengeful response, including murder. If the delusions have bizarre characteristics, such as a belief in alien involvement, then this is more typical of a schizophrenia-like illness than of delusional disorder. Delusional disorder does not appear to have any overlap with schizophrenia or bipolar disorder in terms of causation or inheritance, but can respond to antipsychotic medication.

Information Box 6.2e-I

Psychosis: comments from a Chinese medicine perspective

In Chinese medicine, the features of psychosis are embraced by the syndromes of Dian Kuang (withdrawal and mania), Kuang Zhang (manic condition) and Chi Dai (feeble mindedness). The patterns that can be associated with these syndromes include: Obstruction of the Orifices of the Heart by Phlegm, Damp Phlegm, Fire, Blood Stagnation and Qi Stagnation. In chronic psychosis there can be Depletion of Yin from Excessive Heat leading to a Mixed picture of Yin Deficiency with Internal Heat.

Although in most cases the patterns are Mixed conditions, Empty conditions can account for the negative symptoms and depression seen in the psychoses. These include Blood, Qi and Kidney Yang Deficiency, Heart Blood and Spleen Qi Deficiency, and Spleen and Kidney Yang Deficiency.

Flaws and Lake (2001) suggest that the origin of these patterns is a combination of constitutional Deficiency or Imbalance (excess of Yin or Yang) and expression of excessive emotions (leading to Qi Stagnation, Congealing of Phlegm, Fire and Blood Stagnation).

Part I: Organic psychiatric disorders

The organic psychiatric disorders are those syndromes that can be explained in terms of a clearly understandable problem in brain function or damage to the structure of the brain. There will be a clear link between the onset of the change in function of the brain and the appearance of symptoms, which means that the symptoms can be attributed directly to the physical problem in the brain. Although the current psychiatric classification separates the organic from the functional psychiatric disorders, as more becomes known about disordered brain function in the functional conditions, the demarcation between the two is becoming more arbitrary.

Dementia

'Dementia' is a term derived from the Latin words meaning 'out of mind'. It is used medically to refer to a number of conditions in which there is reduced mental functioning in a wide range of domains as a direct result of long-term change in brain structure. In the dementias, the physical problem can be located predominantly in the cortex of the brain. The cortex is the outer layer of the brain, which is responsible for the higher mental functions such as thinking, memory, insight, speech, inhibition of socially inappropriate behaviour, processing of sensory information and purposeful movement. There is a range of causes of dementia, each of which has a specific physical causation and correspondingly characteristic range of symptoms.

A diagnosis of dementia is made when it can be demonstrated that, in a fully conscious person, new learning is impaired and there has been progressive decline in intellect, movement, speech, recognition of sensory information and performing complex activities. Usually, dementia is a clinical diagnosis made without the need for confirmatory tests, although further tests can help to clarify the underlying cause. However, it is essential that reversible causes of confusion are excluded from the diagnosis (e.g. alcoholism, thyroid disease, normal pressure hydrocephalus). If there is any impairment of consciousness, the diagnosis should not be made, as this is more characteristic of a drug-induced state or a metabolic disorder. Severe depression in elderly people can also mimic dementia.

In most forms of dementia the onset is gradual, with the exception of the second most common cause, which is cerebrovascular disease. In this case the cause of the cortical damage is multiple areas of infarction of the brain, and these generally tend to develop very rapidly.

The most striking and universal aspect of dementia is memory impairment. In general, short-term memory is most profoundly affected initially, although long-term memory will also be eroded as the condition progresses.

Sometimes it appears as if memories are being erased in the opposite order in which they were laid down, and the patient becomes fixated on people and events from their early life. There is also increasing difficulty in complex tasks such as writing, addition, getting dressed and conversation. Physical movements can become more clumsy, and gait unsteady. Urinary and faecal incontinence can develop. There is also gradual disinhibition of normal social control, and the patient becomes impulsive and emotionally unstable. There may be marked emotional or aggressive outbursts.

The different forms of dementia and the Chinese medicine correspondences are described in Chapter 4.1f.

Confusional states and delirium

'Delirium' is a term used to describe a particular organic syndrome in which clouded consciousness is the central feature. The term 'acute confusional state' is synonymous with 'delirium'. Consciousness can be impaired by degrees, and in the most extreme form would manifest as coma. In its more subtle forms there may be difficulty in sustaining attention, disorientation and some memory impairment.

Apart from confusion, other features of delirium include an abrupt onset and fluctuating intensity of symptoms hour by hour. Hallucinations (especially visual in nature) can occur, as can persecutory delusions and misread visual images (illusions) (e.g. the curtains appearing to be like a threatening man in black). Agitation and anxiety can be common emotional components of delirium.

Impairment of consciousness has a wide range of causes, including head injury, stroke, brain infections, inadequate oxygen and glucose, the effect of drugs (and drug withdrawal) and the toxins that build up in chronic diseases. In contrast to dementia, if the cause is treated the delirium will subside. Children and elderly people are much more prone to delirium than the rest of the population. It has been estimated that this state affects up to 20% of elderly people admitted to a general hospital.

Some of the features of delirium are comparable to the symptoms of schizophrenia, but key differences are the fluctuating consciousness and the predominantly visual illusions and hallucinations in delirium.

The most important aspect of the treatment of delirium is elucidation of the cause. If the cause is not obvious, a range of tests (including full blood count, kidney and liver function, thyroid function, blood glucose, chest X-ray and infection screens) may be performed. A reversal of the cause (e.g. treatment of a urinary infection) can result in a remarkable resolution of the delirium with a rapidity that may appear close to miraculous to the carers of the patient. Only in very extreme cases will medical sedation be used, as sedative drugs can exacerbate the depression in consciousness However, the benzodiazepines are routinely used in the treatment of acute alcohol withdrawal to prevent the appearance of the confusional state known as 'delirium tremens' (the DTs).

Part II: Personality disorders

The mental health disorders so far described generally develop either in adolescence or in adult life. For each of the diagnoses so far studied, it would be possible to find cases in which the patient had a history of what would be called 'normal' mental health before the disorder developed. In such cases one might

> **Information Box 6.2e-II**
>
> **Dementia and confusion: comments from a Chinese medicine perspective**
>
> From a Chinese medicine perspective, the dulled thinking and clouding of consciousness that appear in dementia and confusional states correspond to Shen Deficiency and Obstructed Shen, respectively, although it is possible that both of these pathologies of the Shen will coexist in both types of organic disorder.
>
> Shen Deficiency can result from Deficiency of Kidney Essence, Kidney and Spleen Yang, Kidney Yin, and Qi and Blood.
>
> The Shen can be obstructed by the Pathogenic Factors of Phlegm, Phlegm, Damp, Fire and Blood Stagnation.

expect that external biological factors, psychological factors or social factors might have played some part in the development of the condition. Two examples of disorders developing in a person with previously normal mental health would be the case of post-traumatic stress disorder following a car accident and a case of depression following childbirth.

However, in many other cases, it might be clear that a vulnerability to conditions such as obsessive–compulsive disorder, panic disorder, depression or schizophrenia might have been apparent in the form of certain personality traits dating as far back as infancy. For example, a person with obsessive–compulsive disorder might have a long-standing history of obsessive behaviour and magical thinking from early childhood, and a person with panic disorder might have always tended to be fearful and anxious in social situations.

When certain personality traits are so extreme as to lead to a vulnerability to mental health disorder, or to cause problems for the patient in the context of their relationships, work or recreation, the term 'personality disorder' is used. It must be remembered that the personality disorders listed below are common, affecting an estimated 10% of the population, and so it might be argued that to define 10% of the population as disordered is logically flawed. However, the classification of extreme personality traits can prove a useful tool, in that it can help with the understanding of the causation of certain mental illnesses.

By definition, a personality disorder, like personality itself, is deeply engrained and enduring, and dates back to early childhood. It is believed that personality disorder is either inherited, or is the result of pervasive psychological influences that deeply affected development early in life. Personality disorder is believed to be very resistant to treatment (and in the recent past was considered by some psychiatrists to be untreatable), but in many cases long-term psychotherapy of some form may be of significant benefit. However, the talking therapies are the most expensive and difficult to provide, so currently in the UK the bulk of patients with a diagnosable personality disorder are unlikely ever to receive this ideal form of treatment for their condition.

Personality disorders were first categorised by the German psychiatrist Schneider in the 1930s, and this classification is recreated in ICD 10. DSM IV classifies personality disorders slightly differently, as it groups its 11 main forms of disorder into three clusters, each of which share similar characteristics.

The DSM IV clusters are:

- Cluster A (characterised by odd or eccentric behaviour):
  - paranoid personality disorder
  - schizoid personality disorder
  - schizotypal personality disorder.
- Cluster B (characterised by dramatic, explosive, erratic or emotional behaviour):
  - antisocial personality disorder
  - borderline personality disorder
  - histrionic personality disorder
  - narcissistic personality disorder.
- Cluster C (characterised by anxious, fearful, dependent, or introverted behaviour):
  - avoidant personality disorder
  - dependent personality disorder
  - obsessive–compulsive personality disorder
  - passive–aggressive personality disorder.

These categories are considered in turn below.

Paranoid personality disorder

Paranoid personality disorder is characterised by a belief that other people are threatening, devious and untrustworthy. Jealousy and contempt for others are also features. A person with a paranoid personality disorder tends to read hidden, demeaning or threatening meanings into benign remarks or events, hold grudges for a long time and avoids intimate relationships. They may perceive benign comments or reactions from other people as attacks on their character or reputation. They may be in the habit of making formal complaints. Particularly when in positions of power they can consider others as beneath them.

A paranoid personality disorder is associated with a vulnerability to paranoid psychosis, anxiety and depression.

People with this personality disorder do not tend to ask for help, and of course the development of a trusting therapeutic relationship will be difficult. Ideally, intensive psychotherapy is the treatment of choice.

Schizoid personality disorder

A schizoid type is a person who has little desire to form relationships, has a restricted range of emotional expression (flattened affect), and chooses to spend their time in solitary activities and introspective thinking. They also may demonstrate little or no drive to seek out sexual experiences.

In this personality disorder, there also seems to be an indifference to the praise or criticism of others, so giving the impression of a striking self-sufficiency together with oddness, suspiciousness or emotional coldness.

A schizoid personality disorder is associated with a vulnerability to schizophrenia or delusional disorder.

The ideal treatment could be sensitively supervised group therapy, but someone with this sort of personality disorder is unlikely to seek treatment.

Schizotypal personality disorder

As is true for the schizoid type, the schizotypal personality disorder is characterised by a solitary lifestyle and difficulties with close personal relationships. However, in addition to the schizoid aspects, strange speech, odd beliefs and eccentric behaviour are manifest. There may be suspicion and magical thinking, but the person does not meet the diagnostic criteria for schizophrenia. Often there is extreme discomfort in social company, possibly driven by paranoid fears.

A schizotypal personality disorder is associated with a vulnerability to anxiety, depression and episodes of psychosis.

Treatment is very difficult because of the problems the patient has in communicating with others and in forming relationships, but in some cases a cognitive–behavioural approach can help the person modify some of their more stigmatising behaviours. Antipsychotic medication may be of benefit in other cases.

Antisocial personality disorder

In this disorder, the person has a lifelong tendency to behaviour that appears to show total disregard for the needs and rights of others. Aggressive outbursts, lying, stealing and vandalism will have become apparent from early childhood, and from teenage years the child with this disorder will be in conflict with authority and the law. Remorse for this antisocial behaviour is lacking. Impulsivity is characteristic, and features of attention-deficit hyperactivity disorder are commonly present. It has been estimated that 65–75% of convicted criminals in US prisons could be given this diagnosis.

By definition, the diagnosis should not be made in children. The term 'conduct disorder' is used to describe antisocial behaviour in children.

A psychopath is a person who would qualify for the diagnosis of antisocial personality disorder, but has additional particularly chilling characteristics. A psychopath will indulge in violent and sadistic behaviour that is planned, purposeful and emotionless. The person will have an arrogant sense of elevated self-worth, and may even initially appear to be charming and charismatic. This is the diagnosis that would be applied to serial rapists or killers. However, psychopaths may find more 'acceptable' outlets for their sadism by attaining positions of political power or by joining the armed forces.

An antisocial personality disorder is associated with a vulnerability to substance abuse and depression.

Group therapy may be the most appropriate treatment choice for a person with this disorder, and may be more effective if the group consists solely of people with this diagnosis. Often the person has never had the opportunity to form a close emotional relationship and thus the therapeutic relationship can be very challenging, but if it can be established it may have a powerful impact on the patient. It is unlikely that psychopaths will be able to respond significantly to therapy, and imprisonment in a secure unit is the most positive possible treatment option.

Borderline personality disorder

Borderline personality disorder (BPD) is the most prevalent of the personality disorders, affecting an estimated 1–2% of the general population. It occurs in women twice as often as it does in men. It is characterised by a triad of long-standing emotional instability, impulsive and unpredictable behaviour, and poor self-image. The person with BPD may feel unclear about their identity, or their life direction. Mood swings are common, and relate to the feelings of low self-esteem. The mood is profoundly affected by relationships, and fears of rejection or abandonment. Relationships can be stormy, with 'acting out' being a common feature. Close attachments may be made far too quickly, followed rapidly by deep disappointment and relationship breakdown.

Lack of joy or depression is the background mood, and although there can be sudden changes in mood (to anger, anxiety or euphoria), the patient with BPD may often return to suicidal ideation. The risk of suicide is significant, with up to 10% eventually dying as a result of suicide. Self-harm, binge eating and substance abuse are also very common in BPD.

Although it is a common disorder, and one that accounts for 20% of psychiatric hospital admissions in the USA and one that is a significant cause of suicide deaths, BPD is not readily diagnosed. Often, on the surface, a person with BPD may seem to be functioning relatively normally, and it is only those who are closest to them who experience the consequences of their mood swings and impulsive behaviour.

It is believed that the tendency to BPS is inherited, but in some cases a dysfunctional family background may be causative.

BPD is associated with a vulnerability to substance abuse, eating disorders (especially bulimia and obesity), anxiety and depression, suicide and psychosis.

The treatment of choice is intensive psychotherapy, in which the person with BPS is encouraged to explore the emotional roots to their impulsive and often damaging behaviour.

Histrionic personality disorder

'Histrionic' is a term used to describe overdramatic, almost theatrical, behaviour. In this personality disorder, the affected person demonstrates exaggerated emotional responses and attention-seeking behaviour. This personality type is uncomfortable whenever they are not the centre of attention. They may use overdramatic speech and affected appearance to draw attention to themselves. There may be sexually seductive behaviour, and a tendency to consider emotional relationships to be closer than they actually are.

The emotions and behaviour of this personality type may be extremely affected by other people's behaviour and by external circumstances. Stormy interactions may be a consequence of an intense need for life to be less mundane than it is perceived to be. Illnesses and aches and pains are overdramatised, and their lives may be presented as if they are always in crisis. A person of the histrionic type is likely to blame other people and circumstances as the cause of their life's problems.

A histrionic personality disorder is associated with a vulnerability to conversion disorder, somatisation disorder and depression.

In contrast to the other personality disorders, a histrionic type may readily present to a medical practitioner for support and affirmation. However, they may be resistant to change because of the tendency not to take responsibility for the way in which they react to the world around them. Ideally, intensive psychotherapy would be the most appropriate therapy for this disorder. Antidepressant medication can also be a helpful adjunct to therapy.

Narcissistic personality disorder

'Narcissism' is the term used to describe an overemphasised belief in one's own importance. In the narcissistic personality disorder this belief is accompanied by an extreme sensitivity to criticism. The narcissistic person will be preoccupied with fantasies of success, power or attractiveness, and may fabricate stories of past achievement and ongoing projects. There is a desire to relate to special and successful people, and a belief that more ordinary people are without value. The appearance is of someone who lacks empathy and who is arrogant and self-important. It follows that there is a tendency to exploit other people to meet calculated ends. In some cases this exploitation can be severe, and may involve extortion of money or planned harm to another person's well-being. If a narcissistic type experiences challenge or criticism, there can be extreme emotional outbursts or cold withdrawal.

A narcissistic personality disorder is associated with a vulnerability to depression and psychosis.

As is true for all the personality disorders, psychotherapy would be the treatment of choice, although it may be difficult to encourage the person to accept the need for therapy. Group therapy, in which the affected person is confronted with the reactions of others in a safe environment, might prove to be an appropriate treatment option.

Avoidant personality disorder

A person with an avoidant personality type will tend to be anxious and fearful of social situations, with the consequence that they appear very shy and may tend to avoid activities that involve contact with others. They are particularly anxious in the context of new relationships, and prefer to make contact with people who are very familiar to them. In stark contrast to the isolated stance of a person of a schizoid type, the avoidant personality will be acutely sensitive to criticism, and fears social rejection. The isolation that can result from this fear is in fact the opposite of the safe closeness that a person with the avoidant personality desires.

Often, it can be recognised that many of these avoidant traits have been apparent from very early infancy, thus strongly suggesting an inherited tendency to this form of extreme shyness. Undoubtedly, negative experiences such as abuse in childhood can also result in social fearfulness in later life. It is likely that in most cases both biological and psychological factors have contributed to this personality type.

The avoidant personality disorder is associated with a vulnerability to social phobia, depression and anxiety.

Medical treatment, such as SSRI antidepressants and minor tranquillisers, may help the person cope with feelings of low self-esteem and anxiety. However, long-term psychotherapy is the ideal treatment choice, particularly as people with the avoidant tendency are likely to be very keen to uncover the roots of their anxiety and to try to deal with their fears.

Dependent personality disorder

In the dependent personality disorder there is an excessive need for the support of others in meeting emotional and physical needs. A dependent type will tend to cling to known relationships and rely on those around them to help them to make decisions and to sort out problems. They may feel extreme anxiety if these relationships are threatened, and may choose to suffer abuse within relationships rather than challenge the emotional status quo. They may avoid the possibility of being alone and may become preoccupied with fears of being abandoned.

The dependent personality disorder is associated with a vulnerability to low mood and depression.

Psychotherapy may be of benefit in encouraging a person of this type to make their own choices in life. Cognitive–behavioural therapy might be an appropriate mode of treatment.

Obsessive–compulsive personality disorder

It is important to make the distinction between obsessive–compulsive personality disorder (OCPD) and the previously discussed condition obsessive–compulsive disorder (OCD). The ritualistic (obsessive) behaviour seen in OCD, and so often the cause for mental distress, is not the hallmark of OCPD. OCPD is characterised by a perfectionistic attitude to life and an extreme need to control and order events. It is more common in men than in women.

A person with OCPD will have very high personal standards and a preoccupation with attending to rules. They are often high achievers. They may become disturbed if their standards cannot be attained by themselves or others, or if the rules are broken. They may find it difficult to delegate, and may have difficulty in forming close relationships. They may also find it difficult to be generous or to throw things away.

In contrast to the other disorders of personality, a person with OCPD may be able to function well in life without recourse to less healthy coping strategies such as recreational drugs or self-harm. The condition to which they are most vulnerable is depression.

There may be a good response to psychotherapeutic techniques that challenge the seemingly fixed value systems in OCPD.

Information Box 6.2e-III

Personality disorders: comments from a Chinese medicine perspective

The personality disorders describe enduring tendencies in the ways in which a person can respond to the world. In this way they do share some parallels with the understanding in Five Element Constitutional Acupuncture that each person has a characteristic pattern of emotional responses, which may be described in terms of their 'Constitutional' or 'Causative' factor. For each of the personality types there are features that seem to reflect imbalance in one or more of the Five Elements (Wood, Fire, Earth, Metal and Water). For example, the need of the dependent personality for support and encouragement might speak of an imbalance in the Earth element, and the desire for attention and physical affection of the histrionic personality type might reflect an imbalance in the Fire element.

A further parallel is that the personality types can be seen in terms of the way in which they embody a vulnerability to certain mental health disorders. Likewise, according to Five Element Constitutional Acupuncture, the constitutional types also correspond to the vulnerability to particular patterns of disease.

Passive–aggressive personality disorder

In this personality disorder there is a long-term tendency to resist having to take responsibility or to be compliant to the demands of others. However, instead of outright confrontation, the passive–aggressive response is to appear to comply, and even to show willing, but then to sabotage the action by inefficiency or forgetfulness. The person may appear sullen and resentful, and particularly so if their behaviour is challenged. There can be stormy outbursts. Others are usually blamed for life's problems.

The passive–aggressive personality disorder is associated with a vulnerability to low mood, depression and substance abuse.

Psychotherapy may be of benefit in encouraging a person of this type to make their own choices in life. Cognitive–behavioural therapy might be an appropriate mode of treatment.

Part II: Learning disability

Learning disability (formerly termed 'mental retardation') is defined as an enduring state of low intellectual functioning that has persisted since childhood. Intelligence can be assessed in terms of the intelligence quotient (IQ), in which, by definition, an average person would score 100. In learning disability the IQ is more than two standard deviations below this mean value (i.e. less than 70). As well as reduced intellectual functioning, there may be impairments in other developmental areas, such as impairment of motor skills or speech. Learning disability affects 1–3% of the UK population.

Learning disability may first become apparent when a child fails to attain the normal developmental milestones in language, motor function and social skills. A lack of the expected levels of curiosity of childhood may be noticed, and also the fact that infantile behaviour persists beyond the times when it would normally be expected to be reducing.

Table 6.2e-I The known causes of learning disability

Cause type	Specific causes
Trauma	Birth trauma (intracranial haemorrhage or lack of oxygen before, during or after birth) Head injury
Chromosomal abnormalities	Down syndrome Fragile X syndrome Prader Willi syndrome
Genetic abnormalities	Phenylketonuria Galactosaemia Hunter syndrome Rett syndrome
Infections in childhood	Congenital rubella Meningitis and encephalitis Cytomegalovirus (CMV) and toxoplasmosis (congenital) *Listeria* Human immunodeficiency virus (HIV)
Metabolic disorders in infancy	Congenital hypothyroidism Raised levels of bilirubin Hypoglycaemia Malnutrition
Effects of toxins in the fetus or in infancy	Alcohol and other recreational drugs Mercury Lead

In only 25% of cases of learning disability can a specific cause be identified. In all other cases, the cause is unclear, and may be the result of a combination of inherited and environmental factors. There is a clear link between learning disability of unspecified cause and poverty and low socioeconomic class. Some of the known causes of learning disability are summarised in Table 6.2e-I.

Treatment of learning disability

It is now recognised that early recognition of possible learning disability can enable the initiation of early intervention. Maximising educational and social intervention at an early stage in development can dramatically improve the outlook for children who have features of learning disability. As is the case for all children, a stimulating, safe and loving environment can have positive effects on development in all domains.

Young children with early features of learning disability need a particular emphasis on stimulation, because they tend to have less of the natural curiosity that provides most children with the stimulation they need to develop intellectually.

The emphasis on treatment is to enable individuals to reach their full potential and, ideally, to attain the social skills required for independent living.

Information Box 6.2e-IV

Learning disability: comments from a Chinese medicine perspective

From a Chinese medicine perspective, learning disability might result from a combination of constitutional Deficiency, in particular of Kidney Essence, and Obstruction of the Shen, for example by Phlegm, Phlegm Damp or Heat. Just as it is recognised that early intervention in terms of social and educational input can increase the chances of an individual reaching their full potential, so it makes sense that early intervention in terms of Chinese medicine treatment might well have an impact on the outcome of a child with early features of learning disability.

Throughout childhood the individual will need repeated assessment so that the most appropriate educational environment can be chosen, and also so that any coexisting mental health disorders, such as anxiety and depression, can be diagnosed and treated. It is clear that the outcome in terms of personal fulfilment and independence in adulthood is strongly related to the level of intervention and support the individual receives during childhood.

Long-term problems in learning disability include social isolation and an inability to appropriately meet basic needs, such as shelter, nutrition, hygiene and friendship. In such cases the ideal solution would be some sort of sheltered lifestyle, such as a group residential home or community. As well as state-funded residential communities in the UK, there are independent communities, such as the Rudolf Steiner inspired

Table 6.2e-II Red Flags 44b – mental health disorders: psychosis, personality disorder and learning disability

Red Flag	Description	Reasoning
44.1	**Suicidal thoughts**: with features that suggest serious risk: old age, male sex, social isolation, concrete plans in place for how to do it.	This symptom may not be volunteered by a person suffering from depression. It is alright to ask something like 'Have you ever thought life is not worth living?' Such a thought does not necessarily signify serious risk, but if present should lead you to question further about features that suggest seriousness of intent and a high-risk social situation. High-risk factors include old age, male sex, isolation or marital separation, and plans in place about how to do it If you have any concerns that your patient is at serious risk of suicide you should discuss your concerns with the GP. This is a situation when it may be appropriate to breach your normal practice of confidentiality
44.2	**Hallucinations, delusions** or other evidence of **thought disorder** together with evidence of **deteriorating self-care** and **personality change**	These are all features of a psychosis such as schizophrenia. Suicide risk is high Referral has to be considered if you recognise that the patient or other people are at serious risk of harm if you do not disclose the patient's condition. As it may be very difficult for you to fully assess this risk, it is advised that, unless you are absolutely sure of the patient's safety, you should refer them to professionals who are experienced in the treatment of mental health disorders Referral in such a situation may result in the serious outcome of the patient being detained in hospital against their will under a section of the Mental Health Act. As this may be a situation in which you may need to breach patient confidentiality, you may wish to seek prior advice from your professional body about how to proceed
44.3	**Features of mania**: increasing agitation, grandiosity, pressure of speech and sleeplessness with delusional thinking	Mania is a feature of bipolar disorder, and is a form of psychosis that carries a high risk of behaviour that can be both socially and physically damaging to the patient. Suicide risk is high Referral has to be considered if you recognise that the patient or other people are at serious risk of harm if you do not disclose the patient's condition. As it may be very difficult for you to fully assess this risk, it is advised that, unless you are absolutely sure of the patient's safety, you should refer them to professionals who are experienced in the treatment of mental health disorders Referral in such a situation may result in the serious outcome of the patient being detained against their will in hospital under a section of the Mental Health Act. As this may be a situation in which you may need to breach patient confidentiality, you may wish to seek prior advice from your professional body about how to proceed

Continued

Table 6.2e-II Red Flags 44b – mental health disorders: psychosis, personality disorder and learning disability—Cont'd

Red Flag	Description	Reasoning
44.4	Evidence of an organic mental health disorder: e.g. **confusion, deterioration in intellectual skills, loss of ability to care for self**	Organic mental health disorders are, by definition, those that have a medically recognised physical cause, such as drug intoxication, brain damage or dementia. They are characterised by confusion or clouding of consciousness, and loss of insight. Visual hallucinations may be apparent, as in the case of delirium tremens (alcohol withdrawal) Referral has to be considered if you recognise that the patient or other people are at serious risk of harm if you do not disclose the patient's condition. As it may be very difficult for you to fully assess this risk, it is advised that, unless you are absolutely sure of the patient's safety, you should refer them to professionals who are experienced in the treatment of mental health disorders Referral in such a situation may result in the serious outcome of the patient being detained against their will in hospital under a section of the Mental Health Act. As this may be a situation in which you may need to breach patient confidentiality, you may wish to seek prior advice from your professional body about how to proceed
44.5	**Severe depression/obsessive-compulsive disorder or anxiety**: if not responding to treatment and seriously affecting quality of life	In certain cases of minor mental health disorder the symptoms of depression, obsessive thoughts or anxiety can be so overwhelming as to be disabling. Referral needs to be considered for psychiatric or psychological support if these symptoms appear to be seriously affecting quality of life (e.g. the patient is unable to leave their home)
44.7	**Features of autism in a child:** slow development of speech, impaired social interactions, little imaginative play, obsessional repetitive behaviour	Remember that mild degrees of autism may not be diagnosed until the child reaches secondary school age. Refer if you are concerned that the child is demonstrating impaired social interactions (aloofness), impaired social communication (very poor eye contact, awkward and inappropriate body language) and impairment of imaginative play (play may instead be dominated by obsessional behaviour such as lining up toys or checking), as early diagnosis can result in the child being offered extra educational and psychological support
44.9	**Postnatal psychosis**	Refer straight away if you suspect the development of postnatal psychosis (delusional or paranoid ideas and hallucinations are key features) as this condition is associated with a high risk of suicide or harm to the baby

Self-test 6.2e

Psychoses, personality disorders and learning disability

1. What is the defining feature of a psychosis?
2. Schizophrenia and bipolar disorder are the two broad categories of functional psychoses. List three differences in the symptoms of these two disorders.
3. List three differences between the two major categories of organic psychiatric disorder, dementia and delirium.
4. What are the primary features of the following personality disorders:
   - borderline personality disorder
   - avoidant personality disorder
   - schizoid personality disorder.
5. List five important causes of learning disability.

Answers

1. The defining feature of a psychosis is that it is a mental health disorder in which the patient loses contact with reality.
2. - Although it carries a greater stigma, in 25% of cases of schizophrenia there will be a full recovery, whereas bipolar disorder tends to run a more chronic course.
   - The key feature of bipolar disorder is episodes of abnormal mood, whereas in schizophrenia the key feature is thought disorder.
   - Delusions are a common feature of schizophrenia and are often paranoid in nature. In bipolar disorder (mania) they are less common and are more likely to be grandiose in nature.

In schizophrenia thoughts appear to be disconnected, whereas in mania they are connected but tend to move very rapidly on from one to another.

3. • Dementia is progressive and usually gradual in onset. It is irreversible. In contrast, the onset of delirium is often abrupt, its severity tends to fluctuate over time, and it is reversible if the cause can be treated.
   • In dementia the patient remains conscious, whereas in delirium the consciousness is always impaired and will fluctuate over time.
   • Agitation, illusions and visual hallucinations are common features of delirium but are not characteristic of dementia.
4. • Borderline personality disorder is characterised by emotional instability, impulsive and unpredictable behaviour, and poor self-image. It carries a high risk of suicide.
   • Avoidant personality disorder is characterised by extreme shyness, anxiety and avoidance of new social situations. Isolation is a feature, although the affected person will desire closeness.
   • Schizoid personality disorder is characterised by introversion and a desire for solitary activities. The affected person may appear to be relatively immune to the opinion of others, whether negative or positive.
5. In 75% of cases of learning disability no specific cause can be found. Important other causes include physical trauma, either before, during or shortly after birth, chromosomal and genetic abnormalities, metabolic disease and exposure to toxins in early infancy.

Camphill Communities and L'Arche Foundation, in which there is special emphasis on the personal value of each resident and the unique gifts they have to offer the rest of the community.

The red flags of the psychoses, personality disorders and learning disability

Some people with psychoses, personality disorders and learning disability will benefit from referral to a conventional doctor for assessment and/or treatment. Red flags are those symptoms and signs that indicate that referral is to be considered. The red flags of the psychoses, personality disorders and learning disability are described in Table 6.2e-II. This table forms part of the summary on red flags given in Appendix III, which also gives advice on the degree of urgency of referral for each of the red flag conditions listed.

Conclusions

6.3

Chapter 6.3a Red flags of disease: a review

LEARNING POINTS

At the end of this chapter you will be able to:

- discern when a patient should be referred to a conventional doctor for further investigation or treatment
- state the degree of urgency with which referral should be made
- describe the practicalities of making a referral of a patient who presents with red flags of serious disease.

Estimated time for chapter: 60 minutes.

Introduction

Throughout the study of the various diseases considered so far, the red flags of disease have been systematically introduced. In this chapter the rationale for describing certain clusters of symptoms and signs as red flags is clarified. The chapter continues with some guidance on how to prioritise patients who present with any combination of these warning symptoms and signs, and on how to refer patients to conventional medical practitioners. A summary of the red flags in a format designed for quick reference in clinical practice is given in Appendix III.

What is a red flag of disease?

The red flags listed in this text have been defined from the perspective of a practitioner of complementary medicine. Red flags are those symptoms and signs that, if elicited by a complementary medical practitioner, merit referral to a conventional doctor. Referral is indicated because the presence of red flags indicates the possibility of a condition that may not respond fully to complementary medical treatment and/or which may benefit from conventional diagnosis, advice or treatment.

In summary, referral may be considered for the following four broad reasons:

- to enable the patient to have access to medical treatment that will benefit their condition
- for investigations to exclude the possibility of serious disease
- for investigations to confirm a diagnosis and help guide treatment
- for access to advice on the management of a complex condition.

It is important to clarify at this stage that the red flags indicate those potentially serious conditions in which the patient would be in need of further tests, advice or treatment. Complementary medical practitioners vary greatly in their opinions about the benefits of medical treatment. For this reason, some readers of this text may not agree that the presence of a particular red flag need be seen as an indication of referral. However, there is a powerful argument that patients are ideally offered the freedom of choice between treatment options. Referral for a medical opinion offers patients the opportunity to learn about the conventional medical perspective of their condition and thus the freedom to make an informed choice about its future management.

There are very few examples of when complementary medicine would not be beneficial to someone who is also receiving conventional investigation or treatment for a condition. Therefore, referral of a patient in response to red flag symptoms or signs does not mean that complementary medical treatment need be discontinued.

The red flags as guides to referral

Red flags are guides to referral, not absolute indicators. Often, the red flags described in this text specify a fixed, measurable point at which referral should be considered; for example, high fever (especially if over 40°C) not responding to treatment within 2 hours in a child. Of course, in reality, disease falls somewhere along a spectrum that bridges the state of being of little concern and one of being of serious concern. A disease does not suddenly become serious once a fixed point has passed. Moreover, what might constitute a red flag in one individual may be of less concern in someone of a stronger constitution.

Bearing in mind the potential flexibility in the interpretation of red flag syndromes, there may be a case when the conclusion is that referral is unnecessary even though a red flag is present. Conversely, if a nagging uncertainty persists in a clinical situation, even if the patient does not fit the criteria for any of the red flags, it is safest to trust your clinical instincts and refer. The important thing is that there is an awareness of these indicators of possible serious disease, and that in every case time has been taken to consider their relevance for patients in the given clinical situation.

Prioritisation of red flags

The various red flags merit different responses from the practitioner according to the nature of the underlying condition of which they may be an indication. To aid with decision-making in the clinical situation, the red flags listed in this text are assigned to one or more of three categories of urgency:

- *Non-urgent*: a non-urgent referral means that the patient can be encouraged to make a routine appointment with the medical practitioner (GP), which would ideally take place within 7 days at the most.
- *High priority*: a high-priority referral means that the patient should be assessed by a medical practitioner on the same day. This can be either as a home visit or at the medical practice.
- *Urgent*: an urgent referral is for those situations when the patient requires immediate medical attention, and this may mean summoning an on-call doctor or calling the paramedics to the scene. ,

The summaries of red flags that make up Appendix III indicate which category(ies) of urgency best fits each red flag. Again, this categorisation is simply a guide to the degree of urgency rather than a fixed directive on the appropriate response in a particular clinical situation.

How to respond to red flags

The response to a red flag in a clinical situation depends very much on what degree of urgency the response merits. In this part of the chapter, the advice given relates to the practicalities of referral to a GP or emergency hospital department within the UK National Health Service (NHS).

Non-urgent red flags

Some red flags are indicators of possible serious disease, and yet the patient does not require urgent treatment, even if the disease actually is present. An example of this is a patient who has features of anaemia, including pallor, breathlessness and palpitations on exertion. Anaemia can have serious underlying causes (e.g. chronic gastrointestinal bleeding, pernicious anaemia), some of which cannot be expected to respond fully to complementary medicine. In a case of anaemia, the patient obviously requires further investigation and, depending on the outcome of those investigations, may require medical treatment. However, if the symptoms have been developing over the course of weeks to months, the patient does not need to be seen by a doctor on the same day.

Another example of a non-urgent red flag is the child who has symptoms that indicate occasional bouts of mild asthma. In this case referral is recommended more for confirmation of diagnosis, and so that the patient can have access to medical advice about how to manage a potentially serious condition, rather than simply for treatment. It will be obvious that in such a situation the child does not need to be seen urgently.

Most of the red flags of cancer have been prioritised as of non-urgent priority. This is because such features usually have taken weeks to develop, and a delay of 1 or 2 days is not critical in the course of most cancers. In the UK, the NHS referral system is structured so that the patient demonstrating red flags of cancer is seen by a hospital specialist within 2 weeks of referral by their GP, so to be seen by the GP within only a few days of referral would be ideal in order to minimise the total wait. Of course, there will be some situations in which you will wish to make a high-priority referral for patients showing features of cancer, either because of rapidity of progression of symptoms, or in order to allay anxiety for the patient.

Those red flags that have been categorised as non-urgent will require non-urgent referral. What this means is that, in these situations, it can be suggested to the patient to make a non-urgent appointment with their GP. This means that the patient will be seen within the next few days. In this situation a letter of referral can be prepared, although this may not be necessary if the patient is capable of communicating the essential information. A letter can either be taken to the doctor by the patient (the most reliable route) or can be sent by post to the practice (more likely to be delayed or go astray). A guide to writing letters of referral to doctors is to be found in Chapter 6.3c.

High-priority red flags

Some of the red flags are indicators of serious disease, and these merit seeking a medical opinion on the same day. This is because there is a possibility that the condition of the patient might deteriorate rapidly without treatment. An example of a high-priority case is the situation of haemoptysis (coughing up blood) in a man who has lost 2 stone in weight over the past few months (strong indicators of lung cancer or tuberculosis). In this case, the potential for serious blood loss or the possibility of contagiousness makes the referral a high priority.

In high-priority situations it may be best practice to speak to the patient's medical doctor. It is appropriate in such cases to telephone the patient's practice to confirm a time in that day when you can talk to one of the doctors. After discussion, if the doctor agrees with your assessment of urgency, a same-day appointment for the patient can be made. Alternatively, it may be more appropriate that the patient makes this referral themselves, and they can be advised to request a same-day appointment with their doctor.

In such situations it is good practice to give the patient a letter describing the clinical findings and concerns to take to their doctor before they leave your clinic. In a high-priority case, a hand-written referral letter on headed notepaper is acceptable (see Chapter 6.3c).

Urgent red flags

In some cases red flags indicate that the patient requires urgent medical assessment. If you are absolutely sure that the patient needs this, it is appropriate to dial 999 (911 in the USA) to request an ambulance to take the patient to hospital. A less dramatic option is to ring the patient's practice and ask to speak to a doctor urgently in order to get his or her advice about referral to hospital. If there is some uncertainty, the doctor may choose to visit the patient first, or ask for them to come to the practice to be seen before an ambulance is called.

In those urgent cases in which you are unlikely to meet with the examining doctor, it is good practice to hand write the reason for referral in a letter that is either taken with the patient to the hospital or given to the patient's doctor when he or she arrives (see Chapter 6.3c).

The summary of red flags of disease: Appendix III

The red flags of disease are summarised in Appendix III. In the first part of this appendix (Section A), the tables of red flags are presented according to physiological system. Each red flag is labelled according to priority of referral:

*	non-urgent referral
**	high-priority referral
***	urgent referral

For many of the red flags listed, the labelling indicates a range of degrees of priority (e.g. */**). For these red flags the precise level of priority depends on other characteristics of the individual case, which should become clear according to the particular clinical situation.

Section B in Appendix III presents the red flags according to symptom keywords to enable easy reference in a clinical situation.

Section C in Appendix III summarises the high-priority and urgent situations in which first-aid management is indicated, and gives some guidance on first-aid treatments. This guidance is intended to supplement the periodic updates of first-aid training that it is advisable for all complementary medical practitioners to undergo.

Chapter 6.3b Withdrawing from conventional medication

LEARNING POINTS

At the end of this chapter you will be able to:
- describe the ways in which the body might respond to the withdrawal of a long-term medication
- categorise a drug according to the ease with which it can be withdrawn
- guide a patient through the process of drug withdrawal using an approach that is both safe and respectful of the prescribing doctor.

Estimated time for chapter: 90 minutes.

A review of the action of drugs on the body

This first section of this chapter on withdrawal from conventional medication reviews the physical and energetic effects that drugs are understood to have on the body. These effects were first described in Chapters 1.2c and 1.3b.

The physical effects of drugs on the body

The range of physical effects that drugs can have on the body were introduced in Chapter 1.2c, and are summarised in Table 6.3b-I.

The energetic effects of drugs on the body

It was explained in Chapter 1.3b that drugs can affect the energetics of the body in one or more of the following ways: cure, suppression, drug-induced disease and placebo. Table 6.3b-II illustrates the predominant energetic effect that may be associated with therapeutic results for each of the nine categories of drugs grouped by physical action in Table 6.3b-I. Table 6.3b-II does not mention the placebo effect, as this is likely to have some positive impact to some degree in all therapeutic prescriptions.

The three energetic effects that are most relevant to the withdrawal of prescribed medication are those of cure, suppression and drug-induced disease. When a complementary medical practitioner is faced with a patient who wants to withdraw from conventional medication, it is valuable first to take some time to consider which of these three effects may be most relevant for the patient.

Withdrawal from suppressive medication

Chapter 1.3b proposes that suppressive drugs are those that treat the manifest symptoms of a condition without dealing with the root cause. One drug that is suppressive according to this definition is salbutamol, which when inhaled can be remarkably effective in relieving an attack of asthma. Salbutamol is known to act by means of stimulating the cellular

Table 6.3b-I The categorisation of drugs according to the nine modes of physical action

Category	Mode of action of drug	Example
1	Replaces a deficient substance that is normally obtained from the diet	Iron (ferrous sulfate) in iron-deficiency anaemia
2	Replaces a deficient substance that is normally produced by the body	Insulin in diabetes mellitus
3	Kills or suppresses the growth of infectious agents (microbes and other life-forms that cause infection)	Penicillin in meningitis
4	Counteracts the damage caused by toxins	Acetylcysteine infusion in paracetamol overdose
5	Toxic to rapidly dividing human cells, in particular to cancer cells	Vincristine used in cancer chemotherapy
6	Specifically stimulates the immune response by the introduction of an antigen	Polio vaccine
7	Artificially stimulates natural bodily functions	Clomifene used to stimulate ovulation
8	Suppresses natural bodily functions	Corticosteroids used to suppress the immune response
9	Other drugs that directly counteract the symptoms (manifestation) of a disease process rather than its root cause	Digoxin in heart failure; paracetamol in headache

Table 6.3b-II Energetic interpretations of the therapeutic effects of drugs according to the nine modes of drug action

Category	Mode of action of drug	Energetic interpretation of therapeutic effect
1	Replaces a deficient substance that is normally obtained from the diet	Usually cure (when it targets the root cause) Can be suppression Most side-effects are due to drug-induced disease
2	Replaces a deficient substance that is normally produced by the body	Usually cure (when it targets the root cause) Can be suppression
3	Kills or suppresses the growth of infectious agents	Cure, when full clearance of the pathogen occurs in a previously healthy individual Suppression, if the infection is the expression of a Pathogenic Factor already present or when the pathogen is not cleared
4	Counteracts the damage caused by toxins	Cure
5	Toxic to rapidly dividing human cells	Suppression
6	Specifically stimulates the immune response by the introduction of an antigen	Drug-induced disease, and possibly Suppression (of the future expression of a Pathogenic Factor)
7	Other drugs that artificially stimulate natural bodily functions	Drug-induced disease or suppression
8	Suppresses natural bodily functions	Drug-induced disease or suppression
9	Other drugs that directly counteract the symptoms of a disease process	Suppression

receptors (beta receptors) in the bronchi and bronchioles, which normally respond to the action of the hormones adrenaline and noradrenaline. By acting at a chemical level, this drug induces a bodily change, in this case relaxation of the smooth muscle that encircles the lining of the small airways in the lungs. This is how salbutamol causes relief of symptoms. However, by suppressing the asthma, the stressor that has caused the asthma attack, which may actually be a combination of diverse factors such as environmental triggers and emotional disturbance, has not been removed. With symptomatic treatment such as salbutamol, the stressor is likely to remain, and so may possibly cause more subtle or intransigent symptoms at a later date.

It makes sense then, that when suppressive medication is withdrawn, suppressed symptoms may well return. This can occur almost immediately, as would be the experience of the asthmatic who becomes wheezy once he or she has come to the end of their supply of salbutamol. However, this return of symptoms can be delayed. For example, following the withdrawal of some treatments, such as at the conclusion of cancer treatment, the suppressed symptoms (in this case the cancer) do not return immediately, and may even not return at all. According to the theory of suppression, this is explained by the supposition that the original imbalance is still likely to be present, but is now expressed in a different way in the body, such as in the form of depression, or that the imbalance has been rectified by a different means, such as modification of harmful lifestyle factors. A move towards greater balance, therefore, may be accompanied by a recurrence of the original symptoms at a later date. However, a subsequent move towards balance need not always result in recurrence of the original symptoms.

It is important to acknowledge that this idea of suppression springs from complementary medical theory. In contrast, the conventional medical view is that when a drug causes suppression of symptoms this has no lasting deleterious effect. The idea that an imbalance can be pushed away from the surface only to emerge in a different part of the body is not considered within the conventional medical approach.

From an energetic perspective, replacement therapy is an unusual example of a long-term prescription drug. In the case of some forms of replacement therapy (e.g. insulin in type 1 diabetes), the patient cannot survive without the drug. Although the replacement therapy certainly suppresses symptoms, it has been argued in this text that it cannot be described as energetically suppressive. Because there is no doubt that replacement therapy always returns a patient to a more balanced state, then it has to be described as curative in nature.

To summarise, withdrawal from a suppressive drug might be expected from a holistic perspective to have the following consequences: recurrence of the original symptoms either immediately or at a later date, or persistence of the original imbalance expressed in some way at a deeper level. In some cases there might be no symptoms because of total resolution of the original imbalance, but this would only be expected if the patient had been making some positive emotional and lifestyle changes while taking the drug.

Withdrawal from medication that causes drug-induced disease

Most drugs also have side-effects that are unrelated to the condition which they are prescribed to treat. For example, inhaled salbutamol has a range of short-term side-effects, including tremor, palpitations and tachycardia. These side-effects can be explained in terms of the action of the drug in stimulating the beta receptors in other parts of the body, including the skeletal muscles and the heart muscle. These effects would occur in asthmatics and non-asthmatics alike. These effects are an example of drug-induced disease. They are not manifestations of suppression. If the drug is withdrawn, it would be expected that these less beneficial manifestations of drug-induced disease would, in most cases, subside.

However, there is one particular aspect of drug-induced disease that may lead to persistent problems for the patient and this is the development of drug dependence.

Drug dependence

It is recognised that there are some drugs that cause the body to change in such a way that the patient comes to be reliant on the presence of that drug for a 'balanced existence'. What this means is that, if the drug is withdrawn, the patient will experience a range of symptoms which, at least temporarily, will disturb their normal ability to cope with the stresses of everyday living. This effect is known as 'drug dependence'.

Drug dependence may manifest primarily in the physical body. For example, withdrawal from certain types of antihypertensive medication can lead to a dangerous rise in blood pressure. It is as if the body has 'forgotten' how to control blood pressure within a relatively safe range. This type of dependence is termed 'physical dependence'.

Other drugs seem to have effects that are more pronounced in the emotional and mental realms. For example, withdrawal from nicotine can lead to a syndrome of psychological symptoms, including cravings for nicotine, irritability, insomnia and anxiety. This aspect of dependence is termed 'psychological dependence'.

In reality, the distinction is not that clear-cut. Withdrawal from drugs of dependence will usually lead to a constellation of physical and psychological symptoms.

Addiction

'Addiction' is a term that is often used interchangeably with 'dependence'. Medically speaking, the term 'addiction' is used more precisely to mean a state of dependence that leads to 'drug-seeking behaviour' on withdrawal of the drug. A person who is addicted to a drug may spend a significant proportion of their time and effort in ensuring that the drug is in steady supply. Drugs of addiction are those that induce a powerful state of psychological dependence.

The mechanism of drug dependence

To understand what is happening to the body in drug dependence it is helpful to consider the chemical changes that might occur in response to a drug. Conventional pharmacology describes the response of the body to a drug in terms of adaptation. Many drugs act by mimicking the action of one or more of the natural chemicals of the body. These natural chemicals include the hormones and neurotransmitters that connect with receptor proteins on the surface of certain cells to effect a physiological change. The drug salbutamol acts in this way, as does cortisone (an artificial corticosteroid hormone).

If a drug is present in the body for some time, in many cases the body adapts to its presence by reducing the production of the natural chemical that the drug is mimicking. For example, in the case of a long-term prescription of cortisone, the adrenal cortex ceases to produce the normal amounts of natural corticosteroids. In fact, the tissue of the adrenal cortex actually becomes wasted in someone who is taking a long-term prescription of cortisone. This adaptation is potentially fatal if the artificial cortisone is withdrawn suddenly. The shrunken adrenal cortex is no longer able to respond rapidly to produce the level of corticosteroids necessary for a healthy response to stress. From an energetic perspective, this bodily change is a clear example of drug-induced disease.

Other drugs stimulate the body to counteract their effects by increasing the number of protein receptors on the cell membranes of the tissues at which the drug is acting. This means that more drug is required to have the same effect as time goes on. This situation, known as 'tolerance', is very important to understand from the perspective of drug withdrawal. If tolerance to the drug has developed, then on withdrawal the normal levels of the body chemicals that act at those tissues will be insufficient to effect a healthy response. Opiates (including morphine and heroin) are drugs that are known to induce a state of tolerance. Whether used medicinally for pain relief, or illicitly for their psychological effects, increasing doses of opiates are required over time to generate the same effect. It is well recognised that opiates mimic natural body chemicals, including the endorphins. As tolerance develops, it is believed that the numbers of cellular endorphin (opiate) receptors in the body increase. On withdrawal, the body is simply unable to produce sufficient quantities of natural endorphin to stimulate the increased numbers of receptors in the body, and the complex syndrome of opiate withdrawal is experienced.

Tolerance is, of course, a particular aspect of drug dependence. Once a person has become tolerant to a drug, withdrawal is very likely to lead to unpleasant symptoms. The development of tolerance is another example of drug-induced disease.

Recovery from drug dependence

The time for recovery from the physiological imbalances induced in drug dependence depends very much on the drug concerned. For example, it is generally accepted that recovery in acute withdrawal from alcohol and opiates occurs in a relatively short time scale of about 2 weeks, whereas recovery from a long-term prescription of a minor tranquilliser such as diazepam may take many more weeks. The time scale of the prescription is another important factor to take into consideration. The longer the body has been exposed to a drug, the more it will have adapted to accommodate that drug. This is why it is safe for a patient to withdraw suddenly from a short course of corticosteroids (less than 1 week), but if the course has lasted for weeks to months the withdrawal must be extremely gradual.

Social reasons for drug dependence

So far drug dependence has been described in terms of the physiological adaptation to the chemical of the drug. However, in many cases of drug dependence there some far more complex factors in the equation. In particular, cultural and social factors play a profound role in dependence to 'recreational drugs'. This role is, by its very nature, difficult to explore or quantify. Although a heroin addict can withdraw physically from the habit over a period of a few days, an extreme vulnerability to returning to the habit remains for much longer, and sometimes for life. This suggests that the addict is left with a lasting belief that the drug has something to offer, and particularly so in certain settings. Animal experiments have suggested that a brief exposure to certain recreational drugs can lead to a lasting state of depletion of certain neurotransmitters in the brain. This physical phenomenon might explain, at least in part, the persistent state of vulnerability experienced by some drug users following withdrawal from a drug of addiction.

Drug rehabilitation programmes aim to work at reducing this vulnerability. Such programmes take place in a setting that separates the former addict from the factors that might increase their tendency to return to using the drug. A rehabilitation programme often begins with a short period of medical support during the time of physical withdrawal from the drug, followed by weeks to months in which the former addict is encouraged to find a way of living that avoids those triggers that might lead to a return to the habit.

Although social factors might play a less significant role in the withdrawal from most prescribed medication, it is worth considering that they may be important in some cases. The use of a prescribed drug may, in some cases bring rewards that are additional to the relief from symptoms. The possibility of an additional, less obvious benefit resulting from a treatment in this way is conventionally referred to as 'secondary gain'. Reinforcement in the sick role and feelings of protection are two examples of the additional rewards, or secondary gain, that a prescription might bring.

When to consider withdrawal from medications

The possible negative consequences of drug withdrawal just discussed can be seen to result from two distinct processes. The first is the recurrence of symptoms. In the case of curative treatment, the recurrence of symptoms reflects the fact that cure has not taken place and the drug has been withdrawn too early. In the case of suppressive treatment, it is suppressed symptoms that reappear. In some situations these symptoms may be tolerable and responsive to positive lifestyle change, but in others they may be so severe as to overwhelm the patient.

The second process is the appearance of new symptoms as a consequence of a particular form of drug-induced disease known as 'drug dependence'. In this case the symptoms of drug withdrawal can be profound, and in some cases life threatening.

It will be clear from this summary that withdrawal from medication is a process that needs to be managed with care. There are indeed many situations in which withdrawal is a perfectly safe prospect. However, the complementary medical practitioner needs to be familiar with those situations in which it may not be reasonable to consider withdrawal from medication at all, and with those situations in which close medical supervision would be advisable. The remainder of this chapter is concerned with the practicalities of recognising those situations when it is safe to withdraw from medication and, if it is recognised to be safe, supporting a patient through the process of withdrawal.

Withdrawing from prescribed medication: a practical approach

The basic principles

When considering withdrawal from long-term medication it is important to consider some basic principles:

- If the treatment is curative in nature do not consider withdrawal.
- Withdrawal from suppressive medication is very likely to result in recurrence of the symptoms of the original condition, unless the patient has been able to make positive changes in lifestyle or emotions.
- Long-term adaptation of the body to the drug may give rise to an unpleasant withdrawal syndrome.
- In some cases either the recurrence of the original symptoms or the withdrawal syndrome carries serious health consequences.
- There may be other social or cultural factors in the equation that have to be considered.

Categorisation of drugs for withdrawal

Bearing the above-listed principles in mind, the various types of drugs can be categorised according to the main effects that can be expected on their long-term withdrawal. The categories are:

(i) The underlying condition is not serious. Recurrence of symptoms is likely; there is no withdrawal syndrome.
(ii) The underlying condition is not serious. Recurrence of symptoms is likely; the withdrawal syndrome is unpleasant, but does not seriously threaten health.
(iii) Withdrawal may have serious physical or mental health consequences, either because the underlying condition is serious, or because the withdrawal syndrome is dangerous.
(iv) Replacement therapy. Withdrawal will result in serious ill-health or death.

This categorisation of the individual classes of drugs (ordered by the chapter in which they appear in the *British National Formulary* chapter) is given in Appendix IV. This appendix is designed to be a reference aid for use in clinical practice.

Practical aspects of withdrawing from medication

Now that the principles that underlie an approach to drug withdrawal have been clarified, the practical aspects of helping patients to withdraw from medication can be explored.

Knowing when not to withdraw from medication

When considering withdrawal from conventional medication, a fundamental question to ask is 'How much will the patient benefit from withdrawal from medication at the current time?' It may be that the answer to this question leads the practitioner to the conclusion that this is not the time to consider such a change.

Even for Category (i) medications, withdrawal will necessarily result in some physical change in the body. Symptoms of the original condition are likely to recur, and will need to be dealt with. The patient needs to be prepared for this change and willing to make the necessary changes to their lifestyle that will prevent recurrence of the original condition. If the drug is suppressive in nature, any residual symptoms that remain before withdrawal is initiated can only be expected to worsen on withdrawal, even if only temporarily. Therefore, ideally, it needs to be clear that the patient has been making good progress on the treatment before a reduction in medication is contemplated. If not, it may be wise to defer withdrawal until residual symptoms have subsided.

This consideration is even more important for Category (ii) and (iii) drugs. Withdrawal from these medications will result in additional distressing symptoms, as well as recurrence of the original symptoms. The patient needs to be in a good state to prepare for the inevitable period of physical and emotional imbalance that will occur on withdrawal.

Withdrawal from Category (iv) medication should not, in general, be contemplated. This is absolutely the case if the replacement therapy is a substance that is normally produced by an organ whose function has failed totally. An example of this is insulin replacement therapy in type 1 diabetes mellitus. In the case of patients who are taking replacement therapy to support a failing organ, there is a possibility that complementary medical treatment can enable them to reduce the dose of medication. An example of this is the prescription of thyroxine in autoimmune hypothyroidism. However, in general, in such cases it is not usually necessary to be proactive in the reduction of medication. The dose of medication is balanced against the bodily requirements as measured by medical tests. If the body no longer requires such a high dose, the tests will indicate this, and the doctor will reduce the dose accordingly.

Withdrawal from medication: preparatory stages

In all cases of withdrawal from medication it is important to check that the patient is clear about the reasons for withdrawal, and is keen for the process to occur. To make a good decision the patient needs to be equipped with information about the advantages and disadvantages of medication, from both an alternative and a conventional medicine point of view.

If the patient is clear about the pros and cons relating to taking medication and definitely wants to come off the medication, the next stage is to ensure that the patient has the support of their doctor in this process. Most doctors are also keen to reduce medication, and are only reluctant not to if they believe there will be a worsening in the patient's condition as a result. In many cases, it is appropriate simply for the patient to make an appointment with their doctor to explain that they wish to cut down on their medication. You may wish also to give your patient a supporting letter to take to the doctor, although in most cases of withdrawal from Category (i) and (ii) medication this should not be necessary.

Most doctors, if they can see that the patient's symptoms are improved and that the patient is positive about making the change, will give the patient advice about how to set about the withdrawal process. For the complementary medical practitioner this is the ideal situation; the patient can be supported through the process, but the professional responsibility for withdrawal rests with the doctor who initiated the prescription.

It is unwise to set about withdrawal from Category (iii) medication without the patient having the support of their doctor. Table IV-3 in Appendix IV indicates that medical supervision is deemed to be essential for the withdrawal of all classes of drug in this category. In such cases it is appropriate for the complementary health practitioner to write to the patient's doctor to demonstrate awareness of the health consequences of withdrawal, and to indicate a commitment to monitor and support the patient through the withdrawal process. Guidance on how to write a letter on this topic is given in Chapter 6.3c.

Speed of withdrawal

Some drugs can be withdrawn abruptly, as long as the patient is in robust health and is prepared for the consequences of withdrawal. Drugs that can be withdrawn abruptly are those that are given for non-serious conditions and that do not induce a state of physical or emotional dependence. A return of the original symptoms is the main problem for the patient withdrawing from drugs that fit this description. These drugs fall exclusively into Categories (i) and (ii), and are indicated by a single asterisk (*) in the Tables IV-1 and IV-2 in Appendix IV.

Other drugs need to be withdrawn more slowly. Slow withdrawal will allow the return of the original symptoms to be more gradual, and the symptoms of any withdrawal syndrome to appear less abruptly. Slow withdrawal is very important in situations in which the previous condition has serious emotional or physical features. In general, it is also best that drugs which induce a state of dependence are withdrawn gradually.

However, not all drugs which induce dependence should be withdrawn slowly. For example, current medical advice is that people who are addicted to alcohol should withdraw abruptly, and then weather the storm of the inevitable withdrawal period with the aid of alternative physical and emotional support. For some drugs that are highly addictive, gradual withdrawal is less effective than abrupt withdrawal, probably because the drug's continued presence during the withdrawal process can stimulate an easy return to the original 'dose'.

Slow withdrawal of most of the Category (i) and (ii) drugs (indicated in Tables IV-1 and IV-2 by a double asterisk (**)) can take place over the course of 2-4 weeks. In slow withdrawal it is advisable not to cut down the dose initially by more than one-third at a time, and to reduce by less if this is possible. The next step down should be made only when the patient has adjusted to the reduced dose, and when withdrawal symptoms have abated. For those drugs indicated by a treble asterisk (***) in the tables in Appendix IV, for example long-term hypnotics or opiates, the reduction should be even more gradual, with a longer time interval between dose reductions. Full withdrawal may require a few months in some cases.

In many cases medication is given in tablets of fixed dose at prescribed times of day. When the dose is reduced, the frequency must not be reduced. Instead the amount given at each time interval needs to be gradually cut down. For example, if the dose is 400 mg three times daily (t.d.s.), a possible first reduction might be to 300 mg t.d.s.

Sometimes gradual dose reduction is limited by a tablet of a fixed size. If lower dose tablets are available, the doctor might be willing to prescribe these. If not, most tablets can be cut in half and then into quarters to aid the gradual reduction process. Even better is for the patient to switch to a liquid preparation of the medication so that doses can be measured using a dosing syringe. Reducing the dose can become confusing for a patient who is used to a certain routine of taking tablets. Therefore it is good practice to prepare a written schedule for the patient, which contains clear instructions about how the dose should be reduced.

Order of withdrawal of medication

Many people are concurrently taking a number of prescribed drugs. It is always safest to focus on withdrawing only one medication at a time so that if any withdrawal symptoms appear it is clear exactly what has caused them.

Withdrawal from Category (i) medication

Category (i) medication is prescribed to suppress unpleasant symptoms. It does not induce a significant state of drug dependence. Table IV-1 in Appendix IV indicates that all Category (i) medications can either be withdrawn abruptly (*) or gradually over a relatively short period of time (**).

When discussing the withdrawal of a Category (i) medication with a patient, it is important to ascertain the previous symptoms of the underlying condition. The patient needs to be advised that the symptoms may well recur after withdrawal, and may even be more severe for some time during the withdrawal process. The return of symptoms is less likely to be as severe if the patient has been making good progress on the treatment and has attended to those lifestyle factors that have been identified as contributing to the root cause of the condition.

Drugs marked with a single asterisk (*) can be withdrawn abruptly. Drugs marked with a double asterisk (**) should be withdrawn gradually (see the section above entitled Speed of withdrawal). Ideally, the patient is encouraged to inform their GP of their decision to stop taking their medication.

Withdrawal from Category (ii) medication

Withdrawal from Category (ii) medication is characterised not only by a return of the symptoms of the original condition, but also by the features of a withdrawal syndrome. With drugs that induce a state of physical dependence (see Table IV-2), the withdrawal syndrome may manifest in the form of a reappearance of the original symptoms. For example, withdrawal from a stimulant laxative may result in a period of constipation, which temporarily may even be more severe than the original condition. Withdrawal from a drug that induces psychological dependence will result in the appearance of symptoms of emotional imbalance, including anxiety, irritability and sleeplessness. Cravings for the drug may be very strong.

The withdrawal of a Category (ii) medication should follow the same stages as described above for Category (i) medication. However, complementary medical treatment in the withdrawal period will also have to address the symptoms of a withdrawal syndrome. It may be helpful for the patient to have prepared in advance some strategies for coping with these additional symptoms. For example, withdrawal from a stimulant laxative may require an intermediate period of taking another form of laxative. Emotional symptoms might be countered by approaches similar to those advised for people who give up smoking. Strategies such as taking up a programme of gentle exercise, planning a range of activities to distract from cravings, and use of herbal substitutes might all be considered.

Withdrawal from Category (iii) medication

Withdrawal from Category (iii) medication (see Table IV-3 in Appendix IV) again follows the same principles as described for Category (i) medication. However, Category (iii) medication has either been prescribed for a serious medical condition or may result in a dangerous withdrawal syndrome. For these reasons withdrawal from such medications should always be undertaken with the oversight of the patient's doctor.

In some cases the doctor may be reluctant to help the patient to withdraw from the drug. If this is the case, it may help if the complementary medical practitioner writes a letter to the doctor, giving their professional viewpoint (see Chapter 6.3c). If the doctor can be assured in this way that treatment has brought about a positive change in the patient's condition, and that the patient has the ongoing support of their practitioner, then he or she may agree to start reducing the medication.

There are some drugs in this category that are unlikely to be ever withdrawn by a doctor without there being a very marked improvement in symptoms. This is because the threat to physical and mental health from withdrawal would be considered to be too severe to take the risk of withdrawal. These drugs are indicated with a quadruple asterisk (****).

Self-test 6.3b

Withdrawing from conventional medication

1. You have been treating a 55-year-old man for hypertension for the past 3 months. He is currently taking a beta blocker called atenolol. Since you have been seeing him, he has lost a stone in weight and has cut down on salt in his diet. His blood pressure has gradually fallen from 160/105 to 150/95 mmHg since he has started treatment. He is keen to come off his atenolol.
   (i) According to the tables in Appendix IV, in which category of medication is atenolol?
   (ii) What are the key stages in the withdrawal process from this drug?
   (iii) Is now the right time to withdraw?
2. You have a new patient who is a 25-year-old student. She asks you about withdrawal from her antidepressant medication, citalopram. She has been taking this for 6 months now. Before she started taking the drug she felt quite down and anxious at college, but since being on it she feels much more confident. She definitely does not want to stay on the medication.
   (i) According to the tables in Appendix IV, in which category of medication is citalopram?
   (ii) What are the key stages in the withdrawal process from this drug?
   (iii) Is now the right time to withdraw?
3. You have been treating an elderly gentleman for some months now. He is pleased to find that, since treatment, the aches in his hips and knees are much better, and he is much more mobile. You suggest he might consider reducing his dose of painkiller, a non-steroidal anti-inflammatory drug (NSAID) called naproxen. The gentleman is reluctant to do this because he is concerned that it might trigger a flare-up.
   (i) According to the tables in Appendix IV, in which category of medication is naproxen?
   (ii) What are the key stages in the withdrawal process from this drug?
   (iii) Is now the right time to withdraw?

Answers

1. (i) Atenolol is a beta blocker. This is a Category (iii) medication.
   (ii) The key stages are:
   - check that this is the right time for withdrawal
   - ensure that the patient is prepared for the consequences of withdrawal
   - ask the patient to discuss withdrawal with his doctor
   - if necessary, send a supporting letter to the patient's doctor indicating the reasons for withdrawal
   - for Category (iii) drugs, ensure that the doctor oversees the withdrawal process.

   (iii) This is not the right time to withdraw. Although the patient has made good progress, he is still hypertensive. Withdrawal from beta blockers is very likely to be followed by a rise in blood pressure. The doctor would not agree to withdrawal of the drug at this time.
2. (i) Citalopram is an selective serotonin reuptake inhibitor (SSRI) antidepressant. This is a Category (ii) medication.
   (ii) The key stages are:
   - check that this is the right time for withdrawal
   - ensure that the patient is prepared for the consequences of withdrawal
   - ask the patient to discuss withdrawal with her doctor
   - if necessary, send a supporting letter to the patient's doctor indicating the reasons for withdrawal
   - prepare for a gradual withdrawal.

   (iii) This is possibly not the right time to withdraw. You have not had an opportunity to assess how 'well' your patient is on citalopram. You might suggest that she attends for a few treatments before attempting withdrawal, so that she gets to as balanced a state as possible before she starts to reduce the dose of the medication.
3. (i) Naproxen is a non-steroidal anti-inflammatory drug (NSAID). This is a Category (i) medication.
   (ii) The key stages are:

- check that this is the right time for withdrawal
- ensure that the patient is prepared for the consequences of withdrawal
- ask the patient to discuss withdrawal with his doctor
- if necessary, send a supporting letter to the patient's doctor indicating the reasons for withdrawal
- prepare for a gradual withdrawal.

(iii) Although the patient is uncertain about withdrawal, he is in a good position to cut down his medication, because his symptoms have improved so much. You could reassure him that the worst that could happen is that the original symptoms might recur and he may need to return to his original dose. Withdrawal will not risk a worsening of the underlying condition. Ideally, you can encourage him to cut down his dose gradually, so that if symptoms do return they will do so gradually. This means that you will have time to deal with them with treatment. Naproxen tablets are scored, which means that they can be cut in half (this information is given in the *British National Formulary*). You might suggest that the first reduction is to take half a tablet in the morning and the usual dose at night for a few days, before then halving the evening dose.

Chapter 6.3c Communicating with conventional medical practitioners

LEARNING POINTS

At the end of this chapter you will be able to:

- recognise when it is appropriate to make contact with the conventional practitioners who share the care of your patients
- choose an appropriate method of communication when it is necessary to make contact
- compose a letter to a conventional practitioner according to a conventionally accepted style.

Estimated time for chapter: 60 minutes.

Introduction

It is good for both patient care and interprofessional relationships that complementary medical practitioners maintain contact with the conventional medical practitioners who are involved in the ongoing healthcare of their patients. The reasons for communicating include referral of red flags of serious disease, discussions about changes in treatment and acknowledgement of referrals from conventional medical practitioners. Moreover, if the communication is made in a way that is both valid in terms of patient care and respectful of the professional to whom it is directed, it can only serve to improve the ongoing relationship between complementary and conventional medical practitioners. In this way it can serve to promote the ideal of integrated healthcare.

Choice of method of communication

There are three methods by which a complementary medical practitioner might choose to communicate with a conventional medical doctor about a patient. By far the most commonly used and convenient method is to allow the patient to do the communicating by making an appointment with his or her doctor. Alternatively, the practitioner can telephone the practice or hospital to speak to the patient's healthcare professional in person. The most formal approach is to write a letter. These three approaches are considered below in turn.

Using the patient as the communicator

The most clinical situation in which it most likely that it may help for the patient to communicate something about a complementary health consultation with their doctor is when a non-urgent red flag has been identified. An example of this is the situation when an elderly patient mentions that he has been more thirsty than usual for the past 3 months and has been passing large amounts of urine (red flag of type 2 diabetes). In this situation the patient needs to be advised to make an appointment with his doctor so that the possibility of serious disease can be excluded or confirmed.

At the appointment the patient can then explain to the doctor that their complementary practitioner is concerned about their symptoms and that, for example, there is a possibility of diabetes. In many such situations a letter is not necessary.

Patients may also be the communicators when they have decided they want to withdraw from a Category (i) or (ii) medication. A confident patient can simply go to his doctor to say, for example, 'I would like to see how I cope without my beclometasone inhaler as I have no symptoms now. How do you advise that I set about stopping it?'

As long as it is clear that the necessary information can be communicated effectively by the patient, this is the most empowering option for them.

Speaking to the doctor in person

Speaking to the patient's doctor in person is the preferred mode of communication either if the patient needs to be referred urgently or if there is a matter of some complexity that needs to be discussed. Most doctors would be very happy to discuss a problem concerning a patient over the telephone (e.g. 'Mrs. Jones, who lives alone, seems to have been getting progressively more confused. Are you aware of this?'). Whenever possible, it is important to ensure that the patient is told in advance what is going to be said, to ensure that there is no breach of confidentiality.

It is normal in UK general practice that there is a system whereby doctors will make telephone consultations on request, usually at a particular time of the day. Moreover, in a situation of high urgency the duty doctor may be contacted straight away. The practice receptionist is trained to discern which calls merit urgent handling. If the call is made after office hours, it will be transferred to an 'on-call' doctor when the practice telephone number is called. It is important to bear in mind that the doctor who is contacted may not know the patient, although in office hours he or she will have access to the patient's records.

Communicating by letter

A letter is often an appropriate method of referring patients with complex circumstances and also of communicating clinical information about a patient in a non-urgent situation. It is not appropriate if information is required from the doctor, as the process of writing a reply is inconvenient for a busy doctor and delays may be incurred if the letter is typed. If a problem needs to be discussed, such as Mrs. Jones' confusion, the telephone is the best medium.

A letter is most useful when it either precedes or accompanies a patient who has made an appointment with the doctor. The letter can then communicate the additional information which it may be important to impart. Letters are also the recognised means of communication for indicating that a referral from a doctor has been accepted by the complementary practitioner, and also to inform the doctor about the progress of a patient who has been treated following a referral.

The structure and content of the communication

Whenever a referral is made, clear and succinct information needs to be imparted to the medical practitioner. Whether by spoken word or by letter, this is best done in a structured way, and with the information offered in an order that is familiar to the doctor. If it is necessary to communicate by telephone, it is worthwhile for the complementary medical practitioner to prepare the information to be imparted in a systematic way before making contact. The list of the categories of information summarised below can be a useful *aide memoire* to ensure that no important details are omitted from a telephone call or letter. Reference to this list will also help ensure that all the necessary information is given in a logical order. General practitioners and hospital doctors tend to be overburdened with paperwork, and so it is important that telephone calls and referral letters offer information in a brief and accessible format. It helps to organise the information into short, bulleted statements, and to keep a letter to less than one page in length.

In the UK there is legislation designed to protect the rights of patients to have sensitive information about them stored in a safe way. The Data Protection Act 1998 requires a practitioner to register if they intend to keep electronic records of sensitive information about patients. This is not necessary if electronic copies of letters are deleted once the letters have been printed out, in which case paper copies can be kept for the patient records.

Information to include when communicating about a patient to a medical practitioner

- *Patient identifiers*: full name, date of birth and address. All three are required for medical records.
- *Brief summary of reason for referral*: in one sentence. For example: 'I'd be grateful if you could assess this 28-year-old man who tells me he has had three episodes of nocturnal bedwetting'.
- *More detailed history of the main complaint*: A brief synopsis of the key events in the history of the main complaint, including:
  - symptoms: describe the symptoms as described by the patient
  - signs: describe any findings (including relevant negative findings such as 'blood pressure was normal') from your clinical examination.
- *Drug history*: summarise the medication the patient is currently taking (including contraceptives and non-prescribed medication such as indigestion remedies).
- *Social history*: list any relevant lifestyle factors (e.g. smoking, alcohol use) and occupational factors which might have impacted on the current condition.
- *Summarise what is wanted of the medical practitioner*: For example: 'I am concerned that this man might be experiencing nocturnal seizures, and would value your opinion on whether he needs further investigations'.
- *If appropriate, take the opportunity describe how you have been treating the patient*: a referral is a good opportunity to explain more about what complementary medicine involves. It is probably best not to use too much professional jargon in a referral, but a couple of sentences on why the patient is having complementary therapy and how they are benefiting can do no harm.

Important additional points that apply to letters

The important points to follow when structuring letters are:

- *Headed notepaper*: this should include the practitioner's name, professional title and qualifications, address, telephone number(s), fax number, email address and website address.
- *Date*: the date of the letter is essential.

Table 6.3c-I is a simple guide to the basic information required in a professionally headed letter.

Choice of language

It will help with all communications if the practitioner aims to match the medical use of professional language as much as possible, and to avoid using complementary medical terminology, which may be misinterpreted or dismissed as meaningless.

Table 6.3c-I A guide to the basic information required on a professionally headed letter

Dr George Jackson	Jane Goodson RGN LicAc MBAcC
The Springs Surgery	Traditional Chinese Medicine
Reading RG2 3DD	The Willows Clinic
	Reading RGI IOU
	Tel: 01189 222222, Fax: 01189 222223
	jgoodson@acupuncture.com
	12 April 2010

Dear Doctor Jackson

Re: . . . Include all patient identifiers here (i.e. name, address and date of birth) . . . .

Contents of letter . . . .

Yours sincerely

Jane Goodson

Confidentiality

Although letters between conventional health professionals are often written and sent without the express permission of the patient, it is advisable whenever possible to ensure that the patient is happy for you to be writing to another professional about them, even if they have been referred to you by that professional. A helpful hint is to always write a letter that you would be prepared for the patient to read. There should be very few situations in which you wish to give information to the doctor without the patient knowing about it.

Sample letter formats

Tables 6.3c-II to 6.3c-V give sample letter formats as a guide for letter design.

Acceptance of referrals from medical practitioners

It is good practice to acknowledge a formally referred patient by sending a letter to the referring doctor after the first consultation (Table 6.3c-II). In this letter it is conventional practice to thank the referring practitioner for the referral, and then to summarise your diagnosis and treatment plan.

After the last consultation, it is good practice to send a letter in which the patient's response to treatment is summarised in terms of reduced symptoms and improvement in daily activities (Table 6.3c-III).

Referring patients to medical practitioners

A standard format is advised for the referral of patients who merit the opinion of or treatment from a conventional practitioner (Table 6.3c-IV). In such a letter it is important to clearly describe the red flags that are of concern. A medical diagnosis is not required in such a letter, as the red flags will usually speak for themselves.

In urgent situations a hand-written letter is perfectly acceptable. Hand-written letters should be structured in exactly the same way as typed letters.

Communicating about management of patients

A complementary medical practitioner is not obliged to inform a patient's GP of their treatment. However, to do so appropriately is likely to promote good relationships between the professions in general. It is reasonable that the more complementary medical treatment impinges on a disease that is also being managed by a doctor, the more appropriate it would be to communicate about the treatment and its progress. There is less need for a structured letter in this situation (Table 6.3c-V).

Table 6.3c-II
Acceptance of a referral: sample letter

Dear Dr Jackson

Thank you for referring John Smith for treatment of recurrent migraine. I saw him in my clinic today.

History

Recurrent unilateral headaches felt over the left eye and temple which are associated with blurred vision and nausea.

Headaches worse at weekends.

Frequency of headaches increasing over the last 6 weeks associated with stress at work. He currently suffers a headache most weekends.

Alcohol: at least 40 units/week (wine).

Smoking: non smoker.

Examination

Overweight (BMI 35).

Full red complexion.

BP 140/100.

Medication

Pizotifen 1 mg daily.

Ibuprofen and paracetamol during acute attacks.

Diagnosis

My diagnosis, based on his history, physical examination, and pulse and tongue examination, is that he has features of a syndrome recognised in Traditional Chinese Medicine which is likely to respond to acupuncture treatments, together with some modifications to his diet and stressful lifestyle. The raised blood pressure is consistent with this diagnosis.

Treatment plan

Eight acupuncture treatments at weekly intervals.

I have advised him to reduce alcohol, and also the fatty and spicy food in his diet. He is also likely to benefit from gentle exercise and a less stressful approach to his working day.

I would hope that with treatment he may be able to reduce his need for pizotifen, which makes him feel drowsy in the day, and he may discuss this with you in due course, assuming he makes good progress.

Yours sincerely

Jane Goodson

Lesson 6.3d Ethical issues

LEARNING POINTS

At the end of this lesson you will:

- understand some of the ethical implications of dealing with a patient who is concurrently undergoing conventional medical treatment
- be able to describe how you would manage, in a professional manner, a clinical situation that gives rise to an ethical dilemma.

Estimated time for chapter: 20 minutes.

Introduction

This final chapter is concerned with some of the broader issues that specifically relate to the situation of a complementary therapist who is offering therapy to a patient who is concurrently undergoing treatment from a conventional medical practitioner.

The chapter begins by considering two general principles to which all practitioners would be wise to adhere. These are being attentive to keeping clear contemporaneous records, and being prepared to seek professional advice in any situation in which there is ethical uncertainty.

Table 6.3c-III
Discharge summary: sample letter

Dear Dr Jackson

Thank you for referring John Smith for treatment of irritable bowel syndrome. This was causing debilitating attacks of pain and diarrhoea on a daily basis.

I have now seen him for the last of six fortnightly appointments.

Diagnosis

Constitutional weakness of his digestion, which is further weakened by certain dietary components such as raw foods, fatty foods and dairy products.

Ongoing stress from problems in current relationship also a contributory factor.

Treatment plan

Acupuncture to strengthen the constitutional weakness, with points to reduce the tension which he is experiencing.

Reduction of dairy products and raw foods in his diet.

Outcome

By the third treatment, the frequency and severity of attacks was reducing.

Currently he only gets mild attacks at less than weekly intervals.

Feels more able to confront the issues in his relationship, and feels less frustrated.

Future treatment

In view of his excellent response, regular but infrequent treatments could be sufficient to keep his symptoms under control. He knows to contact me should he require further treatment.

Yours sincerely

Jane Goodson

To conclude the chapter, three broad areas in which ethical dilemmas are common are explored. These are maintaining good interprofessional relationships, advising patients on their medical treatments, and maintaining confidentiality.

Ethical issues: general points

The importance of clear records

It is a cardinal rule that should an ethical dilemma arise in practice clear documentation of all relevant issues is made at the time in the case notes. In particular, details should be recorded concerning the treatment and its rationale, any advice given, what has been discussed with the patient, and the date. A practitioner's records are always used in an investigation of possible professional misconduct. If the records can demonstrate that the practitioner was following good practice as defined by their professional body in their dealings with a patient who has subsequently made a complaint, the practitioner is unlikely to be disciplined.

For example, a practitioner could ensure that a clear record was made of the fact she had clearly discussed the pros and cons of withdrawing from tranquillisers with a patient. In particular, she could clarify that she described the possible consequences of a severe withdrawal syndrome and suggested that the patient discuss withdrawal with her GP. If the patient later makes an official complaint that she did suffer from severe symptoms 'as a result of advice given by her therapist', the fact that a discussion about possible complications was clearly recorded at the time will stand in the practitioner's favour (should the complaint come before an investigating committee).

For this reason, it is essential that practitioners never make alterations to clinical records at a later date, even if what is written down is accurate. If it is necessary to add extra information to earlier records, it should be dated with the date of the addition. Altered records that are not dated as such will be seen as falsified by an investigating committee. It is important to note that even 'tidying' records, by reproducing in better writing an exact copy of original records, is enough to cast doubt on their authenticity.

If in doubt, seek advice

If a practitioner has any uncertainties about a particular case in practice, or if a complaint has been made about an aspect of treatment, it is wise for them to consult either the professional

Table 6.3c-IV
Referral letter: sample letter

Dear Dr Jackson

I would be grateful if you could see John Smith with regard to unexplained back pain and weight loss.

I am treating him with acupuncture, but in view of his symptoms I believe he needs further investigations.

History

2 years of increasing low back pain, which first came on while digging.

In recent months pain has been constant, and not responsive to simple painkillers.

5 weeks ago he booked an appointment with me for pain relief.

Loss of 3 kg over the past year.

Poor appetite.

Night sweats and exhaustion over the past 3 months.

Examination

Pale, thin, general muscle wasting.

Abdominal exam: no obvious organ enlargement.

Very tender over the body of L3 vertebra with associated muscle spasm.

Medication

Co-codamol 1-2 tablets up to 4 times a day.

Treatment plan

I intend to see Mr Smith on a weekly basis. My treatments will involve gentle stimulation of acupuncture points to boost the depleted energy, and the use of points local to L3 to minimise pain.

This treatment would be entirely complementary to any treatment you may decide that he requires.

Many thanks for your help.

Yours sincerely

Jane Goodson

Table 6.3c-V
Letter communicating about shared management of patients

Dear Dr Jackson

I have been treating John Smith with acupuncture for the past year. Over this time the treatment has been focused on managing his problems of long-standing anxiety and depression. He has made considerable progress, and is now expressing a desire to reduce, and eventually stop, his regular dose of amitriptyline 100 mg daily which he has been taking for 5 years.

It is my opinion that, since commencing treatment, his mood has progressively become more stable and his anxiety is far less restrictive to his daily activities. He can now go shopping alone to town without a feeling of panic, for example. He now has no unbroken nights of sleep.

Continued acupuncture treatment is therefore likely to support him through a period of gradual withdrawal from amitriptyline. Mr Smith is aware that the withdrawal process may have to be over the course of a few months. Throughout this time I will be seeing him regularly to monitor whether there is recurrence of his old symptoms.

I have asked him to make an appointment to discuss this with you, and if possible to plan with you how he can start gradually to reduce his dosage.

Yours sincerely
Jane Goodson

conduct officer of their professional body or their insurer before taking further action.

Maintaining good relationships with professional colleagues

It is an ethical responsibility for all health practitioners to ensure that they act in the best interests of their patient at all times, and this requires a complementary medical practitioner to ensure that, whenever possible, their care is truly complementary to medical treatment that is being offered concurrently. However, situations may arise in which the conventional medical advice patients may have been given conflicts in some way with complementary medical wisdom.

In this situation, any therapeutic advice offered to the patient must be given to the patient with great circumspection so that it is not understood to denigrate the conventional medical advice. This means that every effort should be made to ensure that the advice and treatment which is offered is based on unbiased research of the topic. Ideally, advice given about complementary therapy should be consistent with the views of the professional body to which the practitioner belongs, and if it is not, the practitioner should make this fact clear to the patient. If any advice or comment is offered about conventional medical treatment, it is the ethical duty of the practitioner to ensure that they are very knowledgeable about that treatment.

It is also important to bear in mind that whatever a patient says about their doctor is a personal view, and is not necessarily representative of what actually happened in a consultation. Therefore, it is wise not to collude with the patient and criticise the practitioner openly on the basis of what the patient alone has told you.

If a practitioner has serious concerns about what has been learned from the patient about the professional conduct of a medical practitioner, it is wise first to discuss this situation in confidence with the professional conduct officer of their professional body. If, following this discussion, it is agreed that a complaint is merited, this should be directed to the complaints manager of the employer of the practitioner, such as the practice manager at a general practice, the local primary health care trust complaints officer or the registering body of the practitioner (e.g. the General Medical Council is the registering body for doctors in the UK).

Helping a patient to reduce or change medical treatment

It is important for a complementary medical practitioner to bear in mind when discussing withdrawal from conventional medication that this could be construed as undermining the considered opinion of another professional. It is wise to make efforts to ensure that this is not what the patient or the prescribing doctor perceives. In most cases it is likely that the patient will be supported by their doctor in their desire to reduce medication.

If a patient requests support in making a change in medication which is against the advice of their medical doctor, it is important to ensure that the patient fully understands the risks and benefits, and that what has been explained to them about such risks and benefits is clearly documented.

To give balanced advice in this situation, it is essential that the practitioner has access to clear and up-to-date information on the risks and benefits of withdrawal from the treatment from a conventional perspective. If it is possible, the advice of another conventionally trained professional should be sought.

Maintaining confidentiality

All healthcare practitioners have a duty to keep all information concerning their patients, medical or otherwise, entirely confidential. Such information should be released only with the explicit consent of the patient. This also applies to any views formed about the patient during consultations. To this end, when communicating with a doctor about a shared patient, it is advisable for practitioners to inform the patient in advance about the content of the letter or conversation, to ensure that they have given full consent to the information to be disclosed.

However, there are times when patient confidentiality needs to be breached. This should only be done when the practitioner is convinced it is in the best interests of the patient or of society at large. For example, there might be genuine concern that an elderly person is becoming too confused to look after themselves, whereas the patient insists he is managing perfectly well. In this instance it could be appropriate to make a telephone call to the patient's GP to check that the practice is aware of the home situation of the elderly person.

If it is decided that it is in the best interests of the patient or to the wider community to disclose information about a patient, clear records should be made of how that decision was made. If a practitioner has any uncertainties about whether or not to disclose confidential information, it is wisest to discuss the situation first, in confidence, with their professional body. It must be emphasised that disclosure without consent is a very serious matter, and unless there is a serious risk of injury or harm to the public it can be very difficult to justify. For example, even suicide threats are not usually thought to be a serious enough reason to disclose unless the means suggested may impinge on other people (e.g. driving a car recklessly or jumping off a shopping centre roof). Therefore, if there is any uncertainty about whether disclosure would be appropriate, it is wisest once again for the practitioner to consult in confidence with the professional conduct officer of their professional body.

References and further information

GENERAL SOURCES

Physiology

Waugh, A., Grant, A., 2006. Ross and Wilson: anatomy and physiology in health and illness, tenth ed. Churchill Livingstone, Edinburgh.

Clinical medicine, surgery and pharmacology

British Medical Association, Br. Med. J. Available http://www.bmj.com

British Medical Association and the Royal Pharmacological Society of Great Britain, 2009. British national formulary 58. Available at: http://www.bnf.org

Collier, J., Longmore, M., Brinsden, M., 2006. Oxford handbook of clinical specialities. Oxford University Press, Oxford.

Ellis, H., Calne, R., Watson, C., 2006. Lecture notes: general surgery, eleventh ed. Blackwell Publishing, Oxford.

Kumar, P., Clark, M., 2005. Clinical medicine, sixth ed. Elsevier Saunders, Edinburgh.

Longmore, M., Wilkinson, I., Turmezei, T., Cheung, C.K., 2008. Oxford handbook of clinical medicine. Oxford University Press, Oxford.

National Institute for Health and Clinical Excellence (NICE), http://www.nice.org.uk

Oxbridge Solutions Ltd, A general practice notebook. Available at: http://www.gpnotebook.co.uk

Chinese medical viewpoint

Cheng, X.N., 1990. Chinese acupuncture and moxibustion. Foreign Languages Press, Beijing.

Larre, C., Schatz, J., Rochat de la Vallee, E., 1986. Survey of traditional Chinese medicine. L'Institut Ricci de Paris, Paris.

Maciocia, G., 1989. The foundations of Chinese medicine. Churchill Livingstone, Edinburgh.

Maciocia, G., 1994. The practice of Chinese medicine. Churchill Livingstone, Edinburgh.

The Simple Questions (Suwen) is an ancient Chinese text that forms part of the Yellow Emperor's Inner Canon, from which Maciocia has drawn a lot of his conclusions about Chinese Organ functions. It is one of the classical texts on which the whole of Chinese medicine theory is based.

One reference to this text is: Veith, I., (Trans.), 1994. The Yellow Emperor's Classic of Internal Medicine, revised ed. University of California Press, Berkeley, CA.

The nomenclature of acupuncture points

Deadman, P., Al-Khafaji, M., Baker, K., 1998. A manual of acupuncture. Journal of Chinese Medicine Publications, Kingham.

Patient information websites

The following are excellent sources of patient information, covering symptoms, causes, diagnosis, treatment options and lifestyle advice. Each also includes links to other web information sources.

NHS Institute for Innovation and improvement, CKS (clinical knowledge summaries). Available at: http://cks.library.nhs.uk/home

Egton Medical Information Systems Limited, Patient UK. Available at: http://www.patient.co.uk

STAGE 1

Chapter 1.2a

Lissauer, T., Clayden, G., 1997. The illustrated textbook of paediatrics. Mosby, Philadelphia, PA.

Possible scientific basis for a holistic body–mind interpretation

Pert, C., 1999. Molecules of emotion: why you feel the way you feel. Pocket Books, New York.

Chapter 1.2b

Drug nomenclature

Information on the recommended International Non-proprietary Names (rINN) system, http://www.who.int/medicines/services/inn/en/index.html

Adverse effects of drugs

Information on the problems resulting from the early release of the Merck product Vioxx, http://www.vioxx.com

Chapter 1.3a

Gascoigne, S., 2000. The clinical medicine guide: a holistic perspective. Jigme Press, Clonakilty.

Chapter 1.3b

The concept of suppression

Hahnemann, S., 1999. The chronic diseases: theoretical part B. Jain Publishers, New Delhi.

Energetic actions of foods

Flaws, B., Wolfe, B., 1983. Prince Wen Hui's cook: Chinese dietary therapy. Paradigm Publications, Taos, NM.

STAGE 2

Chapter 2.1c

British Medical Association and the Royal Pharmacological Society of Great Britain, 2009. British National Formulary 58, Section 4.7: Analgesics. Available at: http://www.bnf.org

Chapter 2.1d

Gascoigne, S., 2000. The clinical medicine guide: a holistic perspective. Jigme Press, Clonakilty.

Vaccination

Department of Health, 2007. Immunisation against infectious disease 2006: The Green Book. Department of Health, London. Available at: http://www.dh.gov.uk/en/Publicationsandstatistics/Publications/PublicationsPolicyAndGuidance/DH_079917

Chapter 2.1e

Complementary medicine

Gascoigne, S., 2000. The clinical medicine guide: a holistic perspective. Ch. 5. Jigme Press, Clonakilty.

Chapter 2.2c

British Medical Association and the Royal Pharmacological Society of Great Britain, 2009. British National Formulary 58, Section 6.3 Corticosteroids. Section 10.1.3 Drugs that suppress the rheumatic disease process. Available at: http://www.bnf.org

Chapter 2.2d

British Medical Association and the Royal Pharmacological Society of Great Britain, 2009. British National Formulary 58, Sections 2.8 and 2.9 Anticoagulants and antiplatelet drugs. Available at: http://www.bnf.org

Patient information leaflets on prevention and treatment of DVT

http://cks.library.nhs.uk/dvt_advice_for_travellers

http://cks.library.nhs.uk/patient_information_leaflet/Deep_vein_thrombosis

Chapter 2.3a

British Medical Association and the Royal Pharmacological Society of Great Britain, 2009. British National Formulary 58. Ch. 8. Available at: http://www.bnf.org

Patient information leaflets on cancer

http://cks.library.nhs.uk/information_for_patients/all_leaflets_by_subject/cancer

Other relevant websites

The following websites are rich in information. Patients need to be advised that information on complementary therapies given on patient information websites is often likely not to be well supported by evidence for effectiveness.

Cancer Research UK – patient information, http://www.cancerhelp.org.uk

Macmillan Cancer Support – advice on conventional therapies, self-help and also some guidance on complementary therapies, http://www.cancerlink.org

MD Anderson Cancer Center, The University of Texas –introduction to complementary treatments and summary of clinical evidence supporting their effectiveness in cancer treatment, http://www.mdanderson.org/departments/CIMER

National Cancer Institute, USA – detailed information for health professionals on cancer and its treatment, http://www.cancer.gov

The Cure Research Foundation – advice on complementary treatments and clinics, http://www.cancure.org

Chapter 2.4d

Maciocia, G., 1989. The foundations of Chinese medicine. Ch. 32. Churchill Livingstone, Edinburgh.

STAGE 3

Chapter 3.1a

Flaws, B., Wolfe, B., 1983. Prince Wen Hui's cook: Chinese dietary therapy. Paradigm Publications, Taos, NM.

Healthy eating

Food Standards Agency, UK, http://www.food.gov.uk

US Food and Drugs Administration, Revealing trans fats, http://findarticles.com/p/articles/mi_m1370/is_5_37/ai_109906683/?tag=content;col1

Chapter 3.1b

Gray, D., Toghill, P., 2001. An introduction to the symptoms and signs of clinical medicine. Ch. 6. Arnold, London.

Chapter 3.1c

Gastro-oesophageal reflux disease (GORD)

RefluxAdvice – a UK website for medical professionals giving up-to-date guidance on the management of GORD, http://www.refluxadvice.co.uk/index.php

Dyspepsia

National Institute for Health and Clinical Excellence, 2004. Dyspepsia: managing dyspepsia in adults in primary care – guidelines on the medical management of dyspepsia. Available at: http://www.nice.org.uk/guidance/CG17

Patient information leaflets

Digestive system (including dyspepsia, reflux, peptic ulcer disease, coeliac disease, Crohn's disease, ulcerative colitis and haemorrhoids). http://cks.library.nhs.uk/information_for_patients/all_leaflets_by_subject/gastrointestinal_digestive_system

Cancers of the digestive system, http://cks.library.nhs.uk/information_for_patients/all_leaflets_by_subject/cancer

Healthy eating

The UK Food Standards Agency, UK – healthy eating advice, http://www.eatwell.gov.uk

Chapter 3.2a

Larre, C., Schatz, J., Rochat de la Vallee, E., 1986. Survey of traditional Chinese medicine. L'Institut Ricci de Paris, Paris.

Hypertension

British Hypertension Society, http://www.bhsoc.org

Williams, B., Poulter, N.R., Brown, M.J., et al., 2004. British Hypertension Society guidelines for hypertension management, 2004 – BHS IV: summary. Br. Med. J. 328, 634–640.

Chapter 3.2b

Gray, D., Toghill, P., 2001. An introduction to the symptoms and signs of clinical medicine. Ch. 4. Arnold, London.

Chapter 3.2d

Calculating coronary risk

British Hypertension Society – a simple risk calculator (calculations require accurate levels of blood lipids) can be downloaded from, http://www.bhsoc.org/Cardiovascular_Risk_Charts_and_Calculators.stm

Academic papers

Barker, D.J., Osmond, C., 1988. Low birth weight and hypertension. Br. Med. J. 297 (6641), 134–135.

Vasan, R.S., Larson, M.G., Leip, E.P., et al., 2001. Impact of high normal blood pressure on the risk of cardiovascular disease. N. Engl. J. Med. 345, 1291–1297.

Williams, B., Poulter, N.R., Brown, M.J., et al., 2004. The BHS Guidelines Working Party. British Hypertension Society guidelines for hypertension management, 2004 – BHS IV: summary. Br. Med. J. 328, 634–640.

Wolf-Maier, K., Cooper, R.S., Banegas, J.R., et al., 2003. Hypertension prevalence and blood pressure levels in 6 European countries, Canada, and the United States. JAMA 289 (18), 2363–2369.

World Health Organization, International Society of Hypertension Writing Group, 2003. World Health Organization (WHO) International Society of Hypertension (ISH) statement on management of hypertension. J. Hypertens. 21 (11), 1183–1192.

Chapter 3.2e

Clinical medicine

National Institute for Health and Clinical Excellence, 2003. Chronic heart failure. Management of chronic heart failure in adults in primary and secondary care. Clinical Guideline CG5. Available at: http://www.nice.org.uk/nicemedia/pdf/CG5NICEguideline.pdf

Academic papers

Sofi, F., Cesari, F., Abbate, R., Gensini, G.F., Casini, A., 2008. Adherence to Mediterranean diet and health status: meta-analysis. Br. Med. J. 337, a1344.

Chapter 3.2g

Safety of acupuncture

British Acupuncture Council, 2006. Guide to safe practice. British Acupuncture Council, London.

National Institute for Health and Clinical Excellence, 2008. Guidance on prophylaxis against infective endocarditis. Antimicrobial prophylaxis against infective endocarditis in adults and children undergoing interventional procedures. Clinical Guideline CG64. Available at: http://www.nice.org.uk/nicemedia/pdf/CG64NICEguidance.pdf

Patient information leaflets

Cardiovascular conditions (including angina, arrhythmias, coronary heart disease, hypertension, heart failure and varicose veins). http://cks.library.nhs.uk/information_for_patients/all_leaflets_by_subject/cardiovascular_heart_blood_vessels

Chapter 3.3b

Gray, D., Toghill, P., 2001. An introduction to the symptoms and signs of clinical medicine. Ch. 5. Arnold, London.

Chapter 3.3c

Clinical medicine

National Institute for Health and Clinical Excellence, 2008. Prescribing of antibiotics for self-limiting respiratory tract infections in adults and children in primary care. Clinical Guideline CG69. Available at: http://www.nice.org.uk/Guidance/CG69

National Institute for Health and Clinical Excellence, 2009. Amantadine, oseltamivir and zanamivir for the treatment of influenza (review of existing guidance No. 58). Available at: http://www.nice.org.uk/guidance/index.jsp?action=byID&o=11774

Chapter 3.3d

Clinical medicine

British Thoracic Society and Scottish Intercollegiate Guidelines Network (BTS/SIGN), 2008. British guideline on the management of asthma: a national clinical guideline. Available at:http://www.brit-thoracic.org.uk/ClinicalInformation/Asthma/AsthmaGuidelines/tabid/83/Default.aspx

Patient information leaflets

Allergic conditions (including asthma, hayfever and rhinitis)http://cks.library.nhs.uk/information_for_patients/all_leaflets_by_subject/allergy

Conditions of the ear, nose and throat (including common cold, sore throat, sinusitis, tonsillitis, epiglottitis, quinsy and cancer of the larynx)http://cks.library.nhs.uk/information_for_patients/all_leaflets_by_subject/ear_nose_and_throat

Respiratory conditions (including asbestosis, bronchiolitis, bronchitis, cancer of the lung, COPD, flu, pleurisy, pneumonia and tuberculosis)http://cks.library.nhs.uk/information_for_patients/all_leaflets_by_subject/respiratory_chest_lungs

Section 3.4

Patient information leaflets

Haematological conditions (including anaemia, leukaemia, lymphoma, myeloma and shock). http://cks.library.nhs.uk/information_for_patients/all_leaflets_by_subject/haematology_blood_lymph

STAGE 4

Chapter 4.1a

Myers, T.W., 2001. Anatomy trains: myofascial meridians for manual and movement therapists. Churchill Livingstone, Edinburgh.

Mayor, D.F., 2006. Electroacupuncture: A practical manual and resource. Churchill Livingstone, Edinburgh.

Chapter 4.1b

Gray, D., Toghill, P., 2001. An introduction to the symptoms and signs of clinical medicine. Ch. 20. Arnold, London.

Chapter 4.1c

British Medical Association and the Royal Pharmacological Society of Great Britain, 2009. British National Formulary 58, Section 4.7 Analgesics. Available at: http://www.bnf.org

Chapter 4.1d

Risks of hormone replacement therapy

Million Women Study Collaborators, 2003. Breast cancer and hormone replacement therapy in the Million Women Study. Lancet 362, 419.

Writing Group for the Women's Health Initiative Investigators, 2002. Risks and benefits of estrogen plus progestin in healthy postmenopausal women. J. Am. Med. Assoc. 288, 321–333.

Chapter 4.1e

Complementary medicine

Legge, D., 1997. Close to the bone: the treatment of musculoskeletal disorder with acupuncture and other traditional Chinese medicine, second ed. Sydney College Press, Woy Woy, NSW.

Simons, D.G., Travell, J.G., 1999. Travell and Simon's myofascial pain and dysfunction: the trigger point manual, vols. 1 and 2, Wilkins and Wilkins, Baltimore, OH.

Patient information leaflets

Musculoskeletal system (including arthritis, bursitis, bone cancer, osteoporosis, gout, Paget's disease and sciatica). http://cks.library.nhs.uk/information_for_patients/all_leaflets_by_subject/musculoskeletal_joints_muscles_bones

Arthritis

Arthritis Foundation – a UK patient support network, http://www.arthritis.org

Arthritis Research Campaign – a UK organisation dedicated to education about arthritis and the promotion of the results of research into arthritis, http://www.arc.org.uk

Chapter 4.3c

National Institute for Health and Clinical Excellence, 2007. Urinary tract infection: diagnosis, treatment and long-term management of urinary tract infection in children. Available at: http://www.nice.org.uk/guidance/CG54

National Institute for Health and Clinical Excellence, 2008. Chronic kidney disease. Clinical Guideline CG73. Available at: http://www.nice.org.uk/guidance/CG73

National Institute for Health and Clinical Excellence, 2008. Type 2 diabetes: the management of type 2 diabetes (update). Clinical Guideline CG66. Available at: http://www.nice.org.uk/guidance/CG66

Scottish Intercollegiate Guidelines Network, 2008. Diagnosis and management of chronic kidney disease. Available at: http://www.sign.ac.uk/guidelines/fulltext/103/index.html

Patient information leaflets

Urinary system (including glomerulonephritis, kidney cancer, urine infections, kidney stones and chronic kidney disease). http://cks.library.nhs.uk/information_for_patients/all_leaflets_by_subject/urology_kidney_bladder_prostate

Kidney disease

National Kidney Federation – information for patients, http://www.kidney.org.uk/Medical-Info

STAGE 5

Chapter 5.1c

Gascoigne, S., 2001. The clinical medicine guide: a holistic perspective. Jigme Press, Clonakilty.

Chapter 5.1d

Matthews, D., Beatty, S., Dyson, P., King, L., Meston, N., Pal, A., et al., 2008. Diabetes: the facts. All the information you need straight from the experts. Oxford University Press, Oxford.

National Institute for Health and Clinical Excellence, 2008. Type 2 diabetes: the management of type 2 diabetes (update). Clinical Guideline CG66. Available at: http://www.nice.org.uk/guidance/CG66

Patient information leaflets

Endocrine disorders (including thyroid disease, diabetes, Addison's disease and Cushing's disease). http://cks.library.nhs.uk/information_for_patients/all_leaflets_by_subject/endocrine_metabolic_diabetes

Other websites

Diabetes UK – information for patients, http://www.diabetes.org.uk/Guide-to-diabetes/Introduction-to-diabetes

Food Standards Agency – Eat Well, Be Well, http://www.eatwell.gov.uk

The GI Diet Guide –information about low glycaemic index foods and recipes, http://www.the-gi-diet.org

The Pituitary Foundation, www.pituitary.org.uk.

Thyroid UK – information for patients, http://www.thyroiduk.org

Chapter 5.2c

Hormone replacement therapy

Maciocia, G., 1998. Obstetrics and gynaecology in Chinese medicine. Churchill Livingstone, Edinburgh.

Royal College of Obstetricians and Gynaecologists, 2004. Hormone replacement therapy and venous thromboembolism. Guideline 19. RCOG, London.

The Million Women Study – evidence for the long-term risks of hormone replacement therapy, http://www.millionwomenstudy.org/publications

Chapter 5.2d

Information on sexual health for the general public

NHS Choices – information on sexual health, including guidance on safe sexual practice, http://www.nhs.uk/Livewell/Sexualhealth/Pages/Sexualhealthhome.aspx

The theory of the candida syndrome

Truss, C., 1985. The missing diagnosis. Missing Diagnosis Inc., Birmingham, AL.

Chapter 5.2e

Long-acting, reversible contraception

National Institute for Health and Clinical Excellence, 2005. Long-acting reversible contraception: the effective and appropriate use of long-acting reversible contraception. Clinical Guideline CG30. Available at: http://guidance.nice.org.uk/CG30

Chapter 5.2f

Infertility.

National Institute for Health and Clinical Excellence, 2004. Fertility: assessment and treatment for people with fertility problems. Clinical Guideline CG11. Available at: http://www.nice.org.uk/guidance/CG11

Chapter 5.2g

Endometriosis

Royal College of Obstetricians and Gynaecologists, 2006. The investigation and management of endometriosis. Available at: http://www.rcog.org.uk/womens-health/clinical-guidance/investigation-and-management-endometriosis-green-top-24

Heavy menstrual bleeding

National Institute for Health and Clinical Excellence, 2007. Heavy menstrual bleeding. Clinical Guideline CG44. Available at: http://www.nice.org.uk/CG44niceguideline

Ovarian cancer

Gascoigne, S., 2001. Homeopathic use of platinum in ovarian cancer. In: The clinical medicine guide: a holistic perspective. Jigme Press, Clonakilty Ch. 18.

Maciocia, G., 1998. Obstetrics and gynaecology in Chinese medicine. Churchill Livingstone, Edinburgh.

Patient information leaflets

Contraception, http://www.cks.nhs.uk/information_for_patients/all_leaflets_by_subject/contraception

Sexual health, http://www.cks.nhs.uk/information_for_patients/all_leaflets_by_subject/sexual_health

Women's health, http://www.cks.nhs.uk/information_for_patients/all_leaflets_by_subject/womens_health

Other websites

Endometriosis UK – information for patients, http://www.endometriosis-uk.org

Human Fertilisation & Embryology Authority – guide for patients, http://www.hfea.gov.uk/22.html

Infertility Network UK – information for patients, http://www.infertilitynetworkuk.com

Chapter 5.3a

Physiology of conception

Wilcox, A.J., Dunson, D., Day Baird, D., 2000. The timing of the 'fertile window' in the menstrual cycle: day specific estimates from a prospective study. Br. Med. J. 321, 1259–1261.

Preconceptual advice

West, Z., 2001. Summary of advice from a Chinese medicine perspective. In: Acupuncture in pregnancy and childbirth. Ch. 1. Churchill Livingstone, Edinburgh.

Chapter 5.3b

Ultrasound scanning: an alternative viewpoint

Gascoigne, S., 2001. The clinical medicine guide: a holistic perspective. Ch. 4. Jigme Press, Clonakilty.

Oats, J., Abraham, S., 2004. Llewellyn-Jones fundamentals of obstetrics and gynaecology. Mosby, Philadelphia, PA.

Chapter 5.3c

Greer, I., Cameron, I., Kitchener, H., Prentice, A., 2001. Mosby's color atlas and text of obstetrics and gynaecology. Mosby, Philadelphia, PA.

Llewellyn-Jones, D., 1999. Fundamentals of obstetrics and gynaecology. Ch. 12. Mosby, Philadelphia, PA.

Maciocia, G., 1998. Obstetrics and gynaecology in Chinese medicine. Chs 31–33. Churchill Livingstone, Edinburgh.

Chapter 5.3d

Llewellyn-Jones, D., 1999. Fundamentals of obstetrics and gynaecology. Ch. 11. Mosby, Philadelphia, PA.

Maciocia, G., 1999. Obstetrics and gynaecology in Chinese medicine. Churchill Livingstone, Edinburgh.

West, Z., 2001. Acupuncture in pregnancy and childbirth. Ch. 10. Churchill Livingstone, Edinburgh.

Patient information

Nausea and vomiting in pregnancy. http://www.cks.nhs.uk/nausea_vomiting_in_pregnancy

Chapter 5.3e

Maciocia, G., 1998. Obstetrics and gynaecology in Chinese medicine. Churchill Livingstone, Edinburgh.

West, Z., 2001. Acupuncture in pregnancy and childbirth. Chs 5–7. Churchill Livingstone, Edinburgh.

Chapter 5.3f

Medications contraindicated in lactation (complete list)

British Medical Association and the Royal Pharmacological Society of Great Britain, 2009. British National Formulary 58. Appendix 5. Available at: http://www.bnf.org

Patient information leaflets

Pregnancy, http://www.cks.nhs.uk/information_for_patients/all_leaflets_by_subject/pregnancy

Other websites

HER Foundation – hyperemesis research, http://www.hyperemesis.org/

National Childbirth Trust, UK, http://www.nctpregnancyandbabycare.com/home

Chapter 5.4a

Lissauer, T., Clayden, G., 2007. Illustrated textbook of paediatrics, third ed. Mosby, Philadelphia, PA.

Scott, J., Barlow, T., 1999. Acupuncture in the treatment of children. Eastland Press, Vista, CA.

Chapter 5.4b

Lissauer, T., Clayden, G., 1999. Illustrated textbook of paediatrics. Ch. 2. Mosby, Philadelphia, PA.

Chapter 5.4c

Lissauer, T., Clayden, G., 1999. Illustrated textbook of paediatrics. Chs 6 and 7. Mosby, Philadelphia, PA.

Scott, J., Barlow, T., 1999. Acupuncture in the treatment of children. Eastland Press, Vista, CA.

Chinese medicine interpretation of the stages of development of the fetus

West, Z., 2001. Acupuncture in pregnancy and childbirth. Ch. 2. Churchill Livingstone, Edinburgh, p. 27.

The Barker Hypothesis

West, Z., 2001. The work of Professor David Barker on the long-term consequences of fetal health is summarised. In: Acupuncture in pregnancy and childbirth. Ch. 3. Churchill Livingstone, Edinburgh.

Chapter 5.4d

Benensen, A.S., 1995. The control of communicable diseases manual. American Public Health Association (APHA), Washington, DC.

Department of Health, Welsh Office, Scottish Office Department of Health, DHSS (Northern Ireland), 1996. Immunisation against Infectious Disease. HMSO, London.

Lissauer, T., Clayden, G., 1999. Illustrated textbook of paediatrics. Mosby, Philadelphia, PA.

Scott, J., Barlow, T., 1999. Acupuncture in the treatment of children. Eastland Press, Vista, CA.

Chapter 5.4e

Leach, P., 1997. Your baby and child. Penguin, London.

Lissauer, T., Clayden, G., 1999. Illustrated textbook of paediatrics. Mosby, Philadelphia, PA.

Scott, J., Barlow, T., 1999. Acupuncture in the treatment of children. Eastland Press, Vista, CA.

Patient information leaflets

Childrens health. http://www.cks.nhs.uk/information_for_patients#-325248

Asthma: treatment guidelines

British Thoracic Society, 1997. The British guidelines on asthma management. 1995 review and position statement. Thorax 52 (Suppl. 1), S1–S2.

Psychiatric developmental and behavioural disorders

Bloch, S., Singh, B.S., 1998. Foundations of clinical psychiatry. Melbourne University Press, Melbourne.

STAGE 6

Chapter 6.1b

Bull, P.D., 1996. Lecture notes on diseases of the ear, nose and throat. Blackwell Science, Oxford.

Graham-Brown, R., Burns, T., 1996. Lecture notes on dermatology. Blackwell Science, Oxford.

James, B., Chew, C., Bron, A., 1997. Lecture notes on ophthalmology. Blackwell Science, Oxford.

Kumar, P., Clark, M., 2005. Clinical medicine, sixth ed. Saunders, Edinburgh.

Chapter 6.1c

Graham-Brown, R., Burns, T., 1996. Lecture notes on dermatology. Blackwell Science, Oxford.

Kumar, P., Clark, M., 2005. Clinical medicine, sixth ed. Elsevier Saunders, Edinburgh.

Scott, J., Barlow, T., 1999. Acupuncture in the treatment of children. third ed. Eastland Press, Vista, CA, p. 348.

Chapter 6.1d

Bates, W.H., 1981. The Bates method for better eyesight without glasses. Owl Books, New York.

International Myopia Prevention Society, http://www.myopia.org

James, J., Chew, C., Bron, A., 1997. Lecture notes on ophthalmology. Blackwell Science, Oxford.

Kumar, P., Clark, M., 2005. Clinical medicine, sixth ed. Elsevier Saunders, Edinburgh.

Maciocia, C., 1994. The practice of Chinese medicine. Ch. 29. Churchill Livingstone, Edinburgh.

Xinnong, C., 1987. Chinese acupuncture and moxibustion. Ch. 18, Section IV. Foreign Languages Press, Beijing.

Chapter 6.1e

Bull, P.D., 1996. Lecture notes on diseases of the ear, nose and throat, eighth ed. Blackwell Science, Oxford.

Kumar, P., Clark, M., 2005. Clinical medicine, sixth ed. Elsevier Saunders, Edinburgh.

Maciocia, G., 1994. The practice of Chinese medicine. Ch. 11. Churchill Livingstone, Edinburgh.

Xinnong, C., 1987. Chinese acupuncture and moxibustion. Foreign Languages Press, Beijing, pp. 482–483.

Chapter 6.2a

Classification systems for mental health disorders

World Health Organization, 1992. The ICD-10 classification of mental and behavioural disorders: clinical descriptions and diagnostic guidelines. WHO, Geneva.

American Psychiatric Association, 1994. DSM IV: Diagnostic and statistical manual of mental disorders, fourth ed. APA, Washington, DC.

Definition of the mind

Pearsall, J., Trumble, B. (Eds.), 1996. Oxford English reference dictionary. Oxford University Press, Oxford.

Biochemical basis of emotions

Pert, C., 1999. Molecules of emotion: why you feel the way you feel. Pocket Books, New York.

Definition of mental health disorder

American Psychiatric Association, 1994. DSM IV: Diagnostic and statistical manual of mental disorders, fourth ed. APA, Washington, DC.

Psychological causes of mental health problems

Lissauer, T., Clayden, G., 1999. Illustrated textbook of paediatrics. Mosby, Philadelphia, PA.

Bloch, S., Singh, B. (Eds.), 1994. Foundations of clinical psychiatry. Melbourne University Press, Melbourne.

Chinese medicine understanding of mental health problems

Flaws, B., Lake, J., 2001. Chinese medicine psychiatry: a textbook and clinical manual. Blue Poppy Press, Boulder, CO.

Maciocia, G., 1994. The practice of Chinese medicine. Ch. 9. Churchill Livingstone, Edinburgh.

Chapter 6.2b

Bloch, S., Singh, B.S., 1994. Foundations of clinical psychiatry. Melbourne University Press, Melbourne.

Classification of mental illness

World Health Organization, 1992. The ICD-10 classification of mental and behavioural disorders: clinical descriptions and diagnostic guidelines. WHO, Geneva.

American Psychiatric Association, 1994. DSM IV: Diagnostic and statistical manual of mental disorders, fourth ed. APA, Washington, DC.

Chapter 6.2c

Mental Health Act 1983 and Mental capacity Act 2008

Mind – clear summaries of these important Acts. http://www.mind.org.uk/help/information_and_advice

Treatments

British Medical Association and the Royal Pharmacological Society of Great Britain, 2009. British national formulary 58. Ch. 4. Available at: http://www.bnf.org

Gascoigne, S., 2001. The clinical medicine guide: a holistic perspective. Ch. 16. Jigme Press, Clonakilty.

Goffman, E., 1961. Asylums. Doubleday, New York.

Laing, R.D., 1966. The politics of experience and the bird of paradise. Penguin, London.

Livitnoff, S., 2001. Better Relationships. Vermilion Press, London.

Livitnoff, S., 2001. Sex in loving relationships. Vermilion Press, London.

National Institute for Health and Clinical Excellence, 2009. Schizophrenia. Core interventions in the treatment and management of schizophrenia in adults in primary and secondary care. Clinical Guideline CG82. Available at: http://www.nice.org.uk/nicemedia/pdf/CG82NICEGuideline.pdf

Ross, J., 2002. The mood cure. Thorsons, London.

Chapter 6.2d

Beck, A.T., Rush, A.J., Shaw, B.F., Emery, G., 1979. Cognitive therapy for depression. Guildford, New York.

Bloch, S., Singh, B.S., 1994. Foundations of clinical psychiatry. Melbourne University Press, Melbourne.

Hamilton, M., 1960. A rating scale for depression. J. Neurol. Neurosurg. Psychiatry 23, 56–62.

Puri, B.K., 2000. Saunders pocket essentials of psychiatry, second ed. WB Saunders, Philadelphia, PA.

Chapter 6.2e

Flaws, B., Lake, J., 2001. Chinese medicine psychiatry: a textbook and clinical manual. Blue Poppy Press, Boulder, CO.

Hicks, A., Hicks, J., Mole, P., 2005. Five element constitutional acupuncture. Churchill Livingstone, Edinburgh.

National Institute for Health and Clinical Excellence, 2009. Schizophrenia. Core interventions in the treatment and management of schizophrenia in adults in primary and secondary care. Clinical Guideline CG82. Available at: http://www.nice.org.uk/nicemedia/pdf/CG82NICEGuideline.pdf

National Institute for Health and Clinical Excellence, 2006. Bipolar disorder. The management of bipolar disorder in adults, children and adolescents, in primary and secondary care. Clinical Guideline CG38. Available at: http://www.nice.org.uk/nicemedia/pdf/CG38niceguideline.pdf

Learning disability

Camphill communities, http://www.camphill.org.uk

L'Arche Communities, http://www.larche.org.uk

Treatment of children with learning disability, see, Scott, J., Barlow, T., 2006. Acupuncture in the treatment of children. Treatment of children with learning disability, see. Eastland Press, Vista, CA.

Patient information websites

Cruse Bereavement Care, http://www.crusebereavementcare.org.uk

Mind – support network for patients and carers, http://www.mind.org.uk

PsychNet UK – mental health and psychology directory, further information on all the important psychological disorders and links to patient support groups, http://www.psychnet-uk.com

Chapter 6.3a

Ali, N., 2005. Alarm bells in medicine. Blackwell, Oxford.

Hopcroft, K., Forte, V., 2003. Symptom sorter, third ed. Radcliffe, Oxford.

Chapter 6.3b

Gascoigne, S., 1998. Prescribed drugs and the alternative practitioner. Ch. 3. Energy Medicine Press.

British Medical Association and the Royal Pharmacological Society of Great Britain, 2009. British National Formulary 58, Sections 2.8 and 2.9 Anticoagulants and antiplatelet drugs. Available at: http://www.bnf.org

Chapter 6.3c

British Acupuncture Council, 2004. Code of Professional Conduct. British Acupuncture Council, London.

Index

Note: Page numbers followed by *b* indicate boxes, followed by *f* indicate figures and followed by *t* indicate tables.

A

C

D

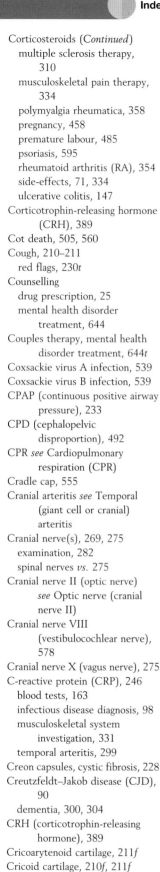

E

F

H

I

M

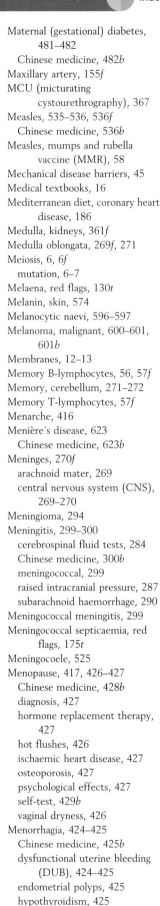

N

O

P

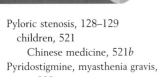

U

V

W

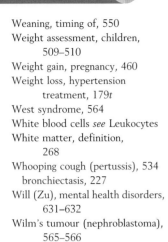